AMERICAN CANCER SOCIETY
TEXTBOOK OF CLINICAL ONCOLOGY

AMERICAN CANCER SOCIETY TEXTBOOK OF

CLINICAL ONCOLOGY

ARTHUR I. HOLLEB, MD   DIANE J. FINK, MD   GERALD P. MURPHY, MD

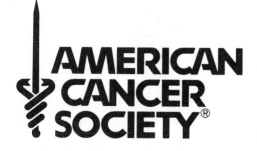

The American Cancer Society, Inc., Atlanta, GA 30329

Published 1991. First edition 1991
Printed in the United States of America

94 93 92   5 4 3 2 1

Library of Congress Cataloging in Publication Data

American Cancer Society textbook of clinical oncology / Arthur I.
    Holleb, Diane J. Fink, Gerald P. Murphy.
        p.   cm.
    Includes bibliographical references.
    Includes index.
    ISBN 0-944235-07-7
    1. Cancer.   2. Oncology.   I. Holleb, Arthur I., 1921-
II. Fink, Diane J.   III. Murphy, Gerald P.   IV. American Cancer
Society.   V. Title: Textbook of clinical oncology.
    (DNLM: 1. Neoplasms.   QZ 200 A5127)
RC261.A677 1991
616.99′4—dc20
DNLM/DLC   91-4642
for Library of Congress   CIP

CONTENTS

PREFACE

The *American Cancer Society Textbook of Clinical Oncology* is the product of the combined efforts of 50 of the leading cancer experts in the United States. The Society assembled this distinguished group of authors to create a new, more comprehensive text for medical students and for physicians working in, or interested in, oncology; a text that addresses not only the treatment of the disease, but also the related issues that are keys to a multidisciplinary approach to cancer care.

In the time that has elapsed since the publication of the last edition of this text's predecessor, *Clinical Oncology: A Multidisciplinary Approach*, the body of knowledge relative to cancer has grown dramatically. The range of issues affecting the cancer patient has expanded, and there has been an explosion in biological knowledge as it relates to cancer treatment. A medical text was needed that would take into account this rapid growth in the science of treatment as well as how clinical issues relate to research. Thus, the American Cancer Society felt that a more comprehensive treatment of the various forms of the disease was required rather than a revision of our former oncology text. For this reason, the American Cancer Society undertook publication for the first time of its own new textbook, one that would embrace the entire body of knowledge relative to oncology and the issues critical to cancer control.

In addition to timely, in-depth discussions of the pathology, etiology, and nature of cancer, the scope of this new text has been broadened to reflect the increased specialization within medicine and the team approach to patient care. And, in keeping with the emerging understanding that health care must be a partnership between physicians and patients, theories of lifestyle factors and preventive measures have been addressed, as have the areas of social work, sexuality, and rehabilitation.

Because of the skill and knowledge of our authors and their broad base of experience in both research and clinical practice, it is our anticipation that the *American Cancer Society Textbook of Clinical Oncology* will be recognized as a definitive work in oncology, one that will be of great educational value to medical students, physicians, and nurses in the United States and elsewhere.

Arthur I. Holleb, M.D.
Diane J. Fink, M.D.
Gerald P. Murphy, M.D.

INTRODUCTION

Arthur I. Holleb, M.D.

Arthur I. Holleb, M.D.
Consultant, Medical Affairs Department
American Cancer Society
Larchmont, New York

As a professional education document, the purpose of this American Cancer Society book is to accomplish certain objectives by providing the reader with not only the basics about cancer, but also with up-to-date information about the disease from recognized experts in their respective fields.

The American Cancer Society traces its origins to 1913, when a group of 10 physicians and five laymen met in New York City and founded the American Society for the Control of Cancer. Its stated purpose at the time was to "disseminate knowledge concerning the symptoms, treatment, and prevention of cancer; to investigate conditions under which cancer is found; and to compile statistics in regard thereto." Later renamed the American Cancer Society, it is today one of the oldest and largest voluntary health agencies in the United States, comprising 2.2 million American volunteers united to conquer cancer through balanced programs of research, education, patient service, and rehabilitation.

The American Cancer Society, Inc. is organized as a National Society, with 57 chartered Divisions and 3,170 Units. A 206-member House of Delegates provides representation from the 57 geographic Divisions and additional representation on the basis of population. It elects, and is governed by, a Board of Directors of 124 voting members, half of whom are members of the medical or scientific professions.

The National Society is responsible for overall planning and coordination. It also provides technical help and materials to Divisions and Units, administers programs of research, medical grants, and clinical and nursing fellowships, and carries out public and professional education on the national level.

The 57 Divisions are governed by members, both medical and lay people, of Divisional Boards of Directors in all the states plus five metropolitan areas, the District of Columbia, and Puerto Rico. The Units are organized to cover the counties in the United States. There are thousands of community leaders who direct the Society's programs at this level.

The Society maintains its priorities and goals through activities developed by the departments of Research, Professional Education, Public Education, Public Information, Epidemiology and Statistics, Service and Rehabilitation, Public Affairs, and Crusade.

Details of every American Cancer Society program can be obtained by writing to the appropriate Department at the National Headquarters, located at 1599 Clifton Road, N.E., Atlanta, GA 30329.

Knowledge and understanding about cancer, its early detection, its prompt diagnosis, and its adequate treatment will assuredly lead to further increases in survival rates. Rehabilitation of the person treated for cancer will improve the quality of his or her life. Of course, the use of measures that can prevent cancer, whenever possible, are ideal goals. These are the objectives this book strives to accomplish.

Cancer is a group of diseases characterized by the uncontrolled growth of abnormal cells that spread from the anatomic site of origin. This spread, if uncontrolled, invades vital organs and results in death. However, many cancers can be cured if they are detected early and treated promptly; others can be controlled for many years with a variety of treatment approaches.

Cancer is most often treated by surgery, radiation therapy, chemotherapy, and hormones. More recently, immunotherapy was added to the therapeutic armamentarium. Cancer occurs at any age. It results in the death of more children ages 3 to 14 than any other disease. Also, it strikes more frequently in older people. According to the American Cancer Society, in the 1980s there were more than 4.5 million deaths due to cancer, almost 9 million new cancer cases, and about 12 million people under medical care for cancer in the United States.

More than 6 million Americans alive today have had a history of cancer; most, but not all, of the 3 million of them who were diagnosed five or more years ago can be considered cured. "Cure" is defined as having no evidence of recurrent cancer while simultaneously having the same life expectancy as a person who never had cancer. For most forms of cancer, five years after treatment with no signs of recurrence is a good statistical mark for continued survival, although there still can be an attrition rate beyond that time. In fact, for some of the more aggressive forms of cancer which frequently are fatal in a short period of time, a 3-year survival may be considered approaching a cure. Others cancers may require much longer periods of time after treatment to be considered cured.

During the year of this text's publication, more than 1 million people will be diagnosed as having cancer. This estimate of incidence is based upon data from the National Cancer Institute's Surveillance, Epidemiology and End Result (SEER) Program (1984-1986). Nonmelanoma skin cancer and carcinoma *in situ* are not included in the statistics. For example, more than 600,000 cases of nonmelanoma skin cancer occur annually.

At the turn of this century very few people with major cancers had much hope of long-term survival. More than 50 years ago, in the 1930s, less than 1 in 5 persons with cancer was alive five years after treatment. In the 1940s it was 1 in 4, and in the 1960s it was 1 in 3.

Today, 40%, or 4 out of 10 persons who develop cancer, will be alive five years after treatment. The improvement from 1 in 3, to 4 in 10 represents 69,000 people in 1990 alone. This 40% figure is the "observed" survival rate. Taking into consideration normal life expectancy (e.g., dying of heart disease, accidents, and so forth) 50% will be alive five years after treatment. This is the "relative" survival rate, a more accurate measure of success in the treatment of cancer.

In 1989 about 42,000 people with cancer died who might have been saved by earlier detection and prompt treatment. This figure emphasizes the need for more programs of public and professional education. In 1989, an estimated 510,000 people in the United States died of cancer—1,400 people every day, or about one death from cancer every minute.

Except for lung cancer, the age-adjusted cancer death rates for major anatomic sites are leveling off, and in some cases declining. "Age-adjusted" is a method used to make valid statistical comparisons by assuming the same age distribution among different groups being compared.

Not all cancers can be prevented using our present state of knowledge; however, some can. Most cancers of the lung are caused by cigarette smoking, and most skin cancers are caused by excessive exposure to direct sunlight. Those cancers caused by occupational and/or environmental factors can be prevented by eliminating or reducing contact with carcinogenic agents.

In the chapters that follow, the reader will be presented with information about how cancer develops; the principles of cancer biology; general trends in screening asymptomatic people; diagnosis and treatment; approaches to modern medical technology; the principles of oncologic specialties; prevention and causation of cancer; the special roles of smoking, nutrition, and viruses; specific types and anatomic sites of cancer; medical emergency situations that occur in cancer patients; AIDS-related cancer; rehabilitation, supportive care, pain control, psychosocial management, and sexuality issues; the remarkable recent advances in diagnostic imaging; and other topics of vital interest to the student of oncology.

No textbook can be complete unto itself; therefore the reader is encouraged to make use of the extensive lists of references following each chapter to expand on the information presented.

Cancer control is a rational pursuit. Considerable progress has been made over the years for many types of cancer and even more progress can be anticipated in the future. Basic scientists are describing the present as the "golden years of cancer research"—an era filled with more promise than at any other time in the past.

The more we educate people about cancer, the more it will come out of the closet. Less and less will there be a cry of anger and resentment against the heavens or fate; the "Why me?" or the "Why has God done this to me?" syndrome will fade. That sense of shame and self-blame when cancer strikes will lessen, and cancer will be looked upon as an illness like any other, not as a social disgrace or stigma.

Oncologists are designing treatment so that patients can live with dignity and respect, not merely exist. More often, the patient is being given what I like to call an "ego prosthesis." In the future, there will be greater and more open communication about cancer between patients, families, and physicians; more truth telling, fewer charades and conspiracies of silence.

It is our hope that this textbook will assist physicians in their communications with other physicians and with their cancer patients, and result in a higher level of mutual understanding.

Chapter 1

CANCER STATISTICS AND TRENDS

Lawrence Garfinkel, M.A.

Lawrence Garfinkel, M.A.
Special Consultant in Epidemiology and Statistics
American Cancer Society
New York, New York

INTRODUCTION

Statistical data play an integral role in evaluating the scope of the cancer problem and the results of cancer control efforts. The most important cancer data sources come from mortality statistics, published annually in the United States by the National Center for Health Statistics of the Department of Health and Human Services. The most recent reports are published about three years prior to the current year (U.S. Public Health Service 1930-1986). Mortality rates are computed according to the number of persons per 100,000 population estimated by the Census Bureau.

Incidence data (the number of new cases reported in a year) are not published for the entire country. Although many states have their own registries to report cases, the figures most often used are from the SEER program (Surveillance, Epidemiology and End Results) of the National Cancer Institute (NCI). This population-based program covers four states, Puerto Rico, and five metropolitan areas and comprises an estimated 12% of all the cancer cases in the United States (NCI 1973-1986).

Estimates of the number of new cases and deaths in 1990 by sex and site are made by American Cancer Society (ACS) staff by projecting trends from published mortality and incidence data.

LEADING CAUSES OF DEATH

Heart diseases are the most common causes of death in the United States and account for 36.4% of all deaths. Next is cancer, which in 1986 accounted for 22.3%. While death rates from heart diseases, stroke, and a number of other diseases have been decreasing over the past generation, the percent of deaths due to cancer rose from 16.8% in 1967 to 22.3% in 1986.

PREVALENCE OF CANCER

Cancer is a disease of aging: 66% of cancer deaths occur after age 65. As the U.S. population ages, cancer death rates have to be statistically adjusted for age to observe trends and to make appropriate comparisons. The age-adjusted cancer death rate per 100,000 population in 1930 was 143; 152 in 1940; 157 in 1950; and 171 in 1986. Lung cancer was the major cause for the increase (fig. 1.1). Excluding lung cancer, the cancer death rate shows no increase in males and a long-term decrease in females.

The ACS estimates that in the 1980s, 4.5 million Americans died from cancer. In addition, there were nearly 9 million new cases and about 12 million people were under medical care for cancer. About 30% of persons now living will develop cancer. Over 6 million living Americans have had a history of the disease, and about 3 million of these were diagnosed five or more years ago. Most of these are considered to be cured of cancer.

SURVIVAL RATES

Survival rates from cancer — that is, those who are alive five years after diagnosis — were 1 in 5 in the 1930s; 1 in 4 in the 1940s; and 1 in 3 in the 1960s. In recent years, 4 out of 10 patients survive five years; this is the observed survival rate. In terms of normal life expectancy (when other causes of death are taken into account) 50% are alive after five years; this is called the relative survival rate, and is the figure customarily used.

RACIAL AND ECONOMIC FACTORS

Mortality and incidence rates are higher for blacks than for whites. For example, over a 14-year period, the cancer death rate among black males rose 15% compared with an 8% increase in black females. The cancer incidence rate in blacks increased 15%; in whites 13%. Blacks have 12% lower 5-year survival rates from cancer than whites.

It has become evident that poor people have higher overall cancer rates. The differences in the cancer death rates between blacks and whites can be attributed, in large part, to the relatively higher percentage of socioeconomically disadvantaged among blacks. Poor Americans, regardless of race, have a 10% to 15% lower 5-year survival (Freeman 1989).

STATISTICS FOR DIFFERENT CANCER SITES

Cancer is a family of diseases. The following descriptions characterize the mortality, morbidity, and survival data for cancers of selected sites. Estimates of the number of new cases and deaths in 1990, by site and sex in the United States, are shown in table 1.1 and survival rates appear in fig. 1.2.

LUNG

This is the most common site of cancer in both mortality and incidence, with an estimated 142,000 deaths and 157,000 new cases in 1990. Lung cancer mortality rates rose rapidly from 7 per 100,000 population in 1940 to 47 per 100,000 in 1986. Mortality rates in men increased greatly from 1940-1979, although in the 1980s the rate of increase has been less. The 5-year age-specific rates in younger men (under age 55) have actually decreased. In women a rapid increase comparable to the increase observed in men in the 1940s was seen starting in the mid-1960s. This reflects the fact that women began smoking cigarettes later than did men. Also, many women who started smoking in the 1940s were reaching ages when cancer occurs 20 and 30 years later.

Incidence rates published by SEER show a decrease in lung cancer in men from 86.5 per 100,000 in 1984 to 81.9 in 1986, after a steady rise since 1973. In women the incidence rate continues to increase, from 18.3 in 1973 to 36.4 in 1986.

Overall, only 13% of all lung cancer patients, 12% of males and 16% of females, survive five or more years after diagnosis.

COLON-RECTUM

Cancer of the colon-rectum is second only to lung cancer in both incidence and mortality. For 1990 estimates are that there will be 155,000 new cases (110,000 colon and 45,000 rectum) and 60,900 deaths. The mortality rate has shown a decline, mostly for rectal cancer, while the incidence rate has risen about 1% from 1973 to 1986. The incidence rate in males (61.1 per 100,000) is higher than in females (42.8 per 100,000).

The overall 5-year survival for colon-rectum cancer is 52%. However, when the disease is diagnosed in a localized stage it is 84%. Survival rates for colon cancer increased from 42% in the early 1960s to 54% in recent years. Rectal cancer survival rates for the same period increased from 37% to 52%.

BREAST

In 1990, it is estimated that 150,900 new cases of breast cancer will occur in the United States. About 1 in 10

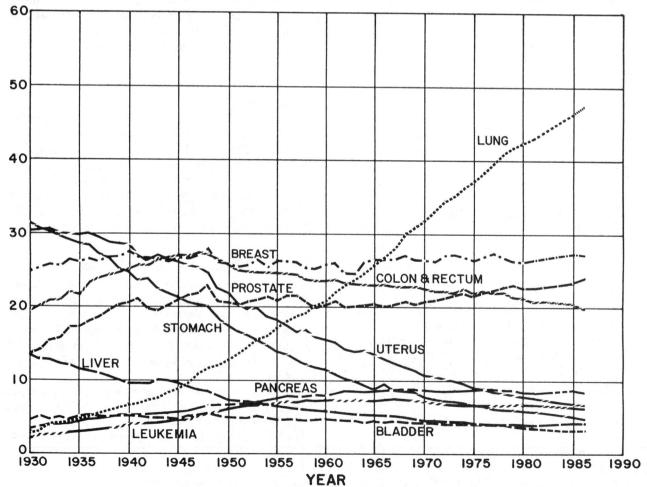

Fig. 1.1. Cancer death rates by site in the United States for the years 1930-1986. The rate for the population is standardized for age on the 1970 U.S. population. Rates are for both sexes combined except for breast and uterus, female population only, and prostate, male population only. (Sources: National Center for Health Statistics and U.S. Bureau of the Census.)

Table 1.1
ESTIMATED NEW CANCER CASES AND DEATHS BY SEX FOR ALL SITES (1990)*

	ESTIMATED NEW CASES			ESTIMATED DEATHS		
	TOTAL	MALE	FEMALE	TOTAL	MALE	FEMALE
ALL SITES	1,040,000*	520,000*	520,000*	510,000	270,000	240,000
Buccal Cavity and Pharynx (ORAL)	30,500	20,400	10,100	8,350	5,575	2,775
Lip	3,600	3,100	500	100	75	75
Tongue	6,100	3,900	2,200	1,950	1,300	650
Mouth	11,500	6,900	4,600	2,500	1,500	1,000
Pharynx	9,300	6,500	2,800	3,800	2,700	1,100
Digestive Organs	236,800	121,300	115,500	122,900	64,600	58,300
Esophagus	10,600	7,400	3,200	9,500	7,000	2,500
Stomach	23,200	13,900	9,300	13,700	8,300	5,400
Small Intestine	2,800	1,500	1,300	900	500	400
Large Intestines ⌐ (COLON-RECTUM)	110,000	52,000	58,000	53,300	26,000	27,300
Rectum ⌐	45,000	24,000	21,000	7,600	4,000	3,600
Liver and Biliary Passages	14,600	7,700	6,900	11,900	6,200	5,700
Pancreas	28,100	13,600	14,500	25,000	12,100	12,900
Other and Unspecified Digestive	2,500	1,200	1,300	1,000	500	500
Respiratory System	173,700	115,000	58,700	147,100	95,900	51,200
Larynx	12,300	10,000	2,300	3,750	3,000	750
LUNG	157,000	102,000	55,000	142,000	92,000	50,000
Other and Unspecified Respiratory	4,400	3,000	1,400	1,350	900	450
Bone	2,100	1,200	900	1,100	600	500
Connective Tissue	5,700	3,000	2,700	3,100	1,500	1,600
SKIN	27,600†	14,800†	12,800†	8,800§	5,700	3,100
BREAST	150,900‡	900‡	150,000‡	44,300	300	44,000
Genital Organs	185,000‡	113,100	71,900‡	54,100	30,600	23,500
Cervix Uteri ⌐ (UTERUS)	13,500‡	—	13,500‡	6,000	—	6,000
Corpus, Endometrium ⌐	33,000	—	33,000	4,000	—	4,000
Ovary	20,500	—	20,500	12,400	—	12,400
Other and Unspecified Genital, Female	4,900	—	4,900	1,100	—	1,100
Prostate	106,000	106,000	—	30,000	30,000	—
Testis	5,900	5,900	—	350	350	—
Other and Unspecified Genital, Male	1,200	1,200	—	250	250	—
Urinary Organs	73,000	51,000	22,000	20,000	12,600	7,400
Bladder	49,000	36,000	13,000	9,700	6,500	3,200
Kidney and Other Urinary	24,000	15,000	9,000	10,300	6,100	4,200
Eye	1,700	900	800	300	150	150
Brain and Central Nervous System	15,600	8,500	7,100	11,100	6,000	5,100
Endocrine Glands	13,600	4,000	9,600	1,750	775	975
Thyroid	12,100	3,200	8,900	1,025	375	650
Other Endocrine	1,500	800	700	725	400	325
Leukemia	27,800	15,700	12,100	18,100	9,800	8,300
Lymphocytic Leukemia	11,600	6,700	4,900	5,200	3,000	2,200
Granulocytic Leukemia	11,500	6,300	5,200	7,600	4,000	3,600
Other and Unspecified Leukemia	4,700	2,700	2,000	5,300	2,800	2,500
Other Blood and Lymph Tissues	54,800	28,900	25,900	28,700	14,900	13,800
Hodgkin's Disease	7,400	4,200	3,200	1,600	1,000	600
Non-Hodgkin's Lymphomas	35,600	18,600	17,000	18,200	9,500	8,700
Multiple Myeloma	11,800	6,100	5,700	8,900	4,400	4,500
All Other and Unspecified Sites	41,200	21,300	19,900	40,300	21,000	19,300

NOTE: The estimates of new cancer cases are offered as a rough guide and should not be regarded as definitive. Especially note that year-to-year changes may only represent improvements in the basic data. ACS six major sites appear in **BOLDFACE CAPS.**

*Carcinoma *in situ* and non-melanoma skin cancers are not included in totals. Carcinoma *in situ* of the uterine cervix accounts for more than 50,000 new cases annually, carcinoma *in situ* of the female breast accounts for about 15,000 new cases annually, and melanoma carcinoma *in situ* accounts for about 5,000 new cases annually. Overall, about 100,000 new cases of carcinoma *in situ* of all sites of cancer are diagnosed each year. Nonmelanoma skin cancer accounts for about 600,000 new cases annually.

†Melanoma only   ‡Invasive cancer only   §Melanoma 6,300; other skin 2,500
(Incidence estimates are based on rates from NCI SEER Program 1983-1986.)

women will develop breast cancer at some time during their lives.

Breast cancer mortality rates have been fairly stable over the past 60 years, at about 27 per 100,000 population. Although incidence rates had also remained stable for many years, since 1980 there has been a 24% increase; from 84.7 to 104.9 per 100,000 in 1986. During the same period, there has been a rapid increase in the percent of women who have mammograms (Gallup Organization 1988), and the two increases may be related.

The 5-year survival rate is 75%, but the rate is 90% for breast cancer cases diagnosed in an early stage. This has also been reflected in the results of an analysis of the Breast Cancer Detection Demonstration Program (BCDDP), a study of 280,000 asymptomatic women offered annual mammograms over a 5-year period. The overall 5-year survival rate for these women was 87% (Seidman et al. 1987).

UTERUS (CERVIX AND ENDOMETRIUM)

The ACS estimates that in 1990 there will be 13,500 new cases of cervical cancer and 33,000 of endometrial cancer. Incidence and mortality rates for cervical cancer have decreased steadily. In 1986 the incidence rate was 8.8 per 100,000 and mortality was 3.2 per 100,000. Much of this decrease is associated with widespread use of the Pap test. At the same time cervical cancers were decreasing, cases diagnosed as carcinoma *in situ* of the cervix have been increasing. The endometrial cancer incidence rate was 21.1 per 100,000 in 1986, and the mortality rate was 3.6. Incidence and mortality rates for endometrial cancer have also decreased, about 2% to 3% per year over the past 25 years. Cervical cancer incidence is twice as high in blacks as in whites; endometrial cancer is 1.5 times as high in whites as in blacks.

The 5-year survival rate for invasive cervical cancer is 67%, but is 88% for cases diagnosed in an early stage. The survival rate for carcinoma *in situ* of the cervix is virtually 100%. The 5-year survival figures for endome-

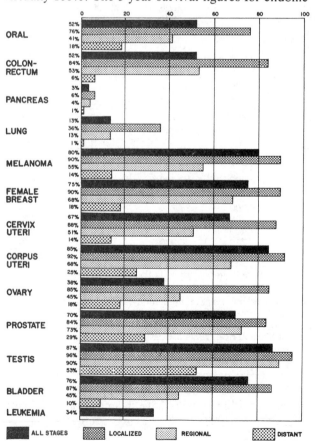

Fig. 1.2. Five-year cancer survival rates for selected sites, adjusted for normal life expectancy. This chart is based on cases diagnosed in 1974-1985. (Source: Cancer Statistics Branch, National Cancer Institute.)

trial cancer are 85% for all cases, and 92% for cases diagnosed as localized.

OVARY

Ovarian cancer accounts for 4% of all cancers in women. In 1990, an estimated 20,500 new cases of ovarian cancer will be diagnosed and about 12,400 women will die of the disease. The incidence rate in 1986 was 12.7 per 100,000 and has changed little over the years. The mortality rate is 7.7 per 100,000 population and has decreased slightly. When treated early, 85% of patients survive five or more years. However, the 5-year survival rate is only 38%, because only 24% are diagnosed early.

ORAL

An estimated 30,500 new cases of cancer of the buccal cavity and pharynx will be diagnosed in 1990, and an estimated 8,350 deaths. The incidence rate for oral cancer was 10.7 in 1986, and has not shown much change over the past 15 years. The mortality rate was 3.1 per 100,000, and has decreased slightly in the past 15 years. Five-year survival rates average 52%, but vary considerably for different sites in the oral cavity: lip 92%; mouth 53%; tongue 42%; and pharynx 32%. The incidence rates are more than twice as high in males than in females, and 1.5 times higher in blacks than whites.

BLADDER

Bladder cancer accounts for 49,000 new cases in 1990, about 7% of all cancers in males, and 3% of cases in females. It is the fourth most common cancer in men and eighth most common in women. The 1986 incidence rate of 16.8 per 100,000 was four times as high in 1986 in males (29.5) than in females (7.5). The rate was nearly twice as high in whites (17.7) as in blacks (9.7). The mortality rate was 3.3 per 100,000. Mortality rates for both sexes have been decreasing.

The overall 5-year survival rate is 75%; it is 87% when diagnosed early, and 43% when diagnosed in a regional stage.

PROSTATE

A total of 106,000 new cases will be diagnosed in 1990. About 1 in 11 men will develop prostate cancer sometime during their lifetime. It has the second highest incidence in men, next to skin cancer. About 30,000 deaths are estimated for 1990, making it the second leading cause of cancer death in men. Eighty-seven percent of cases are diagnosed at age 65 and older. The incidence rate in 1986 was 88.9 per 100,000, an increase of 39% since 1973. Mortality rates have changed very little over the years. Some believe that the pattern of increased incidence with no increase in mortality is attributable to a greater number of latent cancers being diagnosed; diagnosis at an earlier stage; and more successful therapy in early diagnosed cases.

The disease is much more common in blacks than in whites. The incidence rate in 1986 for whites was 87.7

and 123.4 for blacks. Five-year survival rates for prostate cancer have increased in the past 20 years from 48% to 70%. Sixty percent of cases are diagnosed when in a localized stage, which has a 5-year survival rate of 84%.

PANCREAS

Pancreatic cancer is the fifth leading cause of cancer death. About 28,100 new cases will occur in the United States in 1990 and about 25,000 patients will die of it. It is about 1.5 times more common in blacks than in whites. In the past 35 years the death rate rose about 24% in men and 32% in women. The incidence rate in 1986 was 9.3 per 100,000 and the death rate 8.4 per 100,000.

Survival rates for cancer of the pancreas are poor. Only 3% survive five years. Eleven percent are diagnosed in a localized stage, and only 6% of these patients survive five years.

LEUKEMIA

An estimated 27,800 new cases will occur in 1990, about one-half of them acute and the other half chronic. Leukemia strikes many more adults (25,300) than children (2,500) each year. Among adults the most common type (25%) is acute myeloid leukemia (AML), while among children, acute lymphoblastic (ALL) is the most common (76% of cases). The incidence rate for leukemia was 9.3 per 100,000 in 1986, and the mortality rate was 6.4 per 100,000.

The overall 5-year survival rate is 34%, mainly because of poor survival for AML. Over the past 30 years, however, there has been a dramatic improvement in survival of patients with ALL. In the early 1960s about 4% of white patients with ALL survived five years. This increased to 28% in the 1970s, and to 48% in the 1980s. In some medical centers, optimum treatment has raised survival of children with ALL to 75%.

STOMACH

Stomach cancer was the most common type of cancer in 1930; in 1990 it ranked twelfth. An estimated 23,200 new cases and 13,700 deaths will occur in 1990. Mortality rates decreased by 70% in males and 75% in females over the past 35 years. The reason for the decline is not known; some suspect it may be related to changes in the national diet. Survival rates are low, only 16%. In cases diagnosed as localized, the 5-year survival rate is 56%.

SKIN

The ACS estimates that over 600,000 cases of skin cancer will occur in 1990, most of them highly curable basal or squamous cell carcinomas. Malignant melanoma strikes about 27,600 persons a year and causes 6,300 deaths. In 1986 the incidence rate for melanoma was 9.9 per 100,000. It is one of the most rapidly increasing cancers, increasing in incidence by about 4% per year. The mortality rate in 1986 was 2.1 per 100,000. The 5-year survival rate for patients with malignant melanoma is 80%.

OTHER SITES

Kidney cancer, with 24,000 new cases and 10,300 deaths, has shown a 46% increase in mortality rates over the past 30 years. Non-Hodgkin's lymphoma (NHL) has rapidly increased in incidence, from 8.5 per 100,000 in 1973 to 12.6 in 1986, or 48%. It will account for 35,600 new cases in 1990, and 18,200 deaths. Hodgkin's disease (7,400 new cases and 1,600 deaths in 1990) is another cancer in which survival rates have improved greatly, from 40% in the early 1960s to 76% in recent years. Testicular cancer will account for only 5,900 new cases in 1990 and an estimated 350 deaths. Improvement in survival for cancer of the testis has been dramatic; from 63% in the 1960s to 91% in recently diagnosed cases.

CHILDREN'S CANCERS

About 7,600 new cases of childhood cancer (in children under the age of 15) are estimated and about 1,600 deaths, about one-third from leukemia, are estimated for 1990. Cancer is the main cause of death due to disease in children ages 3 to 14. Mortality has decreased from 8.3 per 100,000 in 1950 to 3.5 in 1986. Five-year survival rates vary depending on site: for bone cancer it is 51%; neuroblastoma 55%; brain and central nervous system 57%; Wilms's tumor 81%; and Hodgkin's disease 89%.

GEOGRAPHICAL COMPARISONS

The overall cancer death rate in the United States is 171 per 100,000. It varies among states from a low of 122 in Utah to a high of 220 in the District of Columbia. Cancer death rates are generally higher in New England and the mid-Atlantic states, and lower in the West and Southwest.

Cancer mortality rates vary even more among countries. The highest rates are in the more advanced European countries. Lung, breast, and colon-rectum cancers are higher in more advanced countries, and cervical and stomach cancers are high in Third World countries. Japan has relatively low rates for breast and colon-rectum cancer but high stomach cancer rates; Japan's lung cancer rates are rising rapidly (table 1.2).

REFERENCES

American Cancer Society. 1990. Cancer facts and figures—1990. Atlanta: American Cancer Society.

Freeman, H.P. 1989. Cancer in the economically disadvantaged. *Cancer* 64(Suppl):324-34.

Gallup Organization. 1988. *The 1987 survey of public awareness and use of cancer detection tests.* Princeton, N.J.: The Gallup Organization.

National Cancer Institute. 1989. *Cancer statistics review 1973-1986.* N.I.H. Publication No. 88-2789. Bethesda, Md.: U.S. Dept. of Health and Human Services.

Seidman, H.; Gelb, S.K.; and Silverberg, E. et al. 1987. Survival experience in the breast cancer detection demonstration project. *CA* 37:258-90.

U.S. Public Health Service, National Center for Health Statistics. 1934-1988. *Vital statistics of the United States.* Annual 1930-1986. Washington D.C.: U.S. Government Printing Office.

Table 1.2
CANCER AROUND THE WORLD (1984-1986)
Age-Adjusted Death Rates Per 100,000 Population for Selected Sites for 50 Countries

	All Sites		Oral		Colon and Rectum		Lung		Breast	Uterus		Stomach		Prostate	Leukemia	
	Male	Female	Male	Female	Male	Female	Male	Female	Female	Cervix	Other	Male	Female	Male	Male	Female
UNITED STATES	216.6(26)	140.3(20)	5.0(29)	1.8(13)	24.2(22)	17.5(20)	73.5(12)	26.2(3)	27.4(16)	3.2(40)	3.7(33)	7.4(50)	3.4(50)	23.2(23)	8.3(6)	5.1(11)
ARGENTINA**	196.7(32)	127.1(31)	5.2(29)	1.1(13)	21.1(24)	12.8(33)	50.4(31)	7.2(36)	24.6(23)	5.1(23)	8.4(6)	18.0(33)	8.3(34)	17.2(34)	6.0(35)	4.1(32)
AUSTRALIA	218.2(24)	132.9(25)	6.0(20)	1.8(13)	33.3(6)	21.3(10)	61.4(26)	14.4(14)	25.2(21)	4.0(31)	2.8(47)	12.4(46)	5.6(46)	23.7(20)	8.2(8)	4.9(13)
AUSTRIA	237.5(14)	147.4(12)	6.6(15)	1.2(32)	35.1(3)	20.4(13)	63.4(22)	10.9(16)	27.1(18)	4.6(26)	3.2(44)	28.4(12)	14.2(10)	23.7(20)	7.5(17)	4.6(23)
BARBADOS*	150.7(44)	141.0(18)	8.4(8)	1.4(22)	9.3(42)	6.4(47)	21.4(45)	2.5(50)	28.2(14)	24.8(1)	1.5(50)	14.4(39)	10.3(24)	28.1(6)	6.2(33)	5.3(6)
BELGIUM##	281.2(3)	146.2(15)	4.6(31)	1.3(25)	32.4(7)	20.5(12)	104.1(2)	8.9(26)	32.2(7)	3.6(33)	5.1(21)	18.3(31)	13.3(13)	26.8(8)	7.7(12)	5.2(7)
BULGARIA	166.4(40)	106.1(39)	3.8(36)	0.9(43)	19.2(26)	12.9(31)	47.5(32)	8.4(29)	17.8(35)	4.2(27)	6.5(12)	28.3(13)	16.5(7)	10.5(43)	5.5(36)	3.9(38)
CANADA	224.2(21)	142.2(17)	5.7(23)	1.8(13)	24.7(21)	18.3(19)	73.1(11)	21.9(9)	29.4(13)	3.1(41)	3.5(37)	12.0(47)	5.3(47)	23.7(20)	8.3(6)	4.9(13)
CHILE	189.4(33)	146.3(14)	3.0(42)	0.8(45)	9.3(42)	9.0(39)	28.3(41)	7.7(35)	15.6(39)	15.6(4)	3.3(41)	46.9(4)	20.7(5)	18.8(33)	4.5(42)	4.0(35)
COSTA RICA	214.5(27)	149.8(11)	5.1(26)	2.0(9)	11.5(40)	8.8(40)	22.3(44)	8.3(31)	15.7(38)	15.9(3)	4.4(26)	66.9(1)	34.1(2)	24.4(18)	7.3(19)	4.8(16)
CUBA	170.0(39)	121.6(34)	7.5(11)	2.3(6)	12.7(37)	14.5(25)	52.3(29)	18.3(11)	18.3(31)	6.2(17)	10.5(3)	10.5(49)	5.3(47)	24.5(17)	5.5(36)	4.5(24)
CZECHOSLOVAKIA	289.3(2)	153.2(8)	8.2(9)	1.3(25)	41.2(1)	21.3(10)	93.2(4)	9.8(23)	24.3(24)	6.7(14)	7.8(8)	29.3(11)	14.4(9)	24.5(17)	8.2(8)	5.0(12)
DENMARK	250.9(9)	181.4(1)	4.1(33)	1.7(17)	38.5(2)	25.3(2)	73.0(13)	24.8(6)	34.2(3)	7.3(13)	5.2(20)	14.0(43)	7.1(41)	19.4(28)	9.1(4)	5.6(3)
ECUADOR	124.4(46)	119.2(36)	1.6(49)	1.2(32)	4.6(49)	4.4(49)	10.8(49)	4.2(48)	6.5(49)	9.2(9)	18.7(1)	41.3(5)	28.6(3)	26.7(9)	4.0(45)	3.3(42)
ENGLAND AND WALES	249.4(10)	164.1(4)	3.6(40)	1.7(17)	28.0(14)	20.4(13)	87.1(7)	24.9(5)	36.0(1)	5.7(20)	3.6(36)	20.4(25)	8.8(29)	16.2(35)	6.9(24)	4.4(25)
FINLAND	224.7(20)	124.7(32)	2.6(45)	1.3(25)	17.5(32)	13.0(29)	75.1(10)	8.3(33)	20.2(29)	2.6(44)	3.3(41)	21.8(22)	12.4(18)	22.3(24)	7.6(14)	4.9(13)
FRANCE	269.4(6)	120.1(35)	17.9(1)	1.6(19)	25.2(17)	15.4(24)	57.8(27)	5.6(40)	23.9(25)	2.4(45)	6.1(15)	14.8(36)	6.5(42)	25.6(13)	8.8(5)	5.2(7)
GERMANY, D.R.	216.7(25)	132.8(26)	5.1(26)	1.1(37)	24.8(19)	20.0(16)	66.9(19)	7.0(39)	20.9(28)	7.6(12)	5.5(17)	26.1(14)	12.9(15)	15.8(36)	6.4(29)	4.2(31)
GERMANY, F.R.	241.8(13)	146.9(13)	6.3(18)	1.1(37)	29.8(11)	22.6(4)	64.6(21)	8.9(26)	27.3(17)	4.2(27)	4.7(24)	23.5(19)	12.6(16)	24.8(16)	7.6(14)	4.8(16)
GREECE	188.7(34)	101.1(45)	2.3(47)	0.7(47)	7.7(45)	7.0(45)	62.0(25)	8.4(29)	17.9(32)	1.7(48)	4.3(27)	14.0(43)	7.5(40)	11.9(42)	7.6(14)	4.8(16)
HONG KONG	220.9(22)	122.8(33)	17.3(2)	5.5(2)	19.0(27)	13.5(27)	71.6(14)	32.0(2)	10.6(45)	5.8(19)	2.0(48)	14.4(39)	7.9(35)	3.8(50)	4.3(44)	3.3(42)
HUNGARY	294.9(1)	164.4(3)	13.0(6)	1.9(10)	35.0(4)	24.2(3)	87.6(6)	14.9(13)	26.1(20)	8.5(10)	7.0(9)	34.9(7)	15.8(8)	24.1(19)	9.3(3)	5.5(4)
ICELAND	180.1(37)	140.8(19)	3.0(42)	0.6(48)	15.9(35)	13.0(29)	32.0(37)	22.7(8)	25.1(22)	4.2(27)	3.1(45)	30.5(10)	9.9(26)	30.0(4)	9.6(2)	5.4(5)
IRELAND	230.0(19)	160.7(5)	5.4(24)	2.1(8)	29.5(12)	22.2(5)	69.0(17)	23.0(7)	31.6(10)	3.3(36)	4.1(29)	22.0(21)	10.4(23)	22.0(22)	7.1(22)	4.7(19)
ISRAEL	158.3(42)	127.9(29)	1.9(48)	1.0(40)	19.9(25)	15.9(22)	31.6(38)	10.3(21)	27.9(15)	1.6(49)	3.7(33)	14.2(42)	6.5(42)	12.3(40)	7.7(12)	5.2(7)
JAPAN	198.4(31)	104.1(43)	2.6(45)	0.8(45)	18.2(30)	12.2(35)	38.2(35)	10.5(18)	6.7(48)	2.4(45)	4.2(28)	54.6(2)	25.0(4)	5.1(49)	5.1(38)	3.3(42)
KUWAIT#	139.9(45)	104.4(42)	3.7(38)	2.4(5)	5.6(48)	6.7(46)	31.6(38)	9.6(24)	12.9(43)	3.4(34)	4.2(28)	10.6(48)	6.3(45)	7.7(47)	6.9(24)	7.4(1)
LUXEMBOURG	280.0(4)	150.6(9)	6.8(13)	1.3(25)	30.4(10)	21.5(8)	93.1(5)	11.3(15)	32.6(5)	2.7(42)	6.5(12)	18.6(30)	8.5(32)	25.8(12)	11.5(1)	5.8(2)
MALTA	200.2(30)	131.2(27)	6.8(13)	1.5(20)	18.2(30)	14.2(26)	62.2(24)	5.5(42)	35.5(2)	1.9(47)	6.8(11)	21.7(23)	7.8(37)	14.2(37)	7.9(11)	3.6(40)
MARTINIQUE***	220.1(23)	127.9(29)	15.5(4)	0.0(50)	12.5(38)	7.1(43)	12.5(48)	7.2(36)	26.2(19)	5.6(21)	13.3(2)	25.6(15)	12.6(16)	64.9(1)	3.8(47)	4.4(25)
MAURITUS	113.4(48)	75.5(49)	4.1(33)	1.2(32)	6.1(47)	4.5(48)	26.7(42)	5.2(45)	8.3(47)	6.4(16)	8.5(5)	23.0(20)	6.4(44)	8.6(45)	2.7(48)	3.3(42)
NETHERLANDS	271.2(5)	142.8(16)	2.9(44)	1.0(40)	25.7(16)	19.6(18)	103.8(3)	10.4(19)	32.4(6)	3.4(35)	3.5(37)	14.5(38)	8.8(29)	26.0(11)	7.2(20)	4.7(19)
NEW ZEALAND	230.3(18)	153.7(7)	4.9(30)	1.9(10)	35.0(4)	26.9(1)	64.8(20)	18.1(12)	30.6(13)	5.5(22)	3.4(40)	19.7(26)	8.5(32)	25.4(14)	7.5(17)	5.2(7)
NORTH IRELAND	232.3(16)	153.8(6)	3.9(35)	1.8(13)	31.3(9)	22.0(6)	76.0(9)	20.2(10)	31.8(8)	3.3(36)	3.8(31)	18.3(31)	8.8(29)	20.2(27)	6.5(27)	4.3(28)
NORWAY	202.1(29)	133.9(24)	3.7(38)	1.4(22)	26.9(15)	20.0(16)	38.7(34)	10.4(19)	30.8(12)	4.9(24)	3.3(41)	14.7(37)	9.4(27)	32.3(3)	7.0(23)	4.3(28)
PANAMA	111.6(49)	91.3(48)	3.8(36)	2.8(4)	7.1(46)	7.1(43)	19.7(46)	5.6(40)	10.8(44)	12.2(5)	3.8(31)	18.9(29)	14.1(11)	20.9(26)	5.0(39)	3.1(46)
PERU	73.3(50)	67.5(50)	0.9(50)	0.3(49)	2.8(50)	2.9(50)	7.6(50)	3.2(49)	5.6(50)	7.8(11)	6.4(14)	35.4(6)	13.3(13)	12.5(39)	2.5(49)	1.8(49)
POLAND	246.8(11)	134.1(23)	6.4(17)	1.3(25)	17.5(32)	12.9(31)	80.8(8)	10.3(21)	17.9(32)	9.5(7)	5.4(18)	34.4(8)	13.1(13)	13.4(38)	6.9(24)	4.3(28)
PORTUGAL	178.9(38)	106.1(39)	6.0(20)	1.0(40)	19.0(27)	12.5(34)	30.0(40)	4.8(46)	19.2(30)	2.7(43)	6.9(10)	17.2(34)	17.1(6)	18.9(32)	6.3(30)	4.0(35)
PUERTO RICO**	165.7(41)	102.3(44)	13.2(5)	2.2(7)	11.1(41)	10.2(38)	22.5(43)	9.1(25)	15.9(37)	4.2(27)	4.7(24)	25.5(16)	7.6(38)	26.4(10)	5.0(40)	4.7(19)
ROMANIA*	153.2(43)	99.1(47)	5.4(24)	1.4(22)	11.6(39)	8.5(41)	40.0(33)	7.1(38)	15.2(41)	11.4(6)	5.3(19)	19.2(28)	11.1(20)	9.4(44)	4.6(41)	3.6(40)
SCOTLAND	268.1(7)	175.5(2)	4.5(32)	1.9(10)	29.2(13)	21.8(7)	105.2(1)	33.2(1)	34.0(4)	6.1(18)	3.5(37)	19.2(28)	10.3(24)	19.4(28)	6.3(30)	4.1(32)
SINGAPORE	233.4(15)	134.8(22)	17.1(3)	5.8(1)	22.7(23)	20.3(15)	70.4(16)	25.0(4)	15.3(40)	9.4(8)	2.0(48)	31.2(9)	13.9(12)	5.4(48)	4.4(43)	2.8(47)
SOVIET UNION###	232.3(17)	111.8(37)	7.3(12)	1.2(32)	18.6(29)	13.3(28)	71.5(15)	4.6(47)	14.4(42)	6.5(15)	5.1(21)	48.5(3)	35.0(1)	8.1(46)	6.3(30)	4.0(35)
SPAIN*	207.6(28)	104.7(41)	6.3(18)	0.9(43)	15.0(36)	10.5(37)	50.9(30)	5.3(43)	17.9(33)	1.6(50)	5.8(16)	19.0(31)	11.1(20)	19.0(31)	8.1(10)	4.1(32)
SURINAM**	122.5(47)	100.5(46)	6.0(20)	2.9(3)	8.2(44)	8.5(41)	15.9(47)	5.3(43)	10.3(46)	22.5(2)	4.0(30)	13.2(45)	3.9(49)	19.2(30)	2.2(50)	0.6(50)
SWEDEN	180.5(36)	131.1(28)	3.4(41)	1.3(25)	25.0(18)	15.8(23)	32.5(36)	10.7(17)	22.2(27)	3.3(36)	3.7(33)	14.3(41)	7.6(38)	29.1(5)	6.5(27)	4.4(25)
SWITZERLAND	242.0(12)	138.4(21)	8.2(9)	1.5(20)	31.4(8)	17.0(21)	62.7(23)	8.0(34)	31.7(9)	4.1(31)	5.0(23)	14.3(41)	7.9(35)	33.3(2)	8.1(10)	3.7(39)
URUGUAY	265.3(8)	150.6(9)	8.6(7)	1.3(25)	24.8(19)	21.5(8)	68.7(18)	5.3(43)	31.4(11)	4.8(25)	8.6(4)	24.0(18)	10.5(22)	27.3(7)	7.2(22)	4.7(19)
YUGOSLAVIA**	188.4(35)	108.5(38)	6.5(16)	1.2(32)	16.0(34)	11.7(36)	54.1(28)	8.8(28)	16.0(36)	3.3(36)	8.0(7)	24.7(17)	12.0(19)	12.3(40)	4.0(45)	2.5(48)

NOTE: Figures in parentheses are order of rank within site and sex group. *1984 only; **1984-85 only; ***1985 only; ****1985-86 only; #1984, 1986 only; ##1985-86 only; ###1986 only. (Source: World Health Statistics Annual 1984-1988.)

Chapter 2

THE PATHOLOGIC EVALUATION OF NEOPLASTIC DISEASES

John D. Pfeifer, M.D., Ph.D.
Mark R. Wick, M.D.

John D. Pfeifer, M.D., Ph.D.
Research Fellow in Pathology
Washington University School of Medicine
St. Louis, Missouri

Mark R. Wick, M.D.
Professor of Pathology
Washington University School of Medicine
St. Louis, Missouri

INTRODUCTION

Many physicians think of the pathology laboratory only as an unpleasant area of the medical school in which they were first exposed to museum specimens of human disease, including neoplasia. Accordingly, they too often forget that abnormalities in these mummified or soggy tissues explained many of the physical findings associated with disorders of living human beings. It is advisable to remember Sir William Osler's often-quoted statement on this topic: "To know pathology is to know medicine."

In reality, modern pathology is a dynamic facet of medical practice, through which specialists who are skilled at laboratory analysis actively contribute to the care of living patients. Even the autopsy can accomplish this, because its aim is to serve as a quality assurance measure to be used by clinicians in a prospective educational manner. Other areas of laboratory medicine—including surgical pathology, hematopathology, blood banking, clinical chemistry, and microbiology—are regularly involved in the precise definition of disease and in the monitoring of therapeutic results.

The pathologist's understanding of oncological disorders has progressed far beyond the recognition of abnormal tissues with the microscope, although this is still important in the diagnosis of cancer. Today's laboratory specialist has an integral role in eliminating incorrect differential diagnostic considerations, determining prognostic factors, evaluating treatment outcomes, and otherwise supporting the multidisciplinary care of oncology patients. Recent technological advances have enlarged the scope of such activities significantly, but they must be utilized prudently with knowledge of their specific strengths and weaknesses.

This chapter outlines the general activities of pathologists in this context, and presents a practical introduction to the diverse group of morphological analyses that have an impact on patients with malignant neoplasms. For a more complete exposition, the interested reader is referred to Underwood's excellent text on biopsy interpretation and surgical pathology (Underwood 1987).

INTERACTIONS BETWEEN CLINICIANS AND PATHOLOGISTS

In order for clinicians to make optimal use of the pathologist's services, they must be familiar with the strengths and limitations of the technical procedures employed in the laboratory. Oncologists and surgeons are not merely consumers of pathologic data; rather, they should be interactive participants in the generation of such information. Much of what the anatomic pathologist is able to say about any given case depends upon receipt of pertinent clinical facts, prompt and proper submission of specimens, and adequacy of the tissue sample itself. A rapid and confident pathologic diagnosis is assured only when these factors receive proper attention (Underwood 1987).

Therefore, it is wise for clinicians to consult with the laboratory before scheduling selected invasive diagnostic procedures that will yield pathologic specimens. The physician and pathologist may then discuss the best means of obtaining the tissue; the possible need for frozen sections; special processing requirements; and the role, if any, of adjunctive pathologic analyses in diagnosis and prognosis. For example, if lymphoma is suspected in a patient with lymphadenopathy, it is wiser to undertake an excisional lymph node biopsy instead of fine-needle aspiration; conversely, the latter procedure usually yields adequate tissue in cases of probable metastatic carcinoma. Karyotyping, genotypic analyses, and certain immunohistochemical studies can only be performed on fresh tissue, and are precluded if the specimen is placed in fixative solution before dispatch to the laboratory.

DEFINITIONS OF TUMOR TYPES

Current tumor classification systems (see table 2.1) encompass a multitude of terms that are based on a tumor's biologic behavior, cellular function, histology, embryonic origin, anatomic location, and eponyms. Although it hardly needs mention, nomenclature is important because it is the means by which pathologists communicate a diagnosis, and because specific tumor designations carry specific clinical implications.

Neoplasms (literally, new growths) may be either benign or malignant. They consist of the proliferating tumor cells themselves, and a supportive stroma that contains connective tissue and blood vessels. An abundant stromal collagenic response to a neoplasm (most often to a malignant one) is called *desmoplasia*.

The most important features of a tumor that are used to define it as benign or malignant are its empirically known biologic behavior and its microscopic appearance. Generally, benign neoplasms are innocuous and slowly growing, while malignant lesions often exhibit more rapid proliferation, invade adjacent tissues, and metastasize. Benign neoplasms usually have a bland microscopic appearance while malignant neoplasms often manifest mitotic activity, abnormal nuclear chromatin, cellular pleomorphism, and areas of necrosis. However, exceptions to these generalizations abound. Benign neoplasms can kill the patient if inopportunely located (for example, an ependymoma blocking the

Table 2.1
NOMENCLATURE PERTAINING TO NEOPLASTIC DISEASES*

CELL OR TISSUE OF ORIGIN	BENIGN	MALIGNANT
TUMORS OF EPITHELIAL ORIGIN		
Squamous cells	Squamous cell papilloma	Squamous cell carcinoma
Basal cells	------	Basal cell carcinoma
Glandular or ductal epithelium	Adenoma	Adenocarcinoma
	Cystadenoma	Cystadenocarcinoma
Transitional cells	Transitional cell papilloma	Transitional cell carcinoma
Bile duct	Bile duct adenoma	Bile duct carcinoma (cholangiocarcinoma)
Liver cells	Hepatocellular adenoma	Hepatocellular carcinoma
Melanocytes	Nevus	Malignant melanoma
Renal epithelium	Renal tubular adenoma	Renal cell carcinoma
Skin adnexal glands		
Sweat glands	Sweat gland adenoma	Sweat gland carcinoma
Sebaceous glands	Sebaceous gland adenoma	Sebaceous gland carcinoma
Germ cells (testis and ovary)	------	Seminoma (dysgerminoma)
		Embryonal carcinoma, yolk sac carcinoma
TUMORS OF MESENCHYMAL ORIGIN		
Hematopoietic/lymphoid tissue	------	Leukemia
		Lymphoma
		Hodgkin's disease
		Multiple myeloma
Neural and retinal tissue		
Nerve sheath	Neurilemmoma, neurofibroma	Malignant peripheral nerve sheath tumor
Nerve cells	Ganglioneuroma	Neuroblastoma
Retinal cells (cones)	------	Retinoblastoma
Connective tissue		
Fibrous tissue	Fibromatosis (desmoid)	Fibrosarcoma
Fat	Lipoma	Liposarcoma
Bone	Osteoma	Osteogenic sarcoma
Cartilage	Chondroma	Chondrosarcoma
Muscle		
Smooth muscle	Leiomyoma	Leiomyosarcoma
Striated muscle	Rhabdomyoma	Rhabdomyosarcoma
Endothelial and related tissues		
Blood vessels	Hemangioma	Angiosarcoma
		Kaposi's sarcoma
Lymph vessels	Lymphangioma	Lymphangiosarcoma
Synovium	------	Synovial sarcoma
Mesothelium	------	Malignant mesothelioma
Meninges	Meningioma	Malignant meningioma
TUMORS OF UNCERTAIN ORIGIN		
???	------	Ewing's tumor

* This list is intended only to provide an illustrative introduction to tumor nomenclature. As indicated in the text, the existing terminology is of mixed origins and includes designations derived through a variety of means. (Adapted from: Lieberman, M.W., and Lebovitz, R.M. 1990. Neoplasia. In Kissane, J.M. ed. *Anderson's pathology.* 9th ed. p. 574. St. Louis: C.V. Mosby Co.)

aqueduct of Sylvius, or uterine intravascular leiomyomatosis eventually obstructing the right side of the heart) and some can metastasize (e.g., benign giant cell tumor of bone). Malignant neoplasms, on the other hand, may have a bland, mature cellular microscopic appearance, as seen in small lymphocytic malignant lymphoma.

Malignant neoplasms of epithelial origin are called *carcinomas;* if predominantly glandular or ductal, they are termed *adenocarcinomas;* if derived from a stratified squamous epithelium, they are designated as *squamous cell carcinomas.* Lesions with hybrid features between glandular and squamous carcinomas are known as *transitional cell carcinomas.* Those tumors originating in a specific organ may be named accordingly; for example, *hepatocellular* carcinoma, or *adrenocortical* carcinoma. Malignant neoplasms of mesenchymal origin are termed *sarcomas* (if differentiating towards fat cells, liposarcoma; fibrous tissue, fibrosarcoma; smooth muscle, leiomyosarcoma; blood vessels, angiosarcoma, etc.). Malignant tumors do not necessarily have benign counterparts, and the converse also applies.

Modifying adjectives used in diagnosis often carry prognostic information, as in "poorly differentiated" adenocarcinoma. Neoplasms with biologically ambiguous names are referred to with a precise modifier; for example, *malignant* schwannoma vs. *benign* schwannoma. Nonspecific anatomic names generally should be avoided. To illustrate this point, "bronchogenic" carcinoma could refer to squamous cell carcinoma, adenocarcinoma, small-cell neuroendocrine carcinoma, and other tumor types.

Neoplasms of the hematopoietic system usually have no benign analogues. Consequently, the terms *leukemia* and *lymphoma,* together with appropriate adjectives (e.g., chronic myelogenous leukemia; nodular small cleaved-cell lymphoma) always refer to malignant proliferations. The same generalization applies to the term *melanoma,* which is always used to describe a malignant melanocytic neoplasm.

Finally, time-honored but idiosyncratic eponyms remain. These are used in reference to such neoplasms as Ewing's sarcoma (of uncertain histogenesis), Warthin's tumor (a benign lesion of the salivary glands), and the Brenner tumor (a neoplasm with both benign and malignant forms derived from the surface epithelium of the ovary).

MACROSCOPIC EXAMINATION OF TISSUE SPECIMENS

As a discipline, pathology had its beginnings in the careful gross examination of diseased tissues at the autopsy table. Even before the microscope had come into general use, several disorders were well-recognized at a macroscopic level, including malignant melanomas and various carcinomas. In the current race to introduce new and ever-more-molecular techniques to diagnostic

medicine, it is tempting to forget about the use of the trained observer's eyes and tactile senses. However, these simple tools are crucial to good surgical and pathological practice.

The pathologist grossly examines all resected tumors submitted to the laboratory with several objectives in mind. First, the presence of representative tissue must be confirmed, and the suitability of the specimen for further study is judged. Second, margins of excision are labeled with indelible ink, in order to retain the orientation of the specimen for subsequent histologic analysis. Third, the specimen is opened and sectioned with a scalpel or sharp knife, at which time notes are made on the consistency, color, and extent of the neoplastic growth. By integrating documented macroscopic characteristics with knowledge of the clinical findings, a differential diagnosis may be reached at this stage and appropriate samples taken to resolve it. For example, a soft-tissue tumor of the retroperitoneum may have the gross appearance of a leiomyosarcoma; in order to confirm this interpretation definitively, however, prosected tissues can be placed in special fixative and examined later with the electron microscope. Not uncommonly, macroscopic features alone are sufficient to suggest a final diagnosis. Fig. 2.1 shows an anterior mediastinal tumor from an adult patient, the gross attributes of which are characteristic of thymoma. Along the same lines, the darkly colored mandibular mass from a child in fig. 2.2 is macroscopically typical of a pigmented neuroectodermal tumor.

It is imperative that the pathologist examine *all* of a resected tumor before it is subdivided by the surgeon for other purposes. As an example, portions of neoplasms are often sent directly from the operating room to research laboratories for investigational purposes. However, in cases where careful inspection of the lesional borders is important, it is a disservice to patient care to violate the tissue margins before they can be adequately

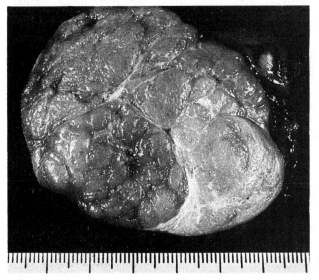

Fig. 2.1. Photograph of resected anterior mediastinal tumor with macroscopic characteristics that are typical of thymoma. These include encapsulation and internal fibrous septation, yielding tumoral nodules with angulated contours.

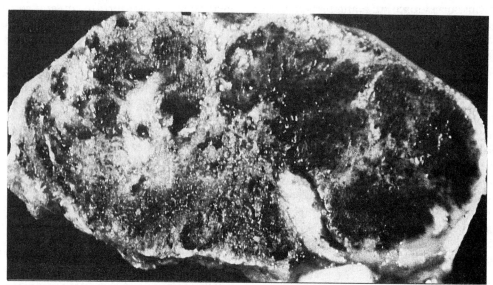

Fig. 2.2. Photograph of pigmented neuroectodermal tumor of infancy, involving the mandible. The appearance of this lesion is virtually diagnostic, in light of its known location and the dense pigmentation that is evident macroscopically.

examined pathologically. For example, a malignant rather than a benign diagnosis is rendered in cases of follicular thyroid lesions or thymic tumors if they invade through the capsular boundaries. Obviously, receipt of a partial specimen in the gross pathology laboratory prevents proper examination of such lesions.

Anatomic orientation of excised tissues should be a routine part of the information submitted to the pathology department. This allows for the precise localization of a tumor that is present at the margin of resection.

HISTOLOGIC STUDY OF HUMAN MALIGNANCIES

In the hands of individuals who have been well-trained in morphologic diagnosis, the light microscope continues to serve as the cornerstone of surgical pathology. With the proviso that the tissue processing requirements have been met, the simple use of the hematoxylin and eosin staining method on paraffin-embedded tissue sections is sufficient to make the diagnosis of most malignant neoplasms. Nonetheless, certain clinical procedures negate the validity of routine light microscopy and should be avoided. For example, vigorous compression of tissue specimens during their procurement, as occurs in some endoscopic biopsies, or extensive use of electrical or thermal cautery in resection procedures severely damages microscopic anatomy and interferes with diagnosis.

Another important aspect of light microscopy relates to the time necessary for proper preparation of stained tissue sections. In order for the morphologic features to be optimally visualized histologically, a minimum period of fixation in formalin (or an alternative mordant) must be obtained. Depending upon the overall size of the specimen, this varies from one to two hours, to more than 12 hours. After fixation, automated dehydration of

the tissues requires several additional hours; subsequent embedding in paraffin, sectioning, and staining processes add still more time for the necessary laboratory procedures (Bancroft and Stevens 1975). This sequence of events is outlined here in order to prevent frustration on the part of clinical physicians, who often wonder why a microscopic interpretation is so long in forthcoming after a specimen has been submitted to the laboratory. A quicker method of histologic examination does exist (the frozen section procedure), but it yields microscopic preparations that are vastly inferior to those procured with conventional processing. For that reason, it is used sparingly.

Once stained microscopic slides have been obtained, the pathologist employs knowledge of histology and cytology to recognize changes related to neoplasia and other diseases. These include assessment of tissue growth patterns, the degree of cellular differentiation, and details that relate to prognosis, such as adequacy of excision. It would, indeed, be fortuitous if a firm diagnosis of cancer were always possible by brief examination of glass slides; unfortunately this is not a realistic expectation, and often there is no substitute for experience, painstaking analysis, and collegial consultation among laboratory physicians on a difficult case.

There are several potential reasons for uncertainty in the interpretation of biopsy or resection specimens. An important cause relates to the natural history of any given pathologic process. A biopsy may be obtained at a time when a neoplastic lesion is not fully developed, and therefore lacks so-called diagnostic histologic features. In addition, treatments such as irradiation or chemotherapy that may have been given before surgical intervention alter the tissue's pathologic characteristics (Underwood 1987). Other lesions that cause a great deal of consternation are the so-called borderline or minimal deviation malignancies. These include epithelial, mesenchymal, and melanocytic proliferations, and are characterized by microscopic features that differ minimally from those of benign neoplasms or reactive processes (Grundmann and Beck 1988).

In the course of arriving at a diagnosis, the pathologist often verbally contacts the responsible clinician to discuss pertinent findings, and a written report is ultimately issued for all specimens. This report should include the tumor type (and grade, if applicable), as well as information that can be used by oncologists to assign a stage to the lesion in cases of malignant neoplasms. Pathologists may be familiar with the biological attributes of some tumors that even experienced oncologists have not encountered. Under these circumstances, a comment may be included in the tissue report on the expected behavior of the lesion, and recommendations for therapy may be given in generic terms. Also, antecedent verbal discussions with clinicians may be distilled into similar suggestions for subsequent management of difficult cases, particularly those that fall into the borderline category.

STAGE AND GRADE

Determination of tumor stage and grade not only offers important prognostic information but also allows for comparison of therapeutic results using various cooperative treatment protocols. Tumor grading is based primarily on the degree of differentiation of the malignant cells (figs. 2.3 and 2.4), and secondarily on an estimate of the growth rate as indicated by the mitotic rate. Because the correlation between histologic appearances and biologic behavior is imperfect, grading criteria vary greatly for different neoplasms. Nonetheless, all grading criteria attempt to describe the extent to which the tumor cells resemble their normal tissue counterparts. Accurate grading is complicated by variations in differ-

entiation from area to area in large tumors, as well as by site-related considerations and changes in tumor biology with time. Tumor stage is based on the size of the primary lesion and the presence of lymph nodal or hematogenous metastasis. The major staging systems in use are the TNM classification (for primary *T*umor size, presence and extent of lymph *N*ode involvement, and distant *M*etastasis) and the AJC (American Joint Committee) system that divides all tumors into stages 0 to IV.

The following examples illustrate the importance in prognosis and treatment of these staging and grading procedures for specific tumors.

Although the morphologic subtype of Hodgkin's disease has an effect on prognosis, tumor burden (stage) appears to be the most important prognostic variable (Spect et al. 1988) given current modalities of therapy. Consequently, the pathologic findings at staging laparotomy (which includes splenectomy and biopsies of liver, retroperitoneal lymph nodes, and bone marrow) have a far greater influence on the choice of treatment than the determination of a specific histologic subtype.

Pathologic examination of squamous cell carcinoma of the uterine cervix is required to define the stage of any given tumor. The clinical significance of the stage is indicated by studies showing less than 1% incidence of pelvic lymph node metastasis in early microinvasive carcinoma (<3 mm depth of stromal invasion), compared with 8.1% in tumors that are 3.1 mm to 5 mm deep. The presence of vascular invasion appears to further increase the risk of nodal metastasis and vaginal recurrence (Ferenczy and Winkler 1987). Patients with stage Ia (occult invasive) carcinoma have a 5-year survival rate of 96%, while patients with stage Ib (frankly invasive) lesions have a survival rate of 86% at the same time point. For cervical squamous carcinoma,

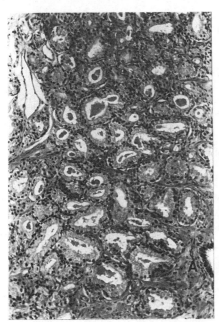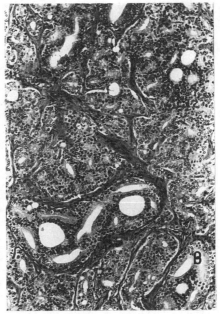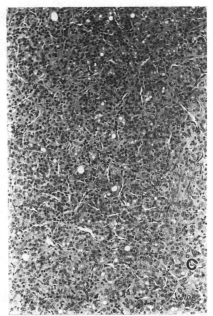

Fig. 2.3. Adenocarcinoma of the prostate. (A) Well differentiated. Note the single, separate, closely spaced uniform glands. (B) Moderately differentiated. Note irregular glands with prominent cribriform epithelium. (C) Poorly differentiated. Note fused glandular epithelium and anaplasia of individual cells.

histologic grade generally has no influence on survival of patients within any staging group.

Adenocarcinoma of the prostate is an example of a tumor for which microscopic grading is strongly correlated with prognosis and response to treatment. The grading system is based on the degree of glandular differentiation and on the *pattern* of growth, as evaluated by low-power microscopic examination (see fig. 2.3). The histologic grade correlates well with clinical stage, as well as with the mortality rate within each stage. A *combination* of microscopic grade and clinical stage provides the best prognostic information (Gleason and Mellinger 1974).

FROZEN SECTIONS

The term "frozen section" is synonymous with an intraoperative microscopic consultation. A sample of fresh tissue obtained at the time of a surgical procedure is frozen by the pathologist; the most widely used method involves rapid cooling in a refrigerated bath of an organic liquid. Histologic sections are then prepared on a cryostat (refrigerated microtome), fixed briefly, stained with hematoxylin and eosin, and examined microscopically. The entire procedure, including thorough histologic study, can usually be accomplished in about 10 to 15 minutes. Proper interpretation requires a complete gross examination of the tissue prior to sectioning and a well-trained, experienced pathologist. Informative, interactive communication with the sur-

geon and an adequate clinical history are also absolutely essential for optimization of this process.

As with all other diagnostic procedures, frozen section consultation has specific indications. In general, these include identification of a tissue; demonstration of the presence and nature of a lesion; definition of the adequacy of surgical margins or the extent of disease; and determination that the excised material is sufficient for diagnosis. Frozen sections should not be used merely to satisfy the surgeon's curiosity, to compensate for inadequate preoperative evaluation or deficiencies in surgical technique, or as a mechanism used to communicate information more quickly to the patient or the patient's family. Also, it is well-known that some diagnoses are so tenuous in this setting that frozen section interpretation is totally inadvisable. For example, it is often impossible to distinguish benign from malignant follicular thyroid tumors or mammary lesions using this technique, even in the best of hands.

Although histopathologic interpretation of cryostat sections is technically limited and more difficult than diagnosis using paraffin-embedded, fixed tissues, frozen sections are highly regarded as a useful means of intraoperative consultation. The accuracy of frozen section diagnosis is commonly reported as being in the range of 94% to 98%, but this figure varies depending on the tissue type and the reason for consultation. Frozen section diagnoses often have a significant influence on the surgical procedure being performed, and hence both surgeons and pathologists must utilize them wisely.

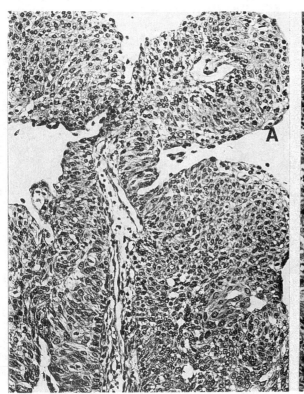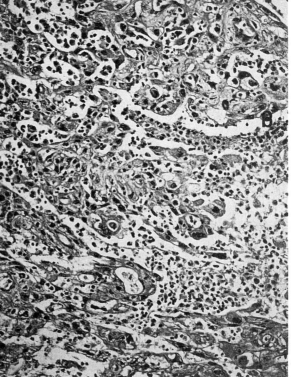

Fig. 2.4. (A) Grade 2/4 transitional cell carcinoma of the renal pelvis. This tumor is composed of relatively uniform cells lacking nuclear pleomorphism, and it demonstrates papillary growth microscopically. (B) Grade 4/4 transitional cell carcinoma of the renal pelvis. The neoplasm demonstrates overt nuclear pleomorphism and anisocytosis, and it lacks papillary differentiation.

CYTOLOGY

Cytology is the science of morphologic examination of individual cells for the purpose of diagnosis. Suitable specimens are collected in one of three basic ways: exfoliation from an epithelial surface (e.g., cervical smears obtained with a spatula or brush; bronchial washings or brushings); aspiration of fluid from body cavities; and fine-needle suction aspiration of solid lesions in the breast, thyroid, salivary glands, lung, prostate, and other organs. The cytologic preparation is then spread on a glass slide and fixed, and can be stained by a variety of methods. The Papanicolaou stain yields the greatest clarity of nuclear detail in most instances. Special investigations (routine histochemistry, immunohistochemistry, static cytometry) also may be carried out on cytologic specimens, but these must be anticipated before sample procurement, and special provisions for such analyses must be implemented.

Although generalizations are difficult, the cytomorphologic evaluation of possible malignancy is predicated on specific features of the cytoplasm and nucleus. The most helpful of these are anisonucleosis, dyskaryosis, and an abnormal nuclear-to-cytoplasmic ratio. Malignant cells show consistent changes in nuclear structure (dyskaryosis) including coarse or dense granularity, hyperchromasia, abnormal nucleoli, and anisonucleosis (marked variation in shape and size); mitotic abnormalities may also be present (fig. 2.5). Anisocytosis, or pronounced variation in cellular size or shape, is seen in malignancies as well. The volumetric nuclear-to-cytoplasmic ratio is increased; most malignant cells have an oversized nucleus that displaces all but a small peripheral zone of cytoplasm. Intercellular cohesion is likewise aberrant; however, carcinomas do retain enough cell-to-cell adhesion to make their cytologic attributes dissimilar from those of mesenchymal neoplasms. Because reactive cellular changes (due to inflammation, infection, irradiation, or cytotoxic chemotherapy) can easily be confused with those of malignant proliferations, a complete clinical history is essential to accurate cytologic diagnosis.

Cytology has a high degree of reliability when morphologic interpretations are performed by experienced, well-trained individuals; nonetheless, an effort should always be made to confirm the diagnosis by conventional biopsy prior to definitive treatment. The reliability of fine-needle aspiration, when compared with open surgical biopsy, continues to be a matter of some controversy.

SPECIAL PATHOLOGIC PROCEDURES

In approximately 10% of all oncology cases, routinely assessed microscopic features of certain neoplasms may be insufficiently conclusive to allow for a firm diagnosis. For example, malignant melanomas and anaplastic carcinomas are maddeningly similar histologically, often mandating the use of electron microscopy or immuno-

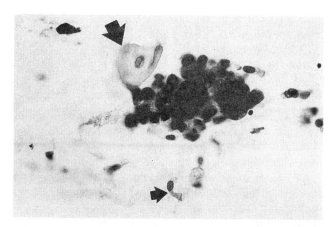

Fig. 2.5. Cytology specimen (bronchial washings) from a 60-year-old woman who had a lung mass. Note the cluster of malignant cells demonstrating pronounced anisocytosis and anisonucleosis. A normal superficial squamous cell is indicated by the large arrow, and a normal ciliated columnar cell by the small arrow.

histochemical studies to separate one from the other through elucidation of submicroscopic, cell lineage-related features (figs. 2.6A and 2.7A). Similarly, spindle-cell sarcomas of soft tissue may resemble one another so markedly that adjuvant analyses are necessary for final diagnosis (fig. 2.8).

Of course, such evaluations require additional time for implementation and interpretation. These techniques merit further discussion, inasmuch as they are utilized widely and provide extremely useful information.

ELECTRON MICROSCOPY

Electron microscopy is performed after tissue is processed in special fixative, embedded in epoxy resin, sectioned thinly ($<1/\mu m$), and impregnated with heavy

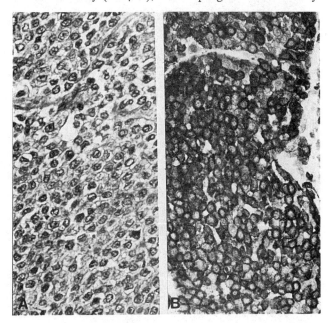

Fig. 2.6. Microscopically indeterminate small-cell neoplasm, metastatic to a cervical lymph node (A). The identity of this tumor as a carcinoma is indicated by immunoreactivity for cytokeratin, an epithelial marker (B).

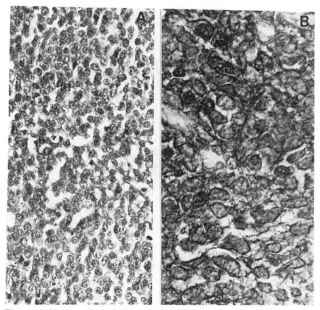

Fig. 2.7. Metastatic lymph nodal neoplasm (A), with histologic features that are virtually identical to those shown in Fig. 2.6A. The two tumors differ in cellular lineage, however, as shown by the immunostain for the melanocytic-specific marker HMB-45 (B). Hence, the final diagnosis in this case was metastatic malignant melanoma.

metals. These allow for differential absorption of a focused electron beam that is passed through the specimen en route to a photographic emulsion plate. The latter provides a pictorial image of intracellular contents, magnified up to 200,000 times or more (Peven and Gruhn 1985). Based on the presence of certain cytoplasmic organelles and other features such as intercellular junctional complexes, the pathologist may be able to distinguish one malignant cell type (e.g., melanocytic) from another (e.g., epithelial) (Gyorkey et al. 1975). Hence, the technique contributes meaningfully to differential diagnosis. Examples of salient electron microscopic findings in human malignancies are provided in table 2.2.

IMMUNOHISTOCHEMISTRY

Practical immunohistochemistry is currently based on an indirect, antibody-enzyme method, known in common parlance as the immunoperoxidase procedure (Hsu et al. 1981). In this technique, frozen or rehydrated deparaffinized tissue is overlaid with a specific, well-characterized primary antibody, directed at an antigen of diagnostic value. After controlled incubation and subsequent removal of the primary reagent, a second

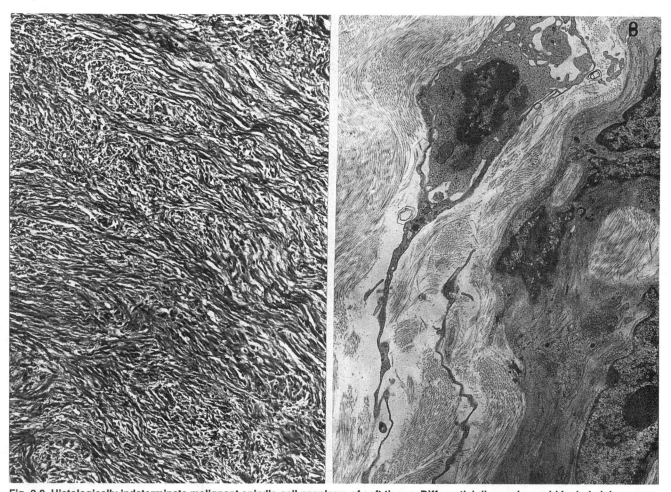

Fig. 2.8. Histologically indeterminate malignant spindle-cell neoplasm of soft tissue. Differential diagnosis would include leiomyosarcoma, fibrosarcoma, and malignant peripheral nerve sheath tumor based on the light microscopic attributes shown here (A). Electron microscopy in the same case shows attenuated, overlapping cytoplasmic processes, indicating the diagnosis of malignant peripheral nerve sheath tumor (B).

Table 2.2
SELECTED ELECTRON MICROSCOPIC FEATURES OF VALUE IN PATHOLOGIC DIAGNOSIS OF NEOPLASMS

FINDING	PREDOMINANT DISTRIBUTION	DIAGNOSTIC USE
Intercellular junctions	Epithelial cells; selected mesenchymal nonlymphoid tumors	Distinction between lymphoma and carcinoma
External basal lamina (pericellular)	Epithelial cells; selected mesenchymal nonlymphoid tumors	Distinction between lymphoma and carcinoma; aids in identification of some soft tissue sarcomas
Intra- or intercellular lumina	Glandular epithelia	Identification of adenocarcinomas
Microvillous core rootlets	Glandular epithelium of alimentary tract	Identification of gastrointestinal origin of metastatic carcinomas
Cytoplasmic tonofibrils	Squamous epithelia	Identification of squamous differentiation in epithelial tumors
Premelanosomes	Melanocytic cells	Identification of melanomas
Neurosecretory granules	Neuroendocrine cells	Identification of neuroendocrine neoplasms
Thick and thin filament complexes	Striated muscle cells	Identification of rhabdomyosarcomas
Attenuated cytoplasmic processes	Schwannian and neural cells	Identification of peripheral nerve sheath or neuronal neoplasms
Thin filament-dense body complexes	Smooth muscle cells	Identification of leiomyomas and leiomyosarcomas
Birbeck granules	Langerhans' cells	Identification of Langerhans' cell proliferations (e.g., "Histiocytosis-X")
Cytoplasmic mucin granules	Secretory glandular epithelium	Distinction between malignant mesothelioma and adenocarcinoma; localization of origin for some adenocarcinomas

antibody with generic specificity for the first is exposed to the tissue sections. The latter antibody may be labeled with biotin, providing a bridge for the subsequent binding of an avidin-biotin-horseradish peroxidase complex which completes the immunochemical assembly (fig. 2.9). The peroxidase enzyme can then be used to catalyze an oxidation-reduction reaction, in the presence of a dye that is precipitated at the site of antibody binding. After a counterstaining procedure designed to highlight morphologic details, the presence of the specific antigen can be visualized at a light

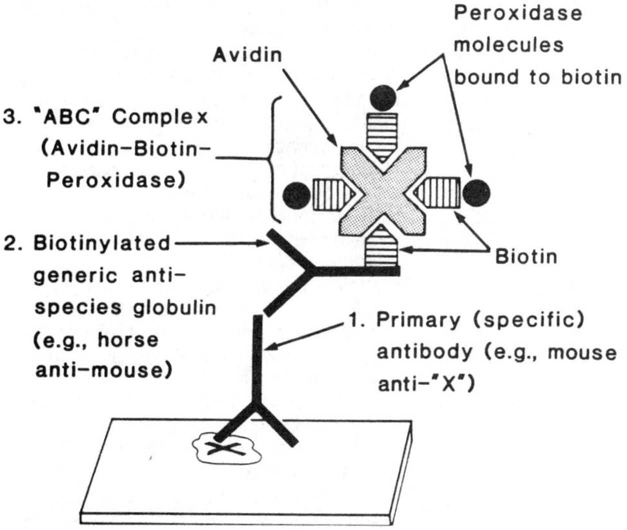

Fig. 2.9. Schematic representation of the avidin-biotin-horseradish peroxidase complex (ABC) technique of immunohistochemistry. A primary antibody to an antigen of interest is incubated with test tissue sections, and followed sequentially by biotinylated secondary antibody and ABC complex. If the primary antibody binds (i.e., if the antigen is present in the tissue), the ensuing sequence of reagent linkages provides the substrate for chromogen localization and light microscopic visibility of the reaction. In this manner, antigens of diagnostic value can be detected in tissue.

microscopic level within the tissue section (figs. 2.6B and 2.7B).

With few exceptions, these determinants are not absolutely tissue- or tumor-specific. Therefore, the immunopathologist must employ panels of primary antibodies in the study of malignant tumors, building an antigenic fingerprint that eventually allows for a final interpretation (Wick 1988). A sampling of commonly assessed antigens is listed in table 2.3. Based on their relative tissue specificities, algorithms (figs. 2.10 and 2.11) can be constructed that enable the resolution of differential diagnostic problems among histologically similar neoplasms.

Neither electron microscopy nor immunohistochemistry is capable of distinguishing benign from malignant tumors. Instead, their principal purpose is to distinguish between microscopic "look-alikes" that have differing prognoses or require dissimilar treatments. Another use for antibody-enzyme staining methods is to localize clinically important tumor markers within tissue sections.

IN SITU HYBRIDIZATION

Two recent advances have allowed for a wider application of *in situ* hybridization (ISH) technology to diagnostic pathology: the labeling of DNA probes by nonradioactive methods, and the development of techniques that permit the direct recognition of endogenous nucleic acid sequences in paraffin-embedded tissue sections and cytologic smears. The use of *in situ* hybridization has several diagnostic advantages. Small tissue fragments and archival material are amenable for use with the method, and the reaction product is localized to specific cells (or even subcellular compartments), facilitating simultaneous evaluation of the histology and the ISH result.

Traditionally, nucleic acid probes were labeled by incorporation of a radioisotope of phosphorus; recently, however, it has been found that biotin can be linked directly to probes by employing biotinylated derivatives of uridine triphosphate (UTP) or deoxyuridine triphosphate (dUTP) during probe synthesis. Importantly, the labeled nucleic acid exhibits denaturation and renaturation kinetics that are equivalent to those of an unsubstituted template. Through the use of avidin that has been complexed to fluorescent marker molecules (fluorescein), chromogenic enzymes (horseradish peroxidase; alkaline phosphatase), or electron-opaque plastic spheres, the biotinylated probe can be detected after *in situ* hybridization. Other methods for nonradioactive labeling of probes include the direct incorporation of fluorochromes or haptens (DeLellis and Wolfe 1987). *In situ* hybridization has been confirmed as a useful aid for diagnosis, for the identification of patient populations at increased risk of developing malignancies, and for the determination of prognosis. Some recently described examples of these applications follow.

In situ hybridization has been widely used in the detection of human papillomaviruses (HPV). Although over 50 variants of this virus have been identified, certain types (16, 18, 31, 33, 35, 39, 45, 51) are correlated with high-grade dysplasias and malignancies of the female genital tract. Because the viral capsid antigen of all types is identical, immunohistochemical techniques are of no value in separating them. However, hybridization with biotinylated or radioactive probes has been used successfully to identify specific HPV types in both Pap smears and biopsy sections (Crum et al. 1986; Pilotti et al. 1989). The results show the value of this method for identifying women with HPV infection who are at risk for progression to uterine cervical carcinoma. In this regard, it is of interest that *in situ* hybridization studies have also identified a predominance of HPV types 6, 11, 16, and 18 in HPV DNA-positive squamous cell carcinomas of the anus (Gal et al. 1988), tongue (deVilliers et al. 1985), penis (Weaver et al. 1989), and lung (Bejui-Thivolet et al. 1990).

Similarly, chronic infection by hepatitis B virus (HBV) is correlated with an increased risk for the development of hepatocellular carcinoma. HBV nucleic acid sequences have been detected by ISH in the liver tissue of some patients who lacked the serologic markers of viral infection (Rijntjes et al. 1985).

The extent of *in situ* hybridization for N-*myc* in neuroblastomas correlates well with the results of Southern blot analysis of this oncogene (Cohen et al. 1988). The importance of this finding lies in the fact that amplification of the N-*myc* oncogene is a seemingly independent prognostic factor associated with rapid progression of neuroblastomas (Seeger et al. 1985).

Table 2.3
SELECTED ANTIGENIC MOIETIES OF DIAGNOSTIC VALUE IN PRACTICAL IMMUNOHISTOCHEMISTRY

ANTIGEN	PREDOMINANT DISTRIBUTION	DIAGNOSTIC USE
Cytokeratin	Epithelial cells	Distinction between lymphoma or melanoma and carcinoma
Epithelial membrane antigen	Epithelial cells	Distinction between melanoma and carcinoma
Leukocyte common antigen	Leukocytes	Distinction between lymphoma, carcinoma, and melanoma
Desmin	Myogenous cells	Identification of myogenic sarcomas
Muscle-specific actin	Myogenous cells	Identification of myogenic sarcomas
Thyroglobulin	Thyroid follicular cells	Identification of certain thyroid carcinomas
Prostate-specific antigen	Prostatic epithelium	Identification of metastatic prostatic carcinomas
Calcitonin	Parafollicular thyroid epithelium	Distinction of medullary thyroid carcinoma from other thyroid tumors
Carcinoembryonic antigen	Endodermally derived epithelium	Identification of certain carcinomas; distinction of mesothelioma and adenocarcinoma
Placental alkaline phosphatase	Placental tissue and germ cell tumors	Screening identification of possible germ cell and trophoblastic tumors
Alpha-fetoprotein	Neoplastic hepatic tissue and selected germ cell tumors	Identification of possible hepatocellular carcinoma, embryonal carcinoma, and endodermal sinus tumor
Beta-human chorionic gonadotropin	Placental tissue; trophoblastic and germ cell tumors	Identification of possible trophoblastic and germ cell tumors
CA 125	Mullerian epithelium	Identification of possible female genital tract carcinomas
CA 19-9	Alimentary tract epithelium	Identification of gastrointestinal and pancreatic carcinomas
Gross cystic disease fluid protein-15	Pathologic mammary epithelium	Identification of metastatic breast carcinomas
HMB-45	Melanocytic cells	Identification of melanomas
Chromogranin-A	Neuroendocrine cells	Identification of neuroendocrine carcinomas
Synaptophysin	Neuroendocrine cells	Identification of neuroendocrine carcinomas and neuroectodermal tumors

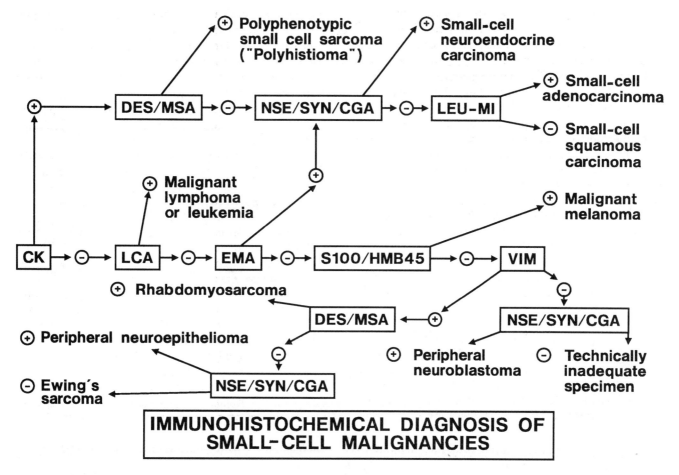

Fig. 2.10. Algorithm for application of immunostains to the differential diagnosis of histologically indeterminate small-cell malignancies. CK = cytokeratin; DES = desmin; MSA = muscle-specific actin; LCA = leukocyte common antigen; EMA = epithelial membrane antigen; NSE = neuron-specific enolase; SYN = synaptophysin; CGA = chromogranin-A: Leu M1 = CD15 antigen; S100 = S100 protein; VIM = vimentin.

DNA PROBE ANALYSIS

Recombinant DNA technology has been applied increasingly in pathology for tumor diagnosis and classification, and also has been used to assess prognosis. In Southern blots, DNA is extracted from cells, denatured, electrophoresed in an agarose gel, and transferred to a filter on which it can be hybridized with a complementary DNA probe. These preparations are used to detect genomic rearrangements, including those of genetic loci which are involved in consistent karyotypic abnormalities of certain tumors. Northern blots, in which RNA is extracted from cells, are employed to detect abnormal gene expression in the absence of gross karyotypic abnormalities, or for the determination of cell lineage on the basis of gene expression. The use of the polymerase chain reaction (PCR) provides a means whereby target nucleic acids may be amplified specifically, resulting in vastly increased sensitivity. This powerful advance in recombinant nucleic acid technology requires only that the nucleotide sequence of at least part of the target DNA is known. Complementary oligonucleotide primers flanking the region of interest are added in vast excess to the target sample, along with DNA polymerase; if the target sequence is present, the primers will hybridize and provide an initiation site for the polymerase to synthesize DNA. After completion of this step, the reaction mixture is heated to denature the nucleic acid, and then cooled to reanneal the reagents; thereafter, another cycle of polymerase-catalyzed synthesis is begun. The 20 to 30 cycles of a typical PCR result in exponential amplification of the target DNA. The application of a heat-stable DNA polymerase enzyme has simplified the technical aspects of PCR greatly and allowed it to be automated (Grody et al. 1989).

HEMATOPOIETIC MALIGNANCIES

Molecular analysis is most widely used in the diagnosis and classification of lymphoid neoplasms. DNA "restriction fragment" sizes change whenever a translocation, inversion, or gene rearrangement occurs in the area detected by a specific probe; this concept has clinical applications in several diagnostic settings in hematopathology (fig. 2.12). These include the distinction of monoclonal from polyclonal lymphoproliferative diseases; detection of rearrangements associated with chromosome translocations in lymphomas and chronic myelogenous leukemias; identification of minimal residual disease during clinical remission; and demonstration

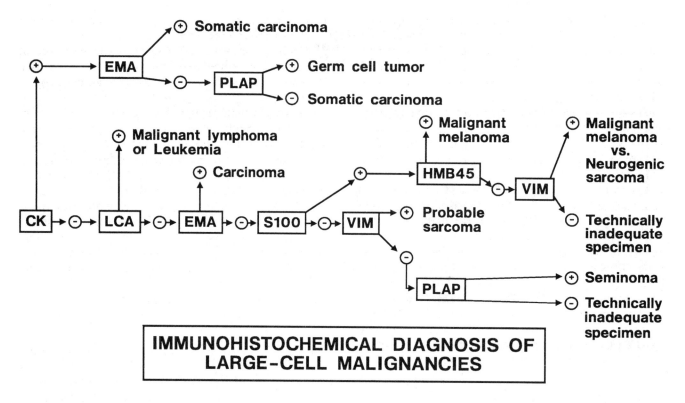

IMMUNOHISTOCHEMICAL DIAGNOSIS OF LARGE-CELL MALIGNANCIES

Fig. 2.11. Algorithm for application of immunostains to the differential diagnosis of histologically indeterminate large-cell malignancies. CK = cytokeratin; EMA = epithelial membrane antigen; LCA = leukocyte common antigen; PLAP = placental alkaline phosphatase; S100 = S100 protein; VIM = vimentin.

of the relationship between a recurrent malignancy and the original clonal population.

A recent study of the diagnostic utility of immunogenotyping in lymphoid proliferations demonstrated that Southern blot analysis (with probes to immunoglobulin heavy chain, immunoglobulin light chain, and a T-cell receptor locus) resolved diagnostic problems in more than 50% of cases where morphology and immunophenotyping yielded indeterminate results (Kamat et al. 1990). Southern blot analysis itself is quite sensitive,

and can detect monoclonality even when the neoplastic proliferation represents only 1% to 5% of the analyzed lymphoid cells (Grody et al. 1989).

Detection of rearrangements associated with chromosome translocations is another well-established role for molecular analysis. For example, over 80% of follicular lymphomas, 20% of diffuse large-cell lymphomas, and approximately 50% of adult undifferentiated lymphomas contain a t(14;18)(q32;q21) translocation in which the *bcl*-2 gene from chromosome segment 18q21

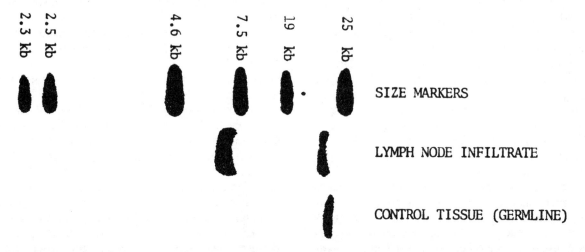

Fig. 2.12. Southern blot of DNA extracted from a lymph node that histologically contained an atypical lymphoid infiltrate (DNA digested with the restriction enzyme EcoR1; immunoglobulin heavy chain J-region probe). A discrete set of detectable restriction fragments is present, indicating that the lymphoid proliferation is monoclonal, and suggesting a diagnosis of malignant lymphoma.

moves into the IgH locus of 14q32. The rearrangements are focused on 18q21, and result in a *bcl*-2/immunoglobulin fusion gene with a chimeric transcript. Thus, a translocation-specific rearrangement unique to neoplastic cells can be identified on Southern blots, and can be used to follow the disease process (Crescenzi et al. 1988). Because PCR is sensitive enough to detect one malignant cell in one million, the technique has been used to identify the subclinical presence of leukemic cells in patients who are in clinical remission (Crescenzi et al. 1988).

Similarly, 95% of chronic myelogenous leukemias (CML) and 13% of acute lymphocytic leukemias (ALL) are associated with a t(9;22) translocation of the C-*abl* oncogene from 9q34 to 22q11, known as the Philadelphia (Ph1) chromosome. Because the translocation breakpoint on chromosome 22 occurs in a very small region (the breakpoint cluster region, *bcr*), detection of the fusion gene (*bcr-abl*) transcript or fusion protein is pathognomonic for CML. The polymerase chain reaction has been used for diagnosis of the Philadelphia translocation, and exceeds the sensitivity of cytogenetic analysis (Kawasaki et al. 1988). In addition, PCR has demonstrated residual chimeric *bcr-abl* transcripts in Ph1-positive CML patients in clinical remission (Lee et al. 1988).

As noted by Lee et al. (1988), the sensitivity of PCR raises several important clinical questions. For example, are leukemic patients who are in remission heterogeneous biologically, or do all of them have quiescent malignant cells with little proliferative potential? The answers to these queries are presently unknown, and this situation illustrates an instance where technology has outstripped the ability to apply its benefits in practice.

HUMAN PAPILLOMAVIRUS INFECTION

A modified PCR reaction has been used to detect HPV types 16 and 18 in routinely processed cervical tissue (Shibata et al. 1988). As noted, the correlation of certain types of HPV with high-grade cervical dysplasia and carcinoma suggests the value of PCR for identification of patients at risk for progression to malignancy. Moreover, PCR has been used to define differences between individual HPV type 16 isolates. Although type 16b was more prevalent in cervical tissue than 16a in one study, the former agent was not found in association with carcinoma cases. In contrast, subtype 16a was identified in approximately 90% of uterine cervical cancers (Tidy et al. 1989).

MALIGNANCIES WITH PROTO-ONCOGENE ABNORMALITIES

The prognostic value of proto-oncogene abnormalities — specifically, gene amplification as detected by Southern blots — has been demonstrated in both neuroblastoma and breast carcinoma. Amplification of the N-*myc* oncogene is associated with advanced stage and rapid progression of neuroblastoma. The estimated 18-month patient survival is 70%, 30%, and 5%, respectively, as related to tumors with one, three to 10, and more than 10 N-*myc* copies (Seeger et al. 1985).

Amplification of the HER-2/*neu* oncogene in breast cancer has been correlated with lymph node metastasis. Patients whose tumors had greater than five gene copies generally have shorter survival periods than those of other women with lesions lacking gene amplification. HER-2/*neu* amplification is believed by some to have greater prognostic value than most currently used predictive factors, including hormone receptor status and primary tumor size (Slamon et al. 1987). There is also preliminary evidence that alteration of the c-*myc* gene (amplification or rearrangement) correlates with poor short-term prognosis in breast cancer cases (Varley et al. 1987). Studies of malignant tumors of the lung, bladder, pancreas, and colon have demonstrated structural alterations in other proto-oncogenes, including members of the *myc* and *ras* gene families, but the significance of these findings is unclear.

CYTOGENETICS

Specific chromosomal abnormalities are consistently associated with certain malignant neoplasms. The application of molecular biological techniques to the detection of such aberrations has defined a new level of cytogenetic analysis. However, in certain situations, routine karyotypic analysis of a tumor is still valuable in diagnosis and determination of prognosis. Specific abnormalities are best known in leukemias and lymphomas, although they have been described in nonhematopoietic tumors as well. The most common structural changes are balanced translocations, deletions, and gene amplifications.

The Philadelphia chromosome is the classic example of a balanced translocation; as noted, it is present in most chronic myeloid leukemias. Because cases lacking the Ph1 chromosome tend to be resistant to therapy and have a less-favorable prognosis (Morris et al. 1986), karyotypic analysis can provide clinically relevant information in the chronic myeloproliferative disorders. Similarly, Ewing's sarcoma (a tumor of bone and soft tissue) consistently harbors the t(11;22) translocation (Whang-Peng et al. 1987). This finding has implications for diagnosis and treatment because most other neoplasms with a histologic resemblance to Ewing's tumor are not associated with the translocation.

In contrast, karyotypic analysis of tumors with chromosomal deletions currently has little role in diagnosis. For example, although molecular techniques have revealed a particular deletion (del13q14) in 95% of patients with hereditary neuroblastoma, karyotypic analyses have done so in only 5% of cases.

The karyotypic manifestations of gene amplification include homogeneously staining regions (HSR) of single chromosomes, and double minutes (DM), which are small, paired extrachromosomal chromatin fragments. The study of HSR and DM in neuroblastoma resulted in the demonstration of a strong correlation between stage, prognosis, and amplification of the N-*myc* oncogene.

FLOW CYTOMETRY

Flow cytometry allows for the rapid quantitative measurement of several cellular characteristics, including DNA content. In flow cytometry, a monodispersed cell sample is stained with appropriate fluorochromes and passed through a flow chamber that has a geometry designed to align the stream of cells so that they are individually struck by a focused laser beam. The scattered light and fluorescent emissions are separated according to wavelength by appropriate filters and mirrors, and directed to detectors which convert them into electronic signals that are analyzed and stored for future display by a computer. The data are displayed as a frequency histogram (number of cells vs. fluorescent energy) for single parameter analysis, or as a scattergraph for multiparametric evaluation. The principle of "gating" (the placement of electronic windows around areas in the frequency distribution so that the computer analyzes data only on cells that fall within the windows) can be used to take full advantage of multiparametric analysis.

The fluorochromes used to stain cells in flow cytometry include compounds that bind stoichiometrically to DNA (propidium iodide, ethidium bromide, or diamidine phenylindole); others which label both DNA and RNA but fluoresce at different wavelengths for each (acridine orange); and those that can be attached covalently to antibodies against cell surface antigens (fluorescein isothiocyanate, Texas red). Simultaneous multiparametric analysis is possible by using two or more fluorochromes that emit at different wavelengths.

In vivo single cell suspensions, such as peripheral blood or bone marrow, can be analyzed easily by flow cytometry. Solid tissues, including lymph nodes and solid tumors, require additional preparation (usually gentle enzymatic, detergent, or mechanical treatment) to achieve a monodispersed sample. Methods have been developed that allow analysis of archival tissue that has been formalin-fixed and embedded in paraffin. Flow cytometric analysis of tumors is performed to identify cellular subpopulations within a specific histologic tumor type, as stratified by stage and grade. These are typically not evident on routine histopathologic examination. To be clinically relevant, the procedure must identify cellular populations whose characteristics are known to influence prognosis or response to treatment.

SURFACE MARKER ANALYSIS

The role of cell surface antigen analysis in the diagnosis of lymphoid and other hematopoietic malignancies is well established. Multiparametric evaluation with a panel of monoclonal antibodies against surface antigens (fig. 2.13 and table 2.4) facilitates classification of different subtypes of lymphoma and leukemia, and has become a routine facet of diagnosis in many medical centers. Some progress has been made in attempts to extend flow cytometric measurements of surface markers to assessments of solid tumors, and in applying the analysis to intracellular constituents, including oncogene products. These can be measured in isolation or compared with DNA content. However, these procedures remain largely experimental.

DNA MEASUREMENTS

Many flow cytometric studies to date have examined DNA ploidy as a prognostic factor. In general terms, very few, if any, malignant tumors have a chromosomal complement that is normal in number and structure. Thus, "diploid range" malignancies conceptually represent a heterogeneous group of lesions with chromosomal abnormalities below the level of resolution of flow cytometry. In addition, a small population of aneuploid cells may not be detected by flow cytometric measurements. Other factors can further complicate the interpretation of poorly controlled flow cytometric studies; some tissues, such as liver, normally contain tetraploid and even octaploid populations (Mendecki et al. 1978). Aneuploid cellular populations also are seen in several benign neoplastic and reactive soft-tissue lesions. Flow cytometric cell-cycle analysis is primarily directed at calculation of the proportion of S-phase cells (the

Table 2.4
REPRESENTATIVE MONOCLONAL ANTIBODIES USED IN FLOW CYTOMETRY OF HEMATOPOIETIC NEOPLASMS
(See fig. 2.13)

Antibody (Cluster Designation)	Specificity	% Positive Cells Gated Region	
		R1	R3
T-Cell Markers:			
CD 3	Pan T cells	57.7	8.3
CD 4	Helper/Inducer T cell subset	25.6	7.4
CD 8	Cytotoxic/Suppressor T cell subset	26.3	7.1
B-Cell Markers:			
CD 19	B Cells	13.7	92.9
HLA-DR	Major histocompatibility complex class II antigen (B cells, activated T cells)	62.4	100.0
Anti-IgM	B cell subset (immunoglobulin heavy chain isotype M)	1.8	37.7
Anti-lambda	B cell subset (lambda light chain)	12.5	68.3

The staining pattern is diagnostic only for the region of the scattergram that contains the atypical lymphocytes (the gated region arbitrarily labeled "R3"). These cells stain positively for HLA-DR, CD 19, and lambda immunoglobulin light chain, consistent with a monoclonal B cell population.

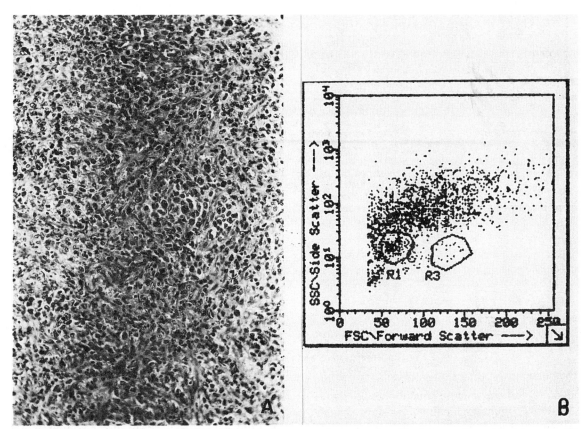

Fig. 2.13. Section of spleen from a 61-year-old woman; the parenchyma is effaced by large, malignant lymphocytes (A). Scattergram of the malignant infiltrate obtained by flow cytometry. Note the presence of two gated regions (arbitrarily labeled R1 and R3); see table 2.4 for the results of multiparametric analysis of R1 and R3.

percentage of cells undergoing DNA synthesis) and is used to identify rapidly dividing neoplasms. However, this approach has been complicated by the discovery of noncycling explanted cells with a DNA content corresponding to those in S-phase.

Consequently, it is difficult to arrive at summary statements regarding the correlation of flow cytometric data with prognosis. Published reports have suggested that some consistent relationships exist in specific forms of neoplasia (Koss et al. 1989; Auer et al. 1989). A careful prospective study of renal cell carcinoma has documented increased survival in patients with tumors having homogeneously diploid or near-diploid DNA content, as opposed to those with an aneuploid DNA profile (Ljungberg et al. 1985). A retrospective study of adenocarcinoma of the prostate demonstrated that only 15% of diploid tumors metastasized or progressed locally, while 75% of tumors with an abnormal DNA pattern did so (Winkler et al. 1988). A relationship between clinical stage and DNA ploidy in prostate cancer has also been documented (Stephenson et al. 1987).

For many other neoplasms, the correlation between DNA content and prognosis is more uncertain. The biologic significance of tumor ploidy and S-phase fractions in breast cancer remains unclear; although aneuploid lesions seem to be associated with a shorter disease-free survival, there is no obvious association between aneuploidy and stage (Visscher et al. 1990).

Similarly, there is no clear pattern of behavior, according to DNA ploidy patterns, that may be discerned in cases of colorectal adenocarcinoma. The exact relationship of tumor ploidy to prognosis has not been established for malignancies of the lung, uterine cervix, head and neck, soft tissue, thyroid, and stomach. In summary, DNA analysis is still in its infancy, and must be approached in a systematic, histologically based fashion.

TUMOR MARKERS

A tumor marker is a biochemical indicator of the presence of a neoplastic proliferation; in clinical usage, this term refers to a molecule that can be detected in serum, plasma, or other body fluids. Sensitive methods of measurement — usually radioimmunoassay (RIA) or enzyme-linked immunosorbent assay (ELISA) — are often required for optimal usefulness. No tumor marker is specific; virtually all are present at low levels in the normal physiological state or in non-neoplastic disease, and any given marker may be seen in conjunction with a variety of different neoplasms. Tumor markers can be divided into two broad categories: tumor-derived moieties, and tumor-associated or host-response markers.

Tumor-derived markers include oncofetal antigens (alpha-fetoprotein [AFP], carcinoembryonic antigen [CEA]); hormones (human chorionic gonadotropin [HCG], human placental lactogen, antidiuretic hormone, parathyroid hormone, calcitonin, insulin-like

Table 2.5
SELECTED TUMOR MARKERS AND THEIR APPLICATIONS IN DIAGNOSTIC MEDICINE

TUMOR MARKER	EXEMPLARY MALIGNANT NEOPLASMS	COMMONLY ASSOCIATED NON-NEOPLASTIC DISEASES
Hormones		
Human chorionic gonadotropin (HCG)	Gestational trophoblastic disease, gonadal germ cell tumors	Pregnancy
Calcitonin	Medullary cancer of the thyroid	
Catecholamines and metabolites	Pheochromocytoma	
Oncofetal Antigens		
Alpha-fetoprotein (AFP)	Hepatocellular carcinoma, gonadal germ cell tumors (especially endodermal sinus tumor)	Cirrhosis, toxic liver injury, hepatitis
Carcinoembryonic antigen (CEA)	Adenocarcinomas of the colon, pancreas, stomach, lung, breast, ovary	Pancreatitis, inflammatory bowel disease, hepatitis, cirrhosis, tobacco abuse
Isoenzymes		
Prostatic acid phosphatase (PAP)	Adenocarcinoma of the prostate	Prostatitis; nodular prostatic hyperplasia
Neuron-specific enolase	Small-cell carcinoma of the lung; neuroblastoma	
Specific Proteins		
Prostate specific antigen (PSA)	Adenocarcinoma of the prostate	Nodular prostatic hyperplasia; prostatitis
Immunoglobulin (monoclonal)	Multiple myeloma	Monoclonal gammopathy of unknown significance
CA 125	Epithelial ovarian neoplasms	Menstruation, pregnancy, peritonitis
CA 19-9	Adenocarcinoma of the pancreas or colon	Pancreatitis; ulcerative colitis

growth factors, catecholamine metabolites); tissue-specific proteins (immunoglobulins, prostate specific antigen [PSA], gross cystic disease fluid protein-15); enzymes (gamma-glutamyl transpeptidase); isoenzymes (prostate acid phosphatase [PAP], placental alkaline phosphatase [PLAP], neuron-specific enolase [NSE]);

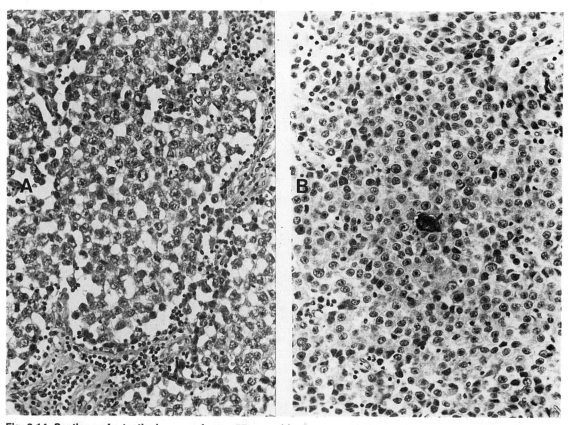

Fig. 2.14. Sections of a testicular mass from a 57-year-old man; preoperative workup demonstrated an increased beta-HCG level in serum. (A) Routine histopathologic examination showed a classic seminoma. Note the uniform malignant cells with abundant, clear cytoplasm, arranged in nests divided by fibrous bands; a lymphocytic stromal infiltrate is present. No trophoblastic elements are noted. (B) Immunohistochemical stain for HCG, demonstrating isolated strongly reactive mononuclear cells, confirming the presence of trophoblastic elements in the tumor.

oncogene products (*src*, N-*myc*, H-*ras*); and various polyamines, sialic acid, and glycolipids.

Tumor-associated (host-response) markers are most often used together with tumor-derived markers. For example, in concert with NSE levels, serum ferritin levels in neuroblastoma have been shown to correlate with stage of disease and response to therapy. Other host-response markers include interleukin-2, tumor necrosis factor, immune complexes, acute phase reactants (C-reactive protein, alpha-2-macroglobulin), and enzymes (lactic dehydrogenase, creatine kinase BB isoenzyme, glutamate dehydrogenase).

No tumor marker has been shown to have a specificity or sensitivity that is adequate for the screening detection of malignancies in the general population. Because of this limitation, the main utility of tumor markers has been in determining the response to therapy; that is, the detection of residual disease or relapse. Useful tumor markers and associated neoplasms are presented in table 2.5. Fig. 2.14 demonstrates that the detection of tumor markers may be accomplished by pathologic examination of tumor tissue itself. Excellent general reviews of these topics have been published recently (Virgi et al. 1988).

Given the lack of specificity of many markers, test panels composed of both tumor-derived and tumor-associated discriminants have been devised. For example, a possible battery of tumor markers for colorectal adenocarcinoma would include CEA, CA 19-9, and PLAP; for small-cell carcinoma of the lung, CEA, NSE, and antidiuretic hormone; and, for adenocarcinoma of the prostate, PAP, PSA, and gamma-seminal protein. More experience is needed to determine if such an approach is clinically useful in patients being screened for malignancy.

SUMMARY

This overview has outlined a number of conventional and recently developed techniques available to the pathologist for use in the evaluation of neoplastic diseases. Knowledge of the potential uses and abuses of these procedures is important for clinical physicians, and helps to assure that patient care is neither hindered through the omission of pertinent studies nor harmed through their misapplication. The cooperation that is required among laboratory physicians and oncologists in the diagnosis and management of oncology patients cannot be overstressed.

REFERENCES

Auer, G.; Askensten, U.; and Ahrens, O. 1989. Cytophotometry. *Hum. Pathol.* 20:518-27.

Bancroft, J.D., and Stevens, A. 1975. *Histopathological stains and their diagnostic uses.* New York: Churchill Livingstone.

Bejui-Thivolet, F.; Llagre, N.; and Chignol, M.C. et al. 1990. Detection of human papillomavirus DNA in squamous bronchial metaplasia and squamous cell carcinomas of the lung by *in situ* hybridization using biotinylated probes in paraffin-embedded specimens. *Hum. Pathol.* 21:111-16.

Cohen, P.S.; Seeger, R.C.; and Triche, T.J. et al. 1988. Detection of N-*myc* gene expression in neuroblastoma tumors by *in situ* hybridization. *Am. J. Pathol.* 131:391-97.

Crescenzi, M.; Seto, M.; and Herzig, G.P. et al. 1988. Thermostable DNA polymerase chain amplification of t(14;18) chromosome breakpoints and detection of minimal residual disease. *Proc. Natl. Acad. Sci. USA* 85:4869-73.

Crum, C.P.; Nagai, N.; and Levine, R.U. et al. 1986. *In situ* hybridization analysis of HPV 16 DNA sequences in early cervical neoplasia. *Am. J. Pathol.* 123:174-82.

deVilliers, E.M.; Weidaurer, H.; and Otto, H. et al. 1985. Papillomavirus DNA in human tongue carcinomas. *Int. J. Cancer* 36:575-78.

DeLellis, R.A., and Wolfe, H.J. 1987. New techniques in gene product analysis. *Arch. Pathol. Lab. Med.* 111:620-26.

Ferenczy, A., and Winkler, E. 1987. Carcinoma and metastatic tumors of the cervix. In Kurman, R.J. ed. *Blaustein's pathology of the female genital tract.* 3rd ed. pp. 218-25. New York: Springer-Verlag.

Gal, A.A.; Saul, S.H.; and Stoler, M.H. 1988. Demonstration of human papillomavirus in anal carcinoma by *in situ* hybridization. *Lab. Invest.* 58:33A.

Gleason, D.F., and Mellinger, G.T. 1974. The Veterans Administration Cooperative Urological Research Group: prediction of prognosis for prostate adenocarcinoma by combined histological grading and clinical staging. *J. Urol.* 111:58-64.

Grody, W.W.; Gatti, R.A.; and Naeim, F. 1989. Diagnostic molecular pathology. *Mod. Pathol.* 2:553-68.

Grundmann, E., and Beck, E. eds. 1988. *Minimal neoplasia.* New York: Springer-Verlag.

Gyorkey, F.; Min, K.W.; and Krisko, I. et al. 1975. The usefulness of electron microscopy in the diagnosis of human tumors. *Hum. Pathol.* 6:421-41.

Hsu, S.M.; Raine, L.; and Fanger, H. 1981. Use of avidin-biotin-peroxidase complex (ABC) in immunoperoxidase staining techniques: a comparison between ABC and unlabeled antibody (PAP) procedures. *J. Histochem. Cytochem.* 29:577-80.

Kamat, D.; Laszewski, M.J.; and Kemp, J.D. et al. 1990. The diagnostic utility of immunophenotyping and immunogenotyping in the pathologic evaluation of lymphoid proliferations. *Mod. Pathol.* 3:105-11.

Kawasaki, E.S.; Clark, S.S.; and Coyne, M.Y. et al. 1988. Diagnosis of chronic myeloid and acute lymphocytic leukemias by detection of leukemia-specific mRNA sequences amplified *in vitro.* *Proc. Natl. Acad. Sci. USA* 85:5698-5702.

Koss, L.G.; Czerniak, B.; and Herz, F. et al. 1989. Flow cytometric measurements of DNA and other cell components in human tumors: a critical appraisal. *Hum. Pathol.* 20:528-48.

Lee, M.S.; Chang, K.S.; and Freireich, E.J. et al. 1988. Detection of minimal residual *bcr-abl* transcripts by a modified polymerase chain reaction. *Blood* 72:893-97.

Ljungberg, B.; Stenling, R.; and Roos, G. 1985. DNA content in renal cell carcinoma with reference to tumor heterogeneity. *Cancer* 56:503-508.

Mendecki, J.; Dillman, W.H.; and Wolley, R.C. et al. 1978. Effect of thyroid hormone on the ploidy of rat liver nuclei as defined by flow cytometry. *Proc. Soc. Exp. Biol. Med.* 158:63-67.

Morris, C.M.; Reeve, A.E.; and Fitzgerald, P.H. et al. 1986. Genomic diversity correlates with clinical variation in Ph1-negative chronic myeloid leukaemia. *Nature* 320:281-83.

Peven, D.R., and Gruhn, J.D. 1985. The development of electron microscopy. *Arch. Pathol. Lab. Med.* 109:683-91.

Pilotti, S.; Gupta, J.; and Stefanon, B. et al. 1989. Study of multiple human papillomavirus-related lesions of the lower female genital tract by *in situ* hybridization. *Hum. Pathol.* 20:118-23.

Rijntjes, P.J.M.; Van Ditzhuijsen, T.J.M.; and Van Loon, A.M. et al. 1985. Hepatitis B virus DNA detected in formalin-fixed liver specimens and its relation to serologic markers and histopathologic features of chronic liver disease. *Am. J. Pathol.* 120:411-18.

Seeger, R.C.; Brodeur, G.M.; and Sather, H. et al. 1985. Association of multiple copies of the N-*myc* oncogene with rapid progression of neuroblastomas. *N. Engl. J. Med.* 313:111-16.

Shibata, D.K.; Arnheim, N.; and Martin, W.J. 1988. Detection of human papillomavirus in paraffin-embedded tissue using the polymerase chain reaction. *J. Exp. Med.* 167:225-30.

Slamon, D.J.; Clark, G.M.; and Wong, S.G. et al. 1987. Human breast cancer: correlation of relapse and survival with amplification of the HER-2/*neu* oncogene. *Science* 235: 177-81.

Specht, L.; Nordentoff, A.M.; and Cold, S. et al. 1988. Tumor burden as the most important prognostic factor in early stage Hodgkin's disease. *Cancer* 61:1719-27.

Stephenson, C.A.; James, B.C.; and Gay, H. et al. 1987. Flow cytometry of prostate cancer: relationship of DNA content to survival. *Cancer Res.* 47:2504-2507.

Tidy, J.A.; Vousden, K.H.; and Farrell, P.J. 1989. Relation between infection with a subtype of HPV 16 and cervical neoplasia. *Lancet* II:1225-27.

Underwood, J.C.E. 1987. *Introduction to biopsy interpretation and surgical pathology.* 2nd ed. New York: Springer-Verlag.

Varley, J.M.; Swallow, J.E.; and Brammar, W.J. et al. 1987. Alterations of either c-*erb*B-2 (*neu*) or c-*myc* proto-oncogenes in breast carcinomas correlate with poor short-term prognosis. *Oncogene* 1:423-30.

Virji, M.A.; Mercer, D.W.; and Herberman, R.B. 1988. Tumor markers in cancer diagnosis and prognosis. *CA* 38:104-27.

Visscher, D.W.; Zarbo, R.J.; and Greenawald, K.A. et al. 1990. Prognostic significance of morphological parameters and flow cytometric DNA analysis in carcinoma of the breast. *Pathol. Ann.* 25:171-205.

Weaver, M.G.; Abdul-Karim, F.W.; and Dale, G. et al. 1989. Detection and localization of human papillomavirus in penile condylomas and squamous cell carcinomas using *in situ* hybridization with biotinylated DNA viral probes. *Mod. Pathol.* 2:94-100.

Whang-Peng, J.; Triche, T.J.; and Knutsen, T. et al. 1986. Cytogenetic characterization of selected small round-cell tumors of childhood. *Cancer Genet. Cytogenet.* 21:185-208.

Wick, M.R. 1988. Immunohistochemistry in the diagnosis of solid malignant tumors. In Jennette, J.C. ed. *Immunohistology in diagnostic pathology.* pp. 161-91. Boca Raton: CRC Press.

Winkler, H.Z.; Rainwater, L.M.; and Myers, R. et al. 1988. Stage D prostatic adenocarcinoma: significance of nuclear DNA ploidy patterns studied by flow cytometry. *Mayo Clin. Proc.* 63:103-12.

Chapter 3

PRINCIPLES OF SURGICAL ONCOLOGY

Timothy J. Eberlein, M.D.
Richard E. Wilson, M.D.[†]

Timothy J. Eberlein, M.D.
Associate Professor of Surgery
Harvard Medical School
Attending Surgeon
Division, Surgical Oncology
Director, Biologic Cancer Therapy Program
Brigham and Women's Hospital
Boston, Massachusetts

Richard E. Wilson, M.D.[†]
Professor of Surgery
Harvard Medical School
Chief, Surgical Oncology
Brigham and Women's Hospital
Boston, Massachusetts

INTRODUCTION

Surgical resection is the oldest form of treatment for cancer. At one time the only effective treatment, it is still the preferred method for many cancers. Presently, more than 60% of patients with cancer are treated surgically, and surgery is used in diagnosis and staging of more than 90% of all cancers.

Surgical treatment has several advantages for the patient. Tumors have no biologic resistance to surgical removal and surgery has no potential carcinogenic effects. The widely accepted concept of "tumor heterogeneity," which might explain treatment failure for other modalities, is not a problem for the surgeon. Surgery can cure a large proportion of undisseminated cancers. Surgical treatment provides the most accurate evidence of the extent of disease, that being pathologic staging, as well as the opportunity to define histologic features of tumor growth.

Surgical treatment also has disadvantages. Resection has no specificity for malignant tissues; that is, normal and neoplastic tissues are destroyed equally. Surgical treatment entails some immediate threat to life and/or significant morbidity, and may result in deformity or loss of function. The surgeon may be required to limit otherwise curative resections in order to avoid damage to vital structures. Finally, cancers that have spread beyond local or regional sites ordinarily are not curable by surgical resection alone.

The era of surgery as a single modality treatment for cancer is over. Patterns of failure studies have led to the recognition that, prior to surgery, many cancers have already seeded metastatic foci not apparent at the time of diagnosis. Therefore, systemic treatment is necessary for the subclinical and undetectable spread of many tumors. Because identification as to which patient may already have systemic disease is now based on rather crude risk factors, optimal treament for both cure and palliation requires individualization of therapy and an approach that uses all therapeutic disciplines capable of improving results. Thus, the surgical oncologist should have a thorough background in the principles of general surgery and be knowledgeable about the most recent advances in the fields of radiation oncology, medical oncology and more recently, immunotherapy.

The surgeon who fails to integrate knowledge from the other disciplines of cancer treatment will be relegated to a role as a technician who, aside from the performance of a selected operation, will have little role in the preoperative planning, postoperative follow-up or integration of multiple therapies for the patient.

The surgeon has a unique perspective in the treatment of cancer, that of being the only member of the multimodality treatment team who routinely sees the tumor *in situ* and can appreciate its patterns of local and regional spread. This makes the surgeon well-suited to apply these principles to newer advances in radiation oncology and immunotherapy. Likewise, the surgeon has a singular responsibility to see to it that removed cancer tissue is studied properly and made available for present and future evaluation and potential therapy.

THE PROBLEM

Cancer is the second leading cause of death for all ages in the United States (*CA* 1990), affecting approximately

---

[†]Deceased.

three out of every four families. Over the last three decades, the number of deaths from cancer for all sites in men has steadily increased, primarily due to the dramatic rise of age-adjusted cancer death rates from lung cancer. Lung cancer deaths in women have increased even further; lung cancer is now the most common form of cancer mortality in women, surpassing even deaths from breast cancer.

In a more positive vein, more Americans survive a diagnosis of cancer today than ever before. Table 3.1 shows the improvement in relative 5-year survival rates from the early 1960s compared to the early 1980s. When adjusted for noncancer causes of death, the 5-year survival rate is 50%.

However, there is still considerable room for improvement. A multidisciplinary approach utilizing cancer prevention, earlier and more accurate diagnosis, and prompt treatment with more effective methods means that many more Americans can be saved from cancer.

HISTORICAL PERSPECTIVE

In ancient times surgery was the obvious first choice of treatment for cancer, since it was thought that the ability to remove the tumor might cure the patient. The earliest discussions of surgical treatment of tumors appear in the *E.S. Papyrus* (ca. 1600 B.C.). The modern era of abdominal surgery began in Colonial America when Ephraim McDowell removed a 22.5-pound ovarian tumor from Mrs. Jane Crawford in December 1809. By modern standards, the procedure was crude and barbaric, but nevertheless effective (the patient survived for 30 years after the operation). This was the first recorded elective abdominal operation and stimulated further developments in surgery (*Surgery in America* 1965).

The early years of surgical treatment for tumors were limited by many obstacles: most cancers were diagnosed in advanced stages, instruments were crude, and antibiotics were unavailable. Furthermore, systematic pathologic evaluation was not available until the early 1900s. Operations were limited in scope because of the inability to perform blood transfusions and the fact that endotracheal anesthesia did not exist. Postoperative care, so necessary for major operations, was very crude

Table 3.1
RELATIVE 5-YEAR SURVIVAL RATES (%)

1960-63		1980-85
60	Melanoma	81
63	Breast (Female)	76
58	Cervix	67
50	Prostate	73
63	Testis	91
40	Hodgkin's disease	76
31	NH lymphoma	51
14	Leukemia	34

(Reprinted with permission from: American Cancer Society [1990].)

Table 3.2
SURGICAL MILESTONES

DATE	PROCEDURE	SURGEON
1809	Excision of ovarian tumor	McDowell
1846	Excision of submaxillary gland	Warren (under ether anesthesia)
1867	Antisepsis	Lister
1881	Gastrectomy	Billroth
1890	Mastectomy	Halsted
1908	Abdominoperineal resection	Miles
1920s	Surgeries for brain tumors	Cushing
1935	Pancreaticoduodenectomy	Whipple

and there was no awareness of fluid and electrolyte balance, volume deficits, and sepsis management.

Three important developments changed the discipline of surgery forever. The first was the introduction of general anesthesia by two dentists, William Morton and Crawford Long. John Collins Warren performed the first major operation under general anesthesia, an excision of a submaxillary gland, at the Massachusetts General Hospital on Oct. 16, 1846. The second development was the practice of antisepsis initiated by Joseph Lister in 1867. Through the use of carbolic acid, surgical treatment was possible with a substantially decreased morbidity and mortality from infection.

Finally, the development of a formal surgical training program, as begun by William S. Halsted at Johns Hopkins University in the late 1890s, was a major stimulus to the growth of the discipline. The impact on American surgery of Halsted and his residents was widespread and long-lasting. Halsted showed that research based on anatomical and physiological principles, often employing animal experimentation, made it possible to develop new operative procedures in the laboratory and apply them in a clinical setting with excellent results. He disseminated a new system of surgery so characteristic that it might be designated a "school of surgery." Thus, with the advent of anesthesia and antisepsis, surgery was made safer and more acceptable. The Halsted method of surgical training set the stage for developing aggressive surgical procedures for cancer treatment.

Table 3.2 lists some milestones in surgical oncology. Most of the pioneers of cancer treatment emphasized meticulous surgical technique and were among the first to elucidate the principles of *en bloc* resection of cancer. Emphasis was increasingly placed on the technical aspects of surgery, such as surgical instruments, retractors and suture material, as well as on refinements in suturing technique, establishment of anatomic boundaries of resection, and the development of most of the major cancer operations still in use.

More recent innovations in cancer surgery include automatic stapling devices, laser surgery, and microsurgical techniques. Major advancements in perioperative patient management and critical care have reduced morbidity and extended the surgeon's ability to perform major operations on cancer patients with good results.

SURGERY TO PREVENT CANCER

Table 3.3 shows some of the syndromes associated with the eventual development of malignancies. The surgeon has a definite role concerning direct surgical intervention for the prevention of cancers. All surgeons should be aware of those patients at high risk and recognize situations in which surgery may prevent subsequent development of malignant disease.

Cryptorchidism is associated with an increased risk of testicular carcinoma. Orchiopexy performed at an early age may reduce the likelihood of the development of this malignancy (Mostofi 1973).

Another disease associated with a high incidence of malignant degeneration is ulcerative colitis. Approximately 40% of patients with diffuse colon involvement due to ulcerative colitis will ultimately die of colon cancer (MacDougall 1964). A colectomy may be indicated when a patient has a greater than 10-year history of ulcerative colitis, although more sophisticated evaluative techniques can reduce the necessity of operation in some patients (Devroede, Taylor, and Sauer 1971).

Patients with the genetic trait for familial polyposis of the colon will also benefit by prophylactic colectomy. If colectomy is not performed in these patients, approximately half will develop colon cancer by age 40 (DeCosse, Adams, and Condon 1977; Moertel, Hill, and Adson 1970).

Patients with multiple endocrine neoplasia MEN-Type 2 are at risk for development of medullary carcinoma of the thyroid. Leukoplakia is a clear risk factor in the development of squamous cell carcinoma of the oropharynx and the vulva. The role of prophylactic mastectomy in the patient at high risk for developing breast cancer is more controversial.

In all of these situations, the surgeon familiar with the syndromes causing high risk for development of malignancies can approximate risk for the patient by using statistical modeling. These estimates are helpful in individualizing the advice given to a patient.

SURGERY AND THE DIAGNOSIS OF CANCER

Correct diagnosis is fundamental to the appropriate treatment of cancer. An accurate diagnosis is based on the histologic findings and depends upon examination of a properly prepared representative tissue sample. Pathology is an interpretative science, so pathologic diagnosis from outside sources must be confirmed by obtaining the slides for review. Because opinions may vary, it may be necessary to obtain tissue blocks and additional biopsies for definitive diagnosis. Surgical techniques for obtaining tissue samples include needle aspiration, core needle biopsy, incisional biopsy, and excisional biopsy.

Needle aspiration refers to obtaining fragments of tumor by suction using a needle and syringe. Using a standard No. 20 or No. 21 needle with a hypodermic syringe, one or two passes are made through the tumor while suction is applied. The advantages of this technique are that it uses readily available materials, it can be performed with local anesthesia or sometimes no anesthesia, and it involves little time or expense. The disadvantages are that it frequently results in disconnected cells and, in most instances, only a cytologic diagnosis rather than a histologic diagnosis. It is not definitive if no cancer is diagnosed, and its use requires the presence of a tumor large enough to make a reliable target and that is not near a major blood vessel or hollow viscera. Cytology cannot distinguish between invasive and noninvasive cancers, and even the most experienced cytologists can mistake inflammatory cells for malignant cells. This error is inherent in cytologic review and accounts for a substantially higher error rate than that of standard histologic diagnosis.

Needle biopsies are performed with specially designed needles (True Cut, Vim-Silverman, Franklin) that can be passed through the skin to retrieve a small core of tissue. This technique can be performed under local anesthesia and also requires little investment of time and relatively little expense. It provides a specimen from which a histologic diagnosis can be made. Its limitations are that it requires special equipment, it is not definitive if only normal tissue is obtained, and it also requires a relatively large target situated away from major blood vessels and hollow viscera.

Incisional biopsy refers to using a scalpel for the removal of a small portion of tumor for diagnosis. It provides a sample for histologic diagnosis and is applicable to both superficial and internal cancers. Often, it can be performed under local anesthesia in an outpatient setting. The disadvantages are the potential sampling error and the theoretical risk of spreading tumor. Incisional biopsy is preferred for the diagnosis of large masses. It is particularly recommended as the method of choice for diagnosis of soft tissue and bony sarcomas, since the definitive surgical procedures to excise sarcomas are so often complex. Incisional biopsies are particularly helpful for tumors over 3 cm in size, and when there is a possible risk of compromise of subsequent surgical excision. Careful technique is essential in order to avoid contaminating new tissue planes with tumor.

Excisional biopsy refers to removal of an entire tumor lesion for diagnosis. It requires local or general anesthesia depending upon the circumstances. Its advantages are that it provides a definitive diagnosis, serves as adequate treatment should the lesion be benign, and involves minimal trauma to the cancer. Its disadvan-

Table 3.3
SYNDROMES ASSOCIATED WITH MALIGNANCY

SYNDROME	MALIGNANCY
Cryptorchid testis	Testicular
Chronic ulcerative colitis	Colon
Familial polyposis	Colon
Multiple endocrine neoplasia (MEN-II)	Thyroid
Leukoplakia	Squamous

tages are that it violates a deeper plane of dissection and may necessitate a wider dissection. This may be critical in certain sarcomas, deeply situated breast carcinomas, and head and neck carcinomas. Excisional biopsy generally is appropriate only for relatively small tumors, and incisions must be carefully placed in order to avoid complicating subsequent treatment.

There is little evidence of differences between incisional and excisional biopsies with respect to tumor spread; however, preparation and planning should be done prior to any surgical biopsy. Needle tracts or scars should be placed carefully in case a subsequent definitive surgical procedure is necessary. Incisions on extremities should, in general, be longitudinal. Care should be taken not to contaminate uninvolved tissue planes during the biopsy. While hemostasis is important in any surgical procedure, it is particularly true of tumor biopsy since hematomas can spread tumor along tissue planes. If more than one lesion is being biopsied, different instruments should be used for each one.

Coordination of the type of biopsy and the amount of tissue taken should be arranged with the pathologist. Electron microscopy, special staining, and special preparation of tissue might be necessary for the accurate diagnosis of selected tumors. Carefully marking a specimen for orientation is very important to the pathologist, and close collaboration between the surgeon and pathologist is paramount. The surgeon must insist that the pathologist receiving the specimen take steps to define the margins of resection.

STAGING OF CANCER

Staging refers to the assignment of cancers to an appropriate category or stage based upon their apparent local, regional, and distant anatomic extent. Stage groups are provided for cancers of similar anatomic sites. Prognosis is closely related to stage. Staging is a convenient means of communication, allowing easy identification of cancers of similar extent and prognostic importance. It condenses detailed descriptions into a manageable classification of comparability and prognosis.

Staging provides a logical means of selecting treatment options. Because cancers disseminated beyond local or regional tissues ordinarily are not curable by surgery alone, appropriate staging is essential in making therapeutic decisions. Additionally, staging provides a method for ensuring comparability of cancers treated by different means when evaluating various treatment methods.

The American Joint Committee on Cancer (AJCC) recognizes five classifications of staging. The *clinical diagnostic stage* uses all information available prior to first definitive treatment, including pathologic confirmation of extent of disease by biopsy or invasive radiographic techniques. This stage is determined by physical examination and other measures such as radiographs or isotopic scans. Although it is relatively inaccurate, it has the advantage of being independent of treatment.

The *surgical evaluative stage* uses all clinical information plus that obtained on surgical exploration. This staging method is often used for a few inaccessible tumors that are not amenable to definitive resection. This stage is determined histologically with information derived from survey biopsies of lymph nodes, bones, and other tissues. While more accurate than clinical staging, it is still based upon limited information because all areas of regional disease may not have been identified. Surgical evaluation may involve such simple procedures as lymph node biopsy or may require more complicated procedures such as thoracotomy, mediastinoscopy, or laparotomy. Intraoperative palpation, and biopsy as necessary, provide additional information. An example of extensive surgical-evaluative staging is that performed for Hodgkin's disease, in which a laparotomy is done to detect clinically occult disease within the abdomen. This procedure includes splenectomy, liver biopsy, and multiple retroperitoneal lymph-node biopsies. The exploration has provided data in the past that resulted in a change of stage in over one-third of the cases. Now, computerized tomography (CT) and magnetic resonance imaging (MRI) scans reduce the number of inaccurately staged patients and limit those that require operative staging.

Postsurgical pathologic staging uses all data available at the time of surgery. It is based upon histological examination of all tissues removed during surgical treatment. Thus, the information is often derived from whole organs and, when an operation has involved a regional node dissection, a number of metastatic nodes often can be defined. However, unless surgical resections have been comparably performed, comparison of cancers cannot be assured.

Retreatment staging is used when restaging is necessary for additional or secondary definitive treatment after a disease-free interval following first treatment. The surgeon must be certain to obtain extensive biopsies in many of these patients. Re-evaluation of receptors in breast cancer tissues, valuable blood studies in other patients, and radiologic imaging are all required to define the stage at the time of recurrence.

Finally, *autopsy staging* is used only when a cancer is first diagnosed at autopsy. The extent of cancer is determined from all tissues available from autopsy examinations. The autopsy stage is highly accurate but by definition cannot help the patient.

There are several systems for cancer staging. The simplest system divides cancers into three categories. *Localized* indicates the cancer is confined to the organ of origin. *Regional* connotes that a spread beyond the organ of origin has occurred, but not to distant sites. This may have occurred by direct growth to adjacent organs or tissues, by metastasis to regional lymph nodes, or by spread to both regional tissues and lymph nodes. *Distant spread* means that there is metastatic disease to locations distant from the organ of origin.

The most widely used, and universally recommended, staging system is the TNM method of the International Union Against Cancer (UICC) and the American Joint

Committee on Cancer (AJCC). Other methods for staging at most sites have been translated into this system. Each cancer is assigned a TNM stage specific to the site of origin. The third edition of the *Manual for Staging of Cancer* has just been published by the AJCC; proper staging is so important that the data form for breast cancer staging has been reproduced in this chapter (fig. 3.1). Cancer staging requires an understanding of the biology of the cancer as well as accurate documentation of the disease extent. This type of data form is representative of those available for each tumor site; the final stage is based on a summation of the TNM identification.

"T" refers to characteristics of the primary tumor in terms of size, skin involvement, ulceration, or other changes. Subscripts 1, 2, 3, and 4 refer to differences in size or other changes. T_0 refers to noninvasive tumors, T_{IS} to *in situ* cancers, and T_X to nondefinable primary lesions. "N" refers to characteristics of regional lymph nodes and localization of those that are involved. "M" refers to distant metastases. A subscript 0 usually indicates the absence and subscript 1 the presence of distant metastases.

Combinations of T, N, and M are grouped to describe tumors of increasing extent of disease into four stages. Clinical findings are distinguished from those based upon histologic information. The final stage should always be calculated on the most accurate data available.

Other staging systems include the Dukes' classification and its modifications for colorectal cancers, the Columbia clinical classification for breast cancers, and the International Federation of Gynecologists and Obstetricians (FIGO) for gynecologic cancers.

SURGERY AND THE TREATMENT OF CANCER

Surgery has always had a pivotal role in the treatment of solid tumors. As a cancer therapy, it has certain advantages over other forms: complete resection of all local and regional disease provides the most complete assessment of the extent of the disease and the most accurate staging; surgery cannot be considered to be carcinogenic; and in general it is not as immunosuppressive as radiotherapy and chemotherapy.

As noted earlier, however, surgery does have disadvantages. Every operation has a potential association with morbidity and mortality. Explorations may be undertaken but resection may not be possible, therefore exposing the patient to the risks of general anesthesia and the pain and discomfort of an operation without tangible benefit except for a more accurate diagnosis. A resection may be curative in only 30% of patients treated with surgery alone because most patients who present with solid tumors already have micrometastases that have spread beyond the primary site.

Documentation of operations and surgical procedures in the treatment of cancer is mandatory. The surgeon is responsible for making accurate, complete, and legible records of the operation, a task best done immediately after the event. Often, the operative note is the only record of the surgeon's observations of the procedure. It is important to document the total extent of involvement of tissue by tumor, all of the tissues that are removed, the surgical margins, and whether in the surgeon's opinion any tumor was not removed. Biopsy evidence of unremoved cancer is very important. Accurate surgical staging of the extent of disease is important and assists in the understanding of tumor biology through use of registries. Often, diagrams filled out by the surgeon right after the operation can provide additional definition of tumor extent as well as indicate the exact procedure performed.

DEFINITIVE SURGICAL TREATMENT

The cardinal principle of curative surgery for cancer is total extirpation of all neoplastic tissue. This principle is based upon the concept that cancerous tissue is capable of unlimited proliferation and growth from a residual of a few cells or even from a single cell. Accurate identification of those patients who may benefit from this type of surgery should be based on the reasonable certainty that all gross and microscopic cancer is confined to local and regional tissue. A surgeon should have a reasonable expectation that all involved tissue can be completely removed with a margin of normal tissue and acceptable morbidity before attempting curative resection. Careful evaluation of the patient's general condition and any other disease is necessary to ensure reasonable safety. Advanced chronologic age, while not a contraindication to surgery, must be a consideration. Careful evaluation of cardiac, pulmonary, hepatic, and renal function is important, especially in the elderly population. Finally, attempts at curative surgery should offer results that are equivalent or superior to other treatment methods in terms of quality of life and life expectancy.

The choice of the definitive operation is individualized and is based upon the stage and type of tumor, the clinical setting, and a thorough understanding of the tumor biology. Complete extirpation of the tumor with a normal margin is often sufficient treatment to completely cure the cancer. Examples include excision of basal cell carcinoma of the skin and wide excision of primary melanoma. Obviously, the surgeon must have a full understanding of the tumor biology in order to plan the extent of surgical resection. The patient, too, should be aware of the surgeon's options for resection and cure.

Frequently, definitive surgical treatment can be conservative and be combined with adjuvant treatments. Re-excision of biopsied primary breast carcinoma with axillary lymph-node dissection and radiation therapy and limb sparing surgery consisting of wide excision of soft tissue sarcomas, also combined with radiation therapy, are examples. These concepts improve the cosmetic and functional results of surgical resections.

The general approach to complete extirpation of cancers should encompass all of the usual general surgical skills, as well as specialized techniques unique to oncologic surgery. Early ligation of blood vessels and

lymphatics and minimal manipulation of the malignant tissue may prevent metastases. *En bloc* resection of the primary tumor and its regional extension to adjacent organs and lymph nodes will reduce the risks of implantation. Frozen section confirmation of adequate tissue margins, if there is concern about microscopic extension

---

BREAST

Data Form for Cancer Staging

Patient identification
Name _____
Address _____
Hospital or clinic number _____
Age _____ Sex _____ Race _____

Institution identification
Hospital or clinic _____
Address _____

Oncology Record

Anatomic site of cancer _____
Histologic type _____
Grade (G) _____
Date of classification _____

Chronology of classification
(use separate form for each time staged)
[ ] Clinical (use all data prior to first treatment)
[ ] Pathologic (if definitively resected specimen available)

Definitions

Primary Tumor (T)
[ ] TX Primary tumor cannot be assessed
[ ] T0 No evidence of primary tumor
[ ] Tis Carcinoma *in situ*: Intraductal carcinoma, lobular carcinoma *in situ*, or Paget's disease of the nipple with no tumor.
[ ] T1 Tumor 2 cm or less in greatest dimension
[ ] T1a 0.5 cm or less in greatest dimension
[ ] T1b More than 0.5 cm but not more than 1 cm in greatest dimension
[ ] T1c More than 1 cm but not more than 2 cm in greatest dimension
[ ] T2 Tumor more than 2 cm but not more than 5 cm in greatest dimension
[ ] T3 Tumor more than 5 cm in greatest dimension
[ ] T4 Tumor of any size with direct extension to chest wall or skin.
[ ] T4a Extension to chest wall
[ ] T4b Edema (including peau d'orange) or ulceration of the skin of breast or satellite skin nodules confined to same breast
[ ] T4c Both T4a and T4b
[ ] T4d Inflammatory carcinoma

Lymph Node (N)
[ ] NX Regional lymph nodes cannot be assessed
[ ] N0 No regional lymph node metastasis
[ ] N1 Metastasis to movable ipsilateral axillary lymph node(s)
[ ] N2 Metastasis to ipsilateral axillary lymph node(s) fixed to one another or to other structures
[ ] N3 Metastasis to ipsilateral internal mammary lymph node(s)

Pathologic Classification (pN)
[ ] pNX Regional lymph nodes cannot be assessed
[ ] pN0 No regional lymph node metastasis
[ ] pN1 Metastasis to movable ipsilateral axillary lymph node(s)
[ ] pN1a Only micrometastasis (none larger than 0.2 cm)
[ ] pN1b Metastasis to lymph nodes, any larger than 0.2 cm
    [ ] pN1bi Metastasis in 1 to 3 lymph nodes, any more than 0.2 cm and all less than 2 cm in greatest dimension
    [ ] pN1bii Metastasis to 4 or more lymph nodes, any more than 0.2 cm and all less than 2 cm in greatest dimension

[ ] pN1biii Extension of tumor beyond the capsule of a lymph node metastasis less than 2 cm in greatest dimension
[ ] pN1biv Metastasis to a lymph node 2 cm or more in greatest dimension
[ ] pN2 Metastasis to ipsilateral axillary lymph nodes that are fixed to one another or to other structures
[ ] pN3 Metastasis to ipsilateral internal mammary lymph node(s)

Distant Metastasis (M)
[ ] MX Presence of distant metastasis cannot be assessed
[ ] M0 No distant metastasis
[ ] M1 Distant metastasis (includes metastasis to ipsilateral supraclavicular lymph nodes)

Stage Grouping

[ ] 0	Tis	N0	M0
[ ] I	T1	N0	M0
[ ] IIA	T0	N1*	M0
	T1	N1*	M0
	T2	N0	M0
[ ] IIB	T2	N1	M0
	T3	N0	M0
[ ] IIIA	T0	N2	M0
	T1	N2	M0
	T2	N2	M0
	T3	N1	M0
	T3	N2	M0
[ ] IIIB	T4	Any N	M0
	Any T	N3	M0
[ ] IV	Any T	Any N	M1

Note: The prognosis of patients with pN1a is similar to that of patients with pN0.

Histopathologic Grade (G)
[ ] GX Grade cannot be assessed
[ ] G1 Well differentiated
[ ] G2 Moderately well differentiated
[ ] G3 Poorly differentiated
[ ] G4 Undifferentiated

Staged by _____ M.D.
_____ Registrar
Date _____

Illustration

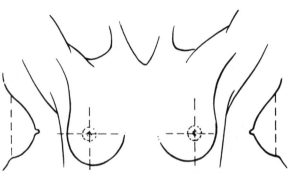

Indicate on diagram primary tumor and regional nodes involved.

Inflammatory
Medullary with lymphocytic infiltrate
Mucinous (colloid)
Papillary
Scirrhous
Tubular
Other
Lobular
   In situ
   Invasive with predominant *in situ* component
   Invasive
Nipple
   Paget's disease, NOS (not otherwise specified)
   Paget's disease with intraductal carcinoma
   Paget's disease with invasive ductal carcinoma
Other

Histopathologic Type

The histologic types are the following:

Cancer, NOS (not otherwise specified)
Ductal
   Intraductal (*in situ*)
   Invasive with predominant intraductal component
   Invasive, NOS (not otherwise specified)
   Comedo

Sites of Distant Metastasis

Pulmonary	PUL
Osseous	OSS
Hepatic	HEP
Brain	BRA
Lymph nodes	LYM
Bone marrow	MAR
Pleura	PLE
Peritoneum	PER
Skin	SKI
Other	OTH

Fig. 3.1. TNM data form for staging of breast cancer.

of tumor, is often helpful. The *en bloc* resection should remove the biopsy tracks and tumor sinuses. Instruments used to remove tumor should be discarded, especially before removing a second specimen.

Table 3.4 shows 5-year survival rates of white patients for some of the cancers that are most curable with surgical excision, if the cancer is localized. Table 3.5 shows some examples of tumors treated surgically, but with a low chance of cure unless the tumor is in a very early stage. Unfortunately, these tumors are also not well treated with alternative modalities and are difficult to identify at a time when they still might be resectable.

PALLIATIVE SURGICAL TREATMENT

Palliative surgery is designed to provide benefit in the absence of cure. Such operations can remove cancers that threaten vital function, relieve intolerable symptoms, produce transient regression, or may be simply prophylactic to prevent the onset of symptoms. Examples include resection or bypass of tumor to prevent obstruction of the intestinal tract, resection of tumor mass to control hemorrhage, or resection to treat perforation of a hollow viscus. Other operations, such as a feeding jejunostomy, may permit nutritional support so that a patient may obtain other modalities of treatment.

SURGICAL TREATMENT TO REDUCE THE BULK OF DISEASE

Resection of bulk disease in selected advanced cancers may improve the ability to control the residual disease. Cytoreductive surgery is of benefit, however, only when other effective treatment modalities are available to control the unresected residual disease. Examples of cancers in which this approach can be used are Burkitt's lymphoma and ovarian carcinoma.

SURGICAL TREATMENT OF METASTATIC DISEASE

In general, patients with a single focus of metastatic disease that can be technically resected with acceptable morbidity should undergo resection. There are obvious exceptions, however. Up to 30% of patients with pulmonary metastases from soft tissue and bony sarcomas may be alive at five years after pulmonary resection.

Table 3.4
5-YEAR CANCER SURVIVAL RATES OF
WHITE PATIENTS (%)
1979-84

SITE	ALL STAGES	LOCALIZED	SPREAD
Colon/Rectum	53	85	38
Melanoma	80	89	39
Breast (Female)	75	90	62
Uterus (Corpus)	83	91	50
Cervix	67	88	43
Bladder	77	88	41
Ovary	37	83	23
Testis	91	98	82

(Reprinted with permission from: American Cancer Society [1989].)

Table 3.5
5-YEAR CANCER SURVIVAL RATES OF
WHITE PATIENTS (%)
1979-84

SITE	ALL STAGES	LOCALIZED	SPREAD
Esophagus	6	13	3
Stomach	16	57	8
Lung	13	33	7
Liver	3	8	2

(Reprinted with permission from: American Cancer Society [1989].)

Similarly, in selected patients with hepatic metastases from colorectal cancer, resection can lead to long-term survival in approximately 25% of patients. Factors to be considered before undertaking surgery for metastatic disease include the tumor's histology, the disease-free interval, the tumor-doubling time, and the location, size, and frequency of metastatic disease.

SURGICAL TREATMENT FOR ONCOLOGIC EMERGENCIES

Surgery for the treatment of oncologic emergencies generally involves hemorrhage, perforation, infection, or possible destruction of vital organs. Patients with advanced cancers are often pancytopenic and therefore present unusual risks and specific needs. Each emergency has to be treated as a unique situation and requires an individualized approach. Care must be taken not to needlessly prolong the patient's suffering.

SURGERY FOR RECONSTRUCTION AND REHABILITATION

For cancer patients, quality of life is an extremely important issue, and surgeons can have a unique and important role in patients' reconstruction and rehabilitation. Transabdominal myocutaneous flaps following modified radical mastectomy, free transfer of tissue following head and neck surgery, and continent ileostomies and sigmoidoscopies are examples of newer surgical techniques that will improve cancer patients' quality of life following definitive therapy.

INTERACTION OF SURGERY WITH OTHER METHODS OF TREATMENT

Surgical resection alone fails to cure almost 70% of cancers, apparently due to residual cancer in regional and distant tissues. This may be in the form of unremoved growths or microscopic primary tumor, micrometastases in unremoved regional lymph nodes, or implantation of cancer cells at the time of primary surgery. Additional metastatic disease may grow at distant sites because of unrecognized occult metastases present at the time of primary surgical treatment. Another potential cause of distant metastases is liberation of tumor cells into the vascular or lymphatic circulation at the time of primary surgical treatment, although most distant seeding of tumor emboli occurs far in advance of any operative procedure.

For some cancers, irradiation to the remaining local and regional tissues, or systemic chemotherapy in conjunction with surgery, has been able to destroy any residual tumor. This results in fewer surgical failures and, in some instances, reduction in the extent of surgical resection necessary for cure.

Table 3.6 shows some tumors in which the benefit of the multimodality approach to therapy has been demonstrated. Wilms' tumor, childhood rhabdomyosarcoma, and nonseminomatous testicular carcinoma are the best examples. Unfortunately, it is obvious from the incidence of the tumors showing no benefit from a multimodality approach that much research needs to be done in order to have an impact on the growth of these tumors.

VASCULAR ACCESS

One of the most common surgical procedures performed on cancer patients has been the implantation of long-term, in-dwelling, central venous catheters. These permanent forms of chronic venous access were initially Hickman catheters; today, totally implantable subcutaneous ports are available. Either single- or double-lumen lines provide access for both venous infusion and blood drawing. The Hickman catheters are designed with Dacron cuffs placed in subcutaneous tunnels, providing a barrier to infection and helping secure the line in place as this area heals. Recent technical developments in percutaneous catheter placement have decreased the operative time and relegated the procedure almost exclusively to an outpatient procedure.

Only three situations, all associated with sepsis, mandate immediate catheter removal. The first is persistent bacteremia despite adequate antibiotic therapy. The second is septic response to catheter infusion. The third is simultaneous exit site and blood cultures showing the same microorganisms. Erythema at the exit site of a Hickman catheter occurs in many patients in the immediate postoperative period and is not an indication for catheter removal. No increase in complications has been noted even when catheters are placed at the time of chemotherapy-induced white cell and platelet nadirs. The ideal time for catheter placement, of course, is prior to initiation of therapy. Any patient facing long-term chemotherapy should be a candidate for placement of either a Hickman catheter or one with a totally implantable subcutaneous port. These catheters make

Table 3.6
MULTIMODALITY TREATMENT

BENEFIT ESTABLISHED	POSSIBLE BENEFIT	NO BENEFIT
Wilms' tumor	Stomach	Colon
Testis	Rectum	Lung
Ovary	Sarcoma	Pancreas
Breast (Female)	Head and neck	Melanoma
Rhabdomyosarcoma (Childhood)	Esophagus	
Anus		

administration of chemotherapy much safer and improve the patient's quality of life.

THE FUTURE OF SURGICAL ONCOLOGY

It is impossible to predict all of the important and meaningful advances in surgical oncology that will be achieved in the next decade. Surgeons must share the responsibility for translating the enormous wealth of research findings to the patient's bedside. Clinical trials of promising treatment approaches will remain the most appropriate method for carrying out this responsibility. The following are several areas under study in which surgeons and surgical oncologists can be expected to be key players.

IMPROVED IDENTIFICATION OF PREMALIGNANT DISEASE

Many syndromes have been described in recent years that define patient populations at relatively high risk of developing invasive cancers. These include such disease states as dysplastic nevi, polyposis of the intestinal tract (primarily the colon and rectum), leukoplakia, and endocrine neoplasia. It is important to define which of the individuals with precancerous lesions will go on to develop malignant ones. Concepts regarding carcinogenesis and the physician's ability to alter or reverse a progressive process will be under intense investigation. Biohazards will be more accurately defined so that specific actions may be taken against them. Magnetic resonance imaging may be used to define abnormal gene products and unusual aberrant cells or serum.

ONCOGENE ACTIVITY

There is already evidence in intraoral cancers that retinoids can reverse oncogene activity. Antiviral agents may alter populations of lymphocytes that have undergone abnormal proliferation, but have not developed specific monoclonal malignancies. As the technology of identifying, stimulating, and depressing oncogene activity grows, so will the ability to alter their biologic activity. Surgeons will have a major role in the tissue procurement, processing, and access procedures required for these kinds of studies.

IMMUNODIAGNOSIS

The field of monoclonal antibody development and marker protein definition has been directed toward earlier diagnosis utilizing immune concepts. The ability to identify ever-smaller quantities of tumor cells in more obscure locations is enhanced by such sophisticated techniques. Surgeons will work with molecular biologists and biochemists to harvest tissues following treatment with such modalities and to provide the antigenic material necessary for the development of these agents. More accurate diagnosis with immune approaches will permit even more selective operative procedures for appropriate patients. Those with no evidence of distant disease might qualify for even more aggressive local procedures, while those with occult metastases might be treated differently.

LASER TECHNOLOGY

The use of the laser as a therapeutic instrument is in its infancy. The potential of its external and internal application as a cutting tool to minimize blood loss, increase the accuracy of tissue dissection, reduce deformity, and speed healing is known. The technology is complex, but this promising tool has captured the enthusiasm of many ophthalmologists and otolaryngologists. Particularly when combined with a more accurate definition of the extent of disease, selected patients might qualify for more limited procedures using laser technology.

PRESURGICAL CHEMOTHERAPY

Traditionally, most chemotherapy when combined with surgery has been given following removal of the primary tumor. This has provided the best chance to treat patients of comparable pathologic stage without sacrificing the opportunity to excise cancers that might not be sensitive to chemotherapy. In the past, the fear has been that such tumors would worsen and possibly become inoperable during the period of delay needed for therapy. Presurgical chemotherapy has been tested recently in testicular and anal carcinoma. In addition, patients with sarcomas have also been treated in some centers with preoperative intra-arterial therapy. Preoperative chemotherapy may be combined in a variety of scenarios with radiation therapy or immune therapy. Each of these concepts will need to be tested in carefully planned clinical trials, and will become the surgical oncologist's responsibility.

CHEMO-RADIOTHERAPY FOR SELECTED CANCERS

The experience with anal cancer has demonstrated the tremendous benefit of chemo-radiotherapy for this lesion (Nigro et al. 1983). Many patients require no surgery, except for preoperative diagnostic biopsies and follow-up evaluative biopsies. Similar approaches with selected new chemotherapeutic agents, radiation sensitizers, and innovative developments in radiation biology may be valuable for other cancers, most notably those of squamous cell origin. Advanced cancers of the cervix and tumors of the head and neck and esophagus may benefit from this approach. However, the surgeon must always be prepared to resect primary tumors that chemo-radiotherapy cannot adequately control.

INTRAOPERATIVE RADIATION THERAPY

Though still in an evaluative phase of development, intraoperative radiation therapy has provided primary therapeutic radiation to local or regional areas after surgical resection. Its obvious advantage is that radiation-sensitive organs, such as bile ducts and hollow viscera, can be moved away from the radiation field and shielded. With the use of new linear accelerators, exact depth of penetration is possible, making the therapy much more accurate. It has the disadvantage of being relatively expensive, and requires that the operating room be shielded with lead.

MONOCLONAL ANTIBODY THERAPY

The specificity of antibodies, once defined for immunodiagnosis, may portend their usefulness as a therapeutic maneuver. The ability to define specific cell populations to be destroyed and to release lethal agents on the surface of identified cancer cells is being aggressively investigated. Either toxic chemotherapeutic substances or radioactive molecules may be released from their bonding site on antibodies and become active eradicators of cancer cells. Repeated treatments may be possible, especially if human monoclonal antibodies are used. As more is understood about the biologic growth of micrometastases, this approach will be increasingly significant in cancer therapy.

IMMUNE THERAPY USING BIOLOGIC RESPONSE MODIFIERS AND LYMPHOCYTES

The present flurry of interest in passive immune therapy using lymphokine-activated killer (LAK) cells and interleukin-2 is just one way that biologic response modifiers could conceivably interact with surgical care. Active specific therapy with defined tumor antigens to stimulate populations of autologous killer cells and passive antibodies, produced either by the patient's own cells or as cross-reacting antibodies defined against other cell populations, may also be beneficial. Since lymphokine-activated killer cell therapy was first introduced (Rosenberg et al. 1985), refinements in this protocol have substantially reduced toxicity and improved efficacy (Schoof et al. 1988; Eberlein et al. 1988). Future work will involve tumor-infiltrating lymphocytes and other biologic response modifiers such as interleukin-4, interleukin-6, tumor necrosis factor, gamma interferon, and alpha interferon. As the immunologic effect of each of these biologic response modifiers is better understood, there will be more awareness of the treatment potentials. For example, this type of immune therapy might be particularly useful following primary surgical therapy in patients with a very high predictable risk of tumor recurrence.

THE SURGICAL ONCOLOGIST

The surgical oncologist differs from his colleagues in general surgery in several respects. With rapid advances in surgery, radiation, medical oncology, and new disciplines such as immunotherapy and hyperthermia, the surgical oncologist is in a critical position to help integrate these approaches to the management of an individual patient. It is likewise critical that the surgical oncologist have special training that makes it possible for him or her to understand these divergent fields and appreciate their potential roles in treatment. The surgical oncologist should take the responsibility for training new residents and educating the general surgical staff of their hospitals and medical schools to better define the concepts and indications of advances in cancer diagnosis and management.

The surgical oncologist should be specially trained to perform unique and complicated surgical procedures, such as resection of soft tissue sarcomas and total pelvic exenteration, not normally performed by the community-based general surgeon. It is expected that general surgeons will perform most of the standard cancer resections, with more complex and less frequently performed procedures being handled by specialists in surgical oncology.

The surgical oncologist should be involved with clinical and basic science research activities in oncology and should help to organize clinical protocols for the study of cancer patients. Management of each patient's care should be coordinated with medical oncologists, radiation therapists, and other disciplines in the practice of medicine as needed, in order to establish the highest possible standards of care for treatment of cancer. Finally, surgical oncologists must lead fellow surgeons who remain the primary treatment source for most patients with malignant disease. Such leadership includes establishment of protocols for research, convincing colleagues that patients should be entered into clinical trials and other studies, helping to explain the results of such trials, and being critical of ineffective or poorly conceived studies. Thus the surgical oncologist will both direct and stimulate better investigation and treatment, and also provide a critical viewpoint as new and innovative management approaches come to the clinical arena.

REFERENCES

American Cancer Society. 1988. *Cancer facts and figures 1988. CA.* 38(1):5-22.

DeCosse, J.J.; Adams, M.B.; and Condon, R.E. 1977. Familial polyposis. *Cancer* 39:267.

Devroede, G.J.; Taylor, W.F.; and Sauer, W.G. 1971. Cancer risk and life expectancy of children with ulcerative colitis. *N. Engl. J. Med.* 285:17.

Eberlein, T.J.; Schoof, D.; and Jung, S. et al. 1988. A new regimen of interleukin-2 and lymphokine-activated killer cells: efficacy without significant toxicity. *Arch. Intern. Med.* 148:2571-76.

Eilber, F.R.; Guiliano, A.E.; and Huth, J. et al. 1985. Limb salvage for high-grade soft tissue sarcomas of the extremity: experience at the University of California, Los Angeles. *Cancer Treat. Symp.* 3:49-57.

MacDougall, I.P.M. 1964. The cancer risk in ulcerative colitis. *Lancet* II:655.

Moertel, C.G.; Hill, J.R.; and Adson, M.A. 1970. Surgical mangement of multiple polyposis and the problem of cancer in the retained bowel segment. *Arch. Surg.* 100:521.

Mostofi, F.K. 1973. Testicular tumors: epidemiologic, etiologic, and pathologic features. *Cancer* 32:1186.

Nigro, N.D.; Seydel, H.G.; and Consideine, B. et al. 1983. Combined preoperative radiation and chemotherapy for squamous cell carcinomas of the anal canal. *Cancer* 51: 1826-29.

Rosenberg, S.A.; Lotze, M.T.; and Muul, L.M. et al. 1985. Observations on the systemic administration of autologous lymphokine-activated killer cells and recombinant interleukin-2 to patients with metastatic cancer. *N. Engl. J. Med.* 313:1485-92.

Schoof, D.D.; Gramolini, B.; and Davidson, D. et al. 1988. Adoptive immunotherapy of human cancer using low-dose recombinant interleukin-2 and lymphokine-activated killer cells. *Cancer Res.* 48:5007-10.

Surgery in America: from the colonial era to the twentieth century, selected writings. 1965. In Earle, A. Scott ed. p. 60. Philadelphia: W.B. Saunders Co.

Chapter 4

PRINCIPLES OF RADIATION ONCOLOGY

Frank R. Hendrickson, M.D.
H. Rodney Withers, M.D., D.Sc.

Frank R. Hendrickson, M.D.
Chairman, Department of Therapeutic Radiology
Rush-Presbyterian-St. Luke's Medical Center
Chicago, Illinois

H. Rodney Withers, M.D., D.Sc.
Professor and Director
Division of Experimental Radiation Oncology
UCLA Medical Center
Los Angeles, California

INTRODUCTION

Following the discoveries by Roentgen and Curie in the late 1890s both roentgen (R) rays and gamma rays from radium were promptly used to treat a variety of diseases, cancers in particular. By the early 1900s clinical evidence had accumulated demonstrating the effects of ionizing radiations on a variety of malignant neoplasms and their injurious effects on many normal tissues (Coutard 1934). As Kramer (1976) stated, "Improvements in the therapeutic ratio can come from either a reduction in normal tissue injury or an increase in the effectiveness of tumor treatment." Understanding how ionizing radiations work and efforts to improve their effectiveness require a grasp of the physical basis of ionizing radiation production and absorption, coupled with an understanding of the biologic processes involved. This information must then be integrated with a clinical understanding of how tumors grow and how normal tissues heal. A malignant neoplasm is a vastly complex entity intimately involved near or within normal tissues or organs. The heterogeneous nature of the cells comprising both the tumor and the normal tissues poses a complex treatment challenge.

THE PHYSICAL BASIS OF RADIATION ONCOLOGY

Ionizing radiations are either electromagnetic or particulate. The electromagnetic radiations consist of x-rays and gamma rays, part of the continuous electromagnetic spectrum that includes radio waves and light. X-rays are produced in a device that accelerates electrons to high energy and then stops them in an appropriate target of tungsten or copper. Part of the stopping energy is dissipated as heat and the rest is converted into x-rays. Gamma rays are emitted from the nucleus of a radioactive isotope. When such an unstable nucleus decays by emitting some particle, the excess energy, above the stable energy level, is emitted as a monochromatic gamma ray. Individual x- or gamma rays differ only in their origin, not in their physical or biological properties. Particulate radiation includes electrons, protons, neutrons, and alpha particles. Electrons are negatively charged particles that can be accelerated to high speed in a variety of machines. Protons and neutrons are some 2,000 times heavier than electrons. Protons can also be accelerated in a machine because they possess a charge. Neutrons are produced by colliding protons or deuterons into an appropriate target material. Alpha particles are some four times heavier yet, and currently are of no particular clinical relevance.

Gamma rays and x-rays are absorbed in tissue by interacting with and dislodging a bound orbital electron. In the energy range generally used in radiation oncology this absorption occurs most frequently by the Compton effect. In this effect an orbital electron is dislodged and given some kinetic energy and the photon scatters in a different direction, depleted of the energy required to overcome the electron's binding potential and the kinetic energy given to the dislodged electron (fig. 4.1). This secondary electron subsequently interacts with other electrons as it traverses the tissues. Protons, neutrons, and alpha particles interact directly with the molecular nucleus, dislodging varying lower-energy nuclear fragments of densely ionizing protons, neutrons, or other nuclear fragments. They do not interact with orbital electrons. These heavier particles deposit energy in a track; the energy deposits are quite close together compared to those produced by photons or electrons

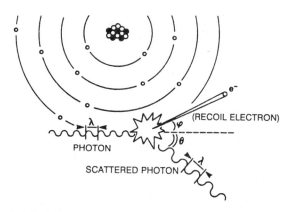

Fig. 4.1. Compton scatter: An energetic short-wave-length photon interacts with an orbital electron, overcoming the electron binding and imparting some kinetic energy that ejects the electron in one direction while the energy-reduced photon scatters in a different direction. The recoil electron will interact with other electrons and gradually lose its kinetic energy. The scattered photon may also react again and give up more energy.

(fig. 4.2). This deposition is called high linear energy transfer (LET) radiation. The biologic effects produced are significantly different from the low-LET radiations of photons and electrons. Conceptually, the disposition of energy at the molecular level is much like skipping stones on water. A light stone thrown with moderate energy will touch the water and deposit energy with long but decreasing distances between each skip as the stone loses energy. Finally, there are several close skips before it sinks. High-LET radiations would be heavier stones requiring even greater energy behind the throw but would still impart a great deal of energy to the water each time they touch, with much less distance between each skip.

The ionizing radiations can be delivered in two ways. In *teletherapy*, the source is some distance from the patient. The long distance is advantageous because the dose is relatively uniform across a given volume and allows for dose-shaping or modifying devices to be interposed between the source and the patient. In *brachytherapy*, the alternative method, the radioactive sources are placed directly into the tumor site. Because of the inverse square law the dose gradient is steep, with a high dose near the sources in the tumor and a much lower dose in the normal tissues further away from the radioactive sources. A combination of teletherapy and brachytherapy is used in the treatment of many common neoplasms.

THE BIOLOGIC BASIS OF RADIATION ONCOLOGY

Prior to the mid-1950s the biologic effects of radiation were measured mainly by lethality to animals, destruction of the germination capabilities of seeds, retardation of growth of plants and their roots, or the observation of the degree of erythematosus reaction on the skin or mucosa (Read 1952). Then in the mid-1950s both *in vivo*

and *in vitro* assay systems were developed in which single mammalian stem cells of both tumor and normal tissue origin could be grown into colonies and counted (Puck and Marcus 1956; McCulloch and Till 1964; Withers 1967). This permitted the quantitation of radiation effects by counting the few surviving cells in tens of thousands, similar to testing the sensitivity of bacterial growth to antibiotics. Over the next three decades a wealth of knowledge arose concerning how the biologic injury is produced and factors that might be manipulated to modify the biologic effect. Injury to DNA is now generally believed to be the primary mechanism by which radiation kills cells (Elkind and Whitmore 1967). Other damage, such as that to membranes and microtubules, may be supplementary mechanisms of cell toxicity (Alper 1979). Membrane injury, for instance, is thought to be important in the interphase death of mature lymphocytes.

The lethal injury to the DNA molecule can occur from direct ionization of the DNA molecule by a scattered electron. This direct effect accounts for perhaps one-third of the injury; most injurious events result from an indirect mechanism of hydroxyl (free) radical production from the ionization of ambient water. Hydroxyl radicals have a lifetime of a few microseconds and therefore cannot migrate long distances (Boag et al. 1975). They are capable of damaging DNA only within the radius of about 100 Å (10 nm). The lifetime, and hence the biologic effectiveness of such radicals, may be

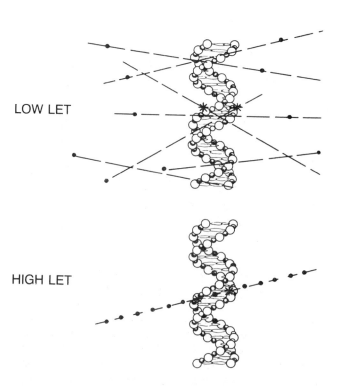

Fig. 4.2. Low-LET radiations produce sparse and widely separated deposits of energy which is inefficient in producing double-strand DNA breaks. High-LET radiations produce a dense track that produces a double-strand break if it hits the DNA molecule.

prolonged by the presence of oxygen or other electron-affinic molecules, such as nitroimidazoles. Conversely, sulfhydryl molecules, which are in varying natural abundance in the nucleus, can scavenge free radicals and hence reduce their biologic effectiveness. High-LET radiations such as neutrons and other heavy particles produce such a densely ionizing track that if they pass through a DNA molecule they produce multiple energy deposits, thereby having a direct effect even in the absence of oxygen (see fig. 4.2). They are also more likely to produce irreparable double-strand breaks.

Radiation dose is recorded as absorbed energy per unit mass. One gray (Gy) is one J/kg, which is 100 rads. Critical to the biologic effect is the specific stem cell exposed. A whole-body dose of 5 Gy would lead to a bone-marrow-failure death within a month, yet the whole-body energy absorbed is less than the energy absorbed by drinking a cup of coffee. It is the specific ionization in critical molecules that produces the devastation. A dose of 3 Gy will produce hundreds of thousands of ionizations in each cell exposed. Each cell will have several thousand single-strand DNA breaks and about 100 double-strand breaks, leading to reproductive cell death in about 90% of the exposed cells; that is, in 10% the damage is either repaired or is to a part of the DNA not essential to reproduction of viable progeny.

The ability to give graded doses of radiation and to quantitate the fraction of cells surviving permits the development of a dose-response curve over several logs of cell kill. The earliest understanding of the dose-response relationships for ionizing radiation comes from studies with bacteria. Bacterial cell survival decreases geometrically with dose; that is, equal dose increments cause a constant proportionate decrease. The dose that reduces survival to 50% will, if doubled, reduce survival to 25%, and, if tripled, to 12.5%, and so forth. When such a relationship is plotted on a logarithmic ordinate for cell survival and a linear abscissa for dose (a so-called semilogarithmic plot), a straight line results. Such a dose-survival relationship reflects a random process of cell killing: 100 lethal lesions distributed randomly throughout 100 equally radiation-sensitive cells will not kill all of them. On average, 37 cells will be spared a lethal lesion, 37 will have one lethal lesion, about 18 will have two, about six will have three, and an occasional one will have four or five such lesions; the total lethal lesion count equals 100. It is immaterial whether a cell is killed by one or more lethal lesions, but the recurring survival of 37% of the survivors for each additional mean lethal dose (100 lethal events in 100 cells) ensures a semilogarithmic relationship between cell survival and dose. The mathematical bent of early radiation biologists caused them to describe the slope of survival curves in terms of the mean lethal dose (D37 or D_0), which reduces survival by one natural logarithm (e-1), rather than D50 (halving dose) or D10 (the dose to reduce survival by one common logarithm, to 10%).

Clinicians generally find it easier to think in terms of halving doses (i.e., D50), analogous to half-lives of randomly decaying radioisotopes, or even in terms of doses that reduce survival to 10% (i.e., by one common base 10 logarithm). However, the nomenclature using natural logarithms is conceptually more elegant and is now established. For rough approximations, a D50 is about 70% of D_0, and D10 is about 2.3 times D_0.

Mammalian cells were relatively radiosensitive, having D_0 values less than one-tenth those for most bacteria. D_0 values for mammalian cells range between about 0.75 Gy and 2 Gy. However, unlike those for bacterial cells, mammalian cell survival curves usually have a shoulder before beginning a logarithmic decline (fig. 4.3). Such a "bending-down" shape implies that cells could accumulate some radiation injury, but that this sublethal injury could be converted to lethal injury by additional irradiation, thus making the additional radiation more effective per unit dose. The general shape of the surviving fraction curve is the same for nearly all cells so evaluated. Normal cell renewal systems of bone marrow, skin, and intestine, as well as a variety of tumor systems both *in vivo* and *in vitro*, show some variations in either the steepness of the dose-response curve or the magnitude of the shoulder. Any differences seem to relate more to the initial slope in the shoulder region of the dose-response curve (Deacon, Peckham, and Steel 1984). These small differences can be amplified by repetitive small dose fractions. For a significant therapeutic ratio to be developed, the relatively minor differences between tumor cells and normal cells must be exploited.

Of clinical relevance is the observation that cells die basically a reproductive death and, hence, do not manifest this until some subsequent attempt at cell division (Thompson and Suit 1969). The major exception to this is the death of mature lymphocytes that occurs during

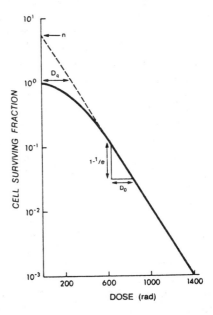

Fig. 4.3. Typical mammalian cell survival curve for low-LET radiation such as x-rays. D_Q = "Quasi-threshold" dose; D_0 = Mean lethal dose; n = Extrapolation. See text for details. (1 rad = 0.01 Gy.)

interphase. The clinical relevance of most cells dying during a subsequent cell division is that slowly proliferating normal tissues and tumors will have delayed response and rapidly growing tumors and tissues will have rapid response. The response rate, however, is not a good predictor of the ultimate effect on the tumor or the probability of tumor control (Suit, Lindberg, and Fletcher 1965). Many slowly growing tumors are highly curable because they have a lesser potential for distant spread, while many promptly responding tumors may regress quickly but regrow quickly if not sterilized. The second clinical consequence of delayed cell death relates to the difficulty in interpreting biopsy specimens secured weeks or months after radiation therapy has been completed. It is not possible to pathologically identify cells destined to ultimately succumb from those destined to regrow (Suit and Gallagher 1964). Even the presence of mitotic figures might only represent the agonal mitosis rather than reproductive integrity.

OXYGEN EFFECT

The biologic effects of ionizing radiations are greatly influenced by the presence of oxygen (Elkind, Swain, and Alescio 1965; Gray et al. 1953). The absence of oxygen conveys a resistance to radiation requiring about three times the dose to produce the same biologic effects. Many early clinicians and radiobiologists had reported that restricting the blood flow to a tissue decreased its radiation response. This was initially thought to be a metabolic effect, but in 1952 Read showed that oxygen sensitized cells through a radiochemical mechanism that enhanced the injury (Read 1952). It is now generally believed that this enhancement occurs by combining oxygen with an unpaired electron in the outer shell of a free radical to yield a peroxide that is more stable and toxic than the free radical itself (Ewing and Powers 1980). Because the lifetime of the free radical is a few microseconds, oxygen must be present in the nucleus at the time of irradiation. Adding oxygen even a microsecond after the exposure produces no sensitization (Boag 1975). This property of an affinity of oxygen for an unpaired electron seems critical to the sensitization and has prompted the development of other electron-affinic, oxygen-mimetic radiosensitizers which are in clinical trial (Brown et al. 1974; Stratford, Sheldon, and Adams 1983). The sensitizing effect of different oxygen concentrations is shown in fig. 4.4. One must be below a partial pressure of 20 mm of mercury (Hg) before significant protection is observed. Most normal tissues have an average oxygen concentration of about 40 mm of Hg and are therefore not protected from radiation injury. Most cancers have areas of poor blood supply harboring many oxygen-deficient tumor stem cells.

The oxygen enhancement ratio (OER, the ratio of doses to produce equal injury in hypoxic cells as in oxic cells) varies with the type of radiation. For very densely ionizing radiations such as alpha particles, or beams of stripped atomic nuclei, the OER may be close to 1. For

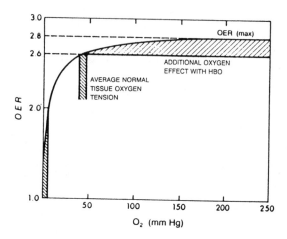

Fig. 4.4. Theoretical curve relating oxygen enhancement ratio (OER) for irradiated mammalian cells to concentration of oxygen. HBO = Hyperbaric (i.e., high pressure) oxygen.

neutrons currently used in clinical radiation therapy the OER is about 1.6 (Withers and Peters 1980). The OER for irradiation with x-rays or gamma rays is around 3.0 for a wide range of cell lines *in vitro* and most tissues *in vivo* (fig. 4.5). At doses greater than 3 Gy this ratio is independent of survival level, i.e., the dose delivered. For doses less than 3 Gy (the shoulder region of the survival curve and the common dose increments, used clinically) the oxygen enhancement ratio may be somewhat less (Palcic and Skarsgard 1984). The clinical relevance of hypoxia protection relates to many solid tumors containing a proportion of cells far enough from a capillary network that they are oxygen deficient, but as yet not necrotic. Several observations suggest that human tumors contain a proportion of hypoxic cells; for example, the pH of venous blood from tumors is usually

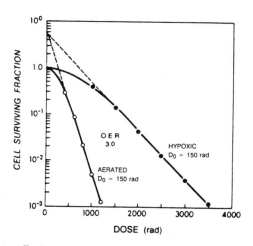

Fig. 4.5. Typical data for survival curves of mammalian cells exposed to x-rays under aerobic and hypoxic conditions illustrating an oxygen enhancement ratio (OER) of 3.0. D_0 = Mean lethal dose. (1 rad = 0.01 Gy.)

lower than from normal tissues, indicating that anaerobic glycolysis occurs within the tumor (Cori and Cori 1925), and the histologic evidence of necrosis that is seen in many tumors (Thomlinson and Gray 1955). Also, the clinical observation of improved results of radiation therapy from treatment with hyperbaric oxygen (Cater and Silver 1960) or after the correction of anemia suggests that hypoxia may limit the curability by standard radiation therapy of some human cancers (Bush et al. 1978). Even a small proportion of cells remaining hypoxic produces a protected subpopulation of tumor stem cells. Despite the probable existence of hypoxic cells within many, if not all, human solid tumors, hypoxia does not appear to be a constant, or a common, cause of failure (Withers and Suit 1974). The most likely reason is that the oxygenation of tumor cells is a dynamic process with cells that were hypoxic one day during radiation therapy being reoxygenated prior to subsequent treatment (Kallman 1972; Thomlinson 1970).

REPAIR

The repair of less-than-lethal intracellular damage produces the clinical observation that larger total doses can be tolerated when the treatment is divided into multiple small fractions. Elkind and Sutton (1959) showed that the shoulder on the surviving fraction curve reflects the accumulation of repairable sublethal damage. The most general biologic phenomenon among those influencing the fractionation response to radiation therapy is the capacity for cellular repair of less-than-lethal injury (fig. 4.6). The repair occurs rapidly. Slowly responding tissues (Barendsen 1982; Thames et al. 1982; Withers et al. 1983) consistently show greater repair capacity than rapidly responding tissues. Slowly responding tissues repair sublethal injury more slowly than rapidly responding tissues, but repair is essentially complete within six to eight hours. A possible explanation of this difference is that the rapidly responding tissues are stressed to undergo cell division, resulting in fixation of the injury rather than its repair. Regardless of the mechanism, the effect is that late responding tissues are spared more by dose fractionation than are acutely responding tissues. Most malignant neoplasms would fall into the acutely responding group as would proliferative normal tissues such as skin, mucosa, and bone marrow. The clinical implication is that large dose fractions are relatively more harmful to late responding tissues; therefore a therapeutic gain may be possible by using the smallest practical dose per fraction for the treatment of all but the slowly proliferating tumors. This may require multiple small fractions every day (Suit, Howes, and Hunter 1977; Thames et al. 1983).

CELL AGE

A growing population of cells is distributed asynchronously throughout the cell cycle. Cells vary in their radiation sensitivity as they traverse the division cycle (Sinclair 1969). Considerable variation is found, particularly in the initial slope of the surviving fraction curve

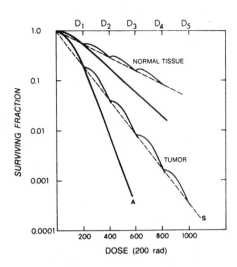

Fig. 4.6. **Cell repair and fractionation effect:** Each repeated fractional dose allows for cell repair of sublethal damage and is expressed by the recapitulation of the shoulder of the survival curve. If 1,000 rad (10 Gy) is given as a divided fractional dose (D_1, D_2, D_3, D_4, D_5) of 200 rad (2 Gy) daily, it achieves a similar degree of cell kill (S on the dashed line) as 600 rad (6 Gy) given in one single exposure. The survival curve for single acute exposures of x-rays is curve A. A differential effect on therapeutic ratio between tumor cells and normal cells increases with divided or fractional doses of radiation. This is displayed by the increasing differences in the slopes of the solid lines (single dose) and dashed lines (fractional dose). (Modified from: Elkind and Whitmore [1967].)

depending upon the cell's age in the cycle (figs. 4.7 and 4.8). For doses in the range of 2 Gy the variation in survival, depending on cell age, may be as great as the variation between oxygenated and hypoxic cells. After such an initial exposure to radiation there will be fewer cells surviving in the sensitive portions of the cycle and more cells surviving in the resistant portion of the cycle. When the relatively resistant survivors resume their progression through the division cycle they will move to more sensitive phases and produce a fluctuating response pattern (Elkind and Sutton 1959). These fluctuations cannot be exploited for clinical gain because the partial synchrony degrades rapidly, at different and uncertain rates in various tissues and tumors.

REPOPULATION

In both tumors and normal tissues, which contain proliferating stem cells, cell division may occur during the course of fractionated radiation therapy. As cells are damaged and die, normal tissues may respond by changing from a steady state to a regenerative pattern of replacing lost cells by recruiting quiescent stem cells into the cell cycle and by shortening the cycle's duration (Ang et al. 1985). This repopulation in normal tissues is beneficial because it reduces the overall injury (fig. 4.9). It may be more important in the early responding normal tissues (skin, mucosa, and bone marrow) and less important in late responding tissues (liver and central nervous system).

Accelerated regeneration of surviving tumor clonogens occurring during radiation therapy was only recently fully appreciated. The most impressive early demonstration of tumor regeneration after irradiation was by Hermens and Barendsen (1969), who showed a rapid exponential increase in clonogen number in a rat rhabdomyosarcoma after a delay equal to about one volume doubling time. The timing of this rapid regeneration in relation to the tumor's regression is also important. Understandably, a clinician observing a tumor to be regressing would not suspect the existence of regeneration among surviving clonogens; however, fig. 4.10 reveals that the initial rapid regrowth among 1% of surviving clonogens occurred during regression. The initial effect on tumor volume of accelerated regrowth by 1% of the tumor cells surviving is not macroscopically evident.

In experiments using a mouse prostate carcinoma, Kummermehr (Kummermehr and Trott 1982) has demonstrated clones containing thousands of regenerating malignant cells easily visible in stained cross sections, while the tumor, consisting mainly of lethally injured, degenerating cells, was still regressing after irradiation. Other evidence for regeneration in experimental animal tumors comes from studies showing an increase in the dose required to control the tumor with increasing overall treatment duration (Suit, Howes, and Hunter 1977).

A clearer picture is emerging of the magnitude of the clinical problem of tumor regeneration during the course of fractionated radiation therapy. Even during the time when the clinical observation is one of tumor regression, the surviving tumor clonogenic cells may be proliferating even more rapidly than before treatment was started (Hermens and Barendsen 1969). This may relate to an improvement in the nutritional status paralleling the reoxygenation status as dead tumor cells are removed. Tumor regeneration appears to be a clinical factor in the treatment of cancers of the head and neck (Knee, Field, and Peters 1985; Maciejewski, Preuss-Bayer, and Trott 1983; Parsons 1984; Wang, Blitzer, and Suit 1985), bladder (Maciejewski 1985), skin (Allen 1984; Hliniak, Maciejewski, and Trott 1983), inflammatory breast cancer (Barker, Montague, and Peters 1980), and melanoma (Choi, Withers, and Rot-

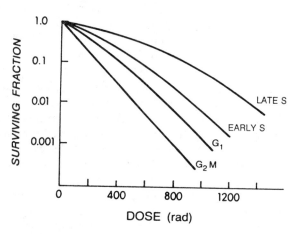

Fig. 4.8. Cell cycle age-response function: The patterns of radiosensitivity change through the cell cycle. This age-response function varies widely among different cell types. Cells in mitosis are almost always sensitive, followed by cells at the G_1/S boundary, while the period of greatest resistance is at late S. M = Mitosis; G_1 = First gap before DNA synthesis; S = DNA synthetic phase; G_2 = Second gap before mitosis; Early S = Early DNA synthetic phase; Late S = Late DNA synthetic phase. (1 rad = 0.01 Gy.)

man 1985). Some clinical implications of tumor regeneration for curative radiation therapy are:

1. Protracting treatment any longer than necessary is likely to be disadvantageous. For example, universal use of 1.8 Gy rather than 2 Gy fractions given five times/week may not be advisable. In general, treatment using 1.8 Gy fractions should be reserved for situations in which acute responses are likely to be severe (e.g., if large areas of mucosa are being treated or if there are additional risk factors, such as chemotherapy, alcohol use, etc.).

2. If a break in treatment is necessary because of acute toxicity, it should be kept as short as tolerable.

3. Planned split-course therapy is inadvisable unless it is part of an accelerated treatment protocol that ultimately shortens the overall treatment duration.

4. For select patients being treated for cure, breaks in

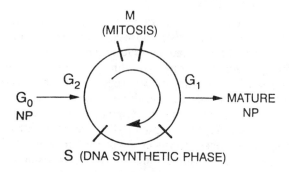

Fig. 4.7. Cell cycle age: The surviving fraction as function of cell cycle age. The radiosensitivity of a cell changes as it moves through the cell cycle, being most sensitive in G_2 and M. G_0 = Resting (quiescent) cell; G = Gaps; G_1 = First gap before DNA synthesis; G_2 = Second gap before mitosis; NP = Nonproliferating (mature cells); M = Mitosis. (Modified from: Hall [1988].)

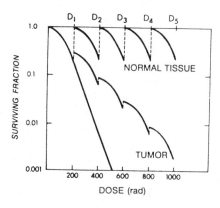

Fig. 4.9. Repopulation: In a rapid renewal system, repopulation or regeneration of cells within the fractional interval occurs. Even if the tumor and normal tissue have the same radiation response, the therapeutic ratio is improved through more rapid regeneration of normal tissue than the tumor. (1 rad = 0.01 Gy.)

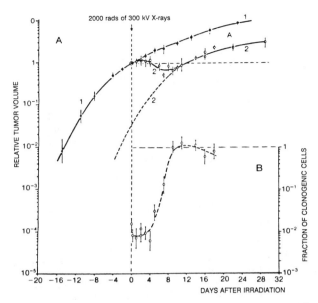

Fig. 4.10. Growth curves for a rat rhabdomyosarcoma and its constituent clonogenic cells after a dose that reduced survival to 1%. The upper curve (1) is for the unperturbed growth of tumors in the rats. The middle curve (2) is for the regression and regrowth of tumors irradiated on day 0 with a dose that reduced cell survival to 1%. The lowermost curve (B) traces the repopulation of the tumor by surviving clonogens. The rapid exponential regrowth of the surviving clonogenic cells occurs, for the most part, while the gross tumor is regressing. (Reprinted by permission from: Hermens and Barendsen [1969].) (1 rad = 0.01 Gy.)

therapy for nonmedical reasons (e.g., machine breakdown, holidays) may sometimes merit "catch-up" treatments, for example, by two treatments on one day (with several hours (e.g., six) between fractionations.

5. Obviously, rapidly growing tumors must be treated quickly. It seems reasonable also to accelerate as much as possible the treatment of those tumors with a high-proliferative index regardless of their pretreatment growth rate. In fact, the treatment of all tumors should be completed as quickly as it is possible to give an adequate dose. All tumors grow, even if they show no markedly regenerative response during treatment.

DOSE FRACTIONATION AND NEUTRONS

Heavy particle therapy is receiving greater interest. Neutrons are the most readily available of these particles and, although they are uncharged, they produce cellular damage through the same free radical mechanism as do x-rays. The difference is that the neutron interacts with the molecular nucleus ejecting other particles and producing ionization in a much denser track (high LET) than do x-rays (see fig. 4.2). Because of the density of these free radicals, neutron irradiation is more likely than x-rays to cause irreparable injury to the double-stranded DNA. The potential biological advantages of neutrons relate to the following factors:

1. They are less dependent on oxygen, with an OER of 1.6 rather than 3. This means that hypoxic tumor cells are less protected from neutron radiation than from standard radiation (Withers 1973).

2. The response of cells to neutrons is less influenced by their position in the cell division cycle, making cells more equally vulnerable regardless of their age. This simplifies the fractionation process because the fraction number and interval are less important (Withers 1985).

3. Because of a greater contribution to cell lethality from single-hit nonrepairable events with neutrons than with x-rays, the cell survival curve is more nearly exponential over a wider dose range. It is also steeper than that for x-rays. Therefore, dose fractionation is of less significance in neutron radiation therapy than in x-ray therapy. Because of the reduced shoulder of the surviving fraction curve there is little repair of sublethal or potentially lethal damage. Clinical observations have suggested that slowly proliferating tumors may have a high relative biologic effectiveness (RBE) for neutrons (Batterman et al. 1981). The preliminary results in treating salivary gland cancers (Saroja et al. 1987), soft tissue sarcomas (Cohen et al. 1987), and prostate cancer (Russell et al. 1987) suggest such a clinical advantage.

CLINICAL CONSIDERATIONS

The treatment of tumors within the body requires that the radiation must pass through some normal tissues that surround them. Cancers also tend to infiltrate into adjacent tissues, thereby requiring treatment of some margin of normal tissue surrounding the known gross tumor. Radiation injures normal tissue as well as tumor tissue, making the treatment goal one of achieving the greatest probability of uncomplicated cure. The consequences of both tumor regrowth and the specific complication must also be considered. If there is an available salvage treatment, a treatment course with lesser risk of normal tissue injury might be prescribed. The magnitude and consequence of the normal tissue complication must also be evaluated. Soft-tissue or bone necrosis might be acceptable in order to improve the probability of cure, but brain-stem or spinal-cord necrosis would not be acceptable as a frequent complication. The radiation therapy dose prescription might be summarized as "giving the maximum dose that the normal tissues can tolerate and praying that it is sufficient to control the tumor." Normal tissues have different tolerances, and the word "tolerance" will have a varied meaning to different physicians and patients. Because normal tissues are more homogenous in their cellular makeup than most tumors, the steepness of the complication-probability curve tends to be greater than the steepness of the tumor-control curve (fig. 4.11).

As in all of biology and therapeutics there is a sigmoid dose-effect relationship. For radiation effects this response curve is steep; small variations in dose have a profound influence on response. The position of the response curve on the dose ordinate is controlled by the number of clonogens in the population and the number that must survive to observe a specific endpoint. Whole-body exposure will produce lethality in 50% of animals if the bone marrow stem cell population is

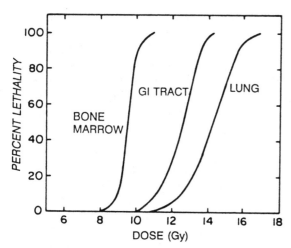

Fig. 4.11. Three different curves indicating percent lethality plotted as a function of radiation dose for the same strain of mouse. The "bone marrow" and "GI tract" curves were obtained using whole-body irradiation and assessing lethality prior to day 30 or prior to day 7 respectively, since death due to GI tract damage occurs earlier than that due to bone marrow failure. The curve labeled "lung" was obtained by assessing lethality 180 days after local irradiation to the thorax. Note the steepness of the dose-response relationship. (1 Gy = 100 rads.)

reduced to about 1%. Cure of a malignant tumor requires having no surviving tumor stem cells. A tumor of 1 cm in size will contain about 10^9 total cells, most of which are viable clonogens; there will also be stroma fibrocytes and vessels and some nonviable tumor cells.

Fig. 4.12 depicts some consequences of this biology (Allen 1984). Once a dose to produce a tumor control probability (TCP) of 15% to 20% is reached, small increases in dose will dramatically increase the TCP. This principle applies equally to chemotherapy. In fact, the dose increase might be achieved by combined treatment, as well as by more of the same treatment (Alper 1979). Curve B has more tumor stem cells than curve A; a greater dose is necessary for any level of TCP for curve B than for curve A. With a given dose of radiation, small tumors will have a higher probability of cure than large tumors or, conversely, for the same probability of cure, smaller tumors require less dose

than larger tumors (Ang et al. 1985). The physical size of a tumor need not parallel its clonogen number. Curve A could be Hodgkin's disease with a large tumor made up mostly of reactive cells. Similarly, curve A could be a large cystic tumor or one with many differentiated cells.

The clinical situation requires understanding of the normal cell response (fig. 4.11) combined with the tumor response (fig. 4.12) in order to understand the therapeutic ratio (fig. 4.13). These curves depict much of the art in radiation therapy by showing that the probability of tumor control must be balanced against the probability of complications in a risk-benefit analysis, which, in a clinical situation, depends on a multitude of factors relating to both the tumor and the host (Withers and Peters 1980). The worst complication of curative therapy is failure to control the cancer.

The curves in fig. 4.13 illustrate a number of points:

1. Improvements in radiation therapy require that the curves for normal tissue and tumor responses be separated further. Increases in biologic effectiveness of therapy must be greater in the tumor than in normal tissues, or normal tissues must be preferentially spared if there is to be a therapeutic gain.

2. In the midrange of tumor control probability, small changes in the biologic effectiveness of therapy can provide substantial changes in outcome. This has two further implications: if a change in treatment produces a modest difference in effect (e.g., of tumor control or of frequency of complications), that change should not be interpreted as a major change in the biologic effectiveness of the dose. Conversely, a small change in a biologically effective dose can translate into a large therapeutic gain or loss.

3. At incidences of effect less than about 10% and greater than about 90%, the changes in effect with changes in biologically effective dose are less dramatic. For example, if the TCP were already 90%, there would be no therapeutic gain from dose increases if there were already an incidence of severe complications of 5% or more.

4. In view of the closeness of dose-response curves for

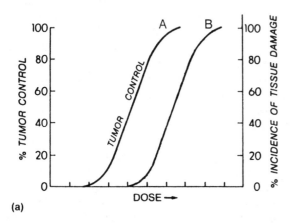

(a)

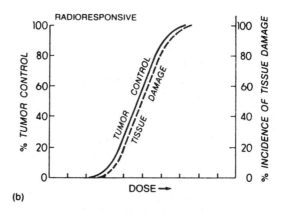

(b)

Fig. 4.12. Tumor response (a and b), combined with normal cell response in fig. 4.11, leads to understanding of therapeutic ratio in fig. 4.13. Probability of tumor control must be balanced against the probability of complications in a risk-benefit analysis.

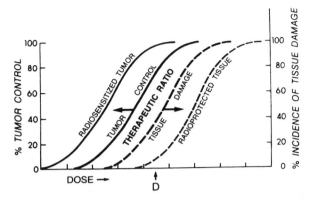

Fig. 4.13. The concept of radiosensitization and radioprotection is based upon the use of agents that can displace either the tumor dose-response curve to the left or the normal tissue damage curve to the right, thereby increasing the therapeutic ratio.

normal tissues and most human tumors, it is inappropriate for the radiation oncologist to produce no complications, though devastating ones such as myelitis should be strenuously avoided. Within the treatment volume, however, injury to normal tissues sufficient to be defined as a complication in some proportions of patients is a prerequisite to good curative radiotherapy for many tumor types and locations.

5. If the tumor-response curve is predominantly to the right of the normal tissue complications curve, other modalities should be used, independently or as adjuvants. For example, the TCP curves for large tumors may lie to the right of those for complications, whereas those for smaller tumors of the same type may be to the left: in this situation a therapeutic gain would result from debulking a large tumor by surgery or chemotherapy. However, a 50% or even 90% debulking is of little value: a 90% reduction in tumor volume represents only one decade reduction in cell number, equivalent to 6 Gy to 8 Gy in 2 Gy fractions.

Often in clinical practice a large volume is treated with a modest dose in an effort to control microscopic disease that might have spread beyond the gross tumor. The treatment volume is then reduced and higher doses are delivered to the more restricted volumes presumed to contain a greater infestation of malignant clonogens. Such restricted volume treatment can be given either with smaller fields of photons, high-energy electrons that will penetrate only a given depth and thereby spare deeper structures, or with an interstitial implant of radioactive sources that will deliver a high dose to a volume restricted by the physical placement of the sources.

KINETICS OF TUMOR RESPONSE

Most tumors, even some slowly growing ones, contain a proportion of rapidly proliferating tumor cells and inflammatory cells that show an early response to irradiation. Although it is important to remember that some respond very slowly, many regress quickly. As with normal tissues, variation in radiosensitivity among

tumor cells cannot be measured by the *rate* of response to irradiation. The tumor's response rate will depend on the proliferation kinetics of the malignant clonogens, the programmed lifetime of terminally differentiated cells within the tumor, and the dead-cell removal rate. Although for a given tumor type the local control rate may be slightly higher for rapidly regressing tumors than for slowly regressing ones, it is not good policy to reduce the total dose because the tumor regresses rapidly (Suit, Lindberg, and Fletcher 1965).

The situation is less clear if a tumor regresses slowly. Slow regression can reflect slow proliferation and cell loss kinetics of the tumor, indicate a mass of residual stroma, or signal treatment failure. Some tumors (prostatic carcinoma, some cases of nodular sclerosing Hodgkin's disease, teratocarcinomas of the testis, some soft-tissue sarcomas, choroidal melanomas, pituitary adenomas, chordomas or glomus tumors) are characteristically slow to regress even though sterilized of clonogens. Sometimes a residual mass persists indefinitely; for example, the cartilaginous stroma of a chondrosarcoma may never resorb even though the tumor never regrows. In addition, a small proportion of most tumor types will regress slowly even though the majority regress quickly. This variability reflects the broad spectrum of tumor proliferation kinetics, even among tumors of the same histology. In view of the heterogeneity of rates of regression among tumors, it is often unnecessary and, worse still, misleading, to obtain early postradiation biopsies of a slowly regressing tumor (Suit, Lindberg, and Fletcher 1965). Biopsies increase the risk of necrosis in heavily irradiated tissues and may result in surgical salvage of a sterilized tumor because sterilized but still living tumor cells are histologically indistinguishable from cells with retained clonogenic capacity (Suit and Gallagher 1964). Biopsy of treated tumors is a matter for clinical judgment. Usually, biopsy should be avoided if the tumor is continuing to regress, and is not often indicated sooner than three months after completion of therapy.

These facets of biologic and clinical response lead to a clearer definition of some commonly used terms. *Cure* does not mean guaranteed immortality, but would better be defined as a removal of the risk of death invoked by the disease that was treated. If the probability of dying returns to that of the general population without a specific disease, on a probability basis that group of patients could be considered as "cured"; any individual patient's immunity to any cause of death is not guaranteed. *Local control* means that the tumor never returned within the local area that was treated. This endpoint is appropriate for any form of local treatment, be it surgical resection or radiation therapy. Because death from distant spread, in the absence of local regrowth, bespeaks the bad nature of the cancer, it should not be the endpoint for evaluating local treatment. *Response* means the tumor showed some decrease in size. A complete response means that the tumor is no longer clinically detectable, but even in the presence of a complete response millions of viable tumor clonogens may remain. A partial response is more than 50% reduction in the tumor area but with some clinical persistence. A partial response, in most clinical situations, may be of some benefit in symptom relief but usually has little or no impact on the duration of survival.

PALLIATIVE TREATMENT (BONE, BRAIN, BLEEDING, AND BLOCKAGE)

A major activity in radiation oncology involves palliative treatment. Where cure is no longer possible, improvement of quality of life is the oncologist's commitment. Such situations do not require tumor sterilization, but only modest reduction in the tumor cell number in order to suppress a distressing symptom. This can generally be accomplished with relatively short courses of radiation therapy and low total doses. As a high therapeutic ratio is not required, the individual fraction sizes can be higher than those used in definitive or adjuvant irradiation programs.

Specific symptoms can be relieved in a number of clinical problems. Reduction in bone pain (Tong, Gillick, and Hendrickson 1982) can be accomplished in the overwhelming majority of patients, and complete relief in half of the patients, with doses in the range of 20 Gy to 30 Gy given in 5 Gy to 10 Gy fractions. The distressing symptoms relating to brain metastases (headaches, convulsions, or specific nerve palsies) can be relieved in a high proportion of patients with doses similar to those for bone pain relief. (Hendrickson 1982). Patients distressed by symptoms related to liver metastases can also receive relief (Prasad, Lee, and Hendrickson 1977). Improved liver function and relief of pain from stretch of the liver capsule usually can be accomplished with doses in the 20 Gy range. Relief is totally independent of the primary tumor site, but the tumor's rate of response and regrowth after its initial regression may be a function of the histology. The control of bleeding from an oozing ulcerative tumor surface requires very modest doses of radiation therapy, regardless of whether the bleeding is from the bladder, bowel, stomach, bronchus, mouth, breast, or other skin surface. The bleeding often stops without any obvious gross tumor regression. It may relate to an improvement in the blood's clotting function secondary to products released in the tissues from the radiation. Obstruction of a conduit such as the esophagus, bile duct, or ureter can often be relieved with local radiation therapy, but a greater degree of tumor regression is needed than for relief of other symptoms. This requires a somewhat higher dose of radiation than what is usually required for other palliative treatment.

COMBINED TREATMENT (SURGERY AND RADIATION THERAPY)

In many situations, radiation therapy alone is inadequate for achieving maximum cure levels. This can be because the

number of tumor stem cells is too large, some or all of the cancer cells are relatively radioresistant, or the tolerance of the contiguous normal tissues is too low. These situations indicate some combination of treatment, including surgical resection and/or the use of varying chemotherapeutic agents with radiation therapy.

The rationale for combining surgery and radiation therapy is the differing mechanisms of the two disciplines. Radiation therapy usually fails at the center of the tumor where the concentration of tumor clonogens is the largest and conditions may be hypoxic. Surgical resection fails because the tumor extends further than the margins of excision, infesting the contiguous tissues with undetectable microscopic foci. Radiation therapy is efficient in the sterilization of the small tumor cell numbers that are well vascularized, and the surgical resection is efficient in removing the bulky necrotic gross tumor masses. These efficiencies lead to the logical combination of radiation and surgery (fig. 4.14) with the major areas of discretion being the optimum sequencing of the two procedures. Radiation given prior to surgery has the advantages of treating undisturbed tissues, with the target volume being well-defined by the clinical knowledge of tumor extent and its likely routes of spread. Even in some tumors that are technically nonresectable, preoperative radiation may reduce the tumor sufficiently to make it removable and occasionally curable. The price paid for preoperative treatment is the loss of precise pathologic definition of tumor extent and the impairment of normal tissue healing at the time

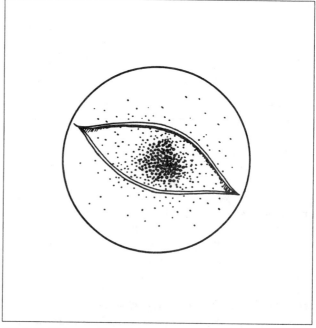

Fig. 4.14. Tissues adjacent to a gross cancer are infested with tumor cells. An excision may remove the visible cancer but the subclinical extensions may remain. Radiation therapy delivered to a larger volume can sterilize the remaining tumor clonogens. The dose necessary is dependent on the number of viable clonogens remaining but is less than that needed to cure a gross cancer.

of subsequent surgery. Preoperative radiation doses are usually modest in order to minimize the healing impairment and to permit the pathologic evaluation with fairly prompt surgery before extensive tumor destruction occurs. Postsurgical radiation has the disadvantage of requiring treatment to all the tissue planes potentially contaminated at the time of surgery. Also, viable tumor cells might have been disseminated beyond the treatment volume at the time of the surgical procedure. Clinical situations may indicate different sequences but such combinations of surgery and radiation therapy significantly improve the local control rate for many advanced cancers. Combined therapy may also improve the cure rate, while at the same time reducing the morbidity associated with more aggressive single-modality treatment.

THE PRINCIPLES OF COMBINING RADIATION THERAPY AND CHEMOTHERAPY

In general, chemotherapy is used either in an adjuvant way to control subclinical disease elsewhere in the body or in an additive way to enhance the local effects of the radiation to achieve a higher rate of local control. Many of the agents will act in both ways. Agents of choice are those whose toxic effects are in organs not included in the radiation target volume. An example is the combination of the cisplatin compounds (Murthy et al. 1987) with radiation therapy for mouth and throat cancers. Here the toxicity of the chemotherapy is primarily hematogenous and renal; the toxicity of the radiation therapy is to the oral mucosa. Previous studies that used bleomycin and methotrexate (Wolf et al. 1987) caused significant added toxicity in the oral mucosa, and did not achieve a therapeutic gain.

In some clinical situations the combined benefits of surgery, radiation therapy, and chemotherapy might be exploited. This has seemed most fruitful in the management of inflammatory breast cancer where each discipline has a significant impact on the disease process, with improved disease-free survival (Barker, Montague, and Peters 1980).

SUMMARY

Both radiation oncology and medical oncology are disciplines based on sound physical and biochemical principles. The nature of cell killing by both ionizing radiations and most chemotherapeutic agents is a random process, with a given dose destroying the reproductive integrity of a given proportion of cells. Therefore, there is no "tumoricidal dose" but only doses that yield a certain probability of cure. Increasing doses will leave fewer surviving cells, and, conversely, the smaller the body burden of tumor clonogens, the greater the likelihood of successful treatment. When radiation doses are divided into multiple fractions there are a variety of biochemical and physiological processes that have an impact on the ultimate magnitude of injury to the tumor and the ability of the body's normal tissue to recover. These include the oxygen status of the tumor cells at the time of radiation, the ability of cells to repair sublethal injury within a short time interval, the partial synchronization of cells by the variation in sensitivity around the cell cycle and, finally and importantly, the repopulation of the stem cells in acutely responding normal tissues, and, unfortunately, a repopulation of tumor clonogens.

The development of a therapeutic ratio of significant tumor control with limited normal tissue injury includes the risk of some level of injury to the patient. More-aggressive treatment increases the probability of tumor control, as well as the probability of serious sequelae. An increase in the probability of tumor control can sometimes be achieved by adroit combinations of surgical resection of the major tumor mass and systemic chemotherapy to control microscopic metastases and to enhance the effect of local radiation therapy. This combined effect also applies to radiation therapy and chemotherapy without surgery.

REFERENCES

Allen, E.P. 1984. A trial of radiation dose prescription based on dose-cell survival formula. *Australas Radiol.* 28:156.

Alper, T. 1979. *Cellular radiology.* London: University Press.

Ang, K.K.; Landuyt, W.; and Rijnders, A. et al. 1985. Differences in repopulation kinetics in mouse skin during split course multiple fractions per day or daily fractionated irradiations. *Int. J. Radiat. Oncol. Biol. Phys.* 10:95.

Barendsen, G.W. 1982. Dose fractionation, dose rate and isoeffect relationships for normal tissue responses. *Int. J. Radiat. Oncol. Biol. Phys.* 8:1981.

Barker, J.L.; Montague, E.D.; and Peters, L.J. 1980. Clinical experience with irradiation of inflammatory carcinoma of the breast with and without elective chemotherapy. *Cancer* 45:625.

Batterman, S.S.; Breur, K.K.; Hart, G.A.M.; and Van Peperzeel, H.A. 1981. Observation on pulmonary metastases in patients after single doses and multiple fractions of fast neutrons and Cobalt 60 gamma rays. *Euro. J. Cancer* 17:539-48.

Boag, J.W. 1975. The time scale in radiobiology. In Nygaard, O.F.; Adler, H.I.; and Sinclair, W.K. eds. *Radiation research.* pp. 9-29. *Proceedings of 5th International Congress of Radiation Research, 1975.* New York: Academic Press.

Brown, B.W.; Thompson, J.R.; and Barkley, H.T. et al. 1974. Theoretical considerations of dose rate factors influencing radiation strategy. *Radiology* 110:197.

Bush, R.S.; Jenkin, R.D.T.; and Allt, W.E.C. et al. 1978. Definitive evidence for hypoxic cells influencing cure in cancer therapy. *Br. J. Cancer* 37(Suppl 3):302.

Cater, D.B., and Silver, I.A. 1960. Quantitative measurement of oxygen tension in normal tissues and in the tumours of patients before and after radiotherapy. *Acta Radiol.* 53:233.

Choi, K.N.; Withers, H.R.; and Rotman M. 1985. Metastatic melanoma in brain: rapid treatment or large dose fractions. *Cancer* 56:10.

Cohen, L.; Hendrickson, F.R.; and Mansell, J. et al. 1987. Response of sarcomas of bone and of soft tissue to neutron beam therapy. *Int. J. Radiat. Oncol. Biol. Phys.* 13:1319-25.

Cori, C.F.R., and Cori, G.T. 1925. Carbohydrate metabolism of tumors: changes in sugar, lactic acid, and CO_2-combining power of blood passing through tumor. *J. Biol. Chem.* 65:397.

Coutard, H. 1934. Principles of x-ray therapy of malignant diseases. *Lancet* II:1-12.

Deacon, S.; Peckham, M.S.; and Steel, C.G. 1984. The radio responsiveness of human tumors and the initial slope of the cell survival curve. *Radiother. Oncol.* 2:317-23.

Elkind, M.M., and Sutton, H. 1959. X-ray damage and recovery in mammalian cells in culture. *Nature* 184:1293.

Elkind, M.M.; Swain. R.W.; and Alescio, T. et al. 1965. Oxygen, nitrogen, recovery and radiation therapy. In *Cellular radiation biology.* pp. 442-46. Baltimore: Williams & Wilkins.

Elkind, M.M., and Whitmore, G.F. 1967. *The radiobiology of cultured mammalian cells.* New York: Gordon and Breach.

Ewing, D., and Powers, E.L. 1980. Oxygen-dependent sensitization of irradiated cells. In Meyn, R.E., and Withers, H.R. eds. *Radiation biology in cancer research.* pp. 143-68. New York: Raven Press.

Gray, L.H., Conger, A.D.; and Ebert, M. et al. 1953. The concentration of oxygen dissolved in tissues at the time of irradiation as a factor in radiotherapy. *Br. J. Radiol.* 26:638.

Hendrickson, F.R. 1982. Management of brain metastases. 1982. In Chang, C.H., and Housepian eds. *Tumors of the central nervous system.* vol. 50. no. 5. New York: Masson.

Hermens, A.F., and Barendsen, G.W. 1969. Changes of cell proliferation characteristics in a rat rhabdomyosarcoma before and after x-irradiation. *Euro. J. Cancer* 5:173.

Hliniak, A.; Maciejewski, B.; and Trott, K.R. 1983. The influence of the number of fractions, overall treatment time and field size on the local control of cancer of the skin. *Br. J. Radiol.* 56:596.

Kallman, R.F. 1972. The phenomenon of reoxygenation and its implication for fractionated radiotherapy. *Radiology* 105:135.

Knee, R.; Field, R.S.; and Peters, L.J. 1985. Concomitant boost radiotherapy for advanced squamous cell carcinoma of the head and neck. *Radiother. Oncol.* 4:1.

Kramer, S. 1976. Research plan for radiation oncology committee on radiation oncology studies. *J. Cancer* 37(2):2031-148.

Kummermehr, J, and Trott, K.R. 1982. Rate of repopulation in a slow and a fast growing mouse tumor. In Karcher, K.H.; Kogelnik, H.D.; and Reinartz, G. eds. *Progress in radio-oncology II.* p. 2299. New York: Raven Press.

Maciejewski, B.; Preuss-Bayer, G.; and Trott, K.R. 1983. The influence of the number of fractions and overall treatment time on the local tumor control of cancer of the larynx. *Int. J. Radiat. Oncol. Biol. Phys.* 9:321.

Maciejewski, B. 1985. Znaczenie liczby frakcji, dawki fakcyjnej i calkowitego czasu leczenia w radioterapii nowotworow w swietle aktualnych pogladow i badan wlasnych. *Nowotwory* 1:32.

McCulloch, E.A., and Till, J.E. 1964. Proliferation of hematopoietic colony forming cells transplanted into irradiated mice. *Radiat. Res.* 22:383.

Murthy, A.K.; Taylor, S.G.; and Showel, J. et al. 1987. Treatment of advanced head and neck cancer with concomitant radiation and chemotherapy. *Int. J. Radiat. Oncol. Biol. Phys.* 13:1807-13.

Palcic, B., and Skarsgard, L.D. 1984. Reduced oxygen enhancement ratio at low doses of ionizing radiation. *Radiat. Res.* 100:328.

Parsons, J.T. 1984. Time-dose-volume relationships in radiation therapy. In Million, R.R., and Cassisi, R.J. eds. *Management of head and neck cancer.* pp. 137-72. Philadelphia: J.B. Lippincott.

Prasad, B.; Lee, M.S.; and Hendrickson, F.R. 1977. Irradiation of hepatic metastases. *Int. J. Radiat. Oncol. Biol. Phys.* 2:129-32.

Puck, T.T., and Marcus, P.I. 1956. Action of x-rays on mammalian cells. *J. Exp. Med.* 103:653-66.

Read, J. 1952. Mode of action of x-ray doses given with different oxygen concentrations. *Br. J. Radiol.* 25:336-38.

Russell, K.J.; Laramore, G.E.; and Krall, J.M. et al. 1987. Eight years experience with neutron radiotherapy in the treatment of stages C and D prostate cancer: updated results of the RTOG 7704 randomized clinical trial. *Prostate* 11:183-93.

Saroja, K.R.; Mansell, J.; and Hendrickson, F.R. et al. 1987. An update on malignant salivary gland tumors treated with neutrons at Fermilab. *Int. J. Radiat. Oncol. Biol. Phys.* 13:1319-25.

Sinclair, W.K. 1969. Dependence of radiosensitivities upon cell age. In *Time and dose relationships in radiation biology as applied to radiotherapy.* p. 97. *Brookhaven National Lab Rep.* 50203 (C-57).

Stratford, I.J.; Sheldon, P.W.; and Adams, G.E. 1983. Hypoxic cell radiosensitizers. In Steel, G.G.; Adams, G.E.; Peckham, M.J. eds. *The biological basis of radiotherapy.* pp. 211-23. Amsterdam: Elsevier.

Suit, H.D., and Gallagher, H.S. 1964. Intact tumor cells in irradiated tissue. *Arch. Pathol.* 78:648-51.

Suit, H.D.; Howes, A.F.; and Hunter, N. 1977. Dependence of response of a C3H mammary carcinoma to fractionated irradiation on fractionation number and intertreatment interval. *Radiat. Res.* 72:440.

Suit, H.D.; Lindberg, R.D.; and Fletcher, G.H. 1965. Prognostic significance of extent of tumor regression at completion of radiation therapy. *Radiology* 84:1100.

Thames, H.D.; Peters, L.J.; and Withers, H.R. et al. 1983. Accelerated fractionation vs. hyperfractionation: rationales for several treatments per day. *Int. J. Radiat. Oncol. Biol. Phys.* 9:127.

Thames, H.D.; Withers, H.R.; and Peters, L.J. et al. 1982. Changes in early and late radiation responses with altered dose fractionation: implications for dose-survival relationships. *Int. J. Radiat. Oncol. Biol. Phys.* 8:219.

Thomlinson, R.H. 1970. Reoxygenation as a function of tumor size and histopathological type. In *Time and dose relationships in radiation biology as applied to radiotherapy.* pp. 242-54. *Brookhaven National Lab Rep.* 50203 (C-57).

Thomlinson, R.H., and Gray, L.H. 1955. The histological structure of some human lung cancers and possible implications for radiotherapy. *Br. J. Cancer* 9:539.

Thompson, L.H., and Suit, H.D. 1969. Proliferation kinetics of x-irradiated mouse L cells studied with time-lapse photography. II. *Int. J. Radiat. Biol.* 15:347.

Tong, D.; Gillick, L.; and Hendrickson, F.R. 1982. The palliation of symptomatic osseus metastases: final results of the study by the Radiation Therapy Oncology Group. *Cancer* 50(5):893-99.

Wang, C.C.; Blitzer, P.H.; and Suit, H.D. 1985. Twice-a-day radiation therapy for cancer of the head and neck. *Cancer* 55:2100.

Withers, H.R. 1967. The dose-survival relationship for irradiation of epithelial cells of mouse skin. *Br. J. Radiol.* 40:187.

Withers, H.R. 1973. The biological basis for high LET radiotherapy. *Radiology* 108:131.

Withers, H.R. 1985. Neutron radiobiology and clinical consequences. *Strahlentherapie* 161:739.

Withers, H.R., and Peters, L.J. 1980. Radiobiology of high LET irradiation (neutrons). In Karcher, K.H.; Kogelnik, H.D.; Meyer, H.J. eds. *Progress in radio-oncology.* Pp. 1-7. Stuttgart: Georg Thieme-Verlag.

Withers, H.R., and Peters, L.J. 1980. Biological aspects of radiation therapy. In Fletcher, G.H. ed. *Textbook of radiotherapy.* 3rd ed. pp. 103-80. Philadelphia: Lea & Febiger.

Withers, H.R., and Suit, H.D. 1974. Is oxygen important in the radiocurability of human tumors? In Friedman, M. ed. *The biological and clinical basis of radiosensitivity.* p. 548. Springfield: Charles C. Thomas.

Withers, H.R.; Thames, H.D.; and Peters, L.J. et al. 1983. Normal tissue radioresistance in clinical radiotherapy. In Fletcher, G.H.; Nervi, C.; and Withers, H.R. eds. *Biological basis and clinical implications of tumor radioresistance.* p. 139. New York: Masson.

Wolf, G.; Strong, E.W.; and Vikram, B. et al. 1987. Adjuvant chemotherapy for advanced head and neck squamous carcinoma. (Head and Neck Contracts Program.) *Cancer* 60:301-11.

Chapter 5

PRINCIPLES OF MEDICAL ONCOLOGY

Michael R. Cooper, M.D.
M. Robert Cooper, M.D.

Michael R. Cooper, M.D.
Senior Clinical Investigator
Clinical Pharmacology Branch
National Cancer Institute
Bethesda, Maryland

M. Robert Cooper, M.D.
Professor of Medicine
Department of Medicine
The Bowman Gray School of Medicine
Wake Forest University
Winston-Salem, North Carolina

INTRODUCTION

Medical oncology is the discipline that specializes in the use of systemic forms of treatment for the management of patients with cancer. This focus on *systemic* therapy distinguishes medical oncology from surgical and radiation oncology, which are best suited for treating localized cancers. In practice, the medical oncologist typically spends less time dealing with issues specifically related to the delivery of chemotherapy and more time confronting the fundamental issues of general oncology: establishment of a tissue diagnosis of malignancy; efficient staging of disease; review of prognosis and various treatment options with the patient and family; effective relief of pain; and coordination of various auxiliary services to ensure that the patient's emotional and social needs are met promptly.

Medical oncology originated in the 1940s when nitrogen mustard was first used to obtain a brief remission in a patient with lymphoma (Gilman 1963). Most of the specialty's major advances—notably in the treatment of childhood acute lymphocytic leukemia (ALL), choriocarcinoma, Hodgkin's disease (HD), testicular carcinoma, and diffuse large cell lymphoma—have followed the introduction and combination of other cytotoxic drugs.

Most cytotoxic drugs are effective in destroying cancer cells because they interfere directly or indirectly with the synthesis or function of nucleic acids. However, chemotherapeutic agents also produce undesirable damage to normal tissues, such as hematologic suppression, mucositis, and hair loss. Many patients also fear the use of these drugs because of their tendency to cause nausea and vomiting. Major advances in understanding the pharmacokinetics and pharmacodynamics of these agents have allowed for less toxicity to normal tissues and have aided the management of chemotherapy-induced nausea and vomiting.

Medical oncology changes rapidly as new agents with entirely different mechanisms of action are introduced. These include interferons, interleukins, hematopoietic colony stimulating factors, growth factor antagonists, and agents capable of inducing cellular differentiation. Medical oncology has also begun to make significant contributions to the treatment of localized disease, as witnessed by the combination of 5-fluorouracil (5-FU) and radiation therapy in the curative therapy of rectal carcinoma—a tumor formerly curable only by radical surgical excision.

The kinetics of tumor growth are important in understanding how chemotherapy may thwart the growth of malignant neoplasms, and why it so often fails to do so. From a clinical standpoint it is most relevant to describe a tumor's growth as that of a whole tissue, but the concepts of tissue growth are built upon observations regarding the growth of individual cells.

CELL CYCLE KINETICS

The familiar model of normal and malignant cell proliferation is the result of studies combining tritiated thymidine (^{3}H-TdR) labeling of cells with autoradiography (Cleaver 1967). Thymidine, the nucleoside precursor of the DNA nucleotide deoxythymidine monophosphate, is essential for the synthesis of DNA; a cell replicating its genome in preparation for mitosis incorporates thymidine into its nucleus. In a typical experiment ^{3}H-TdR is injected into an animal or a patient and fresh tissue is obtained by biopsy at serial intervals thereafter. The tissue so exposed to the isotope is overlaid with a photographic emulsion; the low-energy beta-particles emitted by the tritium have a very short range, so only the silver grains lying directly above labeled nuclei are activated.

Such experiments led to the critical observation that DNA synthesis is not a continuous process from one mitosis to the next, but rather one known as S-phase (Howard and Pel 1951) that occurs during a discrete period of the intermitotic time. The intermitotic time has been subdivided into five phases (fig. 5.1). G_1, the time or "gap" between mitosis and S-phase, is the portion of the cell cycle dedicated to fulfilling the specialized functions of a given cell type. During G_1, the cell's energy is directed toward the synthesis of RNA and protein designed to execute these functions. G_2, the gap between the end of S-phase and mitosis, represents the usually brief time required to organize the nucleus for the events of mitosis. The onset of mitosis (M) is marked by chromosomal condensation and is followed by chromosomal segregation and cell division, yielding two daughter cells. The fifth phase of the cell cycle, G_0, is often depicted as lying outside of the loop connecting one mitosis with the next. This is because cells in G_0 do not respond to the signals that normally prompt initiation of DNA synthesis, in contrast to cells in G_1.

However, cells in G_0 are by no means dead: they continue to synthesize RNA and protein and so may carry out some of the differentiative functions of a particular cell type. They often act as a reserve population of cells that, given the appropriate cues (e.g., increased availability of nutrients), can re-enter the pool of proliferating cells and repopulate a tissue.

Measurement of the duration of the various cell cycle phases is conceptually simple. Because thymidine is either incorporated into DNA or rapidly metabolized and excreted, only those cells that are in S-phase at the time of ^{3}H-TdR administration will develop grains over their nuclei on an autoradiograph. A cohort of cells labeled in S-phase can be followed by obtaining serial biopsies of tissue for autoradiography following the ^{3}H-TdR injection, and by recording the percentage of mitoses that are labeled in each biopsy (Quastler and Sherman 1959). When the percentage of labeled mitoses (PLM) is plotted against the time following ^{3}H-TdR injection, a curve such as that in fig. 5.2 is obtained. Cells that are at the very end of S-phase during ^{3}H-TdR labeling will be the first to produce labeled mitoses; the time that elapses between their exposure to ^{3}H-TdR and the appearance of these first labeled mitotic cells is

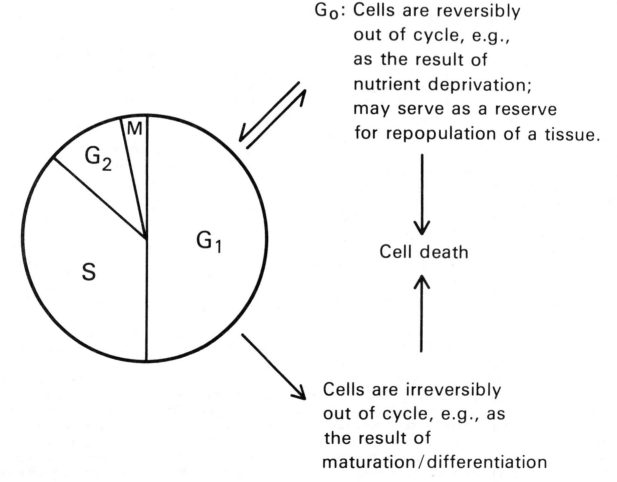

G_0: Cells are reversibly out of cycle, e.g., as the result of nutrient deprivation; may serve as a reserve for repopulation of a tissue.

Cell death

Cells are irreversibly out of cycle, e.g., as the result of maturation/differentiation

Fig. 5.1. Diagrammatic representation of the cell growth cycle, emphasizing the relationships between proliferating cell populations.

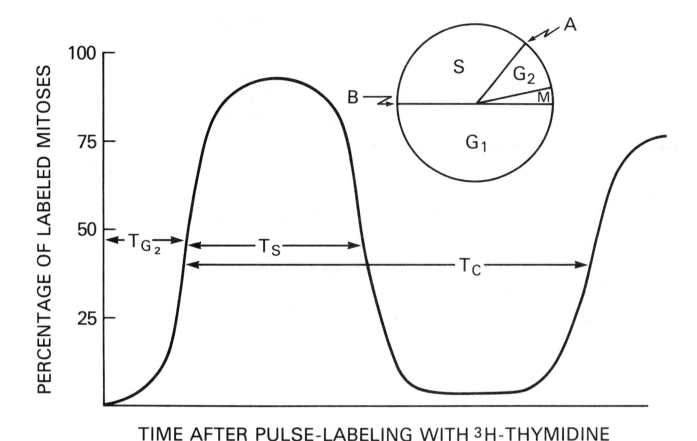

Fig. 5.2. Determination of cell cycle times using the percent labeled mitoses method. Only cells in S-phase become labeled at the time of ³H-thymidine administration. Those cells located at the very end of S-phase (point A) are the first to appear in mitosis, and those just beginning to enter S-phase (point B) are the last to do so. The time lag between ³H-thymidine pulsing and the appearance of the first labeled mitoses represents the time required for cells to pass through G_2. The width of the waves of labeled mitoses gives the duration of S-phase, and the time separating one wave from the next yields the total cell cycle time.

the length of G_2. Cells poised at the beginning of S-phase during labeling are the last to appear in mitosis, so the width of the wave reflects the duration of S-phase (T_s). If tissue samples continue to be examined at later points in time, then subsequent waves of labeled mitoses appear as the daughter cells of those originally labeled pass through mitosis. The time separating the beginning of one wave from the beginning of the next yields the total cell cycle time (T_c).

When the cell cycle kinetics of mammalian cells are examined *in vivo* using the PLM method, the durations of S, G_2, and M phases are found to be remarkably similar—about seven hours, three hours, and one hour, respectively. In most instances there is no significant difference in the duration of these phases between normal and malignant tissues. The longest and most variable phase is G_1, ranging from two to three hours to several days. Surprisingly, the intermitotic time (T_c) for most normal human cells is one to two days, while that of most malignant cells is approximately two to three days (Tannock 1978).

Cell cycle kinetics alone do not adequately describe tumor growth. First, in spite of similar values for T_c, different malignancies have distinctly different growth rates. For example, in acute myelogenous leukemia

(AML) T_c has been estimated at roughly 2.5 days, and in squamous cell carcinoma of the skin T_c has been measured at about 2.0 days (Tannock 1978). Yet AML left untreated results in death within weeks of diagnosis, while squamous cell carcinoma takes a more indolent course usually measured in years. Second, if tumor growth were solely determined by the cell cycle time, then tumors would be expected to double in volume every two to three days. Burkitt's lymphoma can come close to achieving this growth rate, but it is an exception rather than the rule. These incongruities can be resolved by describing tumor growth in the context of a whole tissue.

TISSUE GROWTH KINETICS

Tumors examined as whole tissues clearly show that not all of the cells are proliferating, that is, not all are "in cycle." Proliferating cells are a minority; the remaining bulk of the tumor's cells are in G_0, are differentiated to the point that they no longer have the potential to replicate, or are dead. The fraction of tumor cells that *is* in cycle can be calculated through the use of ³H-TdR autoradiography. The first step is to determine the labeling index (LI), the proportion of cells synthesizing

DNA at the time of exposure to the isotope (or, the proportion of cells that develops labeled nuclei). Then, if T_s and T_c are known for the cells of that tissue, as might be estimated by the PLM method, the fraction of proliferating cells in the tumor—called the growth fraction (GF)—is given by the following relation:

$$GF = LI \times T_c/T_s \times \lambda$$

The labeling index does not by itself give the fraction of proliferating cells, because not all cells that are in cycle will be in S-phase at the time of ^{3}H-TdR exposure; hence the term T_c/T_s to make the correction. The constant λ (always close to 1) is necessary to adjust for the fact that the distribution of cells in different phases of the cell cycle is not strictly equal (each cell going through mitosis yields two daughter cells, so the relative number of cells in each phase of the cell cycle decreases from G_1 to mitosis). The LI for a variety of solid tumors has generally been low, ranging from 1% to 8% (Tannock 1978); the LI of the epithelium of the normal gut is roughly 16%.

In addition to a low growth fraction, most tumors have a high rate of cell loss that further limits their growth rate (Steel 1967). A high percentage of new daughter cells die, in part due to the inherent genetic instability of malignant cells. Tumors also tend to outstrip their vascular supply and develop large areas of ischemic necrosis. Thus, most tumors are *not* what they appear to be on the surface—seething masses of rapidly dividing cells. Yet the nature of tumor growth *is* progressive, so clearly the rate of cell loss ultimately lags behind that of cell production. This imbalance between cell production and cell loss—the fact that tumors are not appropriately checked by the homeostatic mechanisms that maintain a predetermined number of cells in normal tissues—lies at the heart of tumor progression.

The significance of this imbalance is well-demonstrated by comparing acute with chronic myelogenous leukemia (Tannock 1978). Acute myogenous leukemia (AML) is a rapidly progressive disease, killing patients within a matter of weeks to months if left untreated. On the other hand, chronic myelogenous leukemia (CML) usually follows an indolent course over several years. Surprisingly, the LI for myeloblasts in AML is about 5% to 11%, while that for the myeloblasts of CML may be as high as 43%. The difference is that the CML myeloblasts, in all but the terminal stages of the disease, are able to differentiate to more mature progeny (e.g., neutrophils) that have only a brief life span. The AML myeloblasts rarely produce more mature successors and, given their longer life span *vis-à-vis* mature cells, they accumulate rapidly. Even in the terminal phase of CML ("blast crisis"), when the percentage and number of myeloblasts increase rapidly, the LI does not change. The problem at this point in the illness is that the myeloblasts are no longer able to further differentiate and mature, and consequently the tempo of the disease becomes similar to that of AML.

GOMPERTZIAN GROWTH

The growth of a tumor changes drastically through time, a fact that has important implications for cancer treatment in general and for cancer chemotherapy in particular. During the early phases of a tumor's life span both the rate at which cells are produced and the rate at which cells are lost from the tumor are proportional to the number of cells in the tumor at a given time. Since cell number (N) and tumor volume (V) are proportional,

$$\frac{dv}{dt} = (K_P - K_L) \times V$$

where K_P equals the rate constant for cell production and K_L equals the rate constant for cell loss. Rearrangement and integration of the above relation gives the more useful relation

$$V_2 = V_1 e^{(K_P - K_L)(t_2 - t_1)}$$

In short, for a good portion of its life a tumor grows exponentially. This simple exponential relationship allows the doubling time of the tumor (T_D) to be calculated:

$$\frac{\ln 2}{K_P - K_L} = T_D$$

By measuring the time required for a tumor to double in size, it should be possible to estimate how long it took for the tumor to achieve a given size from its beginning as a single cell. Calculations made using tumor-doubling times obtained from measurements in patients would lead to the conclusion that the tumor must have started 10 to 20 years prior to its detection.

Such calculations are fundamentally flawed. With occasional exceptions, by the time a tumor becomes clinically detectable it has achieved a mass of approximately 1 g or 10^9 cells. To reach this size the tumor has already undergone about 30 doublings and its growth is no longer exponential. The additional 10 doublings required to produce 10^{12} cells or 1 kg—the tumor burden at which most patients die—occur much more slowly than the previous 30 doublings and represent a minority of the tumor's growth.

A German insurance actuary named Gompertz developed a mathematical model to describe the relationship between an individual's age and his expected time of death. The asymmetric sigmoidal curve resulting from this model comes close to describing accurately the growth of a tumor over its entire life span (see fig. 5.3). When the Gompertzian equation is used to calculate the time required for a tumor to reach 10^9 cells, it is estimated that most human malignancies originate less than two years prior to their clinical detection. The exact mechanisms influencing the shape of the Gompertzian curve are not well understood, but the slowing of growth in larger tumors is undoubtedly due in part to: hypoxia, as tumors outstrip their fragile vascular supply; decreased availability of nutrients and hormones; accumulation of toxic metabolites; and inhibitory cell-to-cell communication.

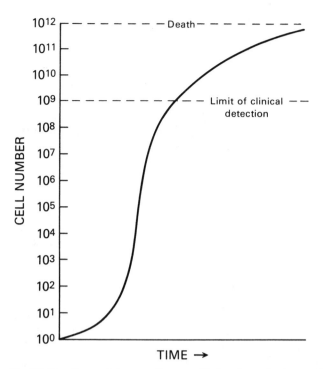

Fig. 5.3. The Gompertzian growth curve. During the early stages of its development a tumor's growth is exponential. But as a tumor enlarges, the growth slows. By the time a tumor becomes large enough to cause symptoms and be clinically detectable, the majority of its growth has already occurred and is no longer exponential.

Given that the majority of chemotherapeutic agents in common clinical use interfere directly with the synthesis or function of DNA, it is not surprising that these drugs are in general more toxic to proliferating cells than to those incapable of replication, or in G_0, and are more effective against tumors with high-growth fractions (Shackney, McCormack, and Cuchural 1978). However, by the time tumors are clinically detectable they lie high on the Gompertzian curve, where their growth fractions are low. If the number of cells in a tumor is reduced by surgical debulking or radiation therapy, then the tumor has been brought to a lower point on the Gompertzian curve. Cells previously in G_0 re-enter the cell cycle, the tumor's growth fraction increases, and its growth rate may be similar to the rate of a tumor that had just attained the same size from a single cell. If effective chemotherapy is available, it would now likely be even more effective against the tumor. This concept of moving tumors down on the Gompertzian curve prior to the delivery of chemotherapy underlies much of the rationale behind adjuvant chemotherapy (Weiss and DeVita 1979), that is, chemotherapy given to patients who have no overt evidence of residual disease following local treatment (such as surgery or radiation therapy for a primary breast cancer), but for whom past experience indicates that similar patients have a high chance of relapse from the presence of undetectable micrometastatic disease.

THE STEM CELL MODEL OF TUMOR GROWTH

A further impediment to effective chemotherapy is the fact that proliferating cells, those that are most vulnerable to the toxic effects of chemotherapy, are not necessarily the cells that must be eliminated in order to eradicate a tumor. Instead, the critical population of cells responsible for a tumor's persistence and growth is often largely in G_0. The reasons for this apparent paradox are found in the stem cell model of tissue growth.

The stem cell model has been most extensively elaborated for the cells of the bone marrow, which are depicted as components of a complex hierarchy. At the top of the hierarchy are relatively undifferentiated cells which have an unlimited capacity for self-replication and for replenishing the marrow with all of its various elements, and yet which have virtually no ability to perform the ultimate functions of the marrow (oxygen transport, hemostasis, and defense against infection). At the bottom are those mature, highly specialized cells (neutrophils, erythrocytes, and platelets) that can execute these tasks but which have no ability to divide and renew themselves. Although the proliferative rates for the immediate descendants of the stem cells tend to be high—the LI index for myeloblasts and myelocytes is 40% and 20%, respectively, and that of early erythroid precursors ranges between 30% and 75% (Tannock 1978)—the stem cells tend to proliferate slowly unless provoked by an appropriate stimulus (e.g., blood loss or infection).

The sluggish proliferation of marrow stem cells has been inferred by observing the extent to which their numbers are reduced by the administration of very high doses of ^{3}H-TdR—a technique dubbed "thymidine suicide." As in ^{3}H-TdR autoradiography, only cells synthesizing DNA (those in S-phase) will accumulate the isotope in their nuclei. However, in the thymidine suicide experiments the doses of ^{3}H-TdR are high enough to be lethal.

The original stem cell assays of bone marrow were performed in mice (Till and McCullouch 1980). A mouse given a sufficiently large dose of radiation will fail to recover hematopoietic function; both the mature cells and the stem cells of the marrow are irrevocably damaged. If, however, this lethally irradiated mouse is transfused with marrow from a nonirradiated syngeneic mouse, its marrow is repopulated and hematopoiesis resumes. The transfused marrow will also establish colonies of hematopoiesis in the spleen, each colony derived from a single stem cell. These spleen cell colonies contain granulocytes, erythrocytes, platelets, and their less mature precursors, so the founding stem cell is referred to as pluripotent, that is, capable of giving rise to cells of all three lineages. When normal bone marrow is exposed to high doses of ^{3}H-TdR and then transfused into a lethally irradiated, syngeneic mouse, the number of spleen colonies formed is reduced only slightly compared to the number obtained with transfusion of marrow not exposed to the isotope. The conclusion is that the marrow's stem cells are not rapidly proliferating; that is, most are in G_0. Yet if the donor marrow is stimulated to proliferate, as might occur if the donor were rendered anemic by phlebotomy, then exposure of that marrow to ^{3}H-TdR before transplantation results in a more pronounced reduction in the number of spleen colonies formed (Becker et al. 1965). The induction of anemia caused the stem cells to move out of G_0 and back into the cell cycle, so that the deficit in erythrocytes might be corrected.

The stem cell model of tissue growth has been extended to describe the growth of nonhematopoietic tissues, including tumors. Several lines of evidence argue in favor of using this model to describe malignant tissues. First, it is well established that nearly all tumors arise from a single, pluripotential, albeit aberrant founding (stem) cell. The possibility that most human tumors are monoclonal is strongly suggested by the unique paraprotein of multiple myeloma; by cytogenetic studies in leukemia (the best example of which is the 9:22 translocation in CML); and by the finding of a single G-6-PD isoenzyme in the tumor cells of women heterozygous at the G-6-PD locus.

Second, tumors, like the bone marrow, contain cells of varying degrees of differentiation. The more differentiated cells have low rates of proliferation and, when transplanted, are incapable of establishing new tumors; the less differentiated cells have higher proliferative rates (just as the LI for myeloblasts is higher than that for myelocytes) and are more efficient at founding new tumors. The more anaplastic tumors tend to have higher growth fractions and follow a more fulminant course if left without effective treatment.

The third point in favor of the stem cell model for tumor growth is the response of some human tumors to radiation therapy. Radiation therapy can cure tumors that arise spontaneously in humans at doses that would be incapable of curing experimental tumors of the same size in mice. The increased sensitivity of the spontaneous human tumors appears to reflect a smaller population of stem cells.

Direct measurement of stem cells in tumors has been accomplished through mouse-spleen colony assays (for example, injection of lymphoma cells into a mouse with the ensuing appearance of lymphoma colonies in the spleen); the enumeration of metastatic lung colonies following the intravenous injection of tumor cells into mice; and tumor colony formation *in vitro* (Hamburger and Salmon 1977). The last method has yielded mixed results in human tumors (Selby, Buick, and Tannock 1983). The impetus for developing of an *in vitro* assay of human tumor stem cells was the hope that it would allow for more rational drug therapy. By noting the effect of varying concentrations of different chemotherapeutic agents on stem cell colony formation, it might be possible to predict which drugs would be most likely to have activity *in vivo*. Unfortunately, such assays are good at predicting which drugs will not be effective, but they fail to predict accurately which drugs will succeed. Nonetheless, the stem cell assay demonstrates that only 1 in 1,000 to 1 in 10,000 cells in a tumor is capable of forming colonies of cancer cells *in vitro*. Although this poor cloning efficiency could be due in part to technical problems related to grow-

ing cells in culture, it is more likely a manifestation of the fact that most cells in a tumor have a very limited potential, if any, for self-renewal.

There is controversy over the proliferative status of stem cells in human tumors. Some studies indicate that they spend less time in G_0 than do their bone marrow counterparts (Shimizu et al. 1982; Minden, Till, and McCulloch, 1978). Nonetheless, the proliferating cells of a tumor—perhaps the cells that respond most dramatically to chemotherapy and yield clinical regression of disease (albeit transient)—are not necessarily the cells that need to be eradicated to effect a cure. Thus, the response of a tumor to a drug is best assessed by measuring the survival of clonogenic or stem cells, not of all tumor cells.

RELATIONSHIPS BETWEEN TUMOR CELL SURVIVAL AND DRUG DOSE

For most of the commonly employed chemotherapeutic agents, the relationship between tumor cell survival and drug dose is exponential, with the number of cells surviving a given dose of drug being proportional to both the dose of the drug and the number of cells at risk for exposure to the drug:

$$dN \propto NdD$$
where N = number of cells in the tumor
and D = dose of drug

or

$$dN = -KNdD$$

where the proportionality constant, $-K$, is introduced with a negative sign since the number of cells decreases with increasing drug dose. Rearranging and integrating the equation above yields the more useful formula:

$$N = N_0 e^{-K(D-D_0)}$$

where the subscript "0" indicates the initial dose and cell number.

A simple exponential relationship implies that the death of a tumor cell is the consequence of a simple interaction between the drug molecule and its target in the cell. Of more immediate clinical relevance, exponential cell killing implies two things: multiple courses of therapy will be needed to eradicate the tumor, since with each dose of drug the same proportion of cells— *not* the same number of cells—is killed; and small changes in the dose of a drug may translate into large changes in cell survival.

For example, assume that at the beginning of treatment a tumor contains 10^{10} cells. If each course of treatment results in the death of 99.9% of these cells, and if 1 log of cell growth occurs between courses of treatment, then five courses of treatment are required to eliminate the last cell (fig. 5.4) This reasoning assumes an ideal situation wherein all cells are equally sensitive to the drug, there are no cells resistant to the drug present at the outset of therapy, and no cells become resistant during therapy. These assumptions are not valid during the treatment of spontaneously occurring human tumors (nonkinetic forms of drug resistance are the major impediment to the successful treatment of human tumors), but the example makes the point that repeated courses of treatment are necessary. It also demonstrates that complete clinical remission, typically achieved when the number of tumor cells falls below 10^9, does not equal a cure; treatment must be continued despite the fact that no overt tumor is present. Continued treatment with potentially toxic drugs when no tumor is clinically evident is difficult for both the patient and the oncologist. Only rarely does the oncologist have the benefit of being able to follow a sensitive and specific tumor marker (e.g., β–HCG in the management of choriocarcinoma) to monitor the effect of treatment beyond the point of complete remission.

The disproportionate increase in cell survival that results from a decrease in drug dose is shown with a simple example. Assume that a tumor before any treatment contains 10^{11} cells. Also assume that the proportionality constant, $-K$, is -5 for the alkylating agent cyclophosphamide when used to treat the tumor. If a dose of 1.5 g of cyclophosphamide is delivered, then the tumor would be left with 5.5×10^7 cells:

$$N = N_0 e^{-K(D-D_0)} \; ; \; N_0 = 10^{11} \text{ when } D_0 = 0$$

$$N = 10^{11} e^{-5\,(1.5-0)} = 5.5 \times 10^7 \text{ cells}$$

What happens if the oncologist chooses to administer 0.75 g of cyclophosphamide instead of 1.5 g?

$$N = 10^{11} e^{-5\,(0.75-0)} = 2.4 \times 10^9 \text{ cells}$$

The result is that a 50% decrease in dose has translated into a 98% increase in cell survival.

Reduction of the dose of a drug given to a patient is often unavoidable because of undue toxicity to normal tissues (e.g., myelosuppression, mucositis). Still, giving drugs in full doses (which implies both the amount and frequency with which a drug is given) is an important goal when treating patients. A retrospective analysis of women receiving adjuvant chemotherapy for stage II, node-positive carcinoma of the breast indicated that those women who received the full dose of scheduled drugs were less likely to develop recurrent disease than those who were given lesser doses (Hryniuk, Levine, and Levin 1986).

Plots of cell survival as a function of drug dose have rarely been constructed for human tumors under treatment *in vivo*. However, such curves have been constructed for animal tumors using the spleen-colony assay or a metastatic lung-nodule assay, and for both animal and human tumor cell lines cultured *in vitro*. These experimental systems measure the survival only of clonogenic tumor cells as a function of drug dose;

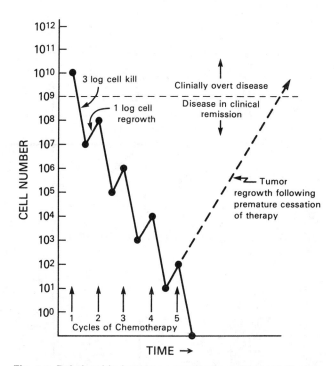

Fig. 5.4. Relationship between tumor cell survival and chemotherapy administration. The exponential relationship between chemotherapy drug dose and tumor cell survival dictates that a constant proportion, not number, of tumor cells is killed with each cycle of treatment. In this example each cycle of drug administration results in 99.9% (3 log) cell kill, and 1 log of cell regrowth occurs between cycles. The broken line indicates what would occur if the last cycle of therapy was omitted: despite complete clinical remission of disease, the tumor would ultimately recur.

clonogenic cells are the cells of interest inasmuch as it is *their* elimination that is necessary for a cure.

In the spleen-colony assay, tumor cells such as those from a murine lymphoma (Bruce et al. 1969) are injected into a lethally irradiated syngeneic mouse following exposure of the tumor cells to varying doses of drug; the number of tumor cell colonies that subsequently appear in the spleen reflects the number of clonogenic cells surviving drug exposure. Some tumors will form metastatic lung nodules following intravenous injection, and stem cell survival can be assayed in this manner as well. The first conclusion to be drawn from such studies and the analogous *in vitro* cell culture assays is that the slope of the cell survival vs. drug dose curve is much steeper for rapidly proliferating cells than for those that proliferate slowly; that is, tumors whose clonogenic cells are more often "in cycle" (not in G_0) are more sensitive to a given dose of drug (Van Patten, Lelieveld, and Kram-Idsenga 1972). Only a handful of drugs—specifically cisplatin, the nitrosoureas, nitrogen mustard, and bleomycin—show little increased toxicity for proliferating cells (Twentyman and Bleehen 1975).

The second conclusion to be drawn from these curves is that some chemotherapy drugs exhibit a plateau in cell killing as dose is further increased (fig. 5.5). Drugs behaving in this manner are those which have their exclusive or major effect during a single phase of the cell cycle, characteristically during S-phase. In order to

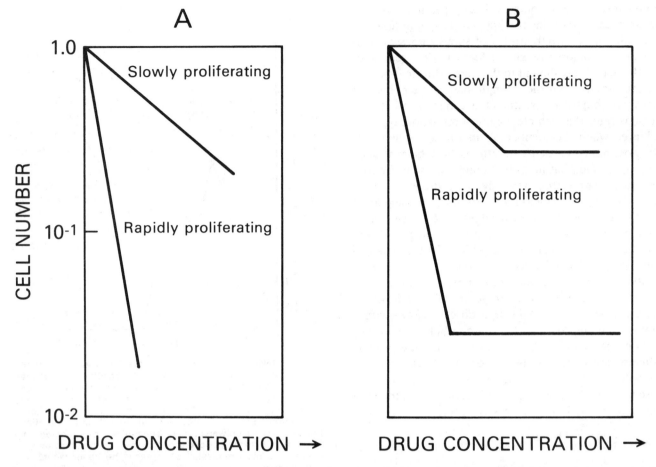

Fig. 5.5. Relationship between the proliferative rate of tumor cells and sensitivity to chemotherapy. (A) Cell populations are briefly exposed to varying concentrations of drug with subsequent determination of clonogenic cell survival. Rapidly proliferating cells, i.e., cell populations with few cells in G_0, are more sensitive to a given dose of drug than are slowly proliferating cells. The drugs used in these experiments are without significant specificity for any one phase of cell cycle. (B) These experiments were performed as in A, but with drugs that are specific for one phase of cell cycle (e.g., S-phase). Again, rapidly proliferating cells are more sensitive to a given dose of drug than are slowly proliferating cells. However, there is now a plateau in survival with increasing drug dose for both types of cell populations. Further decrease in cell survival can be achieved only by prolonging the duration of exposure to drug, allowing more cells to enter the susceptible phase of cell cycle.

increase cell kill beyond the plateau level, the *duration* of exposure must be prolonged to allow more cells in the tumor to enter the susceptible phase of the cell cycle. The antimetabolites—drugs which are structurally similar to normal metabolites and which disrupt cell function by competing with these normal precursor molecules in critical metabolic pathways—are the most notable drugs of this type and include cytosine arabinoside (Ara-C), thioguanine, mercaptopurine, methotrexate, 5-fluorouracil (5-FU), and hydroxyurea. Recognition of the plateau in the cell survival vs. dose curve for antimetabolites has greatly influenced the manner in which several of them are administered to patients.

MECHANISMS OF DRUG RESISTANCE

Given that most chemotherapeutic agents are more toxic to rapidly proliferating tumors, and given that a tumor's proliferative rate increases as its size decreases, it should follow that a tumor, having responded favorably to an initial course of chemotherapy, would become increasingly sensitive to treatment during subsequent

courses of therapy. Unfortunately, this scenario rarely, if ever, transpires. More typically, tumors regress and may become clinically undetectable during the initial courses of chemotherapy, but later resurge with vigor despite continuation of the same therapy. Tumor growth kinetics clearly fail to explain this sequence of events.

Mechanisms other than a tumor's growth fraction or a cell's location in the cell cycle explain why malignancies are resistant to chemotherapy. First, tumor cells may reside in so-called sanctuaries inaccessible to most drugs. The central nervous system (CNS) and testes are often impervious to drugs that distribute freely to other tissues; these are frequent sites of relapse notwithstanding successful treatment elsewhere. A major advance in the treatment of childhood ALL came with the recognition that the meninges were often a site of recurrent disease and that prophylactic treatment of the CNS, either with radiation or intrathecal methotrexate, could increase the chances for cure in those children who had achieved a complete remission with systemic therapy. Second, drug resistance also may seem greater than it is, such as when a drug is incompletely absorbed, is rapidly metabolized and excreted, or when it fails to be completely converted to its active form. In many treatment protocols these forms of pseudoresistance are at least partially circumvented by escalating drug doses until mild normal tissue toxicity occurs. By far the most important forms of drug resistance—the most typical explanations for treatment failure—lie in the genetic and biochemical makeup of malignant cells.

The genetic basis of drug resistance in malignant cells is now well established from several lines of evidence. The same procedures used to prove that bacterial drug resistance arises as a result of spontaneous mutation and subsequent selection (the fluctuation test of Luria and Delbruck) have been applied to tumor cells cultured *in vivo* (Goldie and Coldman 1984). If tumor cells are aliquoted in equal amounts onto media containing equivalent concentrations of a given chemotherapeutic agent, then the number of tumor colonies appearing on each of those media—the progeny of single resistant cells—is equal. The rate of development of drug resistance calculated from such experiments is consistent with known rates of spontaneous mutation—roughly one out of 10^6 to 10^7 cells. Moreover, if the tumor cells are initially plated onto media without drug and allowed to grow to a given size, and if they are thereafter subplated onto media with drug, then the number of colonies appearing in these subcultures varies significantly from one plate to the next. In the drug-free medium there is no selection pressure for drug-resistant cells, so their number varies widely, reflecting the random nature of spontaneous mutation. Other evidence includes the fact that the drug-resistant phenotype may persist despite the absence of drug, and the observation that mutagens may increase the rate with which drug-resistant cells appear. Perhaps most compelling are experiments in which DNA transfer from drug-resistant to drug-sensitive cells confers the drug-resistant phenotype upon the formerly vulnerable cells (Gros et al. 1986).

These arguments most readily apply to drug resistance arising from a point mutation, and on the surface they appear to exclude the idea that drugs may induce resistance to themselves by means other than simply increasing the rate of spontaneous mutation. However, a Lamarckian view of drug resistance has some validity.

If the only force causing tumor cells to become resistant were spontaneous mutation, then a tumor containing 10^9 cells, i.e., one which has just become clinically detectable, probably already contains 10^2 to 10^3 resistant cells (10^9 cells x $1/10^7$ or $1/10^6$). If the rate of spontaneous mutation increases, then the smaller a tumor is, the less likely it is to contain drug-resistant cells. This conclusion makes intuitive sense, but what is not so readily apparent is the exponential relationship between tumor size and the probability of finding drug-resistant cells. Through the use of a mathematical model, Goldie and Coldman (1984) have predicted the following relationship:

$$P_0 = \frac{1}{e \; \alpha \; (N-1)}$$

where P_0 equals the probability of finding no drug-resistant cells within a tumor containing N cells and having a spontaneous rate of mutation α.

This relationship predicts that the curability of a tumor—here equated with the probability of there being no drug-resistant cells—does not decline gradually as the tumor grows larger, but instead decreases precipitously as the tumor approaches a critical size determined by its rate of spontaneous mutation. A tumor containing 10^6 cells and having a spontaneous mutation rate of 10^{-7} stands only a 10% chance of containing drug-resistant cells; but if the tumor is allowed to grow 1.5 logs (to 5×10^7 cells) this chance increases to more than 99%.

The clinical message behind the Goldie-Coldman model is that smaller tumors are easier to cure, and that the best moment for effective treatment is as soon after detection as possible. Delay in treatment, by allowing a modest increase in tumor burden, can result in a large increase in the probability of encountering drug-resistant cells and may so forfeit the patient's chance for cure or at least meaningful disease regression. An extension of the Goldie-Coldman model argues that patients should benefit from the use of multiple, noncross-resistant drugs (effectively decreasing the rate of spontaneous mutation), and also that equally effective, noncross-resistant regimens should be alternated, rather than given sequentially. The use of multiple chemotherapeutic agents in combination has been responsible for much of the success achieved in the treatment of childhood ALL, HD, and testicular carcinoma; single-agent therapy is clearly inferior for the treatment of these malignancies. The superiority of multiple drugs over single agents is not so clear in some of the more common solid tumors, such as colon cancer. The failure of multiple agents in the treatment of these tumors is not so much a failure of the Goldie-Coldman model, but rather a reflection of the inherently high levels of resistance these tumors have to all currently available chemotherapeutic agents. Also, there are practical limits on how far the theoretical advantages of combination chemotherapy can be taken. Two or even three drugs may produce activity against a given tumor, but if they all produce similar normal-tissue toxicities they will be difficult to combine in the clinic. Either the combination will result in excessive morbidity and mortality, or the drug doses will be reduced to levels where none is very effective.

Unfortunately, the problem of drug resistance is a complex one that goes well beyond the simple model of random spontaneous mutation to resistance and subsequent selection. The first level of complexity lies in the ability of some drugs to promote resistance against themselves (the Lamarckian view). Resistance to the antimetabolite methotrexate (MTX) can be effected through several mechanisms (Bertino et al. 1981). An alteration in the cell surface membrane receptor for folates, as might occur by a point mutation, can reduce intracellular levels of MTX and result in less inhibition of the target enzyme dihydrofolate reductase (DHFR). Once MTX enters the cell a number of glutamic acid residues are added to the single glutamic acid moiety that forms one end of the MTX molecule; such polyglutamation, which also occurs with the normal substrate, folic acid, keeps MTX from exiting the cell and yet does not alter its ability to inhibit DHFR.

Decreased polyglutamation of the drug is another potential mechanism for resistance. Although not common, resistance to MTX may also be conferred by an alteration in the structure of the DHFR enzyme so that MTX binds to it less avidly. However, by far the most common form of MTX resistance (at least in experimental tumors and cell lines) is production by the resistant cell of exceedingly large amounts of DHFR through a process known as gene amplification (Schimke 1984). In this process a gene is replicated many times over while the cell is in S-phase. Such amplification is promoted by drugs like methotrexate, which transiently interrupt DNA synthesis in replicating cells. The degree to which the DHFR gene is amplified can be increased by gradually increasing the amount of methotrexate to which tumor cells are exposed. If cells so induced to amplify the DHFR gene are then withdrawn from MTX exposure they may lose some of their resistance to the drug; this phenomenon is related to the loss of amplified DHFR genes located in relatively unstable, poorly conserved extrachromosomal structures called double minutes.

MULTIDRUG RESISTANCE

A second level of complexity is that the development of resistance to one chemotherapeutic agent often results in the coincident development of resistance to other, albeit structurally unrelated ones (Biedler and Riehm 1970). The appearance of the multidrug-resistant phenotype is associated with the expression of a cell surface glycoprotein called P-170 (Juliano and Ling 1976). Cells expressing P-170 tend to manifest increased efflux of the drugs to which they are resistant; there is some evidence implicating P-170 as this so-called drug pump. The multidrug-resistant phenotype is stable even in the absence of exposure to the drugs to which resistance has developed.

Furthermore, the gene encoding the P-170 glycoprotein, called *mdr1*, has been isolated, sequenced, and transferred to a drug-sensitive cell line, so conferring resistance (Gros et al. 1986). Although the phenomenon of multidrug resistance was examined *in vitro*, it likely has relevance for the treatment of spontaneously arising tumors in humans. The P-170 glycoprotein has been identified in a resistant human ovarian cell line (Bell et al. 1985), and the *mdr1* gene has been expressed in some human tumors (Fojo et al. 1987). *In vitro* data indicate that compounds which inhibit calcium entry into cells (e.g., verapamil) interfere with calcium binding to calmodulin, and other drugs that stabilize cell membranes

(e.g., Quinidine) can partially restore drug sensitivity. The use of verapamil to circumvent P-170-associated multidrug resistance has produced initially encouraging results in patients with multiple myeloma and non-Hodgkin's lymphomas. In a small group of patients with these malignancies who had developed clinical resistance to treatment with a chemotherapeutic regimen consisting of vincristine, Adriamycin, and high-dose dexamethasone (VAD), the addition of verapamil to the regimen caused partial tumor regression in a subset (Dalton, Grogan, and Meltzer et al. 1989).

TUMOR CELL HETEROGENEITY

A third layer of drug-resistance complexity emanates from the genetic and phenotypic heterogeneity of human tumors (Schnipper 1986). Despite their common ancestry, it is the rule rather than the exception that tumor cells are diversified both genetically and phenotypically. Tumors, like their normal tissue counterparts, retain some of the originally programmed ability to mature and differentiate.

In the early stages of its growth, a tumor may differ phenotypically only slightly from its tissue of origin, but as it increases in size it characteristically becomes less differentiated or more anaplastic, and more difficult to treat. The genetic material of malignant cells is more unstable than that of normal cells, a fact most grossly manifested by multiple chromosomal defects (breaks, deletions, translocations, inversions, and the evanescent extrachromosomal double minutes) and expressed by higher mutation rates as measured by clonal selection for drug resistance. Chemotherapeutic agents may add to this genetic instability by acting as mutagens themselves. Hence, new subclones of malignant cells appear routinely; those with an increased capacity for self-renewal and proliferation gradually replace the more slowly growing, differentiated cells in the tumor, and drug-resistant clones replace sensitive ones in the face of systemic treatment. Classic examples of disease evolution include: Richter's syndrome, wherein the patient with CLL develops an aggressive diffuse large-cell lymphoma; and the progression of CML, initially an indolent myeloproliferative disorder with a single chromosomal abnormality (the 9;22 translocation), to a more fulminant disease (blast crisis), still accompanied by the 9;22 translocation but heralded by the accumulation of additional chromosomal abnormalities.

STANDARD CHEMOTHERAPEUTIC AGENTS

This chapter does not describe each of the standard chemotherapeutic agents in detail or give specific guidelines for their proper clinical use; this critical information is readily available from several sources (Dorr and Fritz 1980; Skeel 1987; Wittes 1989). Rather, the purpose is to introduce the major classes of cytotoxic drugs, emphasizing their mechanisms of action, pharmacology, and unique toxicities. Selected single agents are described in some detail, either because they are commonly used and important, or because they illustrate the interplay between drug pharmacology and tumor growth kinetics. A classification scheme based upon mechanism of action would be ideal, but in many instances a drug kills tumor cells in several different ways or is effective for reasons not yet well understood. Therefore, drugs are categorized in a conventional format as: (1) alkylating agents, (2) antimetabolites, (3) antitumor antibiotics, (4) plant alkaloids, (5) hormonal agents, or (6) miscellaneous compounds. The recently introduced interferons, interleukins, and hematopoietic growth factors, along with other novel approaches to systemic cancer treatment, are briefly described.

ALKYLATING AGENTS

An alkylating agent, mechlorethamine, was the first nonhormonal cytotoxic drug found to be useful in the treatment of malignant disease. Although structurally diverse, all of the alkylators have or generate via intermediates reactive functional groups that are electron-deficient and which form covalent bonds with electron-rich (nucleophilic) groups in nucleic acids, proteins, and an array of smaller molecules. Despite the wide range of groups with which alkylating agents can form covalent bonds (amino, imidazole, carboxyl, sulfhydryl, and phosphate), the bases in DNA are by far the most important, particularly the electron-rich N-7 position of guanine. DNA alkylation produces a variety of defects—depurination, double- and single-stranded breaks, inter- and intrastrand cross-links—which disrupt (sometimes permanently) DNA replication and transcription. This fundamental alteration in the information coded in the DNA molecule, if it cannot be efficiently repaired, may result in cellular death, mutagenesis, or carcinogenesis. The primacy of DNA base alkylation in mediating these effects is underscored by the heightened susceptibility to alkylating agents of cells known to be deficient in DNA repair enzymes; conversely, an increased ability to repair such damage represents one form of resistance to these drugs. In contrast to the antimetabolites, which interfere with the pathways leading to the synthesis of new DNA (and RNA), alkylating agents react with preformed nucleic acids; thus they tend to be active throughout all phases of the cell cycle. Although most alkylating agents are still more toxic to proliferating than to nonproliferating cells, the distinction is not as pronounced as it is for the antimetabolites. In fact, for a subset of the alkylating agents, the nitrosoureas, the distinction hardly exists (Twentyman and Bleehen 1975). This ability to kill nonproliferating cells makes alkylators attractive drugs to use against tumors with low growth fractions, such as multiple myeloma. Moreover, alkylating agents have an almost infinite number of potential sites in DNA for disruption and, lacking the cell cycle or cell cycle phase specificity of antimetabolites, they do not typically exhibit a plateau in cell survival with increasing dose.

These features make them theoretically attractive drugs to use in testing the notion of drug intensity; that is, the idea that the logarithmic relationship between drug dose and cell survival can be exploited to clinical advantage—as in high-dose chemotherapy followed by bone marrow rescue.

Unfortunately, the same properties that make alkylating agents effective produce a set of unique, long-term toxicities. Their ability to kill the slowly cycling stem cells of tumors also translates into toxicity for the stem cells of the bone marrow. In contrast to the predictable and short-lived myelosuppression of drugs that merely destroy the more mature cells of the marrow (e.g., myeloblasts, myelocytes, metamyelocytes, and neutrophils), alkylators are often responsible for producing delayed, prolonged, and even permanent marrow failure. Stem cell toxicity is also manifested by the frequent development of amenorrhea in women and oligospermia or azoospermia in men, often causing irreversible infertility. Finally, the most feared stem cell toxicity of alkylating agents is their mutagenic and ultimately carcinogenic effect on bone marrow stem cells, culminating in a form of acute myelogenous leukemia that is relatively refractory to treatment. The risk of developing AML is directly proportional to the total dose of drug a patient receives and the length of follow-up; for one group of patients followed for 10 years after completing alkylator therapy for ovarian carcinoma, the risk of AML was as high as 5% to 10% (Greene et al. 1982).

The oldest group of alkylating agents, the nitrogen mustards, includes mechlorethamine (the prototype), melphalan, chlorambucil, cyclophosphamide, and ifosfamide. Mechlorethamine is a highly reactive and unstable molecule, and is liable to cause irritation at the site of injection; its clinical use has become limited to its part in the four-drug MOPP regimen used to treat Hodgkin's disease and, occasionally, other lymphomas. The other nitrogen mustards are derivatives of mechlorethamine; they all contain ring structures that render them more stable and, with the exception of ifosfamide, are available as oral preparations. Chlorambucil has a very narrow spectrum of activity, its use being restricted to the treatment of slowly growing lymphoid neoplasms such as CLL, Waldenstrom's macroglobulinemia, and indolent non-Hodgkin's lymphomas (NHLs). Melphalan has had a role in the treatment of breast and ovarian carcinomas, but it is now used primarily for managing multiple myeloma. Melphalan is notorious for its erratic gastrointestinal absorption; 20% to 50% of an oral dose can be recovered in the feces. Intravenous administration of melphalan can circumvent this problem, but the usual clinical practice is to titrate the oral dose of melphalan to mild hematologic toxicity.

Cyclophosphamide is the most versatile of the alkylating agents and is unique among the nitrogen mustards on several accounts. First, cyclophosphamide is itself inactive, requiring metabolism by the liver to

4-hydroxycyclophosphamide before yielding active alkylating metabolites. Four-hydroxycyclophosphamide (in equilibrium with its acyclic isomer, aldophosphamide) is transported into cells where it spontaneously decomposes into phosphoramide mustard, which has direct alkylating activity, and acrolein, a compound thought to be responsible for the urothelial toxicity of cyclophosphamide. Second, its metabolites have a more selective toxicity for proliferating cells than do other alkylators: prolonged myelosuppression does not occur, cumulative toxicity to the marrow is unusual, and leukemogenesis appears to be less of a problem than with other alkylating agents (Greene et al. 1986). These advantages, coupled with the drug's activity against a broad spectrum of tumors, have made it the most commonly administered alkylating agent.

The peculiar toxicity of cyclophosphamide and its newer analogue, ifosfamide, is an acute, sterile, hemorrhagic cystitis—occurring in up to 10% of patients treated with the drug. The metabolite acrolein is thought to be the culprit. Hemorrhagic cystitis can be largely prevented by simply maintaining a high urine output. However, with high-dose administration of either cyclophosphamide or ifosfamide co-administration of either N-acetylcysteine (Mucormyst) or sodium 2-mercaptoethanesulfonate (Mesna) should be considered. Both are thiol compounds that neutralize acrolein.

The pharmacokinetics of cyclophosphamide have not been fully described because some of its metabolites are difficult to detect in plasma. Nonetheless, it is clear that both the parent compound and its metabolites are excreted by the kidneys. Renal failure results in prolonged blood levels but not usually in increased toxicity—probably because renal clearance of the parent drug is normally low and can be maintained even in patients with marginal renal function. Also, inasmuch as cyclophosphamide requires activation via liver microsomal enzymes, liver dysfunction would likely prompt a change in dose. Systematic data on the influence of renal and hepatic dysfunction upon the choice of dose is lacking, but common sense would at least suggest that cyclophosphamide should be administered in attenuated doses to patients with severe renal failure.

The four other chemical classes of alkylating agents are the nitrosoureas (carmustine, lomustine, semustine, streptozocin); the alkyl sulfonates (busulfan); the triazines (dacarbazine); and the ethylenimines (thiotepa, hexamethylmelamine). The nitrosoureas are distinguished by their lipid solubility, giving them at least a potential role in the treatment of intracranial tumors, and by their lack of cross-resistance with other alkylating agents. Their clinical usefulness has been limited by their tendency to cause more delayed, prolonged, and cumulative myelosuppression than other alkylators. Busulfan, the only alkyl sulfonate in clinical use, has long been employed in the management of chronic myelogenous leukemia. Its utility in CML derives from its rather high degree of selectivity for the myeloid cells of the bone marrow; in some cases it can produce a period of drug-free clinical disease remission, albeit never permanent.

ANTIMETABOLITES

Interest in antimetabolite development followed the discovery that folic acid antagonists were effective in the treatment of childhood ALL. Elucidation of the biochemical pathways leading to DNA and RNA synthesis led to the proliferation of a large number of drugs fashioned to have structural similarity to critical intermediates (metabolites) in these pathways. Antimetabolites function in one of two ways: either they compete with normal metabolites for the catalytic or regulatory site of a key enzyme, or they substitute for a metabolite that is normally incorporated into an important molecule such as DNA or RNA. Because most antimetabolites interfere with nucleic acid synthesis (instead of with preformed nucleic acids, as do the alkylating agents) they have little, if any, effect on cells in G_0 and usually exhibit maximum activity during S-phase. The enzymes that antimetabolites inhibit are more limited in number than the sites potentially available to alkylating agents (i.e., the almost innumerable bases of DNA). Complete inhibition of these enzymes may occur at clinically achievable drug levels, and such relatively complete target inhibition, coupled with specificity for cells in a single phase of the cell cycle, explains the plateau in cell survival with increasing drug dose. Antimetabolites are not associated with delayed or prolonged myelosuppression, and they appear to present a minimal risk of leukemogenesis and/or carcinogenesis— all likely reflections of their impotence against slowly proliferating stem cells.

FOLIC ACID ANALOGUES

A number of folic acid analogues have been produced that inhibit the enzyme dihydrofolate reductase (DHFR); however, only methotrexate (MTX) is in clinical use. DHFR is responsible for the generation of reduced folates, molecules which occupy key positions in nucleic acid synthesis. Reduced folates are required for the transfer of methyl groups during the biosynthesis of purines. Moreover, inhibition of DHFR blocks the production of N^5, N^{10}-methylene tetrahydrofolate, a reduced folate coenzyme that participates with thymidylate synthetase in the conversion of dUMP to dTMP. DNA synthesis ceases as a result of this lack of dTMP and purines.

Plasma methotrexate is about 50% bound to plasma proteins and is eliminated primarily by the kidneys without extensive metabolism. Disappearance of MTX from the plasma is essentially biphasic: the initial distribution phase has a $t\frac{1}{2}$ of two to three hours, while the final phase has a $t\frac{1}{2}$ of eight to ten hours. The terminal phase is prolonged in the face of renal dysfunction. A third phase of elimination, which occurs very slowly, has also been described and is attributed to enterohepatic circulation of the drug. Its excretion by the kidneys can be inhibited by the coadministration of weak organic acids, such as aspirin or penicillin. Aspirin can further compound methotrexate's toxicity by displacing the drug from its binding site on albumin, increasing the concentration of free drug.

The cytotoxicity of methotrexate depends critically upon the duration of tissue exposure to the drug above a certain threshold value rather than on the peak level of drug in the tissue (Bleyer 1978). Irrespective of the duration of exposure to methotrexate, toxicity for many tissues does not occur until the level of drug exceeds 10^{-8} molar. Conversely, exceedingly high levels may be well tolerated by normal tissues provided that exposure is limited to 24 to 36 hours. The availability of a reduced folate "antidote" in the form of 5-formyltetrahydrofolate (leucovorin) allows the duration of methotrexate-induced dTMP and purine depletion to be precisely controlled; the ability to measure serum levels of MTX allows the physician to determine how much leucovorin to give and when leucovorin rescue may be safely discontinued.

An appreciation of these details of methotrexate's pharmacology has allowed the drug to be delivered in doses 10 to 100 times greater than those given conventionally. The major impetus to giving such high doses is the theoretical possibility of so overcoming many forms of MTX resistance: defects in active transport of the drug might be overcome by passive diffusion; increased amounts of DHFR from gene amplification might be more completely inhibited; intracellular levels of the drug might remain high despite decreased polyglutamation; and even enzymes with reduced affinity for MTX might be inhibited. Moreover, high-dose methotrexate followed by leucovorin rescue can achieve tumoricidal drug levels in the CNS and, if properly performed, is without myelosuppression; the latter advantage would allow for more frequent administration of the drug.

These theoretical advantages of high-dose methotrexate with leucovorin rescue explain the regimen's inclusion in a variety of experimental protocols for diseases such as ALL, lymphomas, and tumors of the head and neck. Yet the only disease for which high-dose methotrexate with leucovorin rescue has become standard chemotherapeutic treatment is osteogenic sarcoma. Responses to high-dose methotrexate are rare in patients whose tumors are refractory to conventional doses. The methotrexate resistance of *in vivo* human tumors perhaps has less to do with the mechanisms of resistance cited above, and perhaps more to do with the limited potential of a drug that depends so heavily on DNA synthesis for its toxicity in the treatment of tumors with low growth fractions. The exquisite sensitivity of the rapidly proliferating gestational trophoblastic carcinoma to conventional doses of methotrexate lends additional credence to this argument. Enthusiasm for high doses is also tempered by: (1) the propensity of MTX in high doses to precipitate in the renal tubules (avoided by maintaining a high urine output and by alkalinizing the urine, which requires hospitalization); (2) the tendency of MTX in high doses to significantly

accumulate within third-space fluid compartments (e.g., pleural and peritoneal effusions) and to thereafter slowly diffuse out, producing prolonged exposure to the drug; (3) the need to measure plasma MTX levels; and (4) the enormous expense of leucovorin.

Methotrexate has a wide spectrum of antitumor activity. It is usually curative as a single agent in gestational trophoblastic carcinoma. It is also particularly useful as an intrathecal agent when treating leptomeningeal tumor infiltrates.

PYRIMIDINE ANALOGUES

5-fluorouracil (5-FU). The pyrimidine analogue 5-fluorouracil (5-FU) resembles both uracil and thymidine. Phosphorylation of 5-FU to 5-FUTP allows the analogue to be incorporated into RNA; nuclear processing of mRNA and rRNA is disrupted, and the fraudulent pyrimidine may cause errors in base pairing during RNA transcription. The agent is also converted to 5-FdUMP, a compound that irreversibly inhibits thymidylate synthetase; DNA synthesis is brought to a halt because of thymidine depletion. These two different mechanisms of cytotoxicity allow 5-FU to be active throughout the cell cycle, not just in S-phase. It is given intravenously because of erratic gastrointestinal absorption. When the drug is given as a single IV bolus it has a plasma $t\frac{1}{2}$ of only 10 to 30 minutes, and no drug can be detected in plasma after three hours. However, intracellular levels may persist for hours. Although the bulk of 5-FU is catabolized by the liver, the absence of the enzymes responsible for its catabolism in some colon carcinomas may explain its usefulness in treating gastrointestinal carcinomas.

As a single agent, 5-FU has only modest activity. Recently its effectiveness appears to have been enhanced by the concomitant administration of leucovorin. When 5-FdUMP binds to thymidylate synthetase, it forms part of a ternary complex that also includes N^5, N^{10}-methylenetetrahydrofolate—the normal coenzyme for thymidylate synthetase. Although this ternary complex is covalent, it dissociates with a $t\frac{1}{2}$ of two to three hours in the absence of excess N^5, N^{10}-methylenetetrahydrofolate. High levels of N^5, N^{10}-methylenetetrahydrofolate, derived from leucovorin, produce optimal conditions for the formation of this complex and deter its subsequent degradation. Several clinical trials have yielded evidence to argue that the combination of 5-FU and leucovorin is better than 5-FU alone in the treatment of advanced colon cancer (Grem et al. 1987).

CYTOSINE ARABINOSIDE (ARA-C)

Cytosine arabinoside (Ara-C) differs from deoxycytidine only in its sugar moiety, with arabinose replacing deoxyribose. Ara-C enters cells through a carrier-mediated process shared with deoxycytidine. Once in the cell Ara-C, like deoxycytidine, follows one of two major paths: it is either deaminated to the nontoxic compound Ara-U, or it is sequentially phosphorylated to Ara-CTP, the active form of the drug. Ara-CTP's toxicity arises from its ability to competitively inhibit the binding of the normal substrate, dCTP, to DNA polymerase; DNA synthesis is thereby arrested. Ara-CTP may also be incorporated into DNA and cause defective ligation or incomplete synthesis of DNA fragments. Both effects are consistent with the drug's selective toxicity for cells in S-phase.

Following IV injection Ara-C is rapidly inactivated to Ara-U by cytidine deaminase, an enzyme widely distributed throughout the body. After a single bolus injection, Ara-C has a brief plasma $t^{1/2}$ of only seven to 20 minutes. Such single bolus injections of Ara-C tend to be nontoxic to normal marrow, and ineffective in treating leukemia as well. However, if the drug is given in two divided doses separated by 12 hours, a significant number of patients with leukemia respond. The greater effectiveness of the every-12-hour regimen lies in the fact that the S-phase of AML blast cells lasts approximately 18 to 20 hours. If a leukemia cell is in the cell cycle but not in S-phase at the time of a bolus injection of Ara-C, it escapes toxicity. If the next bolus of Ara-C is not given until another 24 hours have elapsed, the same cell may have already passed through S-phase and so evade the drug's effect altogether. Yet when Ara-C is given on an every-12-hour schedule, no cycling cell can pass through a complete S-phase without being exposed to the drug. If all leukemic cells were in cycle, that is, if none was in G_0, then from a purely kinetic perspective it would be possible to kill all cells by delivering Ara-C as a bolus every 12 hours or as a continuous infusion over the time required to complete one cell cycle. Many leukemia cells are in G_0, so Ara-C must be administered for a longer period of time (5-7 days) to allow as many of these cells as possible to enter the proliferating pool and pass through S-phase.

Most current drug combinations have evolved empirically, and the sequence in which the drugs are given usually reflects little more than an attempt to avoid overlapping toxicities. The sequential use of Ara-C and asparaginase to induce remission in patients with either refractory or relapsed AML is an important exception that shows how the sequence of drug administration can be critical. Asparaginase is an enzyme derived from bacterial sources. When given intravenously it hydrolyzes serum asparagine and deprives leukemia cells of an amino acid they themselves cannot synthesize; normal cells are spared because they generally have the ability to synthesize their own asparagine. When studied in a murine leukemia, pharmacologic antagonism occurred when both drugs were administered concurrently or when the asparaginase preceded delivery of Ara-C (Schwartz, Morgenstein, and Capizzi 1982). Asparaginase depletion shuts down protein synthesis, which inhibits the progression of tumor cells from G_1 to S-phase. Because Ara-C is active only on cells in S-phase, asparaginase pretreatment is protective. However, if asparaginase is given after Ara-C, then synergis-

tic killing of leukemia cells is observed, associated with increased formation of Ara-CTP and Ara-CDNA. Asparaginase treatment lowers the cellular pool of the normal metabolite, dCTP, and so produces less competition for the target enzyme, DNA polymerase. These laboratory observations led to the design of a clinical trial comparing high-dose Ara-C alone to high-dose Ara-C followed by asparaginase, in patients with refractory or relapsed AML (Capizzi et al. 1988). The experimental observations bore fruit: the use of sequential high-dose Ara-C and asparaginase resulted in a 42% complete remission rate while high-dose Ara-C alone achieved a rate of only 12%.

PURINE ANALOGUES

Two guanine analogues are in clinical use: 6-mercaptopurine (6-MP) and 6-thioguanine (6-TG). These two drugs are more alike than they are different, and resistance to one drug usually predicts resistance to the other. Both parent compounds are inactive until they undergo metabolic conversion to their respective monophosphate ribonucleotides — a result of the enzyme hypoxanthine-guanine phosphoribosyl transferase (HGPRTase), whose normal function is to salvage purines for nucleic acid synthesis by adding ribose phosphate to them. The monophosphate nucleotides are capable of inhibiting *de novo* purine synthesis, i.e., the formation of adenylic and guanylic acids from inosinic acid. Further phosphorylation gives rise to the respective triphosphate nucleotides; in the case of 6-TG, conversion to the deoxyribonucleotide allows significant amounts of the drug to be incorporated into DNA, the extent of which correlates with the production of strand breaks and cellular cytotoxicity.

In experimental tumors it has been possible to show that resistance to these two purine analogues can ensue from a deficiency in the activating enzyme HGPRTase. However, leukemia cells are not typically deficient in this enzyme, and other mechanisms of resistance must be important, for example, rapid dephosphorylation of the active nucleotides by a membrane-bound alkaline phosphatase.

The guanine analogues are used almost exclusively for the treatment of leukemias; they have no significant activity against solid tumors. The differences in their catabolism have critical implications in the treatment of leukemia. For example, 6-MP is oxidized to 6-thiouric acid by xanthine oxidase. The concomitant administration of allopurinol, a xanthine oxidase inhibitor used to prevent hyperuricemia and acute uric-acid nephropathy during rapid leukemia cell lysis, may increase the toxicity of 6-MP by impairing its degradation. The dose of 6-MP is therefore reduced by 75% if allopurinol is to be given. The catabolism of 6-TG follows a different pathway and no dose reduction is required in the presence of allopurinol.

Several analogues of adenosine exist, but they have limited clinical utility. Pentostatin (2'-deoxycoformycin) is an adenosine analogue produced by a species of *Streptomyces*. It is a powerful inhibitor of adenosine deaminase (ADA), an enzyme which deaminates adenosine to inosine and deoxyadenosine to deoxyinosine. Accumulation of adenosine and deoxyadenosine is toxic to cells, particularly to those of the lymphoid system, as suggested by the severe lymphopenia of children with congenital ADA deficiency. Pentostatin is probably the most active agent in the treatment of the uncommon hairy-cell leukemia; it also has activity in cutaneous T-cell lymphoma and in CLL.

Fludarabine is a recently tested adenosine analogue that is resistant to deamination by adenosine deaminase; it has been found to be particularly effective in treating CLL.

ANTITUMOR ANTIBIOTICS

The antitumor antibiotics—actinomycin D, the anthracyclines, bleomycin, mitomycin C, and mithramycin—are a structurally diverse group of compounds all derived from various species of *Streptomyces*. They are too cytotoxic to be used as antibacterial agents but they are valuable in treating a broad spectrum of tumors. The anthracyclines are the most widely used antitumor antibiotics in current clinical oncology.

The most commonly encountered anthracycline, doxorubicin, consists of a planar 4-ring anthraquinone attached to an amino sugar, daunosamine. The related compound, daunorubicin, differs from doxorubicin only by the substitution of a methoxy for a methyl group in the anthraquinone ring; it is used almost exclusively in the treatment of acute leukemia.

A good deal of effort has gone into examining the structure-function relationships of doxorubicin and other anthracyclines, first because they are among the most effective antitumor agents available, and second because they produce dose-limiting cardiac toxicity. The clinical benefit of separating the two effects would be substantial.

Complex mechanisms underlie anthracycline cytotoxicity. First, the anthraquinone ring can intercalate between base pairs of DNA; the stability of this complex is enhanced by the attraction of the amino group of daunosamine for the phosphate groups of the DNA backbone. DNA intercalation disrupts DNA replication and RNA transcription, but it is uncertain just how important intercalation is to anthracycline cytotoxicity; DNA is normally organized and folded into chromatin, and perhaps is so protected from this type of drug interaction. Second, anthracyclines can produce single- and double-stranded DNA scission and impair DNA repair. The process of DNA scission may be facilitated by intercalation between base pairs or by an interaction with topoisomerase II. However, a third mechanism capable of generating DNA breaks and many other forms of damage is the creation of free radicals. The quinone ring of the anthracyclines can assume a semiquinone form with an unpaired electron; this species reacts with molecular oxygen (O_2) to generate superoxide (O_2-) which wreaks havoc on a wide variety of cellular structures, including DNA. However, doxorubi-

cin retains toxicity under hypoxic conditions when superoxide radicals cannot be formed (Tannock and Guttman 1981). Finally, anthracyclines tend to bind to almost everything with which they come into contact, and it is possible that they kill cells through disruption of the cell membrane. In fact, in one experimental system where doxorubicin was attached to small beads, cell death occurred despite the drug's inability to enter cells (Tritton and Yee 1982). This gave credence both to the notion of direct membrane disruption and to the importance of free radical formation. Nonetheless, a large body of literature supports the idea that anthracycline toxicity in many systems depends upon the drug's ability to enter cells: witness the phenomenon of multidrug resistance, characterized by increased efflux of anthracyclines, as well as of other natural products, across the cell membrane. As a result of their wide-ranging effects, the anthracyclines are active throughout the cell cycle, although they are most toxic for cells in S-phase or G_2 phase.

The ability to generate free radicals has been implicated in the production of cardiac toxicity. Clinical trials of the free-radical scavengers vitamin E and N-acetylcysteine, which have lessened the cardiac toxicity of doxorubicin in some animal systems, were unsuccessful. However, initial reports of a randomized clinical trial with the EDTA analogue ICRF-187, indicate that this compound can lessen the cardiac toxicity of doxorubicin in humans without altering its antitumor activity (Speyer et al. 1988). ICRF-187 is thought to inhibit free-radical formation by chelating iron. Anthracyclines can bind ferric iron which, when reduced to ferrous iron, can react with O_2 to produce O_2-, H_2O_2, and $OH-$.

Doxorubicin is administered intravenously, is widely distributed in the body, and binds extensively with plasma proteins and other tissues. Plasma clearance of the drug is triphasic: the half-lives of the three phases are 8 to 25 minutes, 1.5 to 10 hours, and 24 to 48 hours, respectively. The second phase is attributed to hepatic metabolism of the drug to yield an active metabolite (doxorubicinol) and a number of metabolites (aglycones) that have no antitumor effect but which may have a hand in causing cardiac and other toxicities. The final phase reflects release of drug from tissue binding sites. Because doxorubicin and its metabolites are excreted via the bile, dosage reduction is mandatory for patients with biliary obstruction.

The damage to heart muscle is a problem whose incidence increases with increasing cumulative dose of drug. As the total dose of doxorubicin approaches 550 mg/m^2 the incidence of chronic congestive heart failure rises from 1% to 4%; above this cumulative dose, the incidence rises dramatically. It is important to monitor patients who receive significant doses of doxorubicin for cardiac toxicity. The gold standard is endomyocardial biopsy. This procedure reflects drug-related myocardial damage in a manner that is linear with dose, but it is neither practical nor widely available. Most commonly the left ventricular ejection fraction (LVEF) is determined by radionuclide cineangiography at serial total doses of the drug, with cessation of doxorubicin therapy if the LVEF drops significantly below its baseline value. It is also important to be aware of the increased risk of anthracycline-induced cardiotoxicity in the presence of other cardiac insults, such as prior mediastinal irradiation, systemic hypertension, or the coadministration of cyclophosphamide or mitomycin C.

PLANT ALKALOIDS

VINCA ALKALOIDS

Extracts of the periwinkle plant, long believed in folklore to have medicinal value, caused myelosuppression in rats and led to the isolation of two active alkaloid anticancer compounds, vincristine and vinblastine. These two compounds are complex, multiringed molecules of nearly identical structure. Vinblastine differs from vincristine only by the substitution of a formyl group for a methyl group at one point in a side chain of the parent molecule; nonetheless, this seemingly minor structural variation results in a very different pattern of toxicity and antitumor activity.

Vincristine and vinblastine share a common mechanism of cytotoxicity: they both bind to the protein tubulin. Tubulin is a dimeric protein that normally polymerizes to form the microtubular apparatus along which chromosomes migrate during mitosis, and which serves as a conduit for neurotransmitter transport along axons. Binding of the vinca alkaloids to tubulin prevents the protein's polymerization. The results are cytotoxicity, manifested by an arrest of cells in metaphase with subsequent lysis; and neurotoxicity, characterized by depressed deep tendon reflexes and paresthesias if mild, and by motor weakness, cranial nerve palsies, and paralytic ileus if severe.

Vincristine's dose-limiting toxicity is its neurotoxicity, and it is uncommon to observe any myelosuppression with conventional doses. Vinblastine, on the other hand, is myelotoxic with less neurotoxicity. Vincristine is an important component of regimens used to induce remission in childhood ALL, and it is used in a variety of combination chemotherapy regimens for other malignancies, especially lymphomas. Vinblastine's major contribution has been to the combination chemotherapy of testicular carcinoma.

The vinca alkaloids are both given by IV injection and display similar pharmacokinetics. Both drugs are extensively bound to proteins, producing rapid biphasic clearance from the plasma as they are distributed into body tissues. The terminal phase of plasma clearance is long, 20 to 30 hours, and reflects elimination of the drugs and their metabolites via the biliary tract. It is common practice to reduce the dose of vincristine or vinblastine in the face of obstructive liver disease.

ETOPOSIDE (VP-16)

Etoposide (VP-16) is a semisynthetic derivative of podophyllotoxin, a cytotoxic drug isolated from the root of the May apple plant, and used for years in the topical treatment of condyloma acuminatum. Like podophyllotoxin and the vinca alkaloids, etoposide causes metaphase arrest. However, unlike these other alkaloids, etoposide dose not inhibit microtubule assembly, apparently due to a sugar moiety absent in the other compounds. Etoposide can, on the other hand, induce strand breaks in DNA, an effect that is likely mediated by its interaction with topoisomerase II.

Etoposide is usually given intravenously because its absorption following oral administration is quite variable. However, larger doses by the oral route can achieve equal systemic effects. The pharmacokinetics of etoposide have not been well sorted out, but it appears that under normal circumstances 40% to 60% of a dose is excreted in the urine as unchanged drug and metabolites. Nonetheless, normal clearance of VP-16 has been described in a patient with end-stage renal disease. Similarly, hepatic dysfunction does not seem to alter the drug's clearance. The only peculiar toxicity of etoposide is its tendency to produce transient hypotension if given by rapid IV injection; this problem is avoided by infusing the drug over 30 minutes or longer.

Etoposide has a wide range of clinical uses. It is a key component of curative combination chemotherapy for nonseminomatous testicular carcinoma. The drug is included in several combination regimens directed toward treating aggressive forms of non-Hodgkin's lymphoma. Etoposide is probably the most active single agent used in small-cell lung cancer.

HORMONES AND HORMONE ANTAGONISTS

Just as the growth of many normal tissues is under hormonal influence, many malignant cells retain a degree of hormonal sensitivity characteristic of their tissue of origin. This is particularly true for carcinomas of the breast, prostate, and endometrium. To date the only clinically useful hormonal manipulations have involved, directly or indirectly, the steroid hormones. Steroid hormones mediate their effects by binding to specific intracellular receptors and, as steroid hormone-receptor complexes, interact with nuclear chromatin to stimulate or repress transcription of specific sequences of mRNA, ultimately modulating cellular function and growth. Manipulation of this sequence of events has produced several important treatment modalities.

Tamoxifen, the most extensively used and perhaps the most important of the hormonal agents, competes with estradiol for binding to a high-affinity estradiol receptor. Tamoxifen's binding to the estrogen receptor does not result in an estrogenic response in most tissues and leaves cells refractory to further estrogen stimulation. A growing body of evidence indicates that the adjuvant (i.e., following local treatment), long-term administration of tamoxifen to postmenopausal women with stage II carcinoma of the breast improves their survival (Stewart 1987). Paradoxically, an older and still effective approach to the palliation of metastatic breast cancer is the use of the synthetic estrogen diethystilbestrol (DES). The explanation of this paradox probably lies in the fact that DES in pharmacologic doses elicits a quite different interaction between steroid hormone, receptor, and nuclear chromatin than do the smaller doses of naturally occurring estrogens.

Depleting a tumor of a steroid hormone may be effected indirectly. Prostate carcinoma is heavily dependent, at least in its early stages, on androgenic stimulation; the disease does not develop in castrated males. Androgen depletion can be achieved directly with orchiectomy, but it can also be produced by administering DES. Although DES may have some slight direct effect on prostate carcinoma, its major effect is to suppress the pituitary's release of luteinizing hormone (LH), which normally stimulates testicular androgen secretion. Neither orchiectomy nor DES is an ideal form of hormonal manipulation: the former approach is emotionally unacceptable for some men, and DES therapy is associated with excessive cardiovascular toxicity. More recently, the development of a group of synthetic gonadotropin-releasing hormone (GnRH) agonists offers an important alternative form of hormonal treatment. At first glance it would seem illogical to use an agent that should elicit increased secretion of LH. The GnRH agonists may initially cause a surge of LH secretion and a consequent flare in the disease, but they eventually desensitize the pituitary to the effects of GnRH by decreasing the number of GnRH receptors. The end result is the same as in therapy with DES: decreased secretion of LH.

The use of high-dose corticosteroids in the treatment of leukemia and lymphomas is effective for different reasons. Lymphoid tumors contain large numbers of cytosolic receptors for corticosteroids, and rather than producing the slow tumor regression typical of other hormonal agents, high-dose corticosteroids have a prompt lytic effect on these cells.

Hormonal therapy causes tumor regression in approximately 30% of patients with endometrial cancer, in 30% to 40% of patients with breast cancer, and in 80% of those with prostate cancer. However, there is no form of hormonal therapy at present that can cure a patient of an established tumor. Tumors regress and on occasion shrink below the limits of clinical detection, and some tumors may respond to a series of different hormonal treatments, but they ultimately become refractory to further hormonal manipulation. With the exception of tamoxifen's use in the adjuvant treatment of postmenopausal women with stage II breast cancer, it has been difficult to show that hormonal therapy even prolongs survival. It is now evident that even hormone-responsive tumors contain from the outset populations of both hormone-dependent and hormone-independent cells. Moreover, the natural history of most tumors is to become increasingly anaplastic (poorly differentiated) and thus less likely dependent on hormonal stimulation for their growth. Still, there is a strong clinical impression that hormonal therapy can be effective, especially when therapy is directed at disease palliation.

MISCELLANEOUS AGENTS

Of all the drugs that fail to fit into a specific category, cisplatin is the most important. Its discovery was fortuitous: during experiments designed to investigate the effect of electrical currents on bacterial growth, growth inhibition occurred in a zone immediately adjacent to platinum electrodes. Cisplatin was found to be the active substance among the numerous platinum compounds in solution. Subsequently, it was found to have substantial activity against a variety of tumors.

Cisplatin (cis-diamminedichloroplatinum II) is an inorganic planar coordination complex, the platinum atom being coordinated to two amine groups on one side and to two chlorine atoms on the other. Cisplatin's cytotoxicity arises from mechanisms similar to those of classic alkylating agents. The chlorine atoms of the complex behave much like those of mechlorethamine, that is, they function as leaving groups, displaced by nucleophils, such as the bases in DNA. In actuality, the chlorine atoms must first be displaced by water molecules, producing a charged platinum complex, prior to nucleophilic addition. Aquation proceeds slowly in the presence of a high Cl^- concentration; theoretically, formation of the active, aquated, charged complex should occur *intracellularly* where the Cl^- concentration is low. As with classic alkylating agents, the preferred site for binding of cisplatin to DNA is the N-7 position of guanine. Because it is bifunctional (having two leaving groups), cisplatin can form interstrand DNA crosslinks, the number of which correlates with the drug's cytotoxicity. The inactive trans-isomer of cisplatin produces DNA-protein crosslinks but cannot form DNA interstrand crosslinks at clinically relevant concentrations. The formation of interstrand crosslinks proceeds slowly and is opposed by enzymatic mechanisms of excision and repair; resistance to the drug may rise from these processes. Cisplatin is most active in G_1 but behaves predominantly in a phase-nonspecific manner.

Cisplatin is given intravenously; in the case of ovarian carcinoma, it is also given intraperitoneally. Upon IV injection, most of the drug (90%) becomes rapidly bound to proteins and is cleared from the plasma slowly. That proportion of a dose which remains as free drug—the active form of cisplatin—is cleared rapidly; 90% of this free drug is cleared from the plasma during the first two hours after injection. Cisplatin is cleared almost exclusively by the kidneys, primarily the result of glomerular filtration. The rate of cisplatin clearance can be accelerated by maneuvers aimed at increasing urinary output, such as saline or mannitol diuresis.

Cisplatin's major dose-limiting toxicity is renal damage; it is a direct tubular toxin, preferentially affecting the proximal straight tubule and the distal and collecting tubules. In addition to a decline in GFR, many patients waste magnesium as a result of tubular dysfunction, occasionally to the point of developing tetany. Acute nephrotoxicity attributable to cisplatin therapy is usually reversible; however, with repeated dosing, cumulative and more permanent damage does occur. Ensuring rapid clearance of the free drug by saline or mannitol diuresis is one way of minimizing nephrotoxicity. Even more protection is needed when very high doses of cisplatin are given. One simple way of providing additional protection is to administer the drug in 3% (hypertonic) saline; this establishes diuresis and generates a high urinary Cl^- concentration that slows the formation of the toxic, charged, and aquated complex in the lumen of the renal tubule. Other toxicities include ototoxicity (tinnitus, high-frequency hearing loss), peripheral neuropathy (usually in the form of a stocking-glove distribution of sensory loss with paresthesias), and relatively severe nausea and vomiting. In contrast to the classic alkylating agents, cisplatin's mild myelotoxicity makes it an ideal drug for many combination regimens.

Cisplatin is the most active single agent against nonseminomatous testicular cancer; when combined with vinblastine and bleomycin (PVB), it is usually curative. Cisplatin is also the most active single agent against ovarian cancer, often accompanied by doxorubicin and/or cyclophosphamide. Other important applications include the treatment of squamous (head and neck) and transitional-cell (bladder) carcinomas, and the treatment of small-cell lung cancer.

STRATEGIES FOR IMPROVING SYSTEMIC CANCER TREATMENT

ADJUVANT CHEMOTHERAPY

When agents are found to produce a high number of palliative responses in overtly metastatic tumors, there will be efforts to use them at an earlier point in the disease, especially as adjuvant therapy. Residual micrometastatic tumors following definitive local therapy should be more susceptible to chemotherapy than the clinically detectable mass for several reasons: a better vascular supply, allowing for better drug penetration; a higher proliferative rate; and a decreased likelihood of drug-resistant cells. This rationale has made a significant impact on the treatment of stage II breast cancer and is being tested in numerous other settings, such as the adjuvant use of 5-FU and leucovorin in colon cancer. The more recent notion of neoadjuvant chemotherapy— given prior to definitive local therapy with surgery or radiation—has a slightly different goal: it strives to shrink locally advanced tumors to the point where they are amenable to local therapy, while at the same time eradicating or at least controlling distant micrometastatic disease.

DOSAGE INTENSIFICATION

The major impediment to exploiting the exponential relationship between dose and cell survival for currently available cytotoxic drugs is the low therapeutic index of these compounds, i.e., their toxicity for normal tissues. By far the most important dose-limiting toxicity for the bulk of these agents is myelosuppression, which places patients at high risk for infection and bleeding. One successful approach to circumventing the prolonged myelosuppression or permanent marrow ablation that results from high-dose chemotherapy is the technique of bone marrow transplantation. The transplanted bone marrow may be allogeneic (from an antigenically distinct individual), syngeneic (from an identical twin), or autologous (from the patient). Allogeneic and syngeneic marrow transplantation following high-dose chemotherapy with or without radiation is being used in the successful treatment of acute myelogenous and lymphocytic leukemias, and in chronic myelogenous leukemia (O'Reilly 1983). Autologous bone marrow transplantation has been effective in treating some intermediate- and high-grade lymphomas (Philip et al. 1987). Efforts are under way to test the potential benefit of high-dose chemotherapy combined with autologous bone marrow rescue in the treatment of more common and typically more resistant solid tumors, such as breast cancer (Eder et al. 1986).

Although allogeneic bone marrow transplantation has an established role in the treatment of some individuals with hematologic malignancies, its use is limited by the need for an antigenically suitable donor and by the phenomenon of graft vs. host disease, which is more severe in older patients. Therefore, a variety of techniques are being investigated for purging a patient's bone marrow of malignant cells *ex vivo* prior to reinfusion. These techniques include exposing the marrow to monoclonal antibodies directed against tumor-associated antigens (TAAs) or by treating it with cytotoxic drugs (Ramsay et al. 1985; Yeager 1986). Alternatively, hematopoietic stem cells may be harvested from peripheral blood, which is less likely to harbor malignant cells. Finally, high-dose chemotherapy is toxic not only to bone marrow, but to other organs as well: hepatic, pulmonary, cardiac, and mucosal toxicities create additional barriers to dose escalation, which may be more difficult to circumvent than myelosuppression.

The delivery of higher doses of chemotherapeutic agents will also likely be facilitated by the use of hematopoietic growth factors, now available in sufficient quantities for clinical trials, thanks to recombinant DNA technology. Although the hierarchical organization of bone marrow is fixed, the relative proportions of each of the components in the hierarchy must be variable in order to meet the body's ever-changing needs, such as the need for increased red cell production with blood loss, or the need for more neutrophils to combat a bacterial infection. Several glycoproteins, known as hematopoietic growth factors, have major roles in orchestrating such responses. The best-described of the hematopoietic growth factors is erythropoietin, a glycoprotein secreted by the kidney in response to diminished O_2 delivery. Erythropoietin acts on the marrow in several ways to enhance O_2 delivery: it induces the most primitive erythroid progenitors to undergo differentiation, it increases hemoglobin synthesis, and it stimulates the release of reticulocytes from the marrow. Erythropoietin's primary use has been in treating the anemia of end-stage renal disease. However, in high doses it can stimulate increased platelet formation, giving it a potential role in ameliorating thrombocytopenia secondary to cytotoxic drugs.

The myeloid growth factors are highly glycosylated proteins like erythropoietin. Instead of behaving like classic hormones on targets distant from their sites of production, they operate in a paracrine fashion: the site of their production and the target cells on which they act are close together. The myeloid growth factors are produced by cells normally found in the bone marrow: stromal fibroblasts and endothelial cells, lymphocytes, and macrophages. These growth factors are also notable for their occasional ability to act on several different progenitor cells and for their somewhat unanticipated ability (by increasing superoxide production of neutrophils or by inhibiting neutrophil migration) to alter the function of the end cell of a given myeloid series. Current thinking suggests that when secreted in the bone marrow, these growth factors act primarily to influence the proliferation and differentiation of progenitor cells, and that when secreted in local sites of inflammation they serve to enhance end-cell function. Four myeloid growth factors—IL-3 (interleukin-3), GM-CSF (granulocyte-macrophage colony-stimulating factor), G-CSF (granulocyte colony-stimulating factor), and M-CSF (macrophage colony-stimulating factor)—have been produced in large quantities by recombinant DNA technology. GM-CSF has been used in high-dose chemotherapy, followed by autologous bone marrow infusion for the treatment of solid tumors. The infusion of this growth factor shortened the duration of neutropenia from 15 to 12 days (Brandt et al. 1988). G-CSF has been used in more conventional settings (e.g., during aggressive chemotherapy for urothelial transitional-cell carcinoma) and likewise has shortened the period of significant neutropenia following cytotoxic drug delivery (Morstyn et al. 1988; Gabrilove et al. 1988).

INTERFERONS

In 1957 the observation was made that it was virtually impossible to infect a mammalian cell with a virus once infection with another virus had been established. The substance responsible for this phenomenon was aptly named interferon. Interferon is now known to be not one but a family of glycoproteins with diverse biologic effects. These molecules are produced normally by leukocytes (IFN−α) or fibroblasts (INF−β) in response to viral infections, or by lymphoid cells in culture that are stimulated by a mitogen (INF−γ). The direct antiviral effect of interferons is not likely to account for their antitumor activity except in benign cellular proliferative diseases where viruses have a direct role, as in juvenile laryngeal papillomatosis and in condyloma acuminatum.

Interferons also inhibit cell proliferation and can cause direct cytotoxicity at high concentrations in tissue culture. Lower concentrations of IFNs have augmented the cytotoxicity of natural killer cells, T-cells, and macrophages; altered antigenic expression on both tumor cells and effector cells; and perturbed oncogene expression and cellular differentiation. Whether any of these more subtle actions contributes to the antitumor activity of INFs *in vivo* is not known. To date interferon, specifically INF−α, has made a significant therapeutic impact only in hairy-cell leukemia (HCL), a rare B-cell lymphoproliferative malignancy. Objective response to INF−α in HCL is as high as 90%, but complete hematologic remission is rare (Golomb 1987). Responses to interferon therapy have also been documented in indolent lymphomas, cutaneous T-cell lymphoma, CML, and in multiple myeloma, but the ultimate role of interferons in these diseases is less clear. Treatment with INF produces a constellation of symptoms reminiscent of viral infection: fever, chills, myalgias, and mild myelosuppression.

INTERLEUKIN-2 (IL-2)

The idea that a tumor cell can be recognized as foreign by the host's immune system is an attractive one, but an idea that is supported by scant *in vivo* evidence. *In vitro*, at least three subsets of mononuclear leukocytes—cytotoxic T lymphocytes, natural killer cells, and activated macrophages—have been shown to effect tumor rejection. In an attempt to exploit this possible endogenous mechanism of tumor cell killing, peripheral blood lymphoid cells from a patient are induced to proliferate *in vitro* using a medium containing T-cell growth factor (a lymphokine also known as interleukin-2); this expanded population of cells is subsequently injected back into the same patient, with the simultaneous IV administration of IL-2. Such treatment with IL-2 and IL-2-activated peripheral blood lymphoid cells, or even with IL-2 alone, has produced definite regression in renal cell carcinoma and melanoma—tumors notoriously refractory to all known forms of therapy short of surgery. Unfortunately, the response rate to IL-2 plus autologous IL-2-activated peripheral lymphoid cells has been low; coupled with the cumbersome, expensive technology required for its use and with its high toxicity, this form of adoptive immunotherapy is not likely to be widely used.

DIRECTED DRUG DELIVERY

A major limitation to the effective use of cytotoxic drugs is their lack of selectivity for malignant cells. Given the dearth of truly tumor-specific agents, several approaches have been taken to more precisely target cytotoxic agents for tumor cells. The most simple and most successful form of directed drug delivery is the instillation of chemotherapeutic agents directly into a body cavity such as the pleural or peritoneal space, if a tumor happens to be limited to the cavity. Few tumors are so confined, but ovarian carcinoma is an important exception. Once ovarian carcinoma extends beyond the ovary's capsule it tends to spread along and, until the most advanced stages of the disease, remain confined to the peritoneal surface. Intraperitoneal administration of cisplatin, the single most effective agent in this disease, can induce a substantial number of responses when the disease has become refractory to systemic cisplatin. Encouraged by these results, intraperitoneal cisplatin therapy for women who have minimal residual disease (lesions <2 mm in diameter) following surgical debulking of tumor has come into widespread use (Myers 1985). Prospective trials of intraperitoneal cisplatin in this setting will hopefully validate the approach.

There have also been attempts to favorably alter drug distribution and uptake by attaching drugs to large molecules such as DNA; by encasing drugs within lipid vesicles (liposomes); or by binding drugs to monoclonal antibodies directed against tumor-associated antigens (TAAs). Tumor cells often have a high capacity for endocytosis, leading to preferential uptake of a drug-DNA conjugate, for example; once inside the cell the drug is released from the DNA by enzymatic cleavage of the bonds joining them. This approach is limited by the instability of drug-DNA complexes, by the difficultly that such large complexes have in penetrating solid tumors, and by the tumor's endocytotic capacity.

Delivering drugs in liposomes causes a preferential distribution of drug to the lungs, liver, and spleen (RES). However, cloaking drugs in liposomes can change the *relative* availability of a drug to different tissues. For example, when doxorubicin was packaged in liposomes and given to mice, there was decreased drug uptake by the heart, reduced cardiac toxicity, and retention of antitumor activity (Rahman et al. 1980).

Attaching drugs to monoclonal antibodies directed against TAAs appears to be plausible, but there are substantial obstacles. First, TAAs are often not tumor specific; less drug is delivered to the tumor, and the drug may end up concentrating in tissues that share the antigen and produce unexpected toxicities. Second, the density of TAAs on cancer cells is often very low; in fact, most tumors cannot be shown to bear any unique antigenic determinants. Finally, the drug-monoclonal antibody complex is usually itself immunogenic, and if successive doses of the complex are given they will eventually be cleared rapidly by the RES.

INDUCTION OF TUMOR DIFFERENTIATION

Given that the progressive growth of tumors is a manifestation of their cells' failure to mature and differentiate, attempts are under way to find agents that might cause malignant cells to "grow up" rather than kill them. The acute promyelocytic leukemia cell line HL60 is susceptible to the induction of differentiation by a number of unrelated compounds including Ara-C, azacytidine, DMSO, and retinoic acids (Sporn, Roberts, and Driscoll 1985). Interestingly, maturation is associated with decreased transcription of the *c-myc* oncogene (Watanabe et al. 1985). The mechanisms whereby these

agents induce differentiation are under intense study; in the case of azacytidine, hypomethylation of DNA may be responsible for altered gene transcription. Efforts are under way to define the potential clinical role of differentiation induction. Oral leukoplakia, a preneoplastic lesion of the oral mucosa, has been treated successfully with 13-cis-retinoic acid (Hong et al. 1986). Trials are under way to assess the role of retinoids in other preneoplastic conditions, for example, metaplasia of the bronchial mucosa and preinvasive cancers, such as recurrent superficial transitional-cell carcinoma of the bladder.

THE FUTURE

Although induction of cellular differentiation is not yet an important weapon in the medical oncologist's armamentarium, it suggests the possibility of a more sophisticated approach to cancer treatment — one that is more discriminating for malignant cells than the current cytotoxic regimens.

Since the mid-1970s there has been an explosion in the understanding of the pathogenesis of cancer, specifically through the discovery of oncogenes. It is now well established that oncogenes are derived from normal genes, called proto-oncogenes, which orchestrate cellular growth and differentiate during the early stages of a person's life. Perturbations of these proto-oncogenes, rarely expressed in the mature individual, allow for their deranged expression as oncogenes, which provoke unbridled and aberrant growth. The protein products of several oncogenes have been identified, and there is hope that they might provide very specific targets for the oncologist. The complex pathways of communication that the oncogene product disturbs are just beginning to be unraveled; there is reason to believe that there will be effective interventions in this area as well.

REFERENCES

Becker, A.J.; McCulloch, E.A.; and Siminovitch, L. et al. 1965. The effect of differing demands for blood cell production on DNA synthesis by hematopoietic colony-forming cells of mice. *Blood* 26:296-308.

Bell, D.R.; Gerlach, J.H.; and Kartner, N. et al. 1985. Detection of P-glycoprotein in ovarian cancer: a molecular marker associated with multidrug resistance. *J. Clin. Oncol.* 3:311-15.

Bertino, J.R.; Dolnick, B.J.; and Berenson, R.J. et al. 1981. Cellular mechanisms of resistance to methotrexate. In Sartorelli, A.C.; Lazo, J.S.; and Bertino, J.R. eds. *Molecular actions and targets for cancer chemotherapeutic agents.* pp. 385-97. New York: Academic Press.

Biedler, J.L., and Riehm, H. 1970. Cellular resistance to actinomycin D in Chinese hamster cells *in vitro*: cross-resistance, radioautographic and cytogenetic studies. *Cancer Res.* 30:1174-81.

Bleyer, W.A. 1978. The clinical pharmacology of methotrexate: new applications of an old drug. *Cancer* 41:36-51.

Brandt, S.J.; Peters, W.P.; and Atwater, S.K. et al. 1988. Effect of recombinant human granulocyte-macrophage colony-stimulating factor on hematopoietic reconstitution after high-dose chemotherapy and autologous bone marrow transplantation. *N. Engl. J. Med.* 318:869-76.

Bruce, W.R.; Mecker, B.E.; and Powers, W.E. et al. 1969. Comparison of the dose- and time-survival curves for normal hematopoietic and lymphoma colony-forming cells exposed to vinblastine, vincristine, arabinosylcytosine, and amethopterin. *J. Natl. Cancer Inst.* 42:1015-25.

Capizzi, R.L.; Davis, R.; and Powell, B. et al. 1988. Synergy between high-dose cytarabine and asparaginase in the treatment of adults. with refractory and relapsed acute myelogenous leukemia: a Cancer and Leukemia Group B study. *J. Clin. Oncol.* 6:499-508.

Cleaver, J.E. 1967. *Thymidine metabolism and cell kinetics.* Amsterdam: North Holland Publishing Co.

Dalton, W.S.; Grogan, T.M.; and Meltzer, P.S. et al. 1989. Drug-resistance in multiple myeloma a non-Hodgkins lymphoma: detection of P-glycoprotein and potential circumvention by addition of verapamil to chemotherapy. *J. Clin. Oncol.* 7(4):415-24.

Dorr, R.T., and Fritz, W.L. 1980. *Cancer chemotherapy handbook.* New York: Elsevier-North Holland.

Eder, J.P.; Antman, K.; and Peters, W. et al. 1986. High-dose combination alkylating agent chemotherapy with autologous bone marrow support for metastatic breast cancer. *J. Clin. Oncol.* 4:1592-97.

Fojo, A.T.; Ueda, K.; and Slamon, D.J. et al. 1987. Expression of a multidrug-resistance gene in human tumors and tissues. *Proc. Natl. Acad. Sci. U.S.A.* 84:265-69.

Gabrilove, J.L.; Jakubowski, A.; and Scher, et al. 1988. Effect of granulocyte colony-stimulating factor on neutropenia and associated morbidity due to chemotherapy for transitional-cell carcinoma of the urothelium. *N. Engl. J. Med.* 318(22):1414-22.

Gilman, A. 1963. The initial clinical trial of nitrogen mustard. *Am. J. Surg.* 105:574-78.

Goldie, J.H.; and Coldman, A.J. 1979. A mathematic model for relating the drug sensitivity of tumors to their spontaneous mutation rate. *Cancer Treat. Rep.* 63:1727-33.

Goldie, J.H.; and Coldman, A.J. 1984. The genetic origin of drug resistance in neoplasms: implications for systemic therapy. *Cancer Res.* 44:3643-53.

Golomb, H.M. 1987. The treatment of hairy-cell leukemia. *Blood* 69:979-83.

Greene, M.H.; Harris, E.L.; and Gershenson, D.M. et al. 1986. Melphalan may be a more potent leukemogen than cyclophosphamide. *Ann. Intern. Med.* 105:360-67.

Greene, M.H.; Boice, J.D.; and Greer, B.E. et al. 1982. Acute nonlymphocytic leukemia after therapy with alkylating agents for ovarian cancer. *N. Engl. J. Med.* 307:1416-21.

Grem, J.L.; Hoth, D.F.; and Hamilton, J.M. et al. 1987. Overview of current status and future directions of clinical trials with 5-fluorouracil in combination with folinic acid. *Cancer Treat. Rep.* 71:1249-64.

Gros, P.; Neriah, Y.B.; and Croop, J.M. et al. 1986. Isolation and expression of a complementary DNA that confers multidrug resistance. *Nature* 323:728-31.

Hamburger, A.W., and Salmon, S.E. 1977. Primary bioassay of human tumor stem cells. *Science* 197:461-63.

Howard, A., and Pelc, S.R. 1951. Nuclear incorporation of P^{32} as demonstrated by autoradiographs. *Exp. Cell Res.* 2: 178-87.

Hryniuk, W.M.; Levine, M.N.; and Levin, L. 1986. Analysis of dose intensity for chemotherapy in early (stage II) and advanced breast cancer. *Natl. Cancer Inst. Monogr.* 1:87-94.

Juliano, R.L., and Ling, V. 1976. A surface glycoprotein modulating drug permeability in Chinese hamster ovary cell mutants. *Biochim. Biophy. Acta.* 455:152-62.

Minden, M.D.; Till, J.E.; and McCulloch, E.A. eds. 1978. Proliferative state of blast cell progenitors in acute myeloblastic leukemia (AML). *Blood* 52:592-600.

Morstyn, G.; Campbell, L.; and Souza, L.M. et al. 1988. Effect of granulocyte colony stimulating factor on neutropenia induced by cytotoxic chemotherapy. *Lancet* I:667-72.

Moscow, J.A., and Cowan, K.H. 1988. Multidrug resistance. *J. Natl. Cancer Inst.* 80:14-20.

Myers, C. 1984. The use of intraperitoneal chemotherapy in the treatment of ovarian cancer. *Semin. Oncol.* 11:275-84.

O'Reilly, R.J. 1983. Allogenic bone marrow transplantation: current status and future directions. *Blood* 62:941-64.

Philip, T.; Armitage, J.O.; and Spitzer, G. et al. 1987. High-dose therapy and autologous bone marrow transplantation after failure of conventional chemotherapy in adults with intermediate-grade or high-grade non-Hodgkin's lymphoma. *N. Engl. J. Med.* 316:1493-98.

Quastler, H., and Sherman, F.G. 1959. Cell population kinetics in the intestinal epithelium of the mouse. *Exp. Cell Res.* 17:420-38.

Rahman, A.; Kessler, A.; and More, N. et al. 1980. Liposomal protection of Adriamycin-induced cardiotoxicity in mice. *Cancer Res.* 40:1532-37.

Ramsay, N.; LeBien, T.; and Nesbit, M. et al. 1985. Autologous bone marrow transplantation for patients with acute lymphoblastic leukemia in second or subsequent remission: results of bone marrow treated with monoclonal antibodies BA-1, BA-2, and BA-3, plus complement. *Blood* 66:508-13.

Schimke, R.T. 1984. Gene amplification, drug resistance, and cancer. *Cancer Res.* 44:1735-42.

Schnipper, L.E. 1986. Clinical implications of tumor-cell heterogeneity. *N. Engl. J. Med.* 314:1423-31.

Schwartz, S.; Morgenstern, B.; and Capizzi, R.L. 1982. Schedule-dependent synergy and antagonism between high-dose I-B-D-arabinofuranosylcytosine and asparaginase in the L5178Y murine leukemia. *Cancer Res.* 42: 2191-97.

Selby, P.; Buick, R.N.; and Tannock, I. 1983. A critical appraisal of the "human tumor stem-cell assay." *N. Engl. J. Med.* 308:129-34.

Shackney, S.E.; McCormack, G.W.; and Cuchural, G.J., Jr. 1978. Growth rate patterns of solid tumors and their relation to responsiveness to therapy: an analytical review. *Ann. Intern. Med.* 89:107-21.

Shimizu, T.; Motoji, T.; and Oshimi, K.; et al. 1982. Proliferative state and radiosensitivity of human myeloma stem cells. *Br. J. Cancer* 45:679-83.

Skeel, R.T. 1987. *Handbook of cancer chemotherapy.* Boston: Little, Brown, and Company.

Speyer, J.; Green, M.; and Ward, C.; et al. 1988. Endomyocardial biopsies (EB) provide additional evidence for ICRF-187 protection against Adriamycin (ADRIA) induced cardiac toxicity (CTOX). *Proc. Am. Soc. Clin. Oncol.* 7:244-64.

Sporn, M.B.; Roberts, A.B.; and Driscoll, J.S. 1985. Principles of cancer biology: growth factors and differentiation. In DeVita, V.T.; Hellman, S.; and Rosenberg, S.A. eds. *Cancer: principles and practices of oncology.* 2nd ed. pp. 49-66. Philadelphia: J.B. Lippincott.

Steel, G.G. 1967. Cell loss as a factor in the growth rate of human tumors. *Eur. J. Cancer* 3:381-87.

Stewart, H.J. et al. 1987. Adjuvant tamoxifen in the management of operable breast cancer: the Scottish Trial. Report from the Breast Cancer Trial Committee. *Lancet* II:171-75.

Tannock, I. 1978. Cell kinetics and chemotherapy: a critical review. *Cancer Treat. Rep.* 62:1117-33.

Tannock, I., and Guttman, P. 1981. Response of Chinese hamster ovary cells to anticancer drugs under aerobic and hypoxic conditions. *Br. J. Cancer* 43:245-48.

Till, J.E., and McCullouch, E.A. 1980. Hematopoietic stem cell differentiation. *Biochim. Biophys. Acta.* 605:431-59.

Tritton, T.R., and Yee, G. 1982. The anticancer agent Adriamycin can be actively cytotoxic without entering cells. *Science* 217:248-50.

Twentyman, P.R., and Bleehen, N.M. 1975. Changes in sensitivity to cytotoxic agents occurring during the life history of monolayer cultures of a mouse tumor cell line. *Br. J. Cancer* 31:417-23.

Van Patten, L.M.; Lelieveld, P.; and Kram-Idsenga, L.K.J. 1972. Cell-cycle specificity and therapeutic effectiveness of cytostatic agents. *Cancer Chemother. Rep.* 56:691-700.

Watanabe, T.; Sariban, E.; and Mitchell, et al. 1985. Human C-*myc* and N-*ras* expression during induction of HL-60 cellular differentiation. *Biochem. Biophys. Res. Commun.* 126:999-1005.

Weiss, R.B., and DeVita, V.T., Jr. 1979. Multimodal primary cancer treatment (adjuvant chemotherapy): current results and future prospects. *Ann. Intern. Med.* 91:251-60.

Wittes, R.E. 1989. *Manual of oncologic therapeutics 1989/1990.* Philadelphia: J.B. Lippincott.

Chapter 6

PRINCIPLES OF TUMOR IMMUNOLOGY

Ronald B. Herberman, M.D.

Ronald B. Herberman, M.D.
Director, Pittsburgh Cancer Institute
Professor, Medicine and Pathology
Departments of Medicine and Pathology
University of Pittsburgh School of Medicine
Pittsburgh, Pennsylvania 15213

INTRODUCTION

The field of tumor immunology encompasses the wide variety of interactions between the immune system and tumors, emphasizing the immune system's role in resisting the development of progressive growth of cancer, and on how it can be manipulated to increase such resistance. Tumor immunology also has important applications in the immunodiagnosis of cancer and the understanding of altered immunologic competence in tumor-bearing individuals.

The main principles of tumor immunology have emerged from extensive studies performed mainly during the last 30 years.

IMMUNE SYSTEM RECOGNITION OF TUMOR CELLS

A wide variety of tumor cells express molecular structures that differ from normal cells of the same individual and can be recognized by one or more components of the immune system. Most of the immunologic discrimination of tumor cells from normal cells has been thought to be due to recognition by the host of *tumor antigens* but in addition, tumor cells have been found to have other, nonantigenic differences that may be recognizable by the natural immune system.

TUMOR ANTIGENS

Most tumor cells have molecular configurations that can specifically be recognized by immune T cells or by antibodies and hence are termed tumor antigens. The most important tumor antigens, in terms of immunodiagnosis or host resistance, have been termed tumor associated antigens (TAAs). They are selectively expressed on tumor cells and are not detectable on normal cells of the same individual. For many years, tumor immunologists sought tumor antigens that would be uniquely present on tumor cells and qualitatively different from antigens on any normal cells, and hence be called tumor specific antigens. However, most antigens on tumor cells that were initially thought to be tumor specific have been found—by more extensive evaluation of a wider range of normal tissues and the use of highly sensitive immunoassays—to be expressed in some circumstances, at least in low amounts, in some normal cells. Thus, the term "TAA" seems more valid. An important subset of TAA is tumor associated transplantation antigens (TATAs), which can induce immunologically specific resistance to tumor growth in the autologous host. The immunologic reactions that allow a host to recognize TATAs and to thereby mediate elimination of the tumor cells appear to closely resemble those that mediate rejection of tissue allografts with weak histocompatibility antigenic differences from the host. Tumor cells also contain many normal cellular antigens, including normal histocompatibility antigens and antigens that are characteristic of the tissue or organ from which the neoplastic cells are derived, or the stage of differentiation of the tumor cells.

Controversy surrounds the issue of whether all or most tumors express TATAs. Although the majority of tumors induced in experimental animals by oncogenic viruses or chemical carcinogens have been shown to have TATAs, some studies of tumors arising spontaneously in aged mice or rats have indicated that most of these spontaneous tumors lacked detectable TATAs (Hewitt, Blake, and Walder 1976). It has thus been argued that most human tumors, which have no known etiology and hence would be considered spontaneous, also lack TATAs (Hewitt 1982). However, there are considerable limitations to such arguments (Herberman 1983). Although there is insufficient evidence about the proportion of human tumors that express TATAs, there is considerable suggestive or circumstantial evidence for the presence of TATAs on many human tumors (Herberman 1983).

For a TAA to function as a TATA, it must be recognized by the host's immune system and elicit immunologic reactivity that results in destruction or at least growth inhibition of the tumor. There are other categories of TAAs, some of which also have considerable practical importance. Any TAA that is recognized by antibodies in the serum of the tumor-bearing host or in the sera of animals immunized against the antigen can potentially be used to discriminate between tumor cells and normal cells, and this may be of value for immunodiagnosis. TAAs that are common to a variety of tumors, at least of the same organ or histological type, are most likely to be useful for diagnostic purposes. Studies in animal model systems have shown that tumors induced by chemical carcinogens and some spontaneous tumors have TATAs that are individually distinct and are not present in other tumors induced by the same agent (Prehn and Main 1957). Such antigens would not be helpful diagnostically, since antibodies against one tumor would not be expected to react with any other tumors. Common TAAs have been identified on many tumors, and even those that are not recognized by the tumor-bearing individual may be readily detected by antibodies elicited in a different species.

NONANTIGENIC DIFFERENCES BETWEEN TUMOR AND NORMAL CELLS

TAAs are the targets for recognition by the components of the classical immune system, the immune T cells and/or antibodies. Also, various components of the natural immune system (e.g., natural killer cells or macrophages) can selectively recognize and react with tumor cells. Although the basis for such recognition is not well understood, it may be due to the expression on tumor cells of a variety of cell-surface molecules in larger quantity or in altered form relative to normal cells. These tumor-associated differences do not seem to be restricted to tumor cells, as virus-infected normal cells or other cells may also be recognized by natural effector cells (Ortaldo and Herberman 1984).

BASIS FOR DIFFERENCES: TUMOR AND NORMAL CELLS

The molecular basis for antigenic or other differences between tumor and normal cells is still not completely understood. Several different mechanisms appear to be involved:

1. Clonally distributed molecules.
Some types of molecules may be highly polymorphic and clonally distributed on normal cells of the population. Because most tumors appear to arise from a single abnormal cell, they may express structurally normal molecules that are characteristic for that clone. The best-known example of this type of TAA is the cell-surface immunoglobulin on malignant B cells. The immunoglobulin genes of normal as well as malignant B cells undergo recombinations that generate clonal diversity, particularly in the region of the antigen-combining sites. Such idiotypic structures provide individually specific antigens on each malignant clone. Monoclonal antibodies to such idiotypic determinants on human B cell lymphoma have been the focus of some attempts at immunotherapy (Meeker et al. 1985).

2. Virus-associated antigens.
Tumors induced by an oncogenic virus, even when they differ in morphologic appearance or arise in different organs, share the same TAAs, some of which may function as TATAs (Habel 1961; Old and Boyse 1964). At least some of these TAAs are determined by new genetic information introduced into the tumor cell by the virus. In other cases the oncogenic virus may induce or alter the expression of oncogenes within the host genome.

3. TAAs of carcinogen-induced tumors.
As noted, tumors induced by chemical carcinogens, ultraviolet irradiation, or other physical agents usually express TATAs that are individually tumor specific. The basis for such induction is not clear, but these agents share the ability to cause mutations in DNA and their TAAs may be due to genetic alterations in normal cellular genes. Progress has been made in determining the physicochemical characteristics of the TATAs on some tumors induced by chemical carcinogens (Srivastava and Old 1988) and such studies may provide new insights into the basis for induction of these antigens.

4. Differentiation antigens.
It has been known for some time that antigens present on normal fetal cells may also be expressed on a variety of tumor cells, regardless of etiology. These have been referred to as oncofetal or carcinoembryonic antigens (Coggin, Ambrose, and Anderson 1970; Ting et al. 1972). With more recent and extensive experience, particularly from the extensive analysis of the specificity of antigens detected by various monoclonal antibodies, it appears that a more general categorization of such antigens might be that of differentiation antigens. Tumor cells often are arrested at a particular point in the pathway of differentiation for the normal cell type from which they arose. They express antigens that are characteristic for that stage of differentiation. Antigens of stem cells or of cells at early stages of differentiation may be rare in adults but frequent in fetuses and therefore may appear to be oncofetal in their distribution. Such differentiation antigens may help to classify certain tumors, particularly those derived from hematopoietic cells, where there has been considerable elucidation of the antigens associated with the stages of development in the various hematopoietic lineages (Foon, Schroff, and Gale 1982).

5. Tissue antigens.
Large amounts of normal tissue or organ-associated antigens may be expressed in tumor cells derived from that tissue. Especially when the normal cells are relatively infrequent, the tissue antigen may appear to be tumor-associated and may only be found to be tissue-associated upon careful examination of the relevant normal cells.

THE IMMUNE SYSTEM'S ROLE IN RESISTING CANCER

Many investigators have proposed that the immune system has a general role in preventing or limiting tumor growth. The central concept, known as the immune surveillance hypothesis, postulates that the immune system is a key factor in resistance against the development of detectable tumors. The first known suggestion along these lines came from Paul Ehrlich in 1909 (Ehrlich 1957); the modern formulation of the hypothesis originated from Burnet (1957) and Thomas (1959). When information about thymus-dependent immunity became known, and particularly when T cells were found to play a central role in homograft rejection, Burnet modified the immune surveillance hypothesis to stress the key role of this effector mechanism in antitumor resistance (Burnet 1970).

The immune surveillance hypothesis has since generated many experimental studies and much discussion and controversy. One of the reasons for the controversy is that the concept leads to a series of predictions; most available evidence relates to tests of one or more of these predictions:

1. Tumor cells have transplantation-type antigens.
2. Resistance against tumors is T-cell dependent and analogous to the homograft reaction.
3. There is a close evolutionary link between malignancy and the development of an immune system with capability for rejection of tumors.
4. Immune depression is associated with, and must precede, development of detectable tumors.
5. A requisite action of carcinogens and/or tumor promoters might be immunosuppression.

The main support for the immune surveillance hypothesis has come from evidence related to prediction No. 4, since naturally occurring or induced immunodepression has been associated with a higher incidence of some types of tumors. In experiments, this has been most clearly demonstrated with tumors induced by oncogenic viruses. Neonatal thymectomy and other forms of immune suppression have been shown to lead to increased susceptibility to polyoma virus-induced tumors in mice (Law 1966) and Marek's disease in chickens (Payne 1972).

Considerable clinical evidence shows that immune deficiency diseases are associated with a much higher incidence of lymphomas and leukemias (Gatti and Good 1971). Allograft recipients of cyclosporine A have an increased incidence (approximately 100-fold) of lymphoproliferative disease or other tumors (Penn and Starzl 1972). Patients with cancer, arthritis, or other diseases who received chemotherapeutic (mainly alkylating) agents have been found to develop a relatively high frequency of subsequent primary malignancies, mainly leukemias and lymphomas (Roberts and Bell 1976). The recent observations of a remarkably high incidence of Kaposi's sarcoma in young adults with acquired immune deficiency syndrome (AIDS) are yet another indication of the association of malignancy with immunodepression.

Although such data support immune surveillance, the original hypothesis had several major problems or limitations:

1. The majority of human tumors associated with immunodepression have been leukemias and lymphoproliferative diseases, rather than a complete array of the common types of malignancy.
2. There has not been a consistent association between immunodepression and tumors (Stutman 1975).
3. Neonatally thymectomized mice have been found to have a decreased incidence of mammary tumors (Yunis et al. 1969), and nude and euthymic mice have similar incidences of spontaneous and carcinogen-induced tumors (Stutman 1975).
4. Most spontaneous tumors of experimental animals lack detectable tumor-associated transplantation antigens (Hewitt, Blake, and Walder 1976).
5. There appears to be an evolutionary dissociation between the development of tumors and the appearance of a sophisticated immune system and T cells (Cooper 1976).

These hypotheses have led to the suggestion (Klein and Klein 1977) that immune surveillance may operate only against tumors induced by oncogenic viruses, which have strong transplantation antigens and for which immune T cells are important in resistance. The major exceptions to the central role of immune T cells in resistance to tumor growth have even led to a counter-theory of immunostimulation (Prehn and Lappe 1971), suggesting that the immune system may have mainly enhancing effects on tumor induction and growth.

A more likely explanation for many of the discordant results is the involvement of a variety of effector mechanisms in host resistance. In the past few years, it has become apparent that natural immunity, as well as specifically induced immune responses, may contribute to host defenses. When T-cell-mediated immunity is viewed as only one of a series of possible host defense mechanisms, the evidence need not be viewed in such a negative light. Target-cell structures other than tumor-associated transplantation antigens might be involved in recognition by other types of effector cells; and in T-cell-deficient individuals, natural immunity might still be functional and capable of resisting tumor growth. This is the basis for an updated immune surveillance hypothesis: transformed cells express surface antigens or other structures that one or more components of the immune system can recognize; one or more components of the natural and/or induced immunological effector mechanisms can eliminate the transformed cells or impede the progression and spread of tumors.

This broader hypothesis leads to a somewhat different set of predictions:

1. Tumor cells have surface structures recognized by one or more effectors.

2. Tumor cells will be susceptible to lysis or growth inhibition by one or more effector mechanisms.

3. One or more of the relevant effector cells should be able to enter the site of tumor growth.

4. Augmentation of relevant effector mechanism(s) will decrease the incidence of tumors or metastases.

5. Depression of relevant effector mechanism(s), either by carcinogen or by immunosuppressive treatment, will increase the incidence of tumors or metastases.

6. Restoration of depressed effector activity will decrease the incidence of tumors or metastases.

In addition to the immune system's postulated role in surveillance against the development of tumors, there is considerable evidence for involvement of both the classical and natural immune responses in host resistance against the progression and metastatic spread of tumors once they arise. In fact, the evidence for an important role of some components of the immune system, e.g., natural killer cells, is much more compelling in regard to antimetastatic effects than for immune surveillance.

The immune system is complex and has several different components that may be important effectors of host resistance against tumors.

THE ROLE OF T CELLS IN HOST RESISTANCE

There is substantial evidence that thymus-dependent immune responses are important in resistance to tumors induced by oncogenic viruses. However, the absence of the thymus has not been associated with increased susceptibility to other types of tumors, suggesting a limited role for T-cell immunity in immune surveillance. Further, the inability to detect tumor-associated transplantation antigens on most spontaneous rodent tumors argues against a major involvement of specific immune responses. Recent evidence indicates, however, the importance of distinguishing between immunogenicity and antigenicity. *Immunogenicity* refers to the ability of a TAA to induce an immune response and appears to depend on the degree of expression of the antigen on the tumor cells as well as on the expression of major histocompatibility complex (MHC) antigens and the host's immunologic responsiveness. Ultraviolet light-induced tumors in mice have been found to express strong TATAs but are usually nonimmunogenic in UV-irradiated animals because of a specific form of immune suppression (Kripke 1981). Some other tumors in mice appear to be nonimmunogenic because they lack expression of MHC antigens. Immunogenicity and MHC antigen expression can be induced by treating the tumor cells with a chemical mutagen or UV irradiation (Gorelik et al. 1985; Peppoloni, Herberman, and Gorelik 1987).

THE ROLE OF MACROPHAGES IN HOST RESISTANCE

Macrophages have been suggested as important factors in antitumor defenses and might be primarily responsible for immune surveillance against tumors (e.g., Hibbs, Chap-

man, and Weinberg 1978; Adams and Snyderman 1979). This possibility is supported by several lines of evidence:

1. Macrophages can accumulate in considerable numbers in a variety of transplantable tumors (Evans 1972) and in many primary tumors (Gauci and Alexander 1975).

2. Macrophages have natural (Keller 1978), as well as the rapidly activatable, ability to lyse or inhibit the growth *in vitro* of a wide variety of transformed cells.

3. Several treatments that can depress the function of macrophages (e.g., silica or carrageenan) have been associated with an increased incidence of tumors and metastases (Norbury and Kripke 1979).

4. Adoptive transfer of *in vitro* or *in vivo* activated macrophages was shown to inhibit the metastatic spread of some tumor cell lines (Fidler 1974; Sones and Castro 1977).

5. Some carcinogens (e.g., methylcholanthrene, acetylaminofluorene) have been shown to depress reticuloendothelial function (Stern 1983).

6. Stimulation of macrophage function by various immunomodulators has been associated with decreased tumor growth or a decreased tumor incidence (Norbury and Kripke 1979).

However, there are some major limitations to such evidence:

1. There is remarkably little evidence that macrophages have cytotoxic activity against primary, freshly harvested tumor cells, as opposed to established tumor cell lines.

2. Silica and carrageenan, and virtually all of the other depressive treatments that have been used, may not be entirely selective in their effects. In fact, they may increase some functions, particularly suppressor activity, by macrophages or other cells (Cudkowicz and Hochman 1979). The treatment effects on tumor growth are not always in the same direction, even with the same tumor. For example, Mantovani et al. (1980) found that treatment of mice with silica or carrageenan increased the incidence of pulmonary metastases but inhibited the growth of primary tumors.

3. The carcinogens shown to depress reticuloendothelial function may also have affected a variety of effector mechanisms, and other carcinogens have had no detectable effects on macrophage or reticuloendothelial function (Zwilling, Filippi, and Chorepenning 1978).

4. In experiments with some transplantable tumors in mice, adoptive transfer of macrophages facilitated the development of metastases rather than conferring resistance to metastasis (Gorelik et al. 1982; Gorelik et al. 1985).

THE ROLE OF NATURAL KILLER (NK) CELLS IN HOST RESISTANCE

Natural killer (NK) cells are a recently defined subpopulation of natural effector cells. They have the morphologic appearance of large granular lymphocytes and a characteristic cell-surface phenotype that distinguishes them from T cells or macrophages (Ortaldo and

Herberman 1984). A group of experts in this research area agree that NK cells are large granular lymphocytes that lack the characteristic cell surface structures of T cells (CD3 and T cell receptors). These cells have spontaneous cytotoxic reactivity against cancer cells and some nonmalignant cells that is not dependent upon or restricted by the MHC. In addition to their spontaneous antitumor reactivity, NK cells secrete a variety of cytokines and also have their cytotoxic reactivity augmented substantially by exposure to cytokines, especially interferons or interleukin-2 (IL-2), or by various biological response modifiers (BRMs) (Ortaldo and Herberman 1984). It has recently become clear that most lymphokine-activated-killer (LAK) cell activity that is generated upon culture of blood or spleen cells with IL2 is attributable to IL-2-activated NK cells (Herberman, Balch, and Bolhuis et al. 1987). LAK cells have very potent cytotoxic activity against most tumor cells, including freshly isolated tumor cells from the autologous or allogeneic solid tumors (Grimm et al. 1982) or leukemias (Adler et al. 1988).

There is substantial evidence for the importance of NK cells in *in vivo* resistance against established tumor cell lines (Gorelik and Herberman 1986). In addition, some evidence conforms to the predictions of the immune surveillance hypothesis:

1. NK cells are able to accumulate at sites of inflammation (Ward, Argilan, and Reynolds 1983) and in small primary as well as transplanted tumors (Gerson 1980).

2. NK cells have a natural and also rapidly activatable ability to lyse a variety of primary autochthonous tumors.

3. NK cells have been shown to have the ability to eliminate metastatic tumor cells and thereby resist tumor spread.

4. An increased tumor incidence (primarily lymphomas) has been found in beige mice with depressed NK activity (Loutit, Townsend, and Knowles 1980); patients with Chediak-Higashi syndrome (Dent et al. 1966); and immunosuppressed transplant recipients (Penn and Starzl 1972). Some carcinogens (urethane, x-irradiation, and dimethylbenzanthracene) have been shown to cause early, profound depression of NK activity (Gorelik and Herberman 1981; Parkinson, Brightman, and Waksal 1981; Ehrlich 1957).

The most convincing data relate to the function of NK cells in host resistance against metastases (Gorelik and Herberman 1986). The observation that NK cells appear to be mainly responsible for the rapid elimination of intravenously inoculated tumor cells provided the initial indication that this effector mechanism might be a very effective control of hematogenous spread of tumors. Experimental support for this possibility first came from the finding that cells from the lung metastases of a transplantable tumor in mice were more resistant to NK activity than were locally growing tumor cells. Further support has been observations that

suppression or augmentation of NK activity of mice was associated with parallel alterations in resistance to artificial metastases produced by intravenous inoculation of tumor cells. The patterns of results obtained in these studies suggested that NK cells may primarily influence metastatic spread by acting during the phase of hematogenous dissemination, presumably by their ability to eliminate rapidly the tumor cells from the circulation of capillary beds. Barlozzari et al. (1983) further confirmed the association between depressed NK activity and increased metastases by showing that selective restoration of NK activity in rats by adoptive transfer of highly purified large granular lymphocytes was accompanied by increased resistance to pulmonary metastases. Similarly, Warner and Dennert (1982) showed that adoptive transfer of a clone of cultured lymphoid cells with NK-like activity protected against development of pulmonary or liver metastases. Immunotherapy studies with transplantable sarcomas in mice, by adoptive transfer of LAK cells, have indicated appreciable antimetastatic effects even when therapy was initiated after pulmonary metastases had occurred (Mule, Shu, and Rosenberg 1985).

Direct evidence for the role of NK cells in immune surveillance is limited and relates mainly to two models of carcinogenesis. The first model provides some indicators of NK cells' role in protecting against urethane-induced lung tumors in mice. In studies in highly susceptible A/J mice, a reduction in NK activity by treatment with cyclophosphamide led to a significantly higher tumor incidence (Gorelik and Herberman 1982). Conversely, adoptive transfer of normal spleen or bone marrow cells, which led to reconstitution of NK activity, inhibited the subsequent incidence of lung tumors. In contrast, spleen cells from urethane-treated donors, which had low NK activity and were unable to restore NK activity in the recipients, had no significant ability to transfer resistance to development of lung tumors (Gorelik and Herberman 1982).

The second carcinogenesis system is the induction of thymic lymphomas by multiple low doses of irradiation of C57BL/6 mice. Tumor development appears to be dependent on a complex series of factors, and it has been difficult to demonstrate a clear contribution of NK cells to the overall process of leukemogenesis (Gorelik et al. 1984). However, NK cells appeared to be involved in protection against the transplantation of preleukemic bone marrow cells from donors that received fractionated doses of irradiation. Warner and Dennert (1982) found that adoptive transfer of cloned cells with NK-like activity, during a 4-week period after the last dose of fractionated irradiation, conferred substantial protection against the development of leukemia. Despite such suggestive positive evidence, a series of other experiments (Gorelik et al. 1984) have indicated that non-NK-related factors seemed to have a more important influence on the incidence of leukemia than did the NK activity levels.

THE ROLE OF ANTIBODIES IN HOST RESISTANCE

In many tumor-bearing and immunized individuals, specific antitumor antibodies can be demonstrated (Ting and Herberman 1976). Antibodies specific for TAAs have been shown to kill tumor target cells in two ways, and there is some evidence that both mechanisms operate *in vivo*. The first way is complement-dependent; IgG and IgM antibodies fix to antigenic sites on target cells and activate the complement cascade. Terminal C8 and C9 components bring about lysis by the classic pathway. The second cytocidal pathway is independent of complement and is known as antibody-dependent cellular cytotoxicity (ADCC). Once antitumor IgG antibody fixes to the target cell membrane, various effector cells with receptors for the Fc portion of IgG, particularly NK cells and macrophages, can then bind to the antibody-coated tumor cells and cause their lysis.

Antitumor antibodies may be detrimental to the host (Ting and Herberman 1976). In experimental situations, antibodies administered before transplantation of tumor or infection by oncogenic virus lead to tumor enhancement (afferent limb-suppression of response) and thus have been termed enhancing antibodies. Other studies suggest that enhancing antibodies attach to the surface of tumor cells, thereby blocking or masking attachment sites for cytotoxic lymphocytes and cytolytic antibodies (efferent enhancement). In some clinical studies, the presence of detectable antibodies or antigen-antibody complexes in the circulation has been associated with the presence of tumor or poor prognosis (Vlock et al. 1988). However, in other clinical studies, high antitumor antibody titers were seen after complete surgical removal of tumor and declining titers were associated with recurrence or metastatic spread (Morton et al. 1970).

CANCER AS MODIFIER OF THE IMMUNE SYSTEM

The presence of cancer can induce antitumor immune responses, involving T cells and/or antibody-producing B cells. In addition, in many situations, tumor-bearing individuals have had more general alterations in their immune system functioning. Usually the direction of modulated immune function in cancer is negative, with depression of a variety of immunologic activities. This has in part been attributable to the release of immunosuppressive factors by the tumor cells (Specter and Friedman 1983) and to the stimulation of suppressor macrophages or T cells (Varesio 1983).

The varied detected deficits in immunologic competence in some tumor-bearing individuals have involved most components of the immune system. These have included decreased cellular immune reactivity, as reflected *in vivo* by delayed cutaneous hypersensitivity tests and *in vitro* by lymphoproliferative responses to mitogens or alloantigens, decreased macrophage responsiveness (Cianciolo and Snyderman 1983), and decreased NK activity. The literature on depressed immunologic competence in tumor-bearers is particularly extensive at the clinical level. The impairments have been most consistent in patients with advanced, metastatic disease, but some studies have detected abnormalities early in the course of disease or in patients with no detectable tumor. In tests for delayed cutaneous hypersensitivity to dinitrochlorobenzene, which involve sensitization by a large dose of antigen, and challenge two weeks later with a low dose, the failure of some cancer patients to be sensitized has been a useful prognostic indicator of unresectable disease or early recurrence after surgery (Eilber and Morton 1970; Pinsky 1978). Decreasing the dose used for sensitization would reveal some defects in patients with early Hodgkin's disease (Eltringham and Kaplan 1973), which had previously only been detected in patients with advanced disease (Young et al. 1972).

In vitro assays of cell-mediated immunity have also been used to look for decreased reactivity in cancer patients and, as with the skin tests, the proportion of patients with localized disease who have had evidence of immune depression has varied considerably. Assays designed to detect subtle alterations in lymphoproliferative responses to mitogens and antigens, and standardization of the procedures for testing and data analysis, have yielded substantial evidence for depression in some patients with localized or early disease (Levy and Kaplan 1974; Stein et al. 1976; Dean et al. 1977; Dean 1979). In one study of lung cancer patients after surgical removal of their tumors, patients with depressed lymphoproliferative responses to the mitogen concanavallin A or in mixed lymphocyte cultures had a significantly reduced disease-free survival (Hersey et al. 1982). More recent studies have suggested that the poor lymphoproliferative responses in some cancer patients may be attributable to a depressed ability to produce IL-2 and for the potential responding T cells to express receptors for IL-2 (Koch et al. 1984; Kikuchi et al. 1988; Kambe et al. 1988). Depressed NK activity levels have also been observed in some cancer patients (Pross, Rubin, and Baines 1982; Hersey et al. 1982; Schantz et al. 1987). In some studies, this has been associated with poor prognosis (Hersey et al. 1982; Schantz et al. 1987). In addition to functional assays, enumeration of the relative proportions and absolute numbers of T and B cells may be useful in immunodiagnosis. In particular, there are indications that many cancer patients, including some with localized disease, have decreased percentages of T-cell subpopulations, as assessed by high-affinity rosette formation with sheep erythrocytes (West et al. 1976) or by flow cytometry with antibodies to CD4+ T cells (Kikuchi et al. 1988).

PRACTICAL APPLICATIONS OF TUMOR IMMUNOLOGY PRINCIPLES

In addition to the contributions of tumor immunology investigations to the overall understanding of the cancer-host interaction biology, there is a variety of potential ways to apply such information and insights to the detection, diagnosis, classification, prognostic assessment, and therapy of cancer.

IMMUNODIAGNOSIS

Immunodiagnosis includes several distinct clinical applications (table 6.1). First, some immunodiagnostic procedures might be useful in the detection of cancer cases by screening general populations or high-risk groups. With patients who have come to a physician with signs or symptoms consistent with, or suggestive of cancer, immunologic assays may aid in distinguishing between patients with cancer and those with benign diseases. Immunodiagnostic procedures can also be used in patients with known cancer, to assist in the classification of the tumor cells and assessment of their lineage and stage of differentiation; in *in vivo* localization of tumor; to determine prognosis; and to monitor patients during the course of disease in order to detect early any recurrences or metastases.

Several criteria constitute a useful immunodiagnostic test for cancer (table 6.2). An obvious point is that the test needs to be able to detect some consistent difference between cancer and noncancer. It is desirable, but not necessary, that the difference be qualitative, i.e., expression of a tumor-specific antigen. The presence of a TAA in cancer patients that was absent in nonneoplastic states, or the loss of a normal component in cancer patients, would be a strong basis for development of a useful diagnostic test. However, quantitative differences between cancer patients and controls could also be sufficient; it would just be necessary to carefully determine the normal range. A good diagnostic test should have a high degree of specificity; there should be very few false-positives, i.e., individuals without cancer who have tests indicating cancer. Also, the test should be very sensitive and have few false-negative results, i.e., be able to detect cancer in a large proportion of cancer patients, including those with small, localized tumors or with small recurrent or metastatic deposits.

A helpful test would be one for initial detection or diagnosis that could localize the tumor mass. A concern that has been raised about detection of occult, clinically undetectable cancer is the difficulty in determining the type of cancer and its location. Clearly, more information than a diagnosis of "cancer, type and site unknown" would be needed for undertaking rational therapy. Specificity for a particular organ site or histologic type

Table 6.1
POTENTIAL APPLICATIONS OF
IMMUNODIAGNOSTIC PROCEDURES

1. Detection-screening of populations and high-risk groups
2. Aid in differential diagnosis of cancer
3. Aid in classification of tumor cells
4. Localization of tumor
5. Assessment of prognosis
6. Monitoring of course of disease and early detection of recurrences or metastases

Table 6.2
CRITERIA FOR USEFUL IMMUNODIAGNOSTIC
TEST FOR CANCER

1. Qualitative or quantitative difference from normal or benign
2. High specificity (low percent of false-positives)
3. High sensitivity (low percent of false-negatives)
4. Organ site specificity for localization

of cancer is important initially, but is not as essential for monitoring previously diagnosed patients.

For detection, it is particularly important that the assay be simple and practical enough for testing large numbers of specimens or individuals. The procedures must be sufficiently well-developed and standardized, so that reproducible results can be obtained in many laboratories. A screening test, which would be given to a high proportion of normal individuals, should present little or no risk to the recipients. The specificity of a screening test is a particularly important factor because the occurrence of an appreciable number of false-positives in a screened population causes psychological, logistic, and economic problems. For example, if the frequency of a given type of a cancer in a population is 0.5% and the frequency of positive tests is 10%, most of the individuals with positive results would be needlessly alarmed and subjected to costly, time-consuming diagnostic procedures.

Tests to be used as diagnostic adjuncts must meet different criteria. These tests should be highly accurate in discriminating between cancer and noncancer in an individual, rather than in showing significant differences between cancer and noncancer groups. False-positive and false-negative results both have serious implications, but an error rate of 5% to 10% in each direction might be considered acceptable. Also, procedures with some risk might be more acceptable in these patients, since the ratio of potential risk to possible benefit is quite different from that in screening general populations.

For immunologic tests to be useful for prognosis or monitoring of cancer patients, they must not only discriminate between individuals with cancer and those without, but also reflect the stage of disease and the presence or absence of small amounts of tumor. The monitoring test needs to be acceptable for repeated use by the patients. There may also be special problems of the assays being affected by the therapy, particularly immunosuppressive therapy.

There are several approaches to take to the immunodiagnosis of cancer (table 6.3). The first approach, the detection of antigenic markers in the tumor-bearing individual, has been used most. Tumor cells may contain antigens that are undetectable or are present in smaller amounts in normal cells. Thus, antibodies in patients' sera, or in the sera of animals immunized against these antigens, can potentially discriminate between tumor cells and normal cells. In order to be useful in immunodiagnosis, the tumor antigens must be common to a variety of tumors, at least those of the same histologic type.

Most immunodiagnostic assays have focused on the detection of circulating tumor markers, with the levels

Table 6.3
IMMUNOLOGIC APPROACHES TO THE
DIAGNOSIS OF CANCER

1. Detection of TAAs, or antigens associated with viruses or with certain organs or tissues
   a. On tumor cells
   b. Circulating in plasma or in secretions
2. Immune competence of cancer patients
3. Immune response to TAAs or to virus-associated antigens
   a. Humoral immunity
   b. Cell-mediated immunity

generally reflecting the amount of tumor present and the metastatic spread of disease. The expression of TAAs or other markers on the tumor cells has been helpful primarily in classifying tumors and discerning their derivation. This may have therapeutic implications, and the application has been most widely used for the leukemias and lymphomas where the surface phenotype has become a standard aspect of assessment (Young et al. 1972). In addition, the loss of some normal antigens, either organ specific (Nairn et al. 1960; Burtin and Clausell 1973) or not, from tumor cells may be useful in immunodiagnosis. For example, loss of blood-group antigens has been correlated with a tendency for metastasis (Davidsohn and Ni 1969; Sheahan, Horowitz, and Zamcheck 1971).

Depression in the cancer patient's immune competence might also be useful diagnostically because deficits in immunologic function or in subpopulations of cells of the immune system have been associated with poor prognosis. Also, there are suggestions that some immunologic assays may be useful in discerning individuals with increased risk of malignancy (Strayer et al. 1984).

Many tumor-associated antigens can elicit an immune response in a tumor-bearing individual. Antigens present in very small amounts can often be recognized by the host and it might therefore be expected that immunologic reactions would be detected while tumors were still small and localized. Both humoral antibodies and cell-mediated immune responses can be measured; sufficiently standardized assays might be more sensitive for detection of the tumor-bearing state than the more usual assays of circulating tumor markers.

With immunodiagnostic assays currently in clinical use, the value of only a small number of tumor markers has been sufficiently demonstrated. However, a larger array is being studied and the list of useful tests may grow, particularly for assessing prognosis and monitoring therapy. This topic has been reviewed (Virji, Mercer, and Herberman 1988).

IMMUNOTHERAPY

The building evidence for the immune system's participation in resistance against the progression and spread of cancer has raised expectations that manipulation of the immune system might also be a valuable treatment. Such optimism has been fostered by the findings that various cytokines and other biological response modifiers can stimulate or augment immunologic reactivity

against cancer (Herberman 1985a). Some species of genetically engineered interferon have had appreciable antitumor effects against experimental tumors and some clinical malignancies (Kirkwood and Ernstoff 1986). Alpha interferon has already been licensed by the United States Food and Drug Administration (FDA) as effective for treatment of hairy-cell leukemia and Kaposi's sarcoma. IL-2, particularly in combination with LAK cells, has been shown to have strong antimetastatic effects against some experimental tumors in mice and rats (Mule, Shu, and Rosenberg 1985). In some cases it has been able to induce cures (Salup, Back, and Wiltrout 1987). Analogous therapy in some patients with advanced cancer, particularly malignant melanoma or renal carcinoma, has induced partial or complete regression of detectable metastatic lesions (Rosenberg et al. 1985). In detailed studies in an experimental tumor model (Salup, Back, and Wiltrout 1987), it appears that optimal results may be achieved by combining cytoreductive therapy by surgery and chemotherapy with the adoptive immunotherapy using IL-2 and LAK cells.

Adoptive therapy with specifically immune T cells and IL-2 may be even more potent than LAK cells and IL-2, with curative effects induced in some experimental tumor models (Greenberg et al. 1988). Recently, promising therapeutic results have been obtained by specific *in vitro* sensitization with irradiated lymphoid tumor cells from mice with growing tumors (Chou et al. 1988). Clinically, tumor-infiltrating lymphocytes from patients with malignant melanoma have been expanded in culture with IL-2 and have appeared to have specific cytotoxic reactivity against the autologous tumor cells (Rosenberg et al. 1988). These IL-2-expanded cells, when transferred to the patients, have induced some complete tumor regressions. Considerably more efforts in adoptive cellular immunotherapy seem warranted, with a focus on defining the effector cells responsible for the therapeutic cells and determining the conditions for optimally generating them and stimulating their antitumor reactivity.

Infusion of monoclonal antibodies against TAAs has been another major approach for the treatment of metastatic cancer. The main strategy has been to combine the antibodies with toxic varieties (either radionuclides, toxins, or drugs). The goal is to have the antibodies selectively carry the toxic agents to the tumor site or sites. Although this form of immunotherapy should eventually be very useful, many technical problems have limited its therapeutic benefits. In addition to the immunoconjugate approach, some antibodies by themselves appear to have promising therapeutic effects. This might be attributed to mechanisms including complement-dependent lysis of tumor cells, interactions with effector cells for ADCC, or immunoregulatory effects such as the induction of anti-idiotypic responses. An example of the therapeutic effects of a monoclonal antibody by itself has come from a study with antibodies to the GD3 ganglioside in human malignant melanoma, with partial regression of tumor in several patients with advanced disease (Houghton et al. 1985).

Other efforts have been directed toward stimulating the host's immune system using a wide variety of immunomodulators. These may be either defined chemical substances or, more frequently, bacterial products such as BCG or OK-432. Although the latter group of agents are usually very heterogeneous and ill-defined, they can induce strong stimulation of various components of the immune system, including antitumor effector mechanisms. BCG, a low-virulence variant of *Mycobacterium tuberculosis,* has been found to be very effective for treatment of superficial recurrent carcinoma of the bladder (Lamm, Thor, and Winters 1981). OK-432, an inactivated form of *Streptococcus pyogenes,* has been used widely in Japan and other countries and appears to be effective for treating malignant effusions and possibly other forms of cancer (Ishida and Hoshino 1985).

Immunotherapy for cancer has had some success to date, but this field is still at a very early development stage. Most of the promising strategies need to be investigated in considerably greater detail, and the optimal doses and conditions for treatment need to be defined. This will require a methodical approach, with close interaction between the *in vivo* studies and detailed *in vitro* evaluation of the effects on the immune system (Herberman 1985b).

REFERENCES

Adams, D.O., and Snyderman, R. 1979. Do macrophages destroy nascent tumors? *J. Natl. Cancer. Inst.* 62:1341-45.

Adler, A.; Chervenick, P.A.; and Whiteside, T.L. et al. 1988. Interleukin-2 induction of lymphokine-activated killer (LAK) activity in the peripheral blood and bone marrow of acute leukemia patients. I: feasibility of LAK generation in adult patients with active disease and in remission. *Blood* 71: 709-16.

Barlozzari, T.; Reynolds, C.W.; and Herberman, R.B. 1983. *In vivo* role of natural killer cells: involvement of large granular lymphocytes in the clearance of tumor cells in anti-asialo GM$_1$-treated rats. *J. Immunol.* 131:1024-27.

Burnet, F.M. 1957. Cancer: a biological approach. *Brit. Med. J.* 1:779-86; 841-47.

Burnet, F.M. 1970. The concept of immunological surveillance. *Prog. Exp. Tumor. Res.* 13:1-27.

Burtin, P., and Clausell, D.T. 1973. Isolation of a human gastrointestinal membrane antigen. *Ann. Immunol.* 124C: 17-26.

Chou, T.; Bertera, S.; and Chang, A.E. et al. 1988. Adoptive immunotherapy of microscopic and advanced visceral metastases with *in vitro* sensitized lymphoid cells from mice bearing progressive tumors. *J. Immunol.* 141:1775-81.

Cianciolo, G.J., and Snyderman, R. 1983. Neoplasia and mononuclear phagocyte function. In Herberman, R.B., and Friedman, H. eds. *The reticuloendothelial system: a comprehensive treatise.* vol. 5. Cancer. pp. 193-216. New York: Plenum Press.

Coggin, J.H. Jr.; Ambrose, K.R.; and Anderson, N.G. 1970. Fetal antigen capable of inducing transplantation immunity against SV40 hamster tumor cells. *J. Immunol.* 105:524-26.

Cooper, E.L. ed. 1976. *Comparative immunology.* Englewood Cliffs, New Jersey: Prentice-Hall.

Cudkowicz, G., and Hochman, P.S. 1979. Do natural killer cells engage in regulated reactions against self to ensure homeostasis? *Immunol. Rev.* 44:13-28.

Davidsohn, I., and Ni, L.Y. 1969. Loss of isoantigens A, B, and H in carcinoma of the lung. *Am. J. Pathol.* 57:307-34.

Dean, J.H.; Connor, R.; and Herberman, R.B. et al. 1977. The relative proliferation index as a more sensitive parameter for evaluating lymphoproliferative responses of cancer patients to mitogens and alloantigens. *Int. J. Cancer* 20: 359-70.

Dean, J.H. 1979. Application of the microculture lymphocyte proliferation assay to clinical studies. In Herberman, R.B., and McIntire, K.R. eds. *Immunodiagnosis of cancer.* pp. 738-69. New York: Marcel Dekker.

Dent, P.B.; Fish, L.A.; and White, J.F. et al. 1966. Chediak-Higashi syndrome: observations on the nature of the associated malignancy. *Lab. Invest.* 15:1634-41.

Ehrlich, P. 1957. Über den jetzigen Stand der Karzinomforschung. In Himmelweit, F. ed. *The collected papers of Paul Ehrlich.* vol. 11. pp. 550-62. London: Pergamon Press.

Eilber, F.R., and Morton, D.L. 1970. Impaired immunologic reactivity and recurrence following cancer surgery. *Cancer* 25:362-67.

Eltringham, J.R., and Kaplan, H.S. 1973. Impaired delayed-hypersensitivity responses in 154 patients with untreated Hodgkin's disease. *Natl. Cancer Inst. Monogr.* 36:107-15.

Evans, C.H. 1972. Macrophages in syngeneic animal tumors. *Transplantation* 14:468-72.

Fidler, I.J. 1974. Inhibition of pulmonary metastases by intravenous injection of specifically activated macrophages. *Cancer Res.* 34:1074-79.

Foon, K.A.; Schroff, R.W.; and Gale, R.P. 1982. Surface markers on leukemia cells: recent advances. *Blood* 60:1-19.

Gatti, R.A., and Good, R.A. 1971. Occurrence of a malignancy in immunodeficiency diseases: a literature review. *Cancer* 28:89-98.

Gauci, C.L., and Alexander, P. 1975. The macrophage content of some human tumors. *Cancer Lett.* 1:20-25.

Gerson, J.M. 1980. Systemic and *in situ* natural killer activity in tumor-bearing mice and patients with cancer. In Herberman, R.B. ed. *Natural cell-mediated immunity against tumors.* pp. 1047-62. New York: Academic Press.

Gorelik, E., and Herberman, R.B. 1981. Inhibition of the activity of mouse NK cells by urethane. *J. Natl. Cancer Inst.* 66:543-48.

Gorelik, E., and Herberman, R.B. 1982. Role of natural-cell-mediated immunity in urethane-induced lung carcinogenesis. In Herberman, R.B. ed. *NK cells and other natural effector cells.* pp. 1415-21. New York: Academic Press.

Gorelik, E., and Herberman, R.B. 1986. Role of natural killer (NK) cells in the control of tumor growth and metastatic spread. In Herberman, R.B. ed. *Cancer immunology: innovative approaches to therapy.* pp. 151-76. Boston: Martinus Nijhoff.

Gorelik, E.; Peppoloni, S.; and Overton, R. et al. 1985. Increase in H-2 antigen expression and immunogenicity of BL6 melanoma cells treated with N-methyl N'-nitro-nitrosoguanidine. *Cancer Res.* 45:5341-47.

Gorelik, E.; Rosen, B.; and Copeland, D. et al. 1984. Evaluation of role of natural killer cells in radiation-induced leukemogenesis in mice. *J. Natl. Cancer Inst.* 72:1397-1403.

Gorelik, E.; Wiltrout, R.H.; and Brunda, M.J. et al. 1982. Augmentation of metastasis formation by thioglycollate-elicited macrophages. *Int. J. Cancer.* 29:575-81.

Gorelik, E.; Wiltrout, R.H.; and Copeland, D. et al. 1985. Modulation of formation of tumor metastases by peritoneal macrophages elicited by various agents. *Cancer Immunol. Immunother.* 19:35-42.

Greenberg, P.D.; Klarnet, J.P.; and Kern, D.E. et al. 1988.

Therapy of disseminated tumors by adoptive transfer of specifically immune T cells. *Prog. Exp. Tumor Res.* 32: 104-27.

Grimm, E.A.; Mazumder, A.; and Zhang, H.Z. et al. 1982. Lymphokine-activated killer cell phenomenon: lysis of natural killer-resistant fresh solid tumor cells by interleukin-2 activated autologous human peripheral blood lymphocytes. *J. Exp. Med.* 155:1823-41.

Habel, K. 1961. Resistance of polyoma virus immune animals to transplanted polyoma tumors. *Proc. Soc. Exp. Biol. Med.* 106:722-25.

Herberman, R.B. 1983. Counterpoint: animal tumor models and their relevance to human tumor immunology. *J. Biol. Resp. Modif.* 2:39-46.

Herberman, R.B. 1985a. Biological response modifiers for the therapy of cancer. *Ann. Allergy* 54:376-81.

Herberman, R.B. 1985b. Design of clinical trials with biological response modifiers. *Cancer Treat. Rep.* 69:1161-64.

Herberman, R.B.; Balch, C.; and Bolhuis, R. et al. 1987. Lymphokine-activated killer cell activity: characteristics of effector cells and their progenitors in blood and spleen. *Immunol. Today* 8:178-81.

Hersey, P.; Edwards, A.; and McCarthy, W. et al. 1982. Tumor related changes and prognostic significance of natural killer cell activity in melanoma patients. In Herberman, R.B. ed. *NK cells and other natural effector cells.* pp. 1167-74. New York: Academic Press.

Hewitt, H.B., Blake, E.R., and Walder, A.S. 1976. A critique of the evidence for active host defense against cancer, based on personal studies of 27 murine tumours of spontaneous origin. *Br. J. Cancer* 33:241-59.

Hewitt, H.B. 1982. Animal tumor models and their relevance to human tumor immunology. *J. Biol. Resp. Modif.* 1:107-19.

Hibbs, J.B., Jr.; Chapman, H.A., Jr.; and Weinberg, J.B. 1978. The macrophage as an antineoplastic surveillance cell: biological perspectives. *J. Reticuloendothel. Soc.* 24:549-70.

Houghton, A.N.; and Mintzer, D. et al. 1985. Mouse monoclonal IgG3 antibody detecting GD3 ganglioside: a phase I trial in patients with malignant melanoma. *Proc. Natl. Acad. Sci.* 82:1242-46.

Ishida, N., and Hoshino, T. 1985. Streptococcal preparation as a potent biological response modifier. *OK-432.* 2nd ed. p. 70. Japan: Excerpta Medica.

Kambe, M.; Mitachi, Y.; and Kanamaru, R. et al. 1988. Responsiveness of peripheral blood lymphocytes from cancer patients and healthy donors to interleukin-2 (IL-2). *Tohoku J. Exp. Med.* 154:101-10.

Keller, R. 1978. Macrophage-mediated natural cytotoxicity against various target cells *in vitro.* I. comparison of tissue macrophages from diverse anatomic sites and from different strains of rats and mice. *Br. J. Cancer* 37:732-41.

Kikuchi, Y.; Kita, T.; and Oomori, K. et al. 1988. Interleukin-2 activity in peripheral blood mononuclear cells of patients with gynecologic malignancies. *Med. Oncol. Tumor Pharmacother.* 5(2):85-90.

Kirkwood, J.M., and Ernstoff, M. 1986. Potential applications of the interferons in oncology: lessons drawn from studies of human melanoma. *Semin. Oncol.* 13:48-56.

Klein, G., and Klein, E. 1977. Rejectability of virus induced tumors and non-rejectability of spontaneous tumors: a lesson in contrasts. *Transplant Proc.* 9:1095-1104.

Koch, B.; Regnat, W.; Solbach, W.; and Lanz, R. et al. 1984. Interleukin-2 production in peripheral blood mononuclear cells of patients with gastrointestinal tumors. *J. Clin. Lab. Immunol.* 13(4):171-78.

Kripke, M.L. 1981. Immunologic mechanisms in UV radiation carcinogenesis. *Adv. Cancer Res.* 34:69-106.

Lamm, D.L.; Thor, D.E.; and Winters, W.D. 1981. BCG immunotherapy of bladder cancer: inhibition of tumor recurrence and associated immune response. *Cancer* 48:81.

Law, L.W. 1966. Studies of thymic function with emphasis on the role of the thymus in oncogenesis. *Cancer Res.* 26: 551-74.

Levy, R., and Kaplan, H.S. 1974. Impaired lymphocyte function in untreated Hodgkin's disease. *New Engl. J. Med.* 290:181-86.

Loutit, J.F.; Townsend, K.M.S.; and Knowles, J.F. 1980. Tumor surveillance in beige mice. *Nature* (London) 285:66.

Mantovani, A.; Giavazzi, R.; and Polentarutti, N. et al. 1980. Divergent effects of macrophage toxins on growth of primary tumors and lung metastasis. *Int. J. Cancer* 25:617-22.

Meeker, T.; Lowder, J.; and Cleary, M.L. et al. 1985. Emergence of idiotype variants during treatment of B-cell lymphoma with anti-idiotype antibodies. *N. Engl. J. Med.* 312:1658-65.

Morton, D.L.; Eilber, F.R.; and Joseph, W.L. et al. 1970. Immunological factors in human sarcoma and melanoma: a rational basis for immunotherapy. *Ann. Surg.* 172:740-49.

Mule, J.J.; Shu, S.; and Rosenberg, S.A. 1985. The antitumor efficacy of lymphokine-activated killer cells and recombinant interleukin-2 *in vivo. J. Immunol.* 135:646-52.

Nairn, R.C.; Richmond, H.C.; and McEntegart, M.G. et al. 1960. Immunological differences between normal and malignant cells. *Br. Med. J.* 2:1335-40.

Norbury, K.C., and Kripke, M.L. 1979. Ultraviolet-induced carcinogenesis in mice treated with silica, trypan blue or pyran copolymer. *J. Reticuloendothel. Soc.* 26:827-32.

Old, L.J., and Boyse, E.A. 1964. Immunology of experimental tumors. *Ann. Rev. Med.* 15:167-95.

Ortaldo, J.R., and Herberman, R.B. 1984. Heterogeneity of natural killer cells. In Paul, W.E.; Fathman, C.G.; and Metzger, H. eds. *Annual reviews of immunology.* vol. 2. pp. 359-94. Palo Alto, Calif.: Annual Reviews, Inc.

Parkinson, D.R.; Brightman, R.P.; and Waksal, S.D. 1981. Altered natural killer cell biology in C57BL/6 mice after leukemogenic split-dose irradiation. *J. Immunol.* 126:1460-64.

Payne, L.N. 1972. In Biggs, P.M.; Dethe, G.; and Payne, L.N. eds. *Oncogenesis and herpes viruses.* pp. 21-37. Lyon: International Agency for Research on Cancer.

Penn, I., and Starzl, T.R. 1972. A summary of the status of *de novo* cancer in transplant recipients. *Transplant Proc.* 4: 719-32.

Peppoloni, S.; Herberman, R.B.; and Gorelik, E. 1987. Lewis lung carcinoma (3LL) cells treated *in vitro* with ultraviolet radiation show reduced metastatic ability due to an augmented immunogenicity. *Clin. Expl. Metastasis* 5:43-56.

Pinsky, C.M. 1978. Skin tests. In Herberman, R.B., and McIntire, K.R. eds. *Immunodiagnosis of cancer.* pp. 722-38. New York: Marcel Dekker.

Prehn, R.T., and Lappe, M.A. 1971. An immunostimulation theory of tumor development. *Transplant Rev.* 7:26-54.

Prehn, R.T., and Main, J.M. 1957. Immunity to MCA induced sarcomas. *J. Nat. Cancer. Inst.* 18:769-75.

Pross, H.F.; Rubin, P.; and Baines, M.G. 1982. The assessment of natural killer cell activity in cancer patients. In Herberman, R.B. ed. *NK cells and other natural effector cells.* pp. 1175-81. New York: Academic Press.

Roberts, M.M., and Bell, R. 1976. Acute leukemia after immunosuppressive therapy. *Lancet* II:768-70.

Rosenberg, S.A.; Lotze, M.T.; and Muul, L.M. et al. 1985. Observations on the systemic administration of autologous lymphokine activated killer cells and recombinant interleukin-2 to patients with metastatic cancer. *N. Engl. J. Med.* 313:1485-89.

Rosenberg, S.A.; Packard, B.S.; and Aebersold, P.M. et al. 1988. Use of tumor-infiltrating lymphocytes and interleukin-2 in the immunotherapy of patients with metastatic melanoma. *N. Engl. J. Med.* 319:1676-80.

Salup, R.R.; Back, T.A.; and Wiltrout, R.H. 1987. Successful treatment of advanced murine renal cancer by bicompartmental adoptive chemoimmunotherapy. *J. Immunol.* 138: 641-47.

Schantz, S.P.; Brown, B.W.; and Lira, E. et al. 1987. Evidence for the role of natural immunity in the control of metastatic spread of head and neck cancer. *Cancer Immunol. Immunother.* 25:141-45.

Sheahan, D.G.; Horowitz, S.A.; and Zamcheck, N. 1971. Deletion of epithelial ABH isoantigens in primary gastric neoplasms and in metastatic cancer. *Am. J. Dig. Dis.* 16:961-69.

Sones, P.D.E., and Castro, J.E. 1977. Immunological mechanisms in metastatic spread and the antimetastatic effect of *C. parvum. Br. J. Cancer* 35:519-26.

Specter, S., and Friedman, H. 1983. Immunosuppressive factors produced by tumors and their effects on the RES. In Herberman, R.B., and Friedman, H. eds. *The reticuloendothelial system: a comprehensive treatise.* vol. 5. Cancer. pp. 315-26. New York: Plenum Press.

Srivastava, P.K., and Old, L.J. 1988. Individually distinct transplantation antigens of chemically induced mouse tumors. *Immunol. Today* 9:78-83.

Stein, J.A.; Adler, A.; and Ben Efran, S. et al. 1976. Immunocompetence, immunosuppression and human breast cancer. I. an analysis of their relationship by known parameters of cell-mediated immunity in well-defined clinical stages of disease. *Cancer* 38:1171-87.

Stern, K. 1983. Control of tumors by the RES. In Herberman, R.B., and Friedman, H. eds. *The reticuloendothelial system: a comprehensive treatise.* vol. 5. pp. 59-153. New York: Plenum Press.

Strayer, D.R.; Carter, W.A.; and Mayberry, S.D. et al. 1984. Low natural cytotoxicity of peripheral blood mononuclear cells in individuals with high familial incidences of cancer. *Cancer Res.* 44:370-74.

Stutman, O. 1975. Immunodepression and malignancy. *Adv. Cancer Res.* 22:261-422.

Thomas, L. 1959. Discussion. In Lawrence, H.S. ed. *Cell and humoral aspects of the hypersensitive state.* pp. 529-30. New York: Harper & Row.

Ting, C.C.; Lavrin, D.H.; and Shiu, G. et al. 1972. Expression of fetal antigens in tumor cells. *Proc. Nat. Acad. Sci.* 69:1664-68.

Ting, C. C., and Herberman, R.B. 1976. Humoral host defense mechanisms tumors. In Richter, G.W., and Epstein, M.A. eds. *International review of experimental pathology.* vol. 15. pp. 93-152. New York: Academic Press.

Varesio, L. 1983. Suppressor cells and cancer: inhibition of immune functions by macrophages. In Herberman, R.B., and Friedman, H. eds. *The reticuloendothelial system: a comprehensive treatise.* vol. 5. Cancer. pp. 217-52. New York: Plenum Press.

Virji, M.A.; Mercer, D.W.; and Herberman, R.B. 1988. Tumor markers in cancer diagnosis and prognosis. *CA* 38:104-26.

Vlock, D.R.; Scalise, D.; and Meglin, N. et al. 1988. Isolation and partial characterization of melanoma-associated antigens identified by autologous antibody. *J. Clin. Invest.* 81:1746-51.

Ward, J.M.; Argilan, F.; and Reynolds, C.W. 1983. Immunoperoxidase localization of large granular lymphocytes in normal tissues and lesions of athymic nude rats. *J. Immunol.* 131:132-39.

Warner, J.F., and Dennert, T.G. 1982. *In vivo* function of a cloned cell line with NK activity: effects on bone marrow transplants, tumor development and metastases. *Nature* (London) 300:31.

West, W.H.; Sienknecht, C.W.; and Townes, A.S. et al. 1976. Performance of a rosette assay between lymphocyte and sheep erythrocytes at elevated temperatures to study patients with cancer and other diseases. *J. Clin. Immunol. Immunopath.* 5:60-66.

Young, R.C.; Corder, M.P.; and Haynes, H.A. et al. 1972. Delayed hypersensitivity in Hodgkin's disease: a study of 103 untreated patients. *Am. J. Med.* 52:63-72.

Yunis, E.J.; Martinez, C.; and Smith, J. et al. 1969. Spontaneous mammary adenocarcinoma in mice: influence of thymectomy and reconstruction with thymus grafts or spleen cells. *Cancer Res.* 29:174-78.

Zwilling, B.S.; Filippi, J.A.; and Chorpenning, F.W. 1978. Chemical carcinogenesis and immunity: immunologic studies of rats treated with methylnitrosourea. *J. Natl. Cancer Inst.* 61:731-38.

Chapter 7

THE CAUSES OF CANCER

John H. Weisburger, Ph.D., M.D.
Clara L. Horn, B.A., M.T.

John H. Weisburger, Ph.D., M.D.
Director Emeritus, Dana Naylor Institute for Disease Prevention
Senior Member, American Health Foundation
Valhalla, New York

Clara L. Horn, B.A., M.T.
Scientific Coordinator
American Health Foundation
Valhalla, New York

INTRODUCTION

The history of medicine and medical research has brought us to the point where many major diseases no longer threaten human life and well-being because of prevention—the definitive cure. Like successes have been achieved in the field of cancer causation. The occupational cause-cancer link first came to public and professional attention with the discovery of scrotal cancer in chimney sweeps and urinary bladder cancer in chemical industry workers. It is now possible to identify potential cancer risks through effective, specific short-term tests. In most industrial countries the risk of cancer related to occupational hazards can be reduced. By current estimates, at most 5% of all cancers can be directly traced to occupation (Wynder and Gori 1977; Doll and Peto 1981; Maltoni and Selikoff 1988; Swanson 1988). The severe contamination of shipyard and insulation workers with asbestos fibers during 1940-1950 in the United States has led to a small increase in the incidence of mesothelioma, and more importantly, an increase in lung cancer among cigarette smokers. Such cases are still becoming mortality statistics now, even though they date to exposure decades ago. Now-corrected adverse working conditions, and a higher proportion of smokers contributed to the higher incidence in that population (Saracci 1986).

Because research has documented that exposure to certain chemicals in the environment has induced cancer in specific organs, environmental pollution is still thought by many, especially lay people, to be a major cause of many forms of cancer (Searle 1984; Efron 1984). Yet, careful research in the last 30 years has shown this concept to be incorrect. Instead, worldwide observations show that lifestyle and lifestyle-related behavior can cause or promote the development of cancer and may account for the many cancers in man. This became clear through examining specific anatomic cancer sites and elucidating the associated etiologic factors and environmental conditions (table 7.1). The etiologic factors are often complex and have distinct properties that act through mechanisms that need careful analysis and evaluation.

Extensive knowledge has accrued through cancer research: (1) on the mechanisms of carcinogenesis as a basis for delineating and classifying risk factors and (2) on the methods for detecting carcinogens in the broadest sense (Searle 1984; Williams and Weisburger 1986; Cooper and Grover 1990). It is fairly certain now that cancer stems from a somatic mutation and once the genetic factors of a cell system have changed, upon several cell duplication cycles the damage generally is not reversible. Environmental chemicals, including those associated with lifestyle, can react with genetic material, especially DNA. This reaction has important functional consequences.

Other agents show no evidence of interaction with DNA, whether investigated through chemical studies or indirect, *in vitro* or *in vivo* bioassays. Such nongenotoxic chemicals with an enhancing effect in cancer causation, under a variety of conditions *in vitro*, in animal models, or in man, may operate by promoting mechanisms or other possible effects (see table 7.2). Thus, it is important to

Table 7.1
DOCUMENTATION IN THE ELUCIDATION OF THE ETIOLOGY OF HUMAN CANCERS

I. Epidemiology
  A. Geographic pathology
  B. Special populations
  C. Time trends
II. Laboratory Studies
  A. Metabolic and biochemical epidemiology—population studies
  B. Model studies in animals
  C. Model studies in cell and organ cultures
  D. Definition of mechanisms
III. Development and Validation of Hypotheses
  A. Established risk factors and their mode of action
  B. Suspected risk factors and their possible role

Table 7.2.
CLASSES OF CARCINOGENIC CHEMICALS

Type	Mode of Action	Example
A. Genotoxic		
1. Direct-acting	Electrophile, organic compound, genotoxic, interacts with DNA	Ethylene imine; bis(chloromethyl) ether
2. Procarcinogen	Requires conversion through metabolic activation by host or *in vitro* to type 1	Vinyl chloride, benzo(a)pyrene, 2-naphthylamine, 2-amino-3-methyl imidazo[4,5-f]quinoline dimethylnitrosamine
3. Inorganic Carcinogen	Not directly genotoxic, leads to changes in DNA by selective alteration in fidelity of DNA replication	nickel, chromium
B. Epigenetic		
4. Solid-state Carcinogen	Usually affects only mesenchymal cells and tissues; physical form vital; exact mechanism unknown, but may increase cell cycling	Polymer or metal foils; asbestos
5. Hormone	Mainly alters endocrine system balance and differentiation; often acts as promoter; usually not genotoxic	Estradiol, diethylstilbestrol
6. Immunosuppressor	Mainly stimulates "virally induced", transplanted, or metastatic neoplasms; usually not genotoxic	Azathioprine, antilymphocytic serum
7. Cocarcinogen	Not genotoxic or carcinogenic, but enhances effect of type 1 or type 2 agent when given at the same time; may modify conversion of type 2 to type 1	Phorbol esters, pyrene, catechol ethanol, SO_2
8. Cytotoxin	Not genotoxic or carcinogenic; above specific dosages kills cells, increases regeneration and cell cycling	Butylated hydroxy anisole; nitrilotriacetate; carbon tetrachloride
9. Promoter	Not genotoxic or carcinogenic, but enhances effect of type 1 or type 2 agent when given subsequently	Phorbol esters, phenol, bile acids, sodium saccharin

define precisely the specific factors associated with each type of human cancer and determine which components have genotoxic properties and which promoting or enhancing agents also play a role (see table 7.3).

For example, the chief cause of cancer of the stomach appears to be genotoxic, as shown by studies of migrants from high-risk to low-risk geographic areas of the world who maintain their risk, and from animal models, where a few doses of a gastric carcinogen lead to gastric cancer (Howson, Hiyama, and Wynder 1986; Weisburger 1987). On the other hand, although tobacco smoke includes a number of low-concentration genotoxic carcinogens, a major effect of tobacco smoke in inducing lung cancer stems from the presence of nongenotoxic, cytotoxic enhancing factors (U.S. Public Health Service 1982; Zaridze and Peto 1986; Hoffman and Hecht 1990). When smoking is stopped, the effect is reversible. Therefore, individuals who stop smoking eliminate the risk factor and have a progressively lower risk of lung cancer; this is in contrast to migrants who maintain their risk in relation to gastric cancer (see table 7.4). Research in breast-cancer models where the level and type of dietary fat play an important promoting role has shown that lowering and adjusting the level and type of

Table 7.3
TYPES OF AGENTS ASSOCIATED WITH HUMAN CANCER ETIOLOGY

Problems or questions to be resolved for each type of cancer

I. Nature of genotoxic carcinogens or mixtures: can be chemical, viral, or radiation
II. Nature of any nongenotoxic promoting or enhancing stimulus: can be chemical or viral
III. Amount, duration of exposure, and potency for each kind of agent
IV. Possibility of inhibition of the action of agents under I or II

fat consumed reduces the extent of mammary carcinogenesis (American Health Foundation 1987).

Each type of human cancer has specific genotoxic carcinogens as causative factors. There also may be powerful enhancing and promoting elements that operate in animal models and most likely in forms of human cancer. These factors will be discussed on the basis of organ site or the mechanisms of action of carcinogens, promoters, and inhibitors in lifestyle-related etiological factors. These factors include the use of tobacco products (smoking, snuff, dipping, or chewing) and nutritional elements as a function of geographic area of residence that affect specific target organs (see tables 7.5 and 7.6).

Table 7.4
IRREVERSIBILITY OR REVERSIBILITY OF CARCINOGENESIS AS A FUNCTION OF ACTION MECHANISM

Type of Cancer	Type and Mode of Action of Carcinogen	Reversibility	Evidence
Glandular, Stomach	Genotoxic from salted, pickled foods	Poor	Migrant studies: maintenance of risk in migrants
Lung	Small amounts of genotoxic carcinogens, polycyclic aromatic hydrocarbons and nicotine-derived nitrosamines, large amounts of phenols, catechols, terpenes, epigenetic cytotoxic enhancing agents	Good	People who stop smoking have progressively lesser risk

Table 7.5
TYPES OF CANCER ASSOCIATED WITH TOBACCO USE

Organ	Additional Factors
Oral cavity, upper GI tract, respiratory tract	Alcohol
Lung	Asbestos, mineral dusts, air pollution
Pancreas	High-fat diet, others?
Kidney, bladder	Diet?
Cervix	Virus?

International, multidisciplinary, and planned studies on the causes of disabling and fatal diseases have provided information on the main factors associated with premature death or disability from coronary heart disease, stroke, and the major types of cancer (Parkin, Laara, and Muir 1988; Joossens, Hill, and Geboers 1985; Wynder and Hiyama 1987; Ziegler, Devesa, and Fraumeni 1986). The causative factors for these chronic diseases are interrelated and effective, simultaneous control can result through research-based reduction of the causes. The complex factors associated with each type of cancer must be analyzed to delineate the elements causing or enhancing the risk for developing the disease. Most human cancers do not stem from intentional or even inadvertent chemical environmental contaminants, so effective prevention means that the real causes of each type of cancer must be identified.

Time trends, worldwide incidence and mortality figures for diverse cancers, the altered risk of migrants from areas of high- to low-incidence, and the analysis of data obtained under controlled conditions in animal models provide clues about the multiple causative factors involved in the main human cancers (see table 7.7). Leads were developed further by laboratory studies of the risk factors under highly controlled experimental conditions. These provided insight into the underlying mechanisms that could be validated further through a multidisciplinary team approach. "Spontaneous" changes in disease incidence or mortality as a function of time, such as the decline of gastric cancer in the United States over the last 50 years, have set the stage for a naturally occurring process that could be examined for clues about causative factors (Howson, Hiyama, and Wynder 1986).

Through controlled laboratory studies of risk factors and other approaches, it has been established that many

of the major cancers are related to lifestyle (see table 7.8). Occupational exposure to chemicals or exposure to drugs has caused some cancers, but the total number is small (Wynder and Gori 1977; Doll and Peto 1981; Swanson 1988; Searle 1984). The term "lifestyle" refers to factors such as cigarette smoking and other tobacco use and the national nutritional customs. Western nutritional traditions have led to a high rate of coronary heart disease and specific types of cancer (e.g., breast, colon, or pancreas), and have contributed to hypertension and stroke. In Japan, particularly northern Japan, the nutritional traditions pose a high risk for hypertensive disease, stroke, and cancers of the stomach, esophagus, or liver. The picture is similar in parts of Latin America.

Insight into disease mechanisms will enable the physician to manage the patient in a manner so that recurrences will usually be minimized. Modern medicine needs to take advantage of the achievements of research in order to reduce "recalls" in the medical field. Good medical management includes advising patients and the general public about currently available means of effective cancer prevention.

MECHANISMS OF CARCINOGENESIS

The concept that chemicals can induce cancer is derived from an understanding of the complex processes of carcinogenesis (Williams and Weisburger 1986; Kocsis, Jollow, and Witmer et al. 1986). The first in a series of essential steps in cancer causation and development (fig. 7.1) is the production of altered DNA in the cell by attack from a reactive form of a carcinogen. This leads to translocation and amplification of proto-oncogenes, specific genes that translate to a distinct expression of the properties of the cells bearing such altered genes (Barbacid 1986; Aaronson, Bishop, and Sugimura et al. 1987; Rich, Hager, and Lopez 1988). A role for an effect on tumor suppressor genes begins to unravel (Sager 1989; Weinberg 1989). Recognition of these effects is the basis for determining through specific rapid, efficient, and economical *in vitro* bioassays whether a given product might induce a mutation in prokaryotic or

Table 7.6
NUTRITIONALLY LINKED CANCERS

Site	Carcinogen From	Promoter From	Mechanism	Inhibitors
Esophagus	Pickled, salted foods	?		Yellow-green vegetables
Stomach	Pickled, smoked foods, nitrate	Salt	Atrophic gastritis	Yellow-green vegetables
Liver	Mycotoxins, nitrosamines	Hepatitis antigen	Cytotoxicity	?
	Senecio alkaloids, hepatitis antigen	Alcohol	Cytotoxicity	
Colon	Fried foods	Fats	Bile acids	Bran fiber, calcium ions, vegetables
Breast	Fried foods	Fats	Hormonal imbalances	Same as above
Prostate	Fried foods?	Fats	Hormonal imbalances	?
Endometrium and ovary	?	Fats	Obesity, estrogen	?

Table 7.7
FACTORS AND POSSIBLE MECHANISMS IN MAIN
EPITHELIAL CANCER CAUSATION AND PREVENTION

Disease	Risk factors	Mechanism	Protective elements	Mechanism
Lung cancer	Cigarette smoking	Complex mixture of genotoxic carcinogens, polycyclic aromatic hydrocarbons and tobacco-specific nitrosamines and risk-determining enhancing, promoting agents; asbestos, air pollutants have strong cocarcinogenic effect	Yellow-green vegetables	Retinoids, β-carotene, other inhibitors
	Occupational	Polycyclic hydrocarbons, coal gas work, bis(chloromethyl)ether, bis(chloroethyl)sulfide, arsenic, nickel, and chromate ores		
Oral cancer	Smoking; tobacco chewing; betel chewing; smoking and alcohol	Carcinogens in tobacco (mainly tobacco-specific nitrosamines), betel nut	Yellow-green vegetables	Retinoids, β-carotene, other inhibitors
Kidney cancer	Smoking; other factors unknown	Carcinogens from tobacco, unknown mechanisms	?	?
	Obesity	Endocrines: fat cells produce estrogens as carcinogens	Weight control/loss	Lowers excessive nonphysiologic estrogen level
Bladder cancer	Bilharzia; schistosomiasis	Carcinogens unknown, increased cell proliferation enhances risk	Yellow-green vegetables	?
	Smoking	Unknown (arylamines?)	Yellow-green vegetables	Retinoids
	Occupational	Arylamines	—	—
Endocrine-related cancers: prostate, breast, ovary	Total dietary fat (saturated + ω-6 polyunsaturated lipids)	Complex multieffector elements: hormonal balances, membrane and intracellular effectors	Monounsaturated oil (olive) ω-3 polyunsaturated oils Medium chain triglycerides Cereal fiber and pectin	Neutral action on hormone metabolism Protective effect in hormone metabolism Caloric equivalent to carbohydrate Affects enterohepatic cycling of hormones
Endometrial cancer	Same as above; excessive body weight	Same as above; fat cells generate estrogen	Same as above; weight control/loss	Same as above; lowers excessive nonphysiologic estrogen levels
Pancreas cancer	Same as endocrine; cigarette smoking	? ?	? ?	? ?
Colon cancer: proximal	?	?	?	?
distal	Same as endocrine-related cancers	Biosynthesis of cholesterol, thence bile acids, and colon cancer promotion including higher cell cycling rates	Cereal fiber Calcium salts	Increases stool bulk; dilutes promoters; lowers intestinal pH Bind bile and fatty acids; lower intestinal cell cycling
Rectal cancer	Alcoholic beverages, especially beer	Increases cell cycling in rectum?	Cereal fiber?	Dilutes effectors by increasing stool bulk
Liver cancer	Mold-contaminated foods	Mycotoxins	Avoid moldy, pickled foods, improve nutrition, more protein, fruits, and vegetables	Lower carcinogen intake
	Some plants	Pyrrolizidine alkaloids		
	Pickled foods	Nitrosamines		
	Chronic virus	Hepatitis B	Vaccination	
	High level of specific alcoholic beverages	Damages liver, risk of cirrhosis potentiates effect of carcinogens	Decrease intake of alcohol	May lower cell duplication rates
	Occupational	Vinyl chloride	Lower exposure	
	Iatrogenic	Some oral contraceptives (infrequent occurrence)		
Nasopharyngeal cancer	Salted, pickled fish	Contains specific nitrosamine?	?	?
	Viral factors	Can increase cell turnover?	Vaccination?	
	Occupational	Wood and leather workers		

Table 7.7 (continued)
FACTORS AND POSSIBLE MECHANISMS IN MAIN
EPITHELIAL CANCER CAUSATION AND PREVENTION

Disease	Risk factors	Mechanism	Protective elements	Mechanism
Esophageal cancer	Salted, pickled food?	Specific nitrosamine	Yellow-green vegetables	Role of vegetables unknown if risk factors present in food (β-carotene, protective element?)
	Alcohol intake + smoking	Alcohol modifies esophageal metabolism of tobacco-specific carcinogens	Yellow-green vegetables	
	Tobacco chewing	Tobacco-specific carcinogens and promoters?	Vegetables?	Same as above
Gastric cancer (intestinal)	Salted, pickled food	Nitrosoindoles, phenolic diazotates	Green-yellow vegetables	Role of vegetables unknown if risk factor present in food
	Geochemical nitrate and salt	Formation of gastric carcinogens, above, in stomach	Green-yellow vegetables, fruits, vitamins C and E	Prevent formation of carcinogen; cellular tissue defenses

eukaryotic cell systems (Williams and Weisburger 1986; Rosenkranz 1988). Also useful is the presence of enzyme systems that repair DNA and provide complementary effective test systems to outline the possible DNA reactivity of chemicals. A specific chemical that displays properties of inducing mutations and DNA repair in a number of cell systems can be labeled genotoxic. Virtually all known human carcinogens are genotoxic; the exception might be the hormone diethylstilbestrol (DES), but newer techniques have found that even estrogens yield genotoxic products (Roy, Weisz, and Liehr 1990). Thus, the determination that a given product is reliably genotoxic signals a potential cancer risk to man, given an appropriate dose and adequate duration of exposure.

Promoters cannot cause cancer without an antecedent cell change. For example, mice with mammary tumor virus (MTV) develop mammary tumors proportional to the level of estrogen administered. Those without MTV do not develop mammary tumors, no matter what dose of estrogen is used (Highman, Norvell, and Shellenberger 1977). The action of promoters requires their presence at high levels for a long time, is reversible, and is often tissue-specific. For example, bile acids are

NEOPLASTIC CONVERSION

NEOPLASTIC DEVELOPMENT AND PROGRESSION

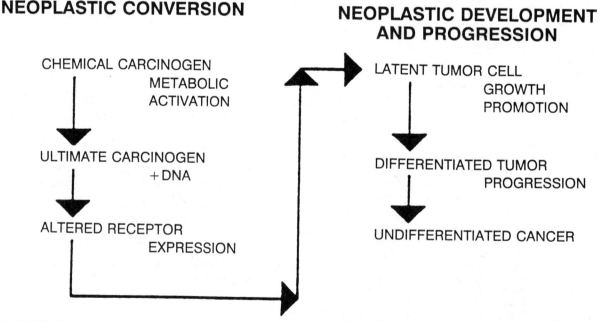

Fig. 7.1. Most types of cancer stem from a complex sequence of steps, schematically outlined. Naturally occurring chemicals related to lifestyle or occupation must undergo metabolic activation (or conversely, be detoxified biochemically, usually the major set of reactions). The resulting ultimate carcinogen, a reactive molecule (and also radiation or oncogenic viruses), interacts with cellular macromolecules, and specifically, with the heritable element, DNA. This altered DNA undergoes further changes during replication, leading to codon (oncogene) rearrangements and amplification. Also involved may be an effect on suppressor genes. This sequence of reactions is the result of "genotoxic" elements. The cells with such abnormal DNA must grow and develop subject to the control of diverse factors at the levels of the cell, organ, tissue, whole animal, or human being, and external environmental elements, including factors bearing on growth promotion or inhibition. The reaction sequence is the result of nongenotoxic, epigenetic events that are highly dose-dependent, with a threshold no-effect dose. Duration of exposure is important.

Table 7.8
POSTULATED CAUSES OF MAIN HUMAN CANCERS

Type	% Total Cases
Occupational Cancer:	1–2
Various organs	
Cryptogenic Cancers	10–15
Lymphomas, leukemias, sarcomas, (cervix?), (virus?)	
Lifestyle Cancers	
1. Tobacco-related: lung, pancreas, bladder, kidney, cervix(?)	34
2. Diet-related — nitrate-nitrite, salt, low vitamins A, C, E	5
(yellow-green vegetables): stomach, esophagus	
Mycotoxins, hepatitis B antigen: liver	
3. High fat, low fiber, low calcium, broiled or fried foods:	37
large bowel, pancreas, prostate, breast, uterus	
Multifactorial	
1. Tobacco and alcohol: oral cavity, esophagus	2
2. Tobacco-asbestos, tobacco-mining, tobacco-uranium-radium: lung, respiratory tract	2
Iatrogenic — radiation, drugs:	1
Different kinds of cancer, dependent on type of agent	
Unspecified sites and actions	7

(Estimates calculated from American Cancer Society. 1990. *Cancer facts and figures.*)

promoters of colon cancer, and saccharin acts as a promoter for cancer of the urinary bladder. The data from standard techniques of health risk analysis involving linear extrapolation of dose-effect experiments focusing on saccharin have been controversial. Extrapolation methods have yielded uninterpretable results because the techniques generally used for genotoxic carcinogens do not apply to promoting agents. New procedures to define the mode of action of epigenetic agents are needed for better epidemiological and biostatistical risk evaluation. Dose-response studies most likely will yield a typical pharmacologic S-shaped response, with a definite no-effect level.

Chemical carcinogens fall into two main groups: genotoxic carcinogens that are DNA reactive, and epigenetic agents that produce some other biological effect as the basis for their carcinogenicity (see table 7.2). Genotoxic carcinogens alter DNA and are mutagenic (Williams and Weisburger 1986; Witmer; Snyder, and Jollow et al. 1990; Rosenkranz 1988). Nongenotoxic carcinogens involve other yet-unclear mechanisms that possibly involve cytotoxicity, chronic tissue injury, hormonal imbalances, immunologic effects, or promotional activity (Butterworth and Slaga 1987). Delineating the role of each agent—genotoxic carcinogen, cocarcinogen, promoter)—in the overall carcinogenic process for specific cancers by uncovering the action mechanisms may be the basis for eventual risk assessment.

Further progress in understanding the mechanisms of carcinogenesis requires information about the nature of the agent—genotoxic or nongenotoxic—associated with the complex, causative factors for each human cancer type (see table 7.3). Reliable information is required on the amount and duration of exposure and, eventually, data on inhibition of the action of carcinogens may lead to effective prevention.

TESTS FOR CHEMICAL CARCINOGENS

Evaluation of human cancer hazards requires detection and quantitation of genotoxic chemicals and other agents that act as promoters or enhancers. If the progression from an initiated cell to a neoplasm is susceptible to external influences, procedures will be needed to detect chemicals affecting that part of the process. Systematic *in vitro* and *in vivo* tests are able to detect and classify chemicals as operating by genotoxic or by epigenetic mechanisms; i.e., whether they play a role in the carcinogenic process by modifying DNA and the genetic apparatus, or by other, usually enhancing, actions. Following is a brief review of efficient approaches to carcinogen bioassay by the "Decision Point Approach" (Williams and Weisburger 1986; table 7.9). The methods used at each point are detailed in a monograph by Milman and Weisburger (1985).

Because virtually all human cancers involve genotoxic carcinogens, their detection is most important. Rapid bioassays have been developed to disclose DNA-reactive carcinogens (Rosenkranz 1988; Milman and Weisburger 1985). Such test systems have several components: one

Table 7.9
DECISION POINT APPROACH IN CARCINOGEN TESTING

A. Structure of chemical
B. *In vitro* short-term tests
   1. Bacterial mutagenesis
   2. Mammalian mutagenesis
   3. DNA repair
   4. Chromosome tests
   5. Cell transformation
Decision Point 1: Evaluation of all tests under A and B.
C. Tests for promoters
   1. *In vitro*
   2. *In vivo*
Decision Point 2: Evaluation of results from stages A–C.
D. Limited *in vivo* bioassays
   1. Altered foci induction in rodent liver
   2. Skin neoplasm induction in mice
   3. Pulmonary neoplasm induction in mice
   4. Breast cancer induction in female Sprague-Dawley rats
Decision Point 3: Evaluation from the beginning plus results from any of the appropriate tests under D.
E. Long-term bioassay
Decision Point 4: Final evaluation of all results available and application to health risk analysis. This evaluation must include data from stages A-C in order to provide the basis for mechanistic considerations.

provides the biochemical activation and detoxification system to mimic as closely as possible the situation prevailing *in vivo* in animals and human beings; the second is the indicator DNA and genetic material; and the third is the transfer of any DNA-reactive metabolite from its site of production to the indicator DNA. A set or battery of select tests provides better evidence about the potential carcinogenic properties of a chemical whether it be synthetic, naturally occurring, or related to human lifestyle activities.

A standard test in any battery is the *Salmonella typhimurium* bacterial mutation assay of Ames (Rosenkranz 1988). This test uses the S9 fraction of a liver homogenate that has the required metabolic capability for converting procarcinogens to reactive products, but has a low capability of detoxifying conjugation reactions. Thus, there could be false-positive results. Several flavones, for example quercetin, are positive in the standard Ames test, but in the presence of detoxification systems, and *in vivo*, these chemicals are negative (Williams and Weisburger 1986).

Freshly explanted hepatocytes, including human liver cells, have a biochemical competence mimicking the *in vivo* situation (Williams and Weisburger 1986). Also, hepatocytes have the indicator DNA in the same cell. A procedure developed by Williams detects DNA damage by carcinogens in hepatocytes. This system should be an essential part of a battery of *in vitro* bioassay systems to detect genotoxic chemicals. The hepatocyte test systems can be modified to use an *in vivo/in vitro* scheme (Rosenkranz 1988).

Other *in vitro* tests include cell transformation and sister chromatid exchange (SCE) (Rosenkranz 1988; Milman and Weisburger 1985; Cooper and Grover 1990). These tests also yield information on possible neoplasm-inducing properties in the broadest sense, but are not specific indicators of DNA-reactivity or genotoxicity. Because SCE can be detected in formed elements from blood, the SCE test could be used to detect possible exposure to harmful chemicals in the workplace. However, the results should be interpreted in light of corollary supporting facts and the possible lack of SCE specificity.

Immunoassays for specific carcinogen-DNA or carcinogen-protein adducts are being developed (Bartsch, Hemminki, and O'Neill 1988; Wogan 1989). Also of interest is a sensitive, widely applicable, novel means of determining the existence of DNA-carcinogen adducts by the 32-P postlabeling technique (Randerath, Randerath, and Danna et al. 1989).

A good approach to tests for promoting potential is based on interference with the function of gap junctions and interruption of intercellular communication in cell culture (Butterworth and Slaga 1987). Chemicals such as certain halogenated hydrocarbons, the antioxidant butylated hydroxytoluene (BHT), or bile acids are positive in this scheme.

The first *in vivo* test for promoters utilized mouse skin, with later studies involving colon, breast, liver, pancreas, and urinary bladder (American Health Foundation 1987; Butterworth and Slaga 1987; Montesano, Bartsch, Vainio et al. 1986). The evaluation of many recent bioassays for carcinogens has shown that a number of environmental chemicals, pesticides such as DDT and chlordane, and solvents such as trichloroethylene or perchloroethylene, usually led to liver neoplasms in the mouse strains, but not so in rats or hamsters. These mouse strains normally display spontaneous liver cancer with a high frequency of activated oncogenes in the neoplasms. When these kinds of compounds or their metabolites were tested for genotoxicity, they were overwhelmingly negative, but they were positive in mammalian cell tests for promoters. Thus, it seems that the finding of tumors in mouse liver was due to the promoting potential of chlorinated hydrocarbons, rather than a carcinogenic effect due to genotoxicity (Williams and Weisburger 1986; Butterworth and Slaga 1987). This mechanistic analysis of any carcinogenicity tests in rodents is important, for it permits sound, science-based extrapolations of risk to man.

If *in vitro* tests yield qualitative evidence that a chemical is a genotoxic carcinogen or a promoter, it is important to secure confirmation *in vivo* and at the same time generate information on potency. Specific rapid *in vivo* tests can accomplish this based on the probable genotoxic or promoting mechanisms of action (Williams and Weisburger 1986; Montesano, Bartsch, and Vainio et al. 1986).

The tests usually take less than one year to complete and include the induction of: abnormal foci in rodent liver; skin tumors in mice; mammary neoplasms in Sprague-Dawley female rats; and pulmonary tumors in sensitive strains of mice. Tests are conducted at a number of dose levels to provide a dose-response curve, relative to a known positive control carcinogen or promoter.

The tests can be designed to yield potency data for genotoxic initiators, relative to suitable known positive control carcinogens, by administering one or a few doses followed by an appropriate promoter. For tests of promoters, a genotoxic carcinogen for a specific target organ is given, followed by the test substance at four to five dose levels. An appropriate positive control promoter given at several dose levels will provide information on relative potency.

Three end points are quantified in these *in vivo* bioassay systems: percent of animals with histopathologically validated lesions; the multiplicity and size of neoplasms; and the expression time from exposure to occurrence of tumor. Overall, the battery of data generated by *in vitro* tests for genotoxicity or promoting potential, with properly designed and limited *in vivo* bioassays most often provides an adequate data base necessary to protect the public. By applying the current understanding of cancer causation, and in the light of data from short-term *in vitro* tests for genotoxicity and possible promoting substances, the standard long-term bioassay in rodents may no longer be essential.

Abbreviated carcinogen bioassay procedures can be

carried out economically to provide data that can forecast potential carcinogenic hazards and analyze health hazards. These rapid tests are as efficient as the cumbersome, time-consuming, and expensive long-term bioassays (Milman and Weisburger 1985; Montesano, Bartsch, and Vainio et al. 1986). Advances in molecular biology may mean further improvement in diagnosing potential cancer risks. For example, some genotoxic carcinogens lead to activation of cellular proto-oncogenes, which may be efficient at determining whether a given chemical could cause cancer (Barbacid 1986; Aaronson, Bishop, and Sugimura et al. 1987; Rich, Hager, and Lopez 1988; Sager 1989; Weinberg 1989). The method of 32-P postlabeling of DNA-carcinogen adducts is a highly sensitive procedure that rapidly generates precise information on such adducts (Randerath, Randerath, and Danna et al. 1989). Better knowledge of the promotion mechanisms may also contribute new test systems for detection of promoters.

LIFESTYLE-RELATED CANCERS

Knowledge about etiologic factors for the prevalent types of human cancer indicates that the use of tobacco products and prevailing nutritional traditions account for the occurrence of those cancers (Parkin, Laara, and Muir 1988; U.S.P.H.S. National Cancer Institute 1988). Tobacco-associated neoplasms and nutritional elements are detailed in other chapters; here the emphasis is on the relevant mechanisms and how they can be applied to risk reduction and prevention (see table 7.7). Because they presumably involve viruses, leukemias and lymphomas of cryptogenic etiology will not be covered in this chapter.

TOBACCO

Although tobacco has been used for centuries, commercially manufactured cigarettes were introduced at the beginning of this century. In the Western world, men became heavy users about the time of World War I and women about the time of World War II (U.S.P.H.S. 1982; Zaridze and Peto 1986; Ernster 1988; Wynder 1988). The custom of smoking cigarettes in Japan and some African countries started somewhat later. On the other hand, the tradition of chewing tobacco and betel nuts has long been practiced in the Asian subcontinent, India, Pakistan, and southern Soviet Union; snuff dipping is more common in Scandinavia (U.S.P.H.S. 1986; Hoffmann and Hecht 1990).

Cigarette smoking is directly associated with emphysema and lung cancer and has been linked with cancers of the pancreas, kidney, urinary bladder, and renal pelvis. It also carries the risk of fatal myocardial infarction (U.S.P.H.S. 1982; Zaridze and Peto 1986; Hoffmann and Hecht 1990; Benowitz 1988). Chewing or dipping of tobacco with or without other ingredients such as betel nut increases the risk for cancers of the oral cavity and esophagus.

The American Cancer Society, American Health Foundation, American Heart Association, American Medical Association, and United States Public Health Service have warned the public about the risks of tobacco use. An impressive decline among the number of men, especially white men, who smoke has occurred in the last 20 years (McGinnis, Shopland, and Brown 1987; Ernster, 1988; U.S.P.H.S. National Cancer Institute 1988; Wynder 1988). In the 1950s, 64% of American men were smokers; currently only 31% smoke. The decline since 1982 in lung cancer rates in white men is a dramatic success for preventive medicine. What would the incidence and mortality of the smoking-related diseases be without this reduction?

CARCINOGENS AND PROMOTERS IN TOBACCO PRODUCTS
Tobacco smoke contains a number of polycyclic aromatic hydrocarbons such as benzo(a)pyrene or dibenzo-(a,h)anthracene that are powerful carcinogens and mutagens (U.S.P.H.S. 1982; Hoffmann and Hecht 1990). Tobacco smoke and unburned tobacco, used for chewing or snuff dipping, also contains several potent nitrosamines, e.g., nitrosonornicotine and related compounds that are produced from nicotine during the tobacco curing process. These compounds are also produced during combustion and *in vivo* from nitric oxides, nicotine, and related alkaloids (Zaridze and Peto 1986; Hecht and Hoffmann 1988; Hoffman and Hecht 1990). In addition, burning tobacco leads to certain carcinogenic heterocyclic amines (Sato, Seino, and Ohka et al. 1977). These chemicals are all genotoxic carcinogens and mutagens that may be keys in the initiation and causation of specific types of cancer.

Tobacco and its smoke contain sizable amounts of cocarcinogens and promoters, such as phenolic compounds and terpenes that are neither carcinogenic nor genotoxic (U.S.P.H.S. 1982; Zaridze and Peto 1986; Hoffmann and Hecht 1990). However, they are major players in the eventual occurrence of lung cancer and account for: the long latent period usually associated with tobacco smoking; the steep rise in disease risk with increasing use of more than 20 cigarettes per day; and the lowered risk of lung cancer upon cessation of smoking through the elimination of the promoting action. The adverse effects of smoking or other tobacco use are highly dose-dependent and are reversible to some extent because of the action of promoters. This science base thus accounts for the fact that cessation by habitual smokers or chewers of tobacco results in a progressively lower cancer risk.

ALCOHOL AS A COCARCINOGEN
Individuals who smoke cigarettes and drink a considerable amount of alcoholic beverages per day are at a high risk of developing cancers of the oral cavity and esophagus. Because alcohol modifies the metabolism of carcinogens in the liver and esophagus (Seitz and Simanowski 1988; Lieber and Garro 1990), it has a role

in the induction of cancer in select organs by increasing the effectiveness of carcinogens, especially in producing increased amounts of reactive ultimate carcinogenic metabolites from procarcinogens in tobacco.

KIDNEY AND BLADDER CANCER

These cancers are considered together even though specific agents may have the property of inducing cancer in either kidney or bladder (U.S.P.H.S. 1982). The main known element yielding both types of cancers is chronic tobacco smoking; however, kidney and bladder cancers are also seen in nonsmokers and the etiologic agents are unknown. Historically, bladder and renal pelvis were targets of high-level occupational exposure to certain aromatic amines such as 4-aminobiphenyl or 2-naphthylamine that were intermediates in the production of dyestuffs (Searle 1984; Maltoni and Selikoff 1988). In most countries these hazardous chemicals are no longer produced, or are manufactured in hermetically sealed vessels that minimize human exposure.

NUTRITION

Many types of cancer have an unequal incidence as a function of where people live (Parkin, Laara, and Muir 1988; Joossens, Hill, and Geboers 1985; Wynder and Hiyama 1987). Pockets of both high and relatively low incidence occur within the same countries. In many instances the geographic site of current or longest residence eventually controls the specific risk for different types of neoplasms. Western diets high in fat, typically 40% of calories, are considered promoters and are correlated with a higher risk for cancers of the large bowel, breast, prostate, ovary, endometrium, and pancreas (American Health Foundation 1987; U.S.P.H.S. 1988; Ip, Birt, and Rogers et al. 1986; Kroes et al. 1986; Rose, Boyar, and Wynder 1986; Furihata and Matsushima 1986; Schiffman 1986) (fig. 7.2). Genotoxic carcinogens in food may be derived from various sources, such as broiled or fried meat and fish (colon or breast cancer); pickled or smoked foods (gastric or esophageal cancer); or contaminant aflatoxins (liver cancer) (see table 7.6).

GENOTOXIC CARCINOGENS

GASTRIC CANCER

Populations at high risk for developing gastric cancer usually have diets including large quantities of dried salted fish, pickled vegetables, and smoked fish and low quantities of seasonal fresh fruits and vegetables. This results in a concomitant lower intake of vitamins C, E, and A (Howson, Hiyama, and Wynder 1986; Weisburger 1987; Joossens, Hill, and Geboers 1985). Descendants of Japanese migrants in Hawaii consume more uncooked vegetables like celery, lettuce, and tomatoes, as well as fresh fruit juices and have a lower gastric cancer risk

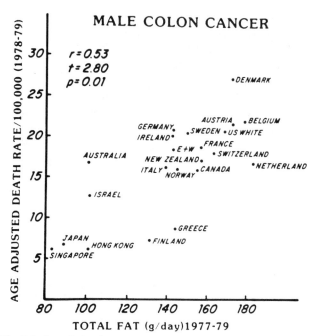

Fig. 7.2. Correlation between per capita consumption of dietary fat and age-adjusted mortality from colon cancer (males). Note the overall relationship of colon cancer risk and total fat, with the important exception of Finland, accounted for by a protective effect of bran cereal fiber intake, customarily eaten in that country, and a high intake of calcium from dairy products. Another apparent exception, Greece, may relate to the use of olive oil. (Data derived from Kurihara, M.; Aoki, K.; and Tominaga, S., eds. 1984. *Cancer mortality statistics in the world.* Nagoya, Japan: University of Nagoya Press; also from a publication prepared by the Basic Data Unit, Statistics Division, Food and Agriculture Organization of the United Nations (FAO). 1984. *Food balance sheets 1979-81 average.* Rome: Food and Agriculture Organization.)

compared with native Japanese. The active carcinogens may be nitroso indoles or diazonium compounds formed from nitrite and specific substrates. Vitamins C and E may block the formation of such agents (Machlin and Bendich 1987). Salt can act as a cocarcinogen in gastric carcinogenesis and also leads to atrophic gastritis, a postulated precursor of cancer (Joossens, Hill, and Geboers 1985). Furthermore, salt appears to be the common element in the stroke-stomach cancer mortality relationship observed as a significant cross-national covariation (figs. 7.3 and 7.4). Lower intake of salted, pickled, and smoked food would lower the risk of gastric cancer, hypertension, and stroke. Decreased use of nitrite-preserved or smoked foods and the increased year-round supply of fresh fruits and vegetables probably accounts for the large decline in gastric cancer in the United States (Howson, Hiyama, and Wynder 1986). The risk factors for esophageal cancer associated with salted and pickled foods and low fresh vegetable and fruit intake in China and other Asian countries are similar (O'Neill, Chen, and Bartsch 1990), although the substrates, distinct types of fish or vegetables preserved by nitrite treatment, are different. In the Hong Kong vicinity, nasopharyngeal cancer is common (Ning, Yu, and Wang et al. 1990). This disease has been induced in rats by feeding them specific types of fish pickled with salt and nitrite; some viral agents may also be involved.

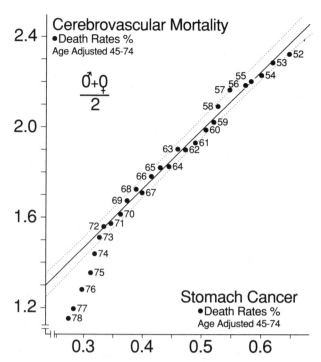

Fig. 7.3. Nutritional customs, specifically the intake of pickled, salted foods and low intake of fresh fruit, vegetables, and milk, are associated with hypertension, cerebrovascular disease, and gastric cancer risk. Progressive changes in nutritional traditions have lowered mortality from gastric cancer and stroke shown in data from seven countries as a function of time, from 1952 to 1978. The greater drop in stroke mortality since 1970 may reflect improved medical management of hypertension. (Reprinted with permission from: Joossens, Hill, and Geboers eds. [1985].)

COLON AND BREAST CANCERS

When fish and meat are broiled or fried certain potent mutagenic compounds are formed; these are potent mutagens according to the Ames assay. The agents also induce DNA repair in hepatocytes in the Williams test for genotoxicity. Several of these mutagens have been structurally identified as heterocyclic amines such as 2-amino-3-methylimidazo[4,5-f]quinoline (IQ) and related compounds (MeIQ and MeIQx), which structurally resemble the known potent colon, mammary gland, and prostate carcinogen, 3,2'-dimethy1-4-amino-biphenyl. In rats, IQ and related heterocyclic amines are potent carcinogens that cause neoplasms in the mammary gland, colon, liver, pancreas, bladder, and other tissues. Frying and broiling, then, may be the sources of carcinogens for these target organs (Weisburger 1987; Furihata and Matsushima 1986; Schiffman 1986; Hatch, Knize, and Healy et al. 1988). However, a recent epidemiologic study in Utah has failed to find an association between cancer and a diet including fried or broiled meat five years prior to a diagnosis of colon cancer (Lyon and Mahoney 1988). One reason may have been that people in Utah display a generally lower risk of colon cancer and a relevant comparison would be between lifelong vegetarians and meat users. Antioxidants such as propyl gallate or BHA, soy protein, and certain indole-containing amino acids (tryptophan and proline) effectively inhibit the formation of these carcinogens during the frying of meat. Such additives may be a practical way to reduce

the formation of heterocyclic amines carcinogens (Jones and Weisburger 1988).

Direct-acting mutagens called fecapentaenes have been observed in the stools of about 10% to 20% of people consuming a typical Western high-fat, low-fiber diet (Schiffman 1986). Fecapentaenes are produced by certain bacteria; bile acids and anaerobic storage stimulate their formation. They display weak carcinogenicity in newborn mice. Carcinogenicity has been questionable at intrarectal-infusion dose levels 10 times higher than those equivalent to the mutagenic activity found in positive humans.

Ketosteroids found in feces, specifically 4-cholesten-3-one, are not mutagenic but induce nuclear aberrations and sister chromatid exchanges upon intrarectal instillation in mice (Bruce 1987). Such positive tests are not sufficient to classify these cholesterol metabolites as genotoxic, and their role in colon carcinogenesis awaits more research data.

LIVER CANCER

The overall incidence of primary hepatocellular carcinoma has declined in the United States in the last 50

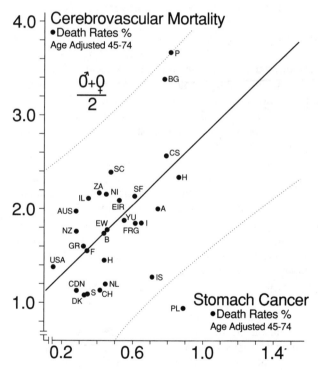

Fig. 7.4. Geographic pathology delineates similar prevalence of risk factors for cerebrovascular mortality and for gastric cancer in specific countries. J = Japan; P = Portugal; BG = Bulgaria; PL = Poland; IS = Iceland; DK = Denmark; S = Sweden; CH = Switzerland; F = France; NL = Netherlands; N = Norway; B = Belgium; EW = England and Wales; YU = Yugoslavia; FRG = West Germany; I = Italy; A = Austria; H = Hungary; CS = Czechoslovakia; SF = Finland; EIR = Ireland; SC = Scotland; NI = Northern Ireland; ZA = South Africa; IL = Israel; GR = Greece; NZ = New Zealand; AUS = Australia; CDN = Canada; USA = United States. Some outliers reflect specific customs; e.g., Iceland with a higher use of smoked foods has a risk factor for gastric cancer but not for hypertension-stroke, which is related to salt use or lack of dairy products. (Reprinted with permission from: Joossens, Hill, and Geboers eds. [1985].)

years (U.S.P.H.S. National Cancer Institute 1988). In parts of Africa, however, it is a major neoplasm affecting men more than women (Parkin, Laara, and Muir 1988). The assumed etiologic factors are dietary, specifically certain genotoxic mycotoxins and liver-specific carcinogens found in plants; and high titers of hepatitis B antigen. However, the relative importance of these factors in the occurrence of liver cancer is not known. Current efforts to vaccinate people against the hepatitis B antigen will delay or perhaps abolish primary liver cancer in the high-incidence countries (Harris and Sun 1987). The mycotoxins are genotoxic carcinogens and exposure to them begins *in utero* and continues throughout life; these conditions favor the occurrence of disease (Searle 1984; Montesano, Bartsch, and Vainio et al. 1986; Wogan 1989; Cooper and Grover 1990). The hepatitis B antigen apparently acts as a cocarcinogen through its cytotoxicity that leads to liver necrosis and chronic regeneration. On the other hand, data indicate that the hepatitis B antigen genome modifies host DNA leading to neoplastic transformation, so that the risk of hepatocellular carcinoma would stem from the additive interaction of two genotoxic carcinogens.

Chronic alcoholic beverage intake induces cirrhosis, a lesion that raises liver cell turnover and acts as an enhancing factor for primary hepatocellular carcinoma with as yet unknown genotoxic carcinogens, perhaps mycotoxins or hepatitis B antigen, or both (Seitz and Simanowski 1988; Lieber and Garro 1990). Those factors may also play a role in the Orient. In addition, salting and pickling may generate certain liver-specific nitrosamines (O'Neill, Chen, and Bartsch 1990).

High-level occupational exposure of reactor cleaners to vinyl chloride has induced angiosarcoma of the liver (Swanson 1988; Searle 1984; Maltoni and Selikoff 1988). Despite the widespread occurrence of low levels of demonstrated rodent liver carcinogens (carbon tetrachloride, trichloroethylene, polychlorinated biphenyls) there are no data that the prevailing low contamination has caused liver cancer in man. In the Western world contamination, especially of water, is frequent yet liver cancer is relatively infrequent.

A small number of benign liver neoplasms has been seen in young women taking oral contraceptives. The mechanism of this is obscure and must be ascribed to a combination of unknown etiologic factors, since the number of cases is small, considering the widespread use of oral contraceptives. However, because of their hemorrhagic nature, these tumors can be fatal.

PROMOTING-EPIGENETIC PHENOMENA

DATA IN HUMANS

Cancers of the breast, prostate, distal colon, pancreas, ovary, and endometrium display a parallel incidence pattern in most countries (Parkin, Laara, and Muir 1988; Joossens, Hill, and Geboers 1985; Wynder and Hiyama 1987; Ip, Birt, and Rogers et al. 1986; Rose,

Boyar, and Wynder 1986). Much of the Western world shows a high incidence of these cancers, but incidence has been low in Japan, China, and the Arctic areas. As nutritional customs become Westernized in those low-risk countries, the frequency of those cancers increases (fig. 7.5). The major environmental lifestyle element associated with disease risk has been the total fat intake, measured in general by fat disappearance data from each region (Simopoulos 1987; Hill 1987). Some exceptions to this correlation have been the key to understanding the underlying mechanisms. Thus, in the Mediterranean region the total fat intake is lower than in other parts of the Western world, but it is highly relevant that the main fat used is olive oil, a non-cancer promoting monounsaturated fat (Ip, Birt, and Rogers et al. 1986; Rose, Boyar, and Wynder 1986). Another key exception is the Arctic population (Eskimos) where the total fat intake is as high as in the West—about 40% to 45% of calories—but the fats and oils are derived from fish and seal and are therefore composed mainly of the protective omega-3 fatty acids (American Health Foundation 1987; Ip, Birt, and Rogers et al. 1986). In Finland, particularly rural areas, there is a high total fat intake, especially of saturated fats, but the colon cancer rate is low and of the same order of magnitude as in

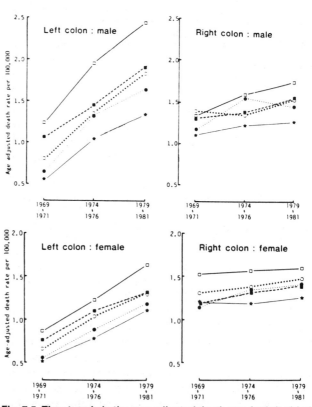

Fig. 7.5. Time trends in the age-adjusted death rate for left-sided and right-sided colon cancer in five areas of Japan: metropolitan cities (□); large cities (■); medium-sized cities (○); small cities (●); counties (*). Note that considerable increases were found for distal colon cancer and only slight changes for proximal colon cancer, documenting the need to examine time trends separately for proximal and distal colon cancer and also rectal cancer. The rapid increase in distal colon cancer appears to be associated with the contemporary rise in fat intake. (Reprinted with permission from: Tajima et al. [1985].)

Japan; the breast cancer rate is also lower compared with Denmark, for example (American Health Foundation 1987; Cummings and Bingham 1987; Rose 1990). The explanation for this is a substantially higher cereal bran fiber consumption.

DATA IN ANIMAL MODELS

For the last 20 to 30 years rats, mice, and hamsters have been available as animal models for studying cancers of the breast, colon, and pancreas. When animals are given a carcinogen that induces cancer in one of these target organs and are fed a nutritional regimen of 10% fat calories, mimicking the situation in the Orient, they invariably display a considerably lower incidence of these neoplasms than when the fat level is equivalent to 40% of calories, mimicking the Western dietary environment (American Health Foundation 1987; Ip, Birt, and Rogers et al. 1986; Cohen 1987). Although a high total fat level increases tumor yield, there have been exceptions. When olive oil or Menhaden oil was used, no significant increase in tumors was noted at any fat level. Thus, these laboratory models fairly reproduce the situation found in the Mediterranean countries in regard to olive oil, or the Arctic countries in regard to fish oils.

MECHANISMS PRODUCING COLON CANCER

This important digestive organ actually represents three distinct segments of the gut. No known mechanisms account for the causes of cancer in the proximal (right side) of the colon and cecum. Colon cancer at that site has a fairly uniform distribution around the world. Where site data are available, the incidence in high-risk regions for proximal colon cancer is only slightly more than the lower-risk areas. The associated risk factors have not yet been delineated. Inclusion of proximal colon cancer in associations between nutrition and colon cancer have led to confusion since proximal colon cancer does not seem to be affected by fat intake, for example (Ziegler, Devesa, and Fraumeni 1986; Weisburger and Wynder 1987).

DISTAL COLON CANCER: ROLE OF FAT

Cancer of the distal (left side) colon and the sigmoid junction, which has a high incidence in the Western world and a much lower incidence in Japan, the Arctic areas, and in Finland, seems to be associated with the type and amount of fat consumed. A high-fat intake pattern controls cholesterol biosynthesis, in turn related to the total bile acid flow, particularly the secondary bile acid level in the intestinal tract. Metabolism by the intestinal flora in part controls bile acid activities and intestinal pH, also a function of several types of fiber and other breakdown products (Rowland 1988). Laboratory experiments have demonstrated that bile acids are not carcinogens. Despite some claims to the contrary, they are not converted to carcinogens, but have been shown to be promoters (American Health Foundation 1987; Weisburger and Wynder 1987). In carcinogenesis, promoters are highly dose dependent. Reducing the concentration of bile acids by lowering fat intake, as is true in Japan by about a factor of 3, appreciably lowers risk. The level of bile acids responds rapidly to the amount of total fat in the diet; decreasing fat intake yields within days a lower bile acid level in the gut, representing a lower promoting potential (Hill 1971; fig. 7.6). This has immediate clinical application, for upon surgical removal of polyps or tumors, patients would be expected to have a much lower recurrence rate if they were on a low-fat diet (Weisburger and Wynder 1987).

ROLE OF FIBER

Finland's lower colon cancer incidence can be explained by the higher cereal fiber intake in the form of porridge and rye bread made from whole grains (American Health Foundation 1987; Joossens, Hill, and Geboers 1985; Cummings and Bingham 1987; Rowland 1988). This results in a greater stool bulk (about 250 g/day) compared with the daily intake in Denmark or the United States (stool about 80 g/day) where such comparative studies have been undertaken. The additional fiber dilutes the concentration of bile acids in the gut and reduces the promoting potential. Other populations, such as lacto-ovo vegetarians or Mormons in Utah who consume appreciable amounts of fat but at the same time eat whole grain cereal foods, likewise have a lower risk for left-sided colon cancer. Other vegetables and fruits provide different types of fiber that do not necessarily increase stool bulk as does cereal, but do so through other mechanisms; thus the frequent intake of various kinds of vegetables and fruits is desirable. Animal models also demonstrate the effects of fat and fiber (American Health Foundation 1987; Sinkeldarn, Kuper, and Boland 1990).

ROLE OF CALCIUM

Wargowich, Newmark, and Bruce (Bruce 1987) first observed the moderating effects of calcium in colon carcinogenesis in animal models. This finding was applied by Lipkin and Newmark (Lipkin 1988; Newmark, Lipkin, and Mareshwari 1990) to the clinical situation among nonpolyposis families at high risk for colon cancer who display a high intestinal cell turnover rate. Increasing their calcium intake dramatically lowered cell turnover rates; thus the mechanisms of carcinogenesis suggest that a proportion of risk can be attributed to cell turnover rates. The lower colon cancer risk seen in Finland may relate to the customary higher intake of calcium-rich dairy products and to the effect of cereal fiber already described. Optimally, an adequate intake of calcium and other desirable micronutrients is obtained through the use of low-fat dairy products, skim milk, and some types of fish, e.g., sardines, in which the bones are normally eaten (Sorenson, Slattery, and Ford 1988).

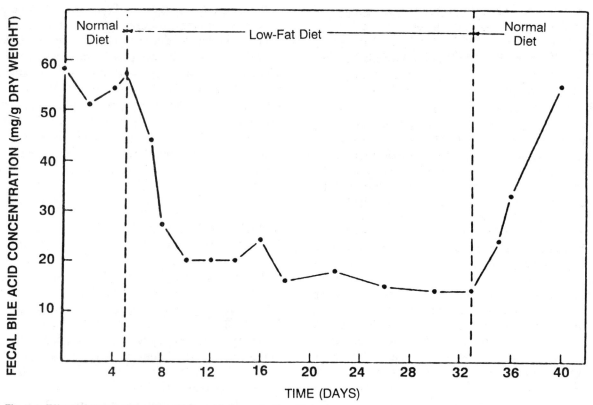

Fig. 7.6. Effect of dietary fat on fecal bile acid concentration. Volunteers on a normal British diet of 100-120 g fat/day were placed on a low-fat diet of less than 30 g fat/day. Note the rapid lowering of the fecal bile acid concentration that remained fairly constant and low throughout the low-fat diet. Upon return to the high-fat normal diet, the fecal bile acid concentration rapidly rose to the previous level (Hill [1971]).

RECTAL CANCER

The incidence and mortality data for rectal cancer need to be reviewed critically on a worldwide basis (Wynder and Hiyama 1987; Ziegler, Devesa, and Fraumeni 1986; Weisburger and Wynder 1987). Only in the last 10 to 15 years has there been general agreement on defining the rectum as constituting the tissue 8 cm from the anal verge, in contrast to the recto-sigmoid area. Little information exists on etiological factors, and virtually nothing is known about any genotoxic carcinogens specifically affecting the rectum. There is some parallelism between the occurrence of rectal cancer and distal colon cancer. However, in the United States the male-to-female ratio for rectal cancer is 1.4:1, but for colon cancer it is about 1:1. Rectal cancer is declining in the United States, but distal colon cancer in men is not. A weak association is noted in international data between distal colon and rectal cancers, possibly due to a promoting element like bile acids common to both cancer sites. This association may be spurious since, unlike the distal colon, the rectum is usually not bathed continuously by the intestinal contents. Some epidemiological studies have associated the intake of alcoholic beverages to rectal cancer (Seitz and Simanowski 1988; Klatsky, Armstrong, and Friedman et al. 1988; Lieber and Garro 1990). Laboratory studies attempting to explore alcohol's role have for the most part been fruitless, but Seitzes' group has found that alcohol stimulates cell cycling in rat rectum. Alcohol would be classified as a cocarcinogen.

PANCREAS CANCER

The worldwide occurrence of pancreatic cancer generally parallels that of colon cancer (Parkin, Laara, and Muir 1988; Wynder and Hiyama 1987), and cigarette smoking has been pinpointed as an additional risk factor. This may partially account for the increase of pancreatic cancer in the United States from 1950 to 1975, in contrast to the unchanging incidence of colon cancer (Wynder 1988). Two distinct animal models, a nitrosamine in the hamster and azaserine in the rat, demonstrate that cancer incidence is proportional to the dietary fat content (Ip, Birt, and Rogers et al. 1986). The mechanisms whereby tobacco smoke and diet account for increased risk are not yet resolved. Although recently a low, chronic intake of NNK, a tobacco-specific nitrosamine, has induced pancreas cancer (Hoffmann and Hecht 1990).

ENDOCRINE-RELATED CANCERS

Breast and prostate cancers are prevalent in the Western world but have considerably lower incidence in Japan and the Arctic countries and intermediate rates in Italy, Greece, and Finland (Parkin, Laara, and Muir 1988; Rich, Hager, and Lopez 1988; Rose, Boyar, and Wynder 1986; Rohan and Bain 1986). Whereas migrants from a lower-risk area for colon cancer, such as Japan, develop the risk of the new place of residence, such as Hawaii or the United States, within the same generation, the increased risk for the endocrine-related cancers is usually found in the offspring of the migrant population (Wynder and Hiyama 1987). Analyses of the difference between breast and colon cancer risks suggest that the time of the endocrine system's differentiation is a critical period, and that external influences such as proper diet can play a major role in controlling relative sensitivity or resistance (Weisburger 1987).

Three different models have been found useful for the study of mechanisms in breast cancer induction (Ip, Birt, and Rogers et al. 1986; American Health Foundation 1987; Cohen 1987). Strains of mice bearing the mammary tumor virus eventually develop breast cancer. When female rats of the Sprague-Dawley and derived strains (Wistar or Buffalo) are given the experimental carcinogen 7,12-dimethylbenz(a)anthracene as a single bolus on day 55, breast cancer is induced within nine months. N-nitrosomethylurea administered IV or parenterally likewise leads to breast cancer, but the regimen is less sensitive to the initial age of exposure since metabolism of the carcinogen is not essential to its action. In all three models, the animals fed a low-fat diet have a lower tumor yield than those that are fed a high-fat diet. These results are obtained with many types of commonly used fats, but exceptions were that Menhaden and olive oils yielded about the same incidence when fed at 20% or 40% fat calories. These models, together with human studies, have been useful in investigating mechanisms (American Health Foundation 1987).

There is presently no useful model to investigate dietary factors in prostate cancer.

The development of cancer in the endocrine-sensitive tissues (breast, ovary, endometrium, and prostate) appears to be related to hormonal control and balance. The entire complex, feedback-controlled interaction between hormones from the pituitary gland, in turn controlled by neuroendocrine hypothalamic stimuli, and the hormones of the ovary, testes, adrenals, thyroid, and liver and kidney concerned with steroid hormone metabolism is being studied. Nutritional factors, particularly fats and proteins, control endocrine metabolism and balance, yet studies have not been able to pinpoint the role of dietary elements in influencing endocrine balances or specific hormone levels in relation to cancer of the endocrine-related organs. Protein hormones have been analyzed by specific radioimmunoassays with specific protein hormones used to generate reagents. The reagents may have been too specific and not representative of the active bioassayable amount of protein hormone. Studies of hormone-binding globulins and specific hormone receptors have revealed that the levels of estrogen and androgen unbound by globulin in the blood may be the factor associated with disease risk. Considering the dramatic incidence variations of these cancers in different countries perhaps attributable to diet, it is surprising that the relationship between diet and endocrine-related causes has not been resolved (Rich, Hager, and Lopez 1988; Ip, Birt, and Rogers et al. 1986; Simopolous 1987; Boyar, Rose, and Wynder 1988).

More recent findings associating lower risk in populations consuming fish oils with specific intracellular effectors in the form of prostaglandin metabolites have drawn attention to important clues accounting for dietary effects. Mechanistic studies in animal models have arrived at these same conclusions as did the investigations in humans. Despite the need to pursue more research on the effect of diet in carcinogenesis and development of invasive metastasizing cancer in the endocrine-related organs, the total information available indicates that a low-risk situation for all of these cancers is one where: (a) the total fat intake is relatively low, about 20% of calories, or the main fat component of the diet is a monounsaturated fat such as olive oil, or the diet is rich in omega-3 polyunsaturated fatty acids as in fish oils, or a combination thereof; (b) an important time frame for a low-fat diet, which in part decides risk, is during the development of the endocrine system at puberty; and (c) a dietary change from high risk to low risk can occur at any age because of the reversibility and flexibility associated with endocrine systems (Prentice, Kakar, and Hursting et al. 1988; Greenwald, Cullen, and McKenna 1987).

ENDOMETRIAL CANCER

In the Western world, many women with severe menopausal symptoms have been treated with pharmacological replacement of estrogen and conjugated estrogen in appreciable doses. During the late 1960s, women on such estrogen replacement therapy were found to be prone to develop endometrial cancer. When the practice of estrogen replacement stopped, the number of women presenting with this condition decreased (Schottenfeld and Fraumeni 1982). This finding confirms the reversibility of hormone promotion at any age. A change in diet toward lower promoting potential would also reduce disease risk in the endocrine-sensitive tissues. Drug manufacturers now are providing estrogen replacement drugs with a considerably lower level of estrogen, which should have a lower cancer-producing risk. Furthermore, the previously used high estrogen level was not balanced by progesterone, which may have played a role in cancer development. Some endocrine preparations that include small amounts of estrogen and progesterone are available and may ameliorate the postmenstrual syndrome, including the risk for osteoporosis, without increasing cancer risk.

Obesity is a major risk factor for endometrial cancer because fat cells readily produce estrogen, itself a key effector in inducing neoplastic disease in the endometrium (Wynder and Hiyama 1987).

CERVICAL CANCER

Cervical cancer, a major cancer in neoplasia in developing countries, has an inverse relationship to socioeconomic status. It appears to be associated with sexual intercourse, often under conditions of poor sexual hygiene, including sex with uncircumcised men. Circumcision and proper sexual hygiene helps in preventing this disease. The causative element may be the Epstein-Barr virus, *Herpes simplex* virus, or human papilloma types of viruses (Koutsky, Galloway, and Holmes 1986; Howley 1987; Knox and Woodman 1988; zur Hausen 1989), or analogous elements. Cigarette smoking appears to increase the risk. (U.S.P.H.S. 1982; Wynder 1988). Early detection through the widespread use of the Pap smear test and prompt treatment have lowered mortality appreciably in the last 50 years. The Pap test also can detect dysplasia (precursors of cancer) which can be treated in order to prevent cancer from developing.

CONCLUSIONS

Carcinogenesis occurs through a number of successive steps, all of which are needed for clinically invasive cancer to develop. Studies in animal models have reproducibly documented this and it seems reasonable to assume that the initiation, development, and progression of human cancers follow such a scheme.

The early lesions are the result of neoplastic changes caused by adequate amounts of genotoxic carcinogens in an occupational setting or specific carcinogens or mixtures associated with lifestyle, including tobacco use or nutritional traditions. Genotoxic carcinogens in tobacco smoke, such as polycyclic aromatic hydrocarbons and the nicotine alkaloid-derived nitrosamines, are associated with respiratory cancer. Nitrosamines, also present in tobacco used for chewing and snuff dipping, affect the oral cavity and esophagus. Genotoxic carcinogens are formed in salted, pickled, or smoked foods, or *in vivo* from nitrate and nitrite, and relate to gastric or esophageal cancer risk, especially when not offset by the presence of vitamin C, vitamin E, or other antioxidants, and nitrite traps. Instead of salting and pickling, we now refrigerate or freeze foods. Fresh fruits and vegetables are now available year-round instead of seasonally, which accounts for the progressive lowering of gastric cancer risk. For other nutritionally linked cancers, research begins to validate the view that the mutagens/carcinogens in fried and broiled foods, with which meat-eating populations have extensive contact, may be associated with the occurrence of colon, breast, or pancreas cancers. Simple, effective means have been developed to decrease the formation of those carcinogens during cooking.

Epigenetic agents (promoters) are major players in the development of many human cancers; they can also be reproduced in animal models for these cancers. Fractions of tobacco smoke contain enhancers and promoters that are essential to the development of respiratory tract cancers. The major promoting element for the nutritionally linked cancers is the level of dietary fat, traditionally 40% to 45% of calories in the Western diet. The mechanism whereby fat translates to risk has been well-outlined for colon cancer where there is a relationship between the amount of fat consumed, the quantity of cholesterol biosynthesized in the liver, and the amount of bile acids in the colon. A reduction of the concentration of bile acids either by a lower intake of dietary fat or by an increased luminal bulk produced by cereal fiber, or both, significantly lowers the incidence of colon cancer. Support for this concept comes from the comparison of the high incidence of colon cancer in the Western world with the low incidence in Japan, where the dietary fat level is 10% to 20% of calories, or the lower incidence in Finland, where the dietary fiber level, and thence stool bulk, is high. In addition, comparative studies of human fecal bile acid concentrations in diverse populations in New York, Finland, Denmark, and Japan provide metabolic evidence relating percent of dietary fat to fecal bile acid concentrations.

Not all fats have identical effects. The omega-6 polyunsaturated lipids, so beneficial in lowering serum cholesterol, are better promoters than mostly saturated fats such as lard or beef fat. On the other hand, monounsaturated oils such as olive oil have little promoting effect, and omega-3 polyunsaturated-rich fish oils appear protective. All of these fats and oils have identical caloric content and caloric availability, so their dramatic difference in promoting breast or colon cancer cannot be explained by calories alone. Dietary restriction experiments have demonstrated a lower breast and colon cancer incidence even when high-fat diets were fed (Lyon, Mahoney, and West et al. 1987; Pariza 1988). It has been known for a long time that dietary restriction depresses cancer development and this has been explained by showing that cell cycling in major organs is reduced by dietary restriction (Albanes and Winick 1988; Lok, Nera, and Iverson et al. 1988; Weindruch and Walford 1988). The importance of cell cycle frequency in controlling the sensitivity of cells to genotoxic carcinogens and in furthering the growth, development, and progression needs greater emphasis. This factor links many previously unrelated phenomena, and its relevance to carcinogenesis is the product of recent research (Weisburger 1987; Lipkin 1988; Albanes and Winick 1988; Ponz de Leon, Roncucci, and Di Donato et al. 1988). Weight control is an important health-promoting, disease-prevention action, but the role of certain lipids in increasing cancer risks is undeniable; this suggests the benefit of limiting intake to 20% of calories.

Bivalent ions such as calcium can bind bile acids, decrease cell cycle time, and may play a role in lowering the colon-cancer risk (Lipkin 1988; Sorenson, Slattery, and Ford 1988; Newark, Lipkin and Maheshwari 1990). Calcium ions are also beneficial in controlling the $Na^+/K^+ + Ca^{++}$ balances that affect hypertension, and the role in preventing osteoporosis is also well known. Excellent sources of calcium are low-fat dairy products, skim milk, or for lactose-intolerant persons, fat-free yogurt. Use of dairy products is favored over calcium preparations alone, since these natural sources provide a balanced Ca/P and vitamin D ratio. All in all, appropriate intake of low-fat dairy products produces several favorable results.

Exercise may offer protection against colon and breast cancer development (Cohen 1987; Weisburger and Wynder 1987; Slattery, Schumacher, and Smith et al. 1988). Because dietary habits and physical activity are often related, controlling for the effect of exercise may provide a truer measure of dietary factors in the etiology of the nutritionally linked cancers.

For the hormone-related cancers, such as breast and prostate, it is not yet known exactly what kind of endocrine balance would favor the growth of neoplastic cells, or what would inhibit such growth. It is also unclear precisely how dietary fat affects endocrine balance and specific hormone receptors. It seems probable that the type and amount of fat, endocrine balances, and receptors are related to these cancers.

All of these elements operate through epigenetic mechanisms; thus their action is dose- and time-dependent. A reduction in effective dose by whatever means would be expected to lead to a rapid lowering of risk and incidence. This may apply even to patients with such diseases in which dietary intervention promises to be an effective adjuvant therapy. Examples of the reversibility of epigenetic phenomena are the lowering of the risk of lung cancer after the cessation of smoking for a number of years, and the rapid decline in the incidence of endometrial cancer when the postmenopausal use of estrogen drugs such as Premarin was discontinued.

The factual information reviewed clearly demonstrates that lifestyle accounts for the majority of human solid cancers. Yet curiously, the public perception and the media are continually suggesting that major cancer risks are associated with food additives, inadvertent food contaminants like pesticides, insecticides, or other agricultural chemicals, air pollution, water pollution, and buildings contaminated with asbestos (Ames, 1989; Samet, 1989; Mossman, Bignon, and Corn et al. 1990). This erroneous public view exerts pressure on state and federal legislatures that, in turn, translates into legislation directing state and federal governments as well as industries to commit large funds, of the order of several hundred million dollars, to remove the majority of this environmental burden. How much progress would have been achieved in cancer research if such funds were available to the preventive research community? Clearly, the public anywhere in the world is entitled to a clean environment, contaminant-free air and water, and an adequate, appetizing food supply. These goals are meritorious by themselves. Yet, the public emphasis often is that the goal of measures to ensure a wholesome environment is cancer prevention. The facts outlined here and documented fully in the literature indicate that the main human cancers are associated with lifestyle, and not to any appreciable extent with environmental contamination. Therefore, if the public believes that changing the environment will protect them against cancer, and thus they elect not to change their lifestyle, we will continue to suffer from important types of cancer. Future efforts by all informed individuals and professions need to direct attention to essential lifestyle changes to achieve the goal of a major reduction of all types of cancer by the year 2000.

Contemporary knowledge recognizes that a dietary change to 20% of fat calories from 40% would go a long way toward lowering the risk of developing colon, pancreas, breast, and prostate cancers, and also ovarian or endometrial cancers if obesity is avoided (American Health Foundation 1987; U.S.P.H.S. 1988; Committee on Diet and Health 1989). Adequate cereal fiber in the diet, by increasing stool bulk and lowering the promoting elements in the gut, would lower the risk for colon cancer. This is particularly important for individuals on a high-fat Western diet, who probably due to genetics maintain a low serum cholesterol, and may be endowed with a high capacity to generate bile acids from cholesterol. Calcium levels and calcium-phosphate ratios, as do caloric restriction and weight loss, control cell division and subsequent cancer development.

For the tobacco-linked cancers, promoters and cocarcinogens are present in tobacco smoke and tobacco in much larger quantities than genotoxic carcinogens. Promoters probably contribute both to the occurrence of cancer after a long latent period and to the reversibility of lung-cancer risk upon smoking cessation. Despite the well-documented hazard of smoking, tragically, women have become heavy smokers (5% of women in 1930, 26.5% in 1987). The rate of lung-cancer deaths for women now exceeds that of breast cancer.

Lifestyle is a factor for preventing disease and for patient survival. Physicians, whose views are greatly respected by patients, ought to provide guidance along the following lines:

1. Don't use tobacco in any form: smoking, chewing, or snuff dipping.

2. Adjust total fat intake to about 20% of calories, and use lipids that pose less risk for heart disease or cancer, such as monounsaturated oils. Consume fish several times a week.

3. Avoid salted, pickled, or smoked foods.

4. Increase intake of cereal bran fiber foods.

5. Increase intake of calcium with low-fat dairy products, skim milk, or low-fat yogurt.

6. Eat more vegetables and fruits, which are excellent sources of vitamins, minerals, and fibers.

7. Avoid obesity and adjust overall energy intake to energy needs.

8. Do regular exercises, but only after a health check-up certifying normal blood pressure and serum cholesterol levels, to ensure cardiovascular patency.

Lifestyle adjustment commensurate with these guidelines is useful for everyone to minimize the risk of chronic disease. It is essential for patients in remission who have had coronary heart disease or cancer to be advised of the need to alter lifestyle as part of therapy.

Much has been learned about the causes of the major diseases in humans in North America and the world. This chapter and other chapters in this book have provided factual background, education, and a glimpse of mechanisms, all of which deal with the most effective means of cancer control: prevention.

REFERENCES

(To limit the number of citations, the list includes only a select guide to the literature. The reader is referred to review serials such as *Advances in Cancer Research, Annual Reviews* series, *Epidemiology Reviews, Cancer Surveys*, and frequent review articles in *Cancer Research, Carcinogenesis*, and the *Journal of the National Cancer Institute*, among others.)

Aaronson, S.A.; Bishop, J.M.; and Sugimura, T. et al. eds. 1987. *Oncogenes and cancer.* Tokyo: Japan Scientific Societies Press.

Albanes, D. and Winick, M. 1988. Are cell number and cell proliferation risk factors for cancer? *J. Nat. Cancer Inst.* 80:772-75.

American Health Foundation. 1987. Proceedings of a workshop on new developments on dietary fat and fiber in carcinogenesis (optimal types and amounts of fat or fiber). *Prev. Med.* 16:449-595.

Ames, B.N. What are the major carcinogens in the etiology of human cancer? Environmental pollution, natural carcinogens, and the causes of human cancer: six errors. In: DeVita, V.T. Jr.; Hellman, S.; and Rosenberg, S.A. eds. *Important advances in oncology 1989.* pp. 237-47. Philadelphia: J.B. Lipincott.

Barbacid, M. 1986. Human oncogenes. In DeVita, V.T. Jr.; Hellman, S.; and Rosenberg, S.A. eds. *Important advances in oncology 1986.* pp. 3-22. Philadelphia: J.B. Lippincott.

Bartsch, H.; Hemminki, K.; and O'Neil, I.K. eds. 1988. Methods for detecting DNA damaging agents in humans: applications in cancer epidemiology and prevention. *I.A.R.C. Sci. Publ. No. 89.* Lyon: International Agency for Research on Cancer.

Benowitz, N.L. 1988. Pharmacologic aspects of cigarette smoking and nicotine addiction. *N. Engl. J. Med.* 319: 1318-30.

Boyar, A.P.; Rose, D.P.; and Wynder, E.L. 1988. Recommendations for the prevention of chronic disease: the application for breast disease. *Am. J. Clin. Nutr.* 48:896-900.

Bruce, W.R. 1987. Recent hypotheses for the origin of colon cancer. *Cancer Res.* 47:4237-42.

Butterworth, B.E., and Slaga, T.J. eds. 1987. Nongenotoxic mechanisms in carcinogenesis. *Banbury Report.* 25:1-397.

Cohen, L.A. 1987. Diet and cancer. *Scientific American* 257: 42-48.

Committee on Diet and Health, Food and Nutrition Board. 1989. *Diet and health: implications for reducing chronic disease risk.* Washington, D.C.: National Academy Press.

Cooper, C.S., and Grover, P.L. eds. 1990. *Chemical carcinogenesis and mutagenesis.* Berlin, Heidelberg, New York: Springer-Verlag.

Cummings, J.H. and Bingham, S.A. 1987. Dietary fibre, fermentation and large bowel cancer. *Cancer Surveys* 6: 601-21.

Doll, R., and Peto, R. 1981. Causes of cancer: quantitative estimate of avoidable risks of cancer in the United States today. *J. Natl. Cancer Inst.* 66:1191-1308.

Efron, E. 1984. *The apocalyptics.* New York: Simon and Schuster.

Ernster, V.L. 1988. Trends in smoking, cancer risk, and cigarette promotion: current priorities for reducing tobacco exposure. *Cancer* 62:1702-12.

Furihata, C., and Matsushima, T. 1986. Mutagens and carcinogens in foods. *Ann. Rev. Nutr.* 6:67-94.

Greenwald, P.; Cullen, J.W.; and McKenna, J.W. 1987. Cancer prevention and control: from research through applications. *J. Natl. Cancer Inst.* 79:389-400.

Harris, C.C., and Sun, T-t. 1987. Multifactorial etiology of human liver cancer. *Carcinogenesis* 5:697-701.

Hatch, F.T.; Knize, M.G.; and Healy, S.K. et al. 1988. Cooked-food mutagen reference list and index. *Environ. Mol. Mutagenesis* 121(Suppl 14):1-85.

Hecht, S.S., and Hoffmann, D. 1988. Tobacco-specific nitrosamines, an important group of carcinogens in tobacco and tobacco smoke. *Carcinogenesis* 9:875-84.

Highman, B.; Norvell, M.J.; and Shellenberger, T.E. 1977. Pathological changes in female C3H mice continuously fed diets containing diethylstilbestrol or 17 beta-estradiol. *J. Env. Pathol. Toxicol.* 1:1-30.

Hill, M.J. 1971. Effect of some factors on the faecal concentration of acid steroids, neutral steroids and urobilins. *J. Pathol.* 104:239-45.

Hill, M.J. 1987. Dietary fat and human cancer (review). *Anticancer Res.* 7:281-92.

Hoffmann, D., and Hecht, S.S. 1990. Advances in tobacco carcinogenesis. In: Cooper, C.S., and Grover, P.L. eds. *Chemical carcinogenesis and mutagenesis I.* pp. 61-102. New York: Springer-Verlag.

Howley, P.M. 1987. Role of papillomaviruses in human cancer. In DeVita, V.T. Jr.; Hellman, S.; and Rosenberg, S.A.; eds. *Important advances in oncology 1987.* pp. 55-74. Philadelphia: J.B. Lippincott.

Howson, C.P.; Hiyama, T.; and Wynder, E.L. 1986. Decline of gastric cancer: epidemiology of an unplanned triumph. *Epidemiol. Rev.* 8:1-27.

Ip, C.; Birt, D.F.; and Rogers, A.E. et al. eds. 1986. Dietary fat and cancer. *Progr. Clin. Biol. Res. 222.* New York: Alan R. Liss, Inc.

Joossens, J.V.; Hill, M.J.; and Geboers, J. eds. 1985. Diet and human carcinogenesis. Amsterdam: Excerpta Medica.

Jones, R.C. and Weisburger, J.H. 1988. L-tryptophan inhibits formation of mutagens during cooking of meat and in laboratory models. *Mutat. Res.* 206:343-49.

Klatsky, A.L.; Armstrong, M.A.; Friedman, G.D. et al. 1988. The relations of alcoholic beverage use to colon and rectal cancer. *Am. J. Epidemiol.* 128:1007-15.

Knox, G. and Woodman, C. 1988. Prospects for primary and secondary prevention of cervix cancer. *Cancer Surveys* 7:377-549.

Koutsky, L.A.; Galloway, D.A.; and Holmes, K.K. 1986. Epidemiology of genital human papillomavirus infection. *Epidemiol. Rev.* 10:122-63.

Kroes, R.; Beems, R.B.; and Bosland, M.C. et al. 1986. Nutritional factors in lung, colon, and prostate carcinogenesis in animal models. *Federation Proc.* 45:136-41.

Lieber, C.S., and Garro, A.J. 1990. Alcohol and cancer. *Ann. Rev. Pharmacol. Toxicol.* 30:219–49.

Lipkin, M. 1988. Biomarkers of increased susceptibility to gastrointestinal cancer: new application to studies of cancer prevention in human subjects. *Cancer Res.* 48:235-45.

Lok, E.; Nera, E.A.; and Iverson, F. et al. 1988. Dietary restriction, cell proliferation and carcinogenesis: a preliminary study. *Cancer Lett.* 38:249-55.

Lyon, J.L. and Mahoney, A.W. 1988. Fried foods and the risk of colon cancer. *Am. J. Epidemiol.* 128:1000-1006.

Lyon, J.L.; Mahoney, A.W.; West, D.W. et al. 1987. Energy intake: its relationship to colon cancer risk. *J. Natl. Cancer Inst.* 78:853-61.

Machlin, L.J. and Bendich, A. 1987. Free radical tissue damage: protective role of antioxidant nutrients. *FASEB J.* 1:441-45.

Maltoni, C., and Selikoff, I.J. eds. 1988. Living in a chemical world: occupational and environmental significance of industrial carcinogens. *Ann. N.Y. Acad. Sci.* 534:1-1045.

McGinnis, J.M.; Shopland, D.; and Brown, C. 1987. Tobacco and health: trends in smoking and smokeless tobacco consumption in the United States. *Ann. Rev. Public Health* 8:441-67.

Milman, H.A.; and Weisburger, E.K. eds. 1985. *Handbook of carcinogen testing*. Park Ridge, NJ: Noyes Publications.

Montesano, R.; Bartsch, H.; and Vainio, H. et al. eds. 1986. Long-term and short-term assays for carcinogens: a critical appraisal. *IARC Sci. Publ. 83.* Lyon: International Agency for Research on Cancer.

Mossman, B.T.; Bignon, J.; and Corn, M. et al. 1990. Asbestos: scientific development and implications for public policy. *Science* 294-301.

Newmark, H.L.; Lipkin, M.; and Maheshwari, N. 1990. Colonic hyperplasia and hyperproliferation induced by a nutritional stress diet with four components of Western-style diet. *J. Natl. Cancer Inst.* 82:491-96.

Ning, J.P.; Yu, M.C.; and Wang, Q.S. et al. 1990. Consumption of salted fish and other risk factors for nasopharyngeal carcinoma (NPC) in Tianjin, a low-risk region for NPC in the People's Republic of China. *J. Natl. Cancer Inst.* 82:291-96.

O'Neill, I.K.; Chen, J.S.; and Bartsch, H. eds. 1990. Relevance to human cancer of nitroso compounds, tobacco, and mycotoxins. *IARC Sci. Publ. 105.* Lyon: International Agency for Research on Cancer.

Pariza, M.W. 1988. Dietary fat and cancer risk: evidence and research needs. *Ann. Rev. Nutr.* 8:167-83.

Parkin, D.M.; Laara, E.; and Muir, C.S. 1988. Estimates of the worldwide frequency of sixteen major cancers in 1980. *Int. J. Cancer* 41:184-97.

Ponz de Leon, M.; Roncucci, L.; Di Donato, P. et al. 1988. Pattern of epithelial cell proliferation in colorectal mucosa of normal subjects and of patients with adenomatous polyps or cancer of the large bowel. *Cancer Res.* 48:4121-26.

Prentice, R.L.; Kakar, F.; and Hursting, S. et al. 1988. Aspects of the rationale for the Women's Health Trial. *J. Natl. Cancer Inst.* 80:802-14.

Randerath, K.; Randerath, R.; and Danna, T.F. et al. 1989. A new sensitive ^{32}P-postlabeling assay based on the specific enzymatic conversion of bulky DNA lesions to radiolabeled dinucleotides and nucleoside 5'monophosphates. *Carcinogenesis* 10:1231-39.

Rich, M.A.; Hager, J.C.; and Lopez, D.M. eds. 1988. *Breast cancer: scientific and clinical progress*. Boston: Kluwer Academic Publishers.

Rohan, T.E. and Bain, C.J. 1986. Diet in the etiology of breast cancer. *Epidemiol Rev.* 9:120-45.

Rose, D.P.; Boyar, A.P.; and Wynder, E.L. 1986. International comparisons of mortality rates for cancer of the breast, ovary, prostate, and colon, and per capita food consumption. *Cancer* 58:2362-71.

Rose, D.P. 1990. Dietary fiber and breast cancer. *Nutr. Cancer* 13:1-8.

Rosenkranz, H.S. ed. 1988. Strategies for the deployment of batteries of short-term tests. *Mutat. Res.* 205:1-426.

Rosenthal, M.B.; Barnard, R.J.; and Rose, D.P. et al. 1985. Effects of a high-complex-carbohydrate, low-fat, low-cholesterol diet on levels of serum lipids and estradiol. *Am. J. Med.* 78:23-27.

Rowland, I.R. ed. 1988. *Role of the gut flora in toxicity and cancer*. London: Academic Press.

Roy, D.; Weisz, J.; and Liehr, J.G. 1990. The 0-methylation of 4-hydroxyestradiol is inhibited by 2-hydroxyestradiol: implications for estrogen-induced carcinogenesis. *Carcinogenesis* 11:459-62.

Sager, R. 1989. Tumor suppressor genes: the puzzle and the promise. *Science* 246:1406-12.

Samet, J.M. 1989 Radon and lung cancer. *J. Natl. Cancer Inst.* 10:745-55.

Saracci, R. 1986. Interactions of tobacco smoking and other agents in cancer etiology. *Epidemiol Rev.* 9:175-93.

Sato, S.; Seino, Y.; and Ohka, T. et al. 1977. Mutagenicity of smoke condensates from cigarettes, cigars and pipe tobacco. *Cancer Lett.* 3:1-8.

Schiffman, M.H. 1986. Epidemiology of fecal mutagenicity. *Epidemiol. Rev.* 8:92-105.

Schottenfeld, D., and Fraumeni, J.F. Jr. 1982. *Cancer epidemiology and prevention*. Philadelphia: W.B. Saunders.

Searle, C.E. ed. 1984. Chemical carcinogens. *Am. Chem. Soc. Monogr. 182.* 2nd ed. vols. 1, 2. Washington, D.C.: American Chemical Society.

Seitz, H.K., and Simanowski, U.A. 1988. Alcohol and carcinogenesis. *Ann. Rev. Nutr.* 8:99-119.

Shamsuddin, A.M.; Elsayed, A.M.; and Ullah, A. 1988. Suppression of large intestinal cancer in F344 rats by inositol hexaphosphate. *Carcinogenesis* 9:577-80.

Simopoulos, A.P. ed. 1987. Diet and health: scientific concepts and principles. *Am. J. Clin. Nutr.* 45(Suppl 1):1015-1407.

Sinkeldam, E.J.; Kuper, C.F.; and Bosland, M.C. 1990. Interactive effects of dietary wheat bran and lard on N-Methyl-N'-nitro-N-nitrosoguanidine-induced colon carcinogenesis in rats. *Cancer Res.* 50:1092-96.

Slattery, M.L.; Schumacher, M.C.; and Smith, K.R. et al. 1988. Physical activity, diet, and risk of colon cancer in Utah. *Am. J. Epidemiol.* 128:989-99.

Sorenson, A.W.; Slattery, M.L.; and Ford, M.H. 1988. Calcium and colon cancer: a review. *Nutr. Cancer.* 11:135-45.

Swanson, G.M. 1988. Cancer prevention in the workplace and natural environment: a review of etiology, research design, and methods of risk reduction. *Cancer* 62:1725-46.

U.S. Dept. of Health and Human Services, Public Health Svc., Report of the Surgeon General. 1982. Smoking and health. *DHEW Publ. No. (P.H.S.) 79-50066.* Washington, D.C.: U.S. Govt. Printing Office.

U.S. Public Health Service. 1986. Health consequences of using smokeless tobacco: a report of the advisory committee to the Surgeon General. *NIH Publ. No. 86-3874.* Washington, D.C.: U.S. Govt. Printing Office.

U.S. Public Health Service. 1988. The Surgeon General's report on nutrition and health. *DHHS (P.H.S.) Publ. No. 88-50210.* Washington, D.C.: U.S. Govt. Printing Office.

U.S. Public Health Service, National Cancer Institute, Division Cancer Prevention and Control. 1988. 1987 annual cancer statistics review. *NIH Publ. No. 88-2789.* Washington, D.C.: U.S. Govt. Printing Office.

Weinberg, R.A. 1989. Oncogenes, antioncogenes, and the molecular bases of multistep carcinogenesis. *Cancer Res.* 49:3713-21.

Weindruch, R.; and Walford, R.L. 1988. *The retardation of aging and disease by dietary restriction*. Springfield, Ill.: Charles C Thomas.

Weisburger, J.H. 1987. Mechanisms of nutritional carcinogenesis associated with specific human cancers. *I.S.I. Atlas of Science: Pharmacology* 1:162-167.

Weisburger, J.H., and Wynder, E.L. 1987. Etiology of colorectal cancer with emphasis on mechanism of action and prevention. In DeVita, V.T. Jr.; Hellman, S.; and Rosenberg, S.A. eds. *Important advances in oncology 1987.* pp. 197-220. Philadelphia: J.B. Lippincott.

Williams, G.M., and Weisburger, J.H. 1986. Chemical carcinogens. In Klaassen, C.D.; Amdur, M.O.; and Doull, J. eds. *Casarett and Doull's toxicology: the basic science of poisons.* 3rd ed. pp. 99-173. New York: Macmillan.

Witmer, C.M.; Snyder, R.; and Jollow, D.J. et. al. 1990. *4th International Symposium Biological Reactive Intermediates.* New York and London: Plenum Press.

Wogan, G.N. 1989. Makers of exposure to carcinogens: methods for human biomonitoring. *J. Am. College Toxicol.* 8:871-81.

Wynder, E.L. 1988. Tobacco and health: a review of the history and suggestions for public health policy. *Publ. Hlth. Repts.* 103:8-18.

Wynder, E.L., and Gori, G.B. 1977. Contribution of the environment to cancer incidence: an epidemiologic exercise. *J. Natl. Cancer Inst.* 58:825-32.

Wynder, E.L., and Hiyama, T. 1987. Comparative epidemiology of cancer in the United States and Japan: preventive implications. *Gann. Monogr. Cancer Res.* 33:183-92.

Zaridze, D.; and Peto, R. eds. 1986. *Tobacco: a major international health hazard. IARC Sci. Publ. 74.* Lyon: International Agency for Research on Cancer.

Ziegler, R.G.; Devesa, S.S.; and Fraumeni, J.F. Jr. 1986. Epidemiologic patterns of colorectal cancer. In DeVita, V.T. Jr.; Hellman, S.; and Rosenberg, S.A. eds. *Important advances in oncology.* pp. 209-32. Philadelphia: J.B. Lippincott.

zur Hausen, H. 1989. Papillomaviruses in anogenital cancer as a model to understand the role of viruses in human cancers. *Cancer Res.* 49:4677-81.

Chapter 8

CANCER PREVENTION

Clark W. Heath, Jr., M.D.

Clark W. Heath, Jr., M.D.
Vice President for Epidemiology and Statistics
American Cancer Society
Atlanta, Georgia

INTRODUCTION

The concept of prevention pervades all activities in cancer management and control. It is common to distinguish between three forms of prevention. *Primary prevention* refers to efforts to reduce or eliminate exposures to carcinogens in order to prevent the initiation or promotion of the fundamental carcinogenic process. *Secondary prevention* includes screening and early detection programs that seek to identify cases early in their development, so that chances for cure are enhanced. *Tertiary prevention* refers to treatment of cancer patients that seeks to prevent undue clinical complications or premature death. This chapter focuses on primary and secondary prevention. Particular attention is given to the principles of epidemiology upon which prevention practices and programs are based.

The importance of prevention concepts in cancer control work is illustrated by the manner in which they have been used in recent years to set national goals for cancer prevention in the United States. Existing knowledge in the fields of cancer risk-control, early detection, and therapy have suggested that overall cancer mortality reduction on the order of 50% is an appropriate goal by the turn of the century (Greenwald and Sondik 1986). This projection apportions mortality reductions as follows: 8% through dietary reduction in fat and increase in fiber, 8% to 15% through reduction in smoking, 3% through early diagnosis and screening, and 10% to 26% through treatment applications.

While these estimates rely on various assumptions that may or may not prove to be correct, they constitute a definable set of targets. They also illustrate the relative weights that current knowledge would assign to different prevention modalities, taking mortality reduction as a particular measure of cancer control progress.

PRINCIPLES OF EPIDEMIOLOGY

The formation of cancer prevention strategies and assessment of progress toward prevention goals rest on two fundamental pieces of knowledge: (1) what is the extent of the cancer problem in terms of numbers of cases, time trends, geographic distributions, and rates of incidence or mortality in different population segments; and (2) what are the causes of cancer, or the determinants of cancer progression, which we would seek to prevent? These two questions are addressed through the discipline of epidemiology. *Descriptive epidemiology,* which examines patterns of disease occurrence in populations, addresses the first; *analytic epidemiology,* which explores etiologic relationships, addresses the second (Schottenfeld and Fraumeni 1982).

DESCRIPTIVE EPIDEMIOLOGY

In describing the characteristics of a disease in a population setting, the epidemiologist calculates rates of disease occurrence: the number of cases per 100,000 population, for example. Rates or frequency measures between different population groups can then be compared. Rates are commonly compared between different points in time, different geographic locations, and different kinds of people — especially those of different age, sex, and racial groups. The differences seen between rates in different population groups, as measured by the three categories of time, place, and person, lead to inferences about the nature of the disease. For example, it could be observed that incidence is decreasing over time, that rates in one country exceed those in another, that rates among whites exceed those in blacks, or that incidence rises with age and with decreasing family income. Because rates for any disease usually vary by several parameters simultaneously (e.g., age, race, geographic location), it is common practice to hold one or more parameters constant while comparing rates with respect to another (for example, age-race-sex adjusted rates in comparisons between different time periods or different geographic locations).

To know the number of cases occurring in any given population, the epidemiologist uses various data sources. Death-certificate registrations are a common source and give rise to mortality rates. Disease registries, drawn from hospital records or physician reports of case diagnoses, yield incidence rates. Conventionally, both the mortality and incidence rates refer to rates of new cases dying or diagnosed within a particular time unit, commonly a year. Alternatively, rates can be calculated in terms of prevalence, or the number of cases existing at a given point in time per unit population, regardless of diagnosis date (prevalence rates).

Tracking disease patterns through examination of rates over time in a given population constitutes disease surveillance. The process of surveillance is fundamental to assessing progress in achieving disease-prevention goals. It involves not merely the collection and analysis of disease-occurrence data, but also the timely communication of those data to persons or groups responsible for conducting programs aimed at disease control and prevention. For cancer, because of its long latency characteristics (intervals of from 10 to 30 years usually exist between cancer initiation and cancer diagnosis), effective surveillance entails tracking not only patterns of case occurrence, but also patterns of risk-factor exposure (e.g., frequencies of smoking, of radiation exposure, of particular diet habits), and of screening or early diagnosis utilization (e.g., Pap testing or mammography).

ANALYTIC EPIDEMIOLOGY

To know that a particular risk factor causes a particular disease is a complex process that usually requires considerable data from various sources. The most direct means for determining causation is to conduct direct exposure experiments, as is done in tests using laboratory animals. Because exposure experimentation is not permissible in human populations, most of what we know concerning human disease causation comes from indirect observations of how risk exposures and disease occurrence interrelate in human populations (patterns of risk and disease), inferences drawn from laboratory experiments using nonhuman test species or *in vitro* test systems, and clinical observations regarding mechanisms of disease progression. It therefore falls to the epidemiologist to evaluate human disease causation through analytic epidemiologic studies in human populations and through integration of those study results with pertinent laboratory and clinical observations.

There are three kinds of analytic epidemiologic studies: prospective or cohort studies, retrospective or case-control (case-referent) studies, and cross-sectional studies. Each seeks to assess the existence and strength of cause-effect relationships through observations regarding disease occurrence in relation to risk-factor exposures in groups of people.

Cohort studies approach this task by comparing prospectively (forward in time) two groups of people: one with documented exposure to a given risk factor (for example, cigarette smoking or ionizing radiation exposure) and one with no such exposure or with exposure of a distinctly lesser degree. These groups are then followed over time, and the extent to which the disease of interest occurs in each group is recorded. If disease frequency in the exposed group distinctly exceeds (that is, to an extent judged to be statistically significant) the frequency in the unexposed group, an etiologic relationship can be suspected between the risk factor and the disease, all other things being equal. The difficulty with epidemiologic studies, however, often comes with keep-ing all other things equal, that is, controlling for competing risk factors or exposures or for so-called confounding factors which may cause the groups being compared to be noncomparable in ways that affect both frequency of risk-factor exposure and frequency of disease occurrence. Such a confounding influence is often encountered, for instance, with respect to socioeconomic differences.

Even if all appropriate adjustments or controls are exercised in the data, a positive risk factor-disease association in a single study is usually not sufficient to justify a final conclusion of causation. Repeated epidemiologic studies, each approaching the question from its own viewpoint, are usually needed, plus evidence from experimental and clinical quarters. If all such evidence points in the same direction and paints an etiologic picture that is biologically coherent and persuasive, then science will usually accept a judgment of causation.

Case-control studies approach the cause-effect question from a different temporal vantage point and hence are often termed retrospective. Such studies start with a series of cases of a particular disease, match them individually or as a group with persons without the disease (controls) — matching by such variables as age, race, or socioeconomic class — and then, through questionnaire interview or review of past records, determine degree or frequency of exposure to the risk factor of interest. If cases display a distinctly increased frequency of exposure compared to controls, an etiologic relationship may be suggested (again, with all other things being equal).

Case-control studies have the advantages of economy of time and resources when compared with cohort studies. They are also better designed for examining questions involving rare diseases. However, they are more prone to the retrospective biases inherent in patient recall.

Cross-sectional studies make risk-factor and disease-frequency comparisons in the same manner as case-control and cohort studies but at particular points in time (usually the present) rather than over periods of time.

PRIMARY PREVENTION

The causes of cancer cover a wide range. Undoubtedly, in any given case, carcinogenesis results from the interaction of multiple risk factors, especially those involving the interplay of host or genetic constitutional factors with external, environmental exposures. The force of environmental causation is evident in the fact that for many cancers (1) large differences in incidence exist between different countries or geographic regions (for example, esophageal cancer); (2) substantial changes have occurred in incidence over time (for example, the rise in lung cancer and fall in stomach cancer in the United States over the past half century), changes that are far too rapid to attribute to genetic alterations; and

(3) incidence level changes in immigrant groups as they move to new cultural settings (for example, cancer patterns among Asian emigrants to Western countries). The magnitude of geographic differences alone has led to the conclusion that perhaps three-quarters of all cancers are theoretically the result of environmental determinants (Doll and Peto 1981). Only about one-third, however, are presently preventable based on existing knowledge and intervention possibilities. The great bulk of this primary prevention forecast rests with the elimination of tobacco use. The remainder is a matter of diet changes, moderation in alcohol use, elimination of occupational exposures, control in man-made radiation sources, control of sexually transmissible infections, and reduction of various environmental exposures such as hormonal medications, sunlight, and air and water pollution.

TOBACCO

The etiologic relationship between cigarette smoking and lung cancer was firmly established in the 1950s through a series of case-control and cohort studies in many different countries. Risk was 10 times greater in current smokers than nonsmokers, and it increased with the number of cigarettes smoked. Studies since that time have demonstrated that cigarette smoking also causes various other forms of cancer, increasing the risk of laryngeal cancer eightfold, oral and pharyngeal cancer fourfold, esophageal cancer threefold, and bladder and pancreatic cancers twofold (U.S. Public Health Service 1989). Pipe or cigar smokers are at increased risk of these same cancers, although with greater emphasis on laryngeal and oral-pharyngeal forms. Users of snuff or chewing tobacco have a fourfold increased risk of oral cancers. Passive exposure to cigarette smoke (sidestream and exhaled smoke) appears to increase risk of lung cancer in nonsmokers who live with smokers.

The epidemiologic evidence from human observations is reinforced by the knowledge of the chemical carcinogenicity of the tars that exist in cigarette smoke, by studies of tobacco carcinogenicity in laboratory animals, and by the observation of precancerous pathologic changes in lung and other tissues studied at autopsy of persons known to be cigarette smokers. The epidemiologic data, in particular, permit estimation of what proportion of particular cancers can be attributable to tobacco use. That proportion overall is about 30%. In men, tobacco use accounts for about 90% of all lung cancers, 75% of all cancers of the mouth, larynx, and esophagus, and about 50% of bladder and pancreas cancers. Proportions among women are somewhat less since tobacco use among women has been substantially less. However, smoking has become increasingly common among women in recent years and rises in the frequency of tobacco-related cancers in women over the next several decades can be expected. Considerable steady progress has been made in reducing tobacco use in the United States so that it is now reasonable to expect that overall rates of tobacco-related cancers will fall perceptibly by the year 2000. For populations in developing countries, however, prospects are less optimistic since promotion of tobacco products is accelerating in parts of the world where cigarette smoking, especially among women, was previously most uncommon.

ALCOHOL

Heavy consumption of ethyl alcohol is largely associated with increases in hepatocellular malignancy as well as cancers of the mouth, esophagus, and upper larynx (Pollack et al. 1984). With regard to liver cancer, this increased risk may relate to alcohol metabolism by liver cells. For other cancers, risk appears to be closely related to cigarette smoking, the effect perhaps being synergistic rather than just additive. Studies of alcohol carcinogenicity in humans, however, are often difficult to interpret because it is common for persons who use alcohol heavily also to use tobacco. The mechanism of alcohol carcinogenicity in tobacco-related cancers may involve either the direct action of alcohol on epithelial tissues or its ability as a solvent to increase the delivery of smoke-derived chemical carcinogens to target tissues.

RADIATION

Some of the earliest knowledge regarding environmental carcinogens relates to ionizing radiation (Walker 1989). Heavy exposures in persons using radium and roentgen rays, prior to awareness of radiation risks, resulted in clear instances of radiation-induced skin cancers and cancers at other sites. Gradually, safeguards were introduced for medical and experimental uses of x-rays and radionuclides, an example of how responsible efforts in primary prevention can be effective. Concerns about risk persist, as does considerable uncertainty regarding the exact extent to which low doses of ionizing radiation contribute to carcinogenesis and genetic damage.

Ionizing radiation encompasses several forms of high-frequency radiation at the upper end of the electromagnetic spectrum (x-rays, alpha, beta, and gamma radiation, and cosmic rays), much of it arising from decay of radioactive elements. Its potential for oncogenicity and genetic change comes from the ability of its energy to cause ionization of molecules within cells. Evidence for radiation carcinogenesis in humans comes from various epidemiologic sources (Shore 1988; Beebe 1982): (1) studies of cancer frequency in persons treated with ionizing radiation for medical purposes (for example, leukemia in men treated with x-rays for ankylosing spondylitis of the spine, breast cancer in women exposed to repeated chest fluoroscopies for pulmonary tuberculosis, and cancers in children who received x-ray treatments for tinea capitis or for an enlarged thymus); (2) studies in Japanese survivors of the atomic bomb explosions in Hiroshima and Nagasaki; and (3) studies of persons exposed to ionizing radiation in occupational settings (for example, lung cancer in uranium miners). In many of these studies, whole-body exposures were involved; in others (especially those in medical settings), exposures of particular organs or tissues. Tissues clearly differ in their degree of radiosensitivity, breast and hematopoietic tissues being particularly sensitive. Nearly every tissue site in the body, however, has been shown (principally in ongoing cohort studies of Japanese atom-bomb survivors) to be subject to increased cancer risk after exposure to increased levels of ionizing radiation. Carcinogenesis is clearly related to tissue dose, although the nature of that relationship is still somewhat speculative, especially at lower-dose ranges. Conservative assumptions based on a linear, no-threshold, dose-response model generally have been used to regulate safety standards. Current controversies with respect to ionizing radiation oncogenesis relate to the possible health significance of low-dose exposures in occupational settings and in populations near nuclear facilities and the degree to which radon exposures from indoor air pollution sources may contribute to lung cancer occurrence (Samet 1989).

Radiation exposure is a fundamental condition of life on earth. Exposure measurements suggest that natural background dosage (from cosmic rays and radioactive elements in the earth's crust and in our own bodies) ranges from about 0.8 mSv to 1.6 mSv per year per person, depending on geologic configurations and elevation above sea level. About another 1.0 mSv are absorbed each year from man-made sources, principally from medical and dental uses. This total background dosage is about equivalent to what is received from a single gastrointestinal series x-ray examination. An estimated 1% of all cancers are attributable to ionizing radiation exposure beyond natural background sources.

Other forms of electromagnetic radiation, of lower frequency than ionizing radiation, have been studied with respect to carcinogenic potential. There is a clear-cut relationship between ultraviolet radiation exposure and skin cancer (American Medical Association 1989) that particularly concerns nonmelanomic forms of skin cancer, but also melanoma to some degree. Skin cancers, largely the result of sunlight exposure, account for about 10% of all cancers and are thus a major target for primary prevention activities.

The oncogenicity of lower-frequency radiation remains speculative. Whereas human epidemiologic and laboratory experimentation data strongly indicate that radiation in the ionizing and ultraviolet frequency ranges causes cancer, neither category of evidence is yet convincing for lower frequencies (Shore 1988). Particular attention has focused on extremely low-frequency radiation such as that generated by electric current passing through electric wire, household appliances, or electric transformers. Epidemiologic studies, seeking to relate such exposures to cancer risk, particularly risk of leukemia and experimental work in laboratories, have to date yielded inconclusive results.

INFECTION

Since early in this century it has been known that both DNA and RNA viruses cause a wide range of animal cancers. Experimental studies, together with the ability to enhance virologic investigations by inbreeding animal strains, made this knowledge possible. Not surprisingly, data were eventually developed showing that a similar range of viruses causes cancer in humans. The earliest human oncogenic virus to be identified was the Epstein-Barr virus (EBV), which is causally associated with African Burkitt's lymphoma and with nasopharyngeal cancer (de The 1979). EBV, a herpesvirus, is a DNA virus that is strongly lymphotropic and cell-bound. It causes infectious mononucleosis and is a widely distributed and commonly latent infection in human populations. Antibody studies show an especially strong association with Burkitt's lymphoma and nasopharyngeal cancer. In the case of Burkitt's lymphoma, EBV infection has been demonstrated, in a cohort study of African children, to precede the development of cancer. In that biologic process, for the African form of the tumor at least, the interaction between EBV infection of lymphoid cells and the intense immunologic disturbance of holoendemic malaria appears to be critical for the emergence of tumor clones.

Infection with another DNA virus, hepatitis B virus (HBV), clearly has been shown to cause hepatocellular carcinoma (hepatoma) in cohort and case-control studies in Oriental populations (Beasley et al. 1981). This tumor is rare in the United States, but it has a high prevalence in developing countries. This prevalence reflects the fact that HBV infection is exceedingly common in these populations, transmission from mother to child at birth being an especially frequent mode of infection. Hepatoma appears to develop when HBV infection is persistent (chronic carrier state). It therefore occurs predominantly in adults who were infected at birth, when immune mechanisms are less well-developed than at older ages, hence permitting persistent and active HBV infection to become established. The existence of widely available and affordable HBV vaccines is an obvious opportunity for a major worldwide primary cancer-prevention program through newborn immunization. The exact mechanism by which HBV causes malignancy is not clear, but it may involve some interaction with chemical carcinogens, such as aflatoxins that are consumed in the diet and are associated epidemiologically with world patterns of liver cancer distribution (Peers et al. 1987).

Herpes simplex virus Type 2 (HSV-2) and human papilloma virus (HPV) are two DNA viruses that have been closely associated with human cancer of the uterine cervix (Corey and Spear 1986; Koutsky, Galloway, and Holmes 1988). Although both viruses cause well-recognized sexually transmitted diseases, proof that they cause cervical cancer has been difficult to establish because of inconsistent findings in serologic and virologic surveys. Certain forms of HPV, however, are known to cause skin warts. The frequent presence of DNA from particular HPV strains in cervical cancer cells makes it likely that the virus eventually will be shown to be a cause of cervix cancer.

One RNA virus, human T-lymphotropic virus Type I (HTLV-I), has been proven to cause a particular form of human leukemia, adult T-cell leukemia-lymphoma or HTLL (Blayney et al. 1983). Evidence for this causative relationship comes from epidemiologic and laboratory observations in southern Japan and in certain Caribbean countries where HTLV-I infection and HTLL are particularly prevalent. HTLV-I belongs to a class of newly discovered human viruses (including the human immunodeficiency virus), which have immunosuppressive properties arising from their effects on lymphocytes. Similar immunosuppressive oncogenic RNA viruses had previously been recognized in animals (for example, the feline leukemia virus).

Nonviral infectious agents have occasionally been shown to cause particular human cancers. These include *Schistosoma hematobium,* which can cause bladder cancer, and *Clonorchis sinensis* (liver fluke), which causes certain forms of liver cancer in the Orient.

DIET

Elements in the human diet have had a clear and considerable impact on cancer risk. Epidemiologic studies correlating dietary differences with cancer-frequency differences in different countries, or within population groups having particular dietary habits, have strongly suggested that high fat levels in the diet are related to increased risk of cancers of the breast and colon, whereas high intake of fruits and vegetables, coupled with low fat intake, leads to lowered risk (Graham 1983). Diet composition is complex and highly intercorrelated, and it is difficult to isolate particular oncogenic causes. This difficulty has led to a wide range of predictions regarding the contribution of diet elements to human cancer causation. While undoubtedly diet's contribution is substantial, the exact extent remains uncertain. In addition to the association of colon and breast cancer risk with high fat intake (and with obesity), evidence has been advanced that high fiber intake may reduce colon cancer risk (American Medical Association 1989).

Particular chemicals may have similar effects. Both vitamin A (beta carotene) and vitamin C appear to have some degree of cancer chemoprevention capacity (Willett et al. 1984). Mutagenic or carcinogenic chemicals may exist naturally in foods (for example, aflatoxins) or may be formed by bacterial action on natural food substrates (for example, the production of nitrosamines from ingested nitrites).

Much concern has focused on food ingredients that have been introduced by man, either in the process of preserving or cooking food, as additives used to enhance food appearance (food coloring), or to protect against pest infestation (Ames, Magaw, and Gold 1987). In many instances, the chemicals have clear oncogenic potential as judged by animal experiments or by other human exposure experiences (for example, certain polycyclic aromatic hydrocarbons introduced during broiling or smoking food and certain pesticides introduced during agricultural processing). Regulations governing food preparation procedures, food additives, and chemical tolerance levels are designed to keep such exposures within acceptable and negligible risk levels. This is a complex, difficult, and expensive area of primary prevention that requires constant attention as new additives are introduced and food markets shift.

MEDICATIONS

Various chemical compounds consumed for medical reasons, either to treat illnesses or to control physiologic functions, can have oncogenic potential. The evidence is clearest for classes of medications used to treat various forms of cancer (Pui et al. 1989). Often such chemotherapeutic agents are themselves carcinogenic (for example, busulfan [Myleran], chlorambucil, cyclophosphamide, and melphalan). That oncogenic risk, of course, as with the use of ionizing radiation in treating cancer, is balanced by the obvious need to provide effective cancer therapy. As such treatments become more successful in extending patient survival, secondary malignancies arising as a result of their use are expected to become more common. As a general cause of cancer, however, such exposures account for only a very small proportion of human tumors.

The use of hormonal preparations as contraceptives and as treatment of various gynecologic conditions has received much epidemiologic attention because of the potential for estrogens to affect risk of breast and female genital cancers. Diethylstilbestrol (DES), a synthetic estrogen preparation, has been shown to be the cause of vaginal cancer in young women whose mothers were treated with the drug during pregnancy to prevent miscarriage (Melnick et al. 1987). The use of exogenous estrogens to relieve menopausal symptoms has been shown to cause increased risk of endometrial cancer (Shapiro et al. 1985). Estrogen-containing oral contraceptive preparations have received particular attention because of their widespread use and because their potential oncogenic effect concerns breast cancer, the most common cancer among women. Evidence that oral contraceptive use increases breast cancer risk has been equivocal, although it now seems likely that a small increased risk may exist for premenopausal tumors (U.K. National Study 1989). Oral contraceptives clearly increase risk of certain rare, benign liver tumors, but at the same time they decrease risk of ovarian cancer. As more is learned about these cancer risks through continued epidemiologic studies, recognition of those risks will need to be balanced against the obvious health benefits of hormonal pregnancy-control methods.

OCCUPATIONAL AND ENVIRONMENTAL EXPOSURES

Some of the earliest and most convincing evidence of chemical carcinogenesis in humans has come from observations made regarding workplace exposures (Rom 1983). Percival Pott's eighteenth-century observation of scrotal skin cancers in chimney sweeps exposed to chimney soot is commonly cited as the earliest such occupational health description. Prior to the mid-twentieth century, occupational exposures to materials later shown to be carcinogenic were often substantial. By virtue of such relatively high-dose exposures, coupled with the ability to document workplace conditions for individual workers through industrial records, both cohort and case-control epidemiologic studies have been able to establish clear evidence of carcinogenesis in occupational settings. Prominent examples include lung cancer and mesothelioma in asbestos workers, hepatic angiosarcomas in vinyl chloride polymerization workers, and myeloid leukemias in workers exposed to benzene used as a solvent in the rubber industry (Austin, Delzell, and Cole 1988). In the case of asbestos exposure, lung cancer risk is greatly increased through synergy with cigarette smoking. The large number of workers exposed in the past to asbestos in various trades (insulation workers, shipyard workers, automotive and construction workers) has made asbestos carcinogenicity a relatively prominent public health issue, intensified by concern for lower-dose exposures in the general public from deteriorating asbestos insulation in buildings. It seems likely that only about 3% to 4% of all human cancers are attributable to occupational exposures, despite higher estimates in the past.

Exposures to chemical carcinogens in the environment have been the subject of much concern and investigation in recent years. Exposure levels in the general environment, however, are generally much lower than those observed in past worksite exposures; hence, documentation of carcinogenicity in human epidemiologic studies has not been clearly established. Examples include various carcinogenic materials in air pollution, halogenated hydrocarbons in drinking water (Cantor et al. 1987), chemicals such as polychlorinated biphenyls and dibenzodioxins from chemical plant emissions or inadequate waste chemical disposal, and pesticide residues in various food products (Hoar et al. 1986; Austin, Keil, and Cole 1989). These general environmental exposures are not likely to be substantial contributors to the overall human cancer burden, despite the alarming circumstances in which they often occur. Occasionally, the exposures can be extensive (for example, the industrial accident at Seveso, Italy, in which dioxin emissions occurred), and it cannot be assumed, even at very low doses, that no carcinogenic effect will occur. Given the man-made, and hence man-controllable, nature of such exposures, their continuous monitoring and control is essential, to the extent that is technically practical. The mechanisms to control occupational and environmental exposures have been established, especially over the past two decades, by means of laws passed in the United States to regulate toxic substances and to safeguard workers' health.

GENETIC FACTORS

The action of environmental carcinogens in tissue is undoubtedly modified by host-genetic constitution. Although genetic factors are not readily addressed in the context of primary prevention, it is important to recognize their influence. For many cancers, familial or inherited patterns are occasionally seen; in some instances the patterns are pronounced (Knudson 1989). At present, the ability to identify the genetic components of carcinogenic risk is limited, as in the case of debrisoquine metabolism in relation to lung cancer risk (Caporaso et al. 1989). As genetic knowledge advances, this aspect of human oncogenesis will become clearer, and genetic studies will begin to have greater relevance for cancer prevention.

SECONDARY PREVENTION

Because primary prevention has only a limited ability to forestall the initiation or promotion of carcinogenesis, reduction of cancer mortality through early diagnosis (i.e., secondary prevention) is of great importance. This approach has been undertaken or suggested for numerous cancer sites (lung, breast, cervix, bladder, colorectal, testis, prostate, mouth) but with clear success only for cervical cancer and breast cancer. Real potential for secondary prevention of colorectal cancers exists but has yet to be clearly demonstrated.

Effective early diagnosis requires an effective screening test that has demonstrated success in reducing mortality when applied in a population setting. Consideration must be given to evaluating the appropriateness of a given screening test and in assessing its performance in practice. The test should be relatively simple, inexpensive, clinically acceptable to people being screened, have negligible side effects, and be evaluable in field trials. The test's sensitivity (ability to identify persons with disease) and specificity (ability to identify persons without disease) are critical. An insensitive test will fail to diagnose actual cases (producing false negatives) while a nonspecific one will mistakenly diagnose disease where none exists (producing false positives). The latter problem can be especially critical if the prevalence of disease is low. The performance of screening tests is commonly assessed in terms of the proportion of positive tests that correctly identify disease (predictive value positive).

Reduction in mortality remains the only true measure of success for a screening or early detection program. Past screening trials have used other measures such as prolongation of patient survival or proportion of diagnoses indicating early stages of disease. Such measures are hard to interpret because of a variety of biases that may exist: lead-time bias, whereby survival appears increased only because early diagnosis advances the date of disease detection; length bias, whereby less aggressive tumors with longer preclinical phases may be more likely to be found during screening; and self-selection bias, whereby people who participate in screening programs may differ from people who do not, in terms of health awareness and education, which in turn may contribute to improved survival.

In the face of such methodologic difficulties, proper assessment of a screening test's effectiveness for early diagnosis and secondary prevention uses reduction in mortality as the definitive endpoint to be achieved and performs the evaluation through a randomized controlled trial. In practice, however, such trials are not easy to conduct, and hence assessments have frequently followed the less-adequate course of incompletely controlled observational studies or purely anecdotal experience.

CERVICAL CANCER

When the Papanicolaou procedure (Pap test) for early cytologic diagnosis of cervical cancer was introduced in the 1950s, no randomized trials were conducted prior to its general application (Koss 1989). As a result, evaluation of the test's effectiveness was conducted through a variety of other epidemiologic approaches. These multiple sources of evaluation have, over time, provided a convincing and consistent body of data to support the idea that use of the Pap test does reduce cervical-cancer mortality. Of particular value have been observations in Scandinavian countries, where quite complete screening coverage was achieved in entire populations in which health-care services and cancer-case surveillance were also quite complete. In such settings, clear reductions in cervical-cancer mortality rates followed institution of screening programs. However, in many populations where screening and health-care services have been less satisfactory, mortality reduction has been less complete, especially among older women of lower socioeconomic class.

BREAST CANCER

When techniques for mammography were developed in the 1960s, the procedure's effectiveness was evaluated in a randomized trial prior to its widescale promotion as a means for reducing breast cancer mortality. This involved a study of about 62,000 women, aged 40 to 64, who were enrolled for health services through the Health Insurance Plan (HIP) in New York. Half of the women received annual mammography and breast physical examinations for four consecutive years, and half received their usual health services. After five years of follow-up, breast cancer mortality among women in the mammography group, who were age 50 and above at the study's start, was more than 50% lower than among the control women. Initially, no mortality reduction was observed in women aged 40 to 49, although after longer follow-up some evidence suggesting a preventive effect has begun to appear. From these findings have emerged present recommendations calling for regular mammographic examinations in all women age 40 and above (American Medical Association 1989). Regular breast self-examination and regular physical examination are also recommended, although their effectiveness in

screening has not been as thoroughly assessed. There was initial concern that, for younger women in particular, cancer risk from mammographic x-ray exposure might outweigh the procedure's preventive benefit. Technical improvements in the radiologic procedure have reduced the exposure dosage so that such health risks are no longer a major concern.

COLORECTAL CANCER

Unlike breast and cervical cancer screening, tests for colorectal cancer have yet to be fully assessed from an epidemiologic point of view (Hardcastle and Pye 1989; Fleischer et al. 1989). Two screening procedures have been proposed: flexible sigmoidoscopy and testing for occult blood in stool. With respect to sigmoidoscopy, questions of its acceptability by asymptomatic persons, as well as concerns about the costs and complexity of the procedure and of subsequent diagnostic studies, especially when initial screening may prove to have been false-positive, have led many people to be cautious about its widespread use in general population screening. Questions about the effectiveness of stool-blood examinations as a screening modality have also been raised, although on different grounds. Although the procedure is inexpensive and relatively simple, it is clearly quite nonspecific with respect to colon cancer detection; positive results are often the result of more common noncancerous conditions. Because bowel cancer is a common form of malignancy and is often not recognized until it has spread widely and survival prospects are poor, it is likely that strong efforts will continue to explore the feasibility of sigmoidoscopy and stool-blood testing as practical approaches to screening and early diagnosis.

REFERENCES

American Medical Association, Council on Scientific Affairs. 1989. Dietary fiber and health. *JAMA* 262:542-46.

American Medical Association, Council on Scientific Affairs. 1989. Mammographic screening in asymptomatic women aged 40 years and older. *JAMA* 261:2535-42.

American Medical Association, Council on Scientific Affairs. 1989. Harmful effects of ultraviolet radiation. *JAMA* 262:380-84.

Ames, B.N.; Magaw, R.; and Gold, L.S. 1987. Ranking possible carcinogenic hazards. *Science* 236:271-80.

Austin, H.; Delzell, E.; and Cole, P. 1988. Benzene and leukemia: a review of the literature and a risk assessment. *Am. J. Epidemiol.* 127:419-39.

Austin, H.; Keil, J.E.; and Cole, P. 1989. A prospective follow-up study of cancer mortality in relation to serum DDT. *Am. J. Public Health* 79:43-46.

Beasley, R.P.; Hwang, L.Y.; and Lin, C.C. et al. 1981. Hepatocellular carcinoma and hepatitis B virus: a prospective study of 22,707 men in Taiwan. *Lancet* II:1129-33.

Beebe, G.W. 1982. Ionizing radiation and health. *Am. Scientist* 70:35-44.

Blayney, D.W.; Blattner, W.A.; and Robert-Guroff, M. et al. 1983. The human T-cell leukemia-lymphoma virus in the southeastern United States. *JAMA* 250:1048-52.

Cantor, K.P.; Hoover, R.; and Hartge, P. et al. 1987. Bladder cancer, drinking water source, and tap water consumption: a case-control study. *J. Natl. Cancer Inst.* 79:1269-79.

Caporaso, N.; Hayes, R.B.; and Dosemici, M. et al. 1989. Lung cancer risk, occupational exposure, and the debrisoquine metabolic phenotype. *Cancer Res.* 49:3675-79.

Corey, L., and Spear, P.G. 1986. Infection with herpes simplex viruses. *N. Engl. J. Med.* 314:686-91; 749-57.

de The, G. 1979. The epidemiology of Burkitt's lymphoma: evidence for a causal association with Epstein-Barr virus. *Epidemiol. Rev.* 1:32-54.

Doll, R., and Peto, R. 1981. The causes of cancer: quantitative estimates of avoidable risks of cancer in the United States today. *J. Natl. Cancer Inst.* 66:1191-308.

Fleischer, D.E.; Goldberg, S.B.; and Browning, T.H. et al. 1989. Detection and surveillance of colorectal cancer. *JAMA* 261:580-85.

Graham, S. 1983. Toward a dietary prevention of cancer. *Epidemiol. Rev.* 5:38-50.

Greenwald, P., and Sondik, E.J. 1986. Cancer control objectives for the nation: 1985-2000. *NCI Monogr. No. 2.*

Hardcastle, J.D., and Pye, G. 1989. Screening for colorectal cancer: a critical review. *World J. Surg.* 13:38-44.

Hoar, S.K.; Blair, A.; and Holmes, F.F. et al. 1986. Agricultural herbicide use and risk of lymphoma and soft-tissue sarcoma. *JAMA* 256:1141-47.

Knudson, A.G. 1989. Hereditary cancers disclose a class of cancer genes. *Cancer* 63:1888-91.

Koutsky, L.A.; Galloway, D.A.; and Holmes, K.K. 1988. Epidemiology of genital human papillomavirus infection. *Epidemiol. Rev.* 10:122-63.

Koss, L.G. 1989. The Papanicolaou test for cervical cancer detection: a triumph and a tragedy. *JAMA* 261:737-43.

Melnick, S.; Cole, P.; and Anderson, D. et al. 1987. Rates and risks of diethylstilbestrol-related clear-cell adenocarcinoma of the vagina and cervix: an update. *N. Engl. J. Med.* 316:514-16.

Peers, F.; Bosch, X.; and Kaldor, J. et al. 1987. Aflatoxin exposure, hepatitis B virus infection and liver cancer in Swaziland. *Int. J. Cancer* 39:545-53.

Pollack, E.S.; Nomura, A.M.Y.; and Heilbrun, L.K. et al. 1984. Prospective study of alcohol consumption and cancer. *N. Engl. J. Med.* 310:617-21.

Pui, C.H.; Behm, F.G.; and Raimondi, S.C. et al. 1989. Secondary acute myeloid leukemia in children treated for acute lymphoid leukemia. *N. Engl. J. Med.* 321:136-42.

Rom, W.N. ed. 1983. *Environmental and occupational medicine.* Boston: Little, Brown.

Samet, J.M. 1989. Radon and lung cancer. *J. Natl. Cancer Inst.* 81:745-57.

Schottenfeld, D., and Fraumeni, J.F. Jr. eds. 1982. *Cancer epidemiology and prevention.* Philadelphia: W.B. Saunders.

Shapiro, S.; Kelly, J.P.; and Rosenberg, L. et al. 1985. Risk of localized and widespread endometrial cancer in relation to recent and discontinued use of conjugated estrogens. *N. Engl. J. Med.* 313:969-72.

Shore, R.E. 1988. Electromagnetic radiations and cancer cause and prevention. *Cancer* 62:1747-54.

U.K. National Case-Control Study Group. 1989. Oral contraceptive use and breast cancer risk in young women. *Lancet* I:973-82.

U.S. Public Health Service. 1989. Reducing the health consequences of smoking: 25 years of progress. A report of the Surgeon General. *DHHS Publ. No. (CDC) 89-8411.*

Walker, J.S. 1989. The controversy over radiation safety: an historical overview. *JAMA* 262:664-68.

Willett, W.C.; Polk, B.F.; and Underwood, B.A. et al. 1984. Relation of serum vitamins A and E and carotenoids to the risk of cancer. *N. Engl. J. Med.* 310:430-34.

Chapter 9

SMOKING AND CANCER

Virginia L. Ernster, Ph.D.
Steven R. Cummings, M.D.

Virginia L. Ernster, Ph.D.
Professor of Epidemiology and Chair
Department of Epidemiology and Biostatistics
School of Medicine
University of California,
San Francisco, California

Steven R. Cummings, M.D.
Associate Professor of Medicine
Department of Epidemiology and Biostatistics
Department of Medicine
School of Medicine
University of California,
San Francisco, California

Supported in part by USPHS grant PO1 CA 13556-18 from the National Cancer Institute, Bethesda, Maryland.

INTRODUCTION

Cigarette smoking is responsible for about one-third of all cancer deaths in the United States, including deaths from cancers of the lung, larynx, oral cavity, pharynx, pancreas, kidney, bladder, and cervix. This century has witnessed an epidemic of lung cancer, first in men then in women, following marked increases in smoking. Recent declines in lung cancer rates in men reflect a decline in men's smoking prevalence over the past few decades, but lung cancer remains the leading cause of cancer death in men and recently surpassed breast cancer as the leading cause of cancer death in women as well. Currently, about 25% to 30% of the U.S. population smoke, with prevalence varying dramatically by sex, age, ethnicity, and socioeconomic status. Efforts to reduce tobacco use in the United States should focus especially on young women, ethnic minorities, and the lower socioeconomic groups.

PART I: SMOKING-RELATED CANCERS AND SMOKING PREVALENCE

CANCERS RELATED TO SMOKING: THE EPIDEMIOLOGIC EVIDENCE

The epidemiologic and other evidence supporting a causal relation between smoking and cancer is overwhelming (U.S. Public Health Service 1964, 1979, 1980, 1981, 1982, 1985, 1986, 1989). An estimated 30% of total cancer deaths are associated with cigarette smoking, making it the leading known preventable cause of cancer.

The proportion of tobacco-related cancers is some-what higher for men than for women, largely reflecting the previously higher smoking rates among men. Moreover, across cancer sites there is great variability in the fraction of deaths attributable to smoking. While smoking bears little relation to cancers of some sites (e.g., colon or prostate), it accounts for as much as 85% of lung cancer cases and lesser though substantial proportions (table 9.1) of cancers of the larynx, oral cavity, esophagus, bladder, and pancreas (U.S. Public Health Service 1982). Smoking contributes to risk of cancers of the kidney, cervix, and other sites, and exposure to the cigarette smoke of others increases the risk of cancer in nonsmokers.

Lung cancer. Since the mid-1950s, lung cancer has been the leading cause of cancer death among men in the United States. In 1987, the annual age-adjusted male lung cancer death rate was 75 per 100,000 population. In 1990, lung cancer accounted for about 34% of all cancer deaths in men. Lung cancer death rates in women have risen approximately five-fold since 1950,

Table 9.1
ESTIMATED PROPORTION OF CANCER MORTALITY ATTRIBUTABLE TO CIGARETTE SMOKING, BY SITE

Site	%
Lung	85
Larynx and oral cavity	50-70
Esophagus	50
Bladder and kidney	30-40
Pancreas	30
Cervix	?
All cancer deaths	30

(Source: United States Public Health Service [1982].)

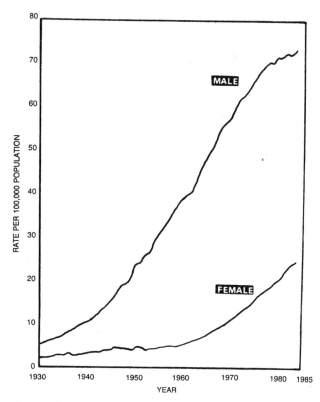

Fig. 9.1. Age-adjusted rates for lung cancer, U.S. males and females, 1930-84 (Silverberg and Lubera 1987).

when the disease accounted for only about 3% of female cancer mortality. By 1987, age-adjusted death rates for lung cancer were slightly higher than those for breast cancer, 28.2 vs. 27.1 per 100,000, respectively. In 1990, lung cancer accounted for an estimated 21% of all cancer deaths in women (fig. 9.1) (National Cancer Institute 1990; Silverberg, Boring, and Squires 1990).

The evidence that smoking is the major cause of lung cancer today comes from a large number of cohort (prospective) and case-control (retrospective) studies in humans, and studies that have monitored lung cancer patterns in populations in relation to smoking habits. This literature and the laboratory evidence for the carcinogenicity of tobacco smoke have been extensively reviewed elsewhere (U.S. Public Health Service 1964,

1979, 1980, 1981, 1982, 1985, 1986; Loeb, Ernster, and Warner et al. 1984). The results of eight prospective studies initiated in the 1950s and 1960s show relative risks of lung cancer of around 10 for males in smokers compared with nonsmokers (table 9.2) (U.S. Public Health Service 1982). Evidence for a dose-response relationship is strong; across studies, risk increases with number of cigarettes smoked, years of smoking, earlier age at onset of cigarette smoking, degree of inhalation, tar and nicotine content of cigarettes smoked, and use of filtered compared to nonfiltered cigarettes. Moreover, risk appears to decrease with number of years since smoking cessation (U.S. Public Health Service 1982; Pathak, Samet, and Humble et al. 1986).

Smoking prevalence patterns and lung cancer mortality are also strongly correlated across populations. Internationally, lung cancer rates vary with levels of cigarette consumption, and special groups within the United States that proscribe cigarette use, notably Mormons and Seventh Day Adventists, have much lower lung cancer rates than do comparison populations that include smokers. Allowing for a lag time of about 20 years, increases in smoking prevalence in the United States were followed by increases in lung cancer mortality, first in men and then in women. British physicians, who have had high smoking cessation rates, have experienced marked declines in lung cancer mortality rates (Doll and Hill 1964).

Recent changes in age-specific lung cancer mortality rates in the United States suggest that future declines in overall lung cancer death rates can be expected, particularly among men, as those birth cohorts who have less exposure to cigarette smoking than their predecessors age (table 9.3). Recent data show a decline in lung cancer mortality rates for men younger than age 55 years, resulting in a plateau of overall age-adjusted rates and presaging a reversal of this century's lung cancer epidemic. Because widespread smoking among women occurred later and the reduction in smoking prevalence has been less marked than for men, overall female lung cancer mortality rates continue to rise. Still, recent mortality data show modest declines in the under-45 age groups (National Cancer Institute 1990).

Table 9.2
LUNG CANCER MORTALITY RATIOS:
PROSPECTIVE STUDIES

Population	Non-Smokers	Smokers	Size	Number of Deaths
British physicians	1.0	14.00	34,000 males	441
	1.0	5.00	6,194 females	27
Swedish study	1.0	7.00	27,000 males	55
	1.0	4.50	28,000 females	8
Japanese study	1.0	3.76	122,000 males	940
	1.0	2.03	143,000 females	304
American Cancer Society 25-state study	1.0	8.53	358,000 males	2,018
	1.0	3.58	483,000 females	439
United States veterans	1.0	11.28	290,000 males	3,126
Canadian veterans	1.0	14.20	78,000 males	331
American Cancer Society 9-state study	1.0	10.73	188,000 males	448
California males in 9 occupations	1.0	7.61	68,000 males	368

(Source: United States Public Health Service [1982].)

Table 9.3
PERCENT CHANGE IN AGE-SPECIFIC LUNG AND BRONCHUS CANCER DEATH RATES, BY SEX, U.S. WHITES 1973-1985

Age	Male	Female
15-34	−20.0	−18.4
35-44	−13.5	−14.3
45-54	− 6.0	− 6.1
55-64	1.1	6.0
65-74	6.3	16.0
75+	12.8	10.7

(Source: National Cancer Institute [1988].)

Recent epidemiologic studies of smoking and lung cancer have addressed diverse issues: (1) the effect of changing cigarette composition on risk; (2) the potential modifying effect of diet on smoking-related risk of lung cancer; (3) the relative effect on risk of duration of smoking, age at initiation, and dose; (4) the nature of the interaction of combined exposures to smoking and occupational or other carcinogens; (5) projections of future lung cancer mortality rates based on trends in smoking prevalence and changing cigarette composition; and (6) the relation of passive smoking to lung cancer risk in nonsmokers.

Several prospective studies, in addition to case-control studies, have reported reduced risks of various cancers, especially lung, for smokers of filtered and lower tar and nicotine cigarettes relative to nonfiltered and higher tar and nicotine cigarettes (U.S. Public Health Service 1981; Stellman 1986). Others have found lower lung cancer risks for smokers with diets relatively high in green and yellow vegetables or beta carotene compared to smokers with diets low in those substances (Colditz, Stampfer, and Willett 1987). However, in all studies, regardless of cigarette type or diet, smokers have much higher lung cancer rates than nonsmokers; thus, quitting smoking is much more beneficial than changing brands or modifying diet. The number of years of smoking appears to be more important than the number of cigarettes smoked per day. It has been stated, for example, that "smoking two packs per day for 20 years is far less hazardous than smoking one pack per day for 40 years" (Peto 1986). Attempts to model the extent of interaction between cigarette smoking and occupational exposures have produced varying results, although the literature is reasonably supportive of a multiplicative effect between smoking and some exposures, most notably asbestos (U.S. Public Health Service 1985; Steenland and Thun 1986; Saracci 1987).

Projections suggest that marked declines in U.S. age-adjusted rates for males can be expected from now on, while rates for females will continue to climb, albeit at an increasingly slower rate, until early into the next century (Brown and Kessler 1988). Lung cancer will probably continue to be the leading cause of cancer death in the United States for the next two decades. Although patterns of smoking and lung cancer elsewhere in the world are not addressed here, it is clear that the increases in smoking prevalence that have occurred later in the less-developed countries are amplifying the lung cancer epidemic abroad, even as it subsides in the United States.

Laryngeal cancer. Smokers have a substantially increased risk of cancer of the larynx, with relative risks reported across studies ranging from 2 to 40; risk increases with amount of smoking. Many studies have also shown particularly elevated risks in individuals who both smoke and drink alcohol, again with dose-response relationships (U.S. Public Health Service 1982; Walter and Iwane 1983; Elwood, Pearson, and Skippen et al. 1984; De Stefani, Corvea, and Orregia et al. 1987). Risk is lower among those who smoke filtered or lower tar cigarettes. Ex-smokers show an inverse relationship between years since smoking cessation and laryngeal cancer risk (U.S. Public Health Service 1982). As female rates for the disease increase, the once-high ratio of male-to-female cases has decreased, which reflects the narrowing of sex differences in smoking (and drinking) prevalence over time.

Laryngeal cancer is relatively uncommon, accounting for an estimated 1.1% of cancer deaths in men and 0.3% in women in 1988 (Silverberg, Boring, and Squires 1990). Most cases are currently attributable to cigarette smoking.

Oral cavity and nasal cancers. A number of anatomic sites are included in the rubric "oral cavity," including the lip, tongue, salivary gland, mouth and gum, and pharynx; different epidemiologic studies vary the combinations of these sites. However defined, across studies smokers have a consistently elevated risk of oral cavity cancer with evidence of a dose-response relationship; risks are much greater for smokers who also drink alcohol. Relative risks of oral cancer associated with cigarette smoking in males have ranged from around 3 (oral cavity) to 6.5 (buccal cavity and pharynx) to 14 (pharynx). Risk appears to decline with cessation of smoking, approximating that of nonsmokers after 16 years (U.S Public Health Service 1982). Oral cancer accounted for an estimated 2.1% of cancer deaths in men in the United States and 1.2% of cancer deaths in women in 1988 (Silverberg, Boring, and Squires 1990). Cigarette smoking is a major cause of the disease. Oral cancer rates in black men have risen dramatically in recent decades, a trend that changes in smoking patterns cannot wholly explain (Stockwell and Lyman 1986).

Only recently have studies of the relationship of cigarette smoking to cancers of the nasal cavity or accessory sinuses been reported. Studies have noted elevated relative risks ranging from 1.8 to 3.0, with increases in risk seen with increasing duration of use and the strongest effects observed for squamous cell carcinomas (Hayes, Karden, and de Bruyn 1987).

Esophageal cancer. Epidemiologic studies of esophageal cancer have consistently demonstrated increased risks of the disease in smokers compared to nonsmokers and clear dose-response relationships. The 25-state prospective study by the American Cancer Society found that male and female smokers aged 45 to 64 had esophageal cancer mortality ratios that were, respectively, 3.96 and 4.89 times those of nonsmokers (Hammond 1966). As is true for cancers of the larynx and oral cavity, there is a strong synergistic effect of cigarette smoking and alcohol use. LaVecchia, Liati, and Decarli et al. (1986) reported a much lower relative risk of developing cancer of the esophagus among smokers of lower tar (<22 mg) cigarettes than smokers of higher tar (>22 mg) cigarettes, 2.9 vs. 8.9, respectively.

Several studies have reported reductions in esophageal cancer risk among ex-smokers compared to continuing smokers (U.S. Public Health Service 1982). In 1988, esophageal cancer accounted for an estimated 2.6% of male cancer deaths, and 1.0% of female cancer deaths (Silverberg, Boring, and Squires 1990); about 50% of overall esophageal cancer mortality is attributable to cigarette smoking (U.S. Public Health Service 1982).

Unlike lung cancer, mortality rates for esophageal cancer among whites have changed little. In blacks, however, rates have increased steadily since 1950. Racial differences in smoking prevalence are too small to account for the differential mortality trends in blacks and whites (Blot and Fraumeni 1987).

Bladder cancer. The relative risk of bladder cancer associated with smoking is about 2 to 3 (U.S. Public Health Service 1982; Piper, Matanoski, and Tonascia 1986). Several studies have shown markedly reduced risks of bladder cancer for ex-smokers compared to continuing smokers (Claude, Kunze, and Frentzel-Beyme et al. 1986; Hartge, Silverman, and Hoover et al. 1987). Dose-response relationship studies have produced less dramatic and less consistent results than for some of the other cancer sites. Bladder cancer is thought to be related to various occupational chemical exposures, and while the nature of any interaction between smoking and occupational exposures in the etiology of bladder cancer is unclear, the independent effect of smoking on risk is well established (U.S. Public Health Service 1985; Schifflers, Jamart, and Renard 1987).

Bladder cancer mortality rates have declined in whites and blacks of both sexes, although incidence rates have increased substantially for black males and modestly for white males and for females of both races (National Cancer Institute 1990). Bladder cancer accounted for an estimated 2.4% of cancer deaths among men and 1.3% among women in 1988 (Silverberg, Boring, and Squires 1990). Perhaps one-third of these deaths are related to cigarette smoking (U.S. Public Health Service 1982), although a recent population-based study from Utah estimated this proportion to be as high as 48.5% (Slattery, Schumacher, and West et al. 1988).

Pancreatic cancer. Studies have consistently found smokers to be at about twice the risk of developing pancreatic cancer as nonsmokers (U.S. Public Health Service 1982). Although studies have reported a dose-response relationship, the gradient with use is minor. At least one large case-control study found no strong evidence of changes in risk with various daily cigarette levels (Mack, Yu, and Hanisch et al. 1986).

Smoking cessation is associated with a reduction in risk approximating that of nonsmokers after about 10 years (Mack, Yu, and Hanisch et al. 1986).

Time trends in pancreatic cancer mortality in the United States, England, and Wales have been positively associated with changes in smoking rates (Weiss and Bernarde 1983; Moolgavkar and Stevens 1981). In recent years (1973-1987), there has been a slight decline in pancreatic cancer mortality rates among white males in the United States, little change among white females and black males, and a 26% increase among black females (National Cancer Institute 1990). Pancreatic cancer accounted for an estimated 4.5% of cancer deaths among men and 5.3% among women in 1990 (Silverberg, Boring, and Squires 1990). About one-third of deaths from the disease are attributable to cigarette smoking (U.S. Public Health Service 1982; Mack, Yu, and Hanisch et al. 1986).

Kidney cancer. Epidemiologic studies have consistently shown an increased risk of kidney cancer among smokers, with the relative risks across studies ranging from about 1.5 to 2.5. Prospective studies also support a moderate dose-response effect. On the other hand, the male-to-female ratio of kidney cancer deaths has increased over time, which would not have been expected on the basis of the later adoption of cigarette smoking by women. In 1989, kidney cancer accounted for an estimated 2.3% of cancer deaths in men and 1.8% in women (Silverberg, Boring, and Squires 1990). The Surgeon General's 1982 report on cancer concluded that cigarette smoking is a "contributory factor" in the development of cancer of the kidney (U.S. Public Health Service 1982).

Cervical cancer. In recent years, various studies in the United States, Canada, and Europe have associated cigarette smoking and cancer of the uterine cervix. This relationship at first drew skepticism, as it was felt that women who smoke may really be at risk due to early age of first intercourse, multiple sexual partners, or other factors already known to be related to cervical cancer. However, when sexual factors are controlled in data analysis, smoking still emerges as an independent risk factor for the disease, associated with relative risks of 1.5 to 2 or greater; there is also evidence of a dose-response effect (Winkelstein, Shillitoe, and Brand et al. 1984; Clarke, Morgan, and Newman 1982; Lyon, Gardner, and West et al. 1983; Trevathan, Layde, and Webster et al. 1983; Brinton, Schairer, and Haenszel et al. 1986). Thus, the dramatic decline in cervical cancer mortality in recent decades, which is attributed to successful screening efforts, has been achieved in spite of underlying increases in the number of women who smoke.

Other female reproductive cancers: breast, ovary, endometrium. Interest in the relation of cigarette smoking to breast cancer has been considerable. Results of the studies to date have been inconsistent. Whereas earlier work and one recent study suggest a protective effect (O'Connell, Hulka, and Chambless et al. 1987), other studies show little or no relation (Rosenberg, Schwingl, and Kaufman et al. 1984; Baron, Byers, and Greenberg et al. 1986; Brinton, Schairer, and Stanford et al. 1986; Stockwell and Lyman 1987). Still others find an increased risk, primarily limited to premenopausal breast cancer (Schechter, Miller, and Howe 1985; Brownson, Blackwell, and Pearson et al. 1988). Although breast cancer incidence rates have recently increased (primarily accounted for by early stage disease and possibly an artifact of more widespread screening), breast cancer mortality rates have been relatively stable over the past several decades. Given time trends in female smoking prevalence, increases in breast cancer mortality rates would have been expected if smoking were an important risk factor. Inconsistent evidence across studies, coupled with the fact that the elevations in relative risk in those studies reporting positive results have been minor, suggests that any effect of smoking on breast cancer risk is likely to be weak (Hiatt and Fireman 1986).

In studies of smoking and ovarian cancer to date, no evidence of an association has appeared, even when potential confounding variables are controlled (Baron, Byers, and Greenberg et al. 1986; Stockwell and Lyman 1987; Franks, Lee, and Kendrick et al. 1987).

Cancer of the endometrium (uterine corpus) is the only cancer for which a number of studies have shown reduced risks for smokers compared to nonsmokers (Baron, Byers, and Greenberg et al. 1986; Stockwell and Lyman 1987; Weiss, Farewell, and Szekely et al. 1980; Lesko, Rosenberg, and Kaufman et al. 1985; Franks, Kendrick, and Tyler et al. 1987; Lawrence, Tessaro, and Durgerian et al. 1987). However, the association may be weak or nonexistent for premenopausal women (Tyler, Webster, and Ory et al. 1985). The finding of a possible protective effect has been of interest to understanding the biologic mechanisms of endometrial cancer, but in the face of the overwhelmingly negative consequences for cancers of other sites and cardiovascular disease and other effects of smoking, no one would recommend smoking as a preventive measure for endometrial cancer.

Anal cancer. A study of anal cancer, which focused on sexual practices and sexually transmitted diseases, reported that current cigarette smoking was a major risk factor for the disease in both heterosexual men (relative risk, 9.4) and in women (relative risk, 7.7). These results were controlled for age, geographic location, and number of lifetime sexual partners (<5 vs. >5) (Daling, Weiss, and Hislop et al. 1987). Anal cancer is very rare and therefore has a minor impact on total cancer mortality. However, the evidence from this work, as well as other work on cervical cancer (Winkelstein, Shillitoe, and Brand et al. 1984), suggests possible interactions between viral factors and tobacco exposure that increase cancer risk. Thus, it may be of considerable interest in understanding the mechanisms of cancer etiology.

INVOLUNTARY SMOKING AND CANCER

In 1986, two major reports on the health consequences of involuntary smoking were issued: one from the National Academy of Sciences entitled *Environmental Tobacco Smoke: Measuring Exposure and Assessing Health Effects* (National Research Council 1986); and the other from the United States Surgeon General entitled *The Health Consequences of Involuntary Smoking* (U.S. Public Health Service 1986). Both concluded that exposure to ambient cigarette smoke causes lung cancer and other diseases in healthy nonsmokers.

Most studies of cancer risk associated with involuntary smoking have focused on lung cancer. Aggregation of data across studies shows significantly elevated summary relative risks. Combining the evidence across 10 case-control studies, Wald et al. recently reported a relative risk of lung cancer in nonsmokers of 1.27 (95% CI, 1.05-1.53) associated with exposure to environmental tobacco smoke and, combining the data from three prospective studies, a comparable relative risk of 1.44 (95% CI, 1.19-1.54) (Wald, Nanchahal, and Thompson et al. 1986). An earlier review reported that five of seven studies providing data by amount of smoking by spouses found evidence of increased risk for nonsmoking women whose husbands smoked heavily compared to those whose husbands were relatively light smokers (Blot and Fraumeni 1986).

Studies of involuntary smoking often pose methodologic difficulties, especially from the standpoint of measuring exposure to others' smoke (Kuller, Garfinkel, and Correa et al. 1986), which has been largely based on questionnaire data regarding the smoking status of household members. This imprecise measure of actual exposure in the home also ignores exposures in the workplace and elsewhere and potentially underestimates the extent of total exposure. Even with these limitations, the general consistency of the studies supports legislative and other efforts to protect nonsmokers from tobacco smoke in the environment.

SMOKING TRENDS

Cigarette smoking is largely a twentieth century phenomenon. Until the 1880s when cigarette production was mechanized, and even into the early part of this century, other forms of tobacco (chewing tobacco, cigars, pipes) were far more popular than cigarettes. The World War I era heralded the widespread adoption of cigarette smoking by men in the United States. At the time, smoking by women was considered morally reprehensible and ordinances forbade smoking by women in public places (Ernster 1985). The double standard began to break down in the 1920s and by World War II

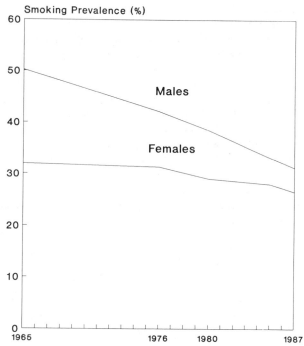

Fig. 9.2. Smoking prevalence in U.S. adults by sex, 1965-1987 (United States Public Health Service 1987; Schoenborn and Boyd [1989]).

cigarette smoking was firmly entrenched among women as well as men (U.S. Public Health Service 1980).

Adults, by sex and ethnicity. Representative national survey data on smoking prevalence have been routinely collected only since the 1950s. However, in 1935 *Fortune* magazine surveyed its readers and found that 52.5% of male respondents and 18.1% of females reported themselves to be cigarette smokers, with much higher percentages of smokers in the under-40 age group than among older respondents in both sexes (The Fortune Survey 1935). Fig. 9.2 shows national data from adults for the period 1965 to 1987. The percentage of current smokers among men declined from 50.2 in 1965 to 31.2 in 1987. Among women the percentage of current smokers declined from 31.9 in 1965 to 26.5 in 1987 (U.S. Public Health Services; Schoenborn and Boyd 1989).

Birth cohort analyses based on data from the Health Interview Survey of 1983 show that lifetime prevalence of cigarette smoking peaked among males born 1920-1929 and among females born 1930-1949 (U.S. Public Health Service 1987). An analysis of smoking exposure by birth cohort took into account the changing composition of cigarettes (i.e., increases in the proportion of filtered cigarettes and declines in tobacco content per cigarette) by examining weight of tobacco consumed per capita over time. The authors concluded that tobacco exposure *per se,* as opposed to number of cigarettes smoked, was greatest for male cohorts born 1911-1920 and for female cohorts born 1921-1940.

Accordingly, male exposure to cigarette tobacco has been declining for at least 35 years and female exposure for at least 20 years (Walker and Brin 1988). By whatever measure, the later adoption of cigarette smoking by women and the more rapid decline in cigarette

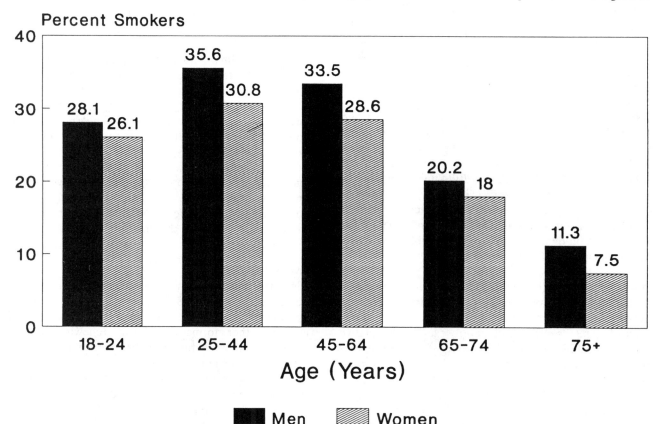

Fig. 9.3. Smoking prevalence among person 18 years of age and over by sex, U.S. 1987 (Schoenborn and Boyd [1989]).

smoking by men have dramatically narrowed the gap between men's and women's smoking rates at every age (fig 9.3) (Schoenborn and Boyd 1989).

Smoking prevalence data for whites and blacks are available since 1965 (table 9.4), when male smoking prevalence rates were higher in black men than in white men but almost identical in black and white women. By 1976, rates for both sexes were higher in blacks (U.S. Public Health Service 1979), a pattern that continues even as rates for all groups have declined. In 1987, the percentage of current smokers among the population 18 years and older was 39.0% in black men compared to 30.5% in white men and 28.0% in black women compared to 26.7% in white women (National Center for Health Statistics 1989).

Data for Hispanic Americans are only recently available. In 1987, 30% of Hispanic men and 18% of Hispanic women smoked (Schoenborn and Boyd 1989). Among male and female children, smoking prevalence rates apparently differ little between Hispanic and non-Hispanic whites, which suggests that the lower risk profile of Hispanic adults may disappear (Greenberg, Wiggins, and Kutvirt et al. 1987).

Differences in smoking prevalence across ethnic groups may in part reflect differences in smoking patterns by socioeconomic status.

Teenagers. The latest published national survey data on overall teenage smoking prevalence are for 1979. Among males ages 12 to 18, the 1979 data revealed a marked decline in smoking prevalence compared to 1970. Prevalence decreased from 18.5% to 10.7% overall; among those aged 17 to 18, the decline was even greater, from 37.3% to 19.3%. Among females aged 12 to 18, the prevalence increased between 1970 to 1974 (from 11.9% to 15.3%) and then declined by 1979 (to 12.7%); however, there was no decline among those aged 17 to 18. By 1979, the percentage of smokers was higher in teenage females than males, a dramatic reversal of the situation in earlier years (U.S. Public Health Service 1980).

Recent studies have focused on high school seniors, based on national surveys conducted annually by investigators at the University of Michigan and published by the National Institute on Drug Abuse (Johnson, O'Malley, and Bachman 1987). They show steady declines in cigarette smoking prevalence among both males and females from 1977 to 1981, followed by vacillations in

rates and much slower declines or even plateaus in rates since that time (fig. 9.4). Those data, too, illustrate the excess prevalence of smoking among females compared to males; for example, 19.8% of females compared to 16.9% of males reported daily use of cigarettes in 1986. The prevalence levels from these surveys probably underestimate teenage smoking in the general population because they do not include school dropouts; cigarette smoking is inversely related to education and is more common among youth who are not college bound (Johnson, O'Malley, and Bachman 1987; McGinnis, Shopland, and Brown 1987).

The National Health Interview Survey, which includes people 18 years and over, reports smoking prevalence rates in the age group 18 to 24 to be 28.1% in men and 26.1% in women (fig. 9.3) (Schoenborn and Boyd 1989). Smoking rates in young women appear to have declined less than in other groups and bear monitoring in the future.

Age at initiation. Data from National Health Interview Surveys and other sources suggest a steady increase over time in the proportion of smokers who begin smoking as teenagers. Today the decision to start smoking is rarely made after reaching adulthood, these data indicate. For the cohort born between 1950 and 1959, fully 88.4% of male smokers and 83.9% of female smokers started the habit before the age of 20 (U.S.

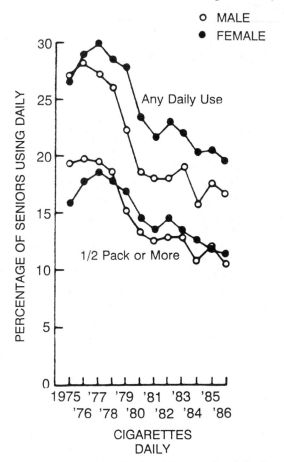

Fig. 9.4. Percent of high school seniors reporting daily cigarette smoking, 1975-1986 (Johnson, O'Malley, and Bachman [1987]).

Table 9.4
SMOKING PREVALENCE BY RACE AND SEX: 1965, 1976, 1987

| | Male | | Female | |
	White (%)	Black (%)	White (%)	Black (%)
1965[a]	51.5	60.8	34.2	34.4
1976[a]	41.2	55.3	31.8	36.8
1987[b]	30.5	39.0	26.7	28.0

[a] Data for adults age 20 and over. (Source: United States Public Health Service [1979].)
[b] Data for adults age 18 and over. (Source: National Center for Health Statistics [1989].)

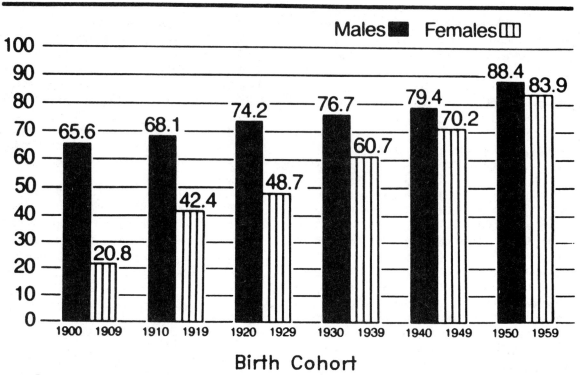

Birth Cohort

Fig. 9.5. Percent of smokers starting before age 20 by birth cohort and sex (United States Public Health Service [1987]).

Public Health Service 1987) (fig. 9.5). Such findings are of concern because studies show that the earlier smoking begins, the greater the amount and duration of use (U.S. Public Health Service 1980, 1987). These data underscore the importance of targeting smoking prevention efforts to children and preteens.

Socioeconomic status. Since at least the 1960s, smoking prevalence has been inversely associated with educational attainment in adult American men; i.e., as years of education increase the proportion of smokers decreases (table 9.5). In 1987, 40.5% of men with less than 12 years of education, 35.9% high school graduates, and 17.4% college graduates were smokers (Schoenborn and Boyd 1989). Among women, the inverse gradient appears more recently, although by the mid-1970s female college graduates had much lower smoking prevalence rates than women with less education (U.S. Public Health Service 1979). In 1987, 30.7% of women with less than 12 years of education, 29.6% high school graduates, and 15.1% college graduates were smokers (Schoenborn and Boyd 1989). Members of the population with grade school or lesser education have generally proven an exception to the patterns, with lower-than-average reported smoking rates.

Smoking rates by occupational status (excluding the farm population and the unemployed) reflect the pattern seen for educational attainment. At least since the mid-1970s, white collar workers as a whole have had lower smoking rates than blue collar workers among both men and women (U.S. Public Health Service 1979). In 1983, 27.9% of males in white collar occupations smoked, compared to 42.7% in blue collar

occupations; among women, only 29.4% of white collar workers smoked, compared to 37.8% of blue collar workers (McGinnis, Shopland, and Brown 1987).

Income, too, is inversely related to smoking prevalence among men earning at least $10,000 per year. Thus, 36.3% of men with family income of $10,000 to $19,999 smoked in 1987 compared to 23.2% with family income of $50,000 or more. Among women with family income of $19,999, 29.8% smoked in 1987 compared to 19.5% with family income of $50,000 or more (Schoenborn and Boyd 1989).

Conclusion: high-risk groups. Efforts to reduce smoking prevalence must aim at the populations currently at highest risk. They should also emphasize the actions most likely to have the greatest impact in reducing exposure to tobacco smoke for the population as a whole, smokers and nonsmokers alike. The demographic characteristics of people who smoke have changed over time. Although male smoking rates still slightly exceed those of women, the gap between the sexes has narrowed dramatically over the years because of more rapid declines in male smoking prevalence.

Table 9.5
SMOKING PREVALENCE BY EDUCATION
MALES AND FEMALES, 1987

	Male (%)	Female (%)
Less than 12 years	40.5	30.7
12 years	35.9	29.6
More than 12 years	22.0	20.3
13-15 years	26.8	24.4
16 years or more	17.4	15.1

(Source: National Center for Health Statistics [1989].)

Table 9.6
EFFECTIVENESS OF PHYSICIANS' ADVICE

Study (Ref.)	Smokers Counseled at Routine Visits	% Quit Intervention (>6 mo)		
Mausner (Mausner, Mausner, and Rail 1986)	Advice	5	No advice	0
Baric (Baric, MacArthur, and Suerwood 1976)	Counseling	14	No counseling	4
Russell (Russell et al. 1976)	Advice and pamphlet	5		
	Brief advice only	3	No advice	0.3
Smokers with Myocardial Infarctions:				
Burt (Burt et al. 1974)	Strong advice and follow-up	62	Usual care	28
Smokers with Risk Factors for Heart Disease:				
Rose (Rose and Hamilton 1978)	15-min. counseling	36	Controls	14

Coupled with increases in smoking prevalence among teenage girls in the 1970s, that has meant that smoking has become an increasingly female behavior. The average age at which people start smoking regularly has declined over time and is currently around 15 years, making smoking initiation an almost exclusively teenage phenomenon. Smoking initiation rates are higher and smoking cessation rates lower among those members of the population with less education. Thus, smoking is now inversely related to socioeconomic status. Finally, smoking rates are currently higher in blacks than whites and show signs of increasing among Hispanic Americans, once a low risk group (especially females).

Programs and community-based campaigns targeted to women, youth (again, especially to females), lower socioeconomic groups, and ethnic minorities should be among the priorities for smoking prevention and cessation efforts. Moreover, legislative and other activities designed to curb smoking in public places should be supported. Successful nonsmoking policies not only protect nonsmokers from the health risks of involuntary smoking but may very well encourage smokers to give up what is increasingly seen as a socially unacceptable behavior. Smoking cessation strategies that the individual physician might attempt with patients in clinical practice are reviewed below.

PART II: THE PHYSICIAN'S ROLE IN SMOKING CESSATION AND PREVENTION

PHYSICIAN COUNSELING ABOUT SMOKING

Is counseling about smoking worthwhile? At least 70% of smokers visit a physician during the course of a year (National Center for Health Statistics 1983), giving physicians the opportunity to advise a large number of smokers about quitting. If only a small percentage of smokers quit as a result of physicians' advice, the total number of quitters would be large.

Most controlled studies suggest that a physician's brief advice to quit smoking will help about 3% to 10% of patients quit (table 9.6). Studies using longer, more intensive interventions with patients who had recent myocardial infarctions or risk factors for heart disease have shown greater effects.

It is important, however, to be realistic about the limitations of physician advice. Most smokers who are advised to quit will continue to smoke, and physicians who expect 100% success will be frustrated.

One analysis (Cummings, Rubin, and Oster, 1989) has found that spending three to five minutes during an office visit advising a smoker to quit is more cost-effective than many other accepted preventive medical practices, even if only 1% of smokers quit (table 9.7). This analysis suggested that a follow-up visit about quitting was similarly cost-effective. Brief advice and extra smoking-related visits are at least as worthwhile as many other accepted preventive medicine practices.

Initial counseling. Advice can be brief and integrated into the usual routines of patient care. There are several steps in counseling smokers to quit (Orleans 1985; Stokes and Rigotti 1988).

Ask about smoking. Only about 40% of smokers who have visited physicians during the previous year recall the doctor advising them to quit smoking (Anda, Remington, and Sienko et al. 1987). Questions can be asked about smoking status when routinely taking other vital signs such as blood pressure.

Ask "Are you interested in quitting?" If the patient is interested, it may be especially worthwhile to develop a plan for the patient. Those who are not immediately interested may be interested later; giving them a booklet about the benefits and methods of quitting may be useful to them if they become interested in quitting.

Boost motivation. Most smokers know that smoking is bad for health in a general way, but they may not believe

Table 9.7
COST-EFFECTIVENESS OF PREVENTIVE PRACTICES*

Cost Per Year of Life Saved ($)	Preventive Practice
2,020	Brief advice about smoking during routine visit (1% quit)
5,051	Follow-up visit about smoking (1% more smokers quit)
4,113	Nicotine gum
11,300	Treating moderate hypertension
24,408	Treating mild hypertension
>65,000	Treatment of hypercholesterolemia

*For middle-aged men

that it is harmful to them. The most effective motivations for quitting are personal, such as symptoms like shortness of breath, pressure from family or coworkers, or dislike of the mess (table 9.8). Trying to scare smokers into quitting by pointing out the increased risk of cancer or heart disease may not work because smokers may believe that they are not vulnerable to those diseases. It is more productive to ask smokers why they might want to quit and find out what reasons are most important to them. A physician can summarize those personal reasons and point out ways that quitting smoking will benefit smokers.

Symptoms due to smoking. Minor symptoms are a very common reason for quitting (table 9.9) and may make smokers feel that they are vulnerable to the effects of smoking. A physician's explanation of how smoking may be the cause of the symptom and how quitting may relieve it or prevent it from worsening may enhance motivation for quitting.

Help the smoker make a plan to quit. Smokers are usually not willing to quit right away, but some will be willing to make a plan for quitting in the near future.

Set a date for quitting. This is an effective focus for the plan to quit. The quit date should be within about one month; dates set further off are often forgotten. Once the date is set, the smoker should tell friends, spouse, and coworkers; these people can provide support for the plan. Sometimes smokers may plan to take a vacation from their usual environment during the first days or weeks after they quit; this can help some smokers temporarily avoid or change the circumstances that they have learned to associate with smoking.

Cold turkey. Having a date to quit smoking means quitting abruptly. Although some smokers prefer to "cut down," most smokers can only cut down to five to ten cigarettes per day, and can go no further. Cutting down and switching to very low nicotine cigarettes can be a prelude to quitting; it might help cut down on the smoker's nicotine need. However, smokers who smoke fewer cigarettes or switch to low (but not ultralow) tar and nicotine cigarettes generally do not reduce their nicotine intake (Benowitz, Jacob, and Yu et al. 1986). Cutting down should only be viewed as preparation for quitting.

Write it down. If the smoker agrees to set a date to quit, writing that date on a prescription pad or writing a

Table 9.8
REASONS SMOKERS QUIT

Health
    Symptoms (more important than fear of fatal diseases)
    Smoking-related illness in friends or relatives
Social/Psychological
    Social pressures from work, friends and family
    To set an example
    Freedom from dependency
    "Messy" or "dirty" habit
Cost

Table 9.9
COMMON SYMPTOMS ATTRIBUTABLE TO SMOKING

Cough
Dyspnea
Sore throat
Respiratory infections
Symptoms of peptic ulcer disease
Esophagitis
Claudication and "poor circulation"
Angina
Wrinkles
Dental and gum disease

brief and informal contract signed by patient and physician will emphasize the physician's interest and remind the smoker of the agreement.

Follow-up. Most smokers who quit relapse within a year, and most relapses happen within the first few weeks (Slitzer and Gross 1988). Follow-up visits to a physician should be encouraged to help prevent relapses and increase quitters' chances of success (Wilson, Wood, and Johnson et al. 1982; Kottke, Battista, and DeFriese et al. 1988).

Obstacles to quitting.

Fear of failing (again). Most smokers have tried to quit smoking at least once before and, having relapsed, may be pessimistic about their chances of succeeding. Smokers can be reassured that this is a normal part of the quitting process; most smokers try to quit several times before they succeed in staying off for good. Previous attempts can be regarded as learning experiences. Answers to questions such as "How did the relapse occur?" and "Did the patient have withdrawal symptoms during previous attempts?" can help in planning the next attempt to quit.

Weight gain. Cigarette smoking increases the body's metabolic rate (Hofstetter, Schuts, and Jequier et al. 1986; Wack and Rodin 1982). Consequently, smokers weigh about five to 10 pounds less than nonsmokers and on average, they gain about five to 10 pounds when they quit. Regular exercise might help control weight and also reduce withdrawal symptoms. Because it can be very difficult to both quit smoking and maintain a rigorous weight loss diet, it is generally better for smokers to quit smoking first and then wait at least one month to begin dieting. Patients concerned about weight gain should be reminded that smoking is much more harmful to health than the extra weight they may gain after quitting.

Spouse, friends, and coworkers who smoke. Quitting is much more difficult if the person must be around other people who are smoking. The sight and smell of other people smoking are stimulants that can trigger a craving for cigarettes; other smokers are generally willing to lend a cigarette. Occasionally, the patient's smoking spouse or roommate is willing to quit on the same day, or at least willing to keep cigarettes and smoke out of the common living or working area. The quitter and smoking spouse, for example, may agree to a "no smoking zone" in the home where smoking, cigarettes, and ash trays are forbidden. The smoker would continue to smoke only in one isolated area of the home.

Stress. Many smokers use cigarettes as sedatives and smoke in response to stressful situations. Consequently, some smokers are reluctant to stop smoking because they are "under too much stress." The smoker could be encouraged to adopt new ways of dealing with stressful situations in place of smoking. Alternatively, during the withdrawal phase, smokers can plan to avoid particularly stressful situations. In counseling smokers about stress, it helps to be specific: what situations are likely to cause stress? what might the smoker do in particular to avoid or minimize stress?

Feelings of added stress during withdrawal from smoking might also be part of the withdrawal syndrome.

Withdrawal symptoms. Most smokers are addicted to nicotine (Gordon, Kannel, and Dawber et al. 1975). Consequently, most smokers who quit experience a typical array of symptoms that include craving for cigarettes, irritability, difficulty concentrating, and sleep disturbances (table 9.10). Some who quit also complain of constipation or diarrhea.

These withdrawal symptoms are transient and generally peak within the first few days after quitting, then gradually abate (U.S. Public Health Service 1988), and generally disappear within a month after quitting. Some smokers, however, may have occasional cravings for cigarettes for months or years after quitting.

During withdrawal, smokers often feel intense cravings for cigarettes that generally last for only a few minutes. Quitters may distract themselves from the craving by taking a walk; chewing on a carrot; closing their eyes; taking slow, deep, controlled breaths; or engaging in some other activity until the feeling passes.

A person who has had severe withdrawal symptoms during previous attempts to quit is likely to have the same types of symptoms again. For these patients, pharmacologic treatments may be especially helpful.

Pharmacologic aids for quitting smoking.

Nicotine gum. When used correctly, nicotine gum produces in the serum nicotine levels of about one-third to one-half of that produced by smoking cigarettes (Benowitz, Jacob, and Savanapridi 1987). It minimizes, but generally does not eliminate, withdrawal symptoms (Fagerstrom

Table 9.10
COMMON WITHDRAWAL SYMPTOMS

Craving
Disorientation
Irritability, lability, and intense emotions
Difficulty concentrating
Insomnia or daytime drowsiness
Dizziness
Constipation or diarrhea

Table 9.11
EFFICACY OF NICOTINE GUM IN MEDICAL PRACTICES

No. of Smokers	% Quit at 1 Year Gum	No Gum	Study (Ref.)
1,983	12	7	Russell (Russell, Merriman, and Edwards 1983)
145	25	9	Fagerstrom (Fagerstrom 1984)
777	10	11	British Thoracic Society (British Thoracic Society 1983)

1988). When combined with behavioral treatments or advice and follow-up about quitting, nicotine gum increases long-term cessation rates (table 9.11).

Nicotine gum is a resin containing 2 mg of nicotine and a bicarbonate buffer; it comes in boxes containing 96 pieces and will cost the patient about $20 to $30 per box. (A 4 mg dose is not available in the United States.) The nicotine is absorbed through the buccal mucosa into the systemic circulation (Benowitz 1986). It is much better absorbed in an alkaline than an acid environment. Although some nicotine is absorbed through the gastric mucosa, most of this is metabolized during its first pass though the liver (Benowitz 1986).

Nicotine gum may be most useful for smokers who are most addicted to nicotine (Jarvik and Schneider 1984). Several questions can provide clues to the degree of a patient's addiction to nicotine (table 9.12). In general, smokers who have had withdrawal symptoms the last time they quit, who smoke within about 30 minutes of waking up in the morning, or who continue to smoke when they are sick, have a stronger addiction to nicotine.

Contraindications to the use of nicotine gum include pregnancy, recent myocardial infarction, and life-threatening arrhythmias (*Physicians' Desk Reference* 1990). Nicotine gum may aggravate coronary disease, peptic ulcers, esophagitis, and peripheral vascular and vasospastic diseases. There are arguments, however, that patients with these conditions would be better off using nicotine gum than continuing to smoke.

The nicotine gum's side effects are generally minor and related to chewing and the effects of nicotine on the gastrointestinal system (table 9.13). Specifically, some users complain of sore jaws, irritation of the mouth, dyspepsia, heartburn, hiccups, and sore throat. Dental appliances (such as bridges and caps) occasionally loosen or deteriorate. A few patients complain of palpitations.

Patients must use the gum correctly in order to get the most benefit and minimize potential side effects (table 9.14). Nicotine gum only relieves withdrawal symptoms; it is important that patients stop smoking first before starting to use the gum regularly (Hughes

Table 9.12
SCREENING QUESTIONS FOR ADDICTION TO NICOTINE

Did you have withdrawal symptoms the last time you quit?
How soon do you smoke after waking up?
Do you continue to smoke when you are sick?
How many cigarettes do you smoke in a day?

Table 9.13
USING NICOTINE GUM

1. Set a date to quit.
2. Start gum only after quitting. Do not smoke and chew.
3. Nicotine is absorbed through the mouth, not the stomach. Therefore, chew slowly. Squeeze just enough to release the "flavor" (each piece should last at least 15 minutes). Pause. Let the nicotine be absorbed.
4. Carry it with you where you used to carry cigarettes.
5. Anticipate. It takes several minutes for the nicotine to reach the blood. Start chewing as soon as you feel a desire to smoke.
6. Continue to carry the gum with you for at least 3 months. Use it until you are confident that you can stay off permanently.

and Miller 1984). This means that nicotine gum should only be prescribed to patients who have a plan to quit. Patients who chew the gum very vigorously may get sore jaws, swallow more nicotine and, consequently, suffer more gastrointestinal symptoms while getting little or no additional nicotine into the systemic circulation (Benowitz 1986). Thus, patients should chew slowly, occasionally, and let the juices of the gum sit in the buccal mucosa while the nicotine is absorbed. Since the risk of relapse is greatest during the first few months, patients should be advised to carry the gum with them where they used to carry their cigarettes for at least three months after quitting.

Most patients discontinue using nicotine gum on their own. The manufacturer recommends that the gum not be used longer than six months (*Physicians' Desk Reference* 1990), but the ideal length of use is unknown. Between 1% and 10% of patients who use nicotine gum beyond one year may have become addicted to it. They may be tapered off the gum by reducing the number of pieces chewed daily, or by substituting regular chewing gum. Some who stop using the gum, however, return to smoking. Although long-term use of nicotine gum may be less harmful than smoking, the safety of such use is not known.

Clonidine.   Clonidine, an alpha-2 adrenergic antagonist that has been used to treat drug withdrawal syndromes, relieves a number of acute withdrawal symptoms in heavy smokers (Glassman, Jackson, and Walsh 1984). One study (Glassman, Stetner, and Walsh et al. 1988) has found that 0.15 mg to 0.30 mg of clonidine per day doubled the short-term (one month) rates of smoking cessation among heavy smokers who also were receiving individual behavioral therapy. The long-term effectiveness of clonidine in medical practice has not yet been studied.

Sedatives.   Although many smokers complain of increased anxiety during withdrawal from cigarettes,

Table 9.14
SIDE EFFECTS OF NICOTINE GUM

Sore jaw
Mouth irritation (rarely, ulceration)
Dyspepsia, heartburn
Hiccups, belching, nausea
Sore throat
Palpitations
Dizziness
Deterioration of dental work

sedatives have not been proven to be effective in helping smokers quit. One randomized blind trial (Glassman, Jackson, and Walsh et al. 1984) found that alprazolam provided marginally better relief of withdrawal symptoms than placebo over a short period of abstinence.

Prevention of relapse.   Many smokers are able to quit for short periods of time but most relapse, generally within the first month (Slitzer and Gross 1988). After one year, as many as 80% return to smoking.

In the first few weeks after quitting, withdrawal symptoms are the most common reason for relapse (Cummings, Jaen, and Giovino 1985). Later on, stressful situations become the most common reason that smokers give for starting to smoke again. Many of those who relapse "borrow" their first cigarette from another smoker (Lichtenstein, Antonuccio, and Rainwater 1977).

When a patient has decided to quit smoking, a physician can suggest a few ways to avoid relapse (table 9.15). In general, smokers should avoid any sources of cigarettes (other smokers, hidden packages of cigarettes, places where they buy cigarettes) and situations that often prompt them to smoke (drinking alcohol, sitting in smoking sections). Self-help booklets generally contain tips about how to avoid relapse.

Follow-up visits.   Studies suggest that follow-up is important in helping maintain abstinence from cigarettes. Three controlled trials (Fagerstrom 1984; Richmond and Webster 1985; Wilson, Wood, and Johnston et al. 1982) have found that among smokers who received advice to quit smoking from a physician, those who also had at least one follow-up visit about smoking were about twice as likely to be abstinent six to 12 months later.

Follow-up visits may be most worthwhile for patients who have made a plan to quit smoking. The first follow-up visit should be scheduled during the period when the patient has the greatest risk of relapse; that is, within two weeks after the quit date. Some patients may benefit from additional visits during the first three months after quitting. Patients who return for follow-up visits will have quit smoking, tried but relapsed, or

Table 9.15
SUGGESTIONS TO PATIENTS
FOR AVOIDING RELAPSES

1. Avoid smokers.
2. If you can't avoid smokers, be assertive:
   *Tell them you are trying to quit
   *Ask them not to smoke near you
3. Throw away *all* your cigarettes, lighters, and ashtrays.
4. Don't go into the place(s) where you bought cigarettes.
5. Avoid places or situations where you usually smoke.
6. Avoid alcohol.
7. Develop other ways of handling stress besides smoking.
8. Use strategies for coping with urges to smoke:
   *Relaxation exercises
   *Deep breathing
   *Distract your attention from smoking
9. Exercise.
10. Plan periodic rewards for yourself for staying off.
11. Enlist the support of others, especially nonsmokers.
12. You can't have "just one."

simply not tried. The approach to each type of patient should vary.

Smokers who have quit. Quitters should be congratulated. The physician can provide support by asking about the problems they have encountered. Often, the best way to help patients solve problems is to ask them if they can think of a potential approach. For patients who are having difficulty, consider scheduling another follow-up visit within one or two weeks.

Smokers who tried but relapsed. These patients should be congratulated for trying and reassured that trying to quit is a prelude to eventual success. In order for the patient to learn from the attempt, it can be helpful to review what specifically happened. For example, asking patients where they got their first cigarettes often uncovers situations (like having lunch with a smoking friend) that could have been avoided. This information can be helpful in planning the next attempt to quit. If withdrawal symptoms were an important barrier, then pharmacologic treatment should be considered for the next attempt. These patients should be offered an opportunity to try again.

Smokers who did not try. Sometimes, unavoidable situations prevent smokers from following through on their plans to quit. Often, the smoker is not yet motivated to quit. It can be useful to review the patients' own reasons for wanting to quit, the benefits they can anticipate, and potential barriers to quitting. These patients should be offered another opportunity to make a plan to quit.

Other follow-up. It may be helpful to call smokers on or shortly after their quit date. Such calls can be made by office staff who are interested in helping smokers quit. If the patient is having difficulty staying off cigarettes, an office visit can be scheduled.

Supportive letters or post cards sent to the smoker on the quit date might serve as a reminder and convey a message of the physician's support.

The pregnant smoker. Because of concerns about the effects of smoking on their unborn children, about 25% of pregnant women quit smoking during their pregnancy (Prager, Malin, and Spiegler et al. 1984). Unfortunately, about 80% resume smoking after giving birth.

Many women are aware of the effects of smoking on the fetus, but a substantial minority either are not aware that smoking is harmful to their child or have only a vague awareness of the problem (Wilner, Secker-Walker, and Flynn et al. 1987).

One randomized trial (Sexton and Hebel 1984) found that individual counseling about how to quit smoking along with monthly supportive telephone calls doubled the rate of cessation (from 20% to 43%) among pregnant smokers. As a result, the birth weight and length of infants among those who were counseled significantly increased. A self-help kit for pregnant women ("Freedom From Smoking for You and Your Baby") is also available from the American Lung Association (see table 9.16).

Organizing a quit-smoking office.

Setting up a system. Physicians have to attend to many problems and responsibilities. They tend to forget about preventive issues, like counseling about smoking, unless the patient brings up the subject or counseling about smoking is made a high priority and is integrated into the office routines, which requires the involvement of the office staff. Make questions about smoking part of routine vital signs; smoking is a risk factor, like blood pressure and weight. Office staff should routinely ask patients whether they smoke. If the office has a stamp or form for filling in vital signs, smoking status should be added to it.

Reminders on the charts of smokers. Physicians often note the patient's smoking status on a problem list, but this is not a very effective reminder to counsel patients. One study (Cohen, Christen, and Katz et al. 1987) found that when a colorful sticker asking "Did you counsel about smoking?" is placed on the patient's record for that visit, physicians were much more likely to discuss smoking and spend more time counseling with their patients.

"Tickler files" of quit days. To remind the staff and physician to call back patients on or just after their dates to quit, the office staff can maintain a small file of quit dates organized by the day of the month. Smokers' cards should be filed by date and should contain their telephone numbers and any other special information, such as whether they received a prescription for nicotine gum.

Honor roll. Some offices post a list of names of smokers who have quit and remained abstinent for at least a month. This quitters' "honor roll" displayed in the office can serve as reinforcement for quitters, physicians, and office staff and might encourage other smokers to quit.

Patient education materials. A number of excellent pamphlets and booklets are available at little or no cost (table 9.16). They provide information on the health risks of smoking, the benefits of quitting, tips for how to quit, and advice about how to avoid relapse.

The American Academy of Family Practice (AAFP) has developed a comprehensive kit of materials for the office that includes reminder stickers and progress notes for patients' charts, audio tapes to instruct physicians and office staff about counseling and using the system, and self-help material for patients (see table 9.16). This comprehensive kit is available to family practitioners through the AAFP. Other programs for physicians are also available (table 9.17).

Table 9.16
SELF-HELP SMOKING CESSATION MATERIALS

Freedom From Smoking in 20 Days. New York: American Lung Association. 1984. 62 pp. Comprehensive self-help manual; provides step-by-step approach to quit smoking in 20 days; includes contract sheet, poster, colorful illustrations, weight control information, and deep breathing and muscle relaxation exercises. American Lung Association 1740 Broadway, New York, N.Y. 10017 ($3.50).

Freedom From Smoking for You and Your Family. New York: American Lung Association. Self-help booklet; discusses preparing to quit smoking, picking a day to quit, quitting for good, and benefits of quitting. A simplified, condensed version of *Freedom From Smoking in 20 Days.* American Lung Association, 1740 Broadway, New York, N.Y. 10017 ($3.50).

Freedom From Smoking for You and Your Baby. New York: American Lung Association. 1987. Ten-day stop-smoking program specifically designed for pregnant women. American Lung Association, 1740 Broadway, New York, N.Y. 10017 ($3.50).

Calling It Quits (two pamphlets). Dallas, Texas: American Heart Association. 1984. 15 pp. and 23 pp., respectively. Pamphlet 1: Concise guide on how to quit smoking; discusses reasons for quitting, setting a target date, and conditioning oneself physically and emotionally to quit smoking for life. Pamphlet 2: Discusses situations that tempt former smokers to resume smoking; suggests ways to cope with difficult situations. American Heart Association, 7320 Greenville Ave., Dallas, Texas 75231 ($1.00).

Cleaning the Air: How to Quit Smoking and Quit for Keeps. Bethesda, Md: National Cancer Institute. 1987. 45 pp. Guide to help smokers think about why they smoke; discusses benefits of quitting, preparing to quit, what to expect. Comical illustrations. Includes list of resources for additional assistance. Office of Cancer Communications, Publications Office, National Cancer Institute, Bethesda, Md. 20892. Telephone: (800) 4-CANCER (Free).

Quit and Win (two booklets). Minneapolis, Minn.: University of Minnesota. 1982. Booklet 1: To help the smoker quit; discusses problems that are likely to face smokers when they quit. Booklet 2: To help former smokers "win the war" against resuming smoking; discusses the urge to smoke and temptations to resume smoking; also addresses withdrawal problems (e.g., tension, restlessness, weight gain), and relapse. Minnesota Heart Health Programs, Stadium Gate 20, 611 Beacon Street, University of Minnesota, Minneapolis, Minn. 55455. Telephone: (612) 624-1818. ($12.75 each).

Quit Smoking Kit. Palo Alto, Calif. Stanford University. 1986. 9 pp. Includes how-to-use guide and heart magnet. Four sections: 1) Get Ready to Quit; 2) Tomorrow's the Day; 3) You've Quit; 4) Staying Free. Health Promotion Resource Center, Stanford Center for Research in Disease Prevention, 1000 Welch Road, Palo Alto, Calif. 94304-1885. Telephone: (415) 723-1000 ($2.90).

Quit For Life (kit). Chapel Hill, N.C.: University of North Carolina. 1987. Designed to help black Americans quit smoking; gives suggestions for preparing to quit, staying smoke-free, and controlling weight after quitting. Smoking and Health Consultants, Inc., University of North Carolina at Chapel Hill, Chapel Hill, N.C. 27514.

A Lifetime of Freedom From Smoking: Maintenance Program For Ex-Smokers. New York: American Lung Association. 1986. 27 pp. Designed to help ex-smokers maintain nonsmoking behavior. Includes suggested daily routine; discusses situations which produce strong cravings for cigarettes and suggests ways to cope with these situations. American Lung Association, 1740 Broadway, New York, N.Y. 10017 ($3.50).

How to Stay Quit Over the Holidays. New York: American Cancer Society. 1985. 44 pp. Self-help pamphlet. Gives hints on how to "stay quit" through the holiday season. American Cancer Society, 1599 Clifton Road N.E., Atlanta, Ga. 30029. Telephone: (404) 320-3333 (Free).

Guidelines for a Weight-Control Component in a Smoking Cessation Program. New York: American Heart Association. 1985. 12 pp. Integrates diet, weight control, and smoking withdrawal. Lists common problems following smoking cessation and possible solutions. American Heart Association, 7320 Greenville Avenue, Dallas, Texas 75231 (Free).

Stop Smoking, Stay Trim. New York: American Lung Association. 1985. 10 pp. Discusses metabolic changes following smoking cessation, weight gain and food cravings. Gives tips for weight control after quitting smoking. American Lung Association, 1740 Broadway, New York, N.Y. 10017 (Free).

Referrals. For patients who are interested in formal smoking cessation programs, a current list of reputable local programs and their telephone numbers should be available in the office. Such listings often are available from local offices of the American Cancer Society or the American Lung Association.

Nonsmoking offices. To set an example, smoking should be prohibited in the office and waiting room. Additionally, waiting areas should be stocked only with magazines that do not carry cigarette advertising.

Other smoking cessation methods. Most smokers who quit and remain abstinent have done so without the aid of physicians or formal programs. Furthermore, in surveys most smokers report they would prefer to try to quit smoking on their own or with the advice of their physician (Schwartz and Dubizky 1967). Only a minority

of smokers are interested in formal groups or other methods. The effectiveness of these methods has been comprehensively reviewed (Schwartz 1987).

Behavioral approaches. Formal smoking cessation programs use a variety of methods. Some programs offer group discussions that share reasons for quitting, tips about how to quit and stay off, and support for quitting. Others may offer individual counseling, behavior modification (such as training the smoker how to cope with situations that lead to relapse), aversive therapy (such as mild electric shock paired with smoking a cigarette), or "rapid smoking" (continuous puffing on cigarettes until the patient develops an aversion to smoking). A well-designed counseling or behavior therapy program can achieve very high (60% to 100%) initial cessation rates and good (20% to 50%) long-term cessation rates among smokers who attend a formal

Table 9.17
SMOKING CESSATION MATERIALS FOR PHYSICIANS

AAFP Stop Smoking Kit. Comprehensive guide for establishing stop-smoking programs in medical offices. Contains self-help booklets for patients, audiotapes for office staff and physicians, stickers and flow sheets for charts, and a manual for the program. American Academy of Family Physicians, 1740 West 92nd Street, Kansas City, Mo. 64114. Telephone: (800) 821-2512 ($50 AAFP members; $75 nonmembers).

A Physician Talks About Smoking (slide series). Designed for physicians and other health professionals who address medical and lay audiences on smoking and health. Slides summarize: 1) cigarette smoking as a risk factor for premature morbidity/mortality; 2) costs of smoking-related disease and death; 3) how cigarettes cause disease; 4) who smokes, how much, and why. Office of Smoking and Health, United States Public Health Service, Rockville, Md 20857. Telephone: (301) 443-1690 (Free).

Clinical Opportunities for Smoking Intervention: A Guide for the Busy Physician. National Heart, Lung, and Blood Institute/American Lung Association/American Thoracic Society. 1986. NIH Publication No. 86-2178. Discusses the role of physicians in helping patients stop smoking; describes specific intervention strategies for the clinical setting; Superintendent of Documents, U.S. Government Printing Office, Washington, D.C. 20402 (Free).

The Physicians Guide: How to Help Your Hypertensive Patient Stop Smoking. National High Blood Pressure Education Program. 1983. NIH Publication No. 83-1271. Designed to help doctors teach their hypertensive patients to quit smoking. Describes the "minimal smoking-cessation procedure," a simple, practical, step-by-step approach that can be integrated into routine office visits (Free).

Clean Air Health Care: A Guide to Establish Smoke-Free Health Care Facilities. Section 1 (Setting the Agenda): Demonstrates that a smoke-free hospitals legal, feasible, and desired by a majority of patients and employees. Section 2 (Implementation): Practical step-by-step guide to developing and adopting a smoke-free policy. Minnesota Coalition for a Smoke-Free Society by the Year 2000, 2221 University Avenue, S.E., Suite 400, Minneapolis, Minn. 55414. Telephone: (612) 378-0902 ($9.75).

program (Health and Public Policy Committee 1986; Mausner, Mausner, and Rial 1986). Many smokers, however, drop out before completing the program. There is no evidence that it is valuable to refer a smoker to a smoking cessation program when they are not interested in that approach.

The nature of smoking cessation programs varies widely among communities. Voluntary agencies, such as the American Cancer Society and the American Lung Association, usually have lists of local smoking cessation programs and may be able to provide information about program methods. In general, programs that include long-term follow-up support are more likely to help patients remain abstinent than programs that offer no such support.

Hypnosis is a popular method for smoking cessation. Studies have found a wide range of effectiveness for hypnotherapy (Schwartz 1987; Health and Public Policy Committee 1986). In general, hypnosis is most effective when there are more sessions, highly motivated subjects, individualized therapy, and follow-up.

It has been claimed that acupuncture treatments can reduce withdrawal symptoms and help smokers quit. The effectiveness of acupuncture in producing long-term smoking cessation, however, has not been adequately evaluated in randomized trials (Health and Public Policy Committee 1986).

Promoting nonsmoking in the community. In addition to helping individual patients quit smoking, physicians can work to restrict smoking in the larger community. As role models, physicians should not smoke and should work toward ensuring that the health care environment in which they work is smoke-free. They can also help to foster a nonsmoking environment in other parts of their communities (restaurants, theaters, church halls, and so on). Physicians often have special opportunities to promote nonsmoking when speaking before community groups or with local media

as well as to testify and vote in support of related legislation and ballot issues. Physicians who sit on the boards of civic and cultural organizations should speak out against any offers of financial support from the tobacco industry. A number of organizations are active in promoting nonsmoking policies, most of which have benefited from physician involvement. These include Americans for Nonsmokers Rights, ASH (Action on Smoking and Health), the Coalition on Smoking and Health, GASP (Group Against Smoking Pollution), DOC (Doctors Oughta Care), and the Advocacy Institute. Many physician societies (e.g., American Medical Association, American Association of Family Practitioners, American College of Obstetrics and Gynecology, American Academy of Pediatrics) have adopted formal resolutions on smoking policy or developed specialized patient programs. Owing to the special credibility conferred by their professional status, physicians can play a pivotal role in efforts to achieve a smoke-free society.

CONCLUSION

Great strides have been made since the 1940s, when a series of magazine advertisements carried the slogan "More Doctors Smoke Camels." Today, smoking among medical students and young physicians is rare, which means that medicine will soon be a virtually nonsmoking profession. Still, about 26% to 30% of the general population in the United States continues to smoke, with several thousand teenagers estimated to be joining the ranks of smokers each day. Lung cancer, an almost entirely preventable disease, remains the leading cancer killer in the United States, and about 30% of cancer deaths overall are currently attributable to cigarette smoking. The challenge of smoking remains a formidable one, and reduction of tobacco use should be a leading priority in cancer prevention.

ACKNOWLEDGMENT

We thank Maureen Morris for her valuable assistance.

REFERENCES

Anda, R.F.; Remington, P.L.; and Sienko, D.G. et al. 1987. Are physicians advising smokers to quit? the patients' perspective. *JAMA* 257:1916-19.

Baric, L.; MacArthur, C.; and Suerwood, M. 1976. A study of health education aspects of smoking in pregnancy. *Int. J. Health Ed.* 19 (Suppl):1-17.

Baron, J.A.; Byers, T.; and Greenberg, E.R. et al. 1986. Cigarette smoking in women with cancers of the breast and reproductive organs. *J. Natl. Cancer Inst.* 77:677-80.

Benowitz, N.C. 1986. Clinical pharmacology of nicotine. *Ann. Rev. Med.* 37:21-32.

Benowitz, N.C.; Jacob, P. III; and Savanapridi, C. 1987. Determinants of nicotine intake while chewing nicotine polacrilex gum. *Clin. Pharm. Therapy* 41:467-73.

Benowitz, N.C.; Jacob, P. III; and Yu, L. et al. 1986. Reduced tar, nicotine, and carbon monoxide exposure while smoking ultralow but not low-yield cigarettes. *JAMA* 256:241-46.

Blot, W.J., and Fraumeni, J.F. Jr. 1986. Passive smoking and lung cancer. *J. Natl. Cancer Inst.* 77:993-1000.

Blot, W.J., and Fraumeni, J.F. Jr. 1987. Trends in esophageal cancer mortality among U.S. blacks and whites. *Am. J. Public Health* 77:296-98.

Brinton, L.A.; Schairer, C.; and Haenszel, W. et al. 1986. Smoking and invasive cervical cancer. *JAMA* 255:3265-69.

Brinton, L.A.; Schairer, C.; and Stanford, J.L. et al. 1986. Cigarette smoking and breast cancer. *Am. J. Epidemiol.* 123:614-22.

British Thoracic Society. 1983. Comparison of four methods of smoking withdrawal in patients with smoking related diseases. *Br. Med. J.* 286:595-97.

Brown, C.C., and Kessler, L.G. 1988. Projections of lung cancer mortality in the United States: 1985-2025. *J. Natl. Cancer Inst.* 80:43-51.

Brownson, R.C.; Blackwell, C.W.; and Pearson, D.K. et al. 1988. Risk of breast cancer in relation to cigarette smoking. *Arch. Intern. Med.* 148:140-44.

Burt, A.; Thornley, P.; and Illingworth, D. et al. 1974. Stopping smoking after myocardial infarction. *Lancet* I: 304-306.

Clarke, E.A.; Morgan, R.W.; and Newman, A.M. 1982. Smoking as a risk factor in cancer of the cervix: additional evidence from a case-control study. *Am. J. Epidemiol.* 115:59-66.

Claude, J.; Kunze, E.; and Frentzel-Beyme, R. et al. 1986. Life-style and occupational risk factors in cancer of the lower urinary tract. *Am. J. Epidemiol.* 124:578-89.

Cohen, S.J.; Christen, A.G.; and Katz, P.G. et al. 1987. Counseling medical and dental patients about cigarette smoking: the impact of nicotine gum and chart reminders. *Am. J. Public Health* 77:313-16.

Colditz, G.A.; Stampfer, M.J.; and Willett, W.C. 1987. Diet and lung cancer: a review of the epidemiologic evidence in humans. *Arch. Intern. Med.* 147:157-60.

Cummings, K.M.; Jaen, C.R.; and Giovino, G. 1985. Circumstances surrounding relapse in a group of recent exsmokers. *Prev. Med.* 14:195-202.

Cummings, S.R.; Rubin, S.M.; and Oster, G. The cost-effectiveness of counseling smokers to quit. *JAMA* 261: 75-79.

Daling, J.R.; Weiss, N.S.; and Hislop, G. et al. 1987. Sexual practices, sexually transmitted diseases, and the incidence of anal cancer. *N. Engl. J. Med.* 317:973-77.

De Stefani, E.; Corvea, P.; and Orregia, F. et al. 1987. Risk factors for laryngeal cancer. *Cancer* 60:3087-91.

Doll, R., and Hill, A.B. 1964. Mortality in relation to smoking: ten years' observations of British doctors. *Br. Med. J.* 1:1399-1410; 1460-67.

Elwood, J.M.; Pearson, J.C.G.; and Skippen, D.H. et al. 1984. Alcohol, smoking, social and occupational factors in the aetiology of cancer of the oral cavity, pharynx and larynx. *Int. J. Cancer* 34:603-12.

Ernster, V.L. 1985. Mixed messages for women: a social history of cigarette smoking and advertising. *N.Y. State J. Med.* 85:335-40.

Fagerstrom, K.O. 1984. Effects of nicotine chewing gum and follow-up appointments in physician-based smoking cessation. *Prev. Med.* 13:517-27.

Fagerstrom, K.O. 1988. Efficacy of nicotine chewing gum: a review. In Pomerlau, O.F., and Pomerlau, C.S. eds. *Nicotine replacement: a critical evaluation.* pp. 109-28. New York: Alan R. Liss.

Franks, A.L.; Kendrick, J.S.; and Tyler, C.W. et al. 1987. Postmenopausal smoking, estrogen replacement therapy, and the risk of endometrial cancer. *Am. J. Obstet. Gynecol.* 156:20-23.

Franks, A.L.; Lee, N.C.; and Kendrick, J.S. et al. 1987. Cigarette smoking and the risk of epithelial ovarian cancer. *Am. J. Epidemiol.* 126:112-17.

Glassman, A.H.; Jackson, W.K.; and Walsh, B.T. et al. 1984. Cigarette craving, smoking withdrawal, and clonidine. *Science* 226:864-66.

Glassman, A.H.; Stetner, M.S.; and Walsh, T. et al. 1988. Heavy smokers, smoking cessation, and clonidine: results of a double-blind randomized trial. *JAMA* 259:2863-66.

Gordon, T.; Kannel, W.B.; and Dawber, T.R. et al. 1975. Changes associated with quitting smoking: the Framingham study. *Am. Heart J.* 90:322-28.

Greenberg, M.A.; Wiggins, C.L.; and Kutvirt, D.M. et al. 1987. Cigarette use among Hispanic and non-Hispanic white school children, Albuquerque, New Mexico. *Am. J. Public Health* 77:621-22.

Hammond, E.C. 1966. Smoking in relation to the death rates of one million men and women. In Haenszel, W. ed. Epidemiological approaches to the study of cancer and other chronic diseases. *Natl. Cancer Inst. Monogr.* 19: 127-204.

Hartge, P.; Silverman, D.; and Hoover, R. et al. 1987. Changing cigarette habits and bladder cancer risk: a case-control study. *J. Natl. Cancer Inst.* 78:1119-25.

Hayes, R.B.; Kardan, J.W.P.F.; and de Bruyn, A. 1987. Tobacco use and sinonasal cancer: case-control study. *Br. J. Cancer* 56:843-46.

Health and Public Policy Committee. 1986. Methods for stopping cigarette smoking. *Ann. Intern. Med.* 105:281-91.

Hiatt, R.A., and Fireman, B.H. 1986. Smoking, menopause, and breast cancer. *J. Natl. Cancer Inst.* 76:833-38.

Hofstetter, A.; Schuts, Y.; and Jequier, E. et al. 1986. Increased 24-hour energy expenditure in cigarette smokers. *N. Engl. J. Med.* 314:79-82.

Hughes, J.R., and Miller, S.A. 1984. Nicotine gum to help stop smoking. *JAMA* 252:2855-58.

Jarvik, M.E., and Schneider, N.G. 1984. Degree of addiction and effectiveness of nicotine gum therapy for smoking. *Am. J. Psychiatry* 141:790-91.

Johnson, L.D.; O'Malley, P.M.; and Bachman, J.G. 1987. *National trends in drug use and related factors among American high school students and young adults, 1975-1986.* Rockville, Md: National Institute on Drug Abuse.

Kottke, T.E.; Battista, R.N.; and DeFriese, G.H. et al. 1988. Attributes of successful smoking cessation interventions in medical practice: a meta-analysis of 39 controlled trials. *JAMA* 259:2882-89.

Kuller, L.H.; Garfinkel, L.; and Correa, P. et al. 1986. Contribution of passive smoking to respiratory cancer. *Environ. Health Perspect.* 70:57-69.

Lawrence, C.; Tessaro, I.; and Durgerian, S. et al. 1987. Smoking, body weight, and early-stage endometrial cancer. *Cancer* 59:1665-69.

LaVecchia, C.; Liati, P.; and Decarli, A. et al. 1986. Tar yields of cigarettes and the risk of oesophageal cancer. *Int. J. Cancer* 38:381-85.

Lesko, S.M.; Rosenberg, L.; and Kaufman, D.W. et al. 1985. Cigarette smoking and the risk of endometrial cancer. *N. Engl. J. Med.* 313:593-96.

Lichtenstein, E.; Antonuccio, D.O.; and Rainwater, G. 1977. *Unkicking the habit: the resumption of cigarette smoking.* Seattle, Wash.: Western Psychological Association.

Loeb, L.A.; Ernster, V.L.; and Warner, K.E. et al. 1984. Smoking and lung cancer: an overview. *Cancer Res.* 44: 5940-58.

Lyon, J.L.; Gardner, J.W.; and West, D.W. et al. 1983. Smoking and carcinoma *in situ* of the uterine cervix. *Am. J. Public Health* 73:558-62.

Mack, T.M.; Yu, M.C.; and Hanisch, R. et al. 1986. Pancreas cancer and smoking, beverage consumption, and past medical history. *J. Natl. Cancer Inst.* 76:49-60.

Mausner, J.S.; Mausner, B.; and Rial, W.Y. 1986. The influence of a physician on the smoking of his patients. *Am. J. Public Health* 58:46-53.

Moolgavkar, S.H., and Stevens, R.G. 1981. Smoking and cancers of bladder and pancreas: risk and temporal trends. *J. Natl. Cancer Inst.* 67:15-23.

National Cancer Institute. 1988. *Annual cancer statistics review including cancer trends: 1950-1985.* U.S. DHHS, PHS. 1990. Cancer statistics review 1973-1987. NIH Publ. No. 90-2789.

National Research Council. 1986. *Environmental tobacco smoke: measuring exposures and assessing health effects.* Washington, D.C.: National Academy Press.

National Center for Health Statistics. 1983. *Physician visits: volume and interval since last visit, United States 1980.* Series 10, No. 144, DHHS, Publ. No. (PHS) 83-1572. Washington, D.C.: U.S. Government Printing Office.

O'Connell, D.L.; Hulka, B.S.; and Chambless, L.E. et al. 1987. Cigarette smoking, alcohol consumption, and breast cancer risk. *J. Natl. Cancer Inst.* 78:229-34.

Orleans, C.T. 1985. Understanding and promoting smoking cessation: overview and guidelines for physician intervention. *Ann. Rev. Med.* 36:51-61.

Pathak, D.R.; Samet, J.M.; and Humble, C.G. et al. 1986. Determinants of lung cancer risk in cigarette smokers in New Mexico. *J. Natl. Cancer Inst.* 76:597-604.

Peto, R. 1986. Influence of dose and duration of smoking on lung cancer rates. In Zaridze, D.G., and Peto, R. eds. Tobacco: a major international health hazard. *IARC Publications No. 74.* pp. 23-33. Lyon: International Agency for Research on Cancer.

Physicians' Desk Reference. 1990. pp. 1070-72. Oradell, N.J.: Medical Economics.

Piper, J.M.; Matanoski, G.M.; and Tonascia, J. 1986. Bladder cancer in young women. *Am. J. Epidemiol.* 123:1033-42.

Prager, J.; Malin, H.; and Spiegler, D. et al. 1984. Smoking and drinking behavior before and during pregnancy. *Public Health Rep.* 99:117-27.

Richmond, R,L., and Webster, I.W. 1985. A smoking cessation programme for use in general practice. *Med. J. Aust.* 142:109-94.

Rose, G., and Hamilton, P.J.S. 1978. A randomized controlled trial of the effect on middle-aged men of advice to stop smoking. *J. Epidemiol. Community Health* 32: 275-81.

Rosenberg, L.; Schwingl, P.J.; and Kaufman, D.W. et al. 1984. Breast cancer and cigarette smoking. *N. Engl. J. Med.* 310:92-94.

Russell, M.A.H.; Merriman, R.; and Edwards, A.R. 1983. Effect of nicotine chewing gum as an adjunct to general practitioner's advice against smoking. *Br. Med. J.* 287: 1782-85.

Russell, M.A.H.; Wilson, C.; and Taylor, C. et al. 1979. Effect of a general practitioner's advice against smoking. *Br. Med. J.* 2:231-235.

Saracci, R. 1987. The interactions of tobacco smoking and other agents in cancer etiology. *Epidemiol. Rev.* 9:175-93.

Schechter, M.T.; Miller, A.B.; and Howe, G.R. 1985. Cigarette smoking and breast cancer: a case-control study of screening program participants. *Am. J. Epidemiol.* 121: 479-87.

Schifflers, E.; Jamart, J.; and Renard, V. 1987. Tobacco and occupation as risk factors in bladder cancer: a case study in Southern Belgium. *Int. J. Cancer* 39:287-92.

Schoenborn C.A., and Boyd, G. 1989. Smoking and other tobacco use: United States, 1987. National Center for Health Statistics. Vital Health Stat 10.

Schwartz, J.L. 1987. *Review and evaluation of smoking cessation methods: the United States and Canada 1978-1985.* U.S. DHHS, NIH Publ. No. 87-2940. Washington, D.C.: U.S. Government Printing Office.

Schwartz, J.L., and Dubizky, M. 1967. Expressed willingness of smokers to try 10 smoking withdrawal methods. *Public Health Rep.* 82:855-61.

Sexton, M., and Hebel, J.R. 1984. A clinical trial of change in maternal smoking and its effect on birth weight. *JAMA* 251:911-15.

Shopland, D.R., and Brown, C. 1987. Toward the 1990 objectives for smoking: measuring the progress with 1985 NHIS data. *Public Health Rep.* 102:68-73.

Silverberg, E., and Lubera, J. 1987. Cancer statistics 1987. *CA* 37:10-11.

Silverberg, E.; Boring C.C.; and Squires T.S. 1990. Cancer statistics, 1990. *CA* 40:9-19.

Slattery, M.L.; Schumacher, M.C.; and West, D.W. et al. 1988. Smoking and bladder cancer: the modifying effect of cigarettes on other factors. *Cancer* 61:402-408.

Slitzer, M.L., and Gross, J. 1988. Smoking relapse: the role of pharmacologic and behavioral factors. In Pomerlau, O.F., and Pomerlau, C.S. eds. *Nicotine replacement: a critical evaluation.* pp. 163-84. New York: Alan R. Liss.

Steenland, K., and Thun, M. 1986. Interaction between tobacco smoking and occupational exposures in the causation of lung cancer. *J. Occupational Med.* 28:110-18.

Stellman, S.D. 1986. Cigarette yield and cancer risk: evidence from case-control and prospective studies. In Zaridze, D.G., and Peto, R. eds. Tobacco: a major international health hazard. *IARC Publications No. 74.* pp. 197-209. Lyon: International Agency for Research on Cancer.

Stockwell, H.G., and Lyman, G.H. 1986. Impact of smoking and smokeless tobacco on the risk of cancer of the head and neck. *Head Neck Surg.* 9:104-10.

Stockwell, H.G., and Lyman, G.H. 1987. Cigarette smoking and the risk of female reproductive cancer. *Am. J. Obstet. Gynecol.* 157:35-40.

Stokes, J., and Rigotti, N.A. 1988. The health consequences of cigarette smoking and the internist's role in smoking cessation. *Adv. Intern. Med.* 33:431-60.

The Fortune Survey. 1935. III: Cigarettes. *Fortune* 12:111-16.

Trevathan, E.; Layde, P.; and Webster, L.A. et al. 1983. Cigarette smoking and dysplasia and carcinoma *in situ* of the uterine cervix. *JAMA* 250:499-502.

Tyler, C.W. Jr; Webster, L.A.; and Ory, H.W. et al. 1985. Endometrial cancer: how does cigarette smoking influence the risk of women under age 55 years having this tumor? *Am. J. Obstet. Gynecol.* 151:899-905.

United States Department of Health and Human Services, Public Health Service, National Center for Health Statistics. 1986. *Health United States 1986.* p. 126, table 41. *DHHS Publication No. (PHS) 87-1232.* Hyattsville, Md: DHHS.

United States Public Health Service. 1987. *Smoking and health: a national status report.* U.S. DHHS, Office on Smoking and Health.

United States Public Health Service. 1986. *The health consequences of involuntary smoking: a report of the Surgeon*

General. Rockville, Md: U.S. DHHS, Office on Smoking and Health.

United States Public Health Service. 1982. *The health consequences of smoking—cancer: a report of the Surgeon General.* Rockville, Md: U.S. DHHS, Office on Smoking and Health.

United States Public Health Service. 1985. *The health consequences of smoking—cancer and chronic lung disease in the workplace: a report of the Surgeon General.* Rockville, Md: U.S. DHHS, Office on Smoking and Health.

United States Public Health Service. 1980. *The health consequences of smoking for women: a report of the Surgeon General.* Rockville, Md: US DHHS, Office on Smoking and Health.

United States Public Health Service. 1979. *Smoking and health: a report of the Surgeon General.* Rockville, Md: US DHEW, Office on Smoking and Health.

United States Public Health Service. 1988. *The health consequences of smoking—nicotine addiction: a report of the surgeon general. Rockville, Md:* U.S. DHHS, Office on Smoking and Health.

United States Department of Health and Human Services, Public Health Service, National Center for Health Statistics. 1986. *Health United States 1986.* p. 126, table 41. DHHS Publ. No. (PHS) 87-1232. Hyattsville, Md: U.S. DHHS.

United States Public Health Service. 1964. *Smoking and health: report of the advisory committee to the Surgeon General of the Public Health Service.* U.S. DHEW, Centers for Disease Control.

United States Public Health Service. 1981. *The health consequences of smoking—the changing cigarette: a report of the*

Surgeon General. Rockville, Md: U.S. DHHS, Office on Smoking and Health.

Wack, J.T., and Rodin, J. 1982. Smoking and its effects on body weight and the systems of caloric regulation. *Am. J. Clin. Nutr.* 35:366-80.

Wald, N.G.; Nanchahal, K.; and Thompson, S.G. et al. 1986. Does breathing other people's tobacco smoke cause lung cancer? *Br. Med. J.* 293:1217-22.

Walker, W.D., and Brin, B.N. 1988. U.S. lung lancer mortality and declining cigarette tobacco consumption. *J. Clin. Epidemiol.* 41:179-85.

Walter, S.D., and Iwane, M. 1983. Re: interaction of alcohol and tobacco in laryngeal cancer. *Am. J. Epidemiol.* 117:639-41.

Weiss, N.S.; Farewell, V.T.; and Szekely, D.R. et al. 1980. Oestrogens and endometrial cancer: effect of other risk factors on the association. *Maturitas* 2:185-90.

Weiss, W., and Bernarde, M.A. 1983. The temporal relation between cigarette smoking and pancreatic cancer. *Am. J. Public Health* 73:1403-1404.

Wilner, S.; Secker-Walker, R.H.; and Flynn, B.S. et al. 1987. How to help the pregnant woman stop smoking. In Rosenberg, M.J. ed. *Smoking and reproductive health.* pp. 215-22. Littleton, Mass: PSG Publishing Co.

Wilson, D.; Wood, G.; and Johnston, N. et al. 1982. Randomized clinical trial of supportive follow-up for cigarette smokers in a family practice. *Can. Med. Assoc. J.* 126:127-29.

Winkelstein, W. Jr; Shillitoe, E.J.; and Brand, R. et al. 1984. Further comments on cancer of the uterine cervix, smoking, and herpes infection. *Am. J. Epidemiol.* 119:1-8.

Chapter 10

DIET AND CANCER

David Kritchevsky, Ph.D.

David Kritchevsky, Ph.D.
Associate Director
The Wistar Institute of Anatomy and Biology
Philadelphia, Pennsylvania
Professor of Biochemistry
University of Pennsylvania
Philadelphia, Pennsylvania

This chapter was supported, in part, by a Research Career Award (HL00734) and a grant (CA 43856) from the National Institutes of Health and by funds from the Commonwealth of Pennsylvania.

INTRODUCTION

The relationship of diet to cancer has been of interest for many years. In 1809, William Lambe published dietary recommendations for cancer prevention (Lambe 1809). More contemporary reviews of dietary factors and cancer have led to guarded conclusions, and rightly so, since cancer may be difficult to diagnose in its early stages. Cancer may be due to various environmental and lifestyle factors and, while diet is part of lifestyle, it is not the sole determinant of outcome.

In an early review of diet and worldwide cancer, Armstrong and Doll (1975) cautioned that the correlations between the two were suggestions for further research and not evidence of a causal relationship. A more recent review of cancer risk in the United States stated that to attribute 30% to 70% of cancers to diet was "highly speculative and chiefly refers to dietary factors which are not yet reliably identified" (Doll and Peto 1981). A special National Academy of Sciences panel reviewed diet, nutrition, and cancer (1982) and made many generalized, but few specific, recommendations. The only definite recommendation was to reduce levels of fat in the diet. Otherwise, the main point of the advice was to follow a well-rounded diet eaten in moderation.

The diet-cancer connection is difficult to examine. Many data from animal experiments are available, but most involve treatment with specific cancer-causing agents. The studies usually end after specific periods of time, and do not record the effects over the animals' life span. Virtually all the studies involve rodents, most often rats or mice. The diets range from commercial to semipurified; the level of component under study can vary broadly. These experiments are useful and may offer clues to areas of concern for humans, but the results must be regarded with caution. Human studies have compared different populations in case-control studies, but most are after-the-fact. Recommendations concerning standardization of protocols for human studies exist (Graham 1981).

The following touches briefly on most areas of diet and cancer, focusing on the two most-discussed topics: fiber and fat.

MACRONUTRIENTS

PROTEIN

Epidemiological evidence has linked diets high in protein with increased risk of cancers of the breast (Armstrong and Doll 1975; Knox 1977; Hems 1977), colon (Gregor, Toman, and Prusova 1969), pancreas (Lea 1961), and prostate (Kolonel et al. 1981). Other studies have not confirmed the observations concerning colon cancer (Bingham et al. 1979; Haenszel et al. 1973; Graham et al. 1978). One difficulty with trying to attribute effects to protein is that intakes of protein and fat are closely correlated in Western diets.

Animal studies with various carcinogens suggest that high protein levels enhance liver tumors induced by aflatoxin (Wells, Aftergood, and Alfin-Slater 1976) or N-acetyl-2 aminofluorene (Morris et al. 1948) or lung tumors induced by dimethylbenzanthracene (DMBA) (Walters and Roe 1964). In general, protein has no effect at or below levels required for optimum growth.

CARBOHYDRATES

The relationship between carbohydrates and cancer has received less attention than that of protein and cancer. Reports have associated an increase in the incidence of liver cancer with a high intake of potatoes (Armstrong and Doll 1975), and have correlated gastric (Modan et al. 1974) and esophageal cancer (DeJong et al. 1974) with a high intake of starch. One study has linked high intake of refined sugar with an increased incidence of breast cancer (Hems 1978).

Sucrose has no effect on spontaneous tumors of rats (Friedman et al. 1972) or mice (Roe, Levy, and Carter 1970). Some researchers have found sucrose to enhance incidence of DMBA-induced mammary tumors in rats (Hoehn and Carroll 1978), but others have not confirmed their findings (Klurfeld, Weber, and Kritchevsky 1984).

The data relating carbohydrates to tumors in men or mice are limited.

FIBER

Fiber is a generic term that describes dietary components that are not broken down during the digestive process. Originally, fiber was defined as plant cell-wall material, but it has been expanded to include other plant fractions such as plant gums, algal polysaccharides, and man-made materials such as methyl cellulose. With the exception of lignins, fiber is carbohydrate in nature. Fiber may be insoluble (cellulose, wheat bran) or soluble (pectin, guar gum). The substances lumped under the designation "dietary fiber" have unique chemical structures and individual physiological effects.

The modern "fiber era" in the United States may have begun with the paper of Burkitt et al. (Burkitt, Walker, and Painter 1974) suggesting that eight conditions common in the United States, but rare in Africa, were due to lack of dietary fiber. In 1971, Burkitt had found a possible correlation between diets low in fiber and increased incidence of colon cancer.

The relation of fiber or fiber-rich foods to colon cancer in humans can be examined through ecological (correlational) epidemiology or through a comparison of cases with matched controls. A recent review of the health-related effects of dietary fiber (Pilch 1987) offers compendia of both types of studies. The document lists a number of studies, the majority of which suggest a beneficial association. Five of the studies are based on the same FAO data on 37 countries. Others are related to one or two countries or different regions of one country. The researchers studied cereals, crude fiber, fiber-rich foods, nonstarch polysaccharides, and fruits and vegetables. The findings include 15 protective correlations, one risk-enhancing, and six no correlation. Examination of retrospective case-control data showed that eight studies suggested a protective role, eight found no effect, and six found risk-enhancement. The mechanisms are "complex and difficult to unravel" (Ziegler, Devesa, and Fraumeni 1986). One difficulty lies in the fact that correlations are made with fiber-rich foods rather than specific fibers. In the case of fruit, for instance, fiber or specific minerals or vitamins could be responsible for the effects. Attempts at cross-correlation are in order.

A few specific examples demonstrate the types of data collected in studies. Comparisons of Danes and Finns showed the latter to exhibit considerably less colon cancer despite a diet high in meat, protein, and fat (Jensen, MacLennan, and Wahrendorf 1982). Researchers considered dietary carbohydrates, fiber, and saturated fat to be protective factors (table 10.1). A

Table 10.1
VARIABLES CORRELATED WITH GRADIENT OF LARGE BOWEL CANCER IN DENMARK AND FINLAND

Negatively Correlated	Positively Correlated
Carbohydrate	Alcohol
Cereals	Fecal bile acid concentration
Protein	
Saturated fat	
Starch	
Total dietary fiber	

(From: Jensen, MacLennan, and Wahrendorf [1982].)

disparity in incidence of colorectal cancer between the native Maori and white New Zealanders is hard to explain. The Maori exhibit declining cancer incidence even though their diet is increasingly Westernized, while rates in other New Zealanders increase steadily (Smith, Pearce, and Joseph 1985). Tests conducted in 1959, 1970, and 1974 compared Japanese, British, and Scandinavian populations. On the average, these groups were found to have similar intakes of nonstarch polysaccharides, but the risk of colon cancer was much lower among Japanese than among the two European populations. Studies of various South African populations have found that the rural and urban blacks have virtually no colon cancer, colored and Indians have low rates of colon cancer, and whites have a high incidence. Still, Walker et al. (1986) found that the three groups ingested similar amounts of fiber (21 $\pm$ 1 g/day).

Fiber may fulfill a number of functions that may account for its protective effect against colon cancer. It dilutes colonic contents, thus reducing the possibility of contact between carcinogens and mucosa, and it may protect by reducing fecal pH (Ziegler, Devesa, and Fraumeni 1986). It also reduces levels of fecal mutagens (Reddy et al. 1987) and reduces the concentration of fecal bile acids (Jensen, MacLennan, and Wahrendorf 1982). However, the disparities in results of studies clearly suggest the involvement of other mechanisms. A clarification of the different mechanisms of action and synthesis of the data into a unified picture require future work.

The interpopulation studies and data on migrant populations (immigrants from areas of low colon-cancer incidence to those of high colon-cancer incidence begin to exhibit more colon cancer) continue to offer suggestive data that relate to overall lifestyle, or specifically to fiber intake. Allusion to fiber in general confounds the data because a specific fraction may be responsible for the observations, due to the chemical diversity of dietary fiber. Most high-fiber regimens are also low-fat and low-calorie regimens, so the effects of fat and calories must be considered as well.

Despite the disappointment of not finding a quick solution, work in the area of fiber and cancer is proceeding vigorously. The data are too provocative to be abandoned without finding the reason or reasons for the dichotomy in the epidemiological findings.

While colon cancer has occupied center stage in studies of fiber-cancer interplay, some research relates to cancers at other sites. Studies in Poland (Jedrychowski and Popiela

1986) and Japan (Tominaga, Ogawa, and Kuroishi 1982) have related gastric cancer to high fiber intake. Research in Canada (Risch et al. 1985) did not reveal this relationship. Lung, breast, and cervix cancers have been inversely correlated with fiber intake (Hirayama 1985; Lubin, Wax, and Modan 1986; Kromhout 1985). These findings may be due to greater intake of fruits and vegetables and may be related to beta-carotene and vitamin A intake rather than to fiber (Byers et al. 1984; Winn et al. 1984; Byers et al. 1983).

Animal studies (almost all carried out in rats and mice using chemical carcinogens) yield even more confusing results. Investigators test animals of different strain and gender, different carcinogens and routes of administration, and commercial or semipurified diets. In general, wheat bran exerts a protective effect (Pilch 1987) that, interestingly, extends to male (Barbolt and Abraham 1978) but not to female (Barbolt and Abraham 1980) rats. Studies of 1,2-dimethyl-hydrazine (DMH) cellulose (Klurfeld et al. 1986), carrageenan (Arakawa et al. 1986), and corn, rice, and soy brans (Barnes et al. 1983) revealed that these enhance carcinogenesis in rats. Brans (Clapp et al. 1984) and Metamucil, a soluble fiber (Toth 1984), seem to enhance carcinogenesis in mice.

These findings do not mean that dietary fiber is unimportant. Even though the results *vis-à-vis* colon cancer are not consistent, fiber plays an important physiological role. The best recommendation for fiber intake is 10 g to 13 g per 1,000 calories consumed (Pilch 1987).

FAT AND ENERGY

Research has shown a positive correlation between dietary fat and several of the cancers (colon, breast, and prostate) prevalent in developed countries that are not the prevalent cancers among the populations of underdeveloped countries. Berg (1975) suggested that the cancers of developed countries might be due to general overnutrition rather than to any specific nutrient.

Fat provided 32% of food energy in the American diet of 1909 to 1913. Its contribution rose to about 40% in 1957. The ratio of animal fat to vegetable fat was 2.33 in 1957 to 1959, 1.86 in 1967-69, and 1.38 in 1984. The ratio of energy from saturated fatty acids, oleic acid, and linoleic acid is about 2.7 to 2.8:1. Cholesterol intake has fallen from 548 mg/day in 1957 to 1959 to 481 mg/day in 1984 (Roper and Marston 1986). In the period from 1949-1951 to 1984-1986, age-adjusted cancer death rates (all sites) increased by 30% in men and decreased by 6% in women. The breast cancer mortality rate in women rose by 5% in that time and colorectal cancer mortality was the same in men and fell by 29% in women. At the same time, mortality from lung cancer rose by 236% in men and 450% in women (American Cancer Society 1990). Epidemiological study of dietary fat and cancer does not yield a simple correlation with these figures (Mettlin 1986). The report on diet, nutrition, and cancer of the National Academy of Sciences (1982) suggested a reduction of fat intake to about 30%

of calories but stated that the available data did not provide a strong basis for the recommendation.

When plotting age-adjusted death rates from breast cancer in women (1973) against total dietary fat availability (9 g/person/day in 1964 to 1966), Carroll (1980) obtained a scattergram that could be interpreted as a straight-line relationship. However, wide differences in mortality existed at selected levels of fat availability, and large differences in fat availability were seen at selected mortality rates. Thus, Iceland (15 deaths per 100,000) and Ireland (26 deaths per 100,000) both had fat availability of 136 g/day; Mexico (5 deaths per 100,000) and Trinidad and Tobago (17 deaths per 100,000) both had fat availability of 58 g/day; Israel and New Zealand (both with death rates of 25 per 100,000) had available 96 g and 157 g of fat/day, respectively.

Miller (1986), in a discussion of the epidemiology of fat and breast cancer, stated that firmer evidence is needed to justify major diet shifts. Kolonel and LeMarchand (1986) stated, "thus, at the present time, one cannot firmly conclude that dietary fat either promotes or has no effect on colon carcinogenesis in humans."

The dichotomy between Maori and white New Zealanders extends to dietary fat as well as to fiber (Smith, Pearce, and Joseph 1985). A recent Belgian study concluded that there is a relationship between dietary oligosaccharides, not fat, and risk of colorectal cancer (Tuyns, Hallterman, and Kaaks 1987). In a review of world data, MacLennan (1985) found no relationship between fat and gastrointestinal or prostate cancer. A study of British nuns showed no relation between either fat or meat and breast or colorectal cancer (Kinlen 1982). A recent Swedish study (Rosen, Nystrom, and Wall 1988) also found no evidence of a correlation between fat and either breast or colorectal cancer. Studies in Israel (Barry et al. 1986) and France (Macquart-Moulin et al. 1986; Berta et al. 1985) have found no relation between dietary fat and colon cancer, and data for Hawaiian Japanese men (Stemmermann et al. 1985) have revealed a negative correlation between saturated fat intake and colon cancer for this group.

A study of almost 90,000 American nurses has shown no correlation with levels of dietary fat and risk of breast cancer (Willett et al. 1987), but because the population followed an American diet (30% to 40% of calories from fat), a difference might have emerged in groups with lower fat intake. Data from the National Health and Nutrition Examination Survey (NHANES) show no correlation between breast cancer and fat intake (Jones et al. 1987). Similarly, researchers in Greece (Kastomyanni et al. 1986) and Hawaii (Hirohata et al. 1987) have found no correlations between breast cancer and dietary fat. On the other hand, investigators in Israel (Lubin, Wax, and Modan 1986) and Canada (Hislop et al. 1986) have found positive correlations between dietary fat and breast cancer.

Endometrial (Villani et al. 1986; Savona-Ventura and Grech 1986) and uterine (Zema, Guminski, and Banasik 1986) cancers have been positively correlated with fat intake, but lung cancer has not (Heilbrun, Nomura, and Stemmermann 1984; Byers et al. 1984). Some researchers have suggested a possible relationship between prostate cancer and low fat intake (Heshmat et al. 1985).

One particular nutrient, milk, is worth mentioning. In one of the earliest epidemiological studies of colon cancer, Stocks and Karn (1933) found a negative correlation with dairy food. The comparative study of Danes and Finns also found that intake of milk and saturated fat is among the negative risks for colon cancer (Jensen, MacLennan, and Wahrendorf 1982). In Sweden, milk was found to be a negative risk for colon cancer (Rosen et al. 1988).

The difficulties of correlating animal data are already clear, but some results deserve mention. High-fat diets enhance tumors of the colon (Bird and Bruce 1986), breast (Sylvester, Ip, and Ip 1986), and pancreas (Roebuck 1986). Unsaturated fat enhanced colon cancer when azoxymethane (ADM) was given subcutaneously (Reddy and Maruyama 1986; Sakaguchi et al. 1984) but not when nitrosomethylurea (NMU) was administered intrarectally (Nauss et al. 1984). Trans-unsaturated fat is less cocarcinogenic than cis fat when rats are given ADM (Reddy, Tanaka, and Simi 1985) but not when they are given DMH (Watanabe, Koga, and Sugano 1985). Unsaturated fat promotes more chemically induced mammary tumors than does saturated fat (Carroll and Khor 1971; Gabor and Abraham 1986). Fish oil does not strongly promote either colon (Reddy and Maruyama 1986) or mammary (Jurkowski and Cave 1985) tumors, but these oils are relatively low in the essential fatty acid content required for optimal tumor growth (Ip, Carter, and Ip 1985).

The role of caloric restriction in tumorigenesis merits serious consideration. Fat-containing diets are calorically dense; this property may link fat intake and cancer risk.

Moreschi (1909) showed that underfeeding mice significantly reduced the growth of transplanted sarcomas. In many studies, Tannenbaum showed that caloric restriction inhibited the growth of spontaneous and induced tumors in mice (Tannenbaum 1945a; Tannenbaum 1945b). Researchers have reviewed much of this early work (White 1961; Kritchevsky and Klurfeld 1986).

A 40% restriction of caloric intake significantly inhibits the growth of induced mammary or colon tumors even when the calorically restricted rats ingest twice as much fat as the controls (Kritchevsky, Weber, and Klurfeld 1984; Kritchevsky, Weber, and Buck 1986). With these caloric restrictions, saturated fat is less of a tumor promoter than is unsaturated fat (Kritchevsky and Klurfeld 1987). Rats fed 5% fat *ad libitum* exhibit higher tumor incidence (65% vs. 30%) and greater average tumor weight (4.2 g vs. 1.5 g) than rats fed a diet containing 26.7% fat but with a 25% restriction in calories (Kritchevsky and Klurfeld 1987; table 10.2). Research indicated no difference in tumor incidence between rats fed 5% or 20% fat when both groups had the same level of caloric restriction (Thompson et al.

Table 10.2
EFFECT OF FAT LEVEL AND 25% CALORIC RESTRICTION ON EXPERIMENTAL TUMORIGENESIS IN RATS

Diet	Tumor Incidence	Tumor Multiplicity	Tumor Weight (g)
Ad libitum			
5% Corn oil (12.4)[i]	65	1.9 ± 0.3	2.0 ± 0.7
26.7% Corn oil (32.7)[i]	85	3.0 ± 0.6	2.3 ± 0.7
20% Corn oil (41.1)[i]	80	4.1 ± 0.6	2.9 ± 0.5
Restricted			
20% Corn oil (43.1)[i]	60	1.9 ± 0.4	0.8 ± 0.2
26% Corn oil (53.5)[i]	30	1.5 ± 0.3	1.4 ± 1.0
Significance[+]	a	b	b

(From: Kritchevsky and Klurfeld [1987].) Tumors induced by a single oral administration of 7,12-dimethylbenz(a)anthracene.
[i]Percent of calories.
[+]a = $p < 0.005$; b = $p < 0.0001$.

1985). In a review of 82 experiments involving caloric restrictions and tumors in mice, Albanes (1987) found a direct relationship between caloric restriction and tumor growth inhibition.

Several investigations have suggested a possible role for caloric intake in tumorigenicity in humans (Bristol et al. 1985; Potter and McMichael 1986; Lyon et al. 1987). Lyon et al. (1987) concluded that "total energy intake must be evaluated before attempting to assign a causal role to any food or nutrient postulated to play a role in colon cancer." A study of colon cancer in three socioeconomic groups in Hong Kong revealed that the most affluent group had twice the tumor incidence of the least affluent (Hill, MacLennan, and Newcombe 1987). Even though they ingested more fiber and vitamins, they also ingested more total calories. Inhibition of energy intake may be one way in which dietary fiber influences colon cancer (Kritchevsky 1986). A small reduction in available energy will have much greater impact on persons eating a low-caloric diet than on those on a higher-caloric Western diet.

MICRONUTRIENTS

VITAMINS

Epidemiologic estimates of vitamin A intake usually derive from data on ingestion of yellow and green vegetables, rich in beta-carotene, a precursor of vitamin A. Whether the published information refers to vitamin A or beta-carotene is difficult to distinguish because people use the terms interchangeably. Vitamin A intake (through vitamin supplements, vitamin-rich foods, or beta-carotene) appears to be inversely related to lung cancer in Norway (Bjelke 1975), Singapore (MacLennan et al. 1977), England (Gregor et al. 1980), and the United States (Mettlin, Graham, and Swanson 1979). One study found an inverse relationship between vitamin A supplements and lung and other cancers (Smith and Jick 1978); another discovered an inverse association between lung cancer and intake of foods rich in beta-carotene but not between lung cancer and vitamin A intake (Shekelle et al. 1981)

Research has inversely associated vitamin A or beta-carotene with cancers of the larynx (Graham et al. 1981), esophagus (Wynder and Bross 1961; Mettlin et al. 1981), stomach (Graham, Schotz, and Martino 1972; Haenszel et al. 1972), prostate (Schuman et al. 1982), and bladder (Mettlin, Graham, and Swanson 1979). Milk is a good source of vitamin A, so its negative relation to some cancers may be due, in part, to its content of this vitamin.

Retinoids, another group of compounds related to vitamin A, also appear to reduce cancer growth (Sporn 1983; Bollag and Hartman 1983; Watson and Moriguchi 1985).

Several studies report an inverse association between intake of vitamin C or citrus fruit and gastric cancer (Higginson 1966; Haenszel and Correa 1975; Bjelke 1978). Vitamin C hinders the formation of nitrosamines by blocking the reaction between nitrite and amines, and this is thought to be the basis of its protective action. Vitamin C intake has also been correlated inversely with esophageal cancer (Cook-Mozaffari 1979), laryngeal cancer (Graham et al. 1981), and cervical cancer (Wassertheil-Smoller et al. 1981); however, the correlation was not found in relation to colon cancer (Jain et al. 1980).

There is no epidemiologic evidence relating to the effects of vitamin E or other vitamins on cancer. Many of the animal data have been reviewed recently (Leonard et al. 1986).

MINERALS

Selenium exists in both organic (selenocystine) and inorganic (selenite, selenate) forms. Shamberger et al. (Shamberger and Frost 1969; Shamberger and Willis 1971; Shamberger, Tytko, and Willis 1976) found an increased incidence of cancer, especially of the gastrointestinal and genitourinary tracts, in U.S. states with low selenium levels in forage crops. Selenium levels are lower in sera of cancer patients than in controls (Shamberger et al. 1973). On the other hand, a positive correlation was reported between colorectal cancer and selenium levels in drinking water (Jansson et al. 1975). Many animal studies indicate that selenium at dietary levels of 0.5 to 6 μg/g (micrograms per gram) plays a protective role against chemically induced tumors. Selenium is an element for which there is a small difference between necessary levels and toxic levels and it should be administered with care. Presently, no good evidence supports its use as an anticancer compound.

Iron deficiency has been associated with Plummer-Vinson syndrome which is, in turn, associated with increased risk for esophageal cancer (Wynder et al. 1957; Larsson, Sandstrom, and Westling 1975). Otherwise few epidemiological or experimental data relate iron to cancer.

Epidemiological data concerning the role of zinc in cancer are sparse and indirect. In animals, studies show that zinc both retards and enhances carcinogenesis.

Zinc deficiency retards the growth of transplanted tumors (Petering, Buskirk, and Crim 1967), but enhances the growth of chemically induced tumors (Fong, Swak, and Newberne 1978).

While there are some data on the roles of copper, cadmium, arsenic, and lead in cancer (reviewed in the article by the Committee on Diet, Nutrition and Cancer 1982), not enough observations exist to permit definitive conclusions.

Molybdenum deficiency in the soil has been associated with an increased incidence of esophageal cancer in Africa (Burrell, Roach, and Shadwell 1966) and China (Yang 1980). Research shows a correlation between esophageal cancer and low levels of molybdenum in drinking water in the United States (Berg, Haenszel, and Devesa 1973). However, there are not enough data to allow judgment on the role of molybdenum in cancer.

There has always been some interest in the role or roles of metals in carcinogenesis (Stocks and Davies 1964), but this area has not received the attention that the macronutrients have. With the great general interest in nutrition and cancer, more work on micronutrients will be forthcoming.

Work and interest in diet and cancer have stimulated many groups to issue various dietary suggestions. Generally they all recommend, in one guise or another, maintenance of ideal weight, reduction to some degree of fat intake, and increase of vegetable, fruit, and cereal intake; in short, moderation. More analytical data are needed on foodstuffs (influence of age, preparation), and more work on nutrient interactions is indicated. Uniform experimental and epidemiological protocols are needed, as well as a measure of restraint in interpreting experimental findings.

REFERENCES

Albanes, D. 1987. Total calories, body weight and tumor incidence in mice. *Cancer Res.* 47:1987-92.

American Cancer Society. 1990. *Cancer facts and figures.* Atlanta: American Cancer Society.

Arakawa, S.; Okumura, M.; and Yamada, S. et al. 1986. Enhancing effect of carrageenan on the induction of rat colonic tumors by 1,2-dimethylhydrazine and its relation to beta-glucuronidase activities in feces and other tissues. *J. Nutr. Sci. Vitaminol.* 23:481-85.

Armstrong, B., and Doll, R. 1975. Environmental factors and cancer incidence and mortality in different countries with special reference to dietary practices. *Int. J. Cancer* 15:617-31.

Barbolt, T.A., and Abraham, R. 1978. The effect of bran on dimethylhydrazine-induced carcinogenesis in the rat. *Proc. Soc. Exp. Biol. Med.* 157:656-59.

Barbolt, T.A., and Abraham, R. 1980. Dose-response, sex difference, and the effect of bran in dimethylhydrazine-induced intestinal tumorigenesis in rats. *Toxicol. Appl. Pharmacol.* 55:417-22.

Barnes, D.S.; Clapp, N.K.; and Scott, D.A. et al. 1983. Effects of wheat, rice, corn, and soybean bran on 1,2-dimethylhydrazine-induced large bowel tumorigenesis in F344 rats. *Nutr. Cancer* 5:1-9.

Berg, J.W. 1975. Can nutrition explain the pattern of international epidemiology of hormone-dependent cancer? *Cancer Res.* 35:3345-50.

Berg, J.W., and Burbank, F. 1972. Correlations between carcinogenic trace metals in water supplies and cancer mortality. *Ann. N.Y. Acad. Sci.* 199:249-64.

Berg, J.W.; Haenszel, W.; and Devesa, S.S. 1973. In *Diet nutrition, and cancer.* pp. 10-17. Washington, D.C.: National Academy Press.

Berry, E.M.; Zimmerman, J.; and Peser, M. et al. 1986. Dietary fat, adipose tissue composition, and the development of carcinoma of the colon. *J. Natl. Cancer Inst.* 77:93-97.

Berta, J.L.; Coste, T.; and Rautureau, J. et al. 1985. Diet and rectocolonic cancers: results of a case-control study. *Gastroenterol. Clin. Biol.* 9:348-53.

Bingham, S.; Williams, D.R.R.; and Cole, T.J. et al. 1979. Dietary fiber and regional large-bowel cancer mortality in Britain. *Br. J. Cancer* 40:456-63.

Bird, R.P., and Bruce, W.R. 1986. Effect of dietary fat levels on the susceptibility of colonic cells to nuclear-damaging agents. *Nutr. Cancer* 8:93-100.

Bjelke, E. 1975. Dietary vitamin A and human lung cancer. *Int. J. Cancer* 15:561-65.

Bjelke, E. 1978. Dietary factors and the epidemiology of cancer of the stomach and large bowel. *Aktuel. Ernahrungsmed. Klin. Prax. Suppl.* 2:10-17.

Bollag, W., and Hartman, H.R. 1983. Prevention and therapy of cancer in animals and man. *Cancer Surveys* 2:293-314.

Bristol, J.B.; Emmett, P.M.; and Heaton, K.W. et al. 1985. Sugar, fat and the risk of colorectal cancer. *Br. Med. J.* 291:1467-70.

Burkitt, D.P. 1971. Epidemiology of cancer of the colon and rectum. *Cancer* 28:3-13.

Burkitt, D.P.; Walker, A.R.P.; and Painter, N.S. 1974. Dietary fiber and disease. *JAMA* 229:1068-74.

Burrell, R.J.W.; Roach, W.A.; and Shadwell, A. 1966. Esophageal cancer in the Bantu of the Transkei associated with mineral deficiency in garden plants. *J. Natl. Cancer Inst.* 36:201-14.

Byers, T.; Marshall, J.; and Graham, S. et al. 1983. A case-control study of dietary and non-dietary factors in ovarian cancer. *J. Natl. Cancer Inst.* 71:681-868.

Byers, T.; Vena, J.; and Mettlin, C. et al. 1984. Dietary vitamin A and lung cancer risk: an analysis by histologic subtypes. *Am. J. Epidemiol.* 120:769-76.

Carroll, K.K. 1980. Lipids and carcinogenesis. *J. Environ. Pathol. Toxicol.* 3:253-71.

Carroll, K.K., and Khor, H.T. 1971. Effect of level and type of dietary fat on incidence of mammary tumors induced in female Sprague-Dawley rats by 7,12-dimethylbenz(a)anthracene. *Lipids* 6:415-20.

Clapp, N.K.; Henke, M.A.; and London, J.F. et al. 1984. Enhancement of 1,2-dimethylhydrazine-induced large bowel tumorigenesis in BALB/c mice by corn, soybean and wheat brans. *Nutr. Cancer* 6:77-85.

Committee on Diet, Nutrition, and Cancer. 1982. *Diet, nutrition and cancer.* Washington, D.C.: National Academy Press.

Cook-Mozaffari, P. 1979. The epidemiology of cancer of the esophagus. *Nutr. Cancer* 1:51-60.

Correa, P.; Haenszel, W.; and Cuello, C. et al. 1975. A model for gastric cancer epidemiology. *Lancet* II:58-60.

DeJong, U.W.; Breslow, N.; and Hong, J.G.E. et al. 1974. Aetiological factors in oesophageal cancer in Singapore Chinese. *Int. J. Cancer* 13:291-303.

Doll, R., and Peto, R. 1981. The causes of cancer: quantitative estimates of avoidable risks of cancer in the United States today. *J. Natl. Cancer Inst.* 66:1191-1308.

Fong, L.Y.Y.; Swak, A.; and Newberne, P.M. 1978. Zinc deficiency and methylbenzyl-nitrosamine-induced esophageal cancer in rats. *J. Natl. Cancer Inst.* 61:145-50.

Friedman, L.; Richardson, H.L.; and Richardson, M.E. et al. 1972. Toxic response of rats to cyclamates in chow and semisynthetic diets. *J. Natl. Cancer Inst.* 49:751-64.

Gabor, H., and Abraham, S. 1986. Effect of dietary menhaden oil on tumor cell loss and the accumulation of mass of a transplantable mammary adenocarcinoma in BALB/c mice. *J. Natl. Cancer Inst.* 76:1223-29.

Graham, S. 1981. Working group I: epidemiology-lipid-related studies, summary of deliberations. *Cancer Res.* 41:3733.

Graham, S.; Dayal, H.; and Swanson, M. et al. 1978. Diet in the epidemiology of cancer of the colon and rectum. *J. Natl. Cancer Inst.* 61:709-14.

Graham, S.; Mettlin, C.; and Marshall, J. et al. 1981. Dietary factors in the epidemiology of cancer of the larynx. *Am. J. Epidemiol.* 113:675-80.

Graham, S.; Schotz, W.; and Martino, P. 1972. Alimentary factors in the epidemiology of gastric cancer. *Cancer* 30:927-38.

Gregor, A.; Lee, P.N.; and Roe, F.J.C. et al. 1980. Comparison of dietary histories in lung cancer cases and controls with special reference to vitamin A. *Nutr. Cancer* 2:93-97.

Gregor, O.; Toman, R.; and Prusova F. 1969. Gastrointestinal cancer and nutrition. *Gut* 10:1031-34.

Haenszel, W.; Berg, J.W.; and Segi, M. et al. 1973. Large-bowel cancer in Hawaiian Japanese. *J. Natl. Cancer Inst.* 51:1765-79.

Haenszel, W., and Correa, P. 1975. Developments in the epidemiology of stomach cancer over the past decade. *Cancer Res.* 35:3452-59.

Haenszel, W.; Kurihara, M.; and Segi, M. et al. 1972. Stomach cancer among Japanese in Hawaii. *J. Natl. Cancer Inst.* 49:969-88.

Heilbrun, L.K.; Nomura, A.M.; and Stemmermann, G.N. 1984. Dietary cholesterol and lung cancer risk among Japanese men in Hawaii. *Am. J. Clin. Nutr.* 39:375-79.

Heshmat, M.Y.; Kaul, L.; and Kovi, J. et al. 1985. Nutrition and prostate cancer: a case-control study. *Prostate* 6:7-17.

Hems, G. 1978. The contributions of diet and childbearing to breast-cancer rates. *Br. J. Cancer* 37:974-82.

Higginson, J. 1966. Etiological factors in gastrointestinal cancer in man. *J. Natl. Cancer Inst.* 37:527-45.

Hill, M.J.; MacLennan, R.; and Newcombe, K. 1979. Diet and large bowel cancer in three socioeconomic groups in Hong Kong. *Lancet* I:436.

Hirayama, T. 1985. A large scale cohort study on cancer risks by diet with special reference to the risk-reducing effects of green-yellow vegetable consumption. *Int. Symp. Princess Takamatsu Cancer Res. Fund* 16:41-53.

Hirohata, T.; Nomura, A.M.Y.; and Hankin, J.H. et al. 1987. An epidemiologic study on the association between diet and breast cancer. *J. Natl. Cancer Inst.* 78:595-600.

Hislop, T.G.; Coldman, A.J.; and Elwood, J.M. et al. 1986. Childhood and recent eating patterns and risk of breast cancer. *Cancer Detect. Prev.* 9:47-58.

Hoehn, S.K., and Carroll K.K. 1978. Effects of dietary carbohydrate on the incidence of mammary tumors induced in rats by 7,12-dimethylbenz(a)anthracene. *Nutr. Cancer* 1:27-30.

Ip, C.; Carter, C.A.; and Ip, M.M. 1985. Requirement of essential fatty acid for mammary tumorigenesis in the rat. *Cancer Res.* 45:1997-2001.

Jain, M.; Cook, G.M.; and Davis, G. et al. 1980. A case-control study of diet and colorectal cancer. *Int. J. Cancer* 26:757-68.

Jansson, B.; Seibert, G.B.; and Speer, J.F. 1975. Gastrointestinal cancer: its geographic distribution and correlation to breast cancer. *Cancer* 36:2373-84.

Jedrychowski, W.A., and Popiela, T. 1986. Gastric cancer in Poland: a decreased malignancy due to changing nutritional habits of the population. *Neoplasma* 33:97-106.

Jensen, O.M.; MacLennan, R.; and Wahrendorf, J. 1982. Diet, bowel function, fecal characteristics, and large bowel cancer in Denmark and Finland. *Nutr. Cancer* 4:5-19.

Jones, D.Y.; Schatzkin, A.; and Green, S.B. et al. 1987. Dietary fat and breast cancer in the National Health and Nutrition Examination Survey 1 Epidemiologic Follow-up Study. *J. Natl. Cancer Inst.* 79:465-71.

Jurkowski, J.J., and Cave, W.T. Jr. 1985. Dietary effects of menhaden oil on the growth and membrane lipid composition of rats' mammary tumors. *J. Natl. Cancer Inst.* 74:1145-50.

Kastomyanni, K.; Trichopoulos, D.; and Boyle, P. et al. 1986. Diet and breast cancer: a case-control study in Greece. *Int. J. Cancer* 38:815-20.

Kinlen, L.J. 1982. Meat and fat consumption and cancer mortality: a study of strict religious orders in Britain. *Lancet* I:946-49.

Klurfeld, D.M.; Weber, M.M.; and Buck, C.L. et al. 1986. Dose-response of colonic carcinogenesis to different amounts and types of cellulose (CEL). *(Abstr.) Fed. Proc.* 45:1076.

Klurfeld, D.M.; Weber, M.M.; and Kritchevsky, D. 1984. Comparison of dietary carbohydrates for promotion of DMBA-induced mammary tumorigenesis in rats. *Carcinogenesis* 5:423-25.

Knox, E.G. 1977. Foods and diseases. *Br. J. Soc. Prev. Med.* 31:71-80.

Kolonel, L.N.; Hankin, J.H.; and Lee, J. et al. 1981. Nutrient intakes in relation to cancer incidence in Hawaii. *Br. J. Cancer* 44:332-39.

Kolonel, L.N., and LeMarchand, L. 1986. The epidemiology of colon cancer and dietary fat. *Proc. Clin. Biol. Res.* 222:69-91.

Kolonel, L.N.; Nomura, A.M.Y.; and Hirohata, T. et al. 1981. Association of diet and place of birth with stomach cancer incidence in Hawaii Japanese and Caucasians. *Am. J. Clin. Nutr.* 34:2478-85.

Kritchevsky, D. 1986. Diet, nutrition, and cancer: the role of fiber. *Cancer* 58:1830-36.

Kritchevsky, D., and Klurfeld, D.M. 1986. Influence of caloric intake on experimental carcinogenesis: a review. *Adv. Exp. Med. Biol.* 206:55-68.

Kritchevsky, D., and Klurfeld, D.M. 1987. Caloric effects in experimental mammary tumorigenesis. *Am. J. Clin. Nutr.* 45:236-42.

Kritchevsky, D.; Weber, M.M.; and Buck, C.L. et al. 1986. Calories, fat and cancer. *Lipids* 21:272-74.

Kritchevsky, D.; Weber, M.M.; and Klurfeld, D.M. 1984. Dietary fat versus caloric content in initiation and promotion of 7,12-dimethylbenz(a)anthracene-induced mammary tumorigenesis in rats. *Cancer Res.* 44:3174-77.

Kromhout, D. 1985. Analyses of food consumption data to nutrients, foods and both. *Int. Congr. Ser.* 685:253-57.

Lambe, W. 1809. *Report on the effects of a peculiar regimen on scirrhous tumors and cancerous ulcers.* London: J. Mawman.

Larsson, L.G.; Sandstrom, A.; and Westling, P. 1975. Relationship of Plummer-Vinson disease to cancer of the upper alimentary tract in Sweden. *Cancer Res.* 35:3308-16.

Lea, A.J. 1961. Neoplasms and environmental factors. *Ann. Roy. Coll. Surg. Engl.* 41:432-38.

Leonard, T.K.; Mohs, M.E.; and Ho, E.E. et al. 1986. Nutrient intakes: cancer causation and prevention. *Prog. Food Nutr. Sci.* 10:237-77.

Lubin, F.; Wax, Y.; and Modan, B. 1986. Role of fat, animal protein, and dietary fiber in breast cancer etiology: a case-control study. *J. Natl. Cancer Inst.* 77:605-12.

Lyon, J.L.; Mahoney, A.W.; and West, D.W. et al. 1987. Energy intake: its relation to colon cancer risk. *J. Natl. Cancer Inst.* 78:853-61.

MacLennan, R. 1985. Fat intake and cancer of the gastrointestinal tract and prostate. *Med. Oncol. Tumor Pharmacother.* 2:137-42.

MacLennan, R.; DaCosta, J.; and Day, N.E. et al. 1977. Risk factors for lung cancer in Singapore Chinese, a population with high female incidence rates. *Int. J. Cancer* 20:854-60.

Macquart-Moulin, G.; Riboli, E.; and Cornee, J. et al. 1986. Case-control study of colorectal cancer and diet in Marseilles. *Int. J. Cancer* 38:183-91.

Mettlin, C. 1986. Methodological issues in epidemiologic studies of dietary fat and cancer. *Prog. Clin. Biol. Res.* 222:3-15.

Mettlin, C.; Graham, S.; and Swanson, M. 1979. Vitamin A and lung cancer. *J. Natl. Cancer Inst.* 62:1435-38.

Mettlin, C.; Graham, S.; and Priore, R. et al. 1981. Diet and cancer of the esophagus. *Nutr. Cancer* 2:143-47.

Miller, A.B. 1986. Dietary fat and the epidemiology of breast cancer. *Prog. Clin. Biol. Res.* 222:17-32.

Modan, B.; Lubin, F.; and Barrell, V. et al. 1974. The role of starches in etiology of gastric cancer. *Cancer* 34:2087-92.

Moreschi, C. 1909. Relation of nutrition to tumor growth. *Z. Immunitatsforsch* 2:651-75.

Morris, H.P.; Westfall, B.B.; and Dubnik, C.S. et al. 1948. Some observations on carcinogenicity, distribution, and metabolism of N-acetyl-2-aminofluorene in the rat. *Cancer Res.* 8:390.

Nauss, K.M.; Locniskar, M.; and Sondergaard, D. et al. 1984. Lack of effect of dietary fat on N-nitrosomethylurea (NMU)-induced colon tumorigenesis in rats. *Carcinogenesis* 5:255-60.

Petering, H.G.; Buskirk, H.H.; and Crim, J.A. 1967. The effect of dietary mineral supplements of the rat on the antitumor activity of 3-ethoxy-2-oxobutyraldehyde bis (thiosemicarbazone). *Cancer Res.* 27:1115-21.

Pilch, S.M. ed. 1987. *Physiological effects and health consequences of dietary fiber.* Bethesda, Md: FASEB.

Potter, J.D., and McMichael, A.J. 1986. Diet and cancer of the colon and rectum: a case-control study. *J. Natl. Cancer Inst.* 76:557-69.

Reddy, B.S., and Maruyama, H. 1986. Effect of different levels of dietary corn oil and lard during the initiation phase of colon carcinogenesis in F344 rats. *J. Natl. Cancer Inst.* 77:815-22.

Reddy, B.S., and Maruyama, H. 1986. Effect of dietary fish oil on azoxymethane induced colon carcinogenesis in male F344 rats. *Cancer Res.* 46:3367-70.

Reddy, B.S.; Sharma, C.; and Simi, B. et al. 1987. Metabolic epidemiology of colon cancer: effect of dietary fiber on fecal mutagens and bile acids in healthy subjects. *Cancer Res.* 47:644-48.

Reddy, B.S.; Tanaka, T.; and Simi, B. 1985. Effect of different levels of dietary trans fat or corn oil on azoxymethane-induced colon carcinogenesis in F344 rats. *J. Natl. Cancer Inst.* 75:791-98.

Risch, H.A.; Jain, M.; and Choi, N.W. et al. 1985. Dietary factors and the incidence of cancer of the stomach. *Am. J. Epidemiol.* 122:947-59.

Roe, F.J.C.; Levy, L.S.; and Carter, R.L. 1970. Feeding studies on sodium cyclamate, saccharin, and sucrose for carcinogenic and tumor-promoting activity. *Food Cosmet. Toxicol.* 8:135-45.

Roebuck, B.D. 1986. Effects of high levels of dietary fat on the growth of azaserine-induced foci in the rat pancreas. *Lipids* 21:281-84.

Roper, N.R., and Marston, R.M. 1986. Levels and sources of fat in the U.S. food supply. *Prog. Clin. Biol. Res.* 222:127-52.

Rosen, M.; Nystrom, L.; and Wall, S. 1988. Diet and cancer mortality in the counties of Sweden. *Am. J. Epidemiol.* 127:42-49.

Sakaguchi, M.; Hiramatsu, Y.; and Takada, H. et al. 1984. Effect of dietary unsaturated and saturated fats on azoxymethane-induced colon carcinogenesis in rats. *Cancer Res.* 44:1472-77.

Savona-Ventura, C., and Grech, E.S. 1986. Endometrial adenocarcinoma in the Maltese populations: an epidemiologic study. *Eur. J. Gynaecol. Oncol.* 7:209-17.

Schuman, L.M.; Mandell, J.S.; and Radke, A. et al. 1982. Some selected features of the epidemiology of prostatic cancer: Minneapolis-St. Paul, Minnesota, case control study 1976-1979. In Magnus, K. ed. *Trends in cancer incidence: causes and practical implications.* pp. 345-354. Washington, D.C.: Hemisphere Publishing Co.

Shamberger, R.J., and Frost, D.V. 1969. Possible protective effect of selenium against human cancer. *Can. Med. Assoc. J.* 100:682.

Shamberger, R.J.; Rukovena, E.; and Longfield, A.K. et al. 1973. Antioxidants and cancer I: selenium in the blood of normals and cancer patients. *J. Natl. Cancer Inst.* 50:863-70.

Shamberger, R.J.; Tytko, S.A.; and Willis, C.E. 1976. Antioxidants and cancer VI: selenium and age-adjusted human cancer mortality. *Arch. Environ. Health* 21:231-35.

Shamberger, R.J., and Willis, C.E. 1971. Selenium distribution and human cancer mortality. *CRC Crit. Rev. Clin. Lab. Sci.* 2:211-21.

Shekelle, R.B.; Liu, S.; and Raynor, W.J. et al. 1981. Dietary vitamin A and risk of cancer in the Western Electric Study. *Lancet* II:1185-89.

Smith, A.H.; Pearce, N.E.; and Joseph, J.G. 1985. Major colorectal cancer aetiological hypotheses do not explain the mortality trends among Maori and non-Maori New Zealanders. *Int. J. Epidemiol.* 14:79-95.

Smith, P.G., and Jick, H. 1978. Cancers among users of preparations containing vitamin A. *Cancer* 42:808-11.

Sporn, M.B. 1983. Retinoids and cancer: introduction. *Cancer Surveys* 2:221-22.

Stemmermann, G.; Nomura, A.M.; and Heilbrun, L.K. et al. 1985. Colorectal cancer in Hawaiian Japanese men: a progress report. *Natl. Cancer Inst. Monogr.* 69:125-31.

Stocks, P., and Davies, R.I. 1964. Zinc and copper content of soils associated with the incidence of cancer of the stomach and other organs. *Br. J. Cancer* 18:14-24.

Stocks, P., and Karn, M.K. 1933. A cooperative study of the habits, homelife, dietary, and family histories of 450 cancer patients and an equal number of control patients. *Ann. Eugen. (London)* 5:237-80.

Sylvester, P.W.; Ip, C.; and Ip, M.M. 1986. Effects of high dietary fat on the growth and development of ovarian-dependent carcinogen-induced mammary tumors in rats. *Cancer Res.* 46:763-69.

Tannenbaum, A. 1945a. The dependence of tumor formation on the degree of caloric restriction. *Cancer Res.* 5:609-15.

Tannenbaum, A. 1945b. The dependence of tumor formation on the composition of the calorie restricted diet as well as on the degree of restriction. *Cancer Res.* 5:616-25.

Thompson, H.J.; Meeker, L.D.; and Tagliaferro, A.R. et al. 1985. Effect of energy intake on the promotion of mammary carcinogenesis by dietary fat. *Nutr. Cancer* 7:37-41.

Tominaga, S.; Ogawa, H.; and Kuroishi, T. 1982. Usefulness of correlation analysis in the epidemiology of stomach cancer. *Natl. Cancer Inst. Monogr.* 62:135-40.

Toth, B. 1984. Effect of Metamucil on tumor formation by 1,2-dimethyl-hydrazine dihydrochloride in mice. *Food Chem. Toxicol.* 22:573-78.

Tuyns, A.J.; Hallterman, M.; and Kaaks, R. 1987. Colorectal cancer and intake of nutrients—oligosaccharides are a risk factor, fats are not: a case control study in Belgium. *Nutr. Cancer* 10:181-96.

Villani, C.; Pucci, G.; and Pietrangeli, D. et al. 1986. Role of diet in endometrial cancer patients. *Eur. J. Gynaecol. Oncol.* 7:139-43.

Walker, A.R.; Walker, B.F.; and Walker, A.J. 1986. Fecal pH, dietary fiber intake, and proneness to colon cancer in four South African populations. *Br. J. Cancer* 53:489-95.

Walters, M.A., and Roe, F.J.C. 1964. The effect of dietary casein on the induction of lung tumors by the injection of 9,10-dimethyl-1,2-benzanthracene (DMBA) into newborn mice. *Br. J. Cancer* 18:312-16.

Wassertheil-Smoller, S.S.; Romney, S.L.; and Wylie-Rosett, J. et al. 1981. Dietary vitamin C and uterine cervical dysplasia. *Am. J. Epidemiol.* 114:714-24.

Watanabe, M.; Koga, T.; and Sugano, M. 1985. Influence of dietary cis- and trans-fat on 1,2-dimethylhydrazine-induced colon tumors and fecal steroid excretion in Fischer 344 rats. *Am. J. Clin. Nutr.* 42:475-84.

Watson, R.R., and Moriguchi, S. 1985. Cancer prevention by retinoids: role of immunological modification. *Nutr. Res.* 5:663-75.

Wells, P.L.; Aftergood, L.; and Alfin-Slater, R.B. 1976. Effect of varying levels of dietary protein on tumor development and lipid metabolism in rats exposed to aflatoxin. *J. Am. Oil Chem. Soc.* 53:559-62.

White, F.R. 1961. The relationship between underfeeding and tumor formation, transplantation, and growth in rats and mice. *Cancer Res.* 21:281-90.

Willett, W.C.; Stampfer, M.J.; and Colditz, G.A. et al. 1987. Dietary fat and risk of breast cancer. *N. Engl. J. Med.* 316:22-28.

Winn, D.M.; Ziegler, R.G.; and Pickle, L.W. et al. 1984. Diet in the etiology of oral and pharyngeal cancer among women from the Southern United States. *Cancer Res.* 44:1216-22.

Wynder, E.L., and Bross, I.J. 1961. A study of etiological factors in cancer of the esophagus. *Cancer* 14:389-413.

Wynder, E.L.; Hultberg, S.; and Jacobsson, F. et al. 1957. Environmental factors in cancer of the upper alimentary tract: a Swedish study with special reference to Plummer-Vinson (Paterson-Kelly) syndrome. *Cancer* 10:470-87.

Yang, C.S. 1980. Research on esophageal cancer in China: a review. *Cancer Res.* 40:2633-44.

Zema, B.; Guminski, S.; and Banasik, R. 1986. Study of risk factors in invasive cancer of the corpus uteri. *Neoplasma* 33:621-29.

Ziegler, R.G.; Devesa, S.S.; and Fraumeni, J.F. Jr. 1986. Epidemiologic patterns of colorectal cancer. In DeVita, V.T. Jr.; Hellman, S.; and Rosenberg, S.A. eds. *Important advances in oncology.* Philadelphia: J.B. Lippincott.

Chapter 11

PROPERTIES OF VIRUSES ASSOCIATED WITH HUMAN CANCER

Fred Rapp, Ph.D.

Fred Rapp, Ph.D.
Professor and Chairman
Department of Microbiology and Immunology
The Pennsylvania State University
College of Medicine
Hershey, Pennsylvania

INTRODUCTION

The possibility that viruses can cause cancer was a hotly debated hypothesis for over 70 years before being resolved during the last two decades. The turn-of-the century observations that leukemia of chickens (Ellerman and Bang 1908) and sarcomas of fowl (Rous 1911) could be caused by filtered material (free of cells and bacteria) from sick animals were widely disputed and ignored by many scientists, physicians, and oncologists. Subsequent observations demonstrated that similar agents could cause neoplastic disease in a wide variety of animal species, but these were thought to be largely laboratory artifacts with no relevance to naturally occurring human or animal cancers. Later, these observations led to studies involving the genes of viruses required to transform a normal cell into one with a malignant phenotype. Many investigators were able to isolate a variety of viral gene products required to initiate or maintain the transformed state of mammalian cells.

Most of the DNA-containing animal viruses have tumorigenic properties, but only one of the RNA-containing virus groups, the retroviruses, shares this ability. The long mystery of how RNA-containing viruses could transform cells heritably was partially solved upon the discovery that they contained the gene for an RNA-dependent DNA polymerase (reverse transcriptase) and were, therefore, able to make a DNA copy of their RNA that could be circularized and incorporated into the host genome (Baltimore 1970; Temin and Mitzutani 1970). Thus, a common mechanism for malignancy by all viruses could be postulated.

There have been many studies concerning the molecular events underlying virus-induced or associated malignancy, but the viral role in "natural" neoplasia is a more formidable question. Early studies linking a variety of DNA-containing viruses to a number of human neoplasia through epidemiologic methods helped to transform this area of scientific endeavor from the theoretical to the practical. Thus, studies linking Epstein-Barr virus with Burkitt's lymphoma (Epstein, Achong, and Barr 1964) and nasopharyngeal carcinoma (Klein 1979); hepatitis B virus with primary hepatocellular carcinoma (London 1983); and more recently, human papillomaviruses with a variety of human cancers (McCance 1986; zur Hausen 1977), particularly those of the cervix and genitalia, have spurred investigations into the role these viruses play and the possible cofactors mediating the neoplastic process.

The recent isolation of human herpesvirus 6, also called HBLV (Salahuddin, Ablashi, and Markham 1986), from peripheral blood leukocytes of lymphoma patients has added further medical implications to this field. The isolation of human retroviruses (Poiesz et al. 1980), human T-cell leukemia viruses I and II (HTLV-I, HTLV-II), has fulfilled the prediction of hard-core tumor virologists that retroviruses, counterparts of those in animals, would be found in human neoplasms. The role viruses play in weakening immunologic defenses against neoplasms has been greatly, although regrettably, strengthened by the discovery (Barre-Sinoussi et al. 1983; Popovic et al. 1984) of the human immunodeficiency virus (HIV), the known cause of acquired immune deficiency syndrome (AIDS). The role of viruses, such as the newly isolated lentiviruses (a retrovirus subgroup), represents a complex interaction between viruses that affect the immune response and those that cause neoplastic disease. Research during the next decade should go a long way toward unravelling such interactions at the level of the biological host and may be useful in developing means of effective treatment or prevention of some common cancers.

HERPESVIRUSES

There are six known human herpesviruses that are suspected agents in human neoplasia. Although tumors have been produced by herpesviruses, herpes simplex virus (HSV) types 1 and 2 (HSV-1, HSV-2), Epstein-Barr virus

(EBV), human cytomegalovirus (HCMV), and human herpesvirus 6 (HHV-6), originally isolated from peripheral blood leukocytes of patients with lymphoproliferative disorders (Salahuddin et al. 1986), have been associated with tumor production in humans by either epidemiologic studies or direct virologic techniques (McDougall et al. 1984; Rapp and Robbins 1984; zur Hausen 1983). The sixth human herpesvirus, varicella-zoster virus (VZV), has transformed cells *in vitro* (Yamanishi et al. 1981), although it has yet to be associated with *in vivo* malignancies.

All of the herpesviruses have an essentially similar structure: a DNA-containing icosahedral nucleocapsid enveloped by one or more lipid bilayers (see fig. 11.1). For an in-depth review of herpesviruses, see Roizman (Roizman 1982, 1983, 1985). All herpesviruses contain double-stranded DNA, have a characteristic genome size and antigenic constitution, are sensitive to ether, and are morphologically similar when examined by electron microscopy. HHV-6 is distinguishable by its host range, antigenic characteristics, and *in vitro* biological effects (Salahuddin et al. 1986). Southern blot

analysis demonstrated that a 9.0-kilobase restriction fragment of HHV-6 DNA does not hybridize with the DNAs of HSV, EBV, VZV, or HCMV and restriction fragments from these herpesviruses do not hybridize to HHV-6 DNA. This indicates that HHV-6 is distinct from the other herpesviruses; however, a region of the HHV-6 genome appears to have considerable nucleotide similarity with HCMV (Efstathiou et al. 1988).

Infection by herpesviruses usually progresses from an acute phase to the establishment of the virus in a state of latency during which the viral agent persists in blood or nerve cells and may be repeatedly activated, causing disease recurrence. The pathology of recurrent disease may or may not be similar to that of the primary infection. Both primary and recurrent infections usually result in the shedding of virus, which poses the risk of infectivity that may occur even during latent periods when the host lacks overt signs of disease.

Four of the human herpesviruses — HSV-1, HSV-2, EBV, and HCMV — cause this progression of primary, latent, and recurrent disease (see table 11.1). VZV causes chicken pox as the primary infection and, later in

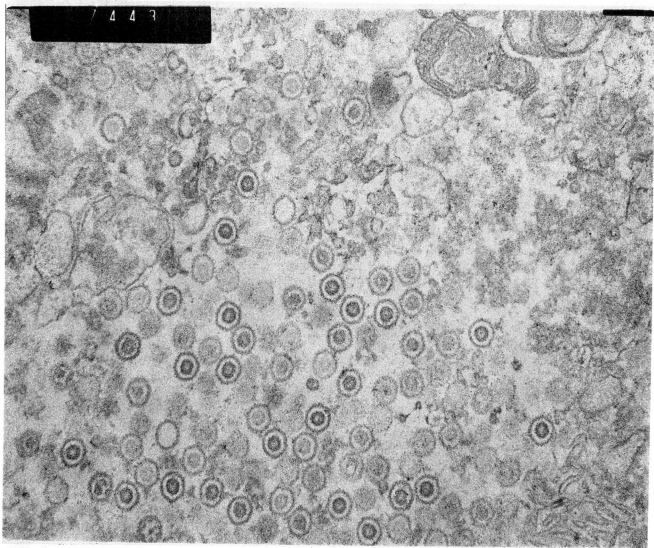

Fig. 11.1. Structure of intracellular herpesviruses as seen by electron microscopy.

life, causes shingles as the recurrent disease. So far HHV-6 has been isolated from patients with lymphoproliferative and hematologic disorders (Salahuddin et al. 1986) and has been identified as the causative agent for exanthem subitum, a common disease of infancy (Yamanishi et al. 1988). It may be more ubiquitous than originally perceived.

Table 11.1
DISEASES DUE TO HUMAN HERPESVIRUSES

Herpes simplex virus type 1	Acute herpetic gingivostomatitis
	Recurrent herpes labialis
	Keratoconjunctivitis
	Herpes genitalis
	Neonatal encephalitis
	Neonatal herpetic septicemia
	Primary herpetic dermatitis
	Eczema varicelliform herpeticum
	Kaposi's sarcoma
	Traumatic herpes
	Herpetic encephalitis in adults
	Trigeminal neuralgia
	Carcinoma of lip?*
	Cervical carcinoma?
Herpes simplex virus type 2	Herpes genitalis
	Neonatal encephalitis
	Neonatal herpetic septicemia
	Acute herpetic gingivostomatitis
	Recurrent herpes labialis
	Keratoconjunctivitis
	Primary herpetic dermatitis
	Eczema varicelliform herpeticum
	Kaposi's sarcoma
	Traumatic herpes
	Herpetic encephalitis in adults
	Trigeminal neuralgia
	Cervical carcinoma?
	Carcinoma of lip?
Cytomegalovirus	Cytomegalic inclusion disease
	Mononucleosis-like syndrome
	Pneumonia in immunosuppressed patients
	Cancer of the prostate?
	Kaposi's sarcoma?
Epstein-Barr virus	Infectious mononucleosis
	Burkitt's lymphoma
	Nasopharyngeal carcinoma?
Varicella-zoster virus	Chicken pox
	Shingles
	Ophthalmic zoster
	Varicella pneumonia
	Congenital abnormalities
	Hemorrhagic varicella
	Encephalitis
Human herpesvirus type 6	Exanthem subitum
	Lymphoproliferative and hematologic disorders

* Signifies neoplastic diseases associated with virus agent.
(Reprinted with permission from McGraw-Hill and modified.)

HERPES SIMPLEX VIRUSES

Both HSV-1 and HSV-2 cause the same disease syndrome, although HSV-1 is generally associated with orofacial infection and HSV-2 with genital infection. Types 1 and 2 originally were differentiated by serologic techniques. The two viruses share approximately 50% base sequence homology of their DNAs, with type 1 composed of 69% guanine plus cytosine, and type 2 composed of 71% guanine plus cytosine. HSV DNA is large (100×10^6 d), and has an extremely complex structure and function. The molecular biology has been reviewed by Roizman (1979) and Roizman and Jenkins (1985).

In 1971, hamster embryo fibroblasts were transformed to tumorigenicity by HSV-2 after the virus was rendered nonlytic by ultraviolet irradiation (Duff and Rapp 1971). Hamster cells also can be transformed by HSV-1; subsequently, other researchers morphologically transformed mouse, rat, chicken, and human cells with HSV-1. Temperature-sensitive mutants of HSV have also transformed cells. In these studies, transformed cell foci were established when cell cultures were held at a temperature that did not allow virus replication.

During HSV infection, normal disease progression destroys cells, which then can no longer be transformation targets. Defective or incapacitated HSV particles are probably needed to initiate transformation; normal host defense mechanisms also may affect virus replication.

Both HSV-1 and HSV-2 have been associated with human carcinomas. HSV-1 has been implicated in a rare tumor, squamous cell carcinoma of the lip, but further studies are needed to define its role in the disease. More substantive data have connected HSV-2 infection with cervical cancer (zur Hausen 1983); table 11.2 summarizes the evidence concerning HSV-2 as a possible etiologic agent.

Epidemiologic research forms most of the evidence associating HSV-2 in the etiology of cervix cancer: early age of first sexual intercourse, sexual promiscuity, and low socioeconomic status have been linked to the disease. Rigoni-Stern (1842) was the first to observe the low incidence of cervical cancer among cloistered nuns and unmarried women in Italy. In contrast, there is a positive correlation between cervical cancer and a large total number of sexual partners. Prostitutes are at a higher risk for cervical cancer; a positive correlation for increased rates of penile cancer in promiscuous males has also been noted (zur Hausen 1983). These observations suggest that an infectious organism, probably transmitted sexually, may be the causative agent in the

Table 11.2
STATUS OF ASSOCIATION OF HERPES SIMPLEX VIRUS TYPE 2 (HSV-2) WITH CERVICAL CANCER

- Conflicting epidemiology of virus isolation and anti-HSV-2 antibodies
- Failure to detect a specific set of virus antigens in cultured tumor cells
- Failure to detect HSV-2 DNA in the majority of cervical carcinoma biopsies
- Transformation in culture of normal cells to malignancy by HSV-2
- Failure to detect HSV-2 mRNA in carcinoma *in situ* and cervical dysplasia
- Controversy over induction of cervical carcinoma in mice by intravaginal administration of inactivated HSV-2

development of cervical carcinomas. Secondary factors, such as cigarette smoking, have recently been reported as increasing the cancer risk twofold (Clarke, Morgan, and Newman 1982; Wigle, Mao, and Grace 1980; Winkelstein 1977; Wright et al. 1978).

Seroepidemiologic studies have shown that a higher incidence of cervical cancer is associated with HSV-2 infection (Nahmias et al. 1970; Rawls et al. 1968). Such studies initially centered on the level of antibodies detected in women with cervical cancer compared with matched case controls. They revealed both higher titers and higher levels of antibodies to HSV antigens in the affected women. These findings were supported by other investigators until a major study involving thousands of women in Czechoslovakia failed to correlate the incidence of cervical cancer with HSV infection (Vonka et al. 1984).

Other investigators have tried to demonstrate direct biologic evidence of HSV antigens in malignant tumors. Data from studies on EBV and other tumor viruses in host systems have shown the presence of virus nucleic acids in tumors. Frenkel and her colleagues (Frenkel et al. 1972) attempted to measure reassociation of DNA from a cervical biopsy with a radioactively labeled HSV-2 DNA probe by DNA-DNA hybridization. However, HSV-2 DNA was detected in only one cervical carcinoma biopsy. Follow-up investigations by Frenkel and others yielded very few positive reports (zur Hausen 1983), but valid technical reasons make detection of HSV-2 DNA difficult. Studies involving both adenoviruses and papovaviruses show that DNA-DNA hybridization techniques may not be sensitive enough to detect the minute quantity of DNA needed for a transforming gene. In these investigations, as little as 1% to 1.5% of the HSV genome (1 to 1.5 x 10^6 d of DNA) was sufficient for transformation. Further analysis of two additional cervical biopsies by Frenkel and coworkers revealed subgenomic rearranged portions of the HSV-2 DNA (Manservigi et al. 1986).

Other investigations have assumed that any biologically relevant HSV-2 DNA sequence would affect a tumor cell via transcription into messenger RNA (mRNA) and into protein gene products (Jenkins and Howett 1984). These studies have sought to detect HSV-specific mRNA in biopsy material. Jones and associates (1979) and McDougall and colleagues (1980) demonstrated 60% positive hybridization of an HSV-2 DNA probe to cervical biopsies of dysplasia and carcinoma *in situ* using a radioactively labeled HSV-2 DNA probe to mRNA in biopsy cryostat sections. Controls hybridized only rarely to the HSV-2 probe, and simian virus 40 (SV40) DNA probes and radioactively labeled lambda bacteriophage failed to hybridize to the biopsy sections. While HSV-2 specific sequences were not found in invasive cervical carcinoma at that time, a later study by McDougall and colleagues (1982) reported positive findings. These conflicting results could indicate the limitations in detection capabilities. Also, invasive

carcinomas may not require the continued presence of virus genetic information.

Other studies have suggested that HSV-2 mRNA sequences can be detected in invasive cervical carcinoma biopsies. Use of *in situ* hybridization has yielded a statistically increased number of grains on autoradiographies (Eglin et al. 1981; Eizuru et al. 1983), although the hybridization levels were very low compared with previous reports.

Attempts have also been made to identify a subset of HSV sequences that might be responsible for *in vitro* and probable *in vivo* transformation (Spear 1983; Tevethia 1985). Transformation has been accomplished with inactivated virus preparations, and tumor formation is potentiated by transfection with intact HSV DNA. Either extensive shearing of the virus DNA, or treating the DNA with certain restriction endonucleases prior to transfection, can abolish the transformation potential. These two methods apparently introduce cuts into essential transforming genes, but not all restriction enzymes accomplish this. It is possible that transfection with purified DNA fragments can potentiate tumor formation.

Camacho and Spear (1978) were able to demonstrate morphologic transformation by transfecting hamster cells with the XbaI-F restriction fragment of HSV-1, which maps between 0.30 and 0.45 from the left-hand side of the HSV DNA genome and corresponds to the region coding for two virus glycoproteins. However, inoculation of syngeneic newborn hamsters with these transformed cells failed to cause tumor formation and HSV-1 glycoproteins were not identified in the cells. It has yet to be determined whether these cells represent true HSV-1 transformants.

Using the BglI-N fragment of HSV-2 DNA, Reyes and colleagues (1979) also demonstrated morphologic transformation of hamster cells; this fragment is located between 0.582 and 0.682 on the HSV-2 DNA map. Rodent cells have been transformed using increasingly smaller fragments of DNA; however, upon examination the cells failed to reveal a unique subset of HSV DNA sequences (Galloway and McDougall 1983). These data may indicate a "hit-and-run" mechanism for cell transformation by HSV-2 (Galloway and McDougall 1983; Hampar et al. 1976; Hampar et al. 1980; Skinner 1976), but details of such a mechanism have yet to be defined.

Investigations of HSV-2's capacity to cause tumor formation in mice after intravaginal inoculation have been controversial. Initial studies by Wentz and his associates (1975) demonstrated *in vivo* development of cervical carcinoma with repeated exposure to inactivated HSV-1 or HSV-2. Although follow-up investigations by Wentz and colleagues (1981) and Chen and colleagues (1983), in the People's Republic of China, supported these findings, a subsequent double-blind study using 1,000 mice (Meignier et al. 1986) reported failure to induce cervical cancer after exposure to HSV-1 or HSV-2. In cases where dysplasia developed, a correlation with insertion of vaginal tampons was shown, regardless of whether the tampons were impregnated with virus or control solution. Because of its scope, the study represents a major contradiction to previous reports.

Efforts to clarify the role of HSV-1 and HSV-2 in cervical cancer have been explored through cell transformation, seroepidemiologic studies in human populations, isolation of antigenic sequences in human malignancies, and tumor formation in animals following virus exposure. Results of many of these attempts to define a causative role for HSV-2 in cancer have conflicted. Such controversy involving viruses of pandemic distribution warrants continued investigation to define the role of herpes simplex viruses in human neoplasia. It is doubtful that these viruses can cause human cancer by themselves; cofactors appear to be necessary.

EPSTEIN-BARR VIRUS

The discovery of Epstein-Barr virus (EBV) was the result of investigation into Burkitt's lymphoma (BL), a malignant lymphoma of the jaw, in African children. Denis Burkitt, a British surgeon in Uganda, reported that the occurrence of this particular jaw tumor was clustered in specific climatic areas in which malaria was endemic. The children of foreign missionaries stationed in these areas also were afflicted. Similar malignancies have been identified only rarely in other areas of the world. While BL most commonly affects the lower jaw, involvement of the upper jaw, thyroid, liver, kidney, and ovaries has been reported.

In attempting to culture tumor cells, a lymphoblastoid cell line was established that could be grown indefinitely. Herpes-like particles were discovered in BL tumor cells during research to identify the disease's etiologic agent (Epstein et al. 1964). Subsequent studies demonstrated that EBV particles were shed from some of these cell lines and that supernatants from the cultures could transform normal human leukocytes to immortalized lymphoblastoid lines (Nadkarni et al. 1969). Additional follow-up studies have verified the transforming capability of EBV in lymphocytes from human adults and infants, and from several animal species.

The association of EBV with infectious mononucleosis (IM) was uncovered unexpectedly during a large-scale investigation into the relationship between the virus and tumor formation (Epstein and Achong 1979). While carrying out experiments in the laboratory of Gertrude and Werner Henle, a research technician contracted IM and simultaneously developed antibody specific for EBV (Henle and Henle 1979a).

The clinical course of IM varies from subclinical to a prolonged syndrome with recurrent fatigue and fever. Serologic evaluation reveals a nonmalignant proliferation of certain lymphocytes, which at times can be suggestive of acute lymphocytic leukemia. The proliferative response is limited and resolves during recovery. IM is usually transmitted by direct contact with salivary secretions (primarily through kissing), as infectious EBV is shed into oropharyngeal secretions (Henle and Henle 1979b). Epidemiologic investigations reveal that EBV infection is ubiquitous, infecting children in lower socioeconomic areas prior to adolescence and those in higher socioeconomic levels during adolescence.

Three types of antigens have been found in EBV-infected individuals: early antigen (EA) is found shortly after infection has occurred; the second type consists of virus structural or capsid antigens (VCA); and the third type is a nuclear antigen (EBNA) associated with transformation. The virus-shedding capacity has been associated with cells containing VCA (Kieff et al. 1983). EBNA consists of several proteins assembled in a complex structure. In a lymphoblastoid culture, only a few cells are EA or VCA positive, while all cells contain EBNA, a finding that parallels the papovavirus T antigen.

Among EBV strains identified, an important distinction can be made between two of them. P3J-HR-1 was isolated from a patient with BL, is capable of superinfecting EBV lymphoblastoid cell lines and inducing antigen synthesis, but is unable to transform umbilical cord leukocytes (Miller et al. 1974; Ragona, Ernberg, and Klein 1980). A second strain, B95-8, readily transforms cord lymphocytes but cannot induce EA synthesis and was isolated from marmoset lymphoblastoid cells which were transformed by an IM isolate. King and colleagues (1982) identified a region of DNA in P3J-HR-1 that is deleted from strain B95-8; this region accounts for approximately 15% of the genome involved in coding for an EBNA protein.

The EBV-human cancer association is supported by numerous studies; evidence of an etiologic role for EBV in BL is summarized in table 11.3. Also, EBV has been associated with nasopharyngeal carcinoma (NPC) (Klein 1979), a tumor concentrated geographically in southern China. EBV is strongly implicated in the etiology of NPC by direct biologic studies and epidemiologic research; genetic factors also may predispose an individual to develop this disease. Simons and colleagues (1974) determined that persons possessing two HLA-related antigens, A2 and B Sin2, are at increased risk for developing NPC, but the correlation only exists

Table 11.3
EVIDENCE FOR ETIOLOGIC ROLE OF EPSTEIN-BARR VIRUS (EBV) IN BURKITT'S LYMPHOMA (BL)

- Association of virus particles, antigens, and nucleic acids with tumor tissues
- Presence of the virus in BL afflicted regions
- Increased anti-EBV antibody in BL patients
- Transformation *in vitro* to immortality of human lymphocytes by EBV shed from BL tumor tissue
- Proliferative response of infectious mononucleosis (IM) patient lymphocytes
- Transformation *in vitro* to immortality of human B lymphocytes by EBV
- Induction of malignant lymphoma in nonhuman New World primates by EBV infection

(Reprinted with permission from McGraw-Hill.)

in the southern Chinese population. The precise role of HLA antigens in the development of NPC has yet to be determined.

EBV also can infect B lymphocytes, resulting in immortalized lymphoblastoid lines (Gerber, Whang-Peng, and Monroe 1969; Henderson et al. 1977) that contain EBV DNA and express EBNA. In contrast, uninfected B lymphocytes cannot replicate. A small percentage of latently infected cells express a surface antigen termed lymphocyte-derived membrane antigen (CYDMA). The antigen's exact nature has not been fully defined, but it has been demonstrated that CYDMA permits cells to be lysed by T lymphocytes from donors immune to EBV (Svedmyr and Jondal 1975).

EBV also may play a role in the formation of B-cell lymphomas, as evidenced by observations in nonhuman primates. Research with New World primates, such as marmosets, has shown that B-cell lymphomas have developed following EBV infection (Miller 1979). Agents genetically and biologically related to EBV are ubiquitous in baboons and Old World primates (Falk et al. 1976; Gerber et al. 1969; Gerber et al. 1976). In the Soviet Union, a baboon colony which is latently infected with the EBV-related agent, herpesvirus papio, shows a high incidence of malignant B-cell lymphomas (Rabin et al. 1977).

HEPATITIS B VIRUS

Hepatitis refers to an inflammation of the liver caused by chemical or viral agents. At least three viruses cause acute hepatitis, resulting in hepatitis A, hepatitis B, or hepatitis C (non-A, non-B hepatitis) (World Health Organization 1977; *Zinsser Microbiology* 1984). Hepatitis A is an acute infection only and does not become chronic. The etiologic agent is currently thought to be a small RNA-containing virus. Transmission of hepatitis A is primarily via the oral/fecal route and the incubation period is relatively short, about 30 days.

Hepatitis B is characterized by an incubation period of approximately 60 days. An acute infection results, which may later become chronic. Chronic hepatitis B infections may or may not be accompanied by acute liver disease. Krugman and associates (1967) reported that a long-incubation hepatitis resulted in individuals exposed to serum from patients with a like hepatitis. Boiling the serum prior to administration rendered it noninfectious and capable of immunizing patients. Currently, hepatitis B is known to be transmitted through blood or blood products, although transmission by other routes can occur; for example, chronically infected women can transmit the disease to their newborns (World Health Organization 1977). The high number of chronic infections in Third World countries is largely a result of such perinatal transmission.

The pathology of non-A, non-B hepatitis is similar to that of hepatitis B, but the etiology is not yet well defined.

Blumberg and colleagues (1965) discovered an antigen while screening thousands of blood samples for genetic variation of serum proteins that reacted with serum antibodies from an American hemophiliac. The antigen was recovered from the serum of an Australian aborigine and further studies (Blumberg et al. 1967; Okochi and Murakami 1968; Prince 1968) indicated that the antigen was rare in North America but more common in Asia and Africa. The "Australia antigen" is now designated hepatitis B surface antigen (HBsAg), and is considered diagnostic for hepatitis B. The nature of HBsAg and structure of the hepatitis B virus have been described in detail.

Hepatitis B virus (HBV) consists of an infectious particle known as the "Dane particle" (Dane, Cameron, and Briggs 1970) (see fig. 11.2). The particle is an enveloped virus with an average diameter of 42 nm and a core structure containing a double-stranded, circular DNA and a virus-specific DNA polymerase (Robinson 1977). Naked cores, obtained from Dane particles treated with lipid solvents, possess antigenicity referred to as the core antigen or HBcAg (Hoofnagle, Gerety, and Barker 1975). The core is composed of about three proteins, with the DNA polymerase possessing its own specificity, HBeAg (Magnius and Espmark 1972). Dane particles circulate in the blood of individuals suffering from either acute or chronic hepatitis, and HBcAg is found in the nucleus of infected liver cells.

The HBsAg is composed of spheres (22 nm) or filaments (22 nm wide and 100 nm to 700 nm long) and is found in blood and other body fluids of infected individuals (Robinson and Lutwick 1976a; Robinson and Lutwick 1976b). In contrast to Dane particles, these subunits of virus particles are found in much higher concentrations in the blood (10^{12}/mL) and in the cytoplasm of infected liver cells. Antibody to HBsAg will agglutinate these subunits and Dane particles, but not the core structures.

Serologic evaluations have revealed several characteristics about patients who are positive for HBeAg (HBeAg$^+$). Such antigenicity has only been identified in patients with HBsAg (Magnius et al. 1975), who also show evidence of increased numbers of Dane particles as well as greater HBV polymerase activity (Magnius et al. 1975; Nielson, Dietrichson, and Juhl 1974). Patients with HBeAg are more likely to have active liver involvement and a greater infectivity capability. In addition, mothers with HBeAg$^+$ blood are more likely to transmit the disease to their newborn infants.

Infection with HBV and the resulting chronic liver disease have been associated with the development of primary hepatocellular carcinoma (PHC) (see table 11.4). Liver damage may also be caused by environmental factors such as alcohol, nitrosamines, aflatoxins and cycads, which may in turn affect the incidence of PHC in populations with hepatitis B.

Primary liver carcinomas represent as much as 30% of the malignancies in Asia and Africa, but only 1% or 2% of those in Europe and the Americas (London

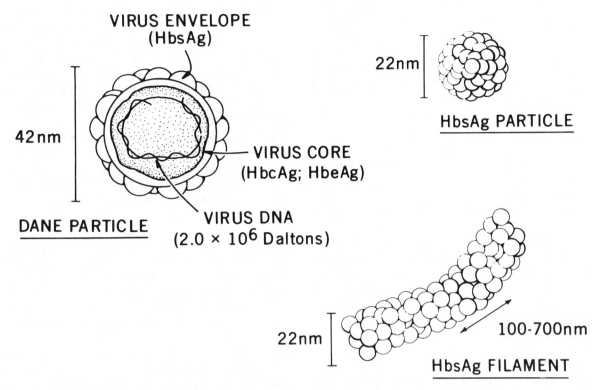

Fig. 11.2. Major structural elements found in the blood of patients with hepatitis B. The Dane particle represents the infectious virion and is an enveloped DNA virus containing a circular double-stranded DNA molecule with a large gap in one strand and a nick in the other. The nucleocapsid contains a core antigen (HBcAg), HBeAg, and a DNA polymerase. The relative frequency of Dane particles is low when compared with the presence of hepatitis B surface antigen (HBsAg) particles and filaments. HBsAg is present in large amounts in the blood of acutely infected individuals and of HBV carriers. HBsAg-containing human blood serves as a source for preparation of a formalin-inactivated vaccine against HBV infection.

1981). The greatest risk occurs between the ages of 50 and 70, with men two to four times more likely than women to develop liver cancer (London 1983). In clinical studies, cirrhosis was associated with about 75% of liver cell cancers (hepatomas) and from 20% to 50% of duct cell cancers (cholangiomas) (Edmundson and Peters 1977).

Chronic hepatitis B infection is strongly implicated in the PHC etiology (Chien and Vyas 1978; Krugman et al. 1979; Robinson 1977; Stevens et al. 1975; Stevens et al. 1979; Szmuness 1975; Vyas, Cohen, and Schmid 1978; Vyas et al. 1974). In areas where HBV is prevalent, neonatal infection commonly occurs via maternal transmission, resulting in large numbers of lifelong HBV carriers. Familial clustering of cirrhosis, chronic liver disease, and PHC also has been observed in such areas. Controlled investigations have demonstrated an association between active hepatitis B and PHC; the association also is supported by the fact that areas with low HBV rates have low PHC rates.

Evidence of virus involvement in liver biopsies from PHC patients has been established, HBV DNA integrated into liver cell DNA has been identified in several independent investigations (Brechot et al. 1980; Gerin, Shih, and Huyer, 1981; Shafritz and Kew 1981), and virus DNA has been detected integrated into cells of patients with chronic active hepatitis, with or without cirrhosis (Brechot et al. 1982). The precise role of HBV in the etiology and development of PHC has yet to be clarified.

Advances in hepatitis research are hindered by a technology gap—the lack of a cell system to culture and grow HBV. This hampers investigations detailing virus gene expression and defining the exact role of gene products in liver cell transformation and the development of PHC. However, the discovery of a hepatitis virus in the Pennsylvania woodchuck should assist research. This virus is similar physically to HBV and causes a spectrum of disease similar to that in humans.

The development of a vaccine with surface antigen is

Table 11.4
EVIDENCE FOR ASSOCIATION OF HEPATITIS B VIRUS (HBV) INFECTION WITH PRIMARY HEPATOCELLULAR CARCINOMA (PHC)

- Correlation of PHC and HBV carrier state, both in high-PHC and low-PHC incidence areas
- Superimposition of PHC on posthepatic cirrhosis
- HBsAG* and HBcAg* in cells of PHC biopsies
- Identification of integrated HBV DNA in hepatoma cell lines derived from PHC patients
- Familial clustering of HBV carrier state, chronic liver disease, posthepatic cirrhosis and PHC
- Maternal transmission of HBV carrier state to newborns in areas where PHC rate is high
- Evidence that a similar virus/disease complex leads to PHC development in the Pennsylvania woodchuck

*HBsAG = Hepatitis B surface antigen; HBcAG = Hepatitis B core antigen.
(Reprinted with permission from McGraw-Hill.)

another triumph that resulted from evidence that antibody to HBsAG provides immunity to hepatitis B (U.S. Patent Office 1972; London 1983). If effective, the vaccine could reduce the rate of HBV infection and dramatically lower the incidence of chronic liver disease and PHC.

PAPOVAVIRUSES

The name "papova" is derived from the three major virus subgroups: papillomavirus, polyomavirus, and simian vacuolating virus [simian virus 40 (SV40)]. Papovaviruses are nonenveloped and contain a double-stranded, circular, covalently closed and supercoiled DNA (Crawford and Black 1964). There is considerable evidence that members of this group affect cell proliferative control (Gross 1983; Tooze 1980). The polyoma subgroup has been extensively investigated, and the DNA of SV40 has been completely sequenced (Fiers et al. 1978; Reddy et al. 1978). SV40 was originally isolated from monkey cell cultures used in the preparation of poliovirus vaccine, a discovery that initiated investigation into the virus' possible role in human oncogenesis. It has not been established that SV40 has an etiologic role in human tumor development, but the virus has become a model for the study of tumor viruses and transforming genes. SV40 is a prototype virus of the polyoma subgroup because polyomavirus has many properties similar to SV40.

SV40 was first isolated from cultures of rhesus monkey kidney cells (Sweet and Hilleman 1960). It can lyse permissive cells, such as African green monkey kidney cells, and transform a variety of nonpermissive cells (e.g., hamster or other rodent) in culture (Black and Rowe 1963; Rabson and Kirschstein 1962; Shein et al. 1963). Injection of SV40 into some newborn hosts (e.g., hamsters) will result in tumor formation (Eddy, Grubbs, and Young 1964; Rabson, O'Conor, and Kirschstein 1962).

The DNA of SV40 is a supercoiled, circular, double-stranded molecule with an approximate molecular weight of 3×10^6 d. When SV40 infects permissive or nonpermissive cells, the virus adsorbs to and is engulfed by the cell membrane (viropexis), forming a vesicle that then traverses the cytoplasm (Hummeler, Tomassini, and Sokol 1970) before coalescing with the nuclear membrane. This releases the virus into the nucleus where uncoating and replication occur (Barbanti-Brodano, Swetly, and Koprowski 1970). Lytic infection by SV40 generally is divided into early and late periods. The early period refers to events preceding virus DNA replication. Immediately after uncoating, early virus mRNA is transcribed and cellular RNA and DNA synthesis is stimulated (Weil et al. 1974).

Prior to DNA synthesis, several distinct enzymes are induced in infected cells (Eckhart 1968; Kit 1968; Kit et al. 1967; Weil et al. 1967). These enzymes include RNA polymerase, DNA ligase, thymidine kinase, dTMP kinase, dTDP kinase, cytidine kinase, dCMP deami-

nase, CDP reductase, dTMP synthetase, dehydrofolate reductase, and probably others. After early RNA and antigen synthesis, cellular DNA synthesis is induced (Sambrook, Sharp, and Keller 1972; Tooze 1980), at which time the induction of histones and nuclear acidic proteins occurs in addition to mitochondrial DNA replication (Rovera, Baserga, and Defendi 1972; Winocour and Robbins 1970). The induction process appears to depend in part upon the early region of the virus genome. Tegtmeyer (1972) demonstrated that induction relies on a gene A (early gene) function since a functional gene A product is required for initiation of virus DNA synthesis. The gene A product is referred to as the tumor (T) antigen.

In permissive cells, replication of SV40 DNA begins in the nuclei at the same time or shortly after the induction of cellular DNA synthesis (Minowada and Moore 1963). Concurrent with or shortly after viral DNA synthesis, the structural proteins are synthesized. After synthesis of SV40 progeny DNA and structural proteins, assembly and maturation of new virions occur in the nuclei.

SV40 infection of nonpermissive cells (i.e., hamster or mouse) results in interactions similar to those of permissive cells. The virus is adsorbed to the cell and then enters the nucleus. Infection with SV40 can alter cell growth patterns and result in cells that behave as if they are transformed, although the alterations are transient (or abortive) and most cells regain somatic properties after several mitoses. Virus DNA synthesis does not occur. Smith and her colleagues (1970) first observed abortive transformation of 3T3 cells infected with SV40. Such cells can grow in low concentrations of serum. Their altered growth patterns seem to depend on the expression of early virus genes because the altered appearance can be blocked by interferon (Dulbecco and Johnson 1970; Taylor-Papadimitriou and Stoker 1971). The same spectrum of cellular enzymes produced in infected permissive cells is induced by abortive transformation, particularly those enzymes involved in DNA synthesis; cellular DNA synthesis also is induced. Attempts to demonstrate the synthesis of virus DNA or structural antigens in infected nonpermissive cells have consistently failed.

A small percentage of abortively infected cells become stably transformed after undergoing at least one round of mitosis (Rabson and Kirschstein 1962; Todaro and Green 1966b). The transformation fixation can be prevented in abortively transformed cells by adding interferon prior to the S period of the cell cycle; this implies that fixation occurs either in the S or G_2 phase (Todaro and Green 1966a). Several techniques have demonstrated that stably transformed cells have stable integrated virus DNA and all the properties described for abortive transformants.

Using cocultivation (Gerber and Kirschstein 1962) or fusion of SV40-transformed lines and permissive cells in the presence of inactivated Sendai virus (Gerber 1966; Koprowski, Jensen, and Steplewski 1967; Tournier et al.

1967; Watkins and Dulbecco 1967), cell hybrids can be formed from which SV40 can be rescued. From this, it is evident that many SV40-transformed lines contain the equivalent of one complete virus genome. If virus cannot be rescued using these techniques, the transformed cell lines are presumed to contain SV40 DNA lacking complete virus genetic information.

Sambrook and his coworkers (1968) investigated the state of the viral DNA in transformed cells. Because the high molecular weight portion of cellular DNA contains SV40-specific gene sequences and because the association is alkali stable, he concluded that SV40 DNA is covalently integrated into the transformed host cell's DNA. Other investigators have confirmed these results. SV40 DNA also has been detected in various transformed lines by measuring nucleic acid hybridization between virus-specific RNA and the total DNA extracted from the cells (Sambrook et al. 1968; Westphal and Dulbecco, 1968). Similar measurements have been made by hybridizing small amounts of denatured, labeled SV40 DNA with the total DNA extracted from transformed cells (Gelb, Kohne, and Martin 1971; Ozanne, Sharp, and Sambrook 1973). Examinations have revealed that transformed lines contain up to 60 integrated SV40 genomes.

Because of the limited coding capacity of SV40 DNA, investigations have centered on the identification of the transforming genes and gene products. An antigen synthesized early after virus infection and in transformed cells was identified in serum from tumor-bearing hamsters. This tumor (T) antigen can be detected by either immunofluorescence or complement fixation assay. Purification of the T antigen began with Del Villano and Defendi (1970) who reported the first estimated molecular weight at 100,000. Prives and her colleagues (1975) demonstrated that the early 19S SV40 mRNA could direct *in vitro* synthesis of the T antigen. Subsequent investigations have defined two proteins whose synthesis can be directed by 19S early mRNA: a 94,000-molecular weight protein termed large T (T), and a 17,000-molecular weight protein referred to as small t (t) (Rigby and Lane 1983). There are, therefore, two species of mRNA in the 19S early mRNA for large T and small t antigens; both have been mapped and their coding sequences are shown on the SV40 genomic map (see fig. 11.3).

Both large T and small t antigens have been implicated in malignant cell transformation. Large T antigen binds to DNA, with numerous investigations demonstrating specific binding to the origin of SV40 DNA replication. Large T antigen (the virus gene A product) is required for SV40 DNA synthesis; it also controls transcription of the virus' late region, and self-regulates early strand transcription. Table 11.5 presents the T antigen functions (Rigby and Lane 1983).

The isolation of several papovaviruses from human patients raised the question of oncogenicity of a human polyoma subgroup of papovaviruses. One group (typified by the JC isolate) was obtained from biopsies of

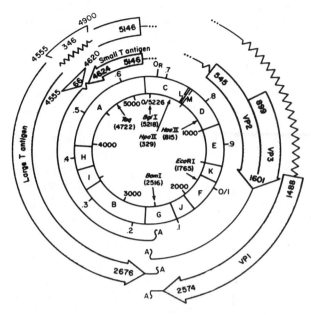

Fig. 11.3. Genomic organization of SV40 adapted from Fiers et al. (1978). Reprinted with permission from Macmillan Journals Ltd.

patients with progressive multifocal leukoencephalopathy (PML), a degenerative disease involving the central nervous system (Padgett and Walker 1976). In culture, JC virus has a very limited host range that grows only in human fetal glial cells. This virus, however, causes transplantable brain tumors in hamsters.

A second human papovavirus, BK virus, was isolated from the urine of an immunosuppressed renal allograft patient (Gardner et al. 1971). BK virus is similar to SV40 and has the capacity for *in vitro* transformation (Tooze 1980). The entire genome of BK virus has been sequenced (Seif, Koury, and Dhar 1979).

The human papovaviruses have not yet been associated with human cancer, although a high prevalence of antibodies to these viruses exists in the human population. Current investigations center on defining an etiologic role for the JC virus in the development of PML. Virtually every PML biopsy shows evidence of papovaviruses, and JC virus infection has been used to produce a PML syndrome in macaques. SV40 fails to cause any

**Table 11.5
PROPERTIES OF LARGE T ANTIGENS***

- Binding to the SV40 origin
- Initiation of viral DNA replication
- Autoregulation of early transcription
- Induction of late viral transcription
- ATPase activity
- Protein kinase
- Adenovirus helper function
- Tumor-specific transplantation antigen
- Target for cytotoxic T cells
- Binding to cellular DNA
- Stimulation of cellular DNA synthesis
- Binding to p53
- Activation of rDNA transcription
- Induction of cellular enzyme synthesis
- Initiation of transformation
- Maintenance of transformation

(*Adapted from Rigby and Lane [1983].)

known disease in its natural host, the cynomolgus monkey, and a similar relationship may exist between man and the human papovavirus.

PAPILLOMAVIRUSES

Papillomaviruses are a subgroup of papovaviruses that cause warts and benign tumors of the skin and other epithelial tissues in man and animals. In humans, these viruses induce plantar, common, and flat warts of the skin; genital warts (both condylomata acuminata and condylomata plana); and laryngeal papillomas of the mucosa. Most warts are benign and frequently regress, but there is increasing concern over the role of papillomaviruses in malignancies. Only a few of these viruses are capable of fibroblast transformation; the most well-understood of these are bovine papillomaviruses (BPV) types 1 and 2.

In the first association of a viral agent with the common human wart, Ciuffo (1907) demonstrated that warts could be transmitted by inoculation of cell-free filtrates from wart tissues. The concept that benign wart lesions could convert into carcinomas was described by Shope (1933) for the cottontail rabbit papillomavirus (CRPV). He demonstrated that a significant percentage of CRPV-induced lesions could progress to metastatic carcinomas (Kidd and Rous 1940; Rous and Beard 1927; Syverton 1952) in infected wild rabbits. The malignant conversion required 12 to 18 months, indicating that secondary environmental or host factors were interacting with the infected tissue. Secondary factors also play a role in the progression of epidermodysplasia verruciformis to carcinoma (Lewandowsky and Lutz 1922). Epidermodysplasia verruciformis is a familial disease characterized by large numbers of skin warts that frequently become malignant if exposed to sunlight. Juvenile laryngeal papillomas, also capable of becoming cancerous, are thought to be transmitted by perinatal infection of children born to mothers with genital human papillomavirus (HPV) infections. At one time x-irradiation was used to ablate laryngeal papillomas, but after long latent periods, many patients developed cancers at the site of the original papilloma. Spontaneous progression is rare and x-irradiation was the required secondary factor (zur Hausen 1977).

HPVs have long been considered the etiologic agents of human warts but they are not well understood because they have not yet been grown in cell culture. Recent advances in molecular biology have allowed extensive typing of papillomaviruses using cloned DNAs. Many virus DNAs can be propagated in bacterial hosts by inserting the 8-kilobase virus DNA molecules into plasmid cloning vectors. While mature virions are not produced, a large amount of virus DNA can be obtained for study. A type of HPV is considered new if analysis by nucleic acid hybridization indicates less than 50% homology with previous isolates (Coggin and zur Hausen 1979). When there is more than 50% homology but differences remain, the virus is considered a subtype. As a result, several previously obscured facts have

been revealed. First, the number of types of papillomaviruses greatly exceeds original estimates. As recently as 1984, 16 types had been identified; now, more than 50 have been described, many of which have identical or overlapping biological targets in the host (see table 11.6). Second, HPVs have been demonstrated in a number of papillomatous lesions involving various human tissues. Third, while more than one type of HPV may cause a lesion, the types may be grouped based on tissue tropism. For example, types 6, 11, 16, 18, 31, 33, and 35 are commonly found in genital warts. Fourth, these viruses have been detected in both common and rare carcinomas, particularly in genital cancers, indicating a possible significant biologic role in human tumors. This concept is supported by the fact that papillomas are recognized histologically as possible precursors to malignant lesions.

The papillomaviruses are a subgroup of the papovaviruses. They are small, nonenveloped DNA viruses with icosahedral symmetry, containing a double-stranded circular genome that is covalently closed and supercoiled. The subgroup contains both human and animal papillomaviruses, CRPV and BPVs being the best-studied. Pfister (1984) has extensively reviewed the virus' biology and biochemistry. The papillomavirus is relatively small, with a DNA molecular weight of approximately 5×10^6 d and a coding capacity for probably less than a dozen proteins. The DNA size is approximately 8 kilobase pairs. By analogy to the rest of the papovaviruses group, the proteins are of two types: early proteins produced prior to the onset of virus DNA replication, and late structural proteins that provide the components for new progeny virions. Little has been accomplished in the area of protein characterization because of the difficulty in obtaining purified populations of papillomaviruses. The proteins of only a few types of HPV have been analyzed, including HPV-1, HPV-2 and HPV-4, HPV-6, HPV-11, HPV-16, and HPV-18 (Androphy et al. 1987; Banks and Crawford 1988; Barbosa et al. 1989; Brown, Chin, and Strike 1988; Brown et al. 1988; Crook et al. 1989; Doorbar and Gallimore 1987; Favre et al. 1975; Garcia-Carranca, Thierry, and Yaniv 1988; Gissman, Pfister, and zur Hausen 1977; Gloss, Chong, and Bernard 1989; Grand et al. 1989; Grossman, Mora, and Laimins 1989; Jenison et al. 1988; Li et al. 1988; Li et al. 1987; Mallon, Wojciechowicz, and Defendi 1987; Orth, Favre, and Croissant 1977; Sato et al. 1989; Schneider-Gädicke et al. 1988; Seedorf et al. 1987; Sekine et al. 1989). Investigation of the HPV proteins must continue in order to fully understand the structure, transmission, and replication of the viruses. Analysis of these proteins may also clarify those which serve as antigenic stimuli in the infected host and which might elicit a protective immune response. Such information is vital to the eventual development of HPV vaccines.

Papillomaviruses are mostly restricted in host range. Only the BPVs seem able to infect cells of different species. Certain types are found in given lesions, but the

Table 11.6
LESIONS COMMONLY ASSOCIATED WITH
VARIOUS HPV TYPES

HPV type	Lesions
1a, b, c	Plantar warts
2a-e	Common hand warts
3a, b	Flat warts/juvenile warts
4	Plantar warts
5a, b	Macules, epidermodysplasia verruciformis patients
6a-f	Condylomata acuminata
	CIN I, II, III*
	VIN I, II, III*
	Laryngeal papillomas
7	Butcher's warts
8	Macules, epidermodysplasia verruciformis patients
9	Warts and macules, epidermodysplasia verruciformis patients
10a, b	Flat warts
11a, b	Condylomata acuminata
	CIN I, II, III
	Laryngeal papillomas
12	Warts and macules, epidermodysplasia verruciformis patients
13	Oral focal hyperplasia (Heck lesions)
14a, b	Skin lesions, epidermodysplasia verruciformis patients
15	Skin lesions, epidermodysplasia verruciformis patients
16	Condylomata acuminata
	CIN I, II, III
	VIN I, II, III
	Bowenoid papulosis
	Malignant carcinoma, cervix and penis
17a, b	Skin lesions, epidermodysplasia verruciformis patients
18	Malignant carcinoma, cervix and penis
19-29	Warts and hyperplastic lesions, epidermodysplasia verruciformis patients
30	Laryngeal carcinoma (rare)
31	CIN; Malignant carcinoma, cervix
32	Oral focal hyperplasia (Heck lesions)
33	Bowenoid papulosis
	CIN; Malignant carcinoma, cervix
34	Bowenoid papulosis
35	CIN; Malignant carcinoma, cervix
36	Actinic keratosis
37	Keratoacanthoma
38	Melanoma
39	Cutaneous lesions
40	Laryngeal carcinoma
41	Flat warts
42	CIN
43	CIN (normal cervical mucosa)
44	CIN (normal cervical mucosa)
45	CIN; Malignant carcinoma, cervix
46	Epidermodysplasia verruciformis (benign)
47	Epidermodysplasia verruciformis (benign)
48	Cutaneous squamous cell carcinoma (isolated)
49	Verruca plana (isolated)
50	Epidermodysplasia verruciformis (benign-isolated
51	CIN; Malignant carcinoma, cervix
52	CIN; Malignant carcinoma, cervix
53	Normal cervical mucosa (isolated)
54	Condyloma acuminatum (isolated)
55	Bowenoid papulosis (isolated)
56	CIN; Malignant carcinoma, cervix
57	CIN; Verruca vulgaris
58	CIN (isolated)

*CIN = cervical intraepithelial neoplasia; VIN = vulvar intraepithelial neoplasia.
(Adapted from McCance [1986] with permission from Elsevier Science Publishers.)

molecular basis of tissue specificity is not understood. Replication occurs in the nucleus of infected cells and virus DNA appears to exist as a stable episome present in high (50 to 200) copy numbers. Papillomavirus replication occurs in the maturing layers of keratinizing epithelium, but this process is not well understood. It is presumed that the virus. infects the basal cells, but the movement of cell progeny into the keratinizing layers may initiate virus production. The initial event in the stratum basale results in increased proliferation. Friedmann and Fialkow (1976) demonstrated that this was a polyclonal event, and isoenzyme analyses of four condylomata acuminata revealed the lesions' multicellular origins. In experimental infections of rabbit skin, detectable levels of virus DNA were present in the stratum granulosum of CRPV-induced papillomas, but were absent in less differentiated skin layers (Orth, Jeanteur, and Croissant 1971). In addition, virus DNA was first detected in the stratum spinosum by *in situ* hybridization of HPV-1-induced human warts (Grussendorf and zur Hausen 1979). Such investigations have shown that most DNA replication occurs in the differentiating layers. However, as low numbers of virus DNA copies per cell would be difficult to detect, they do not exclude the presence of DNA in basal cells. Almeida and coworkers (1962) noted whole virus particles in the stratum spinosum, providing evidence that the full virus replicative cycle is involved during replication in the differentiating layers. Virus aggregates can be seen in keratinized stratum corneum. The molecular mechanism involved is not yet understood, but it can be concluded that increased differentiation, i.e., keratinization, increases the permissiveness of infected cells to HPV infection (see fig. 11.4).

Although propagation of HPV in cell culture has been unsuccessful, a method for the long-term culture of human keratinocytes was developed by Rheinwald and Green (Rheinwald and Green 1975). HPV DNA persisted and replicated in these cultures as a stable episome (La Porta and Taichman 1982) with a high (50 to 200) genome copy number per cell, but mature virions were not found. Inoculation of wart extracts into human skin grafted to hamsters or to the backs of immunoincompetent mice failed to duplicate *in vivo* conditions necessary for wart development, a surprising result because CRPV had successfully transformed rabbit skin grafted onto hamster cheek pouch or onto nude mice (Cubie 1976; Kreider, Bartlett, and Sharkey 1979; Kreider, Haft, and Roode 1971; Pass, Niimura, and Kreider 1973). Infection and transformation of human tissues have been accomplished using xenografts placed beneath the renal capsule of the nude mouse (Kreider et al. 1986; Kreider et al. 1985). Experimental attempts to infect fragments of human uterine cervix, skin, and larynx with extracts containing HPV-11 have been successful. Subsequently, this type could infect human skin grafted to the backs of athymic mice. This model system offers a method for studying the basic process of HPV replication and the interaction of these viruses with host cells.

Cloning virus genomes has enabled DNA sequences to be analyzed, leading to the knowledge that animal

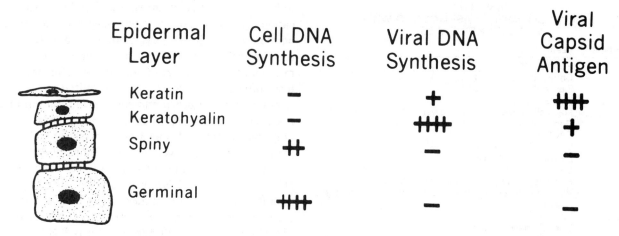

Epidermal Layer	Cell DNA Synthesis	Viral DNA Synthesis	Viral Capsid Antigen
Keratin	−	+	+++
Keratohyalin	−	+++	+
Spiny	++	−	−
Germinal	+++	−	−

Fig. 11.4. Differential localization of cell DNA, viral DNA and viral capsid antigen synthesis in keratinizing epithelium (Kreider and Bartlett [1979]. Reprinted with permission of Academic Press, Inc.)

and human papillomaviruses have a similar genetic organization. BPV-1 is one of the most amenable to study because it forms tumors in laboratory animals and transforms cells in culture (Lancaster and Olson 1982). Both virus particles and cloned virus DNA have been used to transform cells (Howley et al. 1980), and a subgenomic transforming fragment has been defined by detailed examination of this virus (Lowy et al. 1980). The virus DNA sequences have been shown to be multiple and extrachromosomal (Lancaster 1981; Law, Byrne, and Howley 1983) and the virus RNA-coding regions have been detailed using sequence analysis (Chen et al. 1982). This type of molecular biology has greatly advanced understanding of how these viruses function.

The HPV types found in human genital lesions along with the first isolation of each type are listed in table 11.7. HPV-6 was identified and partially characterized in total nucleic acid of a human genital wart (condyloma acuminatum). In the initial report, all six additional condylomata acuminata tested positive for HPV-6. Follow-up investigations in several laboratories demonstrated that this type is common in condylomatous lesions. HPV-11 DNA was originally isolated and cloned from a laryngeal papilloma of a 15-year-old patient. In the initial study, HPV-11 DNA was detected in four of nine laryngeal papillomas. HPV-11 DNA also was detected in a patient with recurrent tracheal and pulmonary papillomatosis and in condylomata acuminata. HPV-16 DNA, cloned from a cervical cancer biopsy, shares some homology with HPV-11 and was originally detected in 61.1% (11 of 18) of cervical cancers from Germany and subsequently isolated from 34.8% (8 of 23) of cervical cancers from Brazil and 28.6% (2 of 7) and 25% (1 of 4) of vulvar and penile carcinomas, respectively. HPV-16 is rare in condylomata acuminata (2 of 33, or 6%), but when detected, HPV-6 or HPV-11 also is present. Subsequent investigations have confirmed that HPV-16 is prominent in uterine cervical carcinomas. Another type, HPV-18, has been cloned from a cervical cancer biopsy. HPV-18 was found in 25% (9 of 36) of cervical

carcinomas from Africa and Brazil, 15.4% (2 of 13) of cervical tumors from Germany, and 10% (1 of 10) penile carcinomas. However, tests failed to detect HPV-18 in 17 cervical dysplasias, 29 genital warts, 8 carcinomas *in situ,* or 15 normal cervical biopsies. Both HPV-16 and HPV-18 DNAs have been detected in several laboratory-maintained cultures of cervical cancer cells. In general, infections with HPV-6 or HPV-11 are virus-positive and contain koilocytotic cells. HPV-16 or HPV-18 lesions do not show a high degree of koilocytosis, but reveal atypia corresponding to cervical intraepithelial neoplasia (CIN) II or III (Crum, Ikenberg, and Richart 1984). These latter lesions demonstrate aneuploid DNA patterns. A recent isolate, HPV-31, cloned from a cervical dysplasia, has been detected in 20% of mild and moderate dysplasias, 6% of invasive cancers, but not in condylomata acuminata. An additional type, HPV-33, cloned from a cervical carcinoma, has been detected in 4% to 8% of genital intraepithelial neoplasms and invasive cervical carcinomas. To date, approximately 90% of all cervical

Table 11.7
HPV TYPES INVOLVED IN GENITAL LESIONS

HPV type	Tissue of Isolation	Original reference
HPV-6	Condyloma acuminatum	Gissmann and zur Hausen (1980)
HPV-11	Laryngeal papilloma	Gissmann et al. (1982)
HPV-16	Cervical carcinoma	Durst et al. (1983)
HPV-18	Cervical carcinoma	Boshart et al. (1984)
HPV-31	Cervical dysplasia	Lorincz et al. (1986)
HPV-33	Cervical carcinoma	Beaudenon et al. (1986)
HPV-34	Bowen's disease (cutaneous)	Kawashima et al. (1986)
HPV-35	Cervical adenocarcinoma	Lorincz et al. (1987)
HPV-39	Penile bowenoid papulosis	Beaudenon et al. (1987)
HPV-40	Penile bowenoid papulosis	de Villiers et al. (1989)
HPV-42	Vulvar papilloma	Beaudenon et al. (1987)
HPV-43	Vulvar hyperplasia	Lorincz et al. (1989)
HPV-44	Vulvar condyloma	Lorincz et al. (1989)
HPV-45	CIN	Naghashfar et al. (1987)
HPV-51	Cervical dysplasia	Nuovo et al. (1988)
HPV-52	CIN	Shimoda et al. (1988)
HPV-54	Condyloma acuminatum	de Villiers (1989)
HPV-55	Bowenoid papulosis	de Villiers (1989)
HPV-56	Cervical dysplasia	de Villiers (1989)
HPV-58	CIN	de Villiers (1989)

Table 11.8
EVIDENCE THAT HPVS ARE INVOLVED IN CERVICAL CANCER

- Knowledge that animal papillomas progress to carcinomas
- Recognition that koilocytotic atypia of the cervix is HPV induced
- Recognition that koilocytotic atypia can progress to carcinoma
- Detection of HPV DNA in a large percentage of dysplasias and cervical carcinomas
- Dysplastic transformation of human tissue after laboratory infection with HPV-11

carcinomas examined under nonstringent hybridization conditions contain HPV-related sequences (Boshart et al. 1984). It is likely that even more HPV types will be associated with these malignancies.

Invasive squamous carcinoma of the cervix is one of the most common cancers of the female genital tract. The suggestion that a transmissible agent may be involved is due to a correlation of this malignancy with promiscuity (zur Hausen 1977). The prevalence of HPVs in the genital tracts of both sexes, and the detection of these viruses in papillomas, dysplasias, and cancers, are evidence that papillomaviruses are likely etiologic agents in the development of genital cancers (see table 11.8) (Pfister 1987). Infection with certain types of HPV may place an individual at higher risk for development of carcinomas. It also is likely that secondary cocarcinogenic factors are critical in the progression of papillomas to carcinomas. As most HPV-induced lesions regress spontaneously, it is doubtful that HPV alone is sufficient for malignancy. In addition, there is a long latent period prior to the development of cancer, i.e., a CIN I lesion may not progress to invasive carcinoma for two to 10 years. The secondary factors capable of effecting the neoplastic progression of warts have yet to be identified.

RETROVIRUSES

The retroviruses contain RNA as their genetic material (see fig. 11.5). Over the past several decades they have been isolated from an enormous number of animal tumors that either occurred naturally, were experimentally induced by chemical carcinogens or radiation, or resulted from the genetic breeding of high tumor-incidence animal strains (Bishop 1978; Coffin 1979). Retroviruses can be transmitted horizontally and vertically, and have been referred to in the literature as "leukoviruses," "C-type RNA viruses," "oncornaviruses," and "RNA tumor viruses." These names refer to characteristics not found in every member of the group and are no longer used. For example, not every retrovirus has been shown to be oncogenic. The term "retrovirus" refers to the fact that the flow of genetic information is reversed from the usual DNA to RNA. Each virus carries, in the virion, the enzyme reverse transcriptase, an RNA-dependent DNA polymerase (Baltimore 1970; Temin and Mitzutani 1970).

Reverse transcriptase allows the single-stranded RNA to replicate through a double-stranded DNA intermediate. The genome RNA is copied into a double-stranded DNA molecule termed the provirus DNA. The provirus DNA may then be integrated into the cell DNA and serve as the template for synthesis of new virion RNA and virus mRNA by host cell RNA polymerase. During synthesis of new virus RNA, the virus mRNA directs concomitant synthesis of virus proteins within the cytoplasm. Subsequently, the nucleocapsid leaves the cell by budding through the cytoplasmic membrane. This sequence usually does not result in cell destruction, making retroviruses ideal tumor viruses.

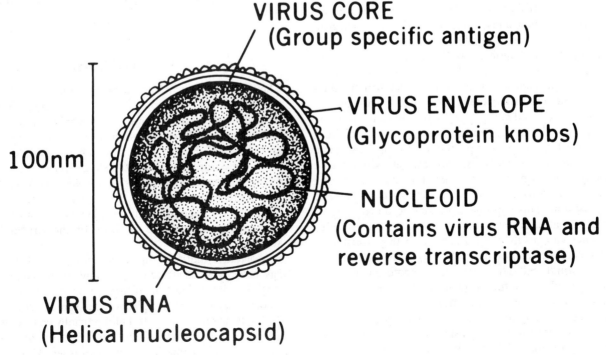

VIRUS CORE
(Group specific antigen)

VIRUS ENVELOPE
(Glycoprotein knobs)

NUCLEOID
(Contains virus RNA and reverse transcriptase)

100nm

VIRUS RNA
(Helical nucleocapsid)

Fig. 11.5. Structure of a typical retrovirus.

The first association of viruses with neoplasia was identified in avian leukemias and sarcomas at the beginning of the twentieth century (Ellermann and Bang 1908; Rous 1911). It is now known that these tumors are caused by retroviruses. Bittner's (1936) isolation of mouse mammary tumor virus from the milk of certain high tumor-incidence mouse strains sparked a huge research effort in the hope of finding counterparts in human tumors. In the 1950s, a retrovirus was linked to leukemia in certain high-incidence strains of mice (Gross 1978). This virus group is known to cause a variety of tumors in connective tissue and in tissues of the hematopoietic and reticuloendothelial systems. The hope of isolating retroviruses from human tumors has been frustrating, especially because their detection in animal tissues was relatively easy and isolation of comparable viruses from human tissues has failed. Their widespread appearance in animal tissues led to hypotheses that retroviruses could be involved in normal biological processes such as gene regulation, somatic cell mutation, and embryonic differentiation.

The study of retroviruses converged with the study of oncogenes when research into DNA and RNA tumor viruses indicated that gene products could convert normal cells to cancer cells. Many of these tumor viruses have transforming genes that can directly alter cell growth patterns in culture and, in some cases, induce tumor formation in animals after inoculation (Tooze 1980). Huebner and Todaro (1969) and Todaro and Huebner (1972) advanced the hypothesis that normal cells might contain covert oncogenes and alleged that factors such as radiation, chemicals, or viruses could derepress or alter oncogenes and result in carcinogenesis at the cellular level. This is now known to be true. Direct-acting oncogenes of retroviruses have cellular counterparts (Bishop 1985; Varmus 1985) whose primary role in oncogenesis may be in altering transcription of cellular growth regulatory genes (Varmus 1987).

Attempts to demonstrate the transfer of cellular oncogenes from cancer cells into normal cells have revealed that such genes can transfer the cancer phenotype, and in certain cases the genes correspond to identical or altered cellular genes that have been transduced into the transforming retroviruses (Weinberg 1985). An hypothesis was postulated for the oncogenic mechanism of the leukemia viruses: retroviruses lack directly transforming oncogenes but contain strong promoter regions capable of influencing cellular gene transcription. This hypothesis was based on the understanding that alteration and/or overexpression of cellular genes can result in an altered growth pattern, and that such genes can be controlled by virus gene regulation. Normal cellular sequences, "proto-oncogenes," can be involved in tumorigenesis. In some cases, the genes can be mutated to alter the function of the resulting protein; in others, gene expression can be altered by chromosomal translocation, mutagenesis, or gene amplification (Bishop 1983; Klein 1981).

A family of human retroviruses, called the human T lymphotropic viruses (HTLVs), was isolated and linked to T-cell abnormalities (Kalyanaraman et al. 1981; Poiesz et al. 1980; Posner et al. 1981; Yoshida, Miyoshi, and Hinuma 1982). The HTLV-I isolate is associated with an aggressive form of adult T-cell leukemia or lymphoma (Kalyanaraman et al. 1981; Poiesz et al. 1980; Yoshida, Miyoshi, and Hinuma 1982). HTLV-II, an infrequent isolate, was discovered in a T-cell variant of hairy-cell leukemia (Kalyanaraman et al. 1982). A third virus, termed human immunodeficiency virus (HIV), causes AIDS (Barré-Sinoussi et al. 1983; Gallo et al. 1984; Popovic et al. 1984; Sarngadharan et al. 1984; Schupbach et al. 1984).

HTLV-I and HTLV-II transform cells in culture, but do not contain direct transforming oncogenes. These viruses probably transform cells by producing a protein factor that inappropriately transactivates transcription of cellular genes involved in growth regulation (Felber et al. 1985; Haseltine et al. 1984; Sodroski, Rosen, and Haseltine 1984). HTLV-I and HTLV-II are important examples of retroviruses involved in human malignancies.

On the other hand, HIVs are cytopathic but not transforming. As they become more virulent in the host, their cytopathology appears to increase (Cheng-Mayer et al. 1988). Their primary effect *in vivo* is to destroy T-cells or their precursors with major spread mediated by macrophages. This induced immunodeficiency results in the increased incidence of a variety of tumors, initially noted with Kaposi's sarcoma. The virus may thus represent a major cofactor for other viruses or carcinogens. Because the primary disease caused by HIV is usually fatal, major efforts are under way to produce effective treatments or vaccines (Walker et al. 1988; Zagury et al. 1988). Such studies should be a catalyst in efforts to control virus-associated human neoplasms.

CONCLUSIONS

The role of viruses in human cancer, once hotly debated as improbable, is now firmly established. Viruses strongly associated with human cancers include hepatitis B, papillomaviruses, Epstein-Barr virus, and HTLV-I and HTLV-II. Fragile associations have been described for herpesviruses, especially HSV-2, HHV-6, and some of the human papovaviruses. The role of HIV in AIDS is striking as its effect on the immune system clearly increases the frequency of neoplasms, many of which are associated with one or more of the viruses listed above.

Molecular methods and recombinant DNA technology have enabled isolation of many of the virus genes that are able, at least in culture, to transform cells from a normal to a malignant phenotype. Some of these gene products have been isolated and partially characterized, although their major effects on initiation or maintenance of transformation remain elusive. This decade should resolve many of the problems concerning the role these proteins have in the neoplastic process and should lead to treatment or prevention of virus-associated cancers.

A more certain way to demonstrate a causal relationship of viruses with a given disease is to prevent the disease by vaccination. Unfortunately, the long latent period of most cancers and the difficulty in evaluating the efficacy and safety of tumor virus vaccines (even precursor protein reagents) make this approach difficult, and improbable in most cases. Attempts to obliterate HBV infection in Third World countries by use of a hepatitis B virus precursor antigen vaccine should yield data over the next 30 to 50 years that may definitely resolve whether this putative tumor virus causes liver cancer. However, the use of this vaccine is justified only because of the massive numbers of individuals afflicted with liver disease caused by hepatitis B virus and not because of its infrequent progression to hepatocellular carcinoma. New and imaginative approaches will be required to resolve cancer causation and to develop new therapies and means of prevention.

ACKNOWLEDGMENTS

The author wishes to thank Pamela Miles, N.P.H., for her help in the orientation of this chapter, Melissa C. Hill and Ann Viozzi for editorial assistance, and Elaine K. Neidigh for secretarial expertise. He also wishes to thank Dr. Mary K. Howett and Dr. Joan Cory for reviewing and improving the sections on the papilloma-viruses and retroviruses, respectively. Special thanks are due to Dr. Karen D. Cockley for improving and strengthening the section on papillomaviruses.

REFERENCES

Almeida, J.D.; Howatson, A.F.; and Williams, M.G. 1962. Electron microscope study of human warts: sites of virus production and nature of the inclusion bodies. *J. Invest. Dermatol.* 38:337-45.

Androphy, E.T.; Hubbert, N.L.; and Schiller, J.T. et al. 1987. Identification of the HPV-16 E6 protein from transformed mouse cells and human cervical carcinoma cell lines. *EMBO J.* 6:989-92.

Baltimore, D. 1970. Viral RNA-dependent DNA polymerase. *Nature* 226:1209-11.

Banks, L., and Crawford. 1988. Analysis of human papillomavirus type 16 polypeptides in transformed primary cells. *Virology* 165:326-28.

Barbanti-Brodano, G.; Swetly, P.; and Koprowski, H. 1970. Early events in the infection of permissive cells with simian virus 40: adsorption, penetration, and uncoating. *J. Virol.* 6:78-86.

Barbosa, M.S.; Lowry, D.R.; and Schiller, J.T. 1989. Papilloma virus polypeptides E6 and E7 are zinc-binding proteins. *J. Virol.* 63:1404-1407.

Barré-Sinoussi, F.; Chermann, J.C.; and Rey, F. et al. 1983. Isolation of a T-lymphotropic retrovirus from a patient at risk for acquired immune deficiency syndrome (AIDS). *Science* 220:868-71.

Beaudenon, S.; Kremsdorf, D.; and Croissant, O. et al. 1986. A novel type of human papillomavirus associated with genital neoplasias. *Nature* 321:246-49.

Beaudenon, S.; Kremsdorf, D.; and Obalek, S., et al. 1987. Plurality of genital human papillomaviruses: characterization of two new types with distinct biological properties. *Virology* 161:374-84.

Bishop, J.M. 1978. Retroviruses. *Ann. Rev. Biochem.* 47:35-88.

Bishop, J.M. 1983. Cellular oncogenes and retroviruses. *Ann. Rev. Biochem.* 52:301-54.

Bishop, J.M. 1985. Viruses, genes and cancer. II: retroviruses and cancer genes. *Cancer* 55:2329-33.

Bittner, J.J. 1936. Some possible effects of nursing on the mammary gland tumor incidence in mice. *Science* 84:162.

Black, P.H., and Rowe, W.P. 1963. SV40-induced proliferation of tissue culture cells of rabbit, mouse and porcine origin. *Proc. Soc. Exp. Biol. Med.* 114:721-27.

Blumberg, B.S.; Alter, H.J.; and Visnich, S. 1965. A new antigen in leukemia sera. *JAMA* 191:541-46.

Blumberg, B.S.; Gerstley, B.J.S.; and Hungerford, D.A. et al. 1967. A serum antigen (Australia antigen) in Down's syndrome leukemia and hepatitis. *Ann. Int. Med.* 66:924-31.

Boshart, M.; Gissmann, L.; and Ikenberg, H. et al. 1984. A new type of papillomavirus DNA, its presence in genital cancer biopsies and in cell lines derived from cervical cancer. *EMBO J.* 3:1151-57.

Brechot, C.; Hadchouel, M.; and Scotto, J. et al. 1980. State of hepatitis B virus DNA sequences in cellular DNA of human hepatocellular carcinoma. *Nature* 286:533-35.

Brechot, C.; Pourcel, C.; and Hadchouel, M. et al. 1982. State of hepatitis B virus DNA in liver diseases. *Hepatology* 2:275-345.

Brown, D.R.; Chin, M.T.; and Strike, D.G. 1988. Identification of human papillomavirus type II E4 gene products in human tissue implants from athymic mice. *Virology* 165:262-67.

Browne, H.M.; Churcher, M.J.; and Stanley, M.A. et al. 1988. Analysis of the L1 gene product of human papilloma virus type 16 by expression in a vaccinia virus recombinant. *J. Gen. Virol.* 69:1263-73.

Camacho, A., and Spear, P.G. 1978. Transformation of hamster embryo fibroblasts by a specific fragment of the herpes simplex virus genome. *Cell* 15:993-1002.

Chen, E.Y.; Howley, P.M.; and Levinson, H.D. et al. 1982. The primary structure and genetic organization of the bovine papillomavirus type 1 genome. *Nature* 299:529-34.

Chen, M.H.; Chang, Y.D.; and Zhi-Hui, L. et al. 1983. Prevention of type 2 herpes simplex virus-induced cervical carcinoma in mice by prior immunization with a vaccine prepared from type 1 herpes simplex virus. *Vaccine* 1:13-21.

Cheng-Mayer, C.; Seto, D.; and Tateno, M. et al. 1988. Biologic features of HIV-1 that correlate with virulence in the host. *Science* 240:80-82.

Chien, D.Y., and Vyas, G.N. 1978. Correlation of the hepatitis B surface and E-antigens. *N. Engl. J. Med.* 299:1253-54.

Ciuffo, G. 1907. Innesto positivo con filtrato di verrucae volgare. *Giorn. Ital. Mal. Veneral* 48:12-17.

Clarke, E.A.; Morgan, R.W.; and Newman, A.M. 1982. Smoking as a risk factor in cancer of the cervix: additional evidence from a case-control study. *Am. J. Epidemiol.* 115:59-66.

Coffin, J.M. 1979. Structure, replication and recombination of retrovirus genomes: some unifying hypotheses. *J. Gen. Virol.* 42:1-26.

Coggin, J.R. Jr., and zur Hausen, H. 1979. Workshop on papillomaviruses and cancer. *Cancer Res.* 39:545-46.

Crawford, L.V., and Black, P.H. 1964. The nucleic acid of simian virus 40. *Virology* 24:388-92.

Crook, T.; Morgenstern, J.P.; and Crawford, L. et al. 1989. Continued expression of HPV-16 E7 protein is required for maintenance of the transformed phenotype of cells co-transformed by the HPV-16 plus EJ-*ras. EMBO J.* 8: 513-519.

Crum, L.P.; Ikenberg, H.; and Richart, R.M. 1984. Human papillomavirus type 16 and early cervical neoplasia. *N. Engl. J. Med.* 310:880-83.

Cubie, H.A. 1976. Failure to produce warts on human skin grafts on "nude" mice. *Br. J. Dermatol.* 94:659-65.

Dane, D.S.; Cameron, C.H.; and Briggs, M. 1970. Virus-like particles in serum of patients with Australia-antigen-associated hepatitis. *Lancet* I:695-698.

Del Villano, B., and Defendi, V. 1970. Preparation and use of an immunosorbent to study the molecular composition of the SV40 T-antigen from hamster tumor cells. *Bacterial Proc. Abst.* 222:118.

De Villiers, E.M. 1989. Human papillomaviruses. In *The Roche Biomedical Laboratories—Roche Diagnostic Systems Reference Chart.* Montclaire, N.J.

De Villiers, E.M.; Hirsch-Behnam, A.; and von Knebel-Doeberitz, C. et al. 1989. Two newly identified human papillomavirus types (HPV 40 and 57) isolated from mucosal lesions. *Virology* 171:248-53.

Doorbar, J., and Gallimore, P.H. 1987. Identification of proteins by the L1 and L2 open reading frames of human papillomavirus 1a. *J. Virol.* 61:2793-99.

Duff, R., and Rapp, F. 1971. Oncogenic transformation of hamster cells after exposure to herpes simplex virus type 2. *Nature New Biol.* 233:48-50.

Dulbecco, R., and Johnson, T. 1970. Interferon-sensitivity of the enhanced incorporation of thymidine into cellular DNA encoded by polyoma virus. *Virology* 42:368-74.

Durst, M.; Gissmann, L.; and Ikenberg, H. et al. 1983. A papilloma virus DNA from a cervical carcinoma and its prevalence in cancer biopsy samples from different geographic regions. *Proc. Natl. Acad. Sci. USA* 80:3812-15.

Eckhart, W. 1968. Transformation of animal cells by oncogenic DNA viruses. *Physiol. Rev.* 48:513-33.

Eddy, B.E.; Grubbs, G.E.; and Young, R.D. 1964. Tumor immunity in hamsters infected with adenovirus type 12 or simian virus 40. *Proc. Soc. Exp. Biol. Med.* 117:575-79.

Edmundson, H.A., and Peters, R.L. 1977. Liver. In Anderson, W.A.D., and Kissane, J.M. eds. *Pathology.* 7th ed. p. 1321. New York: C.V. Mosby.

Efstathiou, S.; Gompels, U.A.; and Craxton, M.A. et al. 1988. DNA homology between a novel human herpesvirus (HHV-6) and human cytomegalovirus. *Lancet* I:63-64.

Eglin, R.P.; Sharp, F.; and MacLean, A.B. et al. 1981. Detection of RNA complementary to herpes simplex virus DNA in human cervical squamous cell neoplasms. *Cancer Res.* 41:3597-3603.

Eizuru, Y.; Hyman, R.W.; and Nahhas, W.A. 1983. Herpesvirus RNA in human urogenital tumors. *Proc. Soc. Exp. Biol. Med.* 174:296-301.

Ellermann, V., and Bang, O. 1908. Experimentalle leukaie bei huhnern. *Zentralbl. bakteriol. Abt. I (Orig.)* 46:595-609.

Epstein, M.A., and Achong, B.G. 1979. In Epstein, M.A., and Achong, B.G. eds. *The Epstein-Barr virus.* pp. 1-459. New York: Springer-Verlag.

Epstein, M.A.; Achong, B.G.; and Barr, Y.M. 1964. Virus particles in cultured lymphoblasts from Burkitt's lymphoma. *Lancet* I:702-703.

Falk, L.; Deinhardt, F.; and Nonomaya, M. et al. 1976. Properties of a baboon lymphotropic herpesvirus related to Epstein-Barr virus. *Int. J. Cancer* 18:798-807.

Favre, M.; Breitburd, F.; and Croissant, O. et al. 1975. Structural polypeptides of rabbit, bovine and human papilloma viruses. *J. Virol.* 15:1239-47.

Felber, B.K.; Paskalis, H.; and Kleinman-Ewing, C. et al. 1985. The pX protein of HTLV-I is a transcriptional activator of its long terminal repeats. *Science* 229:675-79.

Fiers, W.; Contreras, R.; and Haegeman, G. et al. 1978. Complete nucleotide sequence of SV40 DNA. *Nature* 273: 113-20.

Frenkel, N.; Roizman, B.; and Cassai, E. et al. 1972. A DNA fragment of herpes simplex 2 and its transcription in human cervical cancer tissue. *Proc. Natl. Acad. Sci. USA* 69: 3784-89.

Friedman, J.M., and Fialkow, P.J. 1976. Viral "tumorigenesis" in man: cell markers in condylomata acuminata. *Int. J. Cancer* 17:57-61.

Gallo, R.C.; Salahuddin, S.Z.; and Popovic, M. et al. 1984. Frequent detection and isolation of cytopathic retroviruses (HTLV-III) from patients with AIDS and at risk for AIDS. *Science* 224:500-503.

Galloway, D.A., and McDougall, J.K. 1983. The oncogenic potential of herpes simplex viruses: evidence for a "hit-and-run" mechanism. *Nature* 302:21-24.

Garcia-Carranca, A.; Thierry, F.; and Yaniv, M. 1988. Interplay of viral and cellular proteins along the long control region of human papillomavirus type I8. *J. Virol.* 62: 4321-30.

Gardner, S.D.; Field, A.M.; and Coleman, D.V. et al. 1971. New human papovavirus (BK) isolated from urine after renal transplantation. *Lancet* I:1253-57.

Gelb, L.D.; Kohne, D.E.; and Martin, M.A. 1971. Quantitation of SV40 sequences in African green monkey, mouse, and virus-transformed cell genomes. *J. Mol. Biol.* 57:129-45.

Gerber, P. 1966. Studies on the transfer of subviral infectivity from SV40-induced hamster tumor cells to indicator cells. *Virology* 28:501-509.

Gerber, P., and Kirschstein, R.J. 1962. SV40-induced ependymomas in newborn hamsters. I: virus tumor relationships. *Virology* 18:582-588.

Gerber, P.; Nkrumah, F.; and Pritchett, R. et al. 1969. Comparative studies of Epstein-Barr virus strains from Ghana and the United States. *Int. J. Cancer* 17:71-81.

Gerber, P.; Pritchett, R.; and Kieff, E. 1976. Antigens and DNA of a chimpanzee agent related to Epstein-Barr virus. *J. Virol.* 19:1090-99.

Gerber, P.; Whang-Peng, J.; and Monroe, J.H. 1969. Transformation and chromosome changes induced by Epstein-Barr virus in normal leukocyte cultures. *Proc. Natl. Acad. Sci. USA* 63:740-47.

Gerin, J.L.; Shih, J.W.K.; and Huyer, B.H. 1982. Biology and characterization of hepatitis B virus. In Smzuness, W.; Alter, H.J.; and Maynard, J.E. eds. *Viral hepatitis.* p. 49. Philadelphia: Franklin Institute Press.

Gissmann, L.; Diehl, V.; and Schultz-Coulon, H. et al. 1982. Molecular cloning and characterization of human papilloma virus DNA derived from a laryngeal papilloma. *J. Virol.* 44:393-400.

Gissmann, L.; Pfister, H.; and zur Hausen, H. 1977. Human papilloma viruses (HPV): characterization of 4 different isolates. *Virology* 76:569-80.

Gissmann, L., and zur Hausen, H. 1980. Partial characterization of viral DNA from human genital warts (condylomata acuminata). *Int. J. Cancer* 25:605-609.

Gloss, B.; Chong, T.; and Bernard, H.U. 1989. Numerous nuclear proteins bind the long control region of human papillomavirus type 16: a subset of 6 or 23 DNase I-protected segments coincides with the location of the cell-type-specific enhancer. *J. Virol.* 63:1142-52.

Grand, R.J.; Doorbar, J.; and Smith et al. 1989. Phosphorylation of the human papillomavirus type 1E4 proteins *in vivo* and *in vitro. Virology* 170:201-13.

Gross, L. 1978. Viral etiology of cancer and leukemia: a look into the past, present, and future. G. H. A. Clowes Memorial Lecture. *Cancer Res.* 38:485-93.

Gross, L. ed. 1983. *Oncogenic viruses.* 3rd ed. New York: Pergamon Press.

Grossman, S.R.; Mora, R.; and Laimins, L.A. 1989. Intracellular localization and DNA-binding properties of human papillomavirus 18 E6 protein expressed with a baculovirus vector. *J. Virol.* 63:366-74.

Grussendorf, E.I., and zur Hausen, H. 1979. Localization of viral DNA-replication in sections of human warts by nucleic acid hybridization with complementary RNA of human papilloma virus type 1. *Arch. Dermatol. Res.* 264:55-63.

Hampar, B.; Aaronson, S.A.; and Derge, J.G. et al. 1976. Activation of an endogenous mouse type C virus by ultraviolet-irradiated herpes simplex virus types 1 and 2. *Proc. Natl. Acad. Sci. USA* 73:646-50.

Hampar, B.; Boyd, A.L.; and Derge, J.G. et al. 1980. Comparison of properties of mouse cells transformed spontaneously by ultraviolet light-irradiated herpes simplex virus or by simian virus 40. *Cancer Res.* 40:2213-22.

Haseltine, W.A.; Sodroski, J.G.; and Patarca, R. et al. 1984. Structure of 3'-terminal region of type II human T lymphotropic virus: evidence for new coding region. *Science* 225: 419-21.

Henderson, E.; Miller, G.; and Robinson, J. et al. 1977. Efficiency of transformation of lymphocytes by Epstein-Barr virus. *Virology* 76:152-63.

Henle, W., and Henle, G. 1979a. Seroepidemiology of the virus. In Epstein, M., and Achong, B. eds. *The Epstein-Barr virus.* p. 61. New York: Springer-Verlag.

Henle, G., and Henle, W. 1979b. The virus as the etiologic agent of infectious mononucleosis. In Epstein, M., and Achong, B. eds. *The Epstein-Barr virus.* p. 297. New York: Springer-Verlag.

Hoofnagle, J.H.; Gerety, R.J.; and Barker, L.F. 1975. Antibody to hepatitis-B core antigen. *Am. J. Med. Sci.* 270: 179-87.

Howley, P.M.; Low, M.F.; and Heilman, C.A. et al. 1980. Molecular characterization of papillomavirus genomes. *Cold Spring Harbor Conf. Cell Prolif.* 7:233-47.

Huebner, R.J., and Todaro, G.J. 1969. Oncogenes of RNA tumor viruses as determinants of cancer. *Proc. Natl. Acad. Sci. USA* 64:1087-94.

Hummeler, K.; Tomassini, N.; and Sokol, F. 1970. Morphological aspects of the uptake of simian virus 40 by permissive cells. *J. Virol.* 6:87-93.

Jenison, S.A.; Firzlaff, J.M.; and Lanaenberg et al. 1988. Identification of immunoreactive antigens of human papillomavirus type 6b by using *Escherichia coli* expressed fusion proteins. *J. Virol.* 62:2115-23.

Jenkins, F.J., and Howett, M.K. 1984. Characterization of the mRNAs that map in the BglII-N fragment of the herpes simplex virus type 2 genome. *J. Virol.* 52: 99-107.

Jones, K.W.; Fenoglio, C.M.; and Shevchuk-Chaban, M. et al. 1979. Detection of herpesvirus 2 mRNA in human cervical biopsies by *in situ* cytological hybridization. *IARC Sci. Publ.* 24:917-25.

Kalyanaraman, V.S.; Sarngadharan, M.G.; and Bunn, P.A. et al. 1981. Antibodies in human sera reactive against an internal structural protein of human T-cell lymphoma virus. *Nature* 294:271-73.

Kalyanaraman, V.S.; Sarngadharan, M.G.; and Robert-Guroff, M. et al. 1982. A new subtype of human T-cell leukemia virus (HTLV-II) associated with a T-cell variant of hairy cell leukemia. *Science* 218:571-73.

Kawashima, M.; Jablonska, S.; and Favre et al. 1986. Characterization of a new type of human papillomavirus found in a lesion of Bowen's disease of the skin. *J. Virol.* 57:688-92.

Kidd, J.G., and Rous, P. 1940. Cancers deriving from the virus papillomas of wild rabbits under natural conditions. *J. Exp. Med.* 71:469-94.

Kieff, E.; Dambaugh, T.; and Hummel, M. et al. 1983. Epstein-Barr virus transformation and replication. In Klein, G. ed. *Advances in viral oncology.* vol. 3. pp. 133-182. New York: Raven Press.

King, W.; Dambaugh, T.; and Heller, M. et al. 1982. Epstein-

Barr virus DNA. XII: a variable region of the EBV genome is included in the P3HR1-deletion. *J. Virol.* 43:979-86.

Kit, S. 1968. Viral induced enzymes and the problem of viral oncogenesis. *Adv. Cancer Res.* 11:73-221.

Kit, S.; Melnick, J.L.; and Dubbs, D.R. et al. 1967. Virus-directed host response. In Pollard, M. ed. *Perspectives in Virology.* New York: Academic Press.

Klein, G. 1979. Relationship of the virus to nasopharyngeal carcinoma. In Epstein, M., and Achong, B. eds. *The Epstein-Barr virus.* p. 340. New York: Springer-Verlag.

Klein, G. 1981. Role of gene dosage and genetic transpositions in carcinogenesis. *Nature* 294:313-18.

Koprowski, H.; Jenson, F.C.; and Steplewski, Z.S. 1967. Activation of production of infectious tumor virus SV40 in heterokaryon cultures. *Proc. Natl. Acad. Sci. USA* 58: 127-33.

Kreider, J.; Bartlett, G.L.; and Sharkey, F.E. 1979. Primary neoplastic transformation *in vivo* of xenogeneic skin grafts on nude mice. *Cancer Res.* 39:273-76.

Kreider, J.; Haft, H.M.; and Roode, P.R. 1971. Growth of human skin on the hamster. *J. Invest. Dermatol.* 57:66-71.

Kreider, J.; Howett, M.K.; and Lill, N.L. et al. 1986. *In vivo* transformation of human skin with human papillomavirus type 11 from condyloma acuminata. *J. Virol.* 59:369-76.

Kreider, J.; Howett, M.K.; and Wolfe, S.A. et al. 1985. Morphological transformation *in vivo* of human uterine cervix with papillomavirus from condyloma acuminata. *Nature* 317:639-41.

Krugman, S.; Giles, J.P.; and Hammond, J. 1967. Infectious hepatitis: evidence for two distinctive clinical, epidemiological and immunological types of infection. *JAMA* 200: 365-73.

Krugman, S.; Overby, L.R.; and Mushahwar, I.K. et al. 1979. Viral hepatitis, type B: studies on natural history and prevention re-examined. *N. Engl. J. Med.* 300:101-106.

Lancaster, W. 1981. Apparent lack of integration of bovine papilloma virus DNA in virus-induced equine and bovine tumor cells and virus-transformed mouse cells. *Virology* 108:251-55.

Lancaster, W.D., and Olson, C. 1982. Animal papillomaviruses. *Microbiol. Rev.* 46:191-207.

La Porta, R.F., and Taichman, L.B. 1982. Human papilloma viral DNA replicates as a stable episome in cultured epidermal keratinocytes. *Proc. Natl. Acad. Sci. USA* 79: 3393-97.

Law, M.F.; Byrne, J.C.; and Howley, P.M. 1983. Stable bovine papillomavirus hybrid plasmid that expresses a dominant selective trait. *Mol. Cell Biol.* 3:2110-15.

Lewandowsky, F., and Lutz, W. 1922. Ein falleiner bisher nicht beschriebenen hauterkrankung (Epidermodysplasia verruciformis). *Arch. Dermatol. Syph. (Berlin)* 141:193-203.

Li, C-C.H.; Gilden, R.V.; and Showalter, S.D. et al. 1988. Identification of the human papillomavirus E2 protein in genital tract tissues. *J. Virol.* 61:606-609.

Li, C-C.H.; Shah, K.V.; and Seth, A. et al. 1987. Identification of the human papillomavirus type 6b L1 open frame protein in condylomas and corresponding antibodies in human sera. *J. Virol.* 61:2684-90.

London, W.T. 1983. Hepatitis B virus and primary hepatocellular carcinoma. In Klein, G. ed. *Advances in viral oncology.* vol. 3. p. 325. New York: Raven Press.

London, W.T. 1981. Primary hepatocellular carcinoma etiology, pathogenesis, and prevention. *Hum. Pathol.* 12:1085-97.

Lorincz, A.T.; Lancaster, W.D.; and Temple, G.F. 1986. Cloning and characterization of the DNA of a new human papillomavirus from a woman with dysplasia of the uterine cervix. *J. Virol.* 58:225-29.

Lorincz, A.T.; Quinn, A.P.; and Goldsborough, M.D. et al. 1989. Cloning and partial DNA sequencing of two new human papillomavirus types associated with condylomas and low-grade cervical neoplasia. *J. Virol.* 63:2829-34.

Lorincz, A.T.; Quinn, A.P.; and Lancaster, W.D. et al. 1987. A new type of papilomavirus associated with cancer of the uterine cervix. *Virology* 159:187-90.

Lowy, D.R.; Dvoretzky, I.; and Shober, R. et al. 1980. *In vitro* tumorigenic transformation by a defined sub-genomic fragment of bovine papilloma virus DNA. *Nature* 287:72-74.

Magnius, L.O., and Espmark, J.A. 1972. New specificities in Australia antigen positive sera distinct from Le Bouvier determinants. *J. Immunol.* 109:1017-21.

Magnius, L.O.; Lindholm, A.; and Lundin, P. et al. 1975. New antigen-antibody system: clinical significance in long-term carriers of hepatitis B surface antigen. *JAMA* 231:356-59.

Mallon, R.G.; Wojciechowicz, D.; and Defendi, V. 1987. DNA-binding activity of papillomavirus proteins. *J. Virol.* 61:1655-60.

Manservigi, R.; Cassai, E.; Deiss, L.P. et al. 1986. Sequences homologous to two separate transforming regions of herpes simplex virus DNA are linked in two human genital tumors. *Virology* 155:192-201.

McCance, D.J. 1986. Human papillomaviruses and cancer. *Biochim. Biophys. Acta.* 823:195-205.

McDougall, J.K.; Crum, C.P.; and Fenoglio, C.M. et al. 1982. Herpesvirus-specific RNA and protein in carcinoma of the uterine cervix. *Proc. Natl. Acad. Sci. USA* 79:3853-57.

McDougall, J.K.; Galloway D.A.; and Fenoglio, C.M. 1980. Cervical carcinoma: detection of herpes simplex virus RNA in cells undergoing neoplastic change. *Int. J. Cancer* 25:1-8.

McDougall, J.K.; Nelson, J.A.; and Myerson, D. et al. 1984. HSV, CMV and HPV in human neoplasia. *J. Invest. Dermatol.* 83:72S-76S.

Meignier, B.; Norrild, B.; and Thuning, C. et al. 1986. Failure to induce cervical cancer in mice by long-term frequent vaginal exposure to live or inactivated herpes simplex viruses. *Int. J. Cancer* 38:387-94.

Miller, G. 1979. Experimental carcinogenicity by the virus *in vivo*. In Epstein, M., and Achong, B. ed. *The Epstein-Barr virus*. p. 352. New York: Springer-Verlag.

Miller, G.; Robinson, J.; Heston, L. et al. 1974. Differences between laboratory strains of Epstein-Barr virus based on immortalization, abortive infection and interference. Proc. Natl. Acad. Sci. USA 71:4006-4010.

Minowada, J., and Moore, G.E. 1963. DNA synthesis in x-irradiated cultures infected with polyoma virus. *Exp. Cell Res.* 29:31-35.

Nadkarni, J.S.; Nadkarni, J.J.; and Clifford, P. et al. 1969. Characteristics of new cell lines derived from Burkitt lymphomas. *Cancer* 23:64-79.

Naahashfar, Z.S.; Rosenshein, N.B.; and Lorincz, A.T. et al. 1987. Characterization of human papillomavirus type 45, a new type 18-related virus of the genital tract. *J. Gen. Virol.* 68:3073-79.

Nahmias, A.J.; Josey, W.E.; and Naib, Z.M. et al. 1970. Antibodies to herpesvirus hominis types 1 and 2 in humans. II: women with cervical cancer. *Am. J. Epidemiol.* 91:547-52.

Nielson, J.O.; Dietrichson, O.; and Juhl, E. 1974. Incidence and meaning of e-determinant among hepatitis-B antigen positive patients with acute and chronic liver disease. *Lancet* II:913-15.

Nuovo, G.J.; Crum, C.P.; and de Villiers, E-M. et al. 1988. Isolation of a novel human papillomavirus (type 51) from a cervical condyloma. *J. Virol.* 62:1452-55.

Okochi, K., and Murakami, S. 1968. Observations on Australia antigen in Japanese. *Vox Sang* 15:374-85.

Orth, G.; Favre, M.; and Croissant, O. 1977. Characterization of a new type of human papilloma virus that causes skin warts. *J. Virol.* 24:108-20.

Orth, G.; Jeanteur, P.; and Croissant, O. 1971. Evidence for localization of vegetative viral DNA replication by autoradiographic detection of RNA-DNA hybrids in sections of tumors induced by Shope papillomavirus. *Proc. Natl. Acad. Sci. USA* 68:1876-80.

Ozanne, B.; Sharp, P.A.; and Sambrook, J. 1973. Transcription of simian virus 40. II: hybridization of RNA extracted from different lines of transformed cells to the separated strands of simian virus 40 DNA. *J. Virol.* 12:90-98.

Padgett, B.L., and Walker, D.L. 1976. New human papovaviruses. *Prog. Med. Virol.* 22:1-35.

Pass, F.; Niimura, M.; and Kreider, J.W. 1973. Prolonged survival of human skin xenografts on antithymocyte serum-treated mice: failure to produce verrucae by inoculation with extracts of human warts. *J. Invest. Dermatol.* 61:371-74.

Pfister, H. 1984. Biology and biochemistry of papillomaviruses. *Rev. Physiol. Biochem. Pharmacol.* 99:111-68.

Pfister, H. 1987. Human papillomaviruses and genital cancer. *Adv. Cancer Res.* 48:113-47.

Poiesz, B.J.; Ruscetti, F.W.; and Gazdar, A.F. et al. 1980. Detection and isolation of type C retrovirus particles from fresh and cultured lymphocytes of a patient with cutaneous T-cell lymphoma. *Proc. Natl. Acad. Sci. USA* 77:7415-19.

Popovic, M.; Sarngadharan, M.G.; and Read, E. et al. 1984. Detection, isolation, and continuous production of cytopathic retroviruses (HTLV-III) from patients with AIDS and pre-AIDS. *Science* 224:497-500.

Posner, L.E.; Robert-Guroff, M.; and Kalyanaraman, V.S. et al. 1981. Natural antibodies to the human T cell lymphoma virus in patients with cutaneous T cell lymphoma. *J. Exp. Med.* 154:333-46.

Prince, A.M. 1968. An antigen detected in blood during incubation period of serum hepatitis. *Proc. Natl. Acad. Sci. USA* 60:814-21.

Prives, C.; Aviv, H.; and Gilboa, E. et al. 1975. The cell-free translation of early and late classes of SV40 messenger RNA. *INSERM Colloq.* 47:305-12.

Rabin, H.; Neubauer, R.H.; and Hopkins, R.F. et al. 1977. Transforming activity and antigenicity of an Epstein-Barr like virus from lymphoblastoid cell lines of baboons with lymphoid disease. *Intervirology* 8:240-49.

Rabson, A.S., and Kirschstein, R.L. 1962. Induction of malignancy *in vitro* in newborn hamster kidney tissue infected with simian vacuolating virus (SV40). *Proc. Soc. Exp. Biol. Med.* 111:323-28.

Rabson, A.S.; O'Conor, G.T.; and Kirschstein, R.L. et al. 1962. Papillary ependymomas produced in *Rattus (Mastomys) natalensis* inoculated with vacuolating virus (SV40). *J. Natl. Cancer Inst.* 29:765-87.

Ragona, G.; Ernberg, I.; and Klein, G. 1980. Induction and biological characterization of the Epstein-Barr virus (EBV) carried by the Jijoye lymphoma line. *Virology* 101:553-57.

Rapp, F., and Robbins, D. 1984. Cytomegalovirus and human cancer. In Plotkin, S.A.; Michelson, S.; Pagano, J.S.; and Rapp, F. eds. *Birth defects: original articles series, March of Dimes Birth Defects Foundation.* p. 175. New York: Alan R. Liss.

Rawls, W.E.; Tompkins, W.A.F.; and Figueroa, M.E. et al. 1968. Herpesvirus type 2: association with carcinoma of the cervix. *Science* 161:1255-56.

Reddy, V.B.; Thimmappaya, B.; and Dhar, R. et al. 1978. The genome of simian virus 40. *Science* 200:494-502.

Reyes, G.R.; LaFemina, R.; Hayward, S.D. et al. 1979. Morphological transformation by DNA fragments of human herpesviruses: evidence for two distinct transforming regions in herpes simplex viruses types 1 and 2 and lack of correlation with biochemical transfer of the thymidine kinase gene. *Cold Spring Harbor Symp. Quant. Biol.* 44:629-41.

Rheinwald, J.G., and Green, H. 1975. Serial cultivation of strains of human epidermal keratinocytes: formation of keratinizing colonies from single cells. *Cell* 6:331-44.

Rigby, P.W.J., and Lane, D.P. 1983. Structure and function of simian virus 40 large T-antigen. In Klein, G. ed. *Advances in viral oncology.* vol. 3. p. 31. New York: Raven Press.

Rigoni-Stern, D. 1842. Fatti statistia relativi alle malatie cancerose. *G. Dervire. Progr. Pathol. Terap.* 2:507-17.

Robinson, W.S. 1977. The genome of hepatitis B virus. *Ann. Rev. Microbiol.* 31:357-77.

Robinson, W.S., and Lutwick, L.I. 1976a. Virus of hepatitis, type B: 1. *N. Engl. J. Med.* 295:1168-75.

Robinson, W.S., and Lutwick, L.I. 1976b. Virus of hepatitis, type B: 2. *N. Engl. J. Med.* 295:1232-36.

Roizman, B. 1979. Structure and isomerization of herpes simplex virus genomes. *Cell* 16:481-94.

Roizman, B. 1982, 1983, 1985. In Roizman, B. ed. *The herpesviruses.* vols. 1, 2, and 3. New York: Plenum Press.

Roizman, B., and Jenkins, F.J. 1985. Genetic engineering of novel genomes of large DNA viruses. *Science* 229:1208-14.

Rous, P. 1911. A sarcoma of the fowl transmissible by an agent separable from the tumor cells. *J. Exp. Med.* 13:397-411.

Rous, P., and Beard, J.W. 1927. Progression to carcinoma of virus-induced rabbit papillomas (Shope). *J. Exp. Med.* 65: 523-48.

Rovera, G.; Baserga, R.; and Defendi, V. 1972. Early increase in nuclear acidic protein synthesis after SV40 infection. *Nature New Biol.* 237:240-41.

Salahuddin, S.Z.; Ablashi, D.V.; and Markham, P.D. et al. 1986. Isolation of a new virus, HBLV, in patients with lymphoproliferative disorders. *Science* 234:596-601.

Sambrook, J.; Sharp, P.A.; and Keller, W. 1972. Transcription of SV40. I: separation of the strands of SV40 DNA and hybridization of the separated strands to RNA extracted from lytically infected and transformed cells. *J. Mol. Biol.* 70:57-71.

Sambrook, J.; Westphal, H.; and Srinivasan, P.R. et al. 1968. Integrated state of DNA in SV40-transformed cells. *Proc. Natl. Acad. Sci. USA* 60:1288-95.

Sarngadharan, M.; Popovic, M.; and Bruch, L. et al. 1984. Antibodies reactive with human T-lymphotropic retroviruses (HTLV-III) in the serum of patients with AIDS. *Science* 224:506-508.

Sato, H.; Watanabe, S.; and Furuno, A. et al. 1989. Human papilloma virus type 16 E7 protein expressed in *Escherichia coli* and monkey COS-1 cells: immunofluorescence detection of the nuclear E7 protein. *Virology* 170:311-15.

Schneider-Gadicke, A.; Kaul, S.; and Schwarz, E. et al. 1988. Identification of the human papillomavirus type 18 E6 and E6 proteins in nuclear protein fractions from human cervical cells grown in the nude mouse or *in vitro. Cancer Res.* 48:2969-74.

Schupbach, J.; Popovic, M.; and Gilden, R.V. et al. 1984. Serological analysis of a subgroup of human T-lymphotropic retroviruses (HTLV-III) associated with AIDS. *Science* 224:503-505.

Seedorf, K.; Oltersdorf, T.; and Krammer, G. et al. 1987. Identification of early proteins of the human papilloma viruses type 16 (HPV-16) and type 18 (HPV-18) in cervical carcinoma cells. *EMBO J.* 6:139-44.

Seif, I.; Khoury, G.; and Dhar, R. 1979. Genome of human papovavirus BKV. *Cell* 18:963-77.

Sekine, H.; Fuse, A.; and Inaba, N. et al. 1989. Detection of the human papillomavirus 6b E2 gene product in genital condyloma and laryngeal papilloma tissues. *Virology* 170: 92-98.

Shafritz, D.A., and Kew, M.C. 1981. Identification of integrated hepatitis B virus DNA sequences in human hepatocellular carcinomas. *Hepatology* 1:1-8.

Shein, H.M.; Enders, J.F.; and Levinthal, J.D. et al. 1963. Transformation induced by simian virus 40 in newborn simian hamster renal cell cultures. *Proc. Natl. Acad. Sci. USA* 49:28-34.

Shimoda, K.; Lorincz, A.T.; and Temole, G.F. et al. 1988.

Human papillomavirus type 52: a new virus associated with cervical neoplasia. *J. Gen. Virol.* 69:2925-28.

Shope, R.E. 1933. Infectious papillomatosis of rabbits. *J. Exp. Med.* 58:607-24.

Simons, M.J.; Wee, G.B.; and Day, N.E. et al. 1974. Immunologic aspects of nasopharyngeal carcinoma. I: differences in HL-A antigen profiles between patients and control groups. *Int. J. Cancer* 13:122-34.

Skinner, G.R.B. 1976. Transformation of primary hamster embryo fibroblasts by type 2 simplex virus: evidence for a "hit-and-run mechanism." *Br. J. Exp. Pathol.* 57:361-76.

Smith, H.S.; Scher, C.D.; and Todaro, G.J. 1970. Abortive transformation of Balb/3T3 cells by simian virus 40. *Bacteriol. Proc. Abstr.* 217:187.

Sodroski, J.G.; Rosen, C.A.; and Haseltine, W.A. 1984. Trans-acting transcriptional activation of the long terminal repeat of human T lymphotropic viruses in infected cells. *Science* 225:381-85.

Spear, P.G. 1983. Transformation of cultured cells by human herpesviruses. *Int. Rev. Exp. Pathol.* 25:327-60.

Stevens, C.E.; Beasley, R.P.; and Tsui, J. et al. 1975. Vertical transmission of hepatitis-B antigen in Taiwan. *N. Engl. J. Med.* 292:771-74.

Stevens, C.E.; Neurath, R.A.; and Beasley, R.P. et al. 1979. HBeAg and anti-HBe detection by radioimmunoassay: correlation with vertical transmission of hepatitis-B virus in Taiwan. *J. Med. Virol.* 3:237-41.

Svedmyr, E., and Jondal, M. 1975. Cytotoxic effector cells specific for B cell lines transformed by Epstein-Barr virus are present in patients with infectious mononucleosis. *Proc. Natl. Acad. Sci. USA* 72:1622-26.

Sweet, B.H., and Hilleman, M.R. 1960. Vacuolating virus, SV40. *Proc. Soc. Exp. Biol. Med.* 105:420-27.

Syverton, J.T. 1952. Pathogenesis of rabbit papilloma-to-carcinoma sequence. *Ann. N.Y. Acad. Sci.* 54:1126-40.

Szmuness, W. 1975. Recent advances in the study of the epidemiology of hepatitis B. *Am. J. Pathol.* 81:629-49.

Taylor-Papadimitriou, J., and Stoker, M.G.P. 1971. Effect of interferon on some aspects of transformation by polyoma virus. *Nature New Biol.* 230:114-17.

Tegtmeyer, P. 1972. SV40 DNA synthesis: the viral replicon. *J. Virol.* 10:591-98.

Temin, H., and Mitzutani, S. 1970. RNA-dependent DNA polymerase in virions of Rous sarcoma virus. *Nature* 226: 1211-13.

Tevethia, M.J. 1985. Transforming potential of herpes simplex viruses and human cytomegalovirus. In Roizman, B. ed. *The herpesviruses.* vol. 3. pp. 257-314. New York: Plenum Press.

Todaro, G.J., and Green, H. 1966a. Cell growth and the initiation of transformation by SV40. *Proc. Natl. Acad. Sci. USA* 55:302-308.

Todaro, G.J., and Green, H. 1966b. High frequency of SV40 transformation of mouse cell line 3T3. *Virology* 28:756-59.

Todaro, G.J., and Huebner, R.J. 1972. Viral oncogene hypothesis: new evidence. *Proc. Natl. Acad. Sci. USA* 69: 1009-15.

Tooze, J. 1980. *Molecular biology of tumor viruses, parts 1, 2, and 3.* Cold Spring Harbor, New York: Cold Spring Harbor Laboratory.

Tournier, P.; Cassingena, R.; and Wichert, R. et al. 1967. Etude du mecanisme de l'induction chez des cellules de hamster Syrien transformees par le virus SV40. I: proprietes d'une lignee cellulaire clonale. *Int. J. Cancer* 2:117-41.

U. S. Patent Office. 1972. Vaccine against viral hepatitis and process. Blumberg, B.S., and Millman, I. Serial No. 864 filed 10/8/69; patent 36 36 191 issued 1/18/72.

Varmus, H.E. 1985. Viruses, genes and cancer. I: discovery of cellular oncogenes and their role in neoplasia. *Cancer* 55:2324-28.

Varmus, H.E. 1987. Oncogenes and transcriptional control. *Science* 238:1337-39.

Vonka, V.; Kanka, J.; and Jelinek, J. et al. 1984. Prospective study on the relationship between cervical neoplasia and herpes simplex type 2 virus. I: epidemiological characteristics. *Int. J. Cancer* 33:49-60.

Vyas, G.N.; Cohen, S.N.; and Schmid, R. eds. 1978. In *Viral hepatitis*. Philadelphia: Franklin Institute Press.

Vyas, G.N.; Ibrahim, A.B.; and Rao, K.R. et al. 1974. Tolerance to hepatitis-B antigen: hypothesis for its termination with immune-RNA. *Life Sci.* 15:261-66.

Walker, B.D.; Flexner, C.; and Paradis, T.J. et al. 1988. HIV-1 reverse transcriptase is a target for cytotoxic T lymphocytes in infected individuals. *Science* 240:64-66.

Watkins, J.F., and Dulbecco, R. 1967. Production of SV40 virus in heterokaryons of transformed and susceptible cells. *Proc. Natl. Acad. Sci. USA* 58:1396-1403.

Weil, R.; Petursson, G.; and Kara, J. et al. 1967. Interaction of polyoma virus with the genetic apparatus of host cells. In Coleter, J.S., and Paranchych, W. eds. *The molecular biology of viruses*. p. 593. New York: Academic Press.

Weil, R.; Salomon, C.; and May, E. et al. 1974. Simplifying concept in tumor virology: virus specific "pleiotropic effectors." *Cold Spring Harbor Symp. Quant. Biol.* 39:381-95.

Weinberg, R.A. 1985. Action of oncogenes in the cytoplasm and nucleus. *Science* 230:770-76.

Wentz, W.B.; Reagan, J.W.; and Heggie, A.D. 1975. Cervical carcinogenesis with herpes simplex virus type 2. *Obstet. Gynecol.* 46:117-21.

Wentz, W.B.; Reagan, J.W.; and Heggie, A.D. et al. 1981. Induction of uterine cancer with inactivated herpes simplex virus types 1 and 2. *Cancer* 48:1783-90.

Westphal, H., and Dulbecco, R. 1968. Viral DNA in polyoma and SV40-transformed cell lines. *Proc. Nat. Acad. Sci. USA* 59:1158-65.

Wigle, D.T.; Mao, Y.; and Grace, M. 1980. Re: smoking and cancer of the uterine cervix: hypothesis. *Am. J. Epidemiol.* 111:125-27.

Winklestein, W. 1977. Smoking and cancer of the uterine cervix: hypothesis. *Am. J. Epidemiol.* 106:257-59.

Winocour, E., and Robbins, E. 1970. Histone synthesis in polyoma and SV40-infected cells. *Virology* 40:307-15.

World Health Organization. 1977. Report of the WHO Expert Committee on Viral Hepatitis. *Advances in viral hepatitis Tech. Rep. Series 602*.

Wright, N.H.; Vessey, M.P.; and Kenward, B. et al. 1978. Neoplasia and dysplasia of the cervix uteri and contraception: a possible protective effect of the diaphragm. *Br. J. Cancer* 38:273-79.

Yamanishi, K.; Matsunaga, Y.; and Ogino, T. et al. 1981. Biochemical transformation of mouse cells by varicella-zoster virus. *J. Gen. Virol.* 56:421-30.

Yamanishi, K.; Okuno, T.; and Shiraki, K. et al. 1988. Identification of human herpesvirus-6 as a causal agent for exanthem subitum. *Lancet* I:1065-67.

Yoshida, M.; Miyoshi, I.; and Hinuma, Y. 1982. Isolation and characterization of retrovirus from cell lines of human adult T-cell leukemia and its implication in the disease. *Proc. Natl. Acad. Sci. USA* 79:2031-35.

Zagury, D.; Bernard, J.; and Cheynier, R. et al. 1988. A group specific anamnestic immune reaction against HIV-1 induced by a candidate vaccine against AIDS. *Nature* 332:728-31.

Zinsser Microbiology 18th ed. 1984. Joklik, W.K.; Willett, H.P.; and Amos, D.B. eds. Norwalk, Conn.: Appleton-Century Crofts.

zur Hausen, H. 1983. Herpes simplex virus in human genital cancer. *Int. Rev. Exp. Pathol.* 25:307-26.

zur Hausen, H. 1977. Human papillomaviruses and their possible role in squamous cell carcinomas. *Curr. Topics Microbiol. Immunol.* 78:1-30.

Chapter 12

CANCER DETECTION: THE CANCER-RELATED CHECKUP GUIDELINES

Diane J. Fink, M.D.

Diane J. Fink, M.D.
Group Vice President for Cancer Control
American Cancer Society
California Division
Oakland, California

Special thanks are given to Dr. David Eddy for his pioneering work in developing the 1980 Cancer-Related Checkup Guidelines, to Robert V. P. Hutter, M.D., chairman, and to the volunteer members of the National Advisory Committee on Cancer Prevention and Detection, who contributed significantly to the American Cancer Society's continued surveillance of new developments in cancer detection.

INTRODUCTION

In 1980, the American Cancer Society (ACS) published cancer-related checkup guidelines for early detection in asymptomatic persons (ACS 1980). The ACS has since monitored their impact on cancer detection and has evaluated emerging data and new technologies. These guidelines served as the "gold standard" for cancer detection during the 1980s. This paper serves to update the guidelines based on experience over the last 10 years.

Changes in the guidelines have been surprisingly few. They involve greater precision in wording to clarify the role of digital rectal examinations to include evaluation of the prostate, specify the frequency of mammography for breast cancer detection in women 40 to 49 years of age, define detection follow-up for colorectal cancer in high-risk persons, and modify the original advice for the periodicity of the Pap test for cervical cancer detection, sigmoidoscopy for colorectal cancer detection, and chest x-ray for lung cancer. The role of cancer detection recommendations in national cancer control activities is to provide detection protocols to the public and physicians.

Four major concerns were stressed in the development of the guidelines. First, evidence must exist that the test or procedure is medically effective in finding cancer early enough to influence cancer morbidity and/or mortality. Second, the medical benefits must outweigh the risks. Third, the cost of each test must be reasonable in terms of expected outcome. Fourth, the recommended actions must be practical and feasible (ACS 1980).

To be practical, the cancer detection test must be adopted into the existing American health care delivery system. Data for many detection tests are evolving, so decisions often need to be based on incomplete evidence. Keeping these factors in mind, the guidelines represent logical approaches to sensible, useful cancer detection.

As stated in the 1980 ACS publication, the recommendations are for "the early detection of cancer — the search for early cancer in asymptomatic persons on an individual basis." The recommendations are intended "to help individual physicians and their asymptomatic patients select the best early detection protocol for the individual's personal needs."

The Cancer-Related Checkup Guidelines are not intended for the evaluation of persons who have signs or symptoms of cancer. Such persons require careful diagnostic workup to determine the cause of their complaint or complaints.

The Cancer-Related Checkup Guidelines can provide information to public policy makers who need to decide on conducting large population screening programs financed by public funds. Having one set of guidelines for persons seeing their own physicians and another for those who use publicly funded cancer-screening facilities and programs is confusing and generates different standards of medical care.

NEED FOR COMMON GUIDELINES

An important issue surfacing since the 1980 guidelines publication has been the variation in cancer detection guidance provided by health professional organizations and societies. There have been differences in interpretation of existing incomplete data for cancer detection techniques. To promote cancer prevention and detection by community health providers, especially primary-care physicians, a December 1986 workshop attended by representatives of the leading medical organizations, the Congress, the health insurance industry, and selected experts in cancer control was held to explore ways to change health provider behavior.

The workshop participants determined that the most significant need was for uniform guidelines from all major health professional organizations issuing cancer detection recommendations (McKenna and Fink 1988). Currently, the ACS and the National Cancer Institute (NCI) have similar recommendations and have joined together in promoting common guidelines.

COST

The other major consideration was the need to address the cost and sources of payment for cancer detection tests, particularly the most expensive ones such as screening mammography and sigmoidoscopy. Technical advances, community activities, corporate/industry initiatives, and legislative action have all helped make cancer-related checkups more available to Americans, regardless of their ability to pay. These initial efforts must be continued and will need the cooperation of both the public and the public health professionals.

DEFINITIONS

To facilitate understanding of the cancer-related checkup, the ACS adopted the following definitions:

Screening: the search for disease in asymptomatic people. An *asymptomatic* person is one who does not have symptoms or who does not recognize the symptoms as being related to the disease. Once an individual has had a positive screening test, or once signs or symptoms have been identified, further tests are considered diagnostic, not screening.

Detection: the discovery of an abnormality in an asymptomatic or symptomatic person.

Diagnostic Evaluation: the evaluation of a patient who has signs or symptoms suggestive of disease for the purpose of determining the actual existence and nature of the disease.

BACKGROUND INFORMATION

The current status of cancer detection and the Cancer-Related Checkup Guidelines are covered here, as is evidence on medical effectiveness, risks, costs, and practical considerations of tests and procedures for breast, colorectal, lung, and cervical cancer detection. The assessment of tests and procedures for early cancer detection is a complex process and important background information describing issues, the evaluation of early detection tests and procedures, and experimental biases reprinted in part from the original document (ACS 1980) are included in the appendix.

SUMMARY OF ACS RECOMMENDATIONS

Cancer detection using the ACS's Cancer-Related Checkup Guidelines plays an important role in health promotion by assisting the health professional and the asymptomatic individual in making cancer detection decisions. For each cancer site, specific lists of recommended tests and/or procedures are discussed in terms of patient age and sex. In general, the same guidelines are useful for average and high-risk persons. The exceptions are colorectal cancer guidelines, which provide a separate protocol for high-risk persons. Table 12.1 summarizes the cancer-related checkup; tables 12.2 and 12.3 summarize the cancer-related checkup by the participant's sex.

THE CANCER-RELATED CHECKUP
The ACS recommends a cancer-related checkup in asymptomatic individuals:

Every three years for men and women 20 to 39 years of age.

Every year for men and women 40 years of age and older.

The checkup should always include health counseling about personal risk factors such as tobacco use, sun exposure, sexual practices, other environmental or occupational exposures, and the role of diet and nutrition in developing cancer. The encounter should include explanation of the advantages of self-examination of the breasts, testes, and skin, as well as health-provider examinations for cancer of the oral cavity, thyroid, skin, lymph nodes, testes, prostate, and ovaries. Several specific cancer detection protocols have been designed to discover asymptomatic cancers of the colon and rectum, breast, and cervix (tables 12.4 through 12.6). These examinations are recommended as part of the cancer-related checkup.

COLORECTAL CANCER
A triad of tests is recommended for colorectal cancer detection: digital rectal examination, stool blood tests, and sigmoidoscopy (table 12.6). Evidence from a number of sources indicates that tests for colorectal cancer before the onset of signs and symptoms may improve survival and may reduce mortality.

While awaiting data from studies in progress, accumulating evidence suggests that the use of digital rectal examination, stool blood test, and sigmoidoscopy by physicians and other primary health care providers during patient contacts within the health care delivery system is a sensible, prudent approach for persons at average risk. Persons at high risk for colorectal cancer may require additional testing beginning at an earlier age.

The National Cancer Institute has adopted guidelines for colorectal cancer detection that are identical to the ACS's recommendations.

Table 12.1
SUMMARY OF AMERICAN CANCER SOCIETY RECOMMENDATIONS FOR THE EARLY DETECTION OF CANCER IN ASYMPTOMATIC PERSONS AT AVERAGE RISK

Examination	Sex	Age	Periodicity
Sigmoidoscopy	M and F	Age 50 and older	1 exam every 3 to 5 years
Stool Blood Test	M and F	Age 50 and older	Every year
Digital Rectal Examination	M and F	Age 40 and older	Every year
Pap Test and Pelvic Examination	F	Women who have been sexually active, or have reached age 18 or older	Every year. After 3 or more satisfactory, consecutive, normal annual examinations, the Pap test may be performed less frequently at the discretion of the physician
Endometrial Tissue Sample	F	At menopause; women at high risk*	At menopause
Breast Self-Examination*	F	Age 20 and older	Every month
Clinical Breast Examination	F	20-39 Age 40 and older	Every 3 years Every year
Mammography	F	35-39 40-49 50 and over	Baseline Every 1 to 2 years Every year
Health Counseling** Cancer Checkup***	M and F M and F	20-40 Age 40 and older	Every 3 years Every year

*History of infertility, obesity, failure to ovulate, abnormal uterine bleeding, or estrogen therapy.
**To include counseling about tobacco control, sun exposure, diet and nutrition, risk factors, sexual practices, and environmental and other occupational exposures.
***To include examination for cancers of the thyroid, testicles, prostate, ovaries, lymph nodes, oral cavity, and skin.

BREAST CANCER

Three techniques are recommended to detect breast cancer in asymptomatic women: breast self-examination, clinical breast examination, and mammography (table 12.4). Data from randomized clinical trials and a large-scale demonstration project show that physical examination and mammography, beginning at age 40 in particular, can reduce mortality from breast cancer. The risks of radiation-induced cancer using modern mammographic techniques are considered to be extremely low, if any.

The ACS believes that American women should be offered breast cancer detection examinations according to its Cancer-Related Checkup Guidelines. Examination costs can be reduced. The benefits to the individual woman outweigh any possible risk and may help save many lives. The American College of Radiology, the College of American Pathologists, the National Cancer Institute, and other health professional organizations generally concur in these recommendations. It appears to be time to mount an aggressive national program to incorporate breast cancer detection into the health care of all women, including those who are too poor to pay for their examinations.

CANCERS OF THE CERVIX AND ENDOMETRIUM

The efficacy of regular Pap tests to detect early cervical cancer has been documented by worldwide epidemiologic studies showing dramatic reductions in the inci-

dence and mortality of invasive cervical cancer in screened populations. There are no randomized clinical trials to document the benefit of the Pap test.

Recent review of existing data, including evidence of changing sexual patterns, suggests that all women who have had vaginal intercourse are at risk for cervical cancer. Vaginal intercourse started at an early age and intercourse with multiple partners are factors that place women at high risk for the disease. Human papilloma virus (types 16, 18, 30, and 31) has recently been

Table 12.2
RECOMMENDED GUIDELINES FOR EARLY DETECTION OF CANCER IN ASYMPTOMATIC AVERAGE-RISK MEN

Age	Recommendation
20-39	Cancer-related checkup every 3 years, to include health counseling and examination of the oral cavity, thyroid, lymph nodes, testes, and prostate
40-49	Cancer-related checkup yearly, to include all of the above, plus: — Digital rectal examination with palpation of the prostate, yearly
50 and older	Cancer-related checkup yearly, to include all of the above, plus: — Digital rectal exam with palpation of the prostate, yearly — Stool blood test, yearly — Sigmoidoscopy, every 3 to 5 years

Table 12.3
**RECOMMENDED GUIDELINES FOR EARLY
DETECTION OF CANCER IN ASYMPTOMATIC
AVERAGE-RISK WOMEN**

Age	Recommendation
20-39	*Cancer-related checkup* every 3 years, to include counseling and examination of the oral cavity, thyroid, skin, lymph nodes, and ovaries, plus: — Breast self-examination, monthly — Clinical breast examination, every 3 years — Baseline mammography (35-39 years of age) — Pap test and pelvic examination every year; after 3 or more annual, consecutive satisfactory examinations, the Pap test may be performed less frequently at the discretion of the physician for women who are or have been sexually active or are age 18 or older.
40-49	*Cancer-related checkup* yearly, to include all the above plus: — Digital rectal examination, yearly — Breast self-examination, monthly — Clinical breast examination, yearly — Mammography, every 1 to 2 years — At menopause, endometrial tissue sample in high-risk women
50 and older	*Cancer-related checkup* yearly, to include all of the above, plus: — Stool blood test, yearly — Sigmoidoscopy, every 3 to 5 years — Mammography, yearly

implicated as the venereal factor associated with the development of cervical cancer.

The ACS does not advocate an upper age limit for termination of cervical cancer checkups (table 12.5); any such decision must be made by each woman and her physician. Although data for the early detection of endometrial cancer are still evolving, it now appears prudent to provide endometrial tissue sampling for high-risk women beginning at menopause. High-risk status is defined by infertility, obesity, or failure to ovulate.

Based on the best cancer control strategy, the Pap test is one of the most important examinations for asymptomatic women. Coupled with a pelvic examination, the Pap test is a life-saving procedure.

After deliberations with leading health professional groups, The ACS's Board of Directors in November 1987 adopted the following recommendation for cervical cancer detection:

That all women who are or have been sexually active, or have reached age 18 years, have an annual Pap test and pelvic examination. After a woman has had three or more satisfactory normal annual examinations, the Pap test may be performed less frequently at the discretion of her physician.

A number of leading medical organizations and societies support this recommendation.

The exact interval for screening remains a debate. To provide the best national strategy for cervical cancer detection in women, the debate over frequency of

Table 12.4
**BREAST CANCER DETECTION PROTOCOL IN
ASYMPTOMATIC WOMEN AT AVERAGE RISK**

Age	Recommendation
20-39	Breast self-examination, monthly Clinical breast examination, every 3 years Baseline mammography, 35-39 years of age
40-49	Breast self-examination, monthly Clinical breast examination, yearly Mammography, every 1 to 2 years
50 and older	Breast self-examination, monthly Clinical breast examination, yearly Mammography, yearly

testing may mask the real issue — that every effort must be made to get unscreened women into a regular screening to decrease the remaining burden of this disease, especially in underserved women. That is our challenge.

LUNG CANCER RECOMMENDATIONS

Lung cancer screening with chest x-ray examination and sputum cytology has not been demonstrated by a number of studies to be of benefit in reducing mortality. A new analysis of recent clinical trials has been said to show a benefit when lung cancer is detected by chest x-ray examination rather than symptoms. Clearly the risks, resources, and cost of regular chest x-ray examination and sputum cytology must be evaluated when considering chest x-ray examination for an asymptomatic individual. According to available data, lung cancer mortality is not affected by those techniques when applied to normal-risk persons. The physician and the asymptomatic patient must decide in each case whether screening is warranted, based on the possible benefits and risks. In the person who is at high risk for lung cancer, it may not be prudent to withhold these tests, if the physician judges them to be useful for the patient.

Efforts aimed at primary prevention of lung cancer are, at present, the best hope for reducing the impact of lung cancer. The ACS thus urges physicians and all health professionals to advise their patients — and especially those at high risk — not to smoke. Other national and international experts in disease control have concluded similarly. The Canadian Task Force on the Periodic

Table 12.5
**CERVICAL AND ENDOMETRIAL CANCER DETECTION
PROTOCOLS FOR ASYMPTOMATIC WOMEN**

Population	Recommendation
Cervical Cancer	
Women who are or have been sexually active or are age 18 or older	Annual Pap test and pelvic examination. After 3 or more annual, consecutive, satisfactory, normal examinations, the Pap test may be performed less frequently at the discretion of the physician
Endometrial Cancer	
High-risk women at menopause	Pelvic examination Endometrial tissue sample

Health Examination (CTFPHE 1979), the International Union Against Cancer (UICC 1978), the NCI, and others organizations agree with the ACS's lung cancer detection recommendations.

SELF-EXAMINATION

It appears reasonable and practical to teach asymptomatic, healthy adults to examine certain areas of their bodies. These examinations have not been subjected to rigorous prospective randomized clinical trial analysis, but they are simple and inexpensive ways to help people take part in their own health care and to increase their awareness about changes in their bodies between health professional examinations. Self-examination may be especially helpful for certain segments of the population who cannot easily obtain medical care, e.g., the elderly, the economically disadvantaged, or those who live in remote locations. Self-examination is not, however, a substitute for the recommended checkup guidelines.

CANCER OF THE COLON AND RECTUM

INTRODUCTION

Colorectal cancer is a major public health problem for American men and women. An estimated 157,500 new cases and 60,500 deaths are projected to occur in 1991. Excluding common skin cancers, their combined incidence is third after breast and lung cancer (ACS 1990).

When found and treated at an early, localized stage, the 5-year survival rates are 88% for colon cancer and 80% for rectal cancer. Once the cancer is no longer localized these figures drop to 58% and 47%, respectively. The overall 5-year survival for patients with colorectal cancer is now approximately 55%. This could be increased to 85% if the cancers were detected and treated at a localized stage. This means 50,000 more of those diagnosed annually could be saved (ACS 1991).

Cancers of the colon and rectum are particularly good candidates for early detection. It appears that most of these types of cancer arise from adenomatous polyps and take approximately 10 years to progress to an invasive, more lethal malignant stage (Fenoglio-Preiser and Hutter 1989). Furthermore, 94% of colorectal cancers occur in persons after age 50, so targeting detection by age is important.

HIGHER-RISK STATUS

Certain risk factors need special consideration when planning cancer detection protocols. Factors that increase a person's risk of colon and rectum cancers include a personal or family history in first-degree relatives of polyps or colorectal cancer, a family history of polyposis syndromes, and a personal history of inflammatory bowel disease (ulcerative colitis or Crohn's disease).

Table 12.6
COLORECTAL CANCER DETECTION PROTOCOL FOR ASYMPTOMATIC MEN AND WOMEN

Population	Recommendation
Average Risk	
40-49 years of age	Digital rectal examination, with palpation of the prostate in men, yearly
Age 50 and older	Digital rectal examination, with palpation of the prostate in men, yearly Stool blood test, yearly Sigmoidoscopy, every 3 to 5 years
Higher Than Average Risk	
Persons age 40 and over with a family history of colorectal cancer in 1 or more first-degree relatives	Digital rectal examination, with palpation of the prostate in men, yearly Stool blood test, yearly Barium enema with sigmoidoscopy, or total colonoscopy, every 3 to 5 years
Persons with inflammatory bowel disease or familial polyposis syndromes	Individual evaluation should be based on physician clinical judgment
Persons with a history of colorectal adenomas	Requires more careful examination based on individual clinical judgment
Persons with a history of colorectal cancer	Periodic evaluation of the large bowel and examination for evidence of metastases as determined by the physician
Persons with a history of breast, ovarian, or endometrial cancer	Follow standard ACS recommendations for the detection of colorectal cancer in asymptomatic, average-risk persons

TRIAD OF RECOMMENDED PROCEDURES

The ACS recommends a triad of early detection procedures for average-risk persons: digital rectal examination, proctosigmoidoscopy, and stool blood test (table 12.7). While the value of these techniques is under continuing study, they represent sensible, clinical approaches for detecting colorectal cancer before symptoms develop.

Since the publication of the 1980 cancer-related guidelines, flexible sigmoidoscopy has been used more widely in the United States. Numerous stool blood test kits, including do-it-yourself tests, are now available, and a new stool blood test—the Hemoquant test—has been put into clinical trial (Ahlquist et al. 1985).

The ACS reviewed the use of barium enema and colonoscopy as possible examinations for the early

Table 12.7
AMERICAN CANCER SOCIETY RECOMMENDATIONS FOR COLORECTAL CANCER DETECTION IN ASYMPTOMATIC PERSONS AT AVERAGE RISK

Age	Sex	Recommendation
40-50	M and F	Digital rectal examination, with palpation of the prostate in men, yearly
50 and over	M and F	Digital rectal examination, with palpation of the prostate in men, yearly Stool blood test, yearly Sigmoidoscopy every 3 to 5 years

detection of colorectal cancer in asymptomatic persons, but concluded that these tests are not appropriate for cancer detection in average-risk individuals. Both, however, do play a role in surveillance of high-risk groups and in diagnostic studies of persons with signs or symptoms of colorectal cancer or with positive stool blood tests.

OBSTACLES TO COLORECTAL CANCER DETECTION

A number of obstacles still block the regular acceptance and use of ACS recommendations for early colorectal cancer detection. Based on data from a national ACS study of public attitudes regarding cancers of the colon and rectum, Americans older than 40 tended to ignore these organs and have them checked only infrequently by their physicians (ACS 1983). Furthermore, most study participants incorrectly assumed that the disease is invariably found at an advanced stage and therefore the chances of survival are slim. Many also erroneously regarded a permanent colostomy as the usual result of treatment, while in fact only 15% of rectal cancer patients and very few colon cancer patients require a permanent colostomy following surgery (Enker and DeCosse 1981). On the more optimistic side, participants were eager to receive accurate information about colorectal cancer and were willing to undergo early detection procedures.

A 1984 study of primary care physicians revealed that while physicians recognized the value of early detection, only one-third and 75% of respondents said that they had ever performed sigmoidoscopy and the stool blood test on asymptomatic patients, respectively. Only 18% followed ACS guidelines for sigmoidoscopy, and less than half for the stool blood test (ACS 1985). A repeat primary physicians survey indicated that adherence to ACS guidelines was 23% for sigmoidoscopy and 56% for the stool blood test (ACS 1990) but these physicians said that they did do sigmoidoscopy in about half of their asymptomatic patients and almost 90% used the stool blood test—if not specifically by the guidelines.

The benefit from screening asymptomatic persons with the stool blood test depends on the willingness of both the patient and physician to follow up positive tests with a diagnostic evaluation of the entire colon to determine whether any lesion is present.

One recent study program highlighted the need for further education about compliance. A total of 45,658 people in the Chicago area submitted slide presentations to test for stool blood using the Hemoccult II test (Winchester, Sylvester, and Mobet 1983). Five hundred ninety-one (1.3%) had at least one positive slide test. Fewer than half of those with a positive test who saw a physician had adequate follow-up, such as examination of the entire large bowel. Over 20% of persons with a positive stool blood test had only a second stool blood test and/or a digital rectal examination by their physi-

cians. Six percent of the patients said their physicians ignored the positive stool blood test, and conducted no follow-up examination. The study yielded 22 cancers (4.3% of those who saw a doctor after a positive test) and 53 cases of polyps. This program would obviously have been more effective if physicians had properly investigated all positive stool blood tests, pointing to a need for professional and public education to remedy the situation.

RATIONALE FOR EARLY CANCER DETECTION RECOMMENDATIONS

DIGITAL RECTAL EXAMINATION

The inspection of the anal region and palpation on the perineal and sacrococcygeal areas are integral to cancer detection for colorectal cancer. In men, palpation of the prostate during the digital examination is also crucial.

This procedure is so time-honored and time-tested that no formal studies of efficacy have been considered necessary, although one study indicates its usefulness. A multiphasic health screening study conducted by the Kaiser Health Foundation randomly selected plan members who were divided into study and control groups. Study group members were offered a battery of tests including digital rectal examination and sigmoidoscopy (Dales, Friedman, and Collen 1979). During 11 years of follow-up, the screened group had a lower cumulative mortality from colorectal cancer than the controls (2.3 vs. 5.2 deaths per 1,000 members). Although this study was not designed to test the specific effects of various colorectal detection techniques, digital rectal examination may have contributed to the decrease in mortality.

Digital rectal examination is safe, and its cost, as part of a general examination, is relatively low, making any potential benefit worthwhile. It is therefore recommended annually for patients over 40. The only known risks are the patient's emotional reaction, the cost of false-positive results, and the sense of security from false-negative findings. There are no data on the frequency of these risks.

SIGMOIDOSCOPY

Rigid sigmoidoscopic examinations date from the 1920s. Instrumentation has since improved, but surprisingly few studies have evaluated the new technology and its use in the periodic physical examination. The benefits of sigmoidoscopy were suggested in 1960 in a large study involving more than 26,000 men and women over 45 years of age, conducted by the Preventive Medicine Institute-Strang Clinic in New York City (Hertz, Deddish, and Day 1960). About 10% of the participants had minimal symptoms. Periodic rigid sigmoidoscopy detected 58 cancers; 60% were found by sigmoidoscopy, and another 17% were found by barium enema after sigmoidoscopy detected a polyp or noted blood in the bowel lumen. Eighty-one percent of the cancers were localized (Dukes' stage A or B or ASCC stage I or II).

In the 50 patients followed for 15 years or more, the survival rate was close to 90%, or double the expected 10-year rate. However, this study did not have a control group and is subject to several biases.

The Kaiser Health Foundation multiphasic health examination study in the screened vs. control groups demonstrated lower cumulative mortality from colorectal cancer (2.3 vs. 5.2 deaths per 1,000 members) over a 16-year period (Dales, Friedman, and Collen 1979). A recent review of this study examined the cancers arising in the distal 20 cm of the large bowel wall within reach of the rigid sigmoidoscope. The cumulative incidence during the 18-year follow-up was 50% lower in the screened group than in the control group. A higher proportion of screened group tumors were discovered in the localized stage (Selby and Friedman 1989). Only 31% of the screened group had sigmoidoscopy during the first 10 years of the study, while 26% of the control group had at least one. Most of the tumors in each group were diagnosed due to symptoms.

The value of sigmoidoscopy may be related to the removal of polyps. Gilbertson and associates at the University of Minnesota followed more than 18,000 patients over age 45 for up to 25 years using rigid sigmoidoscopy. All adenomatous polyps were removed (Gilbertson 1974). At the end of the surveillance period, only 15% of the anticipated number of cancers were found, suggesting that proctosigmoidoscopy had effectively prevented cancer by facilitating the discovery and removal of premalignant lesions. In addition, all the cancers detected were localized; after 21 years of follow-up, no patient had died of colorectal cancer.

PATIENT COMFORT

The value of rigid sigmoidoscopy has been decreased by poor patient acceptance combined with a relatively low rate of physician application. According to surveys by the ACS, most people are unwilling to undergo the discomfort of the procedure, and few return for follow-up examinations.

The more comfortable flexible scopes, which are available in 60 cm and 35 cm lengths, may increase public and physician acceptance of sigmoidoscopy. The 60 cm flexible scope requires more training and examination time (8 to 15 minutes); the 35 cm scope appears to offer advantages over both rigid and 60 cm flexible sigmoidoscopes. Proficiency with the 35 cm scope is possible in minimal examination time with little patient discomfort. The average length of insertion with the 35 cm scope is 27 to 30 cm; the average examination time is about four to six minutes. It is reasonable to encourage physician training in flexible sigmoidoscopy, considering that many believe flexible sigmoidoscopes should gradually replace rigid ones.

Perforation rates have been estimated by Eddy to be 0.0125% for the rigid sigmoidoscope, 0.02% for the 35-cm flexible sigmoidoscope, and 0.045% for the 60-cm flexible sigmoidoscope (Eddy 1990).

CHANGE IN CANCER DETECTION GUIDELINES

The benefit-risk ratio of sigmoidoscopy supports its inclusion in the periodic cancer-related checkup. In 1988, the ACS modified its original guidelines for sigmoidoscopy to recommend the examination every three to five years, beginning at age 50. The inclusion of two annual sigmoidoscopic examinations did not appear to be justified in terms of yield and cost; therefore, this requisite was eliminated.

Although there is still some controversy over the duration of the transformation period for colorectal cancer, it appears to be many years. An estimated 94% efficacy rate can be achieved using sigmoidoscopy every three to five years. This period reduces the financial burden of an annual program and makes the procedure more acceptable to patients.

The initiation of sigmoidoscopic examination in average-risk persons at age 50 is determined by the age-specific incidence rates of the disease. There are not enough cases in persons under age 50 to justify the risks and costs.

STOOL BLOOD TEST

The testing of stool for occult blood was popularized by Greegor, who used the impregnated guaiac slide to find blood in the stool of asymptomatic individuals (Greegor 1967). The methodology has been refined over the years. The controversies surrounding the use of the stool blood test have recently been reviewed (Simon 1985).

Blood in the stool can result from a wide variety of both benign and malignant conditions. The stool blood test is not specific for cancer, but evidence suggests that stool blood testing in asymptomatic individuals can detect cancer or polyps. About half of colon cancers lie beyond the reach of standard sigmoidoscopes. The shift of cancer toward the right colon is a recent phenomenon, and therefore there is much interest in using the stool blood test to detect cancer throughout the colon.

Studies of the stool blood test are being carried out in New York (Winawer et al. 1980), Minnesota (Gilbertson et al. 1980), England (Hardcastle 1986), and Sweden (Ekiland, Carlson, and Johnson 1985). A fifth study is beginning in Denmark. The Memorial Sloan-Kettering Cancer Center-Strang Clinic study in New York City is not a randomized trial. The study and control groups were selected by calendar periods. Both groups had rigid sigmoidoscopy; the study group had stool blood testing, while the control group did not. The Minnesota program randomly assigned volunteer participants to study and control groups. The Swedish study targeted the 60- to 64-year age group. The English study selected candidates from lists of family practitioners. Definitive results are not yet available from these studies, but the disease has been consistently diagnosed at an earlier stage among those screened.

In the Minnesota study, over 45,000 volunteer participants age 50 years or more were assigned to a control group; two study groups are tested for occult bleeding every one or two years. Early results included compliance with stool blood testing of 75% and more favorable early stage cancer detected. Definitive findings from the current studies may not be available until 1995 or 2000.

LIMITATIONS

The limitations of the stool blood test have recently been described (Simon 1985; Gnauck, MacRae, and Fleischer 1984; Knight, Fielding, and Battista 1986). The false-negative rate for the stool blood test may be as high as 30%. Because colorectal cancers and polyps bleed intermittently, a negative stool blood test does not rule out colorectal cancer. Moreover, prolonged storage (more than 4 to 6 days) of the slide after preparation can cause a weakly positive test to revert to negative (Gnauck, MacRae, and Fleischer 1984). The test should not be used as a prescreening test for sigmoidoscopy or digital rectal examination.

PATIENT PREPARATION

Preparation for the stool blood test must include guidance concerning pretest diet. A positive reaction depends on phenolic oxidation of guaiac in the presence of hemoglobin. Dietary compounds found in vegetables and meat with peroxidase-like activity can interfere with the test. Oral iron medications can result in false-positive reactions. Vitamin C intake also inhibits the test reaction.

The ACS recently evaluated dietary preparation for the stool blood test. Table 12.8 outlines reasonable dietary recommendations that can be followed by healthy adults with minimal discomfort or disruption of family eating patterns.

FOLLOW-UP OF POSITIVE TESTS

Any benefit from the stool blood test depends on proper follow-up of positive tests. Because neoplasms may bleed intermittently, a positive stool blood test, if done

---

Table 12.8
AMERICAN CANCER SOCIETY RECOMMENDATIONS FOR DIETARY PREPARATIONS FOR THE STOOL BLOOD TEST

The following dietary guidelines should be initiated at least 48 hours prior to collection of the first stool sample and continued until the final stool sample has been collected:

Do not take vitamin C supplements.

Do not take oral iron medication.

Do not take multivitamins containing vitamin C or iron.

Avoid foods with high peroxidase activity, such as broccoli, turnips, cantaloupes, cauliflower, radishes, horseradish, and parsnips.

Do not eat red meat. Poultry and fish may be eaten.

Do not take aspirin or non-steroidal anti-inflammatory drugs. Aspirin substitutes such as acetaminophen may be used.

The value of added dietary fiber for the stool blood test has not been established at this time. Most advice on dietary preparation has included bran in the diet, but its value is unproven.

Table 12.9
AMERICAN CANCER SOCIETY RECOMMENDATIONS FOR FOLLOW-UP TO THE STOOL BLOOD TEST

1. All persons presenting for colorectal cancer detection screening should be carefully evaluated for risk factors and signs or symptoms of colorectal cancer by a physician or by a qualified health care personnel under the supervision of a physician. Persons with signs or symptoms of colorectal cancer should not be enrolled in screening programs. Instead, such individuals should receive diagnostic evaluation to determine the presence or absence of colorectal cancer or related pathology such as adenomas.

2. A diagnostic evaluation must be initiated if the stool blood test is positive. A positive stool blood test, if done according to these recommendations, should not be repeated, since bleeding may be intermittent.

3. The stool blood test should not be used as the sole examination for colorectal cancer detection or as a prescreening test for sigmoidoscopy or digital rectal examination. Persons with a negative stool blood test should also have sigmoidoscopy and digital rectal examination.

---

according to usual recommendations, should not be repeated. Instead, if any single test is positive, diagnostic evaluation should follow and may include barium enema, colonoscopy, or both.

Diagnostic evaluation after a positive stool blood test must include examination of the entire large bowel. Guidelines for the suggested follow-up of a stool blood test are given in table 12.9.

Several tests are now commercially available, as are over-the-counter preparations. The yield from do-it-yourself tests is not known, nor is the reliability of self-read vs. laboratory-read test results. Therefore, caution is advised when using these newer products.

COST AND USE OF RESOURCES

The important question of cost for colorectal cancer detection has only recently been studied seriously but is becoming increasingly important as health care expenditures are being more intensively surveyed by the ACS. Eddy and Neuhauser have examined costs of screening for colorectal cancer (Eddy 1986; Prescott, McPherson, and Bell 1980). Eddy has projected various strategies for colorectal cancer detection in high-risk individuals based on cost.

The workup of a patient with a positive stool guaiac slide test can take several days and may cost over $1,000, depending on the protocol followed. However, even if the bleeding is not caused by cancer, its discovery may still have significant benefit, such as the discovery of a premalignant adenomatous polyp. In a study of 81 patients with positive tests, 12% had cancer, 55% had polyps, and 19% had diverticulosis (Winawer et al. 1977).

Cost considerations must include direct costs of detection tests (stool blood tests, sigmoidoscopy, and digital rectal examination) as well as indirect costs, such as follow-up examinations for patients with positive tests. The direct costs of detecting colorectal cancer in asymptomatic people depend on the setting. A digital rectal examination is relatively inexpensive if the patient is in the office for other reasons, but the examination can cost $20 to $30 if a special office visit is required. A series of six stool guaiac slide tests is inexpensive, usually costing patients less than $10. Rigid sigmoidoscopies, when performed as independent procedures, usually cost about $50; flexible procedures cost more.

Indirect costs are also present, especially when the detection examination is part of a community-based program. Costs to run a program include resource personnel, such as receptionists, and time for contacting patients and persuading noncompliant subjects (Simon 1985). Additional indirect costs are incurred from media and public education activities.

Other hidden costs that also influence the cost of colorectal cancer detection include patient time and inconvenience, including time lost from work for follow-up tests.

Emotional stress of patients undergoing follow-up examinations is important in test-positive subjects. A false sense of security in test-negative people may cause delay or failure to seek attention when symptoms appear.

BREAST CANCER

INTRODUCTION

Cancer of the breast is the most common cancer in American women and the second most common cause of death due to cancer (second now only to lung cancer). An estimated 175,000 new cases are expected in the United States in 1991 (ACS 1991). Breast cancer will develop in 1 out of 9 women. An estimated 44,800 deaths are expected in 1991 (44,500 females and 300 males).

The 5-year survival rate for localized breast cancer has risen from 78% in the 1940s to 91% today. If breast cancer is not invasive or is *in situ*, the survival rate approaches 100%. If the cancer has spread regionally, however, the survival rate falls to 69%.

The proportion of cases usually found without lymph node involvement at the time of diagnosis is 53%. When breast cancer detection includes screening mammography, more than 75% of all breast cancers detected show no evidence of nodal involvement.

SCREENING TESTS

The 1980 checkup guidelines recommended that a triad of tests be used at appropriate ages for breast cancer detection in asymptomatic women: breast self-examination, clinical breast examination, and mammography (ACS 1980). Of these techniques, mammography was able to find very small breast cancers, even before they could be palpated by the most experienced examiner.

From the 1985 ACS survey, it was learned that only about half of primary care physicians *ever* ordered screening mammography for their asymptomatic patients. Only 11% followed the ACS guidelines. Physicians who did not use this screening mammography cited cost, lack of knowledge about benefits, and radiation exposure as barriers. Some physicians also believed that mammography was not necessary unless there was a family history of breast cancer. These findings are in contrast to their use of clinical breast examination and teaching of breast self-examination techniques. The majority of physicians said that they perform these procedures on a majority of asymptomatic women.

By 1989 almost all physicians said they would order mammography for their asymptomatic patients and 37% said that they followed the ACS guidelines. In the intervening years significant educational programs were conducted for women and health professionals nationwide by the ACS and other organizations (ACS 1990).

The radiation exposure during modern mammographic testing is extremely low, making the risk of radiation-induced breast cancer minimal, if not nonexistent (NCRP 1986).

Two randomized clinical trials (Shapiro et al. 1981; Tabar et al. 1985) and a recent large demonstration project (Baker 1982), show a significant reduction in mortality from breast cancer when mammography was included in the screening examination. The benefit was found not only in women over the age of 50 but also in those 40 to 49 years of age (Baker 1982). Therefore, in 1983, the ACS changed its guidelines for asymptomatic women age 40 to 49 years, recommending screening mammography every one to two years (ACS 1985). The baseline mammogram between ages 35 to 39 years is for clinical comparison to future examinations.

OTHER IMAGING TECHNIQUES

The role of other breast cancer imaging techniques—thermography, diaphanography, and ultrasound—was recently reviewed by the ACS's National Advisory Committee on Cancer Prevention and Detection and the National Board of Directors. The board concluded that these procedures do not have sufficient proven value at this time to justify their routine use in screening for breast cancer in asymptomatic women. None should be considered a substitute for mammography or physical examination or as a preliminary screening procedure to identify asymptomatic women suitable for mammography. None eliminates the need for biopsy or breast aspiration when indicated by physical examination. Use of these procedures adds cost to the breast cancer screening procedure without increasing benefit.

Magnetic resonance imaging (MRI) and computerized tomography (CT) have not been tested adequately to determine whether they will have a future role in breast cancer detection.

BREAST CANCER DETECTION GUIDELINES

The ACS's breast cancer detection guidelines (table 12.10) are intended for asymptomatic women only. Women with symptoms (a persistent lump or thickening, dimpling, skin irritation, nipple retraction, nipple scaling, discharge, bleeding, or breast pain) must undergo a thorough diagnostic evaluation. In symptomatic patients, mammography is indicated as a valuable diagnostic tool before biopsy, not as a screening technique. A biopsy is indicated in patients with positive findings on physical examination (such as localized mass), even if the mammogram is normal.

Table 12.10
AMERICAN CANCER SOCIETY RECOMMENDATIONS
FOR BREAST CANCER DETECTION IN
ASYMPTOMATIC WOMEN AT AVERAGE RISK

Age	Recommendation
20-39	Breast self-examination, monthly Clinical breast examination, every 3 years Baseline mammography, for patients 35 to 39 years of age
40-49	Breast self-examination, monthly Clinical breast examination, yearly Mammography, every 1 to 2 years
50 and older	Breast self-examination, monthly Clinical breast examination, yearly Mammography, yearly

RISK FACTORS

In an analysis of 570,000 American women, known breast cancer risk factors (older than age 50, personal or family history of breast cancer, nulliparity, or first child after age 30) were present in only one-fourth of all women with breast cancer (Seidman, Stellman, and Mushinski 1982). Thus, from a clinical standpoint, all American women should be considered at risk for breast cancer and candidates for the ACS's breast cancer detection recommendations.

REDUCING BARRIERS

Since the 1980 guidelines were published, a number of important advances have helped reduce the barriers to breast cancer detection, especially the use of screening mammography.

LOWER RADIATION DOSE

Surveys indicate that almost all the image receptors now used for screening mammography are either film/screen or xeromammography (FDA 1986). When properly performed, either technique can provide good images with x-ray doses of 0.01 Gy or less for two views of each breast. This is an improvement from 10 years ago when industrial film screen was more commonly used and equipment delivered higher radiation doses.

During the mid-1970s, questions were raised about the radiation doses used in screening mammography and the possibility of inducing breast cancer by radiation. Studies linking radiation exposure and breast cancer (in atomic bomb survivors, women treated for acute mastitis with x-rays, and women with tuberculosis exposed to repeated chest fluoroscopy) involved subjects who were exposed to doses much higher than those used today in screening mammography. No known case of breast cancer has yet been traced to the use of screening mammography. Modern mammography technology provides a favorable benefit-risk ratio in women age 40 and older when the image quality is maintained using a 2-view examination of each breast with a dose of 0.01 Gy or less (NCRP 1986).

COST

Cost has been regarded as a deterrent to the use of screening mammography by both physicians and women. The examination may cost $100 or more in many communities. Recent changes specifically targeted to screening have made it possible to provide quality screening mammography at costs well below the national average.

In 1986, the ACS sponsored a workshop to review strategies for lowering the cost of screening mammography (Dodd, Fink, and Bertram 1987). The workshop participants identified a number of approaches to provide screening mammography at a lower cost. Most important, *screening* mammography in asymptomatic women must be distinguished from *diagnostic* mammography used to evaluate women with breast cancer signs and/or symptoms. Diagnostic mammography may require special views and a significant amount of the radiologist's time to properly identify the breast lesion or other breast pathology. Screening mammography separates women with breast pathology radiographically from those who have none. To achieve lower costs, screening mammography requires batch processing, minimal radiologist time, and a high volume of women screened. Costs as low as $27 for 2-view mammograms are possible using these methods.

A number of recent community demonstration projects sponsored by the ACS have offered lower-cost screening mammography (usually $40 to $50) for limited periods. Participating hospitals and mammography facilities agree to these lower costs to help stimulate community awareness about mammography for the detection of early breast cancer (Fink 1989).

Even if the costs of screening mammography were significantly decreased, the payment would remain a personal burden for many women because most health insurance policies do not provide coverage for screening examinations. Stimulated by the ACS, other professional organizations, concerned health professionals, and the public, legislative action has taken place across the United States to provide insurance coverage for screening mammography. Currently a number of states have enacted legislation to provide this coverage, usually as part of health insurance plans. It remains to be seen how the health insurance industry and corporate America will respond to the growing interest in coverage for cancer prevention and detection, particularly breast cancer detection; recent trends are encouraging.

A particularly vexing aspect of the cost issue is provision of screening mammography for economically disadvantaged women who often cannot pay for even the necessities of daily living. Their medical care for acute health problems tends to be sporadic and disorganized. To recruit these women into programs for breast cancer detection will require ingenuity by the health care system. Screening mammography is vital to all women of appropriate age regardless of their ability to pay for the examination and for follow-up of abnormal findings. Recent legislation to implement breast and cervical cancer detection through the Centers for Disease Control and states may be of assistance in reaching underserved women.

The importance of a high-quality, low-dose mammogram is critical in providing breast cancer detection. Assuring quality involves increasing the radiologist's ability to provide mammography as well as increasing the quality of the mammographic image. Until recently, mammography was not part of the board examinations in diagnostic radiology. The American College of Radiology (ACR) has moved quickly to provide a large number of educational courses for the practicing radiologist.

The quality of the mammographic image is also important for optimal screening. The ACR has organized an accreditation program for facilities offering mammography. This innovative program reviews radiation levels and image quality and provides advice for modification when needed. Practicing radiologists can contact the ACR to request the accreditation review. A new home study course from the ACR supported by an ACS grant offers practicing radiologists the opportunity to increase their skills for mammography.

RATIONALE FOR BREAST CANCER DETECTION

MAMMOGRAPHY AND
CLINICAL BREAST EXAMINATION

A number of studies indicate the effect of mammography and clinical breast examination for breast cancer detection in asymptomatic women. The most widely cited is the randomized trial conducted by the Health Insurance Plan (HIP) of New York (Shapiro et al. 1981). The study, initiated in 1964, was intended to evaluate breast cancer detection by annual clinical breast examination and mammography in women 40 to 65 years of age. Approximately 62,000 women were randomly assigned to two groups: a study group that was offered an annual detection examination including an initial examination, and a control group. About 67% of the study group accepted the invitation for an initial screening; a large proportion returned for re-examinations (Shapiro 1988). The HIP screening program resulted in about a 30% reduction in mortality from breast cancer during the first 10 years of follow-up for study group women age 50 and older. At 18 years, the reduction was 25%. The favorable effect appeared later in women age 40 to 49 years compared to older women, not appearing until 10 years of follow-up. By 18 years follow-up a similar effect was seen in women 40 to 49 years of age as in those 50 to 59 years of age.

More recently, a randomized controlled trial was conducted in Sweden (Tabar, Fagerberg, and Gad et al. 1985). The study included 160,000 women who were divided into a study group and a control group. Women in the study group were offered a single-view mammogram approximately every two years. Over a 7-year follow-up period, breast cancer mortality was one-third lower in the study group than in the control group, primarily among women age 50 and older.

A large cancer screening demonstration program was mounted by the ACS and the NCI. The Breast Cancer Detection Demonstration Project (BCDDP) was initiated in 1973 to promote the results of the HIP study to physicians and women. By 1975, 29 community projects were organized across the United States, and 280,000 women were enrolled.

Each woman was screened annually for five years with a history, physical examination, and mammography. Thermography was used for the first few years of the study, but was discontinued because it proved to be of low sensitivity and specificity. Breast self-examination was taught and encouraged throughout the project. The BCDDP showed that one-third of the 3,500 cases diagnosed were minimal cancer (noninfiltrating, less than 1 cm in size). More than 75% of all cancers detected showed no evidence of lymph node involvement. Clinical breast examination and mammography found cases not detected by breast self-examination, but the role of mammography in detection was greater. Mammography alone found 40% of all cases, compared to 10% found by clinical breast examination (Baker 1982). A more recent analysis compared the BCDDP outcome with SEER data. Exceptionally high survival rates were found in cases detected through mammography alone. Benefit was seen in women age 40 to 49 years as well as in those over 50 (Seidman et al. 1987).

A number of other studies add to the experience of these three important investigations. In the Netherlands, two case-control studies are under way. In Nijmegem, women age 30 to 65 years were offered participation in annual screening with single-view mammography (Verbeen, Stratman, and Hendricks 1987). Early results show an odds ratio of 0.48, indicating a 50% reduction in breast cancer mortality as related to screening mammography. No benefit has yet been seen in women younger than 50 years.

In Utrecht, women between the ages of 50 and 64 years, and later 40 to 49 years, were offered periodic screening with clinical breast examination and mammography at shorter intervals than the Nijmegem project. The so-called DOM project thus far has results available for women 50 years of age and older that show favorable odds ratios for breast cancer mortality (Collette et al. 1987).

A randomized trial in Canada involving 90,000 women was designed to answer whether annual screening with mammography and physical examination compared to physical examination alone affects breast cancer mortality in women age 40 to 49 years. The study also sought to determine the additional contribution of screening mammography compared to routine physical examination toward reducing breast cancer mortality in women age 50 to 59 years. Screening examinations have been completed, and most follow-up is under way (National Cancer Institute of Canada 1980).

A United Kingdom study compares trends in breast cancer mortality among eight geographic areas; two test the effect of breast self-examination; two test the effect of screening mammography and clinical breast examination at varying intervals; and four serve as control communities (Progress Report of the UK Trial 1987). Results are expected in several years.

Finally, in Finland, women age 50 and older are recruited through a national population registry and are invited to attend a screening program that involves screening every two years. This program intends to assist the Finnish government in determining long-term policy for breast cancer detection. The situation in Finland allows for full monitoring of the program and provides feedback to a coordinated provider team and the screener (Habemma 1987).

This collective experience should provide further valuable evidence about the benefit of screening mammography and clinical breast examination. The interval for optimal screening and use of risk factors to determine recruitment policy remain unresolved issues.

BREAST SELF-EXAMINATION

Breast self-examination (BSE) has been widely promoted by the ACS and other organizations worldwide as a simple and noninvasive method for women to detect breast cancer. It has been promoted as a method to make women aware of their breasts and to detect any changes as early as possible, since historically most women find their own breast cancers. For women unable to receive medical examinations (either clinical breast examination or mammography) due to lack of access or other socioeconomic reasons, BSE has been advocated as an available and inexpensive option. The ACS recommends that the examination be done monthly; however, only about 25% of women surveyed in 1983 and 1987 seemed to be performing the examination that frequently.

Two recent reviews of BSE (Baines 1985; O'Malley and Fletcher 1987) point out that there has been no randomized trial to determine the effect of BSE on breast cancer mortality. A number of retrospective studies have been reported, producing variable results as to the effect of BSE on detecting early breast cancer (Foster et al. 1978; Senie, Rosen, and Lesser 1981; Constanza and Foster 1984). Studies under way in the United Kingdom and the USSR may yield information about BSE in terms of its effect on breast cancer mortality.

Most studies on the benefits of BSE have centered on BSE practice and the stage of cancer at the time of diagnosis (Foster et al. 1978; Senie, Rosen, and Lesser 1981). One study showed that there were fewer deaths among breast cancer patients who practiced BSE (Constanza and Foster 1984).

To be effective, a woman must know how to perform BSE properly. The content and extent of instruction to improve frequency of performance is not known. Approaches have ranged from simply handing a woman a pamphlet and encouraging her to do monthly BSE; to one-to-one, hourlong training using films, models, pamphlets, and demonstrations; to large group presentations using some or all of the methods (Baines 1987).

A recent trial using a simple teaching technique, giving a woman a BSE pamphlet, showed improved detection by clinical stage at biopsy. While mean tumor diameter was smaller among women receiving the booklet (2.5 cm vs. 3.3 cm), the difference was not statistically significant (Turner et al. 1984). Women who practice regular BSE tend to be younger (below age 40). Women are more likely to do BSE monthly when taught by a health professional, so BSE instruction should be incorporated into routine primary care practice (Baines 1984). A recent study in Canada revealed that BSE calendars were not effective as incentives to improve BSE performance (Baines 1984).

Data on the psychologic effects of BSE and BSE training on women is scarce. Women monitoring BSE could feel more in control of their bodies. However, fear and BSE may also be related. In a nationwide survey, 46% of the women surveyed thought BSE caused them to worry unnecessarily. In the United Kingdom trial of early breast cancer detection, similar numbers of women in BSE teaching and control districts reported concern (20% vs. 16%). In the teaching districts more of the women attending BSE programs reported concern as compared to nonattenders. Thus, it appears that BSE may raise concerns about breast cancer in some women but not in others (O'Malley and Fletcher 1987). (The ACS provides simple instruction for women on how to perform BSE; the pamphlet [ACS 1987] is available in all local ACS offices.)

Despite the need to answer a number of important questions, it appears prudent to continue to recommend BSE as a cancer detection technique while not detracting from the importance of screening mammography and clinical breast examination.

USE OF RESOURCES

The introduction of a breast cancer detection program into the individual physician's practice or into a community screening program is likely to involve the use of significant resources. Breast cancer detection can increase surgical workload; the very small lesions require special techniques for localization. The peak in workload occurs in women in their first screening and then levels off. An important determinant of workload is the ratio of the number of biopsies taken to the number of cancers found.

The costs of detecting breast cancer early are relatively high compared with other screening programs. While the direct cost of a mammogram can be as low as $27, these low costs are achieved only in well-organized screening programs. Mammograms performed by private physicians and radiologists can cost $50 to $100 or more. If 25% of women age 40 to 70 years were screened annually with mammography and physical examination, the costs would be approximately $1.3 billion (Eddy 1989). At present, there are insufficient facilities or personnel to accomplish this task. The cost of a clinical breast examination also varies tremendously, depending on whether it is in a well-organized program with cost-control incentives or in a physician's office. A physician's office visit for a clinical breast examination could cost $10 to $25 or more.

Methods to lower the costs of screening mammography have been fully described in the report of the ACS's Workshop on Screening Mammography (Dodd and Fink 1986).

Swedish investigators sought to determine the cost of screening and follow-up examinations including diagnostic mammography, clinical examinations, aspiration cytology, and screening (Jonsson, Hakansson, and Tabar 1987). They estimated that the cost of screening and follow-up examination was $49 for prevalent cases and $37 for incident cases. The cost per prevalent cancer detected was $7,040 and $12,000 for incident cases. These authors point out that costs will change based on screening intervals selected and women targeted for screening. In Sweden, there are 1,594,000 women age 40 to 74 and 1,132,000 women age 50 to 74. If all women age 40 to 74 were screened annually with a 2-view mammography, the total cost would be $71 million for a screening program including follow-up investigation. If screening were limited to women age 50 to 74 with 90% receiving annual single-view mammography, the cost would drop to $30.5 million.

A recent modelling study analyzed the economic consequences of adding annual mammography to annual clinical breast examination in asymptomatic women age 40 to 49. This study proposed a series of outcomes based on a series of estimates. For example, Eddy suggested that if 35% of women age 40 to 49 were screened annually, the breast cancer mortality would decrease by about 373 deaths (Eddy et al. 1988). In 1984, the cost of screening, workups, continuing care, and treatment was calculated to be $402 million. Eddy does not suggest a blanket recommendation for all asymptomatic women in that age group, but indicates that a flexible policy of "see your physician" might be advisable.

CANCER OF THE CERVIX

INTRODUCTION

In 1991, about 50,000 new cases of cervical cancer *in situ* and 13,000 cases of invasive cervical cancer are expected to occur. The incidence of invasive cancer of the cervix has steadily decreased over the years, while cervical cancer *in situ* has risen slightly in women under 50 in recent years. It is estimated that there will be 4,500 deaths from cervical cancer in 1991 (ACS 1991).

Overall, the death rate from uterine cervix cancer has decreased more than 70% during the last 40 years — mainly due to the Pap test and regular checkups. Finding precursors of invasive cancer of the cervix (cervical dysplasia and carcinoma *in situ*) with the Pap test and cervical cytology has been a major factor in the decreased death rate.

The value of early cancer detection has been nowhere more obvious than in cancer of the cervix. Beginning in the late 1940s, the ACS was instrumental in providing the support necessary to establish numerous cytologic detection programs throughout the United States. Extensive public promotional and educational campaigns, such as "Uterine Cancer Year" and the "Let No Woman Be Overlooked" program, successfully brought the message of early detection to millions of American women. Physician education was an important part of this effort.

RISK FACTORS

The risk factors for cancer of the cervix are early age at first vaginal intercourse and multiple sexual partners. More recently, cigarette smoking was identified as a risk factor. Cervical cancer and precancerous lesions in women may be associated with genital human papilloma virus (HPV).

The role of HPV in cervical dysplasia, also called intra-epithelial neoplasia, is being intensively studied. HPV types 16, 18, 31, and 33 are of specific importance in cervical cancer; HPV infection can be transmitted by a woman's male sexual partner (Barrosso et al. 1987; Richart 1987; Koss 1987). The penile lesions related to HPV infection may be difficult to detect clinically and may be evident only after application of acetic acid.

Thus, all women who have had vaginal intercourse appear to be at risk for cervical cancer. Some physicians are concerned that, because of the changing sexual patterns of increased exposure to multiple partners, many women, regardless of their socioeconomic status, may be at risk. Historically, cancer of the cervix has been more common in lower socioeconomic groups.

BACKGROUND

In 1980, the ACS Cancer-Related Checkup Guidelines suggested the following guidance for women and their physicians:

In women 20 to 65 years of age, or in sexually active women under age 20, a Pap test, at least every three years after two previous, consecutive, satisfactory annual tests, plus a pelvic examination, every three years between 20 and 40 years, and yearly thereafter.

The publication of these guidelines led to much debate among medical groups and physicians about the recommended periodicity of the Pap test. There was essentially no controversy about applying the Pap test; the question that emerged was over how often the test should be done. Although no randomized clinical trials comparing women screened with the Pap test and those not screened were available, a number of studies documented the test's benefits (MacGregor 1986; Fidler, Boyes, and Locke 1968; Walton Report 1976; Guzick 1978; Johanneson, Geirsson, and Day 1978). A number of American medical organizations as well as the ACS recommended a variety of suggested intervals for screening, adding to the confusion.

The advocates of annual Pap smears cited the importance of yearly tests for detecting not only cervical cancer but also other gynecologic and medical problems. There were heated debates among gynecologists and other primary care physicians. Many international studies suggest screening intervals of three to five years with expected benefits to cervical cancer screening. As an example, a study from Milan concluded that invasive cervical cancer could be maximally reduced by screening every three years with only a small proportion of benefit (8%) by intervals of less than 3 years (La Vecchia et al. 1984). A study from Denmark indicated that screening intervals of three to five years confer considerable protection (Olesen 1988).

In the 1984 ACS survey, almost all primary care physicians (94%) reported that they have ordered Pap tests for asymptomatic women, but 75% deviated from Pap test guidelines—reporting that they ordered a Pap test at least once a year (ACS 1985).

NEW RECOMMENDATION

In 1986, the ACS sponsored The Community and Cancer Prevention and Detection workshop for health providers. The major recommendation was for the development of common guidelines among medical organizations to assist physicians in evaluating their patients (McKenna and Fink 1988). To accomplish this, the ACS called together major medical organizations in 1987 to examine cervical cancer detection. The results of that workshop have produced the following revision of the ACS's recommendations for the periodicity of the Pap test for cervical cancer detection (Fink 1988):

That all women who are or have been sexually active, or have reached age 18 years, have an annual Pap test and pelvic examination. After a woman has had three or more consecutive, satisfactory, normal annual examinations, the Pap test may be performed less frequently at the discretion of her physician.

These recommendations have been accepted as policy in identical or similar wording by the NCI, the American College of Obstetricians and Gynecologists, the American Medical Association, the American Academy of Family Physicians, the American Medical Women's Association, and the American Nurses Association.

Recent evidence suggests that the Pap test for women over age 65 may be useful, especially among those who have not participated in regular screening programs. Thus, the ACS's revised guidelines have no upper age limiting screening. Such a decision must be made by the woman and her physician.

In the 1990 follow-up survey of primary care physicians there was a sizeable agreement with the new guideline for Pap testing (from 56% to 70%). Two-thirds of the physicians surveyed were aware of the change. Of the 30% of physicians who do not agree with ACS guidelines, the majority believe that the Pap test should be done annually.

RATIONALE FOR EARLY DETECTION

No randomized controlled clinical trials were conducted on the efficacy of the Pap test before its introduction into clinical practice over 40 years ago. Because of the Pap test's obvious benefits and ethical considerations, it is not feasible at this time to conduct such a trial. Evidence for the efficacy of early cervical cancer detection thus comes from two sources: documentation of the natural history of the disease, and observation of reductions in the incidence and mortality of invasive cervical cancer in large populations following the widespread use of Pap tests.

NATURAL HISTORY OF CANCER OF THE CERVIX

In the great majority of women, carcinoma *in situ* (CIS) persists in a detectable stage for an extended period of time before becoming invasive cancer of the cervix (ICC). The known relationship between CIS and ICC is based on several factors: the finding of CIS at the margins of ICC; the presence of foci of CIS in biopsies of ICC; and the existence of transitional CIS with early stromal invasion. The best information, however, has been obtained from following untreated patients with CIS (Graham, Sotto, and Paloneck 1962; Galvin, Jones, and Tellinde 1952; Davis 1967; Burghardt 1973).

Peterson reports on 127 patients with untreated CIS followed for at least three years and showed that by the tenth year, ICC had developed in about 30% of the women (Peterson 1955; Clemmesen 1971). It is noteworthy that, after one year, only half of the original patients still had CIS. It is believed that at least 20% regressed—all within one year—and that 80% were misdiagnosed. Clemmesen and Paulsen later concluded that at least 40% of patients with carcinoma *in situ* would develop invasive carcinoma (Clemmesen 1971). In 1953, Kottmeier reported on biopsies of 14 patients with clearly documented CIS followed for at least 10 years; ICC developed in eight patients (Kottmeier 1953). Another series of 31 patients with CIS followed for 12 years by curettage or biopsy showed ICC in 80% of women over 30 years. Koss and his colleagues (1963) followed 67 patients with CIS for a minimum of three years and observed 17 regressions (25%) after an initial biopsy, while in the remainder of patients, CIS persisted or progressed to invasion.

How long CIS exists in a stage detectable by Pap test prior to symptoms or progression to invasion is obviously a most important factor in determining the optimal frequency of a cervical cancer detection protocol. In the Walton Report, a Canadian task force estimated that CIS persists for about three decades.

Christopherson analyzed data from a massive screening program in Louisville, Kentucky, and found that the duration of CIS was about 22 years (Christopherson 1980). The consensus from several other investigators appears to be that Pap test-detectable CIS is present for eight to 30 years before progressing to ICC (Richart and Barron 1980; Dunn and Martin 1967; Kashigarian and Dunn 1970). The most recent analysis by Richart and Barron estimated the mean duration of CIS to be 10 years, with a lower limit for CIS transit time of about three years.

Eddy recently reviewed the controversy about the possible change in incidence or natural history of cervical cancer. As he states, several authors have voiced the possibility of an increased frequency of preinvasive cancer in younger women or that there is an etiologically distinct subgroup of lesions that have rapid progression time (so called "fast movers") or both. He points out that data from the Surveillance, Epidemiology, and End Result program (SEER) show a decrease in incidence of invasive cervical cancer from 1975 to 1986 in all age groups but one (80-84 years). For carcinoma *in situ*, incidence increased in only three age groups (15-19 years, 20-24 years, and 80-84 years). He urges caution in making a final conclusion since the increase was observed for only two years and was quite small. He points out that there are several studies that refute the evidence of a "fast moving" group. He presents a modeling technique for a "worst case scenario" which indicates that if the "fast mover" concept is true, then increasing the screening frequency would have marginal gains. Debate on this issue will no doubt continue, but over time data should become available to provide solid information on a strong controversy.

REDUCTION IN INCIDENCE AND MORTALITY

A decrease in the incidence of ICC has been observed in several studies. In Aberdeen, Scotland, McGregor found that the incidence of ICC in women over age 30 was 55 per 100,000 in women screened and 310 per 100,000 in those unscreened (MacGregor 1986). Data from British Columbia showed a similar pattern, with a difference of about 5 per 100,000 screened to 29 per 100,000 in unscreened women over 20 years of age (Fidler, Boyes, and Locke 1968). The Walton Report also described a strong correlation between screening intensity and decreased cervical cancer mortality (Walton Report 1976). Even when socioeconomic variables were considered, the observed decline in mortality strongly correlated with the intensity of screening. Virtually every study showed a reduction in the incidence of ICC, as well as a decrease in cervical cancer mortality, following the initiation of detection programs using cervical cytology (Guzick 1978). In a report from Iceland analyzing an intensive nationwide cervical cancer screening program, the annual mortality rate began to decline during the first few years of screening, and in 1978 was less than half the rate observed prior to screening (Johanneson, Geirsson, and Day 1978). Furthermore, the incidence of stages II, III, and IV cancers also decreased. Most deaths were in women who had never received a Pap test.

RISK OF ERROR

Recent stories in the press have called attention to errors in the reading of a Pap test (*Wall Street Journal* 1987). Misinterpretation of the smear appears to be the test's major risk. It is critical that the physician performing the Pap test obtain an adequate sample for review.

The rate of false-negative and false-positive results is difficult to ascertain. In clinical practice, 20% to 30% seem to be an estimate of the false-negative rate. Sedlis and his colleagues compared two slides taken from the same woman and found evidence of CIS present in only one slide 30% of the time. For dysplasia, the discrepancy occurred in half the patients (Sedlis et al. 1974).

Pathologists may also reach different conclusions on the same slide. Ten cytologists disagreed considerably in 38% of CIS and 44% of ICC.

Tissue specimens may also be misread. Brundell found that a panel of experts to which he referred disagreed in 32% of 728 specimens, and estimated that differences of opinion in histopathologic diagnosis could lead to as many as 150 unjustified hysterectomies among their samples of patients (Brundell, Cox, and Taylor 1973). A recent review of the status of cervical cancer detection emphasizes current needs (Koss 1989).

One of the major crises facing cervical cancer detection is the shortage of cytotechnologists. A recent women's magazine listed cytotechnology as one of the worst careers for a woman. The recruitment and training opportunities must be addressed quickly. The shortage has benefitted those persons in the cytotechnology field in terms of increased salaries—a plus. However, vigilance must be maintained as to what this shortage will do to Pap test costs, which could rise and make this important cancer detection test inaccessible for the women at greatest need—the underserved.

COST AND USE OF RESOURCES

The decision about the regularity of the Pap test must take into account the benefits, the cost of the examination, and the factors related to the health care delivery system. Unfortunately, no information from prospective clinical trials exists to settle the question of periodicity. Decisions must be based on available information.

A period of detectable precancerous changes, which ranges from three to 30 years, precedes invasive cancer. Many of the international studies used screening intervals greater than one year, usually three to five years. Their estimates suggest that Pap tests performed every three years deliver 97% of the efficacy of those taken annually (ACS 1983). However, the acceptance of longer intervals does not take into account the attitudes of women and primary care physicians.

The reliability of the Pap test has been cited as an important factor in determining its frequency. Shortening the screening interval to overcome possible problems with slide interpretation and quality control only adds to an already overburdened system.

Eddy has recently discussed the costs for the Pap test. He reports that while the laboratory charges for the Pap test are low, approximately $3, the total charge for a Pap test range from $34 to $100. These costs are based on a survey of 20 instructors and physicians, including clinic and physician fees.

The most important strategy for the future is to involve women who do not have the Pap test in screening programs because that group has the highest mortality. Many women in the unscreened group are poor, are unable to afford the test, and have limited access to screening programs.

CANCER OF THE LUNG

INTRODUCTION

Cancer of the lung is the second most common cancer in the United States. An estimated 161,000 cases are expected to occur in 1991 (ACS 1991). Its responsibility for a shockingly high number of deaths — 143,000 estimated for 1991—makes it the greatest cancer killer of Americans. In women, lung cancer deaths have surpassed deaths due to breast cancer, which for over 40 years was the number one cause of cancer deaths in women.

Lung cancer treatment over the last 10 years has only slightly improved survival rates. The overall 5-year survival rate is only 13%. The rate is 37% for cases localized to the lung, but only 20% of lung cancers are discovered that early.

Cigarette smoking is the major cause of lung cancer. The American Cancer Society estimates that cigarette smoking is responsible for 85% of lung cancer cases in men and 75% in women — about 83% overall. The cancer death rate for male smokers is double that of nonsmokers, and for female smokers it is 67% higher.

The combined efforts of many organizations, health professionals, government officials, legislators, and public educators have led to a dramatic decrease in the rate of cigarette smoking. Smokers made up 29.1% of the total population in 1987, down from 30.4% in 1985. This is a sign that the significant public health problems related to cigarette smoking may decrease. In the interim, strategies to deal with the significant mortality associated with cigarette smoking continue to vex the U.S. health care delivery system. Prevention and smoking cessation are critical actions that must be promoted to the public. The recent Surgeon General's report on Smoking and Health points out the addictive nature of nicotine and provides guidance for prevention and cessation techniques (U.S. Department of Health and Human Services 1989).

Industrial workers are especially susceptible to lung diseases due to the combined effects of cigarette smoking and exposure to toxic industrial substances, such as fumes from rubber and chlorine and dust from cotton and coal. Exposure to asbestos in combination with cigarette smoking increases an individual's risk for cancer many-fold.

STATUS OF CHEST X-RAY EXAMINATION AND SPUTUM CYTOLOGY

In 1980, the ACS could not find evidence that chest x-ray examinations and sputum cytology for asymptomatic persons, even those at high risk, reduced the mortality from lung cancer (ACS 1980). Therefore, the ACS did not recommend chest x-ray examination or sputum cytology as part of its Cancer-Related Checkup Guidelines. The publication of the guidelines provoked debate among health professionals, many of whom believed that chest x-ray examination was an important intervention for high-risk persons. In the Surveys of Primary Care Physician's Attitudes and Practices in Cancer Detection, over 40% of the physicians surveyed said they offered chest x-rays to asymptomatic persons (ACS 1985; ACS 1990).

The results of four prospective randomized clinical trials have been completed since 1980 (Fontana 1986; Berlin et al. 1984; Melamed et al. 1980; Stitik and Tockman 1978). The ACS has reviewed data from these trials and suggests that physicians and high risk asymptomatic persons determine if chest x-rays are indicated. Screening by x-ray and/or sputum cytology in normal-risk nonsmoking persons does not seem indicated. The major emphasis of intervention continues to be the elimination of cigarette smoking. Physicians must strenuously urge all their patients—especially those at high risk—to stop, or not to start, smoking cigarettes or using tobacco in any form.

RATIONALE FOR EARLY CANCER DETECTION RECOMMENDATIONS

The effects of screening with chest x-ray examination and/or sputum cytology in asymptomatic patients to reduce the overall mortality rate from lung cancer have been studied for many years. For example, the Philadelphia Pulmonary Neoplasm Research Project, begun in 1951, screened over 6,000 men age 45 and older with chest x-ray examination and questionnaires every six months (Boucot and Weiss 1973). Although the study was neither randomized nor controlled, it showed an overall 5-year survival rate of only 8% for newly detected cancers, the same as the national statistic at that time for unscreened patients.

From 1958 to 1961, a population of 14,607 high-risk residents of Veterans Administration Domiciliaries were screened for lung cancer with chest x-ray examination and sputum cytology at approximately 6-month intervals for three years (Lilienfeld et al. 1966). Among a total of 200 lung cancers, only 26% could be resected, and only three patients survived three years (a 6%, 3-year survival rate). This study was not a randomized clinical trial, but the data imply that those procedures were of no value in improving the prognosis of lung cancer in the population studied.

In the South London Cancer Study, another uncontrolled trial, all men age 45 and older who attended the southeast and southwest London Mass Radiography Services between January 1, 1959, and June 30, 1963, were offered semiannual chest x-ray examinations for 1½ years (Nash, Morgan, and Tomkins 1968). In this period, 147 lung cancers were detected, for a discovery rate of about 0.7 per 1,000 man-years of surveillance. Of those 147 cancers, 87 were found by patients in the interval between screening. The 4-year survival rate was only 18%.

A randomized controlled trial conducted in the late 1960s by the Kaiser Health Foundation encouraged 5,000 patients, age 35 to 54, to undergo multiphasic screening that included an annual chest x-ray examination, spirometry, and a medical questionnaire (Dales

1979). A control group was not similarly encouraged but could obtain these services upon request. About 50% of the study group and 20% of the control group had the checkup each year. After 11 years of follow-up, there were 25 deaths from cancer in the study group, compared to 26 in the control group. The trial was not specifically designed to evaluate screening for lung cancer, but it is pertinent that no difference in cancer death was observed.

The Mass Radiography Service in northwest London also carried out a controlled but non-randomized investigation of two populations of English factory workers in the 1960s (Brett 1969). During a 3-year period, the lung cancer survival rate for 29,723 men, age 40 and older, who received chest x-ray examinations every six months was compared to that of a control group of approximately 25,311 men. The 5-year survival rate from lung cancer in the study group was 15% vs. 6% in the control group. The annual mortality from lung cancer was 0.7 per 1,000 in the study population and 0.8 per 1,000 in controls.

In 1971, the National Cancer Institute's Cooperative Early Lung Cancer Detection Program initiated three randomized controlled trials at the Johns Hopkins University Hospital in Baltimore; the Mayo Clinic in Rochester, Minnesota; and the Memorial Sloan-Kettering Cancer Center in New York City (Fontana 1986; Berlin et al. 1984; Melamed et al. 1980; Stitik and Tockman 1978). This was the most comprehensive lung cancer detection study to date.

The three studies had somewhat different study designs. At the Mayo Clinic, sputum cytology and chest x-ray examination were performed every four months, compared to performing them annually. At Johns Hopkins and Memorial Sloan-Kettering, annual chest x-ray examination plus triennial sputum cytology were compared to annual chest x-ray examination only. These projects were not designed to test the value of chest x-ray examination, since both study and control groups received annual examinations, but rather to evaluate the impact of sputum cytology. More than 30,000 men 45 years of age and older who smoked 20 or more cigarettes daily were enrolled in the three programs. The end point was considered to be 5-year survival in the New York study, while the other two used mortality rates.

Results showed that chest x-ray examination can detect presymptomatic early stage lung cancer, particularly of the squamous cell type. An increase in resection rates was seen in the three studies as well, but these apparent improvements were offset with further follow-up. All three studies had similar outcomes: no significant difference existed in all cancer mortality or lung cancer mortality between the two groups, and no significant difference was found between the number of stage III and unresected lung cancers in the dual screen and control groups. At Memorial Sloan-Kettering, the 5-year survival rate in both groups approached 35%, while at Johns Hopkins, the 7-year survival in both groups was 20%.

Two other studies, one from Czechoslovakia (using chest x-ray and sputum cytology) and the other from the German Democratic Republic (using annual chest x-ray), did not show any effect from screening or lung cancer mortality (Kuhik 1986, Ebeling 1987).

The results of these trials "do not justify recommending large-scale radiologic or cytologic screening for lung cancer for normal-risk persons. This type of activity is usually initiated by those who conduct the screening and should benefit the screened by reducing lung cancer mortality. The National Cancer Institute-sponsored screening programs failed to do this" (Fontana 1986).

A more recent analysis of the Hopkins and Memorial data attempted to minimize potential biases by controlling for them in Cox regression analysis or by eligibility considerations. Conclusions drawn were that the impact of chest x-rays on survival may correspond to a 30% reduction in lung cancer mortality in radiology incident screen-detected cases compared to symptomatic cases. Given that only 37% of the cancers were incident screen-detected by chest x-ray, the projected reduction of lung cancer mortality in a population of smokers screened with chest x-ray would be about 11% (Chu, Smart, and Byar 1990). Further discussion of this analytic approach will, no doubt, be necessary to determine clinical implications.

RISKS OF SCREENING

Risks are associated with screening for lung cancer. First, there is the possibility of a carcinogenic effect from the x-ray. Although the radiation delivered by one chest x-ray examination is low, the significance of repeated exposures is unknown.

Sputum cytology carries no direct risk but does have the hazard of false-positive examinations. If the pathologist sees cells suggestive of cancer, a diagnostic workup must be undertaken. If no source for the cells can be found, and the patient shows no further evidence of disease, follow-up of the patient should be continued.

Grzybowski and Coy found that 5.5% of 2,112 screened men had a suspicious chest x-ray examination requiring a diagnostic workup, but only 10 of these (8.9%) had lung cancer (Grzybowski and Coy 1970). The Veterans Administration Lung Cancer Screening Study noted that cancer was suspected on chest x-ray examination in approximately 3% of noncancer patients. Melamed found that almost 100 patients with suspicious findings had to be evaluated for every cancer found (Melamed et al. 1981).

On the initial examination of 6,612 subjects, 34 (0.5%) had a negative chest x-ray examination but positive sputum cytology. Of these, only six (18%) were eventually found to have cancer of the lung, while two had cancer of the larynx.

COST AND USE OF RESOURCES

The follow-up of a suspicious detection examination can be expensive, especially for cytology, when the exact source is unknown. Workup may include hospitalization and bronchoscopy (rigid for inspection and differential bronchial washings, fiberoptic for visualization and bronchial brushings). The costs of such workups are well over $1,000 and may increase significantly as CT and MRI are used. The studies have been done in major medical centers using pulmonologists, pathologists, and radiologists experienced in lung cancer detection techniques. The number and intensity of workups would be expected to increase if these detection examinations were done by less-experienced health professionals.

The costs in resources for chest x-ray examination and sputum cytology are tremendous. The average cost for chest x-ray is approximately $50 and sputum cytology is $60. If all smokers over 40 years in the United States were screened with chest x-ray, the cost in 1988 for screening alone would have approximated $1.5 billion (Eddy 1989). There is good reason to believe that this money could be used more effectively for the primary prevention of lung cancer and to prevent and detect other cancers.

Advocating early detection of lung cancer may give patients a false sense of security in two ways. First, it may lead some people to believe that the disease can be diagnosed and cured through early detection and thereby decrease their interest in smoking cessation. In a recent poll, about seven out of 10 cigarette smokers expressed a belief that there is "a very good chance" or "a fairly good chance" that lung cancer is curable if detected early (Nash, Morgan, and Tomkins 1968). Second, an early detection test can miss a patient who has cancer, and the false reassurance may make him or her less alert to signs and symptoms. There is little evidence that a delay in treatment by a few months would affect survival.

APPENDIX*

DESIGN ISSUES FOR RANDOMIZED CLINICAL TRIALS

ACTING WITH INCOMPLETE INFORMATION

Several factors complicate the design of a cancer early detection program, perhaps the most important of which is the lack of complete information about the benefits or risks of any screening test or procedure. For each recommendation, it would be ideal to have evidence obtained from a randomized, controlled trial (RCT) that the test is effective in reducing morbidity and mortality. Beyond that, for each test there should be controlled comparisons of its costs, risks, and benefits when used in different combinations, in different populations (e.g., age and risk groups), and at different frequencies.

Unfortunately, information is available from only a limited number of clinical tests (for breast and lung cancer). The available evidence for the expected benefits and risks of various early detection protocols is much more circumstantial because it is based on controlled, not randomized, studies; on uncontrolled studies; on seasoned clinical judgment; and on anecdotes. In brief,

if making a recommendation demands proof of effectiveness in the form of randomized, controlled trials (and if the external validity of the RCT is accepted), then the analysis is simple: do nothing except to screen women over 50 for breast cancer.

Unfortunately, this recommendation is not very helpful to the practicing clinician, who realizes that one of four persons will get cancer, that a wait for perfect information is a wait forever, and that decisions must be made today. A missed opportunity to use an effective test can be as harmful and wasteful as a premature decision to use an ineffective test. It is simply impossible to have perfect information before making decisions. At any given time, the clinician must make the best decision he or she can based on available information.

This considerably increases the difficulty of designing an early detection protocol. The results of well-designed and well-conducted controlled trials are comparatively easy to interpret. The other sources of information are less precise and open to misinterpretation.

MULTIPLE OPTIONS

Other factors complicate the analysis. Rarely is a medical procedure obviously worth the risks and cost. The value of most early detection tests depends upon how they are used, in what populations, and at what frequencies. There is a prior reason, for example, to assume that an early detection test should be given annually, or that if more than one test is available to detect a disease, they should all be used at every checkup. Each of the possible combinations has a different medical effectiveness, risk, and cost.

COSTS

Checkups involve time for both patients and clinicians. Equipment and supplies must be purchased. Busy physicians, nurses, and technicians must perform and interpret tests, then do a workup on patients who have positive results. These and other activities related to the cancer checkup use resources that will then no longer be available to other patients with other medical problems.

One measure of the practicality of medical activity is its financial cost. Although this measure does not begin to include all the factors that are important to a medical decision, it provides an index of the resources consumed and, when combined with information about medical benefits and risks, helps in comparing what can be accomplished with different health programs. This is the reason that financial costs of each recommendation are presented. There is no way to determine the dollar value of pain, anxiety, or death, but it is possible to compare the costs of different recommendations designed to reduce that suffering.

VALUES

A further complexity is that no correct answer or perfect cancer control protocol exists. Selection of a single protocol requires comparing an improvement in morbidity and mortality with some risks and costs; the selection will depend on the relative values placed on

---

*Reprinted from: American Cancer Society. 1980. Guidelines for the cancer-related checkup: recommendations and rationale. *CA* 30(4).

those outcomes. For example, which is better: a $1,000 program that delivers 30 days of life expectancy or a $4,000 program that delivers 50 days of life expectancy? The answer will depend on who is asked: what is appropriate for one individual may not be appropriate for a national organization; what is acceptable to one group may not be acceptable to another. Because of these reasons, it is important that these recommendations be considered as only guidelines and not as rules. Individuals, patients, and physicians may interpret the available data differently, may have different priorities, and may logically choose to allocate their resources differently.

COST-EFFECTIVENESS ANALYSIS

Cancer detection protocols are not analyzed for their cost-effectiveness in the sense that they place a value on a human life or trade lives for dollars. However, cost-effectiveness is analyzed in the sense that it searches for the best way to obtain the benefits of early detection with the available resources while reducing costs, risks, and inconvenience. The new recommendations deliver to each individual examined virtually the same benefits as the old recommendations, but far more safely and efficiently. Furthermore, by freeing resources, they make possible a greatly increased benefit to the population as a whole. When coupled with public and professional education programs, the new recommendations should deliver more health at less cost.

POPULATIONS VS. INDIVIDUALS

Another issue is the distinction between the design of a mass screening program and recommendations for individual physicians and patients. When there are insufficient data to justify a broad recommendation that everyone be screened, it may still be advisable for individual physicians to recommend for individual patients a protocol that is identical to the broad recommendations. First, it must be recognized that if any early detection program is recommended for all individuals — whether by the government, the ACS, or practitioners — then what happens to each individual will add up to what happens to the population as a whole. On the other hand, there are important features of an early detection program recommended on an individual basis that may make it acceptable when mass screening is not. The very nature of mass screening, in which recruitment is aggressive and may afford little opportunity for individual communication and quality control, implies that the evidence of benefits is clear-cut and the risks are negligible. If the evidence of benefits is unknown, or suggestive but not proven, or there are significant risks or costs, then a yearly detection test may be appropriate only if delivered on an individual, face-to-face basis. This is necessary so that the benefits and risks can be explained carefully and the administration and follow-up of the test can be monitored closely. For example, the ACS does not believe that sufficient evidence of benefit exists at present to justify a broad recommenda-

tion that asymptomatic people, even smokers, be given annual chest x-ray examinations. However, if the evidence of benefits and risks is carefully explained, some practitioners may quite properly decide to recommend such examinations for selected individuals.

FLEXIBILITY

Finally, the acknowledged inadequacy of the current information base, the rapidity with which cancer control technology changes, and the constant availability of new data make it important to interpret these recommendations as interim guidelines. They are based on the best information available today and should be reviewed as new tests and more information become available.

THE EVALUATION OF EARLY DETECTION TESTS AND PROCEDURES

Two steps are involved in the evaluation of an early detection test. First, its impact must be estimated — the costs, risks, and effect on morbidity and mortality. Then, those outcomes must be compared. Various criteria are used to judge the net effectiveness of an early detection protocol.

Suppose it is possible to accurately measure the outcomes of different programs. How do we select the best? Several measures have been used to determine the value of a test, but unfortunately no single measure is adequate. There is no simple process for determining the cost-effectiveness of a screening test or procedure; both cost and effectiveness are multidimensional phenomena, and there is a constant tension between them. For example, the following are all reasonable measures of the effectiveness of a procedure: change of life expectancy; the probability of curing a patient of his or her cancer; the 5-, 10-, 15-year (or any other interval) survival rate; decrease in morbidity; improvement in quality in life; decrease in earnings lost because of premature death; decrease in disability days; reduction in anxiety; and others. Although there is much overlap, no single measure dominates or contains all the others, nor do they all move in the same direction at once.

Similarly, a screening procedure has many types of costs and risks, such as the direct financial costs of screening, the relative discomfort of a sigmoidoscopy, the morbidity of a workup for a false-positive test, lost time from work, the psychologic costs of a biopsy, and others.

Various measures have been developed to try to summarize the results of experiments and to indicate their value. It is important to understand their strengths and limitations.

ABILITY TO DETECT OCCULT CANCERS

Perhaps the most commonly used criterion is simply whether a test can detect cancers in an asymptomatic population. Finding a cancer in a patient who has no signs or symptoms of disease clearly demonstrates that the diagnosis has been made early. However, it says nothing about the importance of detecting the cancer earlier, the effectiveness of therapy, the risks of the test, the costs, or the resources consumed. An ability to detect occult cancers is necessary but not sufficient. A program designed to include all tests that can detect occult cancers would have a direct financial cost of over $20 billion, about twice the total direct costs of all cancers.

YIELD

The yield of an early detection program is the proportion of persons discovered by the test to have the disease. More formally, it is the prevalence of detectable disease in an asymptomatic population and is controlled by the incidence rate of the disease and the duration of its preclinical stage. Unfortunately, it says little about whether detecting the disease early has any benefit. For example, a disease could be common and serious if left untreated, but the patient almost always seeks care for symptoms while it is still in a curable state (e.g., cancer of the skin). Another disease might be common, and early detection might have a high yield, but there might be no effective treatment. Or the disease might be relatively rare (as in fact most cancers are) and the cost of early detection might have a high yield, but there might be no effective treatment. The disease might be relatively rare, but the cost of early detection for even a low yield might be justified if earlier detection and treatment make a great difference to the few patients found through early detection (e.g., cancer of the cervix). In short, the yield tells us only about the frequency with which a disease is detected; it tells us little about the importance of early detection.

COST-PER-CASE DETECTED

This measure at least combines information about the yield with information about program cost, but it can lead to some obviously incorrect recommendations. For example, the lowest cost-per-case detected is achieved by not screening at all. Any cases not detected will eventually be detected by the patients themselves—at no detection cost.

DETECTING CANCERS IN EARLIER STAGES

It is well-known that patients with cancers detected in earlier stages tend to live longer after diagnosis and treatment than do patients detected with advanced disease. It is also known that screening tends to detect cancers in earlier stages. A simple projection of the fact that with early detection more patients achieve better survival rates would seem to suggest that screened patients live longer. Unfortunately, while the finding of cancers in earlier stages carries a great deal of helpful information, it suffers from several biases.

COMPARISON OF CASE-SURVIVAL RATES

The use of staging information requires making some mathematical projections, but an examination of case-survival rates does not and thus appears to provide even more straightforward evidence of effectiveness. It is frequently observed, for example, that the 2-, 5-, or 10-year survival rates of screened patients are higher than those of unscreened patients. Unfortunately, this measure also suffers from the biases that must be considered before any conclusions can be drawn.

MAXIMIZING HEALTH BENEFITS

It is often stated that the physician's objective should be "to deliver the best medical care possible," implying in the case of early detection programs that every effort should be made to maximize patient survival and life expectancy. The obvious objection to this criterion is that it ignores risks, side effects, and costs. If we really believed it, we would screen with a Pap test every day. This is not done because the costs—which include patient discomfort, lost time, and perhaps some unnecessary conizations and hysterectomies—are too high. As desirable as this maxim sounds, it cannot always be followed in practice.

BENEFIT-COST RATIO

Clearly, one cannot look only at benefits, costs, or risks. Improving one factor worsens another, so they must be considered together, and the best combination selected. The benefit-cost ratio has been offered to help achieve this. This measure, however, suffers from two major problems. First, it must be possible to put all the important outcomes into a single measure, usually dollars. The financial value of pain, disability, and life must be known. While we all do this implicitly in our everyday lives (e.g., when we buy a smoke detector or spend an extra $10 to purchase a sturdier motorcycle helmet), at present we do not know enough to do it explicitly in a fair and consistent manner. The second problem is that depending on whether an outcome is listed as a cost or a benefit, the same program can be determined to have different benefit-cost ratios.

For example, suppose a program with a direct cost of $1,000 delivers an increase in life expectancy worth $2,000 and saves the patient $500 in lost time from work. If the $500 savings is combined with the $1,000 cost to deliver a net cost of $500 ($1,000 minus $500), the benefit-cost ratio is $2,000 to $500, or 4:1. If the $500 savings is listed as a benefit (bringing the total benefits to $2,000 plus $500 or $2,500), the benefit-cost ratio is $2,500 to $1,000, or 2.5:1. The same program has two different ratios.

A balanced evaluation must incorporate all of the important outcomes. Because no single measure of cost-effectiveness exists, designing the best program requires reviewing all the outcomes that occur with each recommendation and identifying the one that delivers the best package. At present there is probably no better way to do this than to study and apply careful personal judgment. However, doing this well requires being as careful, accurate, complete, and consistent as possible.

EXPERIMENTAL BIASES IN EARLY DETECTION PROGRAMS

Complications are encountered when programs are being designed and interpreted. There are countless ways to destroy the value of a study. Most can be spotted easily, but in the analysis of early detection programs, there are four biases that are more subtle.

LEAD TIME BIAS

A test that can detect a condition before it is detectable by other means, that appears to detect cancers in earlier stages, and that delivers higher case-survival rates does not necessarily mean that it will increase the chance for a cure or prolong a patient's life. It is possible that the time of detection and the stage of detection have no effect on the course of disease and that earlier detection only moves forward the time of a patient's diagnosis, without moving back the time of death.

The interval between the moment a condition is actually detected and the moment that condition would have been detected otherwise (by the patient through the observance of signs and symptoms) is known as the lead time. To be effective, early detection must increase the lead time of diagnosis. However, some increase in lead time will automatically result from merely moving up the time of diagnosis, and early detection may increase the length of time that the patient is aware of the disease without prolonging his or her life.

Because of the lead time effect, a comparison of 10-year survival rates in screened or unscreened populations can be misleading. By itself, the earlier diagnosis will increase the interval between a patient's diagnosis and death, which in turn will increase the probability that the patient is alive five or 10 years after the time of diagnosis (the 5- and 10-year survival rates).

PATIENT SELF-SELECTION BIAS

Persons who elect to receive early detection tests may be different from those who do not in ways that could affect their survival from a disease such as cancer. For example, they could be more health conscious; more likely to control risk factors such as smoking, diet, and sexual habits; more alert to the signs and symptoms of disease; more adherent to treatment; or generally healthier. Any of these factors could produce a longer survival from cancer in a way that is independent of early detection, and the observance of better survival in screened patients as compared with the general population could be due more to the selection of patients than to the effect of early detection.

The bias can be accommodated by tracking the survival of all the patients offered early detection tests, including those who reject the offer, and comparing it to the survival of a comparable group not offered early detection. The bias is much more difficult to correct for retrospective studies. A chart review may show that patients diagnosed through early detection have earlier-stage cancers than those who sought care on their own, but it is extremely difficult to identify the patients who were offered but refused an early detection protocol, or the so-called interval cases that were dutifully examined but missed.

LENGTH BIAS

A third problem is that cancers detected by a test in a periodic early detection program tend to have longer-than-average preclinical intervals. Conversely, the interval cases tend to be cancers with shorter preclinical intervals. The preclinical interval is the interval between the time a screening test could detect a cancer and the time a patient would seek care on his or her own initiative because of signs and symptoms in the absence of an early detection protocol. The selection of cancers with long preclinical intervals through early detection examinations is known as the length bias, and it complicates the interpretation of data derived only from a screened population.

The duration of this interval is related to the tumor's growth rate and other biological characteristics and to the patient's awareness of cancer signs and symptoms. Both of these factors can influence how long a patient survives from the time of diagnosis. For example, it may be that tumors with long preclinical intervals have slower growth rates and are less malignant. Thus, compared to control or untested persons, cancers detected at scheduled examinations have longer preclinical intervals that may imply slower growth rates, less malignant tumors, and longer survival. Patients with cancers missed at the early detection examinations but detected by self-examination have shorter preclinical intervals, which may mean faster growth rates and lower survival.

Conversely, the preclinical interval can be longer if a patient delays seeking care. This lengthens the preclinical interval by postponing its end point without changing the cancer's rate of growth. Patients with cancers self-detected between scheduled examinations may have short preclinical intervals because they are very alert to signs and symptoms, and they may have better-than-average prognoses. This was observed in the HIP study, where such patients had better 7-year case-survival rates (57.6%) than the controls (52.3%) (ACS 1980).

OVERDIAGNOSIS

Overdiagnosis is another problem that can confuse the interpretation of data regarding tumor stage at the time of diagnosis and affect case-survival rates in an early detection program. The purpose of early cancer detection examinations is to find cancers when they are small. Unfortunately, there is no sharp boundary early on between nonmalignant and malignant cells as seen under a microscope, and it is quite possible to over-diagnose a noncancerous lesion as a very early cancer. As well as increasing the number of so-called cancers detected, this can inflate the number of cancers detected in the earliest stage, and, because these lesions would never become clinically significant cancers, it can inflate survival statistics. To correct for this possibility, it must be ascertained that all the patients actually have cancer, which is best done by counting cancer deaths in a RCT.

SUMMARY

Because of problems such as lead time, patient selection, length bias, and overdiagnosis, it can be misleading to draw conclusions from knowledge of a tumor's stage at the time of detection to case-survival rates. These biases are eliminated by RCTs in which the mortality in the entire group offered early detection examinations is compared to the mortality of the control group. This is why the RCT is so popular. This type of information is rarely available, however, and estimates of the value of early detection must usually be based on the results of other types of studies. Fortunately, the biases do not mean that such information is useless. Nonrandomized and uncontrolled studies can provide a great deal of information, as can projections from the stage at time of detection, case-survival rates, and other measures. The point is that these outcomes must be interpreted with great care, recognizing the problems and adjusting for them whenever possible.

REFERENCES

Ahlquist, D.A.; McGill, D.B.; and Schwartz, S. et al. 1985. Fecal blood levels in health and disease: a study using Hemoquant. *N. Engl. J. Med.* 312:1412-25.

American Cancer Society. 1980. Guidelines for the cancer-related checkup: recommendations and rationale. *CA* 30:4-50.

American Cancer Society. 1983. Cancer of the colon and rectum: a summary of a public attitude survey. *CA* 33:31-37.

American Cancer Society. 1985. Mammography guidelines 1983: background statement and update for the cancer-related checkup guidelines for breast cancer detection in asymptomatic women age 40-49. *CA* 33:255.

American Cancer Society. 1985. Survey of physician's attitudes and practices in early cancer detection. *CA* 36:97-213.

American Cancer Society. 1987. *Breast self-examination* (pamphlet). New York: American Cancer Society.

American Cancer Society. 1990. Survey of physician's attitudes and practice in early cancer detection. *CA* 40:77-101.

American Cancer Society. 1990. *Cancer facts and figures.* American Cancer Society: Atlanta.

Baines, C.J. 1987. Breast self-examination. In Day, N.E., and Miller, A.B. eds. *Screening for breast cancer.* pp. 85-91. Toronto: Hans Huber.

Baker, L. 1982. Breast Cancer Detection Demonstration Project: five-year summary report. *CA* 32:194-203.

Barrosso, R.; DeBrux, J.; and Croissant, O. et al. 1987. High prevalence of papilloma virus-associated penile intra-epithelial neoplasia in sexual partners of women with cervical intra-epithelial neoplasia. *N. Engl. J. Med.* 317:916.

Berlin, N.I.; Buncher, C.R.; and Fontana, R.S. et al. 1984. The National Cancer Institute Cooperative Early Lung Cancer Detection Program: results of the initial screen (prevalence): early lung cancer detection: introduction. *Am. Rev. Respir. Dis.* 130:S45-S49.

Bogdanich, W. 1987. Lax laboratories: the Pap test misses much cervical cancer through labs' error; cut-rate "Pap mills" process slides using screeners with incentives to rush; misplaced sense of security? *Wall Street Journal* Nov. 21, 1987.

Boucot, K.R., and Weiss, W. 1973. Is curable lung cancer detected by semiannual screening? *JAMA* 224:1361-65.

Brett, G.Z. 1969. Earlier diagnosis and survival in lung cancer. *Br. Med. J.* 4:260-62.

Brundell, M.; Cox, B.S.; and Taylor, C.W. 1973. The manuscript of dysplasia, carcinoma *in situ* and microcarcinoma of the cervix. *J. Obstet. Gynaecol. Br. Comm.* 80:673-79.

Burghardt, E. 1973. *Early histological diagnosis of cervical cancer.* p. 263. Philadelphia: W.B. Saunders.

Canadian Task Force on the Periodic Health Examination. 1979. The periodic health examination. *Can. Med. Assoc. J.* 121:1193-1254.

Christopherson, W. Jan. 5, 1980. Personal communication.

Chu, K; Smart, C.R.; and Byar, D. Analysis of benefits of chest x-rays using data from the randomized lung cancer trials as a prospective study of chest x-ray (unpublished report).

Clemmesen, J., and Poulsen, H. 1971. Report of the Ministry of the Interior, Doc. 3, Copenhagen.

Collette, H.J.A.; Rombach, J.J.; and DeWaard. et al. 1987. An update of the DOM Project for the early detection of breast cancer. In Day, N.E., and Miller, A.B. eds. *Screening for breast cancer.* pp. 17-27. Toronto: Hans Huber.

Constanza, M.C., and Foster, R.C. 1984. Relationship between breast self-examination and death from breast cancer by age groups. *Cancer Det. Prev.* 7:103-108.

Dales, L.G.; Friedman, G.D.; and Collen, M.F. 1979. Evaluating periodic multiphase health checkups: a controlled trial. *J. Cron. Dis.* 32:385-404.

Davis, H. 1967. The biologic status of carcinoma *in situ* of the uterine cervix. *Obstet. Gynecol. Surv.* 22:176-77.

Day, N.E., and Miller, A.B. eds. 1987. Progress report of the UK trial of early detection of breast cancer. In *Screening for breast cancer.* pp. 45-49. Toronto: Hans Huber.

Dodd, G.D.; Fink, D.F.; and Bertram, D.A. 1987. Proceedings of a workshop to lower the costs of screening mammography—1986. *Cancer* 60:1669-1702.

Dunn, J., and Martin, P.L. 1967. Morphogenesis of cervical cancer: findings from San Diego County cytology registry. *Cancer* 20:1899-1906.

Ebeling, K., and Nischan, P. 1987. Screening for lung cancer: results from a case control study. *Int. J. Cancer.* 40:141-44.

Eddy, D.M. 1986. A computer-based model for designing cancer control strategies. *Natl. Cancer Inst. Monogr.* 2:75-82.

Eddy, D.M.; Hasselblad, V.; and McGivney, W. et al. 1988. The value of mammography screening in women under age 50 years. *JAMA* 259(10):1512-19.

Eddy, D.M. 1989. Screening for breast cancer. *Ann. Int. Med.* 111:389-99.

Eddy, D.M. 1990. Screening for colorectal cancer. *Ann. Int. Med.* 113:373-84.

Eddy, D.M. 1990. Screening for cervical cancer. *Ann. Int. Med.* 113:214-26.

Eddy, D.M. 1989. Screening for lung cancer. *Ann. Int. Med.* 111:232-37.

Ekiland, G.; Carlson, V.; and Jonzon, L. 1985. The feasibility of large scale population screening. *Brit. J. Surg.* 72:571.

Enker, W.E., and DeCosse, J. 1981. The evolving surgical treatment of rectum and colon cancer. *CA* 31:66-74.

Fagerberg, C.G., and Tabar, L. 1987. The results of periodic one view mammography screening: randomized controlled trial in Sweden. In Day, N.E., and Miller, A.B. eds. *Screening for breast cancer.* pp. 33-34. Toronto: Hans Huber.

Fenoglio-Preiser, C.M., and Hutter, R.V. 1985. Colorectal polyps: pathology, diagnosis, and clinical significance. *CA* 35:322-44.

Fidler, H.K.; Boyes, D.H.; and Locke, D.K. 1968. The cytology program in British Columbia. *J. Obstet. Gynaecol. Br. Comm.* 75:392-404.

Fink, D.J. 1988. Change in American Cancer Society checkup guidelines for detection of cervical cancer. *CA* 38:128.

Fink, D.J. 1989. Community programs: breast cancer detection awareness. In *Proceedings of the General Motors/ American Cancer Society symposium on breast cancer detection*. Philadelphia: J.B. Lippincott; *Cancer* 64:2639-2718.

Fontana, R.S. 1986. Screening for lung cancer: recent experience in the United States in lung cancer. In Hansen, H.H. ed. *Lung cancer: basic and clinical aspects*. pp. 91-111. Boston: Martinus Nijhoff.

Foster, R.S.; Lang, S.P.; and Costanza, M.C. et al. 1978. Breast self-examination practices and breast cancer stage. *N. Engl. J. Med.* 299:265-70.

Galvin, G.A.; Jones, H.W. Jr.; and Telinde, R.W. 1952. The clinical relationship of carcinoma *in situ* and invasive carcinoma of the cervix. *JAMA* 149:744-49.

Gilbertson, V.A. 1974. Proctosigmoidoscopy and polypectomy in reducing the incidence of colorectal cancer. *CA* 34: 936-39.

Gilbertson, V.A.; McHugh, R.; and Schunon, L. et al. 1980. The earlier detection of colorectal cancer. *Cancer* 45: 2899-2901.

Gnauck, R.; MacRae, F.A.; and Fleischer, M. 1984. How to perform the fecal occult blood test. *CA* 34:134-47.

Graham, J.B.; Sotto, L.S.; and Paloneck, F.P. 1962. *Carcinoma of the cervix*. Philadelphia: W.B. Saunders.

Greegor, D.H. 1967. Diagnosis of large bowel cancer in the asymptomatic patient. *JAMA* 201:943-45.

Grzybowski, S., and Coy, P. 1970. Early diagnosis of carcinoma of the lung: simultaneous screening with chest x-ray and sputum cytology. *Cancer* 25:113-20.

Guzick, D.S. 1978. Efficacy of screening for cervical cancer: a review. *Am. J. Pub. Health* 68:125-34.

Habemma, M. 1987. Design of the Finnish breast cancer screening study. In Day, N.E., and Miller, A.B. eds. *Screening for breast cancer*. pp. 59-62. Toronto: Hans Huber.

Hardcastle, J.D.; Armitage, N.C.; and Chamberlain, J.J. et al. 1986. Fecal occult blood screening for colorectal cancer in the general population: results of a controlled trial. *Cancer* 58:397-403.

Hertz, R.E.; Deddish, M.R.; and Day, N.E. 1960. Value of periodic examinations in detecting cancer of the rectum and colon. *Postgrad. Med.* 27:290-94.

International Union Against Cancer. 1978. In Miller, A.B. ed. Screening in cancer: report on the International Union Against Cancer (UICC). International workshop, Toronto, Canada, April 24-27, 1978. UICC Technical Report Series, Geneva. *UICC* 40:216-61.

Johanneson, G.; Geirsson, G.; and Day, N. 1978. The effect of mass screening in Iceland 1965-1974 on the incidence and mortality of cervical carcinoma. *Int. J. Cancer* 21:418-25.

Jonsson, E.; Hakansson, A.; and Tabar, L. 1987. Cost of mammography screening for breast cancer: experiences from Sweden. In Day, N.E., and Miller, A.B. eds. *Screening for breast cancer*. Toronto: Hans Huber.

Kashigarian, M., and Dunn, J.E. 1970. The duration of intra-epithelial and preclinical squamous cell carcinoma of the uterine cervix. *Am. J. Epidemiol.* 92:211-22.

Kern, W.H., and Zivolich, M.R. 1977. The accuracy and consistency of the cytologic classification of squamous lesions of the uterine cervix. *Acta. Cytol.* 21:519-28.

Kiser, J.F.; Spratt, J.S.; and Johnson, C.T. 1968. Colon perforation occurring during sigmoidoscopic examination and barium enema. *Mo. Med.* 65:969-74.

Knight, K.K.; Fielding, J.E.; and Battista, R.N. 1986. Occult blood screening for colorectal cancer in the general population: results of a controlled trial. *Cancer* 58:397-403.

Koss, L.G. 1987. Cytologic and histologic manifestations of human papilloma virus infection of the female genital tract and their chemical significance. *Cancer* 60:1942.

Koss, L.G. 1989. The Papanicolaou test for cervical cancer detection: a triumph and a tragedy. *JAMA* 261:737-43.

Koss, L.G.; Stewart, F.W.; and Foote, F.W. et al. 1963. Some histological aspects of behavior of epidermoid carcinoma *in situ* and related lesions of the uterine cervix. *Cancer* 16:1160-1211.

Kottmeier, H.L. 1953. *Carcinoma of the female genitalia*. Baltimore: Williams & Wilkins.

Kottmeier, H.L. 1961. Evolution et traitment des epithelioma. *Rev. Fr. Gynec. Obstet.* 56:821-26.

Kubik, A., and Polak, S. 1986. Lung cancer detection: results of a prospective study in Czechoslovakia. *Cancer.* 57: 2427-37.

LaVecchia, C; Franceshi, S.; and S. DeCarli et al. 1984. "Pap" smear and the risk of cervical neoplasia quantitative estimates from a case-control study. *Lancet* II:779-82.

Lilienfeld, A.; Archer, P.G.; and Burnett, C.H. et al. 1966. An evaluation of radiologic and cytologic screening for the early detection of lung cancer: cooperative pilot study of the American Cancer Society and Veterans Administration. *Cancer Res.* 26:2083-2121.

MacGregor, J.E. 1986. Evaluation of mass screening programs for cervical cancer in N.E. Scotland. *Tumor* 62:287-95.

McKenna, R.S., and Fink, D.J. 1988. Proceedings of a workshop on the community and cancer prevention and detection. *Cancer* 61:2363-2406.

Melamed, M.R.; Flehinger, B.J.; and Zaman, M.B. et al. 1981. Detection of true pathologic stage I lung cancer in a screening program and the effect on survival. Presented at the American Cancer Society National Conference on Cancer Prevention and Detection, Chicago, Ill., April 17-19, 1980. *Cancer* 47:1182-87.

Nash, F.A.; Morgan, J.M.; and Tomkins, J.G. 1968. South London lung cancer study. *Br. Med. J.* 2:715-21.

National Cancer Institute of Canada. 1980. National breast cancer screening study gets under way. *J. Can. Med. Assoc.* 122:243-44.

NCRP. 1986. Mammography, a user's guide. *NCRP Report No. 85*.

Olesen, F. 1988. A case control study of cervical cytology before diagnosis of cervical cancer in Denmark. *Int. J. Epidemiol.* 17:501-508.

O'Malley, M.S., and Fletcher, S.W. 1987. Screening for breast cancer with breast self-examination: a critical review. *JAMA* 257:2197-2203.

Peterson, O. 1955. Precancerous changes of the cervical epithelium in relation to manifest cervical carcinoma. *Acta. Radiol. Suppl.* p. 127.

Peterson, O. 1956. Spontaneous course of cervical precancerous conditions. *Am. J. Obstet. Gynecol.* 72:1063-71.

Prescott, N.; McPherson, K.; and Bell, J. 1980. Cost effectiveness of screening for occult blood in the stool: another look (letter). *N. Engl. J. Med.* 303:1306-1307.

Richart, R. 1987. Causes and management of cervical intraepithelial neoplasia. *Cancer* 60:1951.

Richart, R.M., and Barron, B.A. 1980. Screening strategies for cervical cancer and cervical intra-epithelial neoplasia. Presented at the American Cancer Society National Conference on Cancer Prevention and Detection, Chicago, Ill., April 17-19, 1980.

Sedlis, A.; Walters, A.T.; and Bolen, H. et al. 1974. Evaluation of two simultaneously obtained cervical cytology smears. *Acta. Cytol.* 18:291-96.

Seidman, H.; Gelb, S.K.; and Silverberg, E. et al. 1987. Survival experience in the Breast Cancer Detection Demonstration Projects. *CA* 37:258-90.

Seidman, H.; Stellman, S.D.; and Mushinski, M.H. 1982. A different perspective on breast cancer risk factors: some implications of nonattributable risk. *CA* 32:301-13.

Selby, J.V., and Friedman, G.D. 1989. U.S. Preventive Services Task Force: sigmoidoscopy in the periodic health examination of asymptomatic adults. *JAMA* 261:594-601.

Senie, R.T.; Rosen, P.P.; and Lesser, M.L. 1981. Breast self-examination and medical examination related to breast cancer stage. *Am. J. Pub. Health* 71:583-90.

Shapiro, S. 1988. From research on effectiveness to implementation and evaluation of effectiveness. *H.M.O. Practice* 2:166-76.

Shapiro, S.; Venet, W.; and Strax, P. et al. 1981. *Periodic screening for breast cancer: the Health Insurance Plan project, 1963-1986, and its sequelae.* Baltimore: Johns Hopkins University Press.

Shapiro, S.; Venet, W.; and Strax, P. et al. 1988. Current results of breast cancer screening study: the Health Insurance Plan of Greater New York study. In Day, N.E., and Miller, A.B. eds. *Screening for breast cancer.* Toronto: Hans Huber.

Simon, J.B. 1985. Occult blood screening for colorectal cancer: a critical view. *Gastroenterology* 88:820-87.

Stellman, S.D., and Garfinkel, L. 1986. Smoking habits and tar levels in a new American Cancer Society prospective study of 1.2 million men and women. *J. Natl. Cancer Inst.* 76:1057-63.

Stitik, F.P., and Tockman, M.S. 1978. Radiographic screening in the early detection of lung cancer. *Radiol. Clin. North Am.* 16:347-66.

Swinton, N.R. 1971. In Bolt, R.J. Sigmoidoscopy in detection and diagnosis of asymptomatic individuals. *CA* 28:121-22.

Tabar, L.; Fagerberg, C.; and Gad, A. et al. 1985. Reduction in mortality from breast cancer after mass screening with mammography. *Lancet* I:8299.

Turner, J.; Bloney, R.; and Roy, D. et al. 1984. Does a booklet of breast self-examination improve subsequent detection rates? *Lancet* II:237-39.

U.S. Department of Health and Human Services. 1989. *Reducing the health consequences of smoking: 25 years of progress. A Report of the Surgeon General.* DHHS Publication No. (CDC) 89-8411, prepublication version.

U.S. Food and Drug Administration. 1986. Progress about breast cancer. Washington, D.C.: *U.S. Food and Drug Administration Bulletin.*

Verbeen, A.L.M.; Stratman, H.; and Hendricks, H.C.L. 1987. Sensitivity of mammography in Nijmegem women under age 50. In Day, N.E., and Miller, A.B. eds. *Screening for breast cancer.* pp. 29-32. Toronto: Hans Huber.

Walton Report. 1976. Cervical cancer screening programs. *Can. Med. Assoc. J.* 114:1003-31.

Winawer, S.J.; Andrews, M.; and Flehinger. B. et al. 1980. Progress report on controlled trial of fecal occult blood testing in the detection of colorectal neoplasia. *Cancer* 45:2959-64.

Winawer, S.J.; Leidner, S.D.; and Miller, D.G. et al. 1977. Results of a screening program for the detection of early colon cancer and polyps using fecal occult blood testing. *Gastroenterology* 127:1150.

Winchester, D.P.; Sylvester, J.; and Mobet, M.C. 1983. Needs and benefits of mass screening for colorectal neoplasia with the stool grease test. *CA* 33:5-15.

Chapter 13

BREAST CANCER

Edward F. Scanlon, M.D.

Edward F. Scanlon, M.D.
Kellogg Cancer Care Center
The Evanston Hospital
Evanston, Illinois

INTRODUCTION

Cancer of the breast is the most common major cancer in women in the United States; 29% of all malignant tumors arise there. An estimated 150,000 cases of invasive breast cancer will be diagnosed in 1990; one of every 10 American women will develop breast cancer (American Cancer Society 1990). There has been a slowly progressive increase in the incidence (Horm 1988), but the mortality rate has remained stable. Among women, deaths from breast cancer in 1990 will be second only to those from lung cancer, 44,000 vs. 50,000.

In comparing figures from 1979-82 vs. 1985, the Surveillance, Epidemiology, and End Results (SEER) data reflect an increase in detection of early breast cancer (table 13.1), although the increase in regional and distant metastatic cases at initial visit was not statistically significant (Horm 1988).

The maintenance of a stable mortality rate in the face of a rising incidence is due to many factors, especially early diagnosis. However, some clinicians believe that the benefits of early diagnosis (increased survival rates) result mainly from changes in length and lead-time bias.

Breast cancer is probably the most feared cancer in women because of its frequency and its psychological impact. It affects the perception of sexuality and self-image to a degree far greater than any other cancer. Psychological trauma has lessened in recent years because of earlier diagnosis, more treatment options, and greater availability of reconstruction and rehabilitation programs, including psychosocial counseling.

RISK FACTORS

The cause of breast cancer is unknown, but some factors associated with an increased incidence are more widely accepted than others. Assuredly, the incidence increases as women grow older. Cancer of one breast places the patient at greater risk for developing cancer of the other breast. A family history of breast cancer is an important risk factor, especially if the cancer occurred in the mother and the sister, is bilateral, and developed before menopause. Exposure to ionizing radiation is a risk factor, especially if the exposure occurs before age 35. Early menarche and late menopause are associated with a higher incidence, as are nulliparity and first pregnancy after age 30. However, it is not completely clear whether women who intentionally defer pregnancy to a later age have as great a risk as women who have difficulty becoming pregnant. Although controversial, evidence favors the statement that taking birth control pills does not predispose to the development of breast cancer, but certain subgroups (long-term users, selected age groups, or those whose members took oral contraceptive pills with a high estrogen content) may be at greater risk (Olsson, Moller, and Rantsam 1989; Chilvers, McPherson, and Peto et al. 1989). Postmenopausal women who undergo estrogen replacement therapy probably do not have a greater risk for breast cancer, but do have an increased risk for endometrial cancer. Women who have had cancer of the colon, thyroid, endometrium, or ovary have a higher incidence of breast cancer (Dobernack and Garcia 1988). An early first pregnancy, and oophorectomy before age 30 are thought to have protective effects. About 70% of breast cancer patients have no evident risk factor (Seidman, Stellman, and Mushinski 1982).

The incidence of breast cancer is very high among people living in northern Europe, Canada, and the United States. The incidence is much lower in the developing countries, Mexico, and the Orient; this is thought to be due to dietary factors, especially a low total-fat intake.

Wynder has advocated diets with 25% or less of the caloric intake in fat, but has stated that the effects of total caloric intake or of obesity are not as relevant as the specific types and amounts of fat consumed (Wynder 1987). Toniolo stated that during adult life, a reduction in dietary intake of fat and proteins of animal

Table 13.1
INCREASE IN EARLY DETECTION OF BREAST CANCER
1979-81 vs. 1985

Age	Increase in Cases		
	In situ	Localized	Regional
<50	114%	10.8%	10.8%
≥50	176%	38.9%	6.1%

(Source: Horm [1988].)

Table 13.2
RELATIONSHIP BETWEEN BENIGN BREAST TISSUE AND RISK
FOR INVASIVE BREAST CARCINOMA

"Is 'Fibrocystic Disease' of the Breast Precancerous?"

If the pathologic diagnosis "fibrocystic disease" is used at all, or when the preferred terms "fibro-cystic changes" or "fibrocystic condition" are used, the component elements should be specified.

RELATIVE RISK FOR INVASIVE BREAST CARCINOMA BASED ON
PATHOLOGIC EXAMINATION OF BENIGN BREAST TISSUE

No Increased Risk
Women with any lesion specified below in a biopsy specimen are at no greater risk
for invasive breast carcinoma than comparable women who have had no breast biopsy:

Adenosis, sclerosing or florid	Duct ectasia	Hyperplasia, mild (more than	Mastitis (inflammation)
Apocrine metaplasia	Fibroadenoma	2 but not more than	Periductal mastitis
Cysts, macro and/or micro	Fibrosis	4 epithelial cells in depth)	Squamous metaplasia

Slightly Increased Risk (1.5 to 2 Times)*
Women with any lesion specified below in a biopsy specimen are at slightly increased risk
for invasive breast carcinoma relative to comparable women who have had no breast biopsy:

Hyperplasia, moderate or florid, solid or papillary
Papilloma with fibrovascular core

Moderately Increased Risk (5 Times)*
Women with a lesion specified below in a biopsy specimen are at moderately increased risk
for invasive breast carcinoma relative to comparable women who have had no breast biopsy:

Atypical hyperplasia (borderline lesion)
Ductal
Lobular

*Please see Explanatory Notes 4 and 5.

(Courtesy: College of American Pathologists Consensus Meeting [1986].)

origin may contribute to a substantial reduction in the incidence of breast cancer in population subgroups with high intake of animal products (Toniolo et al. 1989). Willett followed 90,000 nurses for four years and con-cluded that a moderate reduction in fat intake by adult women is unlikely to result in a substantial reduction in the incidence of breast cancer (Willett et al. 1987). It is Garfinkel's opinion that, at the present time, data are inadequate to make a definite statement on the rela-tionship of a low-fat diet to the development of breast cancer (Garfinkel 1988).

Alcohol consumption, especially if it is excessive, is probably a risk factor (Willett, Stampfer, and Colditz et al. 1987).

Breast cancer related to a strong family history usually occurs at a younger age, and may occur in women in their 20s. Baseline mammograms at age 25 have been recommended for genetically predisposed women (Lynch 1988).

Certain microscopic findings associated with fibro-cystic change of the breast relate to a higher subsequent incidence of cancer (table 13.2). Naturally, many of these microscopic changes cannot be identified on phys-ical examination.

CANCER OF THE MALE BREAST

Cancer of the male breast and Klinefelter's syndrome are both uncommon, and it is difficult to obtain mean-ingful statistics on their association. Opinions differ as to whether the incidence of carcinoma of the male breast is higher in patients with Klinefelter's syndrome, but it is prudent to follow such patients carefully. The risk of developing breast cancer in patients with Klinefelter's syndrome approached 3% in two series (Evans and Crichlow 1987; Holleb, Freeman, and Far-row 1988), but the overall incidence in males is less than 1% of all breast cancer cases (American Cancer Society 1990). Breast cancer in males usually occurs at an older age than in females (Cutler and Young 1975).

DETECTION/SCREENING

The detection of breast cancer uses three main modalities: breast self-examination (BSE); clinical phys-ical examination; and imaging techniques, primarily mammography. About 90% of all palpable breast can-cers are said to be detected by the patient, but an increasing percentage of all breast cancer detection results from screening procedures that include mammo-grams, which can detect a breast cancer too small to be felt by the most experienced examiner (table 13.3).

BREAST SELF-EXAMINATION (BSE)

Most physicians advocate breast self-examination as a good health practice (fig. 13.1). However, many critics believe that while BSE may account for earlier detec-tion, it has not reduced mortality. Studies to evaluate BSE include a project sponsored by the World Health Organization (WHO) in Leningrad (Semiglazov and Moiseyenko 1987), which is designed as a prospective

Table 13.3
GUIDELINES FOR MAMMOGRAPHY AND BREAST EXAMINATIONS

20 YEARS AND OLDER:
Breast self-examination monthly.

20-40 YEARS OF AGE:
A physician breast examination every three years and an initial mammogram between the ages of 35-40.

40-50 YEARS OF AGE:
Periodic mammography every year or two as determined by your own personal history and your doctor's recommendation. Also, an annual physician breast examination.

OVER 50 YEARS OF AGE:
Annual mammography and an annual physician examination.

(Courtesy: American Cancer Society [1988].)

randomized trial. A previous similar, but nonrandomized, trial in Great Britain found no differences in the outcome of breast cancer treatment between the group that participated in the program of BSE and the control group, which did not (Philips et al. 1984).

In one study in England, women who had been taught BSE and had practiced it had more favorable tumors than the nonpracticing group (tumor size ≤2 cm, 45% vs. 33%; clinical stage I, 42% vs. 27%; and N0 pathological stage, 50% vs. 37%) (Mant et al. 1987).

In a Vermont study, 90% of women doing monthly BSE detected their own breast cancers; 82% of women performing less-frequent BSE did so; and only 54% of the women who claimed they never performed BSE detected their own cancers. More-frequent BSE performance was associated with a more favorable clinical stage and fewer axillary lymph node metastases. The average tumor size was 1.97 cm for those practicing BSE monthly; 2.47 cm for those performing BSE less often; and 3.59 cm for patients never performing it. Half of the patients age 70 to 98 and 16% of those age 28 to 49 reported they had never practiced BSE. Five percent of the older age group and one-third of the younger age group reported performing monthly BSE. Twenty-seven percent of cancer patients never practicing BSE had four or more positive nodes, as compared to 17% for those practicing BSE less often than monthly, and 9% for those who did monthly BSE (Foster et al. 1987). Demonstrations of the BSE technique using younger women as models do not have sufficient impact on older women; nurses who themselves practice BSE regularly are more likely to reinforce the desirability and technique of BSE to their patients (Sawyer 1986).

A separate study of 2,092 women found that those who had practiced breast self-examination had earlier cancer, which was true for both black and white races, all educational and economic levels, all age groups, and

within each period of delay between first symptom and medical consultation. The practice of BSE increased as the educational level rose and diminished as age advanced. A higher percentage of whites than blacks performed BSE (Huguely and Brown 1981).

A Mexican study has demonstrated the importance of repeated reinforcement of the desirability of BSE (Shelley and Lessan 1986). This can easily be done by the doctor during a physical examination because many steps in the two examinations are similar. Certain basic points apply to every adequate breast examination: the examination should be unhurried; all parts of the breast should be examined; the breast should be examined with the patient in both a recumbent and a sitting position; the breast should be in a relaxed position; and visual inspection as well as palpation should be done.

A review of the question of BSE emphasizes the necessity for more carefully controlled trials to evaluate the procedure (O'Malley and Fletcher 1987). However, millions of socioeconomically disadvantaged women are unable to afford a visit to the doctor or a mammogram; for early detection of a breast cancer, all these women have is breast self-examination.

CLINICAL EXAMINATION

Clinical examination (CE) is an important part of the evaluation of the breast. There is no absolute proof at present that it will detect cancers sufficiently early to

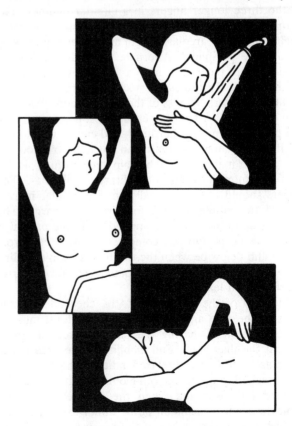

Fig. 13.1. American Cancer Society's recommended procedure for breast self-examination. (Courtesy: American Cancer Society [1987].)

reduce mortality; however, the indirect evidence is much stronger than that for BSE, and is great enough that Miller feels the examinations should not be abandoned (Miller and Baines 1987; Miller 1988). Studies are in progress to evaluate this point. In general, it is difficult to feel lesions smaller than 1 cm in the substance of the breast, but superficial lesions of 0.5 cm or less can be detected. Mammograms miss about 10% to 15% of cancers, some of which are large, so palpation is the only reliable means of early detection in these cases. When possible, CE should be done seven to 10 days after the first day of menstrual flow in premenopausal patients, because breast nodularity and tenderness are least marked at that time. This is especially true in the perimenopausal years.

Changes in skin texture and color can be subtle but significant, so the breast examination should be done in a well-lit room. The examination should be done with the patient both lying and sitting. When the patient is recumbent, her breast should rest easily atop the chest wall; if the breast hangs off to the side, the tissues will be under some tension from the underlying fascia and will be more difficult to examine. Positioning of the breast is best accomplished by having the patient rolled 30 degrees toward the opposite side and supported with a small pillow. Some examiners prefer to examine the breast with the patient's arm over her head, so that the pectoral muscles serve as a platform on which the breast can be palpated.

The breast should be examined by rotating the pads of the three longer fingers in a circular manner. The entire breast should be covered in a spiral fashion, beginning at the areolar margin and gradually working toward the periphery. Alternate methods include the vertical-strip technique and a quadrant-by-quadrant examination. Regardless of technique, the important point is the thoroughness of the examination. Examination of the axillary tail of Spence is best performed with the patient's arm over her head, and cancer developing in the inframammary crease can easily be overlooked. The areolar margin should be palpated carefully, as this is a common location for solitary papillomas. The fingers should next be rolled from the areolar margin toward the nipple to look for nipple discharge. The breast should then be re-examined while the patient is in the sitting position by compressing the breast from above and below between the two hands. Skin dimpling is best detected by having the patient extend her arms overhead and lean forward.

Mobility of the breast should be checked with the arms at the side and again with the pectoral muscles under tension by having the patient forcefully press against the iliac bone. Full mobility of the breast with the muscles tensed and relaxed indicates that a tumor is not attached to the fascia; full mobility with the muscles relaxed but restricted when the muscles are tense indicates some attachment of the tumor to the pectoral fascia; restricted mobility of the breast with the arms relaxed indicates fixation to the chest wall (Scanlon 1984; Scanlon 1987). Fascial fixation does not affect the TNM staging, but chest wall fixation does. Skin dimpling does not affect staging, but skin attachment does.

In one series of 10,000 patients, clinical examination detected 45% of the extant cancers, and 28% of these were minimal lesions (Seidman et al. 1987). In a study of 253 patients who had a palpable mass and a preoperative mammogram, the physical examination was slightly more accurate than the mammogram in indicating the presence of breast cancer. This was true irrespective of the menopausal status of the patient or the location of the tumor within the breast (Sener, Scanlon, and Paige 1977). Studies from Japan, Holland, and Belgium all support the value of clinical examination.

Cardona studied 1,450 cancer cases and evaluated 232 patients who had a false negative impression of cancer based on physical examination (Cardona et al. 1983). Eighty percent of the errors were attributed to misdiagnosis of a cancer as benign, and 20% to nonpalpability due to lesion size and site. In this series the sensitivity of physical examination increased with the increase in lesion size and the patient's age. In a prospective study of 622 patients, Hermansen found the diagnostic accuracy of physical examination to be 0.93; of mammography, 0.96; and of fine-needle aspiration biopsy, 0.96 (Hermansen et al. 1987).

IMAGING

The guidelines of the American Cancer Society and the American College of Radiology recommend that a baseline mammogram should be taken by age 40. Routine mammograms before age 35 are usually not recommended except in women with a strong family history of breast cancer, as the yield is low. Furthermore, the breast tissue in young women is dense and the accuracy of the mammogram is lower, although some radiologists disagree. If the x-ray doses from mammographic screening are carcinogenic, as some critics suggest, this effect would be of concern in women under age 35 (Pochin 1988; Upton 1982). In large screening programs, the yield from mammography in asymptomatic women is about 4 cancers per 1,000 patients screened the first year, which is the prevalence year, and then about 2 cases per 1,000 in subsequent years (Baines 1987). There is no doubt of the very successful results of using mammography to screen for breast cancer in younger as well as in older women (Miller and Baines 1987).

Some critics of screening feel that it results in unnecessary interventions. In a Canadian study (Baines 1987), about 30 women per 1,000 women examined had a surgical diagnostic procedure resulting from the first screen, but by the fifth screen, the rate had dropped to 6 per 1,000. In this trial, there were six benign biopsies for every cancer at the first screen resulting from mammography, and 3.5 benign biopsies for every cancer at the first screen resulting from nonmammography allocations (Baines 1987). In our own cases, 27% of the biopsies done for mammographic indications, and 22% of the biopsies done for a palpable mass, were malignant. These figures correspond to those of most diagnostic programs in the United States and are lower than those reported from European programs. This may be the result of the difficult medical-legal climate in the United States. Fear of a lawsuit may stimulate the earlier performance of a breast biopsy for equivocal changes.

Baines (1987) has emphasized that results from diagnostic evaluations are not comparable to those from screening programs because there will probably be a greater prevalence of cancers in the former group. Diagnostic evaluations are made on symptomatic patients, while screening programs are designed for asymptomatic ones. It is recognized that these criteria are not rigid, and interval cancers detected in a screening program probably are symptomatic.

Skrabanek (1985) has written extensively on the futility of screening for cancer. He states that the evidence that breast cancer is incurable is overwhelming. If a tumor is visible, palpable, or symptomatic, it is too late; if early means premalignant lesions, it is too early. He feels that doctors have become victims of wishful thinking, especially regarding BSE. While Skrabanek's views are not widely accepted, it is important to at least be aware that there are dissenting voices regarding the various screening procedures and the concept of screening as a valid method of reducing deaths from cancer.

An objection to mammographic screening for women under 50 has been that proof that it prolonged life was lacking. After 18 years of follow-up from the New York Health Insurance Program (HIP) study (Shapiro et al. 1988), the figures now show a statistically significant prolongation of life in women under 50 who were screened routinely, as compared to the nonscreened group (table 13.4). The reduction in mortality after mass screening was also demonstrated in a Swedish trial, but only for women over age 50 (Tabar et al. 1985). One study showed a 20% reduction in mortality in the screened group, but only for women over 55 (Anderson et al. 1988).

Mammography is currently the only reliable method of finding a breast cancer before a mass is palpable. These early cases have the best prognosis. There is about a 10% to 15% false-negative rate when breast cancers are examined by mammography; a normal mammogram is not a valid reason to forego a biopsy when it is indicated because of physical findings.

Table 13.4
PERCENTAGE REDUCTION IN DEATHS FROM BREAST CANCER IN THE HIP STUDY

Age at entry	Percent reduction in breast cancer deaths		Year reduction began
	At 5 years	At 18 years	
40-44	(18)	36	9
45-49	(0)	16	6
50-54	65	22	3
55-59	(30)	24	3
60-64	(50)	17	3

Parentheses indicate observations based on 20 or fewer breast cancer deaths in study and control groups combined. (Courtesy: Shapiro et al. [1988].)

By adding the results of two nonrandomized Dutch studies (Collette et al. 1984; Verbeek et al. 1985) to the results of the HIP and Swedish randomized controlled trials, it can be concluded that the key question concerning early detection has been answered, as Moskowitz says, "clearly, unambiguously and beyond doubt. Early detection alters the natural history of this disease" (Moskowitz 1985). Evidence supports the statement that the large-scale application of properly performed and interpreted mammography can result in reduction of mortality from breast cancer by more than 50% in the ever-screened group as compared to the never-screened group (Tabar 1987). The initial large scale project of the benefit of screening mammography by the American Cancer Society (ACS) and the National Cancer Institute (NCI), the Breast Cancer Detection Demonstration Project (BCDDP), has been reported at intervals (Letton and Mason 1986; Eddy, Hassleblad, and McGiveny 1988). In some of those reports, noninvasive lesions exceeded 25% of all the cancers found (Byrd and Hartmann 1988) (table 13.5).

Table 13.5
MODALITY RESULTING IN CANCER DETECTED*

	% of total cancers
M− P−	7
M− P+	6
M+ P+	42
M+ P−	45
	100

*M = mammography; P = physical examination
(Courtesy: Byrd and Hartmann [1988].)

MAMMOGRAPHY

Mammography can be done by a xerogram technique or by a low-dose film method. Xerography has the advantage of being able to examine closer to the chest wall, but low-dose film mammography gives greater detail, in the opinion of many radiologists. Currently, xerogram equipment has more mechanical problems and this can be a difficulty in smaller institutions with a single machine. Most radiologists prefer to use the technique with which they are most familiar.

The acceptable x-ray dose in mammography is 0.01 Gy (1 rad) or less to the center of the breast per 2-view study. With the current optimal film screen mammography, the average midline dose per 2-view study is 0.002 Gy (Feig 1987). Using a linear dose response relationship and assuming there is no threshold, 0.01 Gy per study is presumed to cause 3 extra cancers per 1,000,000 women per year; with the usual screen film dose, it would be 1 cancer per 1,000,000 women per year (Gohagan et al. 1986). Comparable risk factors result from traveling 60 miles by automobile, living in Denver for two months, or 20 minutes of being a 60-year-old man (Upton 1982).

Assuming a baseline mammogram at age 35 to 39 and an annual mammogram after age 40 on 1,000,000 women, as few as 150 or as many as 1,000 radiogenic breast cancers were projected for a screening population over a lifetime, according to one study (Dodd 1988). However, with the current, much-improved mammographic techniques many of these cases could be diagnosed early and at a point when the survival rate would be quite high.

Mammography can sometimes detect ductal carcinoma *in situ* (DCIS) by the appearance of the ducts and the presence of microcalcifications. These microcalcifications will not distinguish between DCIS and other proliferative processes, including intraductal papilloma or intraductal hyperplasia. They can sometimes be confused with the microcalcifications of sclerosing adenosis, although in the latter case, the calcifications are usually more widely scattered (Hall 1986).

ULTRASOUND

Ultrasound (US) has probably been the most-used method other than mammography to determine the presence of preclinical breast cancer. It may be of value, particularly in women with dense breasts, and it is very helpful in differentiating between cyst and solid tumor. One study made a comparison of the size of the breast cancers estimated by physical examination, mammography, and sonography vs. measurements in pathology. Sonography yielded the most accurate determination of breast cancer size, but it was less specific. It has been suggested that US may be useful in the evaluation of tumor response to nonsurgical treatment (Fornage, Toubas, and Morel 1987). Ultrasound does not demonstrate microcalcifications and currently is unacceptable as the primary screening procedure.

OTHER IMAGING METHODS

Magnetic resonance imaging (MRI) has been suggested as a method for detecting breast cancer. In one study of 120 women with both xeromammography and MRI, xeromammography was more accurate in diagnosing cancer (Turner et al. 1988). Moreover, MRI does not demonstrate microcalcifications.

Diaphanography, which uses transillumination of the breast, has been used in some studies to detect early breast cancer. This method is not as effective as mammography and is not widely accepted. A report from Scotland utilizing computerized telediaphanography indicated a sensitivity of 0.94 and a specificity of 0.89 (Bundred et al. 1987).

A combined optical and Doppler US approach to the detection of breast cancer has been reported (Watmough, Moran, and Watmough 1988). It is one of the new approaches in the early detection of breast cancer that has the benefit of no irradiation.

Thermography uses infrared light as a screening tool for breast cancer. It is based on the theory that some cells will produce identifiable hot spots on the screen, which may indicate the presence of malignant tumor. However, benign processes in the breast frequently yield positive results. Furthermore, the temperature of the breast needs to be in equilibrium with the surrounding air, so that the patient will not shiver; the patient should be undressed to the waist in a room with a temperature that supports normal body temperature. Thermography has not proved to be practical or sufficiently accurate, but clinical research continues.

It is important to be aware that screening techniques, when added to mammography, increase the cost considerably, thereby altering the cost-benefit ratio.

DIAGNOSIS

BIOPSY

Originally, biopsies of suspicious, nonpalpable lesions were performed largely by estimation; large amounts of tissue were removed and the lesions frequently were missed. Mammography is now used to localize lesions by injecting small amounts of blue dye or inserting a Kopan's wire into the lesion under x-ray guidance preoperatively. Unless a cancer can be identified grossly in the tissue removed, a specimen mammogram should be done to ensure that the abnormality has been removed. When there is doubt whether the abnormality has been removed, and where no cancer has been identified in the specimen, a repeat mammogram of the breast should be done as soon as the tenderness and the reaction from the biopsy have subsided. Recently, directed aspiration biopsies of nonpalpable lesions have been done using stereotactic equipment or ultrasound (Fornage, Faroux, and Simatos 1987), but further studies are needed to give confidence where the results are negative. If a cyst is thought to be the cause of the mammographic abnormality, but doubt persists, the lesion can be aspirated under US guidance prior to x-ray localization; if fluid is obtained with disappearance of the mass, the biopsy may be cancelled.

Needle aspiration biopsy for a palpable mass can be of two types: fine-needle aspiration biopsy (FNAB) with cytological examination or core-needle or drill biopsy with histological examination. For palpable masses, FNAB is less painful and slightly more accurate than core-needle biopsy, especially for lesions close to the chest wall. In our study of over 6,000 FNAB examinations of worrisome palpable masses, 12% were malignant. False positive results occur rarely. Most surgeons are influenced in their treatment decisions by FNAB, but a negative result should never be a deterrent to further investigation of a suspicious mass (Frable 1983). Occasionally, the cytology can indicate the histological type.

The definitive diagnosis of breast cancer is made by histological examination of tissue obtained by biopsy. Sometimes an adequate specimen can be obtained with a core or drill needle, but more often an operative approach is taken. The biopsy can be incisional when the mass is large, but usually it is excisional. In the upper part of the breast the incision should be circumlinear in the skin lines; in the lower part, a radial incision may be made. A small margin of normal tissue should be removed around the tumor, and the margins of the biopsy should be marked for study by the pathologist. If the tumor is malignant on frozen section, hormone receptors should be determined. A biopsy performed in this way constitutes a lumpectomy and, if the margins are clear, nothing further need be done surgically, if irradiation is the treatment option. The axillary lymph nodes should be treated through a separate incision. The biopsy should not be done with the cautery knife because it distorts the architecture, destroys the margins, and alters the level of hormone receptors (Bloom et al. 1984; Rosenthal 1979; Rosen 1986).

STAGING

Staging of breast cancer serves as a guide for treatment, indicates prognosis, and permits a comparison of different treatment methods. Many staging methods have been described, but the TNM system (table 13.6 A,B,C,D,E) is accepted worldwide.

TREATMENT

Surgical procedures used in the treatment of breast cancer include lumpectomy, partial mastectomy, and quadrantectomy; and subcutaneous, total, modified-radical, radical, and super-radical mastectomy.

Surgical procedures that remove less than all of the breast tissue in the treatment of infiltrating breast cancers are usually combined with irradiation and dissection or sampling of the axilla. In some cases of noninfiltrating cancers, local excision alone is considered definitive treatment. Studies are in progress to determine the role of local excision alone for lobular carcinoma *in situ* (LCIS) and ductal carcinoma *in situ* (DCIS).

Subcutaneous mastectomy is a procedure in which an attempt is made to remove all of the breast tissue while preserving the overlying skin and the nipple-areolar complex. It almost always is accompanied by reconstruction. The procedure is usually used in women who are at high risk, based on previous biopsy, of developing invasive carcinoma. It is used occasionally in patients who can have no peace of mind due to their perception of an unacceptable risk—a perception caused by a strong family history of breast cancer, precancerous hyperplasia or marked cellular atypia, or for other reasons. The objections to subcutaneous mastectomy stem from the fact that breast tissue occasionally extends farther than is generally believed, and it is difficult to remove all of it through the incisions usually used for this procedure. Furthermore, there is no line of cleavage between the breast tissue and the underside of the areola, so that some breast tissue is left behind in this area. If the breast tissue is shaved too close from the underside of the areola, there is a danger that the nipple and areola will slough, due to inadequate blood supply.

The terms "total mastectomy" and "simple mastectomy" are often used synonymously, but the term "total" is increasingly favored because it implies a more

Table 13.6 A
STAGE GROUPING FOR BREAST CANCER

Stage Grouping

0	Tis	N0	M0
I	T1	N0	M0
IIA	T0	N1	M0
	T1	N1	M0
	T2	N0	M0
IIB	T2	N1	M0
	T3	N0	M0
IIIA	T0	N2	M0
	T1	N2	M0
	T2	N2	M0
	T3	N1	M0
	T3	N2	M0
IIIB	T4	Any N	M0
	Any T	N3	M0
IV	Any T	Any N	M1

Note: The prognosis of patients with pN1a is similar to that of patients with pN0.

(Courtesy: American Joint Committee on Cancer [1986].)

Table 13.6 B
TNM CLASSIFICATIONS

TNM CLASSIFICATIONS
The clinical measurement used for classifying the primary tumor (T) should be the one judged most accurate (*e.g.*, physical examination or mammogram). Pathologically, the tumor size for classification (T) is a measurement of the invasive component. For example, if there is a large *in situ* component (4 cm) and a small invasive component (0.5 cm), the tumor is classified T1a. The size of the primary tumor should be measured before any tissue is removed for special studies, such as for estrogen receptors.

Multiple Simultaneous Ipsilateral Primary Cancers
The following guidelines should be used when classifying multiple simultaneous ipsilateral primary (infiltrating, grossly measurable) carcinomas. These criteria do not apply to one grossly detected tumor associated with multiple separate microscopic foci.

1. Use the largest primary carcinoma to classify T.
2. Enter into the record that this is a case of multiple simultaneous ipsilateral primary carcinomas. Such cases should be analyzed separately.

Simultaneous Bilateral Breast Carcinomas
Each carcinoma should be staged separately.

Inflammatory Carcinoma
Inflammatory carcinoma is a clinicopathologic entity characterized by diffuse brawny induration of the skin of the breast with an erysipeloid edge, usually without an underlying detectable mass. Radiologically there may be a detectable mass and characteristic thickening of the skin over the breast. This clinical presentation is due to tumor embolization of dermal lymphatics. The tumor of inflammatory carcinoma is classified T4d.

Paget's Disease of the Nipple
Paget's disease of the nipple without an associated tumor mass (clinical) or invasive carcinoma (pathologic) is classified Tis. Paget's disease with a demonstrable mass (clinical) or an invasive component (pathologic) is classified according to the size of the tumor mass or invasive component.

Skin of Breast
Dimpling of the skin, nipple retraction, or any other skin change except those described under inflammatory carcinoma (T4b) may occur in T1, T2, or T3 without changing the classification.

complete removal of breast tissue. The axillary tail of Spence extends well up into the axilla; if this portion of the specimen is marked to orient the pathologist, a few of the lower axillary nodes will be removed and become available for study.

The modified-radical mastectomy is defined as the removal of the breast in continuity with the axillary lymph nodes. It has become the standard, definitive operative procedure for invasive breast cancer in most institutions. It produces survival results equal to lumpectomy and radiation therapy.

The classic Halsted radical mastectomy removes the breast, the underlying pectoral muscles, and the axillary contents in continuity. It was the standard surgical procedure for treating breast cancer in the United States until about the 1960s. The modified-radical mastectomy and lumpectomy with irradiation and axillary dissection are replacing the Halsted radical mastectomy in the United States (Wilson et al. 1984). This is because tumors are being diagnosed earlier and treatment results, in the short term, demonstrate the lesser procedures to be equally effective. The Halsted radical mastectomy may be the procedure of choice and especially in cases where the muscle is involved with tumor (Urban 1988; Ferguson et al. 1982; Maddox et al. 1987).

The super, extended, radical mastectomy — the Urban procedure — includes the removal of the internal mammary lymphatic chain in continuity with the breast, pectoral muscles, and axillary lymph nodes. In a few series, the supraclavicular lymph nodes have also been resected. The procedure has been used primarily for carcinomas located in the medial or subareolar areas of the breast. The super-radical mastectomy has not resulted in improved survival, with the possible exception of tumors located in the medial or subareolar areas with axillary lymph nodes positive for metastases. In some series, there has been an improvement in that subgroup, but resection of the internal mammary chain increases the operative time and morbidity. In general, the procedure is not widely used (Lacour et al. 1987; Urban 1988; Maddox et al. 1987).

The axilla is customarily discussed in terms of three levels: level I, lateral to the pectoralis minor; level II, under that muscle; and level III, medial to it. The prognosis worsens as nodes at the higher levels become involved. However, this is a prognostic indicator and does not support the concept that tumor metastases progressively move up the axilla. Some surgeons who believe that any axillary lymph node involvement indicates systemic disease feel that axillary sampling or dissection of level I is adequate treatment of the axilla (Boova, Bonani, and Rosato 1981) because it is unusual for higher levels to be involved when lower levels are not. Other surgeons feel strongly that inadequate dissection of the axilla results in higher recurrence rates (Ferguson 1987).

Table 13.6 C
TNM STAGING

TNM Staging

Primary Tumor (T)

Tx	Primary tumor cannot be assessed
To	No evidence of primary tumor
Tis	Carcinoma *in situ.* Intraductal carcinoma, lobular carcinoma *in situ*, or Paget's disease of the nipple with no tumor
T1	Tumor 2 cm or less in greatest dimension
T1a	0.5 cm or less in greatest dimension
T1b	More than 0.5 cm but not more than 1 cm in greatest dimension
T1c	More than 1 cm but not more than 2 cm in greatest dimension
T2	Tumor more than 2 cm but not more than 5 cm in greatest dimension
T3	Tumor more than 5 cm in greatest dimension
T4	Tumor of any size with direct extension to chest wall or skin
T4a	Extension to chest wall
T4b	Edema (including peau d'orange) or ulceration of the skin of breast or satellite nodules confined to same breast
T4c	Both T4a and T4b
T4d	Inflammatory carcinoma

Lymph Node (N)

Nx	Regional lymph nodes cannot be assessed
No	No regional lymph node metastasis
N1	Metastasis to movable ipsilateral axillary lymph node(s)
N2	Metastasis to ipsilateral axillary lymph node(s) fixed to one another or to other structures.
N3	Metastasis to ipsilateral internal mammary lymph node(s)

Distant Metastasis (M)

Mx	Presence of distant metastasis cannot be assessed
M0	No distant metastasis
M1	Distant metastasis (includes metastasis to ipsilateral supraclavicular lymph nodes)

Table 13.6 D
HISTOPATHOLOGIC TYPES OF BREAST CANCER

HISTOPATHOLOGIC TYPE

The histologic types are the following:

Cancer, NOS (not otherwise specified)
Ductal
    Intraductal (*in situ*)
    Invasive with predominant intraductal component
    Invasive, NOS (not otherwise specified)
  Comedo
  Inflammatory
  Medullary with lymphocytic infiltrate
  Mucinous (colloid)
  Papillary
  Scirrhous
  Tubular
  Other
Lobular
    In situ
  Invasive with predominant *in situ* component
  Invasive
Nipple
    Paget's disease, NOS (not otherwise specified)
    Paget's disease with intraductal carcinoma
    Paget's disease with invasive ductal carcinoma
Other

HISTOPATHOLOGIC GRADE (G)

GX	Grade cannot be assessed
G1	Well differentiated
G2	Moderately well differentiated
G3	Poorly differentiated
G4	Undifferentiated

(Courtesy: American Joint Committee on Cancer [1988].)

Table 13.6 E
DEFINITION OF TNM

DEFINITION OF TNM

Primary Tumor
Definitions for classifying the primary tumor (T) are the same for clinical and for pathologic classification. The *telescoping* method of classification can be applied. If the measurement is made by physical examination, the examiner will use the major headings (T1, T2, T3). If other measurements, such as mammographic or pathologic, are used, the telescoped subsets of T1 can be used.

TX   Primary tumor cannot be assessed
T0   No evidence of primary tumor
Tis* Carcinoma *in situ*: Intraductal carcinoma, lobular carcinoma *in situ*, or Paget's disease of the nipple with no tumor
T1   Tumor 2 cm or less in greatest dimension
      T1a   0.5 or less in greatest dimension
      T1b   More than 0.5 cm but not more than 1 cm in greatest dimension
      T1c   More than 1 cm but not more than 2 cm in greatest dimension
T2   Tumor more than 2 cm but not more than 5 cm in greatest dimension
T4#   Tumor of any size with direct extension to chest wall or skin
      T4a   Extension to chest wall
      T4b   Edema (including peau d'orange) or ulceration of the skin of the breast or satellite skin nodules confined to the same breast
      T4c   Both (T4a and T4b)
      T4d   Inflammatory carcinoma (see definition of inflammatory carcinoma in the introduction)

*Note: Paget's disease associated with a tumor is classified according to the size of the tumor.
Note: Chest wall includes ribs, intercostal muscles, and serratus anterior muscle but not pectoral muscle.

Regional Lymph Nodes

NX   Regional lymph nodes cannot be assessed
      (*e.g.*, previously removed)
N0   No regional lymph node metastasis
N1   Metastasis to movable ipsilateral axillary lymph node(s)
N2   Metastasis to ipsilateral axillary lymph node(s) fixed to one another or to other structures
N3   Metastasis to ipsilateral internal mammary lymph node(s)

NIPPLE DISCHARGE

A clinically significant discharge is spontaneous, persistent, nonlactational, unilateral, and of recent onset, although there are exceptions. In one series, 13% of patients operated on for a variety of nipple discharges had cancer; some of these had negative cytology, normal mammography, and no palpable mass (Leis et al. 1988). A milky, bilateral discharge should lead to the suspicion of a pituitary adenoma (Urban and Egeli 1978). Patients with any type of recent-onset unilateral nipple discharge should be evaluated carefully for carcinoma, although clear, sticky discharge is less worrisome. Cytological examination of the nipple discharge and a mammogram should be performed. An x-ray after injection of a radio-opaque dye into the draining duct at the nipple level occasionally can be helpful. In the presence of a serosanguinous or bloody nipple discharge, careful palpation for a papilloma should be done along the areolar margin in the quadrant indicated by the location of the involved duct on the nipple surface.

Sciotto et al. studied the nipple discharge in 3,600 women out of a series of 50,000 consecutive patients. They noted that a bloody nipple discharge was present in 70% of the cancer cases and that cancer was so uncommon in cases with nonbloody discharge that cytological examination would not be cost-effective (Sciotto, Bravetti, and Cariaggi

1986). However, most other studies are not in agreement with this observation (Leis et al. 1988).

The treatment of bloody nipple discharge without a suspicious lump is excision of the major duct system, with extension for a short distance beyond the areolar margin in the direction of the quadrant suspected of harboring the pathology. The specimen should be carefully examined. In those patients in whom no cause for the bleeding can be found, a missed carcinoma will sometimes express itself later. Such patients need to be followed very carefully for a long period of time. Mastectomy has been suggested by some clinicians for bloody nipple discharge in older women (over age 45 in one series, and over age 60 in another) in whom the cause is not found by major duct excision (Atkins and Wolfe 1964; Seltzer et al. 1970), but this is not generally accepted. Sometimes, during pregnancy, a bloody nipple discharge will appear. If the cytology of the discharge is benign and there is no suspicious palpable lump surgery should be postponed, since the discharge will usually disappear after delivery. However, careful follow-up is essential.

LOBULAR CARCINOMA *IN SITU* (LCIS)

The treatment of lobular carcinoma *in situ* is probably the most controversial of breast-cancer treatment decisions. Some say that LCIS should not be considered as carcinoma and should be referred to as a lobular condition of the breast. Treatment recommendations range from biopsy alone to total mastectomy with contralateral biopsy, to bilateral mastectomy with reconstruction. Part of the controversy stems from the fact, pointed out by Hutter (1984), that the breast is not two organs, but rather one organ with two mounds. The male breast does not contain lobules, so LCIS is confined to females. On average, women with LCIS are five to 15 years younger than those with invasive carcinoma. Most patients are premenopausal, and the tumor is more common in whites than blacks (Hutter 1984; Rosner et al. 1980). The incidence of bilaterality of LCIS is generally reported at about 25%, although there are great variations (Frykberg et al. 1987). Up to 35% of all women with untreated LCIS will eventually develop invasive breast cancer, but this may be equally distributed between the two breasts. In Rosen's series of 99 cases of LCIS treated by biopsy only, 32 developed clinically apparent carcinoma (Rosen, Braun, and Kinne 1980). Thirty-two percent of subsequent ipsilateral carcinomas and 43% of those developing in the contralateral breast were diagnosed 20 or more years after LCIS had been found. The fact that the preponderance of lobular carcinoma develops in the premenopausal period and has a high incidence of hormone receptors in invasive lesions, suggests that hormones play a large role in its development. Lobular carcinoma *in situ* is rarely palpable, and is usually found incidentally in a biopsy for what proves to be a benign condition. Treatment decisions should be based on the understanding that invasive carcinoma may subsequently develop, that the opposite breast is as likely to be involved, and that the young age of the patients puts them at risk for a longer period of time. The treatment options should be discussed fully and frankly with the patient and, in all cases, frequent, careful follow-up is indicated.

DUCTAL CARCINOMA *IN SITU* (DCIS); INTRADUCTAL CARCINOMA

Ductal carcinoma *in situ* (DCIS), also called intraductal carcinoma, is generally thought to be a precursor of invasive ductal carcinoma. However, clinicians agree that not all cases progress; some regard it as a marker only. Data are scant and uncontrolled, but indirect evidence was found (Page et al. 1982) that 28% of the cases where the correct diagnosis of intraductal carcinoma was not made on the original biopsy were followed by invasive cancer at a mean of six years. Rosen found carcinoma in 33% of 30 patients followed an average of 9.7 years after the initial biopsy (Rosen, Braun, and Kinne 1980). Fisher reported 23% of the patients treated by lumpectomy alone had recurrence after a mean follow-up of 39 months (Fisher et al. 1986). However, in those patients who received radiotherapy to the breast after lumpectomy, only 7% recurred in the same time interval. Currently, a randomized trial comparing excision alone with excision and radiotherapy for DCIS is being done.

The diagnosis of intraductal carcinoma will usually be made by finding a palpable lump, discharge from or erosion of the nipple, signifying Paget's disease; or an abnormal mammogram, often showing clustered microcalcifications.

Where there is a nonpalpable tumor and biopsy is performed for microcalcifications alone, over half the tumors will be intraductal carcinoma. Gump studied 70 patients who were diagnosed on biopsy to have DCIS and found a significant difference between those cases in which the DCIS was microscopic only as compared to those cases in which there was a palpable mass or nipple discharge (Gump, Jicha, and Ozello 1987). Unsuspected invasion, residual disease in the specimen after biopsy, disease elsewhere in the breast, or positive nodes, were found only in the group with palpable masses.

The optimal treatment for DCIS has not yet been defined, but total mastectomy with or without reconstruction, or local excision with postoperative x-ray therapy is acceptable. The standard treatment for intraductal carcinoma up to the present time has been total mastectomy. In our own studies, the lower axillary lymph nodes were involved in 2% of the cases and, since low axillary dissection is easily performed with total mastectomy, some nodes should be removed and the specimen marked to aid the pathologist in the laboratory examination. While mastectomy has been the traditional treatment and yields almost a 100% survival rate, it may be permissible to treat these lesions with lumpectomy and x-ray therapy, as results are good and salvage surgery of any recurrence will produce a near 100% cure rate in the carefully followed patient (Schnitt et al. 1988).

Lumpectomy alone is not considered acceptable treatment for DCIS at the present time except within the context of a randomized trial. Cryptic intraductal carcinoma may be present in the contralateral breast in as many as 10% of the patients, so some surgeons advocate biopsy of the opposite breast (Leis et al. 1989).

Lagios has reviewed 79 patients with mammographically detected DCIS less than 2.5 cm in diameter (Lagios et al. 1989). All were treated by local excision only. Ten percent of the patients have developed recurrence near the incision site, and four patients developed invasive cancer and were treated by modified radical mastectomy; three were N0 and one had a single micrometastasis in a lymph node at level I. All patients are currently free of tumor. Recurrence correlated with high nuclear grade and comedo-type necrosis.

INVASIVE CARCINOMA OF THE BREAST

About 70% of all invasive breast cancers are ductal carcinomas, usually with a fibrous reaction. This is usually the type meant by "cancer of the breast"—not otherwise specified (NOS). Other types of breast cancer are sometimes thought to have a better prognosis, but this is usually because they are found at an earlier stage, which may reflect a length bias. Fisher has stated that patients with papillary, mucinous, tubular, and combination tumors lacking an infiltrating-duct component without special features have the best prognosis (Fisher et al. 1980). Medullary, lobular invasive, and combination tumors with an infiltrating-duct component with special features are intermediate; and infiltrating-duct carcinomas without special features have the most ominous prognosis. Fisher agrees, however, that stage for stage, there is little if any difference in prognosis among the various pathological types; prognosis depends upon staging, especially the status of the axillary lymph nodes.

There are two readily accepted methods of treating invasive breast cancer: modified radical mastectomy with or without reconstruction, and lumpectomy with axillary dissection or sampling and postoperative irradiation. Some physicians believe that if the axillary lymph nodes contain metastases, there is systemic disease as well and that the axillary nodes serve only as a marker and prognostic indicator; furthermore, it is the low axillary lymph nodes which will be involved first. For that reason, complete axillary dissection is not necessary and axillary sampling will suffice (Forrest et al. 1974; Boova, Bonani, and Rosato 1981; Veronesi 1987). The opposing view states that all invasive breast cancers have shed cells into the systemic circulation long before the diagnosis can be made, but that the body's natural immune defenses will control these micrometastases up to a certain tumor burden. For that reason, a complete axillary dissection should be done in order to remove a reservoir of cancer cells that could metastasize as well as serve as a more reliable prognostic indicator, since prognosis is predicted by the number of metastatic lymph nodes and their location in the axilla (Danforth et al. 1986). At least in some series, axillary sampling was associated with an inferior result in local disease control compared to axillary dissection (Benson and Thorogood 1986). In general, lumpectomy with axillary sampling or dissection and postoperative irradiation is promoted because it provides an improved cosmetic result by breast preservation.

The contrary view is that mastectomy with reconstruction provides comparable esthetic appearance. When a lumpectomy is performed, the margins of resection should be carefully marked to provide adequate pathologic evaluation as the local recurrence rate is higher when the margins are involved by tumor. All breast biopsies should be performed as lumpectomies, unless the lesion is large and will be treated by mastectomy or the biopsy is done only for microscopic confirmation in an advanced tumor.

Contraindications to lumpectomy or quadrantectomy as the initial treatment include large tumors, especially in a small breast where removal with a margin of normal tissue would distort the breast contour. No good data exist for cancers over 5 cm in diameter, so at present the breast preservation procedure is acceptable for stage I and early stage II cancers. Subareolar lesions are probably not preferentially treated with lumpectomy, since cosmesis is thought to be one of the main considerations in this treatment method and removal of the areolar complex nullifies some of this advantage. Some surgeons feel that this is not a compelling reason. The presence of tumor at the resected margins of the lumpectomy specimen and the presence of extensive intraductal carcinoma are relative contraindications (Harris, Connolly, Schnitt et al. 1985), although this is not accepted by everyone (Wickerham and Fisher 1988). Postoperative irradiation is usually given over a period of five or six weeks and it may be supplemented in the region of the lumpectomy with a booster dose from x-rays, electron beam, or brachytherapy.

At present, 5-year survival rates for patients treated by modified radical mastectomy or by lumpectomy and irradiation are essentially the same (Wickerham and Fisher 1988; Veronesi, Saccozzi, Del Vecchio et al. 1981). The prognosis for patients with *in situ* cancer approaches 100%. Nonpalpable cancers 1 cm or less in diameter with negative lymph nodes which are diagnosed by mammography have a 5-year survival rate of almost 95%. The overall survival rate for cancers with negative nodes is 85% to 90%. The prognosis falls progressively with the number of metastatic lymph nodes. Patients whose specimens contain 10 or more positive lymph nodes have a prognosis about the same as that of untreated cancer. Treatment options should be discussed fully with patients; morbidity, treatment time, cost, and cosmesis must be considered. Recent efforts at immunotherapy have shown promise but require further evaluation. Springer (1989) has reported on the use of the T-antigen for diagnostic as well as treatment purposes.

COMPLICATIONS OF TREATMENT

The late complications of modified-radical mastectomy include lymphedema of the arm, limited or painful shoulder motion, hypertrophy of the operative scar, and a feeling of tightness in the chest. Studies of lymphedema indicate that the fluid retention is confined to the skin and fat and does not involve the muscle. The incidence of lymphedema depends upon how it is defined. If the extremity is measured by water displacement preoperatively and postoperatively, the incidence is very high, but symptomatic lymphedema occurs in about 12% of patients. The weight of the arm, the cosmetic appearance, and the difficulty in wearing short sleeves are annoying. The more serious problems are repeated attacks of cellulitis that sometimes occur in the swollen arm, and the relatively rare development of lymphangiosarcoma (Stewart-Treves syndrome), which has a high mortality rate. Compression treatment can be helpful in the milder cases of lymphedema, but it usually must be continued indefinitely. Numerous operative procedures have been tried, but often fail. Initial efforts with liposuction suggest that it may be beneficial, but longer follow-up will be necessary.

Long-term complications of lumpectomy plus irradiation include persistent edema of the breast and tanning of the skin in the irradiated field; irradiation pneumonitis; lymphedema of the arm; fat necrosis of the underlying breast tissue; telangiectasia of the irradiated skin; a rare incidence of rib fracture, which always heals; and recurrence of the carcinoma in the breast in up to 15% of the patients, which is highest in cases where the x-ray dose was reduced. Local recurrence of cancer following irradiation can be treated with mastectomy with about a 65% 5-year survival rate, so that the total number of survivors in large groups of patients treated by either modified-radical mastectomy or lumpectomy with irradiation are similar. Mastectomy for recurrence following irradiation makes reconstruction more difficult. Some physicians feel that the microscopic picture of sections from the irradiated breast suggest that more time is needed to evaluate the long-term adverse effects (Friedman 1988).

OTHER TREATMENT FACTORS

Locally advanced breast cancer can be treated with preoperative chemotherapy and/or irradiation with a 5-year survival rate of 40% to 50% (Wilson 1987; PDQ 1988). This is a significant improvement, since in the not-too-distant past, these lesions were thought to be incurable and even inoperable.

Breast cancer developing in a woman who is pregnant or lactating was formerly thought to be inoperable, but more recent data indicate that the poor prognosis associated with such tumors is usually the result of late diagnosis. Stage for stage, the results of treatment are similar to other invasive breast cancers (Ribeiro, Jones, and Jones 1986).

Inflammatory breast cancer is defined as a malignant tumor originating in the breast, associated with an erysipeloid type of inflammatory reaction of the skin and involvement of the dermal lymphatics with metastatic tumor. These tumors usually grow rapidly and have a poor prognosis. Induction chemotherapy is given as the initial treatment to try to reduce the tumor size. It is followed by surgery, and sometimes also by irradiation, and subsequently by additional chemotherapy. While the prognosis is still worse than for other types of breast cancer, there is a considerable improvement in treatment for this lesion, which previously was considered inoperable. Five-year survival rates up to 50% have been reported (Wilson 1987).

Radiation therapy is used in the treatment of primary breast cancer with lumpectomy and axillary dissection, and in the treatment of localized post-mastectomy recurrence. It is sometimes used in combination with chemotherapy and surgery in the treatment of advanced localized cancer, and for palliation of symptomatic metastatic breast cancer.

Male breast cancer is best treated with modified radical mastectomy, as these lesions are always subareolar in location and do not have an improved cosmetic result from lumpectomy and irradiation. Cancer of the male breast always develops close to the pectoral fascia, so muscle involvement requiring its resection is more common.

A pessimistic point of view on the treatment of breast cancer has been expressed by Mueller. He states that within a given group at risk, the likelihood of dying is no different in the fifteenth year than in the third year after diagnosis, and the rate of dying is approximately 8% per year in the group at risk. Eighty to 85% of women who die after a diagnosis of breast cancer, do so because of their breast cancer. He concludes that breast cancer treatment should be given only when and where the cancer is known to exist. Treatment should not be proposed as a means of influencing either time of death or cause of death. Measurements of the quality of life should be established and should constitute the only realistic objectives of treatment (Mueller 1987). Most clinicians do not accept this philosophy.

RECONSTRUCTION

Reconstruction of the breast following mastectomy has become popular in recent years. It can be done immediately at the time of mastectomy or delayed until a later time. Silicone gel in a plastic envelope is the most popular artificial insert and is usually placed behind the pectoral muscles, in contradistinction to the insertion between the breast tissue and the muscles in operations for breast augmentation. When reconstruction is planned and the skin is tight or the pectoral muscles are taut, an expander is frequently inserted. Following the operation, fluid is injected into a side port of the expander at weekly intervals, stretching the tissues until the desired size is obtained. At that time, the expander can be replaced by a permanent prosthesis, although some expanders are constructed so that replacement is unnecessary. Myocutaneous flaps are often preferred instead of an artificial prosthesis; the transabdominal myocutaneous (TRAM) or latissimus dorsi flaps are favored. Isolated local recurrence is more difficult to detect under a flap than after insertion of a subpectoral prosthesis, but local recurrence is usually accompanied by distant metastases.

Reconstruction is not for everyone. Many patients prefer to wear one of the wide variety of prostheses available rather than undergo reconstruction.

ADJUVANT TREATMENT

Adjuvant treatment is defined as therapy administered to patients with no demonstrable residual tumor after the initial treatment. Chemotherapy, hormone therapy and, to a lesser extent x-ray therapy, are used most commonly. It is generally agreed that adjuvant therapy is indicated for patients whose axillary lymph nodes contain metastatic tumor; there are still some reservations about routinely treating patients whose specimen does not. The current consensus is that in the node positive group chemotherapy should be given to premenopausal patients and hormone therapy to postmenopausal ones. The results from chemotherapy seem to be best in the group with one to three positive nodes, but all node positive patients should be treated. Patients with 10 or more positive nodes have a prognosis not much different from untreated patients. Combination chemotherapy is superior to single-agent and many different protocols are available (PDQ 1990). Multiple first line drugs are usually used, and treatment programs most often extend for about six months.

The relapse-free survival at 12 years for one entire series of cases treated with Cytoxan, methotrexate and 5-FU (CMF) was 28% for the control group and 40% for the treated group. Corresponding findings for total survival are 38% and 50%. Comparative reduction in tumor mortality (observed vs. expected) was 23% for the entire series and 40% for premenopausal patients; it was 3% for postmenopausal patients (Bonnadonna and Valagussa 1988). In an overview combining the results of all of the trials reported at the Consensus Conference at the National Cancer Institute, a 25% reduction in mortality during the first five years after starting adjuvant CMF was reported (Peto 1985).

Studies suggest that it may be desirable to give tamoxifen (Nolvadex) indefinitely in the postmenopausal, node positive, receptor positive patients (Gottardis, Martin, and Jordan 1985). As an indicator of treatment outcome, progesterone receptor status is most important in predicting the role of adjuvant tamoxifen treatment (Australian and New Zealand BCTG 1986).

Bianco reported that in their series, in receptor-positive patients, tamoxifen significantly reduced the incidence of relapse and deaths compared to the control, or no-treatment, arm in all postmenopausal patients and in premenopausal patients with negative nodes. Tamoxifen added no benefit to premenopausal patients with positive nodes treated with CMF (Bianco et al. 1988). It is not clear that hormone therapy improves the results from chemotherapy alone.

It is not yet certain that concurrent adjuvant treatment cures patients, but it does delay recurrence in many cases and prolongs survival in node-positive patients. In general, the time to recurrence depends on the stage of the tumor, and the treatment of early tumors requires a long interval for complete evaluation.

Some clinicians feel that negative results are published less often, which gives a stronger perception of good results based on a review of the literature. Bonnadonna, in publications from Milan regarding CMF adjuvant therapy in postmenopausal women, reported a recurrence rate at three years of 5% in treated patients vs. 24% in untreated controls. At 10 years after treatment, the figures were 28% for treated patients and 20% for untreated controls (Bonnadonna and Valagussa 1988).

In one controlled clinical trial comparing single-agent to combination adjuvant chemotherapy, the results at 27 months showed such differences that the single-agent arm was stopped. At 62 months, however, the differences were insignificant (Cohen et al. 1982).

The opinions on treatment of patients whose axillary nodes do not contain tumor are not as uniform. Recently the NCI issued a clinical alert stating that all cases of breast cancer, except *in situ* and minimal lesions (i.e., a primary tumor less than 1 cm in diameter and negative axillary lymph nodes), should be treated with adjuvant therapy. Fisher has stated that all patients except the *in-situ* and microinvasive group, should be treated. This announcement has had a mixed reception, because stage I carcinoma cases have a disease-free survival at five years of about 85%, and in those where the primary tumor is less than 1 cm, survival is 90%. Eventually, however, up to 25% of node-negative patients will develop recurrence. Post-menopausal patients with positive receptors, and some with negative receptors, often benefit from tamoxifen, but the value of chemotherapy is controversial in this group. Total survival may not be affected to the same degree as disease-free survival. Some skeptics feel that the results of treatment in the control groups which are used in the comparison in the NCI's clinical alert are worse than those usually seen in node-negative patients and that follow-up time is too short for the results to be valid. Many investigators, therefore, feel that more data need to be made available before a final decision is made. The use of tamoxifen, which is relatively nontoxic, is accepted more widely than the use of adjuvant chemotherapy in the node-negative group, especially in postmenopausal women.

A recent study reviewing this topic proposes that all future trials of adjuvant chemotherapy be standardized and that patients not enrolled in the trials be similarly followed and evaluated (Cascinelli, Greco, and Leo 1988).

A review of the results of 61 randomized trials among 28,896 patients has been done by a collaborative group. It showed a reduction in mortality from the administration of tamoxifen only in women 50 or older, who made up one-fifth of the patients. Reductions of mortality in women under 50 was seen only in the polychemotherapy group and amounted to one-fourth of the patients. There was no demonstrable advantage from administering chemotherapy longer than four to six months. Tamoxifen did not seem to reinforce the value of chemotherapy. In patients with one to three metastatic axillary lymph nodes as compared to those with four or more, the proportional reductions in the annual death rates during the first five years were not different in either the polychemotherapy- or tamoxifen-treated groups. Although the proportional reductions in mortality among women with or without metastatic nodes appeared to be similar, the reduction was not statistically significant in an analysis restricted to patients with negative nodes (Early Breast Cancer Trialists' Collaborative Group 1988).

Currently, the majority opinion for the adjuvant treatment of node negative patients is to treat premenopausal patients with chemotherapy for about six months. Postmenopausal patients should be treated with tamoxifen for at least six months. Patients at high risk for recurrence should be treated, but controversy persists about giving adjuvant treatment otherwise (table 13.7).

TREATMENT OF SYSTEMIC BREAST CANCER

Patients with metastatic cancer who have had adjuvant chemotherapy, as compared to patients who have not, show a higher incidence of central nervous system involvement, a lower response rate to additional chemotherapy, and a shorter survival. These findings may help explain the failure of the improved relapse-free survival seen in many adjuvant chemotherapy trials to result in improved overall survival (Ahmann, Jones, and Moon 1988). These observations essentially are in agreement with an earlier study on the value of prophylactic vs. therapeutic castration in breast carcinoma (Fracchia et al. 1969). Treatment of metastatic disease is usually done with multiple second-line drugs and is continued at least until there is complete remission or failure to respond.

About 60% of primary breast cancers contain estrogen receptors and the levels are usually greater in postmenopausal women than in premenopausal ones. A little more than half of the patients with positive receptors respond to endocrine therapy, and some with negative receptors will do so. If the breast tumor has positive receptors for both estrogen and progesterone, the chances of response are greater. Estrogen receptor and progesterone receptor determinations should be made on all breast cancers.

A wide range of hormonal manipulation is used in treating breast cancer. Some of it is administered as adjuvant therapy for patients whose tumors are at high risk for recurrence; most of it is done for metastases. It can be ablative, such as oophorectomy, adrenalectomy, or hypophysectomy; increasingly, however, medications are used with equal results. Tamoxifen is currently the most popular drug, but aminoglutethimide, megestrol acetate, estrogens, androgens, and other drugs are used (Fletcher 1986).

Table 13.7
RISK FACTORS FOR RELAPSE IN STAGE I BREAST CANCER

1. Negative ER/PgR
2. High S-phase
3. Aneuploidy
4. Large tumor (2 cm)

(Courtesy: McGuire [1986].)

FOLLOW-UP

There are no well-controlled studies on follow-up procedures after treatment of the primary tumor. Most investigators recommend that the patient be seen at 3-month intervals for 18 months to four years, after which patients are usually seen at 6-month intervals for variable periods of time depending on risk factors. Some cases of isolated local recurrence can be controlled for long periods of time, especially in those that appear two or more years after primary treatment. Routine laboratory testing is not worthwhile in the asymptomatic patient (Scanlon et al. 1980). Data suggest that the interval between detection from routine testing and discovery from testing for symptoms is about three months, and there are no data that this time period affects treatment or prognosis.

Patients on protocol studies are placed on a routine testing schedule, since there must be comparable endpoints of the different treatment schedules. Patients being treated for systemic disease may benefit from routine testing, since treatment failure requires switching to a different regimen.

PROGNOSIS

It is generally agreed that the single most important prognostic indicator in breast cancer is the number of involved metastatic axillary lymph nodes. The more nodes involved, the worse is the prognosis, but for practical purposes, patients are usually grouped into those with three nodes or fewer as compared to those with four or more involved nodes. Other unfavorable prognostic factors include perimenopausal status at diagnosis, larger tumor size, infiltrating duct histology, lymphatic and blood vessel invasion, the absence of hormone receptors, aneuploidy, a higher percentage of cancer cells in the S-phase, and certain oncogene translocations such as C-myc, c-erb or HER-2/neu. Skin window reactivity to autologous breast cancer reflects cell mediated immunity (CMI) to a determinant expressed by glycoprotein 55. It can reflect changes in prognosis in the postoperative period in patients who are followed by this procedure (Black et al. 1989). Patients with a single micrometastasis (≤2 mm) have the same prognosis as patients with a single macrometastasis in an axillary lymph node, but the statistical insignificance does not become manifest until 12 years after treatment (Rosen et al. 1981). The strong correlations between tumor receptor content, percent S-phase, and aneuploidy suggest that these measurements in concert are important indicators for the risk of recurrence (McGuire 1986). The absence of hormone receptors in the tumor does not correlate with the likelihood of subsequent metastases, but rather reflects the timing of a recurrence, if it is to occur at all (Aamdal et al. 1984).

Since 1960, more than 3,000 consecutive patients have been treated by lumpectomy by the Marseilles Group (Kurtz et al. 1987). Thirty-five percent of the patients alive and disease-free at 10 years required a second operation for presumed local or regional tumor persistence or recurrence; no residual disease was found in 24% of the operative specimens. Of the patients cured at 10 years, 29% had lost their breast. Patients with lower doses of irradiation were at greater risk for recurrence, but local-regional recurrence had no adverse effect on 10-year survival.

A factor that may influence the results of treatment of the node-negative group is the fact that cryptic lymph-node metastases are frequently overlooked. In one small study lymph nodes that had been reported as negative on routine pathology examination were shown on serial sections to have metastatic tumor deposits in 33% of the cases (Saphir and Amromin 1948). A second study detected metastases in nodes previously reported as negative and additional metastases in positive nodes (Schurman et al. 1990).

The prognosis of patients with 10 or more metastatic nodes is very poor and approaches that of untreated breast cancer. For that reason, it has been suggested that future studies should divide patients into categories of negative nodes, three or fewer positive nodes, four to nine positive nodes, and 10 or more. The heterogeneity of the disease explains some of the variability in reported results of treatment with chemotherapy.

BILATERAL BREAST CANCER

Cancer in one breast is a significant risk factor for the subsequent development of cancer in the other breast, at a rate of about 1% per year. Premenopausal women have almost twice the risk of postmenopausal women. Anaplastic cancers have a higher risk of second cancers, regardless of true prognosis, as compared to histologically low-grade cancers. There is a higher risk in the second breast of those patients who present with multiple primary cancers in the first breast (Leis et al. 1988). The more aggressive monitoring of patients with previous breast cancer, including mammography, probably results in an earlier detection of second breast cancers (Senofsky et al. 1986). In one series of almost 1,000 patients with breast cancer, the second breast contained a synchronous primary cancer in 12.5% and a precancerous mastopathy in 9.8%. In this same series of 143 prophylactic contralateral total mastectomies, 21% had carcinoma and an additional 15% had precancerous lesions, despite a normal physical examination and a negative mammogram; 60% of the cancers were *in situ* (Leis et al. 1988). These clinicians tend to avoid irradiation of the breast for small cancers because of the fear of an increased incidence of cancer in the contralateral breast (Moffat et al. 1988).

PSYCHOSOCIAL ASPECTS

Recently, much attention has been paid to the psychosocial aspects of breast cancer. In the past, a high percentage of women had a marked depression postoperatively, but that situation has improved considerably in recent years. Patients are better informed about breast cancer; many tumors are detected early with a resultant improvement in prognosis; cosmesis is improved because of reconstruction after mastectomy or preservation of the breast by treatment with irradiation; and counseling is available through several groups, including the American Cancer Society.

REFERENCES

Aamdal, S.; Bormer, O.; and Jorgensen, O. et al. 1984. Estrogen receptors and long term prognosis in breast cancer. *Cancer* 53:2525-29.

ACS. 1988. *Cancer facts and figures.* ACS guidelines for breast cancer detection.

ACS. 1987. *Diagram on BSE special touch: participant's guide.* American Cancer Society.

Ahmann, F.R.; Jones, S.E.; and Moon, T.E. 1988. The effect of prior adjuvant chemotherapy on survival in metastatic breast cancer. *J. Surg. Oncol.* 73:116-22.

American Joint Committee on Cancer. 1988. *Manual for staging of cancer.* 3rd ed. pp. 145-48.

Andersson, I.; Aspegren, K.; and Lanzon, L. et al. 1988. Mammographic screening and mortality from breast cancer: the Malmo mammographic screening trial. *Br. Med. J.* 297:943-48.

Atkins, H., and Wolfe, B. 1964. Discharges from the nipple. *Br. J. Surg.* 51:602-606.

Australian and New Zealand Breast Cancer Trials Group. 1986. A randomized trial in postmenoapual patients with adjuvant breast cancer, comparing endocrine and cytotoxic therapy given sequentially or in combination. *J. Clin. Oncol.* 4:186-93.

Baines, C.J. 1987. The Canadian National Breast Screening study: current status. In Paterson, H.G., and Lees, A.W. eds. *Fundamental problems in breast cancer.* pp. 25-27. Boston: Marcus Nijhoff.

Benson, E.A., and Thorogood, J. 1986. The effect of surgical technique on local recurrence rates following mastectomy. *Eur. J. Surg. Oncol.* 12:267-71.

Bianco, A.R.; Gallo, C.; and Marinelli, A. et al. 1988. Adjuvant therapy with tamoxifen in operable breast cancer. *Lancet* II:1095-99.

Black, M.M.; Zachrau, R.E.; and Ashikari, R.H. et al. 1989. Prognostic significance of cellular immunity to autologous breast carcinoma and glycoprotein 55. *Arch. Surg.* 124:202-206.

Bloom, M.D.; Johnson, F.; and Pertshuck, K. et al. 1984. Electrocautery: effects on steroid receptors in human breast cancer. *J. Surg. Oncol.* 25:21-24.

Bonnadonna, G., and Valagussa, P. 1988. Adjuvant chemotherapy for breast cancer. *Sem. Surg. Oncol.* 4(4):250-55.

Boova, R.S.; Bonanni, R.; and Rosato, F.E. 1982. Patterns of axillary nodal involvement in breast cancer: predictability of level one dissection. *Ann. Surg.* 196(6):642-44.

Bundred, N.; Levack, P.; and Watmough, D.J. et al. 1987. Preliminary results using computerized telediaphanography for investigating breast disease. *Br. J. Hosp. Med.* 37(1):70-71.

Byrd, B.F., and Hartmann, W.H. 1988. Breast cancer detection epoch. *Sem. Surg. Oncol.* 4(4):221-25.

Cardona, G.; Cataliotti, L.; and Ciatto, S. et al. Reasons for failure of physical examination in breast cancer detection (analysis of 232 false negative cases). *Tumors* 69(6):531-37.

Cascinelli, N.; Greco, M.; and Leo, E. 1988. Comments on primary and adjuvant treatments of breast cancer. *Eur. J. Cancer Clin. Oncol.* 24:3:487-91.

Chilvers, C.; McPherson, K.; and Peto, J. et al. 1989. Oral contraceptive use and breast cancer risk in young women: U.K. national case-control study group. *Lancet* I:973-82.

Cohen, E.; Scanlon, E.F.; and Caprini, J.A. et al. 1982. Follow-up adjuvant chemotherapy and chemoimmunotherapy for stage II and III carcinoma of the breast. *Cancer* 49:1754-61.

Colin, C. and Gordenne, W. eds. 1985. *Evaluation du Risque de Cancer Mammaire. Chemiotherapie Premiere?* pp. 119-21. Brussells, Belgium: Pierre Mardaga.

Consensus Meeting, Cancer Committee, College of American Pathologists. 1986. Is fibrocystic disease of the breast precancerous? *Arch. Pathol. Lab. Med.* 110:171-73.

Controlled trial of tamoxifen as a single adjuvant agent in management of early breast cancer: analysis at six years by Nolvadex Adjuvant Trial Organisation. 1985. *Lancet* I(8433):836-40.

Collette, H.J.A.; Day, N.E.; and Rombach, J.J. et al. 1984. Evaluation of screening for breast cancer in a nonrandomized study. *Lancet* I:1224-26.

Cutler, J.C., and Young, J.L. 1975. Third national cancer survey: incidence data. *Natl. Cancer Inst. Monogr. 41.*

Danforth, D.N.; Findlay, P.A.; and McDonald, H.D. 1986. Complete axillary lymph node dissection for stage I-II carcinoma of the breast. *J. Clin. Oncol.* 4(5):655-62.

Dobernack, R.C., and Garcia, J.E. 1988. Primary breast cancer in patients with previous endometrial or ovarian cancer. *J. Surg. Oncol.* 37:100-103.

Dodd, G.D. 1989. Personal communication.

Early Breast Cancer Trialists' Collaborative Group. 1988. Effects of adjuvant tamoxifen and of cytotoxic therapy on mortality in early breast cancer. *N. Engl. J. Med.* 319:1681-92.

Eddy, D.W.; Hassleblad, V.; and McGiveny, W. 1988. Value of mammography screening in women under age 50 years. *JAMA* 259:1512-19.

Evans, D.B., and Crichlow, R.W. 1987. Carcinoma of the male breast and Klinefelter's syndrome: is there an association? *CA* 37(4)246-51.

Feig, S.A. 1987. Xero and screen-film: mammography's rival systems. *Diag. Imaging* 27:112-17.

Ferguson, D.J.; Meier, P.; and Karrison, T. et al. 1982. Staging of breast cancer and survival rates: an assessment based on 50 years of experience with radical mastectomy. *JAMA* 248:1337-41.

Ferguson, D.J. 1987. The actual extent of mastectomy: a key to survival. *Pers. Bio. Med.* 30(3):311-23.

Ferguson, D.J.; Meier, P.; and Karrison, T. et al. 1989. A controlled trial of extended radical mastectomy vs. radical mastectomy: 10-year results. *Cancer* 63:188-95.

Fisher, E.R.; Palekan, A.S.; and Redmond, C. et al. 1980. Pathologic findings from the National Surgical Adjuvant Breast Project (Protocol 4) M.D. *AJCP* 73(3):313-20.

Fisher, E.R.; Sass, R.; and Fisher, B. et al. 1986. Pathologic findings from the National Surgical Adjuvant Breast Project (Protocol 6) 1: intraductal carcinoma. *Cancer* 57:197-208.

Fisher, E.R. 1989. Personal communication.

Fletcher, W.F. 1986. Endocrine manipulation in advanced breast cancer. In Najarian, J.S., and Delaney, J.P. eds. *Advances in breast and endocrine surgery.* Chicago: Year Book Medical Publishers.

Fornage, B.D.; Faroux, M.J.; and Simatos, A. 1987. Breast masses: US-guided fine-needle aspiration biopsy. *Radiology* 162:409-14.

Fornage, B.D.; Toubas, O.; and Morel, M. 1987. Clinical, mammographic, and sonographic determination of preoperative breast cancer size. *Cancer* 60:765-71.

Forrest, A.P.M.; Roberts, M.M.; and Preece, P. 1974. The Cardiff-St. Mary's trial. *Br. J. Surg.* 61:766-69.

Foster, R.S. Jr.; Lang, S.P.; and Costanza, M.C. et al. 1987. Breast self examination practices and breast cancer stage. *N. Engl. J. Med.* 299(6):205-70.

Frable, W.J. 1983. Thin needle aspiration biopsy. In Pennington, J.L. ed. *Major problems in pathology.* vol. 14. Philadelphia: W.B. Saunders.

Fracchia, A.A.; Murray, D.R.; and Farrow, J.H. et al. 1969. Comparison of prophylactic and therapeutic castration in breast carcinoma. *Surg. Gynecol. Obstet.* 129:270-76.

Friedman, N. 1988. The effects of irradiation on breast cancer and the breast. *CA* 38(6):368-71.

Frykberg, E.; Santiago, F.; and Betsill, W. et al. 1987. Lobular carcinoma *in situ* of the breast: collective review. *Surg. Gynecol. Obstet.* 164:285-301.

Garfinkel, L. 1989. Personal communication.

Gohagan, J.K.; Darby, W.K.; and Spitznagel, E.L. et al. 1986. Radiogenic breast cancer effects of mammographic screening. *J. Natl. Cancer Inst.* 77(1):71-76.

Gottardis, M.M.; Martin, M.K.; and Jordan, V.C. 1985. Long-term tamoxifen therapy to control transplanted human breast tumor growth in athymic mice. In Salmon, S.E. ed. *Adjuvant therapy for cancer V.* pp. 447-53. Orlando: Grune & Stratton.

Gump, F.E.; Jicha, D.L.; and Ozello, L. 1987. Ductal carcinoma *in situ* (DCIS). *Surgery* 102(5):790-95.

Hall, F.M. 1986. Mammography in the diagnosis of *in situ* breast carcinoma. *Radiology* 168:279-80.

Harris, J.R.; Connolly, J.L.; and Schnitt, S.J. et al. 1985. The use of pathologic features in selecting the extent of surgical resection necessary for breast cancer patients treated with primary radiation therapy. *Ann. Surg.* 201:164-69.

Hermansen, C. et al. 1987. Diagnostic reliability of combined physical examination, mammography, and fine needle puncture in breast tumors. *Cancer* 60:1866-71.

Holleb, A.I.; Freeman, H.P.; and Farrow, J.H. 1968. Cancer of the male breast. *N.Y. State J. Med.* 68:544-53.

Horm, J. 1988. Personal communication.

Huguley, C.M. Jr., and Brown, R.L. 1981. The value of breast self examination. *Cancer* 47:989-95.

Hutter, R.V.P. 1984. Management of patients with lobular carcinoma *in situ* of the breast. *Cancer* 53:798-802.

Kurtz, J.M.; Amalric, R.; and Delouche, G. 1987. The second ten years: long-term risks of breast conservation in early breast cancer. *J. Radiat. Oncol. Biol. Phys.* 13:1327-32.

Lacour, J.; Le, M.G.; and Hill, C. 1987. Is it useful to remove internal mammary nodes in operable breast cancer? *Eur. J. Surg. Oncol.* 13:309-14.

Lagios, M.D.; Margolin, F.R.; and Westdahl, P.R. 1989. Mammographically detected duct carcinoma *in situ. Cancer* 63:618-24.

Leis, H.P. Jr.; Greene, F.L.; and Cammarata, A. et al. 1988. Nipple discharge: surgical significance. *South Med. J.* 81(1): 20-26.

Leis, H.P. Jr.; Greene, F.L.; and Hilfer, S.E.; et al. 1988. Simultaneous primary cancer in the other breast. *Breast Dis.* 1(2):83-96.

Letton, A.H., and Mason, E.M. 1986. Routine breast screening: survival after 10.5 years follow-up. *Ann. Surg.* 203:470-73.

Lynch, H.T. 1990. The family history and cancer control: hereditary breast cancer. *Arch. Surg.* 125(2):151-52.

Maddox, W.A.; Carpenter, J.T. Jr.; and Laws, H.T. 1987. Does radical mastectomy still have a place in the treatment of primary operable breast cancer? *Arch. Surg.* 122:1317-20.

Mant, D.; Vessey, M.P.; and Neil, A. et al. 1987. Breast self examination and breast cancer at diagnosis. *Br. J. Cancer* 55:207-11.

McGuire, W.L. 1986. Prognostic factors in primary breast cancer. *Cancer Surv.* 5(3):527-36.

Miller, A.B., and Baines, C.J. 1987. Letter to the editor. *Can. J. Surg.* 30(3):153-54.

Miller, A.B. 1988. Screening for breast cancer: a review. *Eur. J. Clin. Oncol.* 24:49-53.

Moffat, F.J.; Ketchum, A.S.; and Robinson, D.S. 1988. Breast cancer management of the opposite breast. *Oncology* 2(11): 25-33.

Moskowitz, M. 1985. Do the results of the Swedish Trial, the Dutch case-control study and the Cincinnati breast cancer detection demonstration project tell us anything of importance about the natural history of breast cancer? *Proc. Int. Symp. Senology* Liege, Belgium.

Mueller, C.B. 1987. Cancer of the breast: valid alternatives in the management of early breast cancer. *Ann. Surg.* 20: 183-16.

Olsson, H.; Moller, T.R.; and Rantsam, J. 1989. Early oral contraceptive use and breast cancer among premenopausal women: final report from a study in southern Sweden. *J. Natl. Cancer Inst.* 81:13.

O'Malley, M.S., and Fletcher, S.W. 1987. Screening for breast cancer with breast self examination: a critical review. *JAMA* 57:2196-2203.

Page, D.L.; Dupont, W.D.; and Rogers, L.W. et al. 1982. Intraductal carcinoma of the breast: follow-up after biopsy only. *Cancer* 49:751-58.

PDQ. July 1988.

Peto, R. 1984. Review of mortality results in randomized trials in early breast cancer (editorial). *Lancet* II:1205.

Philips, J. et al. 1984. Breast self examination: clinical results from a population-based prospective study. *Br. J. Cancer* 50(1):7-12.

Pochin, E.E. 1987. Radiation risks in perspective. *Br. J. Radiol.* 60:42-50.

Ribeiro, G.; Jones, D.A.; and Jones, M. 1986. Carcinoma of the breast associated with pregnancy. *Br. J. Surg.* 73: 607-609.

Rosen, P.P.; Braun, D.W.; and Kinne, D.E. 1980. The clinical significance of preinvasive breast cancer. *Cancer* 46:919-25.

Rosen, P.P.; Saigo, P.E.; and Braun, D.W. 1981. Axillary micro- and macrometastases in breast cancer. *Ann. Surg.* 194(5):585-91.

Rosen, P.P. 1986. Letter to the editor. *Ann. Surg.* 204(5): 612-13.

Rosenthal, L.J. 1979. Discrepant estrogen receptor protein levels according to surgical techniques. *Am. J. Surg.* 138: 680-81.

Rosner, E.; Bedwani, R.N.; and Vana, J. et al. 1980. Noninvasive breast carcinoma: results of a national survey by the American College of Surgeons. *Ann. Surg.* 192:139-47.

Saphir, O., and Amromin, G.D. 1948. Obscure axillary lymph-node metastasis in carcinoma of the breast. *Cancer* 1: 238-41.

Sawyer, P.F. 1986. Breast self examination: hospital-based nurses aren't assessing their clients. *Oncol. Nurs. Forum* 13(5):44-48.

Scanlon, E.F.; Oviedo, M.A.; and Cunningham, M.P. 1980. Preoperative and follow-up procedures on patients with breast cancer. *Cancer* 46:977-79.

Scanlon, E.F. 1984. How we do a breast palpation. *Primary Care & Cancer* 4(7):35-42.

Scanlon, E.F. 1987. A photo checklist for a better breast palpation. *Primary Care & Cancer* 7(9):13-20.

Schnitt, S.J.; Silen, W.; and Sadowsky, N.L. 1988. Ductal carcinoma *in situ. N. Engl. J. Med.* 318(14):898-903.

Schurman, S.H.; Sharone, N.; and Goldschmidt, R.A. et al. 1990. Improved detection of metastases to lymph nodes and estrogen receptor determination. *Arch. Surg.* 125:179-82.

Sciotto, S.; Bravetti, P.; and Cariaggi, P. 1986. Significance of nipple discharge: clinical patterns in the selection of cases for cytological examination. *Acta Cytologica* 30(1):17-20.

Seidman, H.; Stellman, S.D.; and Mushinski, M.H. 1982. A

different perspective on breast cancer risk factors: some implications of the non-attributable risk. *CA* 32:5.

Seidman, H.; Gelb, S.K.; and Silverberg, E. 1987. Survival experience in the Breast Cancer Detection Demonstration Project. *CA* 37(5):258-90.

Seltzer, M.H.; Perloff, L.J.; and Kelley, R.I. 1970. The significance of age in patients with nipple discharge. *Surg. Gynecol. Obstet.* 131:519-22.

Semiglazov, V.F., and Moiseyenko, V.M.P. 1987. Current evaluation of the contribution of self examination to secondary prevention of breast cancer. *Eur. J. Epidemiol.* 3(1):78-83.

Sener, S.; Scanlon, E.F.; and Paige, M.L. 1977. Potential accuracy of xeroradiographic examination of the breast with respect to menopausal status and location of pathologic findings. *Breast* 3(3):39-47.

Senofsky, G.M.; Wanebo, H.J.; and Wilhelm, M.C. 1986. Has monitoring of the contralateral breast improved the prognosis in patients treated for primary breast cancer? *Cancer* 57:597-602.

Shapiro, S.; Venet, W.; and Strax, P. 1988. Current results in the Breast Cancer Screening Randomized Trial: the Health Insurance Plan (HIP) of Greater New York Study. In Day, N.E., and Miller, A.B. eds. *Screening for breast cancer.* Toronto: Hans Huber Publishers.

Shelley, J.F., and Lessan, G.T. 1986. Limited impact of the breast self examination movement: a Latin American illustration. *Soc. Sci. Med.* 23(9):905-10.

Skrabanek, P. 1985. False premises and false promises of breast cancer screening. *Lancet* II:316-20.

Springer, G.F.; Desai, P.R.; and Scanlon, E.F. 1989. T and Tn pan carcinoma autoantigens: fundamental and clinical aspects. *Proceedings 7th International Congress of Immunology.* (abstr) Berlin.

Tabar, L.; Fagerberg, G.; and Gad, A. et al. 1985. Reduction in mortality from breast cancer after mass screening with mammography. *Lancet* 985:829-32.

Tabar, L. 1987. Screening for breast cancer: an overview. *Rec. Results Cancer Res.* 105:58-61.

Toniolo, P.; Riboli, E.; and Protta, F. 1989. Calorie-providing nutrients and risk of breast cancer. *J. Natl. Cancer Inst.* 81:278-86.

Turner, D.A. et al. 1988. Carcinoma of the breast: detection with MR imaging vs. xeromammography. *Radiology* 168:49-58.

Upton, A.C. 1982. The biological effects of low-level ionizing radiation. *Scientific American* 246(2):41-46.

Urban, J.A., and Egeli, R.A. 1978. Nonlactational nipple discharge. *CA* 28(3):130-40.

Urban, J.A. 1988. Primary surgical treatment of breast cancer. *Sem. Surg. Oncol.* 4(4):237-43.

Verbeek, A.L.M.; Hendriks, J.H.C.L.; and Holland, R. et al. 1985. Mammographic screening and breast cancer mortality: age specific effects in Nijmegen project. *Lancet* I:865-66.

Veronesi, U.; Saccozzi, R.; and Del Vecchio, M. et al. 1981. Comparing radical mastectomy with quadrantectomy, axillary dissection, and radiotherapy in patients with small cancers of the breast. *N. Engl. J. Med.* 305:6-11.

Veronesi, U.; Rilke, F.; and Luini, A. et al. 1987. Distribution of axillary node metastases by level of invasion: an analysis of 539 cases. *Cancer* 59:682-87.

Watmough, D.J.; Moran, C.; and Watmough, J.A. 1988. Son et Lumiere. *J. Biomed. Engl.* 10:119-22.

Wickerham, D.L., and Fisher, B. 1988. Surgical treatment of breast cancer. *Sem. Surg. Oncol.* 3:226-33.

Willett, W.C.; Stampfer, M.J.; and Colditz, G.A. et al. 1987. Dietary fat and the risk of breast cancer. *N. Engl. J. Med.* 316:22-8.

Wilson, R.E.; Donegan, W.L.; and Mettlin, C. et al. 1982. The 1982 national survey of carcinoma of the breast in the United States by the American College of Surgeons. *Surg. Gynecol. Obstet* 159(4):309-18.

Wilson, R.E. 1987. Recommendations for the surgical management of advanced breast cancer. *Oncology.* 1(3):21-26.

Wynder, E.L. 1987. Amount and type of fat/fiber in nutritional oncogenesis. *Prevent. Med.* 16:451-59.

Chapter 14

LUNG CANCER

L. Penfield Faber, M.D.

L. Penfield Faber, M.D.
Associate Dean, Surgical Sciences and Services
Associate Vice President for Medical Affairs
Rush-Presbyterian-St. Luke's Medical Center
Chicago, Illinois

INTRODUCTION

Lung cancer is a disease of almost epidemic proportion. Approximately 157,000 new cases and 142,000 deaths are estimated for the year 1990. The male-to-female incidence ratio is approximately 2.1:1. Lung cancer represents 20% of new cancers in males and 11% of new cancers in females. It causes 34% of the cancer deaths in males and 21% of the cancer deaths in females. The deaths from lung cancer in women now exceed the expected number of deaths from breast cancer. Despite the continuing efforts of clinicians and researchers who deal with this malignancy, long-term survival has increased only slightly. The overall 5-year survival rate for all patients with lung cancer is 13%, whereas it was approximately 7% in 1963. A major reason for the overall poor prognosis of patients having lung cancer is that only 21% have localized disease when the diagnosis is made. In addition, 50% are considered to be inoperable. The 5-year survival rate for localized disease improves to 37%; with regional lymph node involvement, survival is 33% (Silverberg, Boring, and Squires 1990).

Despite the overall dismal outlook, the clinician must always be aware that there are significantly varying rates of survival related to the stage of the disease, the histology of the lung cancer, and the overall condition of the patient. Early diagnosis and changes in environmental conditions and habits are major factors that will enhance survival of lung-cancer patients.

HISTOGENESIS

All histologic types of bronchogenic carcinoma are thought to originate from the basal cells of the bronchial epithelium; these cells are of endodermal origin. Carcinogenesis occurs when a carcinogen or chemical initiator damages cellular DNA. There is a long latent period from the initial time of exposure to the development of the clinically apparent bronchogenic carcinoma. This period can be as long as several decades. Following DNA damage, there is differentiation into the various histologic types of lung cancer. Many lung cancers demonstrate cellular heterogenicity, which supports the concept of differentiation from a common cell of origin. The reasons for development into the various histologic types of lung cancer will be further elucidated by continual study of the cellular and molecular biology of lung cancer.

RISK FACTORS

TOBACCO

The most significant risk factor for bronchogenic carcinoma is tobacco smoking. The risk of developing lung cancer is 10 times greater in men who smoke and five times greater in women. This risk is increased by the number of years an individual has smoked, the number of cigarettes smoked per day, the length of each cigarette, the depth of inhalation, and the tar content of the cigarettes. Carcinogens identified in the particulate and gas phases of tobacco smoke include nitrosamines, benzopyrenes, benzanthracene, and others in varying concentration. Squamous cell carcinoma and small-cell carcinoma are the common histologic types found in the smoker, but adenocarcinoma and large-cell carcinoma are also related to smoking. The incidence of lung cancer decreases when smoking is stopped and after 15 years of cessation, the incidence of lung cancer approaches that of people who have never smoked.

AGE

Lung cancer in a person under the age of 40 is rare. The incidence increases rapidly after age 50, with 60 years being the average age of onset. Lung cancer is found most frequently in patients 50 to 75 years of age and the incidence is higher in the 65- to 75-year-old group than in the 55- to 64-year-old group.

SCARRING

Bronchogenic carcinoma can be initiated in a scarred area of the lung caused by a prior inflammatory process. The histologic type of a so-called scar cancer is usually adenocarcinoma.

ASBESTOS

Death from bronchogenic carcinoma among asbestos workers is seven times more frequent than in the general population (Selikoff, Hammond, and Seidman 1979). Because of a synergistic carcinogenic effect between smoking and asbestos fibers, this group has a high incidence of lung cancer. Asbestos exposure alone carries a 5-fold increased risk for the development of lung cancer. Asbestos-related lung cancers are more frequently found in the lower lobes and also may originate in multiple sites. Federal guidelines are being developed to minimize exposure to asbestos, and safeguards against asbestos exposure in the workplace have been developed.

OCCUPATION

Various occupations are associated with exposure to agents that may initiate the development of a bronchogenic cancer. These agents include ionizing radiation among uranium and hard rock miners; and coal tars, petroleum, chromates, nickel, arsenic, and mustard gas.

AIR POLLUTION

The urban population may have a slightly increased incidence of lung cancer related to air pollution that contains benzopyrenes and hydrocarbons from automobile exhaust. However, the effect of smoking clouds the issue of air pollution as a strong causative factor.

GENETICS

Lung cancer also occurs in nonsmokers, which raises the question as to other factors that play a role in its development. There are some hereditary conditions that predispose to cancer, although these are not strongly associated with bronchogenic carcinoma. There may be a slight increase in the incidence of lung cancer among the siblings and children of lung cancer patients.

HOST SUSCEPTIBILITY

There is an increased risk of lung cancer in vitamin A-deficient people. Also, the risk of developing a second primary lung cancer is greater in a person who has had an original primary lung cancer successfully treated.

PATHOLOGY

A wide variety of malignant neoplasms arise from the bronchi and pulmonary parenchyma and the great majority of these are epithelial in origin. Histochemistry, immunohistochemistry, and electron microscopy have provided significant new information about the types and classifications of these malignancies. A modified classification of bronchial carcinoma of the World Health Organization (WHO) is shown in table 14.1 (Sobin and Yesner 1981). Bronchogenic carcinoma is categorized into two major groups: non-small cell bron-

Table 14.1
HISTOLOGIC CLASSIFICATION OF LUNG CANCER

I.	SQUAMOUS CELL CARCINOMA Well, moderately, and poorly differentiated
II.	ADENOCARCINOMA Well, moderately, and poorly differentiated Acinar, papillary, and bronchioloalveolar
III.	LARGE-CELL UNDIFFERENTIATED CARCINOMA Giant cell carcinoma Clear cell carcinoma
IV.	NEUROENDOCRINE LUNG NEOPLASMS Carcinoid Atypical (malignant) carcinoid Intermediate-cell neuroendocrine carcinoma Small-cell neuroendocrine carcinoma
V.	MULTICOMPONENT (MULTIDIFFERENTIATED CARCINOMA)
VI.	BRONCHIAL GLAND NEOPLASMS Adenoid-cystic carcinoma Mucoepidermoid carcinoma
VII.	SARCOMAS Lymphomas Carcinosarcomas

chogenic carcinomas (NSCLC) and small-cell lung carcinomas (SCLC).

NON-SMALL CELL LUNG CANCER (NSCLC)

SQUAMOUS CELL CARCINOMA

Squamous cell carcinoma accounts for approximately 35% of all lung cancers. It is closely correlated with a smoking history and is the lung cancer most frequently found in males. The squamous carcinoma frequently originates in a central or hilar location and may cavitate when in a peripheral location.

Squamous malignancies can be classified as to well, moderately, and poorly differentiated. On microscopic examination, the cells are stratified and show intercellular bridges, and individual cells reveal hyperchromatic nuclei with scanty cytoplasm. The well differentiated tumor shows keratin pearl formation, while the poorly differentiated tumor reveals very anaplastic cells with few of the findings of classic squamous cell carcinoma. Examination of the bronchial mucosa adjacent to a squamous cell carcinoma may reveal epithelial cell atypia and possibly even carcinoma *in situ.*

ADENOCARCINOMA

The incidence of adenocarcinoma is increasing and now accounts for approximately 35% of pulmonary malignancies (Vincent et al. 1977). Adenocarcinoma is commonly located in the periphery of the lung and rarely cavitates. The growth rate is more rapid than that of squamous cell carcinoma. These tumors frequently spread through submucosal lymphatics to regional lymph nodes and often metastasize to the brain and other distant organs by vascular invasion.

Histologically, adenocarcinomas show varying degrees of glandular differentiation and may have papillary features. The individual cells have round nuclei with pale-pink cytoplasm. The poorly differentiated cancers show more anaplastic features with an increase in mitoses and a less distinct glandular formation.

The peripheral adenocarcinoma can also arise in an area of parenchymal scar, which has resulted in the term "scar cancer." The scar cancer has the same clinical features and similar prognosis to any adenocarcinoma of the lung.

Bronchioloalveolar carcinomas are adenocarcinomas that account for approximately 5% of all pulmonary malignancies. They can present as a solitary nodule, as multiple nodules, or as a diffuse infiltrate that mimics pneumonia. On microscopic examination, the alveolar carcinomas lie on the alveolar septum with a dense proliferation of cuboidal cells, giving the appearance that the normal pulmonary architecture has been preserved. The solitary nodular form carries an excellent prognosis when excised, but this type of lung cancer is thought to be multicentric in origin and the clinician must maintain long-term follow-up for the appearance of second and even third primaries. The diffuse form is also multicentric in origin and is generally fatal, although surgical therapy when the disease is confined to one lobe may provide some palliation.

LARGE-CELL UNDIFFERENTIATED CARCINOMA

Large-cell undifferentiated carcinomas constitute approximately 15% of pulmonary malignancies. They exhibit no squamous or glandular differentiation. Their location can be either central or peripheral, they tend to disseminate early in their course, and they are associated with a poor prognosis.

The tumor cells are characteristically large when compared to squamous carcinoma and adenocarcinoma. A generous amount of cytoplasm, a central nuclei, and frequent mitosis are histologic features.

NEUROENDOCRINE LUNG NEOPLASMS

The malignant neuroendocrine tumors of the lung consist of the carcinoid, the well-differentiated neuroendocrine carcinoma or atypical carcinoid, the intermediate-cell neuroendocrine carcinoma, and the small-cell neuroendocrine carcinoma (Gould and Warren 1989). Neuroendocrine tumors originate from epithelial cells that synthesize and secrete neuroendocrine markers. These substances include serotonin, norepinephrine, bombesin, calcitonin, ACTH, and antidiuretic hormone. This pathological classification has been facilitated by the development of immunohistochemical staining techniques and electron microscopy. The neuroendocrine neoplasms frequently are associated with the extrapulmonary clinical manifestations of lung cancer.

Carcinoid tumors are low-grade malignant lesions; 75% are located centrally and 25% are located periph-

erally. They occur in young patients, have equal frequency in males and females, and appear as polypoid bronchial tumors. They are highly vascular and can be associated with bleeding from bronchoscopic biopsy. Carcinoids have an excellent long-term prognosis when completely excised, but occasionally can develop regional and distant metastasis.

The well-differentiated neuroendocrine carcinoma is also called the atypical carcinoid. It is usually located in the periphery of the lung and can be misdiagnosed as a stage I peripheral small-cell carcinoma. The histology is similar to the carcinoid tumor, but it further differentiates by showing cellular pleomorphism, areas of necrosis, and mitoses. They do not demonstrate the extensive necrosis and crush artifact that delineate them from the classic small-cell carcinoma. Although surgical resection can be curative, this tumor is more aggressive than the carcinoid and is more frequently associated with regional lymph node metastasis and death. Overall long-term prognosis is favorable.

Intermediate-cell neuroendocrine carcinoma is also referred to as a large-cell undifferentiated carcinoma or large cell-small cell carcinoma. The term "intermediate" refers to the size of the cell and not to the amount of differentiation or clinical course. The cells of this tumor are two times the size of the small-cell carcinoma and have abundant mitoses and cellular pleomorphism. These tumors carry a very poor long-term prognosis. Treatment is similar to that of small-cell lung cancer.

The small-cell neuroendocrine carcinoma is associated with a history of smoking and often presents as a bulky hilar cancer. Approximately 20% occur in the peripheral portion of the lung and metastasize early to regional lymph nodes and distant organs. Their microscopic appearance is that of small, fusiform cells that have hyperchromatic nuclei and scanty cytoplasm; the presence of crush artifact is characteristic. Long-term survival for small-cell neuroendocrine carcinoma is 5%.

BRONCHIAL GLAND NEOPLASMS

The adenoid-cystic carcinoma is the second-most-common tumor of the trachea, but it can also originate in a major bronchus. It is rarely encountered in a peripheral location. It characteristically spreads submucosally and along the extrabronchial lymphatics. The mucoepidermoid carcinoma has varying histologic grades of severity and each grade correlates with prognosis. Both these tumors are histologically similar to their salivary gland counterparts. These tumors usually are located in a major bronchus and are a frequent cause of hemoptysis (coughing up blood) or chronic obstructive pneumonitis.

CLINICAL MANIFESTATIONS

The great majority (88%) of patients with lung cancer have symptoms referable to the primary tumor itself, to intrathoracic extension of the tumor, or to distant metastatic disease. The 12% of patients that are asymptomatic are usually diagnosed by routine chest x-ray (Cromardi et al. 1980) done as a screening procedure for another medical problem. A small group of patients may have symptoms caused by biologically active substances that are secreted by the tumor; these symptoms are termed paraneoplastic syndromes.

Smoking habits, a family history of lung cancer, and occupational or environmental exposure to carcinogens all increase the possibility of lung cancer in the differential diagnosis.

Cough is the most common symptom associated with lung cancer. Most patients attribute their cough to smoking and tend to ignore it, but any change in cough habits is significant and warrants careful investigation. The cough of lung cancer is related to irritation of the bronchial mucosa or mechanical compression of the airway by the tumor. Hemoptysis may be one of several symptoms in 50% to 60% of patients with lung cancer, and is the initial presenting complaint in 30%. Any episode of hemoptysis in a person over 40 should be investigated by chest x-ray and fiberoptic bronchoscopy. Wheezing is an indication of bronchial obstruction and unilateral wheezing is pathognomonic of partial bronchial obstruction. Fever can be a result of localized bronchial obstruction with distal pneumonitis or abscess formation in the lung. Dyspnea (difficulty in breathing) may be related to major bronchial obstruction, hypoxemia related to pulmonary shunting from obstructive atelectasis, pleural effusion, or diaphragmatic paralysis due to tumor invasion of the phrenic nerve.

Spread of the cancer in the ipsilateral thorax can cause other symptoms. Chest pain is related to invasion of the parietal pleural or chest wall, or from parietal pleural irritation secondary to an obstructing carcinoma causing distal pneumonitis. The chest pain of lung cancer is persistent and requires a narcotic for relief. Chest pain associated with an abnormal chest x-ray usually indicates a diagnosis of lung cancer. Hoarseness usually indicates involvement of the recurrent laryngeal nerve and is more common on the left side due to the inferior anatomic course of the nerve around the aortic arch.

Pleural effusions occur in approximately 12% of lung cancer patients (Tandon 1966). Effusions may be related to involvement of the viscera or parietal pleura by the cancer, but can also be caused by mediastinal lymphatic obstruction or obstructive pneumonitis. Whenever a pleural effusion is present in a patient with lung cancer, a diagnostic thoracentesis is mandatory because cancer cells in the fluid are a contraindication to curative surgery. A benign pleural effusion is not a contraindication to surgery, but is associated with a poor long-term prognosis.

An enlargement of the neck with venous distention is caused by compression or invasion of the superior vena cava by carcinoma. The phrenic nerve can be directly involved by the cancer and result in unilateral diaphragmatic paralysis and dyspnea. An elevated diaphragm can be confirmed as being paralyzed by paradoxical motion seen on chest fluoroscopy.

Superior sulcus cancers are located at the apex of the chest. These cancers invade the chest wall and the brachial plexus and produce symptoms of shoulder and arm pain and paresthesias along the distribution of the C-7 or T-1 dermatome (the Pancoast syndrome). The first and second ribs are frequently invaded by the apical tumor. In this case, pain in the shoulder, back, or radiating down the arm is the predominant symptom. Horner's syndrome (ipsilateral lack of sweating of the face, ptosis of the eyelid, and a constricted pupil) is a manifestation of an apical cancer invading the stellate sympathetic ganglion.

Lung cancer can metastasize to any organ of the body and cause specific symptoms related to that organ. However, it commonly metastasizes to the bones, brain, or liver. Headaches, nausea, vomiting, and loss of motor or sensory function are all manifestations of metastatic lung cancer to the brain. Pain is a common presentation of skeletal metastasis. Liver metastases are associated with nonspecific abdominal complaints and weight loss.

The extrapulmonary clinical manifestations of bronchogenic carcinoma (paraneoplastic syndromes) are outlined in table 14.2.

The endocrine syndromes are caused by secretion of a hormone-like substance by the tumor; if the tumor is completely eradicated, the symptoms will disappear. Most of these syndromes are associated with small-cell carcinoma. Hypercalcemia is associated with squamous cell carcinoma, which secretes a parathyroid hormone-like polypeptide. However, hypercalcemia in patients with lung cancer is most frequently due to bony metastasis.

The neuromyopathies are the most frequent of the extrathoracic manifestations of bronchogenic carcinoma. These have been reported in 16% of lung cancer patients, 56% of which had a small-cell cancer (Croft and Wilkinson 1965). Neuromyopathy commonly is present several months prior to the clinical diagnosis of

Table 14.2
PARANEOPLASTIC SYNDROMES ASSOCIATED WITH LUNG CANCER

ENDOCRINE
Antidiuretic hormone excess
Cushing's syndrome
Hypercalcemia
Carcinoid syndrome
Ectopic gonadotropin
NEUROMUSCULAR
Myasthenia-like syndrome
Subacute cerebellar degeneration
Peripheral neuropathy
Myopathy
DERMATOLOGIC
Acanthosis nigricans
Dermatomyositis
SKELETAL
Hypertrophic pulmonary osteoarthropathy
Clubbing
HEMATOLOGIC
Anemia
Intravascular coagulopathy
Leukocytosis
Red cell aplasia
VASCULAR
Thrombophlebitis
Non-bacterial endocarditis

the cancer. The myasthenia-like or Eaton-Lambert syndrome is characterized by weakness of the muscles, particularly those of the pelvis and thighs. Electromyographic studies can differentiate this syndrome from true myasthenia gravis.

Skin lesions associated with lung cancer include acanthosis nigricans, dermatomyositis, scleroderma, and other nonspecific dermatoses.

Clubbing of the fingers, a common finding in patients with lung cancer, is associated with hypertrophic pulmonary osteoarthropathy. This is a painful periostitis with the characteristic radiologic finding of periosteal proliferation of the long bones. There is increased blood flow to the affected extremity that may be due to both humoral and neurogenic factors. Surgical excision of the tumor provides dramatic pain relief and the may cause the clubbing to disappear.

DIAGNOSTIC PROCEDURES

RADIOGRAPHY

CHEST X-RAY

The posteroanterior (PA) and lateral chest x-ray is the simplest way to detect a primary lung cancer. The films can identify a peripheral tumor, tumor size and location, effects of bronchial obstruction, diaphragmatic paralysis, and invasion of the chest wall or mediastinum. Mediastinal lymph nodes greater than 2 cm in diameter can be detected on the plain chest x-ray, but it is an unreliable method for identifying early lymph node metastasis in the mediastinum or hilum. A nodular density may appear to be malignant but it may have been present and unchanged for many years; thus it is mandatory to compare the current chest x-ray with any prior films. Most cancers will double in volume in 18 to 24 months, although a few will be stable for one or two years. If the patient's symptoms are those of an inflammatory process and the chest x-ray supports this diagnosis, a repeat film may be obtained in three to four weeks. If the x-ray abnormality is not significantly decreased in size or gone, further diagnostic studies are warranted. A new chest x-ray abnormality always warrants further evaluation.

COMPUTED TOMOGRAPHY

Computed tomography (CT) is the most accurate radiologic technique for evaluating the mediastinum, mediastinal and hilar lymph nodes, pulmonary parenchyma, and vertebral bodies. It is not as precise for defining chest wall and rib invasion. It has become routine to obtain the CT scan when evaluating a patient suspected of having lung cancer. The CT scan with intravenous infusion of contrast material can highlight invasion or compression of vascular structures. This technique further aids in the identification of abnormal mediastinal lymph nodes. Concomitant imaging of the upper abdomen can delineate metastatic disease in the liver or adrenal glands and is a routine part of the examination.

The CT scan is used to determine the presence of enlarged lymph nodes in the mediastinum. Cancer in mediastinal lymph nodes significantly alters prognosis and this finding is a major determinant of operability. The predictive accuracy of the CT scan in determining the presence of cancer in mediastinal lymph nodes is related to the size of the nodes. Lymph nodes under 1 cm in greatest diameter are considered to be uninvolved for purposes of clinical staging; CT scanning is almost as accurate in identifying mediastinal metastasis as is mediastinoscopy in this instance (Breyer et al. 1984). Diagnostic accuracy of the CT scan in predicting cancer in mediastinal lymph nodes over 1 cm in diameter varies from 60% to 78% (McKenna et al. 1985; Glazer et al. 1984). Lymph nodes that are 1.5 cm or greater in diameter are considered to be positive, and cancer will be found in 85% of patients with nodes of this size (Daley et al. 1984). The CT scan cannot differentiate between inflammatory or granulomatous lymph node enlargement and cannot detect microscopic tumor in small nodes. Biopsy is mandatory to confirm the presence of metastatic cancer, particularly in squamous cell carcinomas that can be associated with enlarged, hyperplastic lymph nodes that do not contain tumor. Lymph nodes in the hilum and aorticopulmonary region are not accurately assessed by CT scanning.

The CT scan can identify major mediastinal invasion, but has difficulty in differentiating minor tumor invasion from contact without invasion. Confluence of the tumor with mediastinal structures and thickened main stem bronchi are both indications of malignant mediastinal involvement (Frederick et al. 1984).

High resolution CT with 1 mm-thick cuts through a solitary pulmonary nodule permits precise delineation of the anatomic characteristics of the nodule and also identifies the presence of calcium, which in various configurations suggests that the lesion is benign. Uniform scanning techniques have been developed to measure the density of the nodule, a finding that can assist in the differentiation between benign and malignant lesions (Zerhouni et al. 1986).

MAGNETIC RESONANCE IMAGING

Magnetic resonance imaging (MRI) has some advantages over CT: it can provide images in both the sagittal and coronal planes, it has the yet-unproven potential of characterizing malignant tissue by spectroscopy, and it does not expose the patient to ionizing radiation. The technique has a low intensity for flowing blood and demonstrates invasion or compression of vascular structures by a tumor. Coronal sections can be advantageous in evaluating the aorticopulmonary window, a weak area for CT, and also the involvement of the brachial plexus by a superior sulcus tumor. At the present time, MRI offers no advantage over CT in precisely defining involvement of mediastinal lymph nodes by cancer (Heelan et al. 1985). Disadvantages of MRI are that small calcifications are not well-delineated and the imaging time to study the entire thorax and upper abdomen is prolonged. Improved technology and spectroscopic research in the identification of malignant tissue may increase the use of MRI for evaluation of lung cancer.

OTHER RADIOGRAPHIC STUDIES

Fluoroscopic examination of the diaphragm will confirm paralysis and phrenic nerve involvement by the cancer. Bronchograms are of no benefit in evaluating a patient with bronchogenic carcinoma; the site of obstruction can be identified, but histologic confirmation is still required. Pulmonary angiography is not indicated to determine operability as evaluation of the pulmonary artery is now accomplished with the CT scan or MRI. The barium esophagogram is indicated when dysphagia is a complaint, as esophageal invasion indicates extension of the cancer into the central mediastinum.

CYTOLOGY

Sputum cytology is positive in 60% to 90% of patients with bronchogenic carcinoma who have an abnormal chest x-ray (Oswald et al. 1971). The higher yields are obtained in patients with central lesions that invade major bronchi and the lower yields are obtained in patients with peripheral lesions. Cytologic accuracy is directly related to the technique of obtaining the specimen and the expertise of the cytopathologist. Pooled, three-day specimens give improved results. Induction is helpful in patients who cannot raise sputum. Induction techniques include inhalation of hypertonic saline or propylene glycol by ultrasonic nebulization.

A positive sputum cytology in a patient with a negative chest x-ray is referred to as an occult carcinoma of the lung. The cytologic examination may have been obtained because of a change in cough habits or hemoptysis. Diagnostic assessment of this patient must include visualization of the oral cavity, hypopharynx, and larynx as the positive cytologic specimen may have originated from a cancer in these locations. A negative examination of the oral pharynx and upper airway then requires a flexible fiberoptic bronchoscopy. All lobar and segmental orifices must be carefully visualized, with bronchial brushing and biopsy obtained from any area of mucosal abnormality. The use of hematoporphyrin derivatives (Hpd) to enhance visualization of the cancer by laser-stimulated fluorescence is rarely required, as careful bronchoscopic examination usually identifies the lesion. If a lesion is not found, bronchoscopy and cytology are repeated at 4-month intervals.

BRONCHOSCOPY

Any patient suspected of having bronchogenic carcinoma should undergo bronchoscopy. The flexible fiberoptic bronchoscope permits evaluation of segmental and subsegmental bronchi, and bronchial brushings and biopsy are more easily obtained than with the rigid bronchoscope. A complete and careful examination of the entire tracheobronchial tree is mandatory, as a second unsuspected primary cancer may be identified and the surgeon must be aware of any anatomic variations when segmental resection or lobectomy is contemplated. There are many subtleties associated with cancer involving the tracheobronchial tree and the endoscopist must be familiar with all of them. These include submucosal vascularity, irregular bronchial folds or corrugation, mucosal thickening, stenosis, indistinct cartilage rings, and loss of circular folds (Oho and Omemiya 1984). These findings are proximal to the site of origin of the cancer and indicate to the surgeon that the resection must be more proximal than the x-ray would indicate.

If a suspicious lesion is identified in any bronchus, both bronchial brushing and biopsy are carried out. A combination of biopsy and brushing increases the diagnostic yield (Kvale, Bode, and Kini 1976). Bronchial washing for cytologic study and the collection of postbronchoscopic sputum have not increased diagnostic accuracy and their routine use is not recommended. In patients with proven bronchogenic carcinoma, a diagnostic accuracy of 85% should be achieved using brushing and biopsy techniques (Zavala 1975).

The indications for diagnostic bronchoscopy in a peripheral lesion include bronchial evaluation prior to surgical resection, an attempt to rule out an inflammatory etiology, and an attempt to establish the diagnosis of carcinoma. It is routine to use the C-Arm fluoroscope to be certain that the forceps or brush is in the lesion. Diagnostic accuracy is lower for peripheral lesions, but a 68% positive result has been achieved using brushing and transbronchial biopsy in lesions greater than 2 cm in diameter (Radke et al. 1979). Diagnostic accuracy for lesions under 2 cm in size is significantly lower. In this instance, transthoracic needle aspiration is the recommended diagnostic procedure.

TRANSTHORACIC NEEDLE ASPIRATION

Transthoracic needle aspiration (TNA) has become an important procedure in the diagnosis of peripheral pulmonary tumors because it has a much higher diagnostic yield than flexible fiberoptic bronchoscopy. A small-bore needle is placed in the central portion of the nodule under fluoroscopic control or by CT guided direction and aspirated material is studied as a cytologic preparation. Complications including hemoptysis, air embolism, and pneumothorax occur in approximately 23% of patients, of which 5% require chest tube drainage (Berquist et al. 1980). Diagnostic accuracy relates to the expertise of the physician performing the biopsy and the experience of the cytopathologist. Rapid processing and interpretation of the cytopathologic material will permit two or three aspirations if the initial aspirate is negative for malignancy. A diagnostic accuracy of 88% has been achieved in patients with subsequently proven bronchogenic carcinoma (Zaman et al. 1986). A diagnosis of benign disease is infrequently established and TNA is therefore less sensitive in its overall accuracy. Sensitivity is 85% and specificity approaches 100%.

There is controversy over the indications for TNA. If the cytologic aspirate is positive for cancer, resection will be carried out; if it is negative, there is still a 15% probability that the lesion is cancer and the resection would still be performed. Therefore, why do the TNA? The clinician must always be prepared to answer this question prior to recommending TNA as a diagnostic procedure. It can be helpful for diagnosis in the patient who will not tolerate thoracotomy, and it is of benefit in establishing diagnosis of a superior sulcus carcinoma prior to radiation treatment. The procedure may also confirm the clinical suspicion of carcinoma in a patient who is reluctant to proceed with thoracotomy or in a patient who has an associated increased operative risk. Transthoracic needle aspiration can also be of significant benefit in the patient with bilateral lesions.

TRANSBRONCHIAL NEEDLE ASPIRATION

Transbronchial needle aspiration (TBNA) is a technique in which a needle is passed through the wall of the trachea or bronchus to obtain cytologic or histologic material. The needle is sheathed so that it can be safely passed through the channel of the flexible bronchoscope. The TBNA procedure can be used in the clinical staging of primary bronchogenic carcinoma by cytologically sampling subcarinal and paratracheal lymph nodes. It can also enhance the diagnostic yield when evaluating submucosal extension and peripheral nodules (Wang 1989). Also, TBNA has proven to be effective in the diagnosis of the Pancoast carcinoma, large necrotic lesions in the bronchus, and highly vascular bronchial adenomas. Complications are rare, but pneumothorax and minor mediastinal bleeding can occur. The application of this technique requires that the endoscopist be skilled in the use of the flexible instrument and also have the complete knowledge of mediastinal and bronchial anatomy to avoid penetration of major vascular structures.

SCALENE NODE BIOPSY

Scalene node biopsy is not recommended as a routine preoperative or staging procedure. Most reports indicate a low yield for scalene node biopsy without the presence of palpable lymph nodes, so the procedure is only recommended for patients with palpable lymph nodes.

BONE MARROW BIOPSY

Bone marrow biopsy is indicated when a diagnosis of a centrally located small-cell carcinoma has been made. It is considered a baseline staging procedure because cancer cells frequently are identified in the marrow.

PULMONARY FUNCTION TESTS

Many patients with bronchogenic carcinoma have chronic obstructive pulmonary disease and are at increased risk for a major resection of lung tissue. Pulmonary function tests that screen for abnormalities provide an indication of increased risk for postoperative pulmonary complications and the need for further studies. A 50% reduction in the predicted forced vital capacity (FEV_1), maximum voluntary ventilation (MVV), or vital capacity (VC) indicates the need for more extensive testing. Arterial blood gas analysis becomes important and a PaO_2 under 65 torr and a $PaCO_2$ over 45 torr are predictors of increased risk. The ability to withstand thoracotomy also relates to the patient's general physical condition, the presence of cardiac or renal disease, and the amount of lung tissue to be removed. Poor pulmonary function tests do not necessarily prohibit a thoracotomy, but the type of resection must be carefully selected and prophylactic measures implemented to minimize complications.

Ventilation and perfusion radionuclide scanning of the lung (V/Q) is of benefit in assessing operability as it measures how much function the lung to be removed is contributing to the patient's ability to breathe. A patient with marginal pulmonary function still may be able to withstand a resection if the V/Q lung scan demonstrates little or no function in the lung tissue to be resected. Following resection, the patient should have an FEV_1 of at least 800 cc to permit satisfactory rehabilitation (Olsen, Block, and Tobias 1974). The V/Q scan is indicated when a pneumonectomy is contemplated and the patient's pulmonary function is marginal. It is not a routine screening procedure.

Accompanying the patient up two flights of stairs is a gross exercise tolerance test that evaluates both pulmonary function and patient motivation. Most patients who can climb two flights of stairs without stopping will tolerate thoracotomy and pulmonary resection.

STAGING

Staging is the determination of the extent of the lung cancer and is mandatory for every patient with this disease. Grouping patients according to stage achieves standardization of reported results and serves as a basis for prognosis. Therapeutic options are dependent upon the clinical stage as determined by the various diagnostic and evaluative procedures.

The TNM classification of staging is used for lung cancer: T refers to the size and extent of the primary tumor, N refers to involvement of lobar and mediastinal lymph nodes, and M refers to metastatic disease. The staging system has gone through several modifications and the current internationally accepted one (see table 14.3) has been developed by the American Joint Committee on Cancer (*Manual for Staging of Cancer*, 3rd ed. 1988; Mountain 1986).

The two methods of staging are clinical staging (CS) and pathologic staging (PS). Clinical staging is based on the anatomic extent of the cancer determined by all diagnostic studies before definitive therapy is started. Pathologic staging is based on the findings at surgery and the histologic examination of the resected specimen,

Table 14.3
AMERICAN JOINT COMMITTEE ON CANCER STAGING FOR LUNG CARCINOMA (3rd ed.)

T = Primary Tumor **N** = Regional Lymph Nodes **M** = Distant Metastasis

PRIMARY TUMOR (T)

TX	Primary tumor cannot be assessed, or tumor proven by the presence of malignant cells in sputum or bronchial washings but not visualized by imaging or bronchosopy
T0	No evidence of primary tumor
Tis	Carcinoma *in situ*
T1	Tumor 3 cm or less in greatest dimension, surrounded by lung or visceral pleura, without bronchoscopic evidence of invasion more proximal than the lobar bronchus *(i.e., not in the main bronchus)
T2	Tumor with any of the following features of size or extent: more than 3 cm in greatest dimension, involves main bronchus, 2 cm or more distal to the carina; invades the visceral pleura; associated with atelectasis or obstructive pneumonitis that extends to the hilar region but does not involve the entire lung
T3	Tumor of any size that directly invades any of the following: chest wall (including superior sulcus tumors), diaphragm, mediastinal pleura, parietal pericardium, tumor in the main bronchus less than 2 cm distal to the carina* but without involvement of the carina; or associated atelectasis or obstructive pneumonitis of the entire lung
T4	Tumor of any size that invades any of the following: mediastinum, heart, great vessels, trachea, esophagus, vertebral body, carina; or tumor with a malignant pleural effusion**

*NOTE: The uncommon superficial tumor of any size with its invasive component limited to the bronchial wall, which may extend proximal to the main bronchus, is also classified T1.

**NOTE: Most pleural effusions associated with lung cancer are due to tumor. However, there are a few patients in whom multiple cytopathologic examinations of pleural fluid are negative for tumor. In these cases, fluid is non-bloody and is not an exudate. When these elements and clinical judgment dictate that the effusion is not related to the tumor, the effusion should be excluded as a staging element and the patient should be staged T1, T2, or T3.

REGIONAL LYMPH NODES (N)

NX	Regional lymph nodes cannot be assessed
N0	No regional lymph node metastasis
N1	Metastasis in ipsilateral peribronchial and/or ipsilateral hilar lymph nodes, including direct extension
N2	Metastasis in ipsilateral mediastinal and/or subcarinal lymph node(s)
N3	Metastasis in contralateral mediastinal, contralateral hilar, ipsilateral or contralateral scalene, or supraclavicular lymph node(s)

DISTANT METASTASIS (M)

MX	Presence of distant metastasis cannot be assessed
M0	No distant metastasis
M1	Distant metastasis

STAGE GROUPING

Occult Carcinoma	TX	N0	M0
Stage 0	Tis	N0	M0
Stage I	T1	N0	M0
	T2	N0	M0
Stage II	T1	N1	M0
	T2	N1	M0
Stage IIIA	T1	N2	M0
	T2	N2	M0
	T3	N0, N1, N2	M0
Stage IIIB	Any T	N3	M0
	T4	Any N	M0
Stage IV	Any T	Any N	M1

surgical margins, and all lymph nodes. The various stages are illustrated in figs. 14.1, 14.2, 14.3, and 14.4.

Survival is directly related to the stage of the lung cancer, as is demonstrated in fig. 14.5. Stage I patients have a significantly greater survival rate than do stage III patients.

CLINICAL STAGING

Besides the previously mentioned diagnostic procedures, clinical staging also includes mediastinoscopy/ mediastinotomy, radiographic scanning for detection of metastatic disease when indicated, and thoracentesis if a pleural effusion is present.

MEDIASTINOSCOPY

Of all lung cancer patients, 30% to 50% who appear to have localized disease within the chest and are candidates for surgical resection will be found to have mediastinal lymph node metastasis. Transcervical medi-

astinoscopy is a procedure in which mediastinal lymph nodes are evaluated and biopsied in order to gain information concerning the proper therapeutic approach to patients with lung cancer. The presence of cancer in mediastinal lymph nodes significantly alters long-term prognosis and has many therapeutic implications. Positive mediastinal lymph nodes are associated with a 5-year survival of 28%, and their presence also increases the likelihood of an incomplete resection (Mountain 1986).

Philosophies vary as to the indications for preoperative mediastinoscopy. Some clinicians advocate it as routine for all patients with proven lung cancer, while others recommend using the criterion of lymph node size as determined by the CT scan. A mediastinal lymph node greater than 1 cm in diameter has the possibility of containing metastatic carcinoma, but a lymph node under 1 cm in diameter has less than a 10% incidence of containing metastatic cancer and therefore mediastinoscopy is not indicated (Daly et al. 1984). Regarding

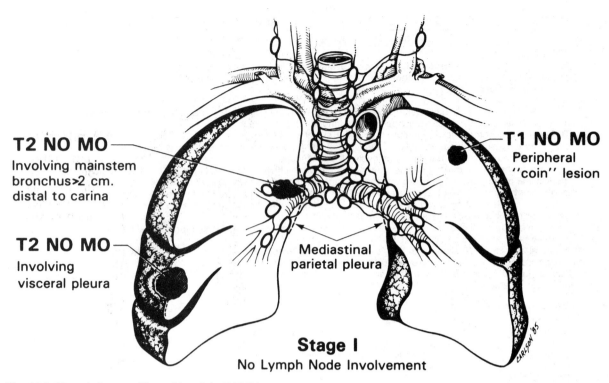

T2 N0 M0

Involving mainstem
bronchus >2 cm.
distal to carina

T2 N0 M0

Involving
visceral pleura

Mediastinal
parietal pleura

T1 N0 M0

Peripheral
"coin" lesion

Stage I
No Lymph Node Involvement

Fig. 14.1. Stage I disease. (From: Mountain [1986].)

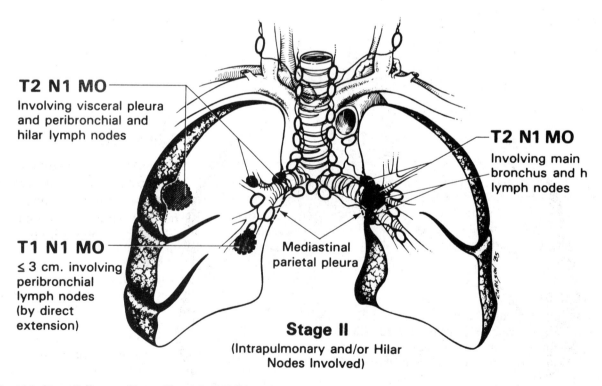

T2 N1 M0

Involving visceral pleura
and peribronchial and
hilar lymph nodes

T1 N1 M0

≤ 3 cm. involving
peribronchial
lymph nodes
(by direct
extension)

Mediastinal
parietal pleura

T2 N1 M0

Involving main
bronchus and h
lymph nodes

Stage II
(Intrapulmonary and/or Hilar
Nodes Involved)

Fig. 14.2. Stage II disease. (From: Mountain [1986].)

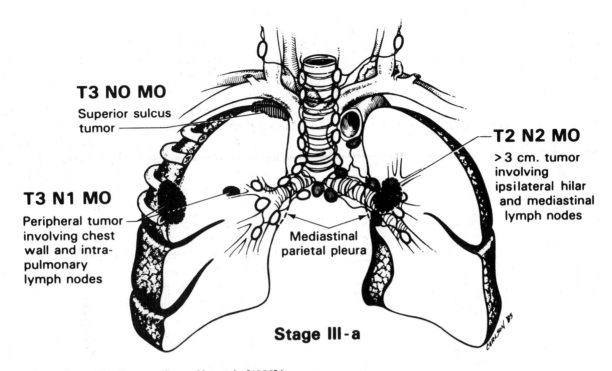

T3 N0 M0
Superior sulcus tumor

T3 N1 M0
Peripheral tumor involving chest wall and intra-pulmonary lymph nodes

Mediastinal parietal pleura

T2 N2 M0
> 3 cm. tumor involving ipsilateral hilar and mediastinal lymph nodes

Stage III-a

Fig. 14.3. Stage IIIA disease. (From: Mountain [1986].)

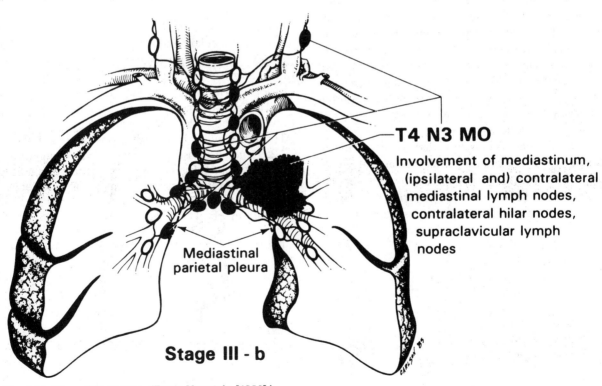

T4 N3 M0
Involvement of mediastinum, (ipsilateral and) contralateral mediastinal lymph nodes, contralateral hilar nodes, supraclavicular lymph nodes

Mediastinal parietal pleura

Stage III - b

Fig. 14.4. Stage IIIB disease. (From: Mountain [1986].)

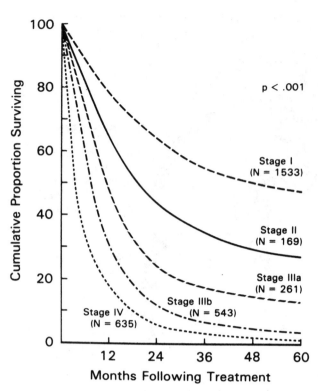

Fig. 14.5. Proportion of patients surviving five years according to clinical stage of disease. (From: Mountain [1986].)

lymph nodes varying from 1 cm to 1.5 cm in diameter, some physicians feel these nodes can be completely resected and the patient will benefit; others feel that routine mediastinoscopy is indicated for this group. The CT scan alone should never be used as an indication of inoperability because infection associated with a cancer can cause lymph nodes to enlarge. Histologic confirmation is always required to deem a patient inoperable based on positive mediastinal nodes.

Findings at mediastinoscopy that clearly indicate inoperability include contralateral mediastinal lymph node involvement, extranodal extension of cancer that precludes a complete resection, superior mediastinal lymph nodes that prevent complete resection, and the histology of small-cell carcinoma. The finding of microscopic cancer in an ipsilateral mediastinal lymph node in which a complete resection can be achieved remains controversial as to whether surgical or nonsurgical therapy is appropriate. Investigational clinical protocols are ongoing to evaluate preoperative chemotherapy and radiation for patients with positive mediastinal nodes and bronchogenic carcinoma (stage IIIA). The benefit of mediastinoscopy in the determination of patients who will benefit from resection has been outlined by Pearson (Pearson et al. 1982). Of 79 patients selected for resection in whom positive mediastinal lymph nodes were documented by mediastinoscopy, the overall 5-year survival was 9%. Increased resectability following negative mediastinoscopy is demonstrated by a curative and complete resection rate of 89% (Coughlin et al. 1985).

When surgical therapy is recommended for a lung cancer patient with positive mediastinal nodes, it is implied that the resection will be complete. A complete resection means free margins, including all disease in the lung and mediastinum. This group of patients is characterized by having T1 or T2 tumors, a normal mediastinum on plain chest x-ray, and no carinal widening seen at bronchoscopy. When postoperative radiation therapy is added, the long-term survival is 30% (Martini and Flehinger 1987).

Lymph nodes accessible for biopsy by mediastinoscopy include bilateral tracheal nodes, anterior subcarinal nodes, and nodes at both the right and left tracheobronchial angles. Lymph nodes inaccessible for biopsy include those located in the anterior mediastinum, aorticopulmonary space, posterior carina, and posterior inferior tracheobronchial areas (see fig. 14.6).

The risk of complications with mediastinoscopy is low, but those that may occur include fatal bleeding. Thoracotomy for hemorrhage was necessary in 0.2% of 1,259 mediastinoscopies performed (Coughlin 1985). Other complications include vocal cord paralysis from damage to the left recurrent laryngeal nerve, pneumothorax, tracheal and esophageal injury, chylothorax, and wound infection.

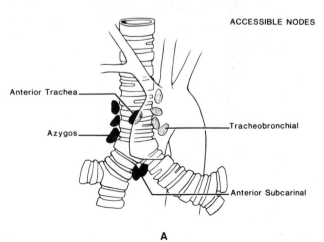

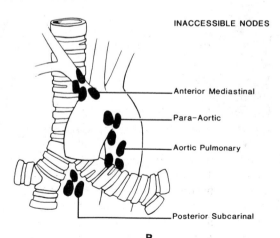

Fig. 14.6. Mediastinal lymph nodes accessible (A) and unaccessible (B) for biopsy by mediastinoscopy.

MEDIASTINOTOMY

Mediastinotomy is a technique used to biopsy enlarged lymph nodes in the left aorticopulmonary space associated with a left upper lobe bronchogenic carcinoma. A transverse incision extending from the lateral edge of the sternum is placed over the second costal cartilage, which is usually excised. The approach can be either intrapleural or extrapleural and a mediastinoscope is inserted through the wound to assist in the visualization of the lymph nodes to be biopsied. Complications with mediastinotomy are greater than those reported for cervical mediastinoscopy and are approximately 9% (Jolly et al. 1973). The use of mediastinotomy as a staging procedure has decreased since Patterson's report describing a group of 37 patients with positive aorticopulmonary nodes that underwent resection and had a 5-year survival rate of 33% (Patterson et al. 1987).

RADIONUCLIDE SCANS

Bone, brain, and liver scans are not obtained in the asymptomatic patient with non-small cell lung cancer. These procedures produce both false-positive and false-negative results and must become more sensitive and specific before their routine use can be recommended. A complete CT scan for lung cancer now includes the upper abdomen to rule out evidence of metastasis to the liver and adrenals. An ultrasound (US) examination can be quite specific for metastatic disease to the liver. The CT scan of the brain with infusion or the MRI has replaced the brain radionuclide scan and is indicated in any patient who has lung cancer and central nervous system symptoms. The gallium scan has varying sensitivity for the detection of metastatic cancer to regional lymph nodes and its use is not recommended. The bone scan is indicated for any lung cancer patient who has bone pain.

THORACENTESIS

Cytologic examination of a pleural effusion should always be done. Malignant cells in the fluid are a contraindication to curative surgical resection. A needle pleural biopsy is usually accomplished at the time of the thoracentesis, as other diseases are often considered in the differential diagnosis.

SMALL-CELL LUNG CANCER (SCLC)

Small-cell lung cancer (SCLC) is separated from the other histologic types due to its rapid growth rate and usually fatal course. Symptoms are of brief duration prior to diagnosis. Eighty percent of SCLC is located centrally and 20% in the periphery of the lung. The paraneoplastic syndromes are more commonly associated with SCLC and occur in about 10% of patients (Bunn and Minna 1985).

Histologic verification of SCLC is mandatory because treatment is significantly different from that of NSCLC. At times, this can be difficult due to a small fiberoptic biopsy or scanty material obtained by aspiration cytology. If the diagnosis is in question, repeat biopsy should be carried out. Staging procedures are of benefit to plan the treatment program, determine eligibility for surgical resection, assess response by stage for results reporting, and to estimate prognosis. Optimal staging techniques in the asymptomatic patient with SCLC also include CT scan of the brain, bone scan, and a bone marrow biopsy. These are frequent sites of metastatic disease in a patient with SCLC.

Small-cell carcinomas produce several biologically active substances including ACTH, ADH, calcitonin, neuron-specific enolase, and others. These products along with carcinoembryonic antigen (CEA) have been investigated as to their usefulness as tumor markers for NSCLC. Advantages of having an active tumor marker would include defining tumor burden, response to therapy, and recurrence (Akoun et al. 1985). However, results are varied and a consistent serum marker has not been identified.

THERAPEUTIC ALTERNATIVES

The primary therapeutic approach differs for NSCLC and SCLC. The primary treatment of NSCLC is surgical, whereas the primary treatment of SCLC is chemotherapy and surgery in very selected instances. Clinical staging and the patient's ability to withstand a surgical resection are the prime determinants for surgical therapy. Clinical staging relates to the local extent of the tumor and the involvement of regional lymph nodes. For example, N1 disease is hilar or lobar lymph node involvement and a complete resection can be accomplished. In patients with N2 disease, which is ipsilateral mediastinal lymph node involvement, the decision for surgery is controversial. Ipsilateral N2 disease can be categorized into two main groups: those that are discovered at the time of thoracotomy by complete lymph node resection and those diagnosed by invasive clinical staging. In N3 disease, contralateral or supraclavicular lymph nodes are involved by metastatic cancer, a finding that makes operation on the patient impossible.

SURGERY

Surgical resection is the treatment of choice for all stage I and stage II NSCLC patients, and also in selected stage III patients. Stage I patients have localized tumors that may involve the visceral pleura or a lobar bronchus without metastasis to regional lymph nodes. The reported actuarial 5-year survival rate for this specific group of patients at three years is 85% (Martini and Beattie 1977). Stage II disease includes tumors that may involve the visceral pleura or a lobar bronchus and have metastasized to the ipsilateral segmental or lobar lymph nodes. Prognosis is worsened by the extension of the tumor to the regional lymph nodes and survival rates for T1N1M0 and T2N1M0 patients are 14% to 39% (Ferguson et al. 1986; Martini et al. 1983). Stage IIIA tumors are locally advanced into the chest wall, diaphragm, or mediastinal pleura; invade a main stem bronchus; and may or may not involve ipsilateral lobar or mediastinal lymph nodes. Tumors invading the phrenic nerve, pericardium, diaphragm, mediastinal pleura, and parietal pleura can be completely resected by an *en bloc* technique. The T3N0 tumors have a favorable prognosis following complete resection; 5-year survival rates of 50% have been reported (Piehler et al. 1982)

Patients with N2 disease can have a 30% opportunity for long-term survival if all nodal disease is completely resected (Sawamura et al. 1985). However, prognosis is decreased to 9% if there is obvious radiologic evidence of enlarged mediastinal lymph nodes prior to thoracotomy (Martini and Flehinger 1987). In selected patients who have positive lymph nodes detected by preoperative mediastinoscopy, a projected survival of 18% has been reported (Coughlin et al. 1985). Prognosis is worsened by extracapsular invasion, more than one N2 nodal station involved (i.e., subcarinal and tracheobronchial), and involvement of superior mediastinal nodes.

Patients with T3N2 disease are considered to be inoperable due to their relatively rare long-term survival (Mountain 1986).

Lobectomy is the standard pulmonary resection for most stage I and stage II lung cancers. Mortality is 2.9% and minimal physical alteration of pulmonary function occurs after resection (Ginsberg et al. 1983). *Sleeve lobectomy* is an alternative procedure to pneumonectomy when the tumor extends from the lobar orifice to the main stem bronchus. When technically feasible, it is the operation of choice as it preserves lung tissue and its long-term results are comparable to those of pneumonectomy (Faber, Jensik, and Kittle 1984). *Pneumonectomy* is required for a large centrally located tumor, involvement of a main stem bronchus, or invasion of the main pulmonary artery. Complications of empyema and bronchial fistula are greater following pneumonectomy, and mortality is 6.2% (Ginsberg et al. 1983). *Sleeve pneumonectomy* is an extended resection for carcinoma involving the tracheobronchial angle, carina, or lower trachea and lung. The airway is reconstituted by anastomosis of the opposite main stem bronchus to the lower trachea. This is a technically demanding procedure and carries an operative mortality of 15% to 20%.

A *limited pulmonary resection* is any resection less than lobectomy. *Segmentectomy* is an anatomic pulmonary resection that includes the bronchus, pulmonary artery and vein, and lung parenchyma to that particular segment or segments. A *wedge resection* is a nonanatomic removal of a peripheral portion of lung parenchyma and can traverse segmental planes. A *limited resection* is only considered when the tumor is identified as a clinical stage I cancer, its diameter is 3 cm or less and, more specifically, the patient's cardiopulmonary status is marginal and salvage of lung tissue is required. Long-term survival of 55% has been reported for segmentectomy (Jensik 1987). For wedge resection the actuarial 2-year survival is 72% (Errett et al. 1985). A limited resection for bronchogenic carcinoma continues to be evaluated as to whether it is an operation of choice and not a compromise. Local recurrence has been reported to be 12% (Jensik 1987) and may be a problem with this type of resection. The benefits of preserving lung tissue is obvious, as the reported mortality with limited resection is 1.4%.

Extended resections include *en bloc* portions of the chest wall (which is usually reconstructed with prosthetic material), vertebral body, left atrium, or diaphragm.

Ipsilateral lymph nodes include subcarinal, lobar, and mediastinal groups and should be completely resected. Their anatomic location is specifically labeled for the pathologist so that precise pathologic staging is possible. Lymph node labeling is done according to Naruke's lymph node map (Naruke et al. 1978).

Contraindications to surgery include extrathoracic metastatic disease; positive contralateral mediastinal and supraclavicular lymph nodes (N3 disease); pleural effusion with positive cytology; paralysis of the left or right vocal cord due to involvement of the recurrent laryngeal nerve; obstruction of the superior vena cava by cancer; and inadequate cardiopulmonary function.

Age is not a contraindication to surgical resection. Many patients over the age of 70 will tolerate the procedure and limited resections, when possible, are advocated for this patient group.

Survival following surgery is directly related to TNM staging, tumor histology, and completeness of resection. Results according to stage are shown in table 14.4 and results according to histology in table 14.5.

Table 14.4
POSTSURGICAL SURVIVAL OF OVER 1,400 PATIENTS ANALYZED BY UNIVERSITY OF TEXAS AND LUNG CANCER STUDY GROUP*

STAGE	TN SUBSET	NUMBER OF PATIENTS	5-YEAR SURVIVAL (%)
I	T1N0	439	69
	T2N0	436	59
	T1N2	67	54
II	T2N1	250	40
III	T3N0	57	44
	T3N1	29	18
	Any N2	168	28

*Postoperative mortality is excluded.
T3N2 disease was not analyzed separately because the numbers were small, but it carries the poorest prognosis (<10%).
(Modified from: Mountain [1986] and Ginsberg, R.J.; Goldberg, M.; and Waters, P.F. 1989. Surgery for non-small cell lung cancer. In Roth, Ruckdeschel, and Weisenberger eds. [1989]).

Table 14.5
ANALYSIS OF SURVIVAL ACCORDING TO STAGE AND HISTOLOGY FROM THE LUNG CANCER STUDY GROUP*

STAGE	SUBSET	CELL TYPE	4-YEAR SURVIVAL (%)
I	T1N0	Squamous cell	85
		adenocarcinoma	72
	T1N1	Squamous cell	80
		adenocarcinoma	63
	T2N0	Squamous cell	65
		adenocarcinoma	60
II, III		Squamous cell	37
		adenocarcinoma	25

*Postoperative mortality is excluded.
(From: Ginsberg, R.J.; Goldberg, M.; and Waters, P.F. [1989]. Surgery for non-small cell lung cancer. In Roth, Ruckdeschel, and Weisenberger eds. p. 196.)

RADIATION THERAPY

Radiation therapy can be an effective form of primary treatment. It is also of benefit in the palliation of hemoptysis, bronchial obstruction, and bone pain from metastatic disease. Radiation therapy is similar to surgery in that it provides local control. Surgery remains the best form of therapy for stage I and stage II NSCLC, and in some patients with stage IIIA disease. Radiation therapy has its own associated complications and it offers no better control of disseminated disease. It should not be considered as a comparable alternative to surgical therapy.

High-dose radiation therapy can sterilize NSCLC as demonstrated in studies evaluating preoperative radiation therapy, where the tumor was sterilized in 46% of the patients using 60 Gy (Bloedorn et al. 1960). Radiation therapy is recommended for patients who are considered inoperable due to the advanced stage of their cancer or for medical reasons. They should have a good performance status and pulmonary functions should be adequate to tolerate any complications of pulmonary fibrosis. In this instance, there is the possibility of cure. High-dose treatment of 60 Gy is given over six to seven weeks and the size of the fields are decreased at the end of the treatment to minimize radiation damage to the normal lung. A 12% 5-year survival has been reported (Cox, Komaki, and Eisert 1980). Local control of the tumor is accomplished in 60% of patients with this treatment program, and symptoms of cough and dyspnea are relieved in the majority of patients. Complications associated with radiation therapy include radiation pneumonitis and fibrosis, esophagitis, pericarditis, and damage to the spinal cord.

Preoperative radiation therapy to shrink the tumor and enhance resectability was demonstrated to be of no benefit in a large, multicenter clinical trial (Warram 1975). Preoperative radiation therapy is recommended for the superior sulcus tumor in order to sterilize its peripheral boundaries adjacent to the brachial plexus and vertebral body. A preoperative dose of 30 Gy to 40 Gy followed by resection can achieve a cure rate of 34% (Paulson et al. 1962).

Radiation therapy is recommended when resected surgical margins are positive for residual cancer; doses of 50 Gy are given.

Prophylactic cranial radiation is recommended by some for patients with small-cell carcinoma and adenocarcinoma because of the high incidence of brain metastasis associated with these histologic types. This treatment remains controversial due to the possible long-term deleterious effects to the brain; its effectiveness has also been questioned (Cox et al. 1981).

Interstitial radiation is the placement of a high-dose radiation source in close proximity to residual cancer, usually along the mediastinum or vertebral body. Gross residual cancer is usually treated with iodine 125 implant seeds. Microscopic residual disease in the mediastinum is treated with iridium 192 inserted into small plastic catheters properly positioned at the time of surgery. The radiation source is left in place for approximately four days and the catheters are then removed. Local control is improved with this technique of radiation, and a 13% long-term survival has been achieved in patients with incomplete resections (Hilaris et al. 1985).

Postoperative radiation therapy has been effective for both squamous and adenocarcinoma cell types (Martini et al. 1983) and is of benefit when resected mediastinal lymph nodes are found to contain cancer (Kirsh and Sloan 1982). However, in a recent report by the Lung Cancer Study Group in a prospective randomized trial of over 200 patients with squamous cell lung cancer and positive regional lymph nodes, survival was not prolonged, but local recurrence was significantly decreased in the group receiving 50 Gy postoperatively (Weisenberger and Gail 1986). It would appear that postoperative radiation therapy decreases the incidence of local recurrence and is therefore indicated when mediastinal lymph nodes are involved by metastatic cancer.

Radical radiation therapy is indicated for patients who are inoperable due to the local extent of their disease or because of their general medical condition. It is also effective when resected tumor margins are positive and there is local recurrence that cannot again be resected. The future investigational aspects of radiation therapy include the study of cell sensitizers, hyperfractionated dose schedules, neutron energy sources, and radiation in combination with chemotherapy.

CHEMOTHERAPY

Chemotherapy is not used as a primary form of treatment for NSCLC, but is recommended for metastatic lung cancer, SCLC, and in clinical trials of adjuvant therapy. Of the numerous chemotherapeutic agents that have been investigated, there is yet to evolve one best drug or combination of drugs for the treatment of NSCLC. Despite the administration of newer drugs in higher concentrations, a complete response can only be achieved in 5% to 10% of patients. These latest regimens are more active in their destruction of cancer cells, but they are also more toxic and their side effects can be fatal. The patients who respond to treatment will usually have improvement in symptoms and their physical activity will be maintained.

There have been several reported trials of combination chemotherapy in the treatment of disseminated NSCLC. The Eastern Cooperative Oncology Group evaluated four different chemotherapeutic regimens in a randomized trial. These drug regimens are listed in table 14.6 and are representative of other, similar studies. Complete and partial response rates for each regimen were MVP, 31%; VDA-P, 25%; VP-P, 20%; and CAMP, 17%. Twelve of 486 patients survived over two years and 18% survived one year; median survival was 24 weeks. Unfortunately, there was no statistically significant difference between the various treatment

Table 14.6
DRUG REGIMENS

COMBINATION	GENERIC NAMES
VP, VDA-P	Vindesine
	Cisplatin
CAMP	Cyclophosphamide
	Doxorubicin
	Methotrexate
	Procarbazine
MVP	Mitomycin
	Vinblastine
	Cisplatin
VP-P	Etoposide (VP-16)
	Cisplatin

programs and no firm recommendation regarding agents of choice could be made (Ruckdeschel et al. 1986). Other studies have shown a somewhat more favorable response rate to etoposide and cisplatin (Finkelstein, Ettinger, and Ruckdeschel 1986). Current drugs active against NSCLC appear to include cisplatin, mitomycin, etoposide, and vindesine. Prognostic factors that favor a long-term response to chemotherapy have been evaluated and they include a good performance status of the patient prior to initiation of therapy, weight loss less than 5% of usual body weight, absence of liver and bone metastasis, and maintenance of physical activity during treatment (Finkelstein, Ettinger, and Ruckdeschel 1986).

The question as to the merits of chemotherapy in relation to survival and cost was evaluated by a recent randomized prospective study in Canada demonstrating that patients treated by chemotherapy lived twice as long as those who received only supportive care. It was also shown that it was more expensive to give the supportive care than it was to administer chemotherapy (Rapp et al. 1988).

Chemotherapy can be given prior to surgery (neoadjuvant therapy) or postoperatively when resected hilar or mediastinal lymph nodes contain metastatic cancer. Improved survival has been reported using a regimen of cyclophosphamide, doxorubicin, methotrexate, and procarbazine (CAMP) in patients with T1N1M0 and T2N1M0 resected NSCLC. Median survival for patients receiving surgery, radiation, and CAMP was 45 months as compared to similar stage patients who only had surgery and a median survival of 13 months (Ferguson et al. 1986). A Lung Cancer Study Group trial has also shown benefit for pathologic stages II and III adenocarcinoma and large-cell carcinoma with the use of cyclophosphamide, doxorubicin, and cisplatin (CAP). Other investigators have not clearly duplicated these results and the routine use of postoperative chemotherapy is not recommended. However, continued participation in randomized prospective trials is recommended.

IMMUNOTHERAPY

Therapeutic trials using various forms of immunotherapy have not been successful. Intrapleural instillation of *bacille Calmette-Guérin* (BCG) did not extend disease-free interval or length of survival in randomized prospective trials. No long-term benefit has been achieved with levamisole and *Corynebacterium parvum*.

Purified tumor antigens derived from lung cancer and mixed with Freund's adjuvant has been used as specific immunotherapy by vaccination for lung cancer. Reported results are divergent and its routine use is not recommended.

TREATMENT OF SCLC

Maximum dose, multiagent chemotherapy is the initial treatment of choice for the centrally located SCLC and also when metastatic disease is present. Active chemotherapeutic agents for SCLC include etoposide, cyclophosphamide, vincristine, vinblastine, doxorubicin, and carboplatin. The majority of combination chemotherapy regimens are given in 3-week cycles over a course of six months. Chemotherapy produces a rapid response; 70% of patients will demonstrate an objective response and 30% will show a complete response (Bunn and Ihde 1981).

Despite a complete or partial response, SCLC tends to recur at its original site and radiation therapy can provide increased local control. Radiation therapy has been advocated to be administered concomitantly with the start of chemotherapy, after chemotherapy is completed, or as a split course between the cycles of chemotherapy. Those patients who demonstrate total eradication of their SCLC should receive prophylactic cranial radiation to minimize the possibility of brain metastasis. Radiation therapy is not recommended for patients with extensive metastatic SCLC.

Surgical therapy following chemotherapy for centrally located lesions or for patients with N2 disease has been evaluated. There were no long-term survivors in this trial and surgery is not recommended for stage III SCLC (Meyer et al. 1984) The peripheral or stage I (T1N0, T2N0) SCLC should be resected. When chemotherapy is given postoperatively, a 50% 5-year survival has been achieved (Shepherd et al. 1983; Shields et al. 1979). Postoperative radiation is recommended if pathologic staging reveals N1 or N2 disease.

NEOADJUVANT THERAPY IN LUNG CANCER

Neoadjuvant is the current terminology for any form of preoperative therapy. Neoadjuvant treatment can consist of radiation alone, chemotherapy alone, or both in combination. This program of treatment is only used for stage IIIA NSCLC patients, as survival in this group remains at 20% to 25% (Pearson et al. 1982). Advantages of a preoperative program of treatment in stage IIIA disease is that the incidence of a complete resection is increased and a theoretical decrease in the occurrence of distant metastatic disease may occur. The disadvantages of preoperative therapy are a delay in surgery if the tumor is not responsive and an increase in postoperative complications. Treatment-related toxicity and mortality are also associated with chemotherapy.

Radiation has not been effective as a form of preoperative treatment (Warram 1975). However, new high-intensity energy sources are again being evaluated.

Chemotherapy combination regimens containing cisplatin do have an effect on NSCLC and they can be of benefit preoperatively in patients with stage IIIA NSCLC. Cisplatin, bleomycin, and mitomycin combination has been effective in a preoperative treatment program for squamous cell carcinoma by achieving a clinical response in 75% (24 of 32) and sterilizing the tumor in three patients (Raut et al. 1984). A well-controlled study using cisplatin, mitomycin, and a vinca alkaloid has demonstrated complete sterilization of the tumor as demonstrated by careful pathologic analysis of the resected specimen in 20% (8 of 41). Survival at three years was 34% with a median survival of 20 months (Martini et al. 1988).

Radiation and chemotherapy both work to effect biologic tumor cell destruction and can be used in combination as neoadjuvant treatment for the following purposes: (1) to increase the effect of the other modality in bulky localized disease; (2) to accelerate response; and (3) to increase the effect of the other modality in marginally responsive tumors. Cisplatin and 5-fluorouracil are synergistic in their action and both are radiation sensitizers. Adding etoposide to this chemotherapeutic regimen in combination with simultaneous split course radiation therapy for stage III NSCLC patients has a reported median survival of 22 months with 36% surviving at four years (Faber et al. 1989). These early results show promise for neoadjuvant therapy for stage IIIA NSCLC.

Conclusions that can be reached about neoadjuvant programs for stage IIIA NSCLC patients are that the use of cisplatin achieves relatively high response rates, resectability rates are increased, morbidity and mortality are acceptable, and the tumor can be sterilized. However, this type of therapy remains experimental and should only be carried out in well-controlled clinical trials.

OTHER TREATMENT APPROACHES

ENDOBRONCHIAL LASER THERAPY

Obstructing primary or secondary cancers frequently cause significant hemoptysis, distal pneumonitis and atelectasis, and death by strangulation. Significant palliation can be achieved if the tumor can be debulked and the airway re-established. Both the carbon dioxide (CO_2) and neodymium-YAG lasers have been utilized for this purpose, but the YAG laser has proven to be the instrument of choice. It burns deeper with optimal hemostasis, so tumor tissue can be debulked more rapidly. The technique of endobronchial tumor removal with the YAG laser is best accomplished through the rigid bronchoscope and requires special technical expertise and knowledge of laser therapy. Outlined indications for YAG laser therapy of endobronchial lesions include (1) a tumor that is unresponsive to conventional

therapy; (2) the ability to identify a distal bronchial lumen by probe or visualization; and (3) the existence of functioning lung tissue distal to the obstruction (Cortese 1986).

PHOTODYNAMIC THERAPY

Photodynamic therapy (PDT) is endobronchial treatment of both small, early cancers and bulky, obstructing lesions by the use of a photosensitizer. This localizes in the tumor and is then activated by visible light, usually the Argon Pump Dye laser. The photosensitizer commonly used is hematoporphyrin derivative (Hpd). PDT has totally eradicated small noninvasive endobronchial cancers for up to five years in 50% of treated patients (Edell and Cortese 1987). This form of treatment is only for a very small and select group of patients, including those with small, early cancers who are deemed inoperable due to medical reasons or in patients with small, multiple cancers. Photodynamic therapy does not eradicate tumors that extend through the bronchial wall or have metastasized to regional lymph nodes.

ENDOBRONCHIAL BRACHYTHERAPY

Endobronchial brachytherapy is the placement of a high-intensity radiation source into the bronchial lumen adjacent to the tumor. A small plastic catheter is placed through the nasopharynx into the involved bronchus with the aid of the flexible fiberoptic bronchoscope. The radiation source is then inserted through the catheter and properly positioned in the center of the cancer. This technique has the advantage of irradiating only a very small field and sparing large areas of surrounding tissue. It is indicated for patients who have recurrent endobronchial cancer and have previously received external radiation therapy. The radiation source is either from remote afterloading units or iridium 192. Prolonged palliation has been achieved by eliminating hemoptysis and bronchial obstruction (Nori, Hilaris, and Martini 1987).

PATIENT FOLLOW-UP

A successfully treated patient with lung cancer should be examined at 3- to 4-month intervals for the first three years and then every four to six months for the rest of his or her life. These patients are at risk for developing a second primary lung cancer and this occurrence should be diagnosed and treated as soon as possible. Metastatic disease will usually appear during the first two years after therapy.

Physical examination includes careful evaluation of the neck for metastatic lymph nodes and auscultation of both lungs. A chest x-ray with frontal and lateral projections is obtained at every visit. Symptoms of cough or hemoptysis may indicate local recurrence in the bronchus, indicating the need for sputum cytology and flexible fiberoptic bronchoscopy.

Recurrent disease can be local or metastatic recurrence from the original cancer, or it can be a new second or even third primary lung cancer. The incidence of a second primary lung cancer occurs at a frequency of 10% (Shields et al. 1978; Martini, Ghosen, and Melamed 1985). To be considered a second or third primary lung cancer, the lesion should be in a separate and distinct lobe, occur three years after the primary resection, and not be associated with distant metastatic disease. Other indicators that the lesion is a second primary are its location in the opposite lung and a differing histologic type.

Clinical staging and diagnosis are accomplished as if the new lesion were a primary lung cancer. Surgical resection is the treatment of choice for a second primary and a cumulative survival of 33% at five years for second primary lung cancer has been reported (Mathisen et al. 1984). Limited resections can be accomplished in patients who have undergone prior pneumonectomy (Kittle et al. 1985). Patients in whom a prior pneumonectomy has been performed require careful preoperative cardiopulmonary physiologic testing to be certain that they will withstand the contemplated surgical procedure.

Solitary metastatic disease to the brain has been successfully treated by surgical excision, with 55% of 41 patients alive at one year (Magilligan et al. 1986).

Multiple nodules of metastatic disease to the brain and metastasis to the bone are treated with radiation, which can achieve successful palliation. Recurrent bronchogenic carcinoma is also treated with a variety of combination chemotherapy programs; this has achieved a response rate as high as 35% with stabilization of the disease in 15% of patients. Toxicity varies with the drugs given, but these regimens are not without serious and complicated side effects. Long-term survival is rare. There is no role for immunotherapy in the treatment of recurrent bronchogenic carcinoma.

SCREENING

Screening techniques utilizing annual chest x-rays and serial 4-month sputum cytology examinations are not cost effective and do not have therapeutic benefit (Fontana and Sanderson 1986; Melamed and Flehinger 1987; Tockman 1986). However, an increased cure rate is predicated upon early detection and the prudent clinician will obtain an annual chest x-ray of the individual who is at high risk for the development of lung cancer either by occupation, genetic background, or smoking history.

REFERENCES

Akoun, G.M.; Scarna, H.M.; and Milleron, B.J. et al. 1985. Serum neuron-specific enolase: a marker for disease extent and response to therapy for small-cell lung cancer. *Chest* 87:39-43.

Berquist, T.H.; Bailey, P.B.; and Cortese, D.A. et al. 1980. Transthoracic needle biopsy: accuracy and complications in relation to location and type of lesion. *Mayo Clin. Proc.* 55:475-81.

Bitran, J.D.; Golam, L.A.G.; and Weichselbaum, R.R. eds. 1988. *Lung cancer: a comprehensive treatise*. Orlando: Grune & Stratton.

Bloedorn, F.G.; Cowley, R.A.; and Cuccia, C.A. et al. 1960. Combined therapy: irradiation and surgery in the treatment of bronchogenic carcinoma. *Am. J. Roentgenol.* 85:875-85.

Breyer, R.H.; Karstaedt, N.; and Mills, S.A. et al. 1984. Computed tomography for evaluation of mediastinal lymph nodes in lung cancer: correlation with surgical staging. *Ann. Thorac. Surg.* 38:215-20.

Bunn, P.A. Jr., and Ihde, D.C. 1981. Small-cell bronchogenic carcinoma: a review of therapeutic results. In Livingston, R.B. ed. *Lung cancer*. pp. 169-208. Boston: Martinus Nijhoff.

Bunn, P.A., and Minna, J.D. 1985. Paraneoplastic syndromes. In DeVita, V.T.; Hellman, S.; and Rosenberg, S.A. eds. *Principles and practice of oncology*. pp. 1797-1842. Philadelphia: J.B. Lippincott.

Cortese, D.A. 1986. Endobronchial management of lung cancer. *Chest* 89(Suppl 4):234S-36S.

Coughlin, M.; Deslauriers, J.; and Beaulieu, M. et al. 1985. Role of mediastinoscopy in pretreatment staging of patients with primary lung cancer. *Ann. Thorac. Surg.* 40:556-60.

Cox, J.D.; Komaki, R.; and Eisert, D.R. 1980. Irradiation for inoperable carcinoma of the lung and high performance status. *JAMA* 244:1931-33.

Cox, J.D.; Stanley, K.; and Petrovich, Z. et al. 1981. Cranial irradiation in cancer of the lung of all cell types. *JAMA* 245:469-72.

Croft, P.B., and Wilkinson, M. 1965. Carcinomatous neuromyopathy: its incidence in patients with carcinoma of the lung and breast. *Lancet* I:184-88.

Cromatie, R.S.; Parker, E.F.; and May, J.E. et al. 1980. Carcinoma of the lung: a clinical review. *Ann. Thorac. Surg.* 30:30-35.

Daly, B.D.T.; Faling, L.J.; and Pugatch, R.D. et al. 1984. Computed tomography: an effective technique for mediastinal staging in lung cancer. *J. Thorac. Cardiovasc. Surg.* 88:486-94.

Delarue, N.C., and Eschapasse, H. eds. 1985. *International trends in general thoracic surgery*. vol. 1. Philadelphia: W.B. Saunders.

Edell, E.S., and Cortese, D.A. 1987. Bronchoscopic phototherapy with hematoporphyrin derivative for treatment of localized bronchogenic carcinoma: a 5-year experience. *Mayo Clin. Proc.* 62:8-14.

Errett, L.E.; Wilson, J.; and Chen, R.C. et al. 1985. Wedge resection as an alternative procedure for peripheral bronchogenic carcinomas in poor risk patients. *J. Thorac. Cardiovasc. Surg.* 90:656-61.

Faber, L.P.; Kittle, C.F.; and Warren, W.H. et al. 1989. Preoperative chemotherapy and irradiation for stage III non-small cell lung cancer. *Ann. Thorac. Surg.* 47:669-77.

Faber, L.P.; Jensik, R.; and Kittle, C.F. 1984. Results of sleeve lobectomy for bronchogenic carcinoma in 101 patients. *Ann. Thorac. Surg.* 37:279-85.

Ferguson, M.K.; Little, A.G.; and Golomb, H.M. et al. 1986. The role of adjuvant therapy after resection of T1N1M0 and T2N1M0 non-small cell lung cancer. *J. Thorac. Cardiovasc. Surg.* 91:344-49.

Finkelstein, D.M.; Ettinger, D.S.; and Ruckdeschel, J.C. 1986. Long-term survivors in metastatic non-small cell lung cancer. *J. Clin. Oncol.* 4:702-709.

Fontana, R.S., and Sanderson, D.R. 1986. Screening for lung cancer: a progress report. In Mountain, C.F., and Carr, D.T. eds. *Lung cancer: current status and prospects for the future*. p. 51. Austin: University of Texas Press.

Frederick, H.M.; Bernardino, M.E.; and Baron, M. et al. 1984. Accuracy of chest computerized tomography in detecting malignant hilar and mediastinal involvement by squamous cell carcinoma of the lung. *Cancer* 54:2390-95.

Ginsberg, R.J.; Hill, L.D.; and Eagan, R.T. et al. 1983. Modern thirty-day operative mortality for surgical resections in lung cancer. *J. Thorac. Cardiovasc. Surg.* 86:654-58.

Glazer, G.M.; Orringer, M.B.; and Gross, B.H. et al. 1984. The mediastinum in non-small cell lung cancer: CT-surgical correlation. *AJR* 142:1101-1105.

Gould, V.G., and Warren, W.H. 1989. Epithelial neoplasms of the lung. In Roth, J.R.; Ruckdeschel, J.C.; and Weisenburger, T.H. eds. *Thoracic oncology.* pp. 77-93. Philadelphia: W.B. Saunders.

Heelan, R.T.; Martini, N.; and Westcott, J.W. et al. 1985. Carcinomatous involvement of the hilum and mediastinum: computed tomographic and magnetic resonance evaluation. *Radiology* 156:111-15.

Hilaris, B.S.; Gomez, J.; and Nori, D. et al. 1985. Combined surgery, intraoperative brachytherapy, and postoperative external radiation in stage III non-small cell lung cancer. *Cancer* 55:1226-31.

Holmes, E.C., and Gail, M. 1986. Surgical adjuvant therapy for stage II and stage III adenocarcinoma and large cell undifferentiated carcinoma. *J. Clin. Oncol.* 4:710-15.

Jensik, R.J. 1987. Miniresection of small peripheral carcinomas of the lung. *Surg. Clin. North Am.* 67(5):951-58.

Jolly, P.; Hill, L.; and Lawler, P. et al. 1973. Paratracheal mediastinotomy and mediastinoscopy. *J. Thorac. Cardiovasc. Surg.* 66:549-56.

Kirsh, M.V., and Sloan, H. 1982. Mediastinal metastases in bronchogenic carcinoma: influence of postoperative irradiation, cell type and location. *Ann. Thorac. Surg.* 5:459-63.

Kittle, C.F.; Faber, L.P.; and Jensik, R.J. et al. 1985. Pulmonary resection in patients after pneumonectomy. *Ann. Thorac. Surg.* 40:294-99.

Kvale, P.A.; Bode, F.R.; and Kini, S. 1976. Diagnostic accuracy in lung cancer: comparison of techniques used in association with flexible fiberoptic bronchoscopy. *Chest* 69:752-57.

Magilligan, D.J. Jr.; Duvernoy, C.; and Malik, G. et al. 1986. Surgical approach to lung cancer with solitary cerebral metastasis: twenty-five years' experience. *Ann. Thorac. Surg.* 42:360-64.

Manual for staging of cancer. 1988. 3rd ed. American Joint Committee on Cancer. Bears, O.H.; Henson, D.E.; and Hutter, R.V.P. et al. pp. 115-21.

Martini, N., and Beattie, E.J. Jr. 1977. Results of surgical treatment in stage I lung cancer. *J. Thorac. Cardiovasc. Surg.* 74:499-505.

Martini, N., and Flehinger, B.J. 1987. The role of surgery in N2 lung cancer. *Surg. Clin. North Am.* 67(5):1037-49.

Martini, N; Flehinger, B.J.; and Zaman, M. et al. 1983. Results of resection in non-oat cell carcinoma of the lung with mediastinal lymph node metastases. *Ann. Surg.* 198:386-97.

Martini, N.; Ghosen, P.; and Melamed, M.R. 1985. Local recurrence and new primary carcinoma after resection. In Delarue, N.C., and Eschapasse, H. eds. *International trends in general thoracic surgery.* vol 1. pp. 164-69. Philadelphia: W.B. Saunders.

Martini, N.; Kris, M.; and Gralla, R. et al. 1988. The effects of preoperative chemotherapy on the resectability of non-small cell lung carcinoma with mediastinal lymph node metastases (N2M0). *Ann. Thorac. Surg.* 45:370-79.

Mathisen, D.J.; Jensik, R.J.; and Faber, L.P. et al. 1984. Survival following resection for second and third primary lung cancers. *J. Thorac. Cardiovasc. Surg.* 88:502-10.

McKenna, R.J. Jr.; Libshitz, H.I.; and Mountain, C.E. et al. 1985. Roentgenographic evaluation of mediastinal nodes for preoperative assessment in lung cancer. *Chest* 88:206-10.

Melamed, M.R.; Flehinger, B.N.; and Zaman, M.B. 1987. Impact of early detection on the clinical course of lung cancer. *Surg. Clin. North Am.* 67(5):909-24.

Meyer, J.A.; Gallo, J.J.; and Ikins, P.M. et al. 1984. Adverse prognostic effect of N2 disease in treated small-cell carcinoma of the lung. *J. Thorac. Cardiovasc. Surg.* 88:495-501.

Mountain, C.F. 1986. A new international staging system for lung cancer. *Chest* 89(Suppl 4):225S-33S.

Naruke, T.; Suemaser, K.; and Ishikawa, S. et al. 1978. Lymph node mapping and curability at various levels of metastasis in resective lung cancer. *J. Thorac. Cardiovasc. Surg.* 76: 832-39.

Nori, D.; Hilaris, B.S.; and Martini, N. 1987. Intraluminal irradiation in bronchogenic carcinoma. *Surg. Clin. North Am.* 67(5):1093-1102.

Oho, K., and Omemiya, R. 1984. Bronchoscopic diagnosis. In Oho, K., and Omemiya, R. eds. *Practical fiberoptic bronchoscopy.* pp. 68-85. New York: Igaku-Shoin.

Olsen, G.N.; Block, J.; and Tobias, J.A. 1974. Prediction of postpneumonectomy function using quantitative macroaggregate lung scanning. *Chest* 66:13-16.

Oswald, N.C.; Hinson, K.F.W.; and Canti, G. et al. 1971. The diagnosis of primary lung cancer with special reference to sputum cytology. *Thorax* 26:623-31.

Patterson, G.A.; Piazza, D.; and Pearson, F.G. et al. 1987. Significance of metastatic disease in subaortic lymph nodes. *Ann. Thorac. Surg.* 43:155-59.

Paulson, D.L.; Shaw, R.R.; and Kee, J.L. et al. 1962. Combined preoperative irradiation and resection for bronchogenic carcinoma. *J. Thorac. Cardiovasc. Surg.* 44:281-94.

Pearson, F.G.; Delarue, N.C.; and Ilves, R. et al. 1982. Significance of positive superior mediastinal nodes identified at mediastinoscopy in patients with resectable cancer of the lung. *J. Thorac. Cardiovasc. Surg.* 83:1-11.

Piehler, J.M.; Pairolero, P.C.; and Weiland, L.H. et al. 1982. Bronchogenic carcinoma with chest wall invasion: factors affecting survival following *en bloc* resection. *Ann. Thorac. Surg.* 34:684-91.

Radke, J.R.; Conway, W.A.; and Eyler, W.R. et al. 1979. Diagnostic accuracy in peripheral lung lesions: factors predicting success with flexible fiberoptic bronchoscopy. *Chest* 76:176-79.

Rapp, E.; Pater, J.L.; and Wellan, A. et al. 1988. Chemotherapy can prolong survival in patients with advanced non-small cell lung cancer: report of a Canadian multicenter randomized trial. *J. Clin. Oncol.* 6:633-41.

Raut, Y.; Hun, N.; and Clovier, J. et al. 1984. Surgery and chemotherapy: a new method of treatment for squamous cell bronchial carcinoma. *J. Thorac. Cardiovasc. Surg.* 88: 754-57.

Roth, J.A.; Ruckdeschel, J.C.; and Weisenberger, T.H. eds. 1989. *Thoracic oncology.* Philadelphia: W.B. Saunders.

Ruckdeschel, J.C.; Finkelstein, D.M.; and Ettinger, D.S. et al. 1986. A randomized trial of the four most active regimens for metastatic non-small cell lung cancer. *J. Clin. Oncol.* 4:14-22.

Sabin, L.H., and Yesner, R. 1981. *Histologic typing of living tumors: International Histologic Classification of Tumors.* Geneva: World Health Organization.

Sawamura, K.; Mori, T.; and Hashimota, S. et al. 1986. Results of surgical treatment for N2 disease. *Lung Cancer* 2:96.

Selikoff, I.J.; Hammond, E.C.; and Seidman, I.T. 1979. Mortality experience of insulation workers in the United States and Canada 1943-1976. *Ann. N.Y. Acad. Sci.* 330:91-116.

Shepherd, F.A.; Ginsberg, R.J.; and Evans, W.K. et al. 1983. Reduction in local recurrence and improved survival in surgically treated patients with small-cell carcinoma of the lung. *J. Thorac. Cardiovasc. Surg.* 86:498-506.

Shields, T.W.; Higgins, G.A. Jr.; and Matthews, M.J. et al. 1979. Surgical resection in the management of small cell carcinoma of the lung. *J. Thorac. Cardiovasc. Surg.* 77:243-48.

Shields, T.W.; Humphrey, E.W.; and Higgins, G.A. et al. 1978. Long-term survivors after resection of lung carcinoma. *J. Thorac. Cardiovasc. Surg.* 76:439-45.

Silverberg, E.; Boring, C.C.; and Squires, T.S. 1990. Cancer statistics, 1990: *CA* 40(1):9-26.

Tandon, R.D. 1966. The significance of pleural effusion associated with bronchial carcinoma. *Br. J. Dis. Chest* 60:49.

Tockman, M.S. 1986. Survival and mortality from lung cancer in a screened population: the John Hopkins Study. *Chest* 89(Suppl 4):324S-25S.

Vincent, R.G.; Pickens, J.W.; and Lane, W.W. et al. 1977. The changing histopathology of lung cancer: a review of 1,682 cases. *Cancer* 39:1647-55.

Wang, K.P. 1989. Flexible bronchoscopy with transbronchial needle aspiration: biopsy for cytology specimens. In Wang, K.P. ed. *Biopsy techniques in pulmonary disorders.* pp. 63-71. New York: Raven Press.

Warram, J. 1975. Preoperative irradiation of cancer of the lung: final report of a therapeutic trial. *Cancer* 36:914-23.

Weisenberger, T.H., and Gail, M. 1986. Effects of postoperative mediastinal radiation on completely resected stage II and stage III epidermoid cancer of the lung. *N. Engl. J. Med.* 315:1377-81.

Zaman, M.B.; Hajder, S.I.; and Melamed, M.R. et al. 1986. Transthoracic aspiration cytology of pulmonary lesions. *Sem. Diag. Pathol.* 3:176-87.

Zavala, D.C. 1975. Diagnostic fiberoptic bronchoscopy: technique and results of biopsy in 600 patients. *Chest* 68:12-19.

Zerhouni, E.A.; Stitik, F.P.; and Siegelmans, et al. 1986. CT of the pulmonary nodule: a cooperative study. *Radiology* 160:319-27.

Chapter 15

COLORECTAL CANCER

Robert W. Beart, Jr., M.D.

Robert W. Beart, Jr., M.D.
Caywood Professor of Surgery
Mayo Clinic Scottsdale
Scottsdale, Arizona

EPIDEMIOLOGY

INCIDENCE

Colorectal cancer is the second most common malignant tumor in the United States. This is in contrast to the low but increasing incidence in Japan and Finland, where there is a high incidence of esophageal and stomach cancers. People from these countries who move to Westernized cultures develop colorectal cancer at rates similar to that of the Western cultures. Approximately 155,000 new cases of colon and rectal cancer will be identified in the United States in 1990 (*CA* 1990).

DEATH RATE

In the United States, there will be 61,000 deaths from colon or rectal cancer in 1990. This compares with 24,000 deaths from cancers of the esophagus, stomach, and small intestine, and 25,000 for cancer of the pancreas. The death rate for colon and rectal cancer is second to that of cancer of the lung (*CA* 1990).

SEX

In the United States, males and females are affected equally. There are some families, however, whose female members seem to demonstrate a genetic propensity to develop colon cancer.

AGE

Mean age of incidence is 62 years; two of three patients are over age 50. With predisposing conditions such as familial polyposis, ulcerative colitis, or family cancer syndrome, cancer appears at an early age. Occasionally the disease is seen in patients in their second or third decade, and the prognosis in this setting reportedly is very poor.

SITE

In recent decades, this disease has been moving toward the right colon (Beart et al. 1983). Currently, 38% of cases occur proximally and 62% distally; previously, the site distribution was 22% proximal and 78% distal. The reason for this apparent change is unclear. Adenocar-cinomas are most commonly located in the colon. Carcinoid tumors are most commonly found in the appendix and in the rectum, and tend to have little propensity to metastasize unless they are larger than 2 cm. In the anal canal, most carcinomas are epidermoid or cloacogenic in type; anal adenocarcinomas are rare (Boman et al. 1984).

ETIOLOGY

PREDISPOSING DISEASES

A number of predisposing conditions for colorectal cancer have been identified (Bresnick et al. 1980). These include:

Familial polyposis. This disease is inherited as an autosomal dominant trait. The adenomatous polyps have a tendency to undergo malignant change when the patient is at a young age, probably because of the number of polyps that develop early. Cancers develop in all parts of the colon about 15 years after the onset of polyposis, which usually occurs around puberty. Typically, a patient develops polyps at age 15, cancer at age 30, and if untreated is dead by age 35 (Bussey 1975).

Chronic ulcerative colitis. Patients who have pancolonic involvement with ulcerative colitis are at an increased risk of developing colon cancer. This risk begins to rise after 10 years of disease and increases at 2% per year thereafter. The cancer risk for less-extensive involvement of the colon is dramatically reduced (Keweuter, Ahlman, and Hulten 1978; DeVrode, Taylor, and Sauer 1971).

Family cancer syndrome. Families who have a propensity to develop uterine, breast, or colon cancer appear to be at high risk for the development of colon cancer and should be identified and screened regularly (Lynch et al. 1973).

CASE FINDINGS AND DIAGNOSIS

Patients who have any of the high-risk factors should be evaluated annually for the presence of malignancy. In some cases, prophylactic colectomy is warranted.

SCREENING

Individuals who are not at increased risk and who have no symptoms should be screened annually beginning at age 40. This should consist of an annual digital rectal examination; for ages 50 and over, additional screening procedures of an annual fecal occult blood test and sigmoidoscopy every three to five years should be performed (Eddy et al. 1987).

BARIUM ENEMA

Barium enema or colonoscopy are indicated if any symptoms are present or if the patient has a history of polyps.

A positive occult fecal blood test needs to be followed up with total gastrointestinal tract evaluation until no clear source is identified. Patients with abdominal symptoms such as pain, cramping, or change of bowel habits should undergo a total colonic evaluation with either a high-quality barium enema or colonoscopy. There are no blood tests that are effective in identifying colonic malignancy.

STAGING

TNM CLASSIFICATION

The TNM (primary tumor, nodal involvement, distant metastasis) system is used to classify colorectal cancers (see table 15.1).

HISTOPATHOLOGY

The vast majority of colon cancers are adenocarcinomas. Carcinoid tumors, sarcomas, lymphomas, adenoacanthomas, melanomas, and other rare tumors have been identified. The grading system utilized refers to Broders' system and defines a degree of differentiation (Spratt and Spuitt 1967).

STAGE GROUPING

DUKES' CLASSIFICATION

The Dukes' classification was first described in 1932 (Dukes 1957) and depends upon the depth of tumor invasion into and through the bowel wall. This classification has been modified several times and is, therefore, confusing when referred to in the literature. The American Joint Committee on Cancer (AJC) classification (tables 15.1 and 15.2) is based upon similar pathologic evaluation and recognizes: superficial tumors without muscular involvement (stage I); invasion through the serosa (stage II); invasion and involve-

Table 15.1
TUMOR (T), NODE (N) CLASSIFICATION
COLON AND RECTAL CANCER

UICC		AJC
T1/pT1	Mucosa or submucosa only	T1
T2/pT2	Muscle or serosa	T2
T3a/pT3a	Extension to contiguous structures	T3
	No fistula	
T3b/pT3b	With fistula	T4
T4/pT4	Extension beyond contiguous structures	T5
N	No regional node involvement	N0
N1	Regional	N1
N4	Juxtaregional	

Table 15.2
STAGE GROUPING
COLON AND RECTAL CANCER

Stage Ia	T1	N0	M0
Stage Ib	T2	N0	M0
Stage II	T3, T4	N0	M0
Stage III	Any T	N1	M0
Stage IV	Any T	N4	M0
	Any T	Any N	M1

ment of regional lymph nodes (stage III); and distant metastasis (stage IV). The N4 category is an International Union Against Cancer (UICC) classification only and recognizes juxtaregional nodal involvement.

METASTATIC SPREAD

Regional lymph nodes are involved in 50% of cases (Wilson and Searlers 1976). Most cancers spread sequentially from the primary tumor to adjacent lymph nodes and then up the mesenteric lymph node chain. Low rectal and anal cancers tend to spread laterally to perineal nodes and may appear in inguinal nodes rather than in retroperitoneal nodes. Distant spread most commonly involves the liver and lungs; rarely are these organs involved without lymph node involvement (fig. 15.1).

PREOPERATIVE EVALUATION AND WORKUP

If patients are poor operative candidates, then computed tomography (CT) scanning is helpful in evaluation of spread. Primary tumors, however, should be removed surgically because local symptoms are incapacitating. Quality of life is improved even in the presence of distant metastasis. In otherwise healthy patients, preoperative staging is rarely necessary. An elevated carcinoembryonic antigen (CEA) level preoperatively suggests metastatic disease (O'Dwyer 1988).

DIAGNOSTIC PROCEDURES

Diagnostic procedures may include a *colonic visualization* using either a high-quality barium enema or colonoscopy. This should be completed preoperatively in order to define the primary tumor and to rule out metachronous lesions.

A number of other procedures may be employed in order to establish a diagnosis. *Rigid sigmoidoscopy* is helpful in evaluating the level of the tumor and predicting whether a colostomy may be necessary. *Cystoscopy and intravenous pyelography* studies are rarely indicated except for very large tumors of the rectum. *Chest x-ray* is necessary only for preanesthetic evaluation. *Liver scans and CT scans* are rarely indicated except for cases where the clinician seeks to confirm a clinical judgment of medical inoperability. *Laboratory tests* should include the usual preoperative evaluations and a CEA measurement. Any evidence of disseminated disease should be confirmed with biopsies, taken during surgery. *Postoperative CEA* should be obtained one or two months

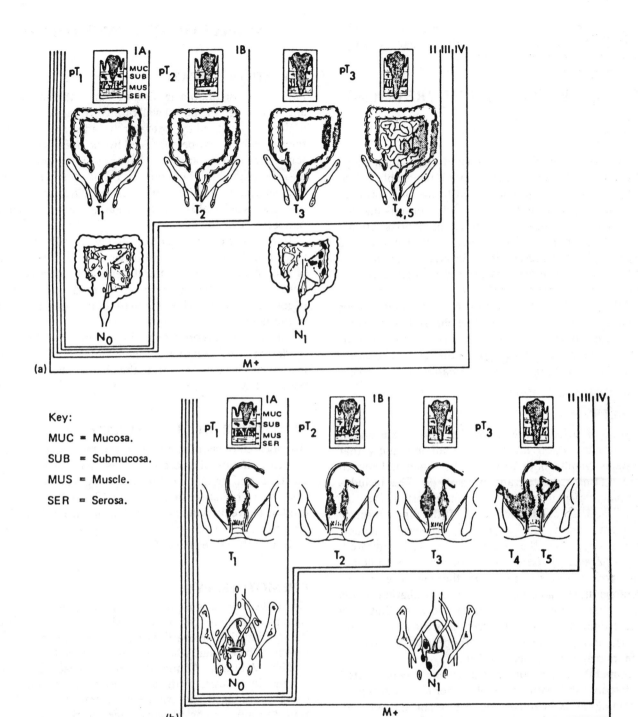

Fig. 15.1. Anatomic staging for (A) colon cancer and (B) rectal cancer. Tumor (T) categories: The depth of penetration is the most important criterion, but for some unknown reason is carried to 5 categories. The order of progression for hollow viscera is a stage for each layer: mucosa, muscle, serosa (T1 to T2 to T3). Extension to extramural structures also characterizes T3, fistula in T4, and adjacent organs T5, which are superfluous. Node (N) categories: The regional nodes are either negative or positive and are confined to the course of the inferior mesenteric artery and vein. Stage grouping: This is awkward but essential. It groups favorable T lesions (T1 and T2) as stage I because of ease of resection. Unfavorable T3 to T5 lesions are grouped in stage II. Positive nodes are stage III and metastases that include nodes beyond the inferior mesenteric are stage IV. AJC vs. UICC classification: The UICC has approximately 4 categories, but confuses the standard categories of visceral organs by lumping muscle and serosal invasion into T2. The UICC T3 (a and b) is equivalent to the AJC's T4 and T5. The UICC's T4 category is quite absurd. It has primary tumor extending to the immediately adjacent organs, which for the AJC, would be a T6. There is an additional UICC N4 category for juxtaregional nodes whereas N2 and N3 are noted as not applicable.

after surgery. A normal level is a favorable sign; elevated CEA strongly suggests occult residual disease.

PRINCIPLES OF SURGICAL TREATMENT

POLYPS

Colon polyps should be evaluated with colonoscopy (Carlsson et al. 1987). Pedunculated, removable polyps should be resected and subjected to histologic evaluation. Malignant polyps with no evidence of stalk involvement and a clean line of resection require no additional therapy. If there is submucosal involvement of the polyps or if the resection line is involved, then the risks of residual or recurrent disease are unacceptably high and further resection is indicated.

Patients who have benign or malignant polyps resected endoscopically should be checked annually for recurrent disease for two years. If no recurrent or residual disease is identified, then they should be examined every two to three years thereafter (Hoff 1987).

CANCERS

Cancers of the colon are removed by a wide resection of the primary lesion together with all mesentery that contains lymph nodes to which the tumor is likely to spread (Enker, Loffer, and Block 1979). This includes the main vascular tree to the colon as well as areas of lymph-node spread in the rectum. If the tumor involves adjacent organs such as the small bowel, bladder, uterus, or ovaries, then *en bloc* resection is indicated. Areas of residual disease should be marked with hemoclips for subsequent radiation therapy. The use of intraoperative radiation therapy or radiation seeds should be considered for residual disease, but only where limited margins of resection occur (Gunderson, Beart, and O'Connell 1987). Inoperable obstructing tumors may be bypassed surgically.

Inoperable obstructing rectal cancers may be treated endoscopically with multiple thermal techniques, including the laser to core out the tumor and leave an open passage. This helps to avoid the need for a colostomy. External beam radiation therapy may also help diminish these tumors.

Local excision of rectal cancers helps to avoid a colostomy for well-differentiated lesions less than 3 cm in size (Heberer et al. 1987). Lesions that do not meet these criteria are best removed with more extensive procedures. One alternative local therapy includes excision and transanal irradiation.

Although radiation therapy and chemotherapy have adjuvant roles in the management of colon and rectal cancer, surgery should be considered the primary treatment, except for small, well-differentiated rectal cancers and anal cancers.

PRINCIPLES OF ADJUVANT THERAPY

RADIATION THERAPY

Patients whose tumors lie within 15 cm of the anal verge and go through the bowel wall or involve regional lymph nodes are benefited by postoperative adjuvant radiation therapy, which may be enhanced by the use of radiation sensitizers (Kliegman 1976). Preoperative therapy may also be valuable, but this has not been as well-documented in the literature (Seseley 1982). Preoperative use would also involve treating many patients unnecessarily.

Radiation treatment requires 40 Gy to 50 Gy for large fields that include the entire pelvis and the bifurcation of the aorta. Shrinking lateral fields may increase the dose delivered. Attention must be paid to minimize exposure of the small bowel and other normal structures in the field.

The role of preoperative, single-dose, low-dose, or moderate-dose radiation remains undefined. Several institutions have an interest in this therapy, but as yet its benefits have not been established.

PALLIATIVE RADIATION THERAPY

Adenocarcinomas of the rectum are moderately sensitive to radiation. Tumors that cause pain or excessive bleeding and cannot be surgically removed will often respond to radiation therapy. Fifty Gy to 60 Gy delivered in six weeks will have a 90% incidence of relieving symptoms. Unfortunately, this usually lasts only six to eight months (Priestman 1977).

CHEMOTHERAPY

As of 1990, there is a proven effective adjuvant chemotherapy regimen for colon cancer (Moertel 1990). Chemotherapy with 5-fluorouracil (5-FU) and metronidazole has proven to be of value when used as a radiation sensitizer.

The Veterans Administration Surgical Adjuvant Group, in a large, controlled randomized group trial using prolonged intermittent intravenous 5-FU, reported no significant advantage in the treatment group. Survival at five years was 49.1% for patients receiving 5-FU and 44.7% for controls (Higgins 1979).

Chemotherapy for palliation results in 20% response rates with 5-FU alone. Combinations have been reported to be more effective but have not proven reliably to be any better than 5-FU alone.

Chemotherapy with 5-FU and immunostimulants (*bacillus Calmette-Guérin* [BCG], methanol extraction residue of BCG [MER-BCG], and levamisole are all nonspecific immunostimulants) have not been found to be reliably effective. One study with 5-FU plus levamisole has proven benefit in advanced cancer and is currently being looked at in the adjuvant setting (Laurie et al. 1988).

CURATIVE TREATMENT

The only curative therapy is surgical resection of the primary tumor and regional mesenteric lymph nodes. Postoperative radiation therapy in tumors dissecting the bowel wall or with positive lymph nodes is recommended.

Advanced or metastatic rectal cancers are best treated with palliative surgery or radiation. Chemotherapy may be an effective radiation sensitizer.

RESULTS OF TREATMENT

As reported in the literature, results for right- and left-sided colon cancer are approximately equal. Of 100 patients with proven colon cancer, 5% will be inoperable for medical reasons or because they refuse surgery; 10% will be unresectable or resectable only for palliation; 2% will die as a result of surgery; 23% will die from associated causes within five years; 2% will be alive with persistent cancer in five years; and 58% will be alive without evidence of disease at five years after the cancer (Cameron, Verdenheimer, and Callan 1979). These statistics are improving through the years (Sugarbaker 1986).

FOLLOW-UP AFTER TREATMENT

Patients with favorable lesions at the time of surgery should have follow-up for a minimum of five years for the primary tumor and then be followed every two to three years. It should be recognized that they are at increased risk from recurrent or new cancers of the colon. The patients should be seen every four months for a history, physical examination, and CEA test (Martin et al. 1977). Any specific symptoms, in addition, should be followed up with appropriate tests. Annually, the patient should have a history, physical examination, CEA measurement, liver function test, chest x-ray, and other tests as indicated by symptoms. Computed tomography scans are helpful in identifying recurrent or residual pelvic disease for rectal cancer. In addition, the colon should be examined either with a high-quality barium enema or colonoscopy annually. These tests should be carried out every four months for two years; every six months for an additional three years; and then annually thereafter. The rationale for the sequence and interval of testing maximizes the identification of tumors at a reasonably early point while minimizing the cost. Patients who are not candidates for additional therapeutic modalities should not be followed aggressively.

If recurrent disease is identified, isolated tumors of distant organs such as liver, lung, or brain should be resected (Robin and Green 1968; *Resection of the Liver for Colorectal Carcinoma Metastases* 1988). Long-term survival is about 40%. Similarly, aggressive management of isolated pelvic recurrences can have a 25% to 40% incidence of cure (Gunderson et al. 1980). Multiple lesions in a single organ have a less-favorable prognosis.

CURRENT AREAS OF CLINICAL INVESTIGATION

The question of whether wider surgical resections are of value, particularly in the pelvis, is under investigation. Currently, it would not appear that wider resections are indicated.

Adjuvant management for rectal cancer centers on radiation therapy, together with the use of various radiation sensitizers and the sequencing of the sensitizers and the radiation therapy.

Adjuvant chemotherapy for colon cancer centers on the use of 5-FU and levamisole and appears to have promise. Recurrent disease can be managed by intraoperative radiation therapy together with surgical debulking. This appears promising as a means of controlling the local disease, with a 25% to 30% long-term survival.

REFERENCES

American Cancer Society. 1990. *CA* 40:9-26.

American Cancer Society. 1980. *CA* 30:208-15.

Beart, R.W.; Melton, L.J.; and Maueta et al. 1983. Trends in right- and left-sided colon cancer. *Dis. Colon Rectum* 26:393-98.

Boman, B.M.; Moulet, C.G.; and O'Connell, M.J. et al. 1984. Carcinoma of the anal canal: a clinicopathological study of 188 cases. *Cancer* 54:114-25.

Bresnick, E. 1980. Colon carcinogenesis: an overview. *Cancer Suppl.* 45:1047-51.

Bussey, H.J.R. 1975. *Familial polyposis coli.* Baltimore: Johns Hopkins University Press.

Cameron, M.C.; Verdenheimer, M.C.; and Callan, J.A. 1979. Colorectal carcinoma: a decade's experience at the Lahey Clinic. *Am. Colon Rectum* 22:4777-79.

Carlsson, G.; Petrelli, N.J.; and Nache, H. et al. 1987. The value of colonoscopic surveillance after curative resection for colorectal cancer. *Arch. Surg.* 122:1261-63.

Chlebowski, R.T.; Nuystrom, S.; and Reynolds, R. et al. 1988. Long-term survival following levamisole or placebo adjuvant treatment in colorectal cancer. *Oncology* 4:141-43.

DeVroede, G.J.; Taylor, W.F.; and Sauer, W.G. 1971. Cancer risk and life expectancy of children with ulcerative colitis. *New Engl. J. Med.* 285:17-21.

Dukes, C.E. 1957. Discussion on major surgery on carcinoma of the rectum, with or without colostomy, excluding the anal canal and including the rectosigmoid. *Proc. Roy. Soc. Med.* 50:1031-35.

Eddy, D.M.; Nugent, F.W.; and Eddy, J.F. et al. 1987. Screening for colorectal cancer in a high-risk population. *Gastroenterology* 92:682-92.

Enker, W.E.; Loffer, U.T.; and Block, G.E. 1979. Enhanced survival of patients with colon and rectal cancer is based upon wide anatomic resection. *Ann. Surg.* 190:350-60.

Gunderson, L.C.; Cohen, A.M.; and Welch, C.W. 1980. Residual, inoperable, or recurrent colorectal cancer: surgical radiotherapy interaction. *Am. J. Surg.* 139:518-25.

Gunderson, L.C.; Beart, R.W.; and O'Connell, M.J. 1987. Current issues in the treatment of colorectal cancer. *Curr. Res. Oncol. Hematol.* 6:223-59.

Heberer, G.; Denedre, H.; and Derninel, W. et al. 1987. Procedures in the management of rectal cancer. *World J. Surg.* 11:499-503.

Higgins, G.A. 1979. Adjuvant radiation therapy in colon cancer. *Int. Adv. Surg. Oncol.* 2:1-24.

Hoff, G. 1987. Colorectal polyps. *Scand. J. Gastroenterol.* 22:769-75.

Keweuter, J.; Ahlman, H.; and Hulten, L. 1978. Cancer risk in ulcerative colitis. *Ann. Surg.* 188:824.

Kliegman, M.M. 1976. Radiation therapy for rectal carcinoma. *Sem. Oncol.* 3:407-13.

Krook, J.; Moertel, C.; and Wiend, H. et al. 1986. Radiation vs. sequential chemotherapy radiation-chemotherapy. *Proc. Am. Soc. Clin. Oncol.* 5:82.

Lynch, H.T.; Guergis, H.; and Swartz, M. et al. 1973. Genetics and colon cancer. *Arch. Surg.* 106:669-75.

Martin, E.W. Jr.; James, K.K.; and Hurtubise, P.E. et al. 1977. The use of CEA as an early indicator for gastrointestinal tumor recurrence and second look procedures. *Cancer* 39:440-46.

Maton, P.N. 1988. The carcinoid syndrome. *JAMA* 260:1602-1605.

Moertel, C.G.; Fleming, T.R.; and Macdonald, J.S. et al. 1990. Levamisole and fluorouracil for adjuvant therapy of resected carcinoma. *N. Engl. J. Med.* 322:352-58.

O'Dwyer, P.T.; Mojzcski, C; and McCabe, D.P. 1988. Reoperation directed by carcinoembryonic antigen level: the importance of a thorough preoperative evaluation. *Am. J. Surg.* 155:227.

Priestman, T.S. 1977. The place of radiation therapy in the management of rectal adenocarcinomas. *Cancer Treat. Rev.* 4:1-12.

Resection of the liver for colorectal carcinoma metastases: a multi-institutional study of ulcerative colitis for resection. *Surgery* 103:278-88.

Robin, P., and Green, J. 1968. *Solitary metastasis.* Springfield: Charles C. Thomas.

Sesely, B. 1982. The place of radiotherapy in the management of rectal adenocarcinoma. *Cancer* 50:2631-37.

Spratt, J.S., and Spuitt, H.J. 1967. Prevalence and prognosis of individual clinical and pathological variables associated with colorectal carcinoma. *Cancer* 20:1976-85.

Sugarbaker, P.H. 1986. Colorectal tumor. In Cameron, J.L. ed. *Current surgical therapy.* vol. 2. pp. 121-22. St. Louis: C.V. Mosby Co.

Wilson, S.M., and Searlers, O.H. 1976. The curative treatment of carcinoma of the sigmoid, rectosigmoid, and rectum. *Ann. Surg.* 183:556-65.

Chapter 16

TUMORS OF THE PANCREAS, GALLBLADDER, AND EXTRAHEPATIC DUCTS

Robert M. Beazley, M.D.

Isidore Cohn, Jr., M.D.

Robert M. Beazley, M.D.
Professor of Surgery
Boston University School of Medicine
Head, Section of Surgical Oncology
University Hospital
Boston, Massachusetts

Isidore Cohn, Jr., M.D.
Professor and Chairman
Department of Surgery
Louisiana State University
School of Medicine
New Orleans, Louisiana

INTRODUCTION

Pancreatic ductal cancer is the second most common gastrointestinal cancer and the fourth leading cause of cancer death in the United States. In 1990 the American Cancer Society predicts that 28,100 new cases will occur (Silverberg, Boring, and Squires 1990). The major obstacle to successful management of this disease is the inability to establish the diagnosis at an early, curable stage. Therefore, most clinical efforts are diagnostic and palliative.

PANCREATIC CANCER

EPIDEMIOLOGY AND NATURAL HISTORY

Pancreatic cancer increases in incidence with age. The tumor registry of Charity Hospital of Louisiana at New Orleans records a peak incidence in the seventh decade, with 82% of patients between 50 and 80 years of age (Gray, Crook, and Cohn 1972). Rarely, the disease has been reported in younger individuals and children.

There is a slight male predominance in pancreatic cancer with males averaging about five years younger at inception than females (65 vs. 70 years) (Waterhouse 1974). This male predominance prevails in both whites and nonwhites. Religious and ethnic studies support an increased frequency among Jews in New York City and in Israel (Newill 1961; Doll, Muir, and Waterhouse 1970). Pancreatic cancer mortality is lower among

Mormons than among nonsmoking white males in both California and Utah (Enstrom 1978).

Pancreatic cancer does not seem to be increased in patients who have chronic pancreatitis, nor is there an increased rate among diabetics. Wynder, however, has shown a significant association of prior diabetes in females (Wynder et al. 1973). In a few patients, a recent onset of diabetes may precede by several months the diagnosis of pancreatic cancer.

Many studies have documented a dose-related association between pancreatic cancer and smoking. Whittemore et al. (1983) studied 50,000 male former college students, attempting to identify factors that might predict an increased risk of pancreatic cancer. A relative risk of 2.6 was determined for those individuals who smoked during their college years.

Dietary factors have been implicated in the causation of pancreatic cancer. In animal studies, dietary fat enhances the experimental production of azaserine-induced pancreatic tumors (Roebuck et al. 1981). Although coffee consumption was believed to be a strong etiologic factor (McMahon et al. 1981), more recent studies have failed to support this observation (Goldstein 1982). Evidence relating alcoholism to pancreatic cancer is weak, but studies in this area are complicated by the difficulty in discriminating between the effects of alcohol and tobacco, substances which are usually used together.

Environmental and occupational association with pancreatic cancer appears in areas where workers are in contact with organic chemicals, particularly coke and coal gas operations, and workers in the betanaphthylamine and benzidine industries (Mancuso and el-Attar 1967). A study by Li et al. (1969) found an increased pancreatic cancer death rate among white male chemists compared with a control group of professional men and the elderly white male U.S. population in general.

Unfortunately, none of these epidemiologic factors is sufficiently specific to define a population at high risk of developing pancreatic cancer.

CLINICAL FEATURES

The clinical features of pancreatic ductal cancer are generally vague and nonspecific; most commonly these are weight loss, jaundice, and abdominal pain. Table 16.1 outlines the frequency of presenting symptoms in 449 patients with pancreatic cancer treated at Charity Hospital of Louisiana at New Orleans (Gray, Crook, and Cohn 1972).

Weight loss, often gradual and progressive, is one of the earliest and most frequently unappreciated symptoms. There is usually several months of patient delay in seeking medical attention, but often an even greater physician delay in establishing the diagnosis. Moosa (1980) found that 70% of patients had been investigated in the hospital within a year prior to the diagnosis. Similar reports of undue diagnostic delay further reflect the difficulty of making earlier diagnoses.

Pain is part of the clinical picture in 70% to 80% of patients. It is most likely to be midepigastric, steady, dull, boring in quality, and usually worse at night. Left-upper-quadrant pain is more common with cancer of the body or tail of the pancreas. A small number of patients will suffer lower abdominal pain. Approximately 15% to 30% of patients have back pain that is aggravated by lying flat and relieved by sitting up and bending forward, or by lying curled in a fetal-type position. The pain is frequently vague and ill-defined, which confuses the examiner and contributes to diagnostic delay. One study documented that two-thirds of the jaundiced patients had experienced abdominal pain for an average of three months prior to the onset of icterus (Douglass and Holyoke 1974).

Jaundice is the third most frequent symptom and, in many instances depending upon tumor location, may be a late symptom. Although usually progressive, spontaneous fluctuation has been documented. Jaundice is commonly accompanied by bothersome pruritus involving the arms, legs, and abdomen that is typically worse in the evening and at night. The pruritus is thought to be related to retained bile salts, since the level of certain bile salts in the skin correlates better with the degree of itching than does the serum bilirubin level. Another theory is that bile salts promote the release of proteases from the surrounding cells, and that the proteases cause itching. However, not all jaundiced patients complain of itching, and, occasionally, itching will precede clinical onset of jaundice. While painless jaundice is still heralded erroneously as the classical symptom of pancreatic cancer, the patient who presents in this manner is the exception.

Nonspecific signs and symptoms of pancreatic cancer include anorexia, which usually accompanies weight loss. Perhaps 10% of patients will present with symptoms of ascending cholangitis, i.e., jaundice, chills, fever, and right-upper-quadrant pain (Charcot's triad). Generally, the biliary tree obstructed by cancer that has not been instrumented is sterile in contrast to that obstructed by biliary calculi. Alteration of bowel habit may occur in the form of diarrhea or steatorrhea resulting from pancreatic insufficiency; more frequently constipation secondary to decreased total food intake may occur. Bloating and flatulence are other nonspecific bowel complaints. Gastric outflow obstruction and vomiting resulting from direct invasion of the pylorus, stomach, or duodenum, or simply functional obstruction, is an unusual symptom. Direct tumor invasion may result in hematemesis or melena; obstruction of the splenic or portal vein may result in esophageal varices and hemorrhage.

Trousseau's sign (migratory thrombophlebitis), while not specific, occasionally heralds pancreatic cancer. Migratory or recurrent thrombophlebitis in the older patient should prompt evaluation for occult cancer, especially that of pancreatic origin, although the syndrome may be associated with cancers of a lung, ovary, uterus, or colon. Thrombophlebitis is most frequent in advanced disease and more common with tumors arising in the body and tail of the pancreas.

Many patients will present with recent-onset diabetes or deterioration of a previously stable diabetic state, presumably as a result of the development of a pancreatic cancer.

Since the Middle Ages melancholia, hypochondria, and hysteria have been thought to originate in the pancreas. Psychiatric disturbances, chiefly depression, are occasionally observed in patients with pancreatic cancer. More than half of such patients will have

Table 16.1
PRESENTING SYMPTOMS OF PANCREATIC CANCER

Symptom	Number of Patients	Percent of Patients (%)	Patients with Resectable Lesions Number	Percent (%)
Weight loss	327	73	48	74
Abdominal pain	293	65	29	45
Jaundice	201	45	45	69
Anorexia	163	36	18	28
Significant GI bleeding	30	7	1	15

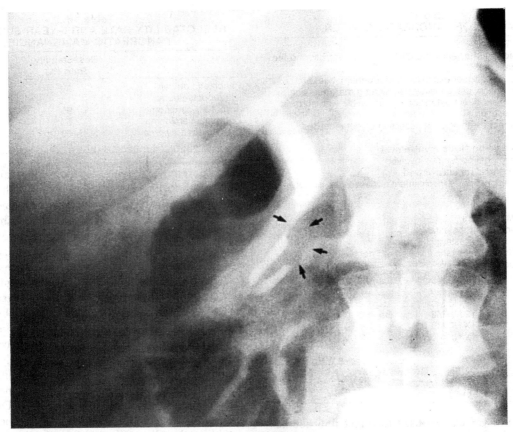

Fig. 16.1. Double-duct sign on endoscopic cholangiopancreatography is the result of simultaneous obstruction of both the common bile duct and pancreatic duct by tumor arising in the head of the pancreas. This sign is highly suggestive of carcinoma but has been reported with pancreatitis.

psychiatric symptoms that precede the physical symptoms by a median interval of six months.

It is easy to understand how difficult it is to arrive at an early diagnosis of pancreatic cancer when there is a broad spectrum of vague and nonspecific symptoms. The physician must maintain a high level of suspicion.

DIAGNOSIS

Early diagnosis is essential to the cure of pancreatic cancer. Because the signs and symptoms of the earliest stages of the disease may be nonspecific, it is not cost-effective to perform an extensive evaluation of every patient. Furthermore, no high-risk population has been identified to warrant screening; there is no inexpensive, sensitive, and specific diagnostic test for early detection.

Moosa (1980) has suggested that a high level of suspicion is appropriate for patients who are 40 years of age or older who present with any of the following clinical features: (1) obstructive jaundice; (2) recent unexplained weight loss greater than 10% of normal body weight; (3) recent unexplained upper abdominal or lumbar back pain; (4) recent vague, unexplained dyspepsia and a normal upper GI investigation; (5) sudden onset of diabetes mellitus without predisposing factors such as family history or obesity; (6) sudden onset of unexplained steatorrhea; (7) an attack of

idiopathic pancreatitis; and (8) if the patient is a heavy smoker, the level of suspicion should be doubled.

Older diagnostic investigations such as GI x-ray series, arteriography, pancreatic function tests, and duodenal drainage and cytology are done infrequently. Currently, the initial diagnostic test of choice in patients suspected of having pancreatic cancer is a computerized tomographic (CT) scan. Ultrasound (US) was the initial diagnostic test of choice a few years ago, but newer, faster scanners have allowed CT scanning to replace it. The advantages of CT scanning are that it is not operator-dependent, it is not limited by stomach or bowel gas, and it will demonstrate liver metastasis (as small as 2 cm) as well as retropancreatic areas for perivascular invasion and lymphadenopathy (Hessel et al. 1982; Levitt et al. 1982). It is also possible to demonstrate dilation of the pancreatic duct and the site of the obstruction in 88% to 97% of instances (Baron et al. 1982; Pedrossa, Casanova, and Rodriguez 1981). Ward reviewed the CT findings in 100 pancreatic cancer patients, most of whom were not jaundiced, and was able to detect a pancreatic mass of 2 cm or larger in more than 95%. Smaller tumors are more difficult to detect with regularity because they may fail to distort the gland's contour (Ward, Stephens, and Sheedy 1983). Furthermore, small lymph nodes, peritoneal seeding, and hepatic metastases (less than 2 cm) may go undetected, rendering CT scans inaccurate in determining resectability in all patients.

Table 16.2
STAGING OF PANCREATIC CANCER

T	**Primary Tumor**	
	T1	No direct extension of the primary tumor beyond the pancreas
	T2	Limited direct extension to duodenum, bile duct, or stomach, still possibly permitting tumor resection
	T3	Further direct extension, incompatible with surgical resection
	TX	Direct extension not assessed or not recorded
N	**Regional Lymph Node Involvement**	
	N0	Regional nodes not involved
	N1	Regional nodes involved
	NX	Regional node involvement not assessed or not recorded.
M	**Distant Metastasis**	
	M0	No distant metastasis
	M1	Distant metastatic involvement
	MX	Distant metastatic involvement not assessed or not recorded

Stage I	T1 N0 M0	Stage II	T3 N0 M0
	T1 NX M0		T3 NX M0
	T2 N0 M0		
	T2 NX M0	Stage III	T1 N1 M0
	TX N0 M0		T2 N1 M0
	TX NX M0		T3 N1 M0
			TX N1 M0
		Stage IV	T-N-M1

(Source: *CA* 31:6 [1981].)

Both CT and US can be used to direct fine needle aspiration biopsies of pancreatic masses and metastatic lesions to aid in establishing cytologic diagnosis and staging. This procedure can be performed on an outpatient basis and may complete the diagnostic evaluation in the inoperable patients.

Endoscopic retrograde cholangiopancreatography (ERCP) is the third test to consider after CT and US. Although more invasive, it allows direct visualization of the ampulla of Vater and the duodenal mucosa and tissue biopsy. Radiological evaluation is possible for both pancreatic and common bile ducts. The highly desmoplastic pancreatic cancer may compress, invade, and obliterate surrounding ductal structures, which can be recognized by irregular, eccentric, or "rat tail" termination of the pancreatic duct, nodular or eccentric stenosis suggesting tumor encasement or the "double duct" sign resulting from a pancreatic tumor that is contiguous to both the common bile duct and the pancreatic ducts (fig. 16.1) (Freeney, Bilbao, and Kalton 1976). There may be interpretation difficulties in differentiating pancreatic cancer and pancreatitis, in which case the history and clinical information may be helpful. Clinical data and cytology obtained at the time of the procedure can lead to an accurate diagnosis 80% to 90% of the time.

Another diagnostic modality is angiography, which may reveal arterial encasement, stenosis, or major venous involvement by avascular pancreatic tumor tissue. Unfortunately, early angiographic changes are subtle, while typical changes are generally associated with more advanced disease. Angiography will also provide the exact anatomy of an aberrant right hepatic artery and thereby permit avoidance of vascular injury during

Table 16.3
RESECTABILITY RATE AND 5-YEAR SURVIVAL OF PANCREATIC MALIGNANCIES

	Resectability Rate (%)	Five-year Survival (%)
Pancreatic ductal adenocarcinoma	10	5
Ampullary carcinoma	95	40
Duodenal carcinoma	50	45
Cystadenocarcinoma	90	40
Islet cell carcinoma	65	35

surgical removal. Angiographic studies are especially useful for localizing islet cell tumors, which are typically homogeneous, well-circumscribed, and have a vascular blush that persists well into the venous phase. Cystadenoma and cystadenocarcinoma are frequently large and thus show significant arterial displacement and areas of intense vascular blushing and avascularity.

A procedure that has some value in diagnostic staging is laparoscopy. Warshaw evaluated a series of 40 patients deemed resectable by both US and CT evaluation; 17 (43%) had metastatic tumors found by laparoscopy, which would have contraindicated a resection. This approach might be especially helpful in staging patients who are candidates for intraoperative radiation therapy as part of their treatment program (Warshaw, Tepper, and Shipley 1986). DiMagno has suggested that a combination of tests may be required to establish the diagnosis in some patients (DiMagno, Malagelada, and Taylor 1977).

STAGING

CT, US, and ERCP have improved significantly the ability to establish a diagnosis in the patient suspected of having pancreatic cancer. In the past five years these modalities have reduced the number of diagnostic laparotomies from 28% to 5%, and at the same time increased the resectability rate in patients undergoing laparotomy from 5% to 21% (Crist, Sitzman, and Cameron 1987; Kummerle and Ruckert 1984; Trede 1985). Increased resectability rates are due to improved preoperative clinical staging. Table 16.2 outlines TNM categories for surgical staging of pancreatic cancer. It is difficult to evaluate past treatment results because of inadequate staging, failure to use the recognized staging system, or the many failures to definitely establish the exact site of tumor origin. Some older studies characterize cancer of the duodenum, ampulla of Vater, lower common bile duct, and pancreas as "periampullary" cancers. Tumors arising in these four areas have vastly different clinical presentations, rates of resectability, and survival. Such staging failures detract from the value of some of the older published studies (table 16.3). Wider use of the recognized pancreatic cancer staging system should help to minimize this confusion.

TUMOR MARKERS

The recent search for a specific tumor marker for pancreatic cancer that might aid in screening and early diagnosis has not yet been successful, although several serological markers are helpful in managing the patient. Hybridoma technology has permitted the development of immunologic tests for detecting tumor associated antigens (TAAs). While the CA19-9 assay was originally developed using an antibody raised against colorectal cancer, Haglund (1986) has found it useful in managing patients with pancreatic cancer. Carcinoembryonic antigen (CEA) is another useful serologic study; when combined with CA19-9, it helps to differentiate benign from malignant pancreatic disease (Steinberg et al. 1986). Beretta et al. have demonstrated that CA19-9 may be used as a marker of early tumor recurrence (Beretta, Malesci, and Zerbi et al. 1987). Pancreatic oncofetal antigen (POA), first described in 1974, is another serological study reported to be elevated in a series of patients with pancreatic cancer. There may be a diagnostic role for this test, but it does not appear to have a place in screening.

Galactosyltransferase isoenzyme II (GTII) is involved in glycoprotein biosynthesis and has been associated with gastrointestinal cancer. Podolsky and associates (1981) concluded that GTII is a useful single test that might be combined with imaging techniques to distinguish benign from malignant pancreatic disease. However, this test is not widely available.

TREATMENT

SURGERY

Surgery continues to be the curative treatment mainstay for cancer of the head of the pancreas. Unfortunately, most patients are not candidates for curative surgery. In the past, 5% to 10% of all patients undergoing laparotomy had resectable lesions; today with improved preoperative staging, this figure has risen to 20% (Crist, Sitzman, and Cameron 1987).

Since 1935, the standard extirpative procedure for cancer of the head of the pancreas has been the Whipple resection or pancreatoduodenectomy (Whipple, Parsons, and Mullins 1935). Between 1935 and 1960 the operation evolved into the current procedure. Figs. 16.2 through 16.7 outline the basic operative steps of the Whipple procedure.

In 1944 Priestly et al. reported the first long-term survival following total pancreatectomy. Since that time total pancreatectomy has had limited popularity in the treatment of pancreatic cancer. More recently Traverso and Longmire (1978) proposed the pylorus sparing pancreatectomy as a modification that might reduce the nutritional problems associated with gastrectomy and vagotomy (fig. 16.8). Whether this innovation will prove to be an adequate cancer operation is yet to be documented.

The results of surgical treatment leave room for considerable improvement. However, recently published papers have reported operative mortality rates in the 2% to 4% range and morbidity rates of 26% to 36% (Crist, Sitzman, and Cameron 1987; Trede 1985; Grace, Pitt, and Tompkins et al. 1986; VanHeerden 1984). These improved statistics (table 16.4) are thought to be the result of better patient selection and the evolution

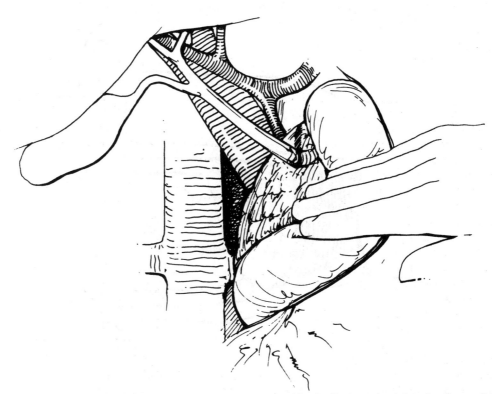

Fig. 16.2. After an initial search for regional tumor spread in the liver, periportal and celiac nodal groups and extension to the base of the transverse colon, a Kocher maneuver is performed. This enables the surgeon to evaluate extension into the duodenum, vena cava, and aorta, as well as to estimate tumor fixation to the portal vein or superior mesenteric artery.

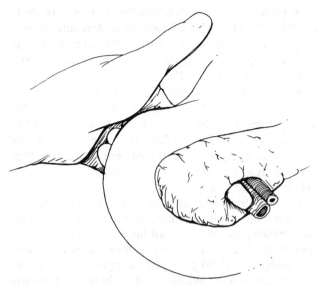

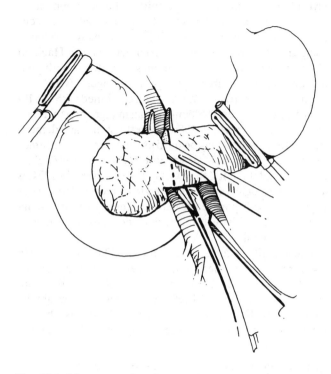

Fig. 16.3. If the lesion appears resectable following the Kocher maneuver, the procedure is continued by exposing the portal vein. Access to the portal vein may be gained by following the middle colic vein to the superior mesenteric at the inferior pancreatic edge. Careful dissection frees the superior mesenteric vein and portal vein from the overlying pancreatic neck. This maneuver is facilitated by the fact that the pancreatic portal vein branches enter the portal vein medially or laterally and that ventrally the vein surface is usually free of venous tributaries. Difficulty with this dissection might indicate tumor involvement. Similarly, portal vein exposure may be obtained by dissection behind the first portion of the duodenum and common bile duct.

Fig. 16.4. After separating the pancreas from the portal vein, carefully protecting the underlying vein, the pancreas is transected.

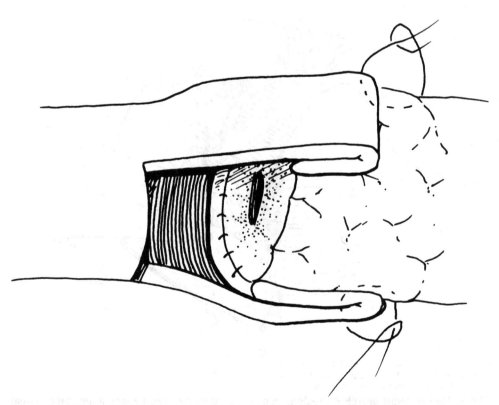

Fig. 16.5. Performance of the pancreaticojejunostomy is a critical step in the Whipple procedure. For the pancreas that is soft or one with a small duct of Wirsung, an end-to-end, two-layer, invaginating type anastomosis is advocated.

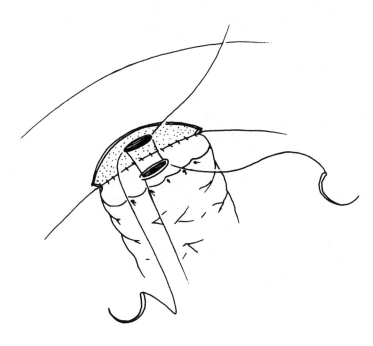

Fig. 16.6. Another approach to pancreaticojejunostomy is the end-to-side anastomosis. This is most easily performed when the pancreatic duct is enlarged, permitting a mucosa-to-mucosa anastomosis, and when the pancreas is firm and fibrous as a result of chronic pancreatitis. This allows sutures to hold more securely.

of the "surgical team approach" at a number of centers. The improvement in operative and postoperative mortality has not been reflected in long-term survival; median survivals in patients with pancreatic cancer undergoing Whipple resection are between 16 and 30

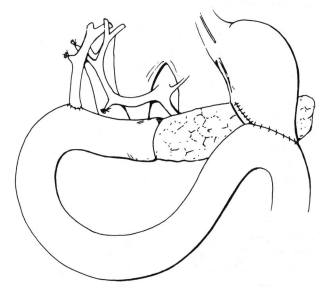

Fig. 16.7. After completing the pancreaticojejunostomy, the common bile duct is anastomosed to the jejunal loop followed by the gastrojejunostomy. It is important to include a vagotomy if a limited gastric resection is accomplished. Also, in order to minimize the risk of stomal ulceration, it is critical that the gastrojejunostomy be placed distal to the biliary and pancreatic anastomoses.

Table 16.4
IMPROVED MORBIDITY AND MORTALITY OF PANCREATODUODENECTOMY

STUDY	YRS	N	MORB(%)	MORT(%)
Crist, Sitzman,	1969-70	41	59	24
and Cameron 1987	1981-86	47	36	2
Grace et al. 1986	1975-79	51	49	10
	1980-84	45	26	2
Trede 1985	1972-84	91	—	1.1
VanHeerden 1984	1951-75	124	—	16
	1976-83	146	36	4.1

months (Connolly et al. 1987; Kellum, Clark, and Miller 1983). Long-term survivals for total pancreatectomy are similar to those of the Whipple procedure.

PALLIATIVE SURGERY

Most pancreatic cancer patients will be candidates for palliative procedures only, chiefly to relieve jaundice and itching and, occasionally, symptoms of gastric outlet obstruction. The biliary tree may be bypassed surgically by anastomosing the jejunum to the distended gallbladder or to the distended common bile duct. Most surgeons prefer the latter, because it eliminates the theoretic potential for tumor obstruction at the cystic duct and recurrence of jaundice that sometimes follows cholecystojejunostomy. Neither procedure (5.5 months) appears to offer a survival advantage (Sarr and Cameron 1984).

Patients with gastric outlet obstruction may get symptomatic relief from a gastrojejunostomy. However, a decision must be made for those who do not have obstructive symptoms at the time of biliary bypass, and who appear likely to survive for more than a few months. If not performed at the time of biliary bypass, approximately 16% will develop outlet symptoms requiring treatment. The operative mortality resulting from the addition of a gastrojejunostomy to a biliary diversion (13%) is not increased over biliary diversion alone (Sarr and Cameron 1984). A recently published retrospective study has concluded that gastrojejunostomy

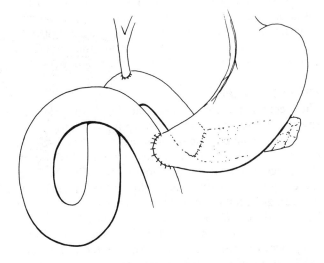

Fig. 16.8. The pylorus sparing pancreatectomy is a recent modification that may reduce some of the nutritional morbidity associated with standard, classical Whipple resection.

provides very little palliation for those with outlet symptoms and is not an effective preventive measure in the asymptomatic patient. This is an area where a prospective randomized trial is needed to determine the procedure's true palliative value (Weaver et al. 1987).

Pain is a troubling symptom of pancreatic cancer that eventually affects most patients during the course of their disease. Transient pain relief is sometimes obtained following decompression of the biliary tree. However, the basis for back pain associated with carcinoma of the pancreas is thought to be related to tumor involvement of the retroperitoneum and afferent nerve fibers around the celiac axis. Bridenbaugh introduced chemical splanchnicectomy as a pain-control technique (Bridenbaugh, Moore, and Campbell 1964). The celiac axis is injected at laparotomy or percutaneously with either 50% alcohol or 6% phenol; this relieves pain in approximately 80% of patients (Flanigan and Kraft 1978). The pain relief obtained by the use of oral methadone has been impressive in this difficult group of patients.

ADJUVANT THERAPY

The poor survival following surgery for pancreatic cancer makes the role of adjuvant therapy an important clinical question. The Gastrointestinal Tumor Study Group (GITSG) has addressed this problem with two controlled studies in which patients received 5-fluorouracil (5-FU, 500 mg/m^2 by infusion) combined with two 20-Gy courses of radiation therapy in individuals receiving curative resection. The median survival for the control group was 10.9 months compared with 21 months for those randomized to treatment. A second confirmative study, without a control arm and using the original control group, had similar findings. The nearly 20% 5-year survival probability and the 2-year survival probability exceeding 40% found in the GITSG adjuvant studies definitely favor a more aggressive approach to the treatment of the early stage of pancreatic cancer and negate the widespread fatalistic approach to this disease. "Further trials attempting to build on this experience are recommended for eligible patients who have undergone a curative resection for pancreatic cancer" (Gastrointestinal Tumor Study Group 1987).

CHEMOTHERAPY

Unresectable pancreatic cancer has been studied extensively with response rates averaging 20% for 5-FU. Other agents, including nitrosoureas, mitomycin-C, and doxorubicin (Adriamycin), have been evaluated, but no single agent appears to be superior to 5-FU. Many of the early studies with combination chemotherapy were discouraging, failing to better the results of 5-FU alone. The Southwest Oncology Group evaluated the combination of mitomycin-C and 5-FU with and without streptozotocin (SMF). In the SMF-treated group, 34% exhibited an objective response compared with 8% of those not receiving the drug. The median survival was deemed to be superior in the responders, but the overall

median survival for both treatment arms was the same (Bukowski, Aberhalden, Hewlett et al. 1980). A GITSG study has confirmed the results of the Southwest Oncology Group in phase II studies when compared with combinations of SMF, doxorubicin, and methyl CCNU (Smith, Stablein, and Schein 1984). These studies appear to show a correlation between objective response and improved survival, suggesting that chemotherapy might be used to assess tumor chemoresponsiveness in patients with unresectable disease.

5-FU has been combined with radiation therapy. A GITSG study reported a longer survival for patients receiving 5-FU and 60 Gy than for patients receiving 5-FU and 40 Gy, although the difference was not clinically significant. Schein concluded that "for the present, radiation therapy plus 5-FU must be regarded as the standard albeit limited therapy for these patients" (Schein 1985).

RADIATION THERAPY

For many years, cancer of the pancreas was thought to be radiation-resistant. With gains in radiation physics, it is now considered radiation-sensitive. There have been a number of radiation cures over the years. The benefits are clearly dose-related; adequate treatment is limited most frequently by the radiation tolerance of surrounding uninvolved vital structures.

Delivery approaches include precision high-dose external beam, interstitial, intraoperative, and adjuvant therapy. Occasionally each of these approaches has been reported effective. Because of factors such as the heterogeneity of patients, stage of disease, performance status, and volume of tumor, it is difficult to draw definite conclusions concerning the effectiveness of radiation therapy. Marking the tumors with metallic clips, which allows precision external beam therapy, will minimize injury to normal structures. Dobelbower and Milligan (1984) used this technique to treat 40 patients, 12 of whom had also received chemotherapy. A 12-month median survival was observed for those who received radiation therapy, and a 15-month survival for those who also received chemotherapy. Two patients survived five years, and one was alive after nine years. Interestingly, 22 of 32 patients initially obtained subjective pain relief from the radiation therapy. Studies by Komaki and colleagues (1980) have confirmed these results.

The implantation of radiation sources directly into pancreatic tumors, introduced in 1934 by Handley, has been performed for many years. More recently, I^{125} seeds have been used for local control in a small number of patients; results were deemed to be equal to those of a Whipple resection with excellent pain relief (Shipley et al. 1980; Syed, Puthawala, and Neblett 1983). However, the data do not indicate better survival than that achievable with external beam radiation therapy.

A number of institutions in the United States and Japan have been evaluating intraoperative radiation therapy in combination with external beam therapy, and in some instances chemotherapy. Some observers believe that local tumor progression in the irradiated field has been affected. However, to date there has been no demonstrated advantage to this approach over that obtainable with external beam irradiation alone (Abe et al. 1980; Sindelar et al. 1983; Shipley et al. 1984; Gunderson et al. 1987).

Interventional radiology has gained a role in patient management through the use of intraluminal radiation sources and the application of brachytherapy directly to the tumor. Strands of nylon tubing containing pellets of iridium[192] may be passed by way of a percutaneous biliary stent through the tumor and left in contact with the tumor for a calculated length of time. This applies very large but localized dosages of radiation to the obstructing tumor mass. Prospective clinical trials are needed to evaluate its effectiveness. Limited experience has shown it to be helpful in patients with malignant obstruction of the bile duct, including that secondary to pancreatic cancer.

OTHER THERAPIES

Several recent papers have suggested that pancreatic cancer may be a sex-hormone-dependent tumor (Benz 1983; Schally, Comaru-Schally, and Redding 1984). A number of phase II studies are under way utilizing tamoxifen and analogues of luteinizing hormone releasing factor (TRP-6L-RH) (Tonnesen and Kamp-Jensen 1986; Gonzalez-Barcena et al. 1986). This avenue of clinical investigation is being taken in Scandinavia and Great Britain and may develop a new direction in the disease management.

ENDOCRINE TUMORS
OF THE PANCREAS

While the vast majority of pancreatic tumors arise from the ductal mucosa, a subset arising from the pancreatic islet produces specific secretagogues that allow tumor classification. The clinical picture and the use of radio-immunoassay classify these lesions into five major tumor types.

INSULINOMA

The most common, insulinoma, was the first islet cell tumor discovered as a secreting neoplasm. It arises from the beta cell and presents with symptoms chiefly related to hypoglycemia. Because of the bizarre nature of such symptoms, the tumor may go unrecognized for a long time. Most insulinoma symptoms are directly related to hypoglycemic effects on CNS function. In general, higher cortical functions are lost first, resulting in apathy, sluggishness, clouding of the sensorium, and abrupt behavioral changes that may progress to coma and seizure. Progression and prolonged hypoglycemic attacks may result in symptoms often thought to be neuropsychiatric. When the symptoms are chronic, the patient learns that relief may be achieved by eating carbohydrate-rich foods. As a result, many of these patients become obese.

DIAGNOSIS AND TREATMENT

The diagnosis of insulinoma rests on the demonstration of Whipple's triad, which includes (1) fast-induced hypoglycemic symptoms; (2) blood sugar less than 50 mg/dL; and (3) relief of symptoms with intravenous glucose administration. After prolonged fasting of as much as 72 hours, further testing is not usually required, but provocative tests may be done that use tolbutamide or glucagon. Elevated serum proinsulin concentrations are highly specific for insulin-secreting tumors of the pancreas (Rubenstein et al. 1973). In addition, C-peptide determinations may aid in the diagnosis in some patients, as well as helping to rule out hypoglycemia resulting from surreptitious use of insulin and establishing the diagnosis of beta-cell hyperplasia or insulinoma in diabetic patients requiring insulin (Rubenstein, Kuzuya, and Horwitz 1977).

Demonstration of tumor hypervascularity, using selective arteriography of the celiac axis, superior mesenteric, and hepatic arteries, may aid in tumor localization. Percutaneous transhepatic portal venous sampling has been reported to be of value in localizing insulinomas and other pancreatic endocrine tumors (Ingemansson et al. 1978).

Approximately 75% of these lesions are solitary. In a collected series, 84% were benign (Stefanini, Carboni, and Patrassi 1974; Edis et al. 1976); 65% of the lesions in the Mayo series were less than 1.5 cm in diameter. Tumors occurring in the tail of the pancreas are best managed by distal pancreatectomy. Approximately 1% of lesions will be found in ectopic locations such as the hilum of the spleen, stomach wall, or small bowel. Use of blood glucose monitoring during surgery and intra-operative use of US may assist in localizing the tumor. Preoperative tumor localization will result in reduced operative time, fewer blind resections when no tumor is located, and possibly a more successful outcome.

Multiple tumors should suggest a multiple endocrine neoplasia, type 1 (MEN-1) syndrome. Approximately 15% of insulinomas are malignant. Local excision of large metastatic deposits and easily accessible tumor masses may be helpful in reducing hypoglycemic episodes. Malignant insulinoma may be treated with SMF and chlorotocin (Herbai and Lundin 1976). Other pharmacologic agents may be used to reduce hypoglycemia, including diazoxide, which directly inhibits the release of insulin by the beta cell, and diphenylhydantoin, which may reduce insulin secretion in roughly one-third of the cases.

GASTRINOMA

Gastrinoma is the second most common endocrine tumor, accounting for approximately 15% to 20% of all islet cell neoplasms. In 1955, Zollinger and Ellison reported the case histories of two individuals with peptic ulceration of the jejunum associated with islet cell tumors of the pancreas. Despite numerous gastric operations, the gastric hyperacidity and peptic ulceration persisted and both patients eventually had total gastrectomies (Zollinger and Ellison 1955). An "ulcerogenic humoral factor of pancreatic islet origin" was thought to be responsible for recurrent peptic ulcerations in Zollinger and Ellison's original paper. In 1960, Gregory and Tracy extracted a gastric secretagogue from an islet cell tumor removed from a patient with Zollinger-Ellison syndrome (Gregory et al. 1960). Repeated studies concluded that the tumor's principal secretagogue was in fact gastrin. In 1962, a Zollinger-Ellison Tumor Registry was established to collect long-term follow-up information relating to this disease. Although once considered rare, more than 2,000 cases have been reported with an estimated incidence of approximately 1 in 1,000,000 people per year. Males tend to predominate, but in the familial-MEN-1 gastrinoma population the sex ratios are essentially equal. The peak incidence occurs between the ages of 40 and 60.

DIAGNOSIS AND TREATMENT

Symptoms are often mild and 80% of patients may have symptoms for more than a year before undergoing surgery. Abdominal pain related to ulceration is seen in about 75% of patients; cramping pain from diarrhea is seen in approximately 15% of patients; and symptoms related to complications such as bleeding, perforation, and obstruction are also seen. Peptic ulceration in a previously operated patient should be considered pathognomonic for Zollinger-Ellison syndrome until proven otherwise. Classic symptoms of Zollinger-Ellison syndrome include: (1) diarrhea in a patient with peptic ulcer disease; (2) peptic ulcer persisting after conventional therapy; (3) recurring ulceration after an adequate ulcer operation; (4) large gastric folds; (5) jejunal ulcers; (6) multiple atypical peptic ulcers; and (7) high gastric acid secretion in excess of 15 mEq/hr.

Diagnostic studies generally reveal abnormalities in nearly every Zollinger-Ellison patient who has not been managed by strict medical control. Gastric acid hypersecretion may be diagnostic; 80% of Zollinger-Ellison patients having a basal acid output greater than 15 meq/hr. The provocative secretin test is useful for stimulating a serum gastrin response and thus establishing the diagnosis of gastrinoma. Secretin infusion will increase both gastric acid secretion and serum gastrin levels, a finding that is unique to the Zollinger-Ellison patient and is not seen in normal individuals, patients with the garden variety peptic ulcer disease, or patients with retained gastric antrum or antral C-cell hyperfunction. Selective visceral arteriography can visualize primary gastrinomas in less than 50% of patients. Tumors larger than 2 cm may be detected by CT scanning, which may also identify thickening of the duodenal wall and liver metastases. Percutaneous transhepatic venous sampling in gastrinoma may help select patients in whom hypergastrinemia is the result of antral C-cell hyperfunction (Glowniak et al. 1982). Occasionally, the endoscopist may localize a gastroduodenal gastrinoma, particularly in the wall of the duodenum, which may be overlooked at the time of abdominal exploration.

Between 1960 and 1975, total gastrectomy and tumor excision, when feasible, was the preferred treatment for Zollinger-Ellison syndrome. When H_2 receptor antagonists were introduced in 1975, pharmacologic treatment replaced surgery. However, to date, no randomized prospective study has been done comparing medical and surgical therapies. Many patients are controlled with H_2 receptor antagonists, but the ideal pharmacologic agent for controlling acid secretion has not become available. Two new drugs, the H_2 blocker famotidine and the proton pump inhibitor omeprazole, hold therapeutic promise. It has been proposed that all patients be followed for a 6- to 12-month period with intense medical management before operation is considered. This will delineate those patients who fail because they are intractable to medical management and who might benefit from a total gastrectomy (Pissaro and Stabaile 1983).

If operation is elected, an attempt must be made to locate resectable gastrinoma tissue, which is not always in the pancreas. Gastrinomas of the duodenal wall may be submucosal and amenable to local excision. A solitary tumor in the tail of the pancreas may be removed by distal pancreatectomy, but this rarely occurs. Even nonresectable gastrinoma patients have had long-term survivals following total gastrectomy. Nearly half the patients recorded with tumor metastases in the Zollinger-Ellison registry survived 10 years following total gastrectomy (Fox et al. 1974).

Streptozotocin, Adriamycin, and 5-FU have been effective in reducing the size of liver metastases and the primary tumor in 75% of patients (Howard 1983).

GLUCAGONOMA

McGavran and colleagues (1966) described a woman with bullous and eczematoid dermatitis of the hands, feet, and legs, as well as diabetes mellitus. She was later found to have liver enlargement as well as a mass in the tail of her pancreas; metastatic pancreatic carcinoma was found. The patient did well for the next eight months, at which time her slides were reviewed and the tumor was interpreted as being of islet cell rather than acinar origin. Partial tumor resection resulted in prompt remission of the dermatitis and marked improvement in her diabetes. Immunoassay showed the presence of large amounts of glucagon in both the tumor and her serum.

Glucagonoma patients also exhibit malnutrition with anemia-hypoproteinemia because of the catabolic glycogenolytic and lipolytic actions of glucagon. The distal pancreas is the most frequent site of tumor origin. Approximately 75% will be malignant, and liver and peripancreatic nodal metastases are common. Most lesions are over 3 cm in diameter.

DIAGNOSIS AND TREATMENT

The clinical presentation of diabetes, dermatitis, significant weight loss, thrombotic complications, diarrhea, and mental changes including depression, should raise the suspicion of glucagonoma. Most patients will have a normochromic, normocytic anemia, hypoaminoacidemia, and hyperglucagonemia. Elevated basal serum levels of glucagon and detectable abnormal large molecular forms of immunoreactive glucagon confirm the diagnosis (Weir 1977). Localization of lesions may be done using CT scan, US, and angiography. Selective venous catheterization is usually unnecessary but may be helpful in selected cases.

Dramatic clinical improvement may follow surgical resection of these lesions, especially in rare instances in which the tumor is localized. The more common situation of metastatic or unresectable tumor may respond to debulking procedures and administration of intravenous diaminotriazenoimidazol carboxamine (DTIC) and SMF. Recently, significant clinical improvement was seen following the administration of synthetic somatostatin (Sohier, Jeanmougin, and Lombrail 1980).

VIPOMA

In 1958, Verner and Morrison described a syndrome characterized by severe diarrhea and hypokalemia in association with islet cell adenoma of the pancreas (Verner and Morrison 1958). A number of patients have since been described in the literature with this syndrome, which is variously referred to as Verner-Morrison syndrome; watery diarrhea, hypokalemia, and achlorhydria (WDHA) syndrome; or pancreatic cholera. In 1973, Bloom et al. reported a new peptide with vasoactive properties that had been isolated from both plasma and tumor in patients with Verner-Morrison syndrome. This peptide is known as vasoactive intestinal polypeptide (VIP) (Bloom, Polak, and Pearse 1973). Clinical signs and symptoms of this tumor usually can be attributed to the pharmacologic actions of vasoactive intestinal polypeptides.

DIAGNOSIS AND TREATMENT

Sixty percent of patients with vipoma are women; the mean age at diagnosis is 47 years. Eighty percent to 90% of the tumors are located in the pancreas, although extrapancreatic sites have been described. The most common, most prominent feature is the profuse and cholera-like diarrhea that may be present for a long time before the diagnosis is made. Because the stools contain a high concentration of potassium, daily potassium losses may be 20 to 25 times normal. A metabolic acidosis often results from large fecal losses of bicarbonate. Profound potassium depletion is reflected by weakness, lethargy, and occasional nephropathy. Antidiarrheal agents are ineffective. About 60% of patients have an abnormal glucose tolerance test and mild hypercalcemia. If hypercalcemia is present, a diagnosis of an MEN-1 syndrome must be considered. Achlorhydria was originally observed with the syndrome; however, most of these patients do produce gastric hydrochloric acid. Aspiration of the gastric contents does not influence the diarrhea. Approximately 80% of patients with Verner-Morrison syndrome have pancreatic tumors, half of which are malignant. The tumors usually have metastasized by the time of the diagnosis.

VIP is a highly specific marker for the Verner-Morrison tumor and should be looked for in patients who have massive diarrhea. Evaluation of markers for other pancreatic tumors should also be done. Patients have the clinical syndrome with low levels of VIP, in which case other serum mediators such as pancreatic polypeptide (PP) and prostaglandin E_2 (PGE_2) may be present. Localization of VIP-secreting tumors is made in essentially the same way as that of other islet cell lesions, i.e., CT scan, selective arteriography, and percutaneous transhepatic portal venography with selective portal venous sampling.

The initial goal is to correct the patient's diarrhea and the resultant dehydration and hypokalemia. This may be accomplished by administering prednisone 40 mg/day or a somatostatin analogue. A resectable tumor mass should be removed, and any metastases should be debulked (Nagorney et al. 1983). If the tumor is not found in the pancreas, the adrenal glands and sympathetic nerve chain should be evaluated carefully. A distal subtotal pancreatectomy is recommended for tumors in the abdominal cavity.

A patient who has inoperable tumor or significant metastatic disease can be treated with SMF alone or in combination with 5-FU. Many tumors will respond to streptozotocin (Moertel, Hanley, and Johnson 1980), and long-term management with somatostatin should also be considered (Ruskone et al. 1982). The patient with a completely excised benign tumor may be cured; some with presumably benign tumors have had recurrence years later. Survival for patients with malignant tumors is about a year.

OTHER PANCREATIC TUMORS

SOMATOSTATIN-SECRETING TUMORS

Another islet-cell tumor of the pancreas is the somatostatin-secreting tumor, which arises in the D cells of the pancreatic islet. Other GI tumors of stomach, duodenal, and jejunal origin may produce somatostatin (Thompson and Marx 1984). Somatostatin inhibits the release of all known gastrointestinal hormones and insulin, and delays gastric emptying. Symptoms generally relate to prolonged exposure to somatostatin and include diabetes, cholelithiasis, diarrhea, steatorrhea, and gastric hypochlorhydria. Presenting symptoms and clinical features may be variable. Only a handful of somatostatin-producing tumors of the pancreas have been described, the majority occurring in women ranging in age from 30 to 84 years. Most tumors were located in the head of the pancreas, were malignant, and had liver metastases at the time of presentation.

CARCINOIDS-ISLET CELL TUMORS

Carcinoids arise from enterochromaffin cells and can occur in most tissues derived from endoderm. Although most abdominal carcinoids arise in the midgut they may arise in the foregut, which includes the pancreas, stomach, and bronchi. Most foregut carcinoids lack the enzyme aromatic L-amino-acid decarboxylase, which converts 5-hydroxytryptophan to 5-hydroxytryptamine (serotonin). The carcinoid syndrome may not be seen or may be atypical (Friesen 1982). In addition to the metabolites of tryptophan, carcinoids of the pancreas may secrete a variety of other polypeptides. These pancreatic tumors are exceedingly rare and are diagnosed because they have a carcinoid morphologic pattern, but many may be polypeptide-producing islet cell tumors.

PANCREATIC POLYPEPTIDE-PRODUCING TUMORS

Pancreatic polypeptide (PP) is found in F cells of the pancreatic islets, and, while its physiologic function is uncertain, it may inhibit exocrine pancreatic secretion and biliary tract motility. An exaggerated plasma PP response following meal stimulation has been associated with the trait for MEN-1 in MEN-1 families (Friesen, Tomita, and Kimmel 1983). Only a handful of PP tumors have been documented, but because there is no typical clinical picture, many more may have been overlooked.

CARCINOMA OF THE BILIARY TRACT

CARCINOMA OF THE GALLBLADDER

In the United States, carcinoma of the gallbladder is the fourth most common GI cancer, representing two-thirds of carcinoma of the extrahepatic biliary tree and approximately 2% to 3% of all cancers. Gallbladder carcinoma is a disease of older people; most patients are in their late 60s and early 70s. There is a slight female predominance, but there is no age difference between males and females (Vaittinen 1970). The incidence of gallbladder carcinoma is higher in white women than in black women (Krain 1972), and 10 times higher in Mexicans, American Indians, and Alaska Natives (Krain et al. 1982). Although the incidence of gallbladder carcinoma in patients with gallstones is low, it is associated with chronic gallstone disease in approximately 70% to 80% of patients. Lund followed 526 patients with gallstones for a long period and found a 1% incidence of carcinoma. The incidence is too low to justify prophylactic cholecystectomy to prevent development of gallbladder carcinoma (Lund 1960). Polk and others have emphasized the occurrence of carcinoma in porcelain (calcified) gallbladders. In 100 collected patients with porcelain gallbladders, Polk found 22 gallbladder carcinomas (Polk 1966). The vast majority of gallbladder carcinomas are adenocarcinomas, most being the scirrhous type, but mucus-secreting papil-

lary forms are also seen. Squamous and mixed adenoepidermoid tumors constitute about 5% of gallbladder carcinomas.

Two staging systems have been proposed for classifying gallbladder carcinomas: a clinical staging classification and a histologic classification (Beltz and Condon 1974; Nevin et al. 1976). Scirrhous carcinoma generally presents with a small, contracted, and thickened gallbladder. In the mucus-secreting type of carcinoma, the gallbladder may be distended and occasionally perforated. Lymphatic spread occurs early to the cystic and common duct lymph nodes, followed by the pancreaticoduodenal nodes behind the duodenum, and to the celiac axis (Shain et al. 1962). Direct invasion of the gallbladder bed as well as the lymphoareolar tissues in the triangle of Calot may occur simultaneously. In the Vaittinen series, 52% of patients had direct extension of infiltrating tumors into the liver (Vaittinen 1970).

DIAGNOSIS

Patients may be asymptomatic or present with significant pain, weight loss, jaundice, and a right-upper-quadrant mass. While right-upper-quadrant distress can be prolonged for years (Vaittinen 1970), a change in character of gallbladder symptoms may herald the development of gallbladder carcinoma.

Ultrasound of the gallbladder may show localized thickening or a mass. Endoscopic retrograde cholangiopancreatography (ERCP) may demonstrate filling defects in the gallbladder or evidence of infiltration of the common bile duct (Ogoshi and Niwam 1977).

Contrast studies of the GI tract may show compression or invasion of the duodenum, stomach, or transverse colon. On percutaneous transhepatic cholangiogram, the segment V intrahepatic bile duct may show an irregular narrowing or be completely obstructed, documenting the liver invasion or significant infiltration of the gallbladder bed (Collier et al. 1984).

CT scanning accurately demonstrates gallbladder abnormalities. Itai, in assessing 27 patients with gallbladder carcinoma, found that 70% had a mass in the gallbladder region, 22% presented with thickening of the gallbladder wall, 15% had intraluminal masses, and 78% had a low-density area adjacent to the tumor. They were able to correctly diagnose 20 of 27 patients, although there was a false positive diagnosis in five patients. Angiography may be helpful in diagnosing gallbladder carcinoma, particularly in the late stages when there is uneven wall thickness and hepatic arterial or portal vein encasement (Itai et al. 1980).

Tissue diagnosis may be made by US- or CT-guided percutaneous fine-needle-aspiration cytology to substantiate the presence of cancer. In some advanced stages, surgical intervention may be avoided.

MANAGEMENT AND RESULTS

The management of gallbladder carcinoma depends largely upon the stage of disease at presentation as described by Nevin et al. (1976). Stage I is an intramucosal lesion, unrecognized at operation and later discovered by the pathologists; stage II involves mucosa and muscularis. Cholecystectomy may be all that is required for stages I and II. Arguments can be made for treating stage II by the so-called extended cholecystectomy (fig. 16.9), additional regional lymphadenectomy combined with a section of adjacent liver and removal of the lymphatic tissue surrounding the bile duct, portal vein, and hepatic artery. Liver resection may be beneficial in stage III, characterized by involvement of all three layers, or stage IV, characterized by involvement of all three layers plus the cystic duct lymph node. Stage V, involvement of liver by direct extension, is not influenced by additional operative procedures.

Adson and Farnell treated 12 patients with gallbladder carcinomas that they deemed resectable. Seven of eight patients who had a simple cholecystectomy died in less than 16 months. Four patients had extended cholecystectomy with liver resection and all four had significant tumor-free survival (Adson and Farnell 1981). Bergdahl evaluated 32 patients deemed to have incidental carcinoma of the gallbladder. Twenty-one of these patients had involvement of all layers of the gallbladder and had a median survival of less than one year. Of the 11 individuals with cancers confined to the mucosa, seven survived five years and four survived 10 years after simple cholecystectomy (Bergdahl 1980).

Wanebo found only 23 of 100 patients with localized gallbladder carcinoma. Only three were long-term survivors, two of whom had only cholecystectomy (Wanebo, Castle, and Fechner 1982). The sole 5-year survivor of the 69 patients reported from Charity Hospital of New Orleans was a patient who had simple cholecystectomy for localized disease (Hamrick et al. 1982).

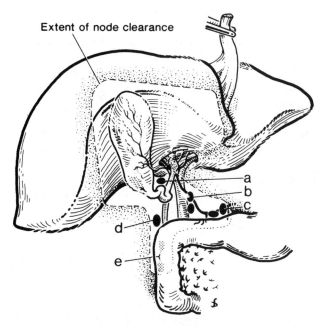

Fig. 16.9. Extended cholecystectomy, including portions of liver segments IV and V and dissection of regional lymph nodes (A-E). (Courtesy: Blumgart, p. 847 [1985].)

Clinically suspected gallbladder carcinoma is not frequently resectable so many of the patients undergo palliative procedures using endoprostheses placed either percutaneously or endoscopically through an obstructed biliary tree. For those patients who are better operative risks, biliary enteric anastomosis may produce good palliation and prolonged relief of jaundice. Bismuth and Corlette found that 39 patients with carcinoma of the liver hilus, the majority of whom had gallbladder carcinoma, experienced an average survival of 30 months after biliary enteric bypass of the type described by Soupault and Couinaud (Soupault and Couinaud 1957).

In patients with advanced cancer, diagnostic laparotomy and biopsy have been superseded in many centers by percutaneous fine-needle-aspiration cytology to make the diagnosis. Chemotherapy has little benefit in advanced cancer or as an adjuvant treatment after surgical resection. A strong theoretical case may be made for postoperative radiation therapy, particularly to avoid local recurrence and as palliative treatment in patients with advanced cancer. Todoroki et al., using dosages in the range of 25 Gy to 30 Gy, treated six patients with carcinoma of the gallbladder and the median survival was about 11 months. Several patients showed cholangiographic evidence of biliary stricture improvements (Todoroki et al. 1980).

Survival in gallbladder carcinoma is quite low and is essentially confined to patients with unsuspected cancers found at cholecystectomy. Piehler and Crichlow found that the overall 5-year survival in more than 6,000 patients was 4.1%, and 1-year survival was 11%. Survival in the occult group was approximately 15% at five years. If the tumor was recognized grossly at the operating table and resected, only 3% of patients survived five years (Piehler and Crichlow 1978).

Less common gallbladder tumors include carcinoids, primary malignant melanoma, and a variety of sarcomas (Anderson, Hughes, and Williamson 1983) including spindle cell sarcomas and rhabdomyosarcomas. The clinical behavior of each of these tumors roughly approximates that of adenocarcinoma.

CARCINOMA OF THE BILE DUCTS

Carcinoma of the bile duct is an unusual lesion that accounts for approximately one-third of tumors arising in the extrahepatic biliary tree. Longmire reported that about 4,500 new cases are seen in the United States annually (Longmire 1976); however, there is some evidence of increasing frequency (Cohn 1978).

Primary carcinoma of the extrabiliary tract has been classified according to anatomical location: the upper third as the confluence of the common hepatic duct; the middle third as the common bile duct between the cystic duct and upper border of the duodenum; and the lower third as that portion of the duct between the upper part of the duodenum and the ampulla of Vater. Cholangiocarcinoma assumes three basic morphologic variants: papillary, nodular, or diffuse. The papillary variety appears most often in the lower third of the common bile duct. The nodular form is generally a small, well-localized mass that occurs most commonly in the middle and upper thirds. The diffuse type presents as marked thickening of the duct wall over an extensive area, with narrowing of the lumen, and mimics sclerosing cholangitis (Weinbren and Mutum 1983).

NATURAL HISTORY

The vast majority of patients with bile duct cancer die within six to 12 months following diagnosis, most frequently of local tumor extension and the secondary effects of obstruction and cholangitis, frequently without distant metastases (Ottow, August, and Sugarbaker 1985). Tumors of the lower biliary tree have the best prognosis, presumably because of technical ease of surgical management. The etiology of cholangiocarcinoma is uncertain; there may be a relationship with ulcerative colitis although the number of documented patients with both lesions is small (Ross, Braasch, and Warren 1973; Roberts-Thompson, Strickland, and Mackay 1973). Development of cholangiocarcinoma has been associated with hepatic fibrosis, polycystic disease, and a poorly drained choledochocyst. In Southeast Asia and the Orient, *Clonorchis sinensis* or *Opisthorchis viverrini* are the most frequent etiologic agents, although they are generally associated with intrahepatic cholangiocarcinoma, rather than extrahepatic sites.

DIAGNOSIS

Tumors of the bile duct may be unrecognized and clinically silent for a long time. Jaundice, which may be intermittent, is the most common presenting symptom. Of 94 patients admitted to London's Hammersmith Hospital with cholangiocarcinoma at the confluence of the hepatic ducts, all "had liver function tests consistent with obstructive jaundice" (Blumgart et al. 1984).

Occasionally, a patient complaining of fever or malaise may have an elevated alkaline phosphatase discovered incidentally in the anicteric state. Pruritus, anorexia, nausea, and vomiting are other signs and symptoms. Thirty-one patients with hilar tumors who underwent either bypass or resection had a median weight loss in excess of 14 pounds (Beazley et al. 1984).

Bleeding and melena are very unusual symptoms of bile duct tumors. Liver enlargement with a smooth liver edge is frequently found. Lower bile duct lesions may give rise to a clinically enlarged gallbladder, but a palpable mass in the right-upper-quadrant should raise the clinical suspicion of gallbladder carcinoma.

The most efficient approach to patients thought to have extrahepatic obstruction secondary to bile duct cancer initially should be US of the liver, gallbladder, and extrahepatic ducts. Dilated intrahepatic radicals, a normal or absent common bile duct, and normal gallbladder strongly suggest a diagnosis of hilar or upper-third bile duct cancer. The next diagnostic procedure should be a percutaneous transhepatic cholangiogram to visualize the intrahepatic ducts and the site of obstruction. Care must be taken to ensure filling of both the right and left sides of the intrahepatic biliary tree, so that operability of tumors at the confluence may be more accurately predicted. The segment V duct should be examined carefully due to its frequent involvement by gallbladder carcinoma but infrequent infiltration by bile duct cancer. CT scanning has not been a major clinical aid in high bile duct tumors but helps in the diagnosis of the lower-third lesions. In most instances the tumor has completely obstructed the bile duct on presentation, and therefore ERCP has a limited diagnostic role because only the distal extent is visualized while knowledge of the tumor's proximal limit is essential for surgical planning.

If the confluence of the hepatic ducts is involved and major resection is being considered, visualization of the portal vein and its branches is mandatory because the extent of the tumor may render curative resection impossible. Late-phase splenoportography will provide information required to make a decision about resectability.

TREATMENT

Surgical resection.   Cancers occurring at or near the confluence have a resectability rate of about 20% (Blumgart et al. 1984). Generally, in this region, liver resection will be required in an attempt to cure. Contraindications to resection include bilateral ductal involvement beyond the second-order hepatic ducts, involvement of the main trunk of the portal vein, bilateral involvement of hepatic arterial or portal venous structures, or a combination of vascular involvement on one side and tumor involvement on the opposite side. Complete tumor excision in the latter situation will result in a poorly vascularized hepatic remnant (Voyles et al. 1983).

For patients considered ineligible for local resection of the confluence because the surgical margins cannot be free of tumor, a palliative resection may be performed and Silastic stenting tubes placed through the subsequent hepaticojejunostomy allowing postoperative brachytherapy (Cameron, Broe, and Zuidema 1982). If resection cannot be done, then the therapeutic options include: (1) biliary diversion, using percutaneously placed stenting tubes through the liver and tumor into the GI tract or surgically placed to exit through the skin in the U-tube fashion; (2) the exoendoprosthesis as described by Voyles (Voyles 1985) (fig. 16.10); or (3) by hepaticojejunostomy to the segment III duct as described by Soupault and Couinaud (1957).

Lower bile duct tumors tend to be papillary and may be visualized by ERCP, which establishes the tumor's site of origin and its extent. These tumors are less frequent than upper lesions but are more easily managed by conventional surgical techniques: local resection with establishment of a hepaticojejunostomy by Roux-en-Y loop or by pancreaticoduodenectomy for intrapancreatic bile duct lesions. Many times these tumors

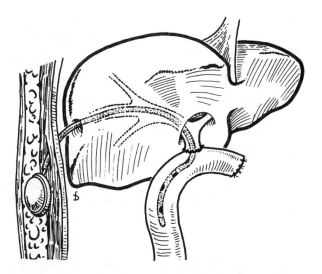

Fig. 16.10. Exoendoprosthesis for stenting lesions of the extrahepatic biliary tree. The proximal end of the tube is buried under the skin in the subcutaneous tissues. It may be attached to a reservoir allowing access for bile sampling or radiologic studies. (Courtesy: Blumgart, p. 847 [1985]; Voyles [1985].)

are not differentiated from more common pancreatic carcinoma. The operative mortality and morbidity for resection of these cancers is considerably lower than for cancer in the hilar region. Blumgart reported 11 patients with mid- or low-bile-duct cancers treated by local resection without mortality, despite the fact that a third of the patients were older than 60. Resectable cancers in this location have a 5-year survival rate of 15% to 20%, not as good as duodenal or ampullary carcinoma but superior to cancer of the pancreas.

Palliative procedures can include local or limited resection without regard for tumor-free microscopic margins and stenting with tubes, percutaneous placement of tubes, or endoscopic placement of transtumoral tubes or stents (Cotton 1982; Cotton 1984; Huibregtse and Tygat 1984). Many mid- or lower-bile-duct cancers can be effectively palliated by proximal biliary enteric anastomosis.

Radiation therapy. The localized nature of bile duct cancer permits the use of radiation therapy for both cure and palliation. Until the last decade, most authors believed that bile duct carcinoma was radiation-resistant (Komaki et al. 1980). Radiation therapy is limited by the tolerance of surrounding normal tissue, but newer specialized techniques such as wedging and shrinking fields have helped minimize risks. Dosages exceeding 40 Gy appear to be required for tumor control (Goebel et al. 1979; Smoron 1977; Pilepich and Lambert 1978; Hanna and Rider 1978). Hishikawa et al. (1983) reported their experience of 25 patients with cancers involving the confluence of common hepatic duct. Although tissue confirmation of cancer was obtained in only six of the 25 patients, there was a mean survival of 9.2 months, and one survived 6.5 years. While no long-term survivals have been reported, the mean survival following external beam radiation therapy

appears to exceed the untreated natural history of this disease.

Intraoperative radiation therapy described by Iwasaki and associates (1977) has the advantage of increased normal tissue tolerance by allowing precise delivery of radiation directly to the tumor exposed at laparotomy. Todorki et al. (1980) treated five patients who had unresectable bile duct cancer with 20 Gy to 30 Gy intraoperatively and the average survival time was 9.5 months. Two patients were reported living 16 and 18 months after therapy. Experience with intraoperative radiation therapy for bile duct cancers has been too limited to definitely evaluate its effectiveness.

Placement of percutaneous bridging tubes through the obstructing biliary tract cancer permits internal radiation or brachytherapy (Molt et al. 1986). Herskovic et al. (1981) used this approach in six patients using the radionuclide iridium (^{192}Ir) by way of catheter and direct-tumor contact. This approach allows a very high dose to be given to a small circumscribed area, minimizing injury to normal tissue. No long-term results have been reported, but the author states that the tumor disappeared in one patient and there was angiographic evidence of tumor reduction in the others. Fletcher and others (1981) demonstrated similar results with an average survival of 12 months. This approach can be used to treat not only hilar cancer but also pancreatic cancer and metastatic cancer that might cause biliary obstruction.

Chemotherapy. The agents employed in treatment of bile duct cancer have been 5-FU and Adriamycin. The latter offers at least a theoretical advantage of excretion in the bile, but no randomized prospective trials have been published. Hall et al. (1979) reported the results in treatment of seven patients who received Adriamycin, carmustine (BCNU), and Ftorafur with median survival of approximately 11 months for those patients in whom complete or partial response was observed. The authors believed that this regimen had some promise in biliary tract cancer. Because these cancers are generally slow growing, and in many instances encased in dense desmoplastic reaction with a relatively limited blood supply, dramatic chemotherapy responses are not expected.

RESULTS

Relatively little information is available concerning the natural history of bile duct carcinoma but series mentioning untreated patients generally record a survival of about three to four months from the time of diagnosis. Blumgart et al. (1988) reported the collected experiences at the Royal Postgraduate Medical School, Hammersmith Hospital, London; Department of Surgery, University of Lund, Sweden; and Department of Surgery, University of Rennes, France, for 48 patients submitted to tumor resection. The operative mortality was 14.5%. More than 20 patients died at a mean of 16 months postoperation. Six survived over three years; five were alive after five years; and three patients lived longer than 10 years. Ten patients averaged a mean postoperation lifespan of 5.5 years; of those, eight had undergone major hepatic resections.

Cameron et al. reported 10 of 27 patients with resectable bile duct cancers. Twenty patients received postoperative radiation therapy. Transhepatic tubes were used in many patients and left in place indefinitely. Survival results of patients having tumor resection and tube placement were about 21 months, comparable to those results obtained by Blumgart and others for local resection without transhepatic stents or radiation therapy. Survival after tubal drainage or percutaneous or endoscopic placement is associated with a 20% to 30% 30-day postoperative mortality and an average survival of three to six months (Cameron, Broe, and Zuidema 1982; Cotton 1982; Cotton 1984; Huibregtse and Tygat 1984).

REFERENCES

Abe, M.; Takahashi, M.; and Yabumoto, E. et al. 1980. Clinical experiences with intraoperative radiotherapy of locally advanced cancers. *Cancer* 45:40-48.

Adson, M.A., and Farnell, M.B. 1981. Hepatobiliary cancer: surgical considerations. *Mayo Clin. Proc.* 56:686-99.

Anderson, J.B.; Hughes, R.G.; and Williamson, R.C.N. 1983. Malignant melanoma of the gallbladder. *Postgrad. Med. J.* 59:390-91.

Baron, R.L.; Stanley, R.J.; and Lee, J.K. et al. 1982. Prospective comparison of the evaluation of biliary obstruction using computerized tomography and ultrasonography. *Radiology* 145:91-98.

Beazley, R.M.; Hadjis, N.; and Benjamin, I.S. et al. 1984. Clinicopathological aspects of high bile duct cancer: experience with resection and bypass surgical treatments. *Ann. Surg.* 199:623-36.

Beltz, W.R., and Condon, R.E. 1974. Primary carcinoma of the gallbladder. *Ann. Surg.* 180:180-84.

Benz, C. 1983. Hormone sensitivity and modulation of chemosensitivity in human pancreatic carcinoma. *Proc. Am. Soc. Clin. Oncol.* 2:39.

Beretta, E.; Malesci, A.; and Zerbi, A. et al. 1987. Serum CA19-9 in the postsurgical follow-up of patients with pancreatic cancer. *Cancer* 60:2428-31.

Bergdahl, L. 1980. Gallbladder carcinoma first diagnosed at microscopic examination of gallbladders removed for presumed benign disease. *Ann. Surg.* 191:19-22.

Bismuth, H., and Corlette, M. 1975. Intrahepatic cholangioenteric anastomosis and carcinoma of the hilus of the liver. *Surg. Gynecol. Obstet.* 140:170-78.

Bloom, S.R.; Polak, J.M.; and Pearse, A.G. 1973. Vasoactive intestinal peptide and watery-diarrhea syndrome. *Lancet* II:14-16.

Blumgart, L.H. 1988. In Blumgart, L.H. ed. *Surgery of the liver and biliary tract.* p. 841. Edinburgh-London-Melbourne-New York: Churchill Livingstone.

Blumgart, L.H.; Hadjis, N.F.; and Benjamin, I.F. et al. 1984. Surgical approaches to cholangiocarcinoma at confluence of hepatic ducts. *Lancet* I:66-70.

Boss, L.P.; Lanier, A.P., and Dohan, P.H. et al. 1982. Cancers of the gallbladder and biliary tracts in Alaskan natives 1970-1979. *J. Natl. Cancer Inst.* 69:1005-1007.

Bridenbaugh, L.D.; Moore, D.C.; and Campbell, D.D. 1964.

Management of upper abdominal cancer pain: treatment with celiac plexus block with alcohol. *JAMA* 190:877-80.

Bukowski, R.M.; Aberhalden, R.T.; and Hewlett, J.S. et al. 1980. Phase II trial of streptozotocin, Mitomycin-C and 5-fluorouracil in adenocarcinoma of the pancreas. *Cancer Clin. Trials* 3:321-24.

Cameron, L.H.; Broe, P.; and Zuidema, G.B. 1982. Proximal bile duct tumor: surgical management with silastic transhepatic biliary stents. *Ann. Surg.* 196:412-18.

Cohn, I. Jr. 1978. Presidential address: gastrointestinal cancer, surgical survey of abdominal tragedy. *Am. J. Surg.* 135:3-11.

Collier, M.A.; Carr, D.; and Hemingway, A. et al. 1984. Preoperative diagnosis and its effect on the treatment of carcinoma of the gallbladder. *Surg. Gynecol. Obstet.* 159: 465-70.

Connolly, M.M.; Dawson, P.J.; and Michelassi, F. et al. 1987. Survival in 1001 patients with carcinoma of the pancreas. *Ann. Surg.* 206:366-73.

Cotton, P.B. 1982. Duodenoscopic placement of biliary prostheses to relieve malignant obstructive jaundice. *Br. J. Surg.* 69:501-503.

Cotton, P.B. 1984. Endoscopic methods for relief of malignant obstructive jaundice. *World J. Surg.* 8:854-61.

Crist, D.W.; Sitzman, J.V.; and Cameron, J.L. 1987. Improved hospital morbidity, mortality and survival after the Whipple procedure. *Ann. Surg.* 206:358-65.

DiMagno, E.P.; Malagelada, J.R.; and Taylor, W.F. et al. 1977. A prospective comparison of current diagnostic tests for pancreatic cancer. *N. Engl. J. Med.* 297:737-42.

Dobelbower, R.R. Jr., and Milligan, A.J. 1984. Treatment of pancreatic cancer by radiation therapy. *World J. Surg.* 8:919-28.

Doll, R.; Muir, C.; and Waterhouse, J. 1970. *Cancer incidence in five continents.* vol. 2. Berlin-Heidelberg-New York: Springer-Verlag.

Douglass, H.D., and Holyoke, E.D. 1974. Pancreatic cancer: initial treatment as the determinant of survival. *JAMA* 229:793-97.

Edis, A.J.; McIlrath, D.C.; and VanHeerden, J.A. et al. 1976. Insulinoma: current diagnosis and surgical management. *Curr. Prob. Surg.* 13:1-45.

Enstrom, J.E. 1978. Cancer and total mortality among active Mormons. *Cancer* 42:1943-51.

Flanigan, D.P., and Kraft, R.O. 1978. Continuing experience with palliative chemical splanchinectomy. *Arch. Surg.* 113: 509-11.

Fletcher, M.S.; Brinkley, D.; and Dawson, J.L. et al. 1981. Treatment of high bile duct carcinoma by internal radiotherapy with iridium-192 wire. *Lancet* II:172-74.

Fox, P.S.; Hofmann, J.W.; and DeCosse, J.J. et al. 1974. The influence of total gastrectomy on survival and malignant Zollinger-Ellison tumors. *Ann. Surg.* 180:558-66.

Freeney, P.C.; Bilbao, M.K.; and Kalton, R.M. 1976. Blind evaluation of endoscopic retrograde cholangiopancreatography (ERCP) in the diagnosis of pancreatic carcinoma: the "double duct" and other signs. *Radiology* 119:271-74.

Friesen, S.R. 1982. Tumors of the endocrine pancreas. *N. Engl. J. Med.* 306:580-90.

Friesen, S.R.; Tomita, T.; and Kimmel, J.R. 1983. Pancreatic polypeptide update: its roles in detection of the trait for multiple endocrine adenopathy syndrome, type 1 and pancreatic polypeptide-secreting tumors. *Surgery* 94:1028-37.

Gastrointestinal Tumor Study Group. 1987. Further evidence of effective adjuvant combined radiation and chemotherapy following curative resection of pancreatic cancer. *Cancer* 12:2006-10.

Glowniak, J.V.; Schapiro, B.; and Vinik, A.I. et al. 1982. Percutaneous transhepatic venous sampling of gastrin: value in sporadic and familial islet-cell tumors and G-cell hyperfunction. *N. Engl. J. Med.* 307:293-97.

Goebel, R.H.; Levene, M.B.; and Weichselbaum, R.R. et al. 1979. Techniques for localized radiation of carcinoma of the biliary tree. *Int. J. Radiat. Oncol. Biol. Phys.* 5:80.

Goldstein, H.R. 1982. No association between coffee and cancer of the pancreas (letter). *N. Engl. J. Med.* 306:997.

Gonzalez-Barcena, D.; Rangel-Garcia, N.; and Perez-Sanchez, P.L. et al. 1986. Response to D-Trp-6-LH-RH in advanced adenocarcinoma of pancreas (letter). *Lancet* II: 154.

Grace, P.A.; Pitt, H.A.; and Tompkins, R.K. et al. 1986. Decreased morbidity and mortality after pancreatoduodenectomy. *Am. J. Surg.* 151:141-49.

Gray, L.W. Jr.; Crook, J.N.; and Cohn, I. Jr. 1972. Carcinoma of the pancreas. *Seventh National Cancer Conf. Proc.* pp. 503-510.

Gregory, R.A.; Tracy, J.H.; and French, J.M. et al. 1960. Extraction of a gastrin-like substance from a pancreatic tumor in a case of Zollinger-Ellison syndrome. *Lancet* I:1045.

Gunderson, L.L.; Martin, J.K.; and Kvols, L.K. et al. 1987. Intraoperative and external beam irradiation +/- 5-FU for locally advanced pancreatic cancer. *Int. J. Radiat. Oncol. Biol. Phys.* 13:319-29.

Haglund, C. 1986. Tumour marker CA125 in pancreatic cancer: a comparison with CA19-9 and CEA. *Br. J. Cancer* 54:897-901.

Hall, W.S.; Benjamin, R.S.; and Murphy, W.K. et al. 1979. Adriamycin, BCNU, Ftorafur chemotherapy of pancreatic and biliary tract cancer. *Cancer* 44:2008.

Hamrick, R.E. Jr.; Liner, F.J.; and Hastings, P.R. et al. 1982. Primary carcinoma of the gallbladder. *Ann. Surg.* 195:270-73.

Handley, N.S. 1934. Pancreatic cancer and its treatment by implanted radium. *Ann. Surg.* 100:215-23.

Hanna, S.S., and Rider, W.D. 1978. Carcinoma of the gallbladder or extrahepatic bile ducts: the role of radiotherapy. *Can. Med. Assoc. J.* 118:59-61.

Herbai, G., and Lundin, A. 1976. Treatment of malignant metastatic pancreatic insulinoma with streptozotocin: review of 21 cases described in detail in the literature and report of complete remission of a new case. *Acta. Med. Scand.* 200:447-52.

Herskovic, A.; Heaston, D.; and Engler, M.J. et al. 1981. Irradiation of biliary carcinoma. *Radiology* 139:219-22.

Hessel, S.J.; Siegelman, S.S.; and McNeil, B.J. et al. 1982. Prospective evaluation of computed tomography and ultrasound of the pancreas. *Radiology* 143:129-33.

Hishikawa, Y.; Shimada, T.; and Miura, T. et al. 1983. Radiation therapy of carcinoma of the extrahepatic bile ducts. *Radiology* 146:787-89.

Howard, J.M.; Collen, M.J.; and Raufman, J-P. et al. 1983. Comparison of the effect of chemotherapy on tumor size, serum gastrin, and gastric acid secretion in patients with Zollinger-Ellison Syndrome (ZES). *Gastroenterology* 84(abstr):1192.

Huibregtse, K., and Tygat, G.N.T. 1984. Endoscopic placement of biliary prosthesis. In Salmon, P. ed. *Advances in gastrointestinal endoscopy.* vol. I. pp. 219-31. London: Chapman and Hall.

Ingemansson, S.; Kuhl, C.; and Larsson, L.I. et al. 1978. Localization of insulinomas and islet cell hyperplasias by pancreatic vein catheterization and insulin assay. *Surg. Gynecol. Obstet.* 146:725-34.

Itai, Y., and Araki, K. et al. 1980. Computed tomography of gallbladder carcinoma. *Radiology* 137:713-18.

Iwasaki, Y.; Ohto, M.; and Todoroki, T. et al. 1977. Treatment of carcinoma of the biliary system. *Surg. Gynecol. Obstet.* 144:219-224.

Kellum, J.M.; Clark, J.; and Miller, H.H. 1983. Pancreaticoduodenectomy resectable malignant periampullary tumors. *Surg. Gynecol. Obstet.* 157:362-66.

Komaki, R.; Wilson, J.F.; and Cox, J.D. et al. 1980. Carcinoma of the pancreas: results of irradiation for unresectable lesions. *Int. J. Radiat. Oncol. Biol. Phys.* 6:209-12.

Kopelson, G.; Harisiadis, L.; and Tretter, P. et al. 1977. Role of radiation therapy in cancer of the extrahepatic biliary system: an analysis of thirteen patients and a review of the literature of the effectiveness of surgery, chemotherapy and radiotherapy. *Int. J. Radiat. Oncol. Biol. Phys.* 2:883-94.

Krain, L.S. 1972. Gallbladder and extrahepatic bile duct carcinoma: analysis of 1,808 cases. *Geriatrics* 27:1111-17.

Kummerle, F., and Ruckert, K. 1984. Surgical treatment of pancreatic cancer. *World J. Surg.* 8:889-94.

Levitt, R.G.; Stanley, R.J.; and Sagel, S.S. et al. 1982. Computed tomography of the pancreas: three second scanning vs. 18 second scanning. *J. Comput. Assist. Tomogr.* 6:259-67.

Li, F.P.; Fraumeni, J.F. Jr.; and Mantel, N. et al. 1969. Cancer mortality among chemists. *J. Natl. Cancer Inst.* 43:1159-64.

Longmire, W.P. Jr. 1976. Tumors of the extrahepatic biliary radicals. *Current Prob. Cancer* 1:1-45.

Lund, J. 1960. Surgical indications in cholelithiasis: prophylactic cholecystectomy elucidated on the basis of long-term follow-up on 526 non-operated cases. *Ann. Surg.* 151: 153-62.

MacMahon, B.; Yen, S.; and Trichopoulos, D. et al. 1981. Coffee and cancer of the pancreas. *N. Engl. J. Med.* 304:630-33.

Mancuso, T.F., and el-Attar, A.A. 1967. Cohort study of workers exposed to betanaphthylamine and benzidine. *J. Occup. Med.* 9:277-85.

McGavern, M.H.; Unger, R.H.; and Recant, L. et al. 1966. A glucagon-secreting alpha cell carcinoma of the pancreas. *N. Engl. J. Med.* 274:1408-13.

Moertel, C.G.; Hanley, J.A.; and Johnson, L.A. 1980. Streptozocin alone compared with streptozocin plus fluorouracil in the treatment of advanced islet-cell carcinoma. *N. Engl. J. Med.* 303:1189-94.

Molt, P.; Hopfan, S.; and Watson, R.C. et al. 1986. Intraluminal radiation therapy in the management of malignant biliary obstruction. *Cancer* 57:536-44.

Moosa, A.R. 1980. *Tumors of the pancreas.* p. 433. Baltimore and London: Williams & Wilkins.

Nagorney, D.M.; Bloom, S.R.; and Polak, J.M. et al. 1983. Resolution of recurrent Verner-Morrison syndrome by resection of the metastatic vipoma. *Surgery* 93:348-53.

Nevin, J.E.; Moran, T.J.; and Kay, S. et al. 1976. Carcinoma of the gallbladder: staging, treatment and prognosis. *Cancer* 37:141-48.

Newill, V.A. 1961. Distribution of cancer mortality among ethnic subgroups of the white population of New York City, 1953-1958. *J. Natl. Cancer Inst.* 26:405-17.

Ogoshi, K., and Niwam, M. 1977. Diagnostic evaluation of ERCP in pancreatic and biliary carcinoma. *Gastroenterol. J.* 12:218-23.

Ottow, R.T.; August, D.A.; and Sugarbaker, P.H. 1985. Treatment of biliary tract carcinoma: an overview of techniques and results. *Surgery* 97:251-62.

Pedrosa, C.S.; Casanova, R.; and Rodriguez, R. 1981. Computerized tomography in obstructive jaundice. I: the level of obstruction. *Radiology* 139:627-34.

Piehler, J.M., and Crichlow, R.W. 1978. Primary carcinoma of the gallbladder. *Surg. Gynecol. Obstet.* 147:929-42.

Pilepich, M.V., and Lambert, P.M. 1978. Radiotherapy of carcinomas of the extrahepatic biliary system. *Radiology* 127:767-70.

Pissaro, E. Jr., and Stabaile, B.E. 1983. Gastrinomas and their management (editorial). *Gastroenterology* 84:1621.

Podolsky, D.P., and McPhee, M.S. et al. 1981. Galactosyltransferase isoenzyme II in the detection of pancreatic cancer: comparison with radiologic endoscopic and serologic tests. *New Engl. J. Med.* 304:1313-18.

Polk, H.C. 1966. Carcinoma in the calcified gallbladder. *Gastroenterology* 50:582.

Priestly, J.T.; Comfort, M.W.; and Radcliffe, J. Jr. 1944. Total pancreatectomy for hyperinsulinism due to an islet cell adenoma: survival and cure at sixteen months after operation, presentation of metabolic studies. *Ann. Surg.* 119:211-21.

Roberts-Thompson, I.C.; Strickland, R.G.; and Mackay, I.R. 1973. Bile duct carcinoma in chronic ulcerative colitis. *Aust. N. Z. J. Med.* 3:264-67.

Roebuck, B.D.; Yager, J.D. Jr.; and Longnecker, D.S. et al. 1981. Promotion by unsaturated fat of azaserine-induced pancreatic carcinogenesis in the rat. *Cancer Res.* 41:3961-66.

Ross, A.P.; Braasch, J.W.; and Warren, K.W. 1973. Carcinoma of the proximal bile ducts. *Surg. Gynecol. Obstet.* 136:923-28.

Rubenstein, A. H.; Kuzuya, H.; and Horwitz, D. L. 1977. Clinical significance of circulating C-peptide in diabetes mellitus and hypoglycemic disorders. *Arch. Intern. Med.* 137:625-32.

Rubenstein, A.H.; Mako, M.E.; and Starr, J.I. et al. 1973. Circulating proinsulin in patients with islet cell tumors. In Malaisse, W.J., and Pirat, J. eds. p. 736. *Diabetes: proceedings of the eighth congress of the International Diabetes Foundation.* Amsterdam: Excerpta Medica.

Ruskone, A.; Rene, E.; and Chargvialle, J.A. et al. 1982. Effect of somatostatin on diarrhea and on small intestinal water and electrolyte transport in a patient with pancreatic cholera. *Dig. Dis. Sci.* 27:459-66.

Sarr, M.G., and Cameron, J.L. 1984. Surgical palliation of unresectable carcinoma of the pancreas. *World J. Surg.* 8:906-18.

Schally, A. V.; Comaru-Schally, A. M.; and Redding, T.W. 1984. Antitumor effects of analogs of hypothalamic hormones in endocrine-dependent cancers. *Proc. Soc. Exp. Biol. Med.* 175:259-81.

Schein, P.S. 1985. Role of chemotherapy in the management of gastric and pancreatic carcinomas. *Semin. Oncol.* 12:49-60.

Shain, R.B.; McDonald, J.R.; and Richards, J.C. et al. 1962. Carcinoma of the gallbladder. *Am. Surg.* 156:114.

Shipley, W.U.; Nardi, G.L.; and Cohen, A.M. et al. 1980. Iodine-125 implant and external beam irradiation in patients with localized pancreatic carcinoma: a comparative study to surgical resection. *Cancer* 45:709-14.

Shipley, W.U.; Wood, W.C.; and Tepper, J.E. et al. 1984. Intraoperative electron beam irradiation for patients with unresectable pancreatic carcinoma. *Ann. Surg.* 200:289-96.

Silverberg, E.; Boring, C.; and Squires, T. 1990. Cancer statistics 1990. *CA* 40:7-24.

Sindelar, W.F.; Kinsella, T.; and Tepper, J. et al. 1983. Experimental and clinical studies with intraoperative radiotherapy. *Surg. Gynecol. Obstet.* 157:205-19.

Smith, F.P.; Stablein, D.M.; and Schein, P.S. 1984. Phase II combination chemotherapy trials in advanced measurable pancreatic cancer. *Proc. Am. Soc. Clin. Oncol.* 3:150.

Smoron, G.L. 1977. Radiation therapy of carcinoma of gallbladder and biliary tract. *Cancer* 40:1422-24.

Sohier, J.; Jeanmougin, M.; and Lombrail, P. et al. 1980. Rapid improvement in skin lesions in glucagonomas with intravenous somatostatin infusion (letter). *Lancet* I:40.

Soupault, R., and Couinaud, C. 1957. Procede nouveaux derivation biliare intrahepatique; la cholangiojejunostomie gauche sans sacrifice hepatique. *Presse Medicale* 65:1157-59.

Stefanini, P.; Carboni, M.; and Patrassi, N. 1974. Surgical treatment and prognosis of insulinoma. *Clin. Gastroenterol.* 3:697-709.

Steinberg, W.M.; Gelfand, R.; and Anderson, K.K. et al. 1986. Comparison of the sensitivity and specificity of the CA19-9 and carcinoembryonic antigen assays in detecting cancer of the pancreas. *Gastroenterology* 90:343-49.

Syed, A.M.; Puthawala, A.A.; and Neblett, D.L. 1983. Interstitial iodine-125 implant in the management of unresectable pancreatic carcinoma. *Cancer* 52:808-13.

Thompson, J.C., and Marx, M. 1984. Gastrointestinal hormones. *Curr. Prob. Surg.* 21:1-80.

Todoroki, T.; Iwasaki, Y.; and Okamura, T. et al. 1980. Intraoperative radiotherapy for advanced carcinoma of the biliary system. *Cancer* 46:2179-84.

Tonnesen, K., and Kamp-Jensen, M. 1986. Anti-estrogen therapy in pancreatic carcinoma: a preliminary report. *Eur. J. Surg. Oncol.* 12:69-70.

Traverso, L.W., and Longmire, W.P. Jr. 1978. Preservation of the pylorus in pancreaticoduodenectomy. *Surg. Gynecol. Obstet.* 146:959-62.

Trede, M. 1985. The surgical treatment of pancreatic carcinoma. *Surgery* 97:28-35.

Vaittinen, E. 1970. Carcinoma of the gallbladder: a study of 390 cases diagnosed in Finland 1953-1967. *Ann. Chir. Gynaecol. Fenn. (Suppl)* 168:1-18.

VanHeerden, J.A. 1984. Pancreatic resection for carcinoma of the pancreas: Whipple vs. total pancreatectomy, an institutional perspective. *World J. Surg.* 8:880-88.

Verner, J.V., and Morrison, A. B. 1958. Islet cell tumor and syndrome of refractory watery diarrhea and hypokalemia. *Am. J. Med.* 25:374-80.

Voyles, C.R. 1985. The exoendoprosthesis in proximal bilioenteric anastomoses. *Am. J. Surg.* 149:81-83.

Voyles, C.R.; Bowley, N.J.; and Allison, D.J. et al. 1983. Carcinoma of the proximal extrahepatic biliary tree radiologic assessment and therapeutic alternatives. *Ann. Surg.* 197:188-94.

Wanebo, H.J.; Castle, W.N.; and Fechner, R.E. 1982. Is carcinoma of the gallbladder a curable lesion? *Ann. Surg.* 195:624-31.

Ward, E.M.; Stephens, D.H.; and Sheedy, P.R. II. 1983. Computed tomographic characteristics of pancreatic carcinoma: an analysis of 100 cases. *Radiographics* 3:547.

Warshaw, A.L.; Tepper, J.E.; and Shipley, W.U. 1986. Laparoscopy in the staging and planning of therapy for pancreatic cancer. *Am. J. Surg.* 151:76-80.

Waterhouse, J.H.H. 1974. *Cancer handbook of epidemiology and prognosis.* p. 126. Edinburgh, London: Churchill-Livingstone.

Weaver, D.W.; Wiencek, R.G.; and Bouwman, D.L. et al. 1987. Gastrojejunostomy: is it helpful for patients with pancreatic cancer? *Surgery* 102:608-13.

Weinbren, K., and Mutum, S.S. 1983. Pathological aspects of cholangiocarcinoma. *J. Pathol.* 139:217-38.

Weir, G.C. et al. 1977. Secretion by glucagonomas of possible glucagon precursor. *J. Clin. Invest.* 59:325-30.

Whipple, A.O.; Parsons, W.B.; and Mullins, C.R. 1935. Treatment of carcinoma of the ampulla of Vater. *Ann. Surg.* 102:763.

Whittemore, A.S.; Paffenbarger, R.S. Jr.; and Anderson, K. et al. 1983. Early precursors of pancreatic cancer in college men. *J. Chronic Dis.* 36:251-56.

Wynder, E.L.; Mabuchi, K.; and Maruchi, N. et al. 1973. Epidemiology of cancer of the pancreas. *J. Natl. Cancer Inst.* 50:645-67.

Zollinger, R.M., and Ellison, E. H. 1955. Primary peptic ulcerations of the jejunum associated with islet cells tumors of the pancreas. *Ann. Surg.* 142:709-28.

Chapter 17

TUMORS OF THE LIVER

Robert M. Beazley, M.D.
Isidore Cohn, Jr., M.D.

Robert M. Beazley, M.D.
Professor of Surgery
Boston University School of Medicine
Head, Section of Surgical Oncology
University Hospital
Boston, Massachusetts

Isidore Cohn, Jr., M.D.
Professor and Chairman
Department of Surgery
Louisiana State University
School of Medicine
New Orleans, Louisiana

INTRODUCTION

In the Western world, liver tumors are relatively unusual but in major regions of Africa and Asia they rank among the most common neoplasms. An estimated 250,000 new cases of hepatocellular carcinoma (HCC) occur yearly worldwide (World Health Organization 1983).

Primary liver tumors are classified as benign or malignant. The benign group are more common and include hemangiomas, adenomas, and focal nodular hyperplasia. In the malignant group, hepatocellular carcinoma (HCC) leads the list, followed by cholangiocellular carcinoma, mixed hepato-cholangiocellular carcinoma, and angiosarcoma. Benign liver neoplasms are important because they must be considered in the differential diagnosis.

BENIGN LIVER TUMORS

HEMANGIOMA

EPIDEMIOLOGY AND ETIOLOGY
Hemangioma is the most common benign liver tumor. It can range in size from a small lesion to a large, giant cavernous hemangioma weighing 5,000 g to 6,000 g. These lesions are considered congenital rather than neoplastic and to date, no one has documented malignant transformation.

Cavernous hemangiomas are usually solitary and may be associated with similar lesions in the skin or other organs, especially in children. Adam has classified any lesion greater than 4 cm as "giant hemangioma" (Adam, Huvos, and Fortner 1970). Giant hemangiomas are usually found in adults with a median age of 45 years (Grieco and Miscall 1978). They tend to develop more frequently in women and at a slightly younger age. Sewell and Weiss (1961) suggested a 6:1 female-to-male ratio, which poses a question concerning a potential causative role for estrogens.

The natural history of liver hemangioma is one of quiet evolution, intravascular thrombosis, sclerosis, and fibrosis in most lesions. Those less than 4 cm seldom become symptomatic.

DIAGNOSIS AND TREATMENT
Lesions may present in several ways, the most dramatic of which is rupture and intra-abdominal hemorrhage; fortunately, this is rare. The most common presentation is by incidental finding on computerized tomography (CT) or ultrasound (US) studies that might have been performed for another problem or to evaluate vague, nonspecific symptoms. Diagnostic evaluation of pain, abdominal mass associated with increasing abdominal distention, abdominal fullness, anorexia, or nausea and vomiting are symptoms that may lead to the discovery of giant hemangioma (Adam, Huvos, and Fortner 1970).

Angiographic studies usually will differentiate hemangioma from other liver lesions because of the characteristic venous pooling and persistent tumor staining throughout the capillary and late venous stages. Magnetic resonance imaging (MRI) has a role in diagnosis. Glazer and colleagues concluded that MRI was extremely sensitive in detecting cavernous hemangiomas because the lesions have a characteristic and consistent MRI appearance and are brighter than most hepatic metastases (Glazer, Aisen, and Francis, 1985). Needle biopsies are not recommended because of a significant risk of life-threatening hemorrhage.

237

Simple observation is sufficient to manage the vast majority of hemangiomas. When lesions are symptomatic, surgery is a treatment option. Depending upon the lesion's size and location, the procedure may range from a minor wedge resection to an extended hepatectomy. Symptomatic patients in whom surgery was contraindicated because of size, multiplicity, or operative risk, have been successfully treated with radiation therapy (Issa 1968). The current surgical consensus is that resection of even large hemangiomas is not indicated in the asymptomatic patient (Foster 1988).

ADENOMAS

EPIDEMIOLOGY AND PATHOLOGY

Liver cell adenomas (LCA) occur most frequently in young females with a history of long-term oral contraceptive use. Three-fourths of these tumors are solitary, usually well-circumscribed and sharply demarcated from surrounding normal liver tissue, although they are not necessarily encapsulated. On cut surfaces they bulge, are light tan to brown in color, and may show areas of necrosis or hemorrhage. Approximately one-third of adenomas show significant hemorrhage with about one-third rupturing into the peritoneal cavity or the liver. Microscopically, they are composed exclusively of uniform, well-developed hepatocytes. There are no bile ducts within the tumor, and bile secretion is not usually seen. The tumors are quite vascular, containing numerous dilated sinusoidal vessels (Christopherson and Mays 1987).

DIAGNOSIS

Patients with LCA generally have an abdominal mass and pain. About one-third have acute abdominal hemorrhage secondary to rupture of the tumor. Table 17.1 compares the presentation of 119 patients with either LCA or focal nodular hyperplasia reported by Blumgart and Berman (Foster 1988).

Alpha-fetoprotein (AFP) is not elevated in patients with liver cell adenoma. While LCAs are clearly visible on US and CT scan, neither test is specific and neither can differentiate them from malignant tumors. Angiography shows a homogeneous lesion of slightly decreased density when compared to normal liver tissue. Often,

Table 17.1
PRESENTING SYMPTOMS OF PATIENTS WITH LIVER CELL ADENOMA (LCA) OR FOCAL NODULAR HYPERPLASIA (FNH)

	LCA (n=71)	FNH (n=48)
Mass	26	24
Intraperitoneal hemorrhage	16	0
Upper abdominal pain without rupture	2	3
Incidental finding at laparotomy	1	41
Incidental radiographic finding	3	3

(Courtesy: Foster [1988].)

CT scanning reveals hemorrhage within the tumor, further suggesting the diagnosis of LCA. Information derived from two or more tests is frequently required to arrive at a diagnosis (Welch et al. 1985).

The potential for spontaneous hemorrhage in LCA makes the safety of percutaneous needle biopsy questionable. Needle biopsies of LCA may be interpreted as normal liver because the hepatocytes within the tumor have a regular pattern and are only slightly larger than normal.

TREATMENT

Most LCA patients will undergo surgical treatment either because of acute hemorrhage or diagnostic uncertainty about the lesion's nature. Small tumors on the edge of the liver and pedunculated ones are easily excised. For asymptomatic, central lesions that would require major resection, the advisability of surgery is questionable, particularly if oral contraceptives are discontinued. Follow-up observation should continue.

For the symptomatic patient with a central lesion, a decision for resection should depend on the symptomatology, whether the patient is taking oral contraceptives, and the surgeon's skill. If resection is not performed, oral contraceptive use and pregnancy should be avoided. Recently, a patient became pregnant after a right hepatectomy for LCA, and subsequently presented with bleeding from a second tumor in the liver remnant. Observed lesions may be easily followed by serial US or CT scans.

FOCAL NODULAR HYPERPLASIA

EPIDEMIOLOGY AND PATHOLOGY

Focal nodular hyperplasia (FNH) tends to occur at a median age of 31 years. The relationship between sex steroids and FNH is not as clear as that for liver cell adenoma. The gross appearance of FNH typically shows a large central scar with radiating, fibrous white bands. This stellate scar shows up on CT scan about 40% of the time (Mattieu et al. 1986). These tumors frequently have a nodular surface and on gross examination may be confused with cirrhosis. Necrosis and hemorrhage are considerably less frequent in FNH than in adenoma, while multicentricity appears to be approximately the same, roughly 20%. Christofferson has proposed two stages for FNH. Firm, small tumors free of hemorrhage and necrosis, and prominent central-stellate scars characterize the quiescent or end phase. He calls a second phase the "active-growth phase" (Christopherson and Mays 1987); these tend to be larger and less firm, and the scar is not as conspicuous. Intratumoral hemorrhage may be present and lead to a misdiagnosis of the lesion as an adenoma. Microscopically, FNH contains well-differentiated hepatocytes arranged in sheets and forming nodules of various sizes. The most characteristic feature is the proliferation of small bile ducts in relation to fibrous septum, usually accompanied by heavy infiltration of lymphocytes.

DIAGNOSIS

These lesions are usually asymptomatic and discovered incidentally. CT scanning may be somewhat more specific than scanning of LCA, because about 40% of FNH have a central scar of low attenuation with intense peripheral enhancement on contrast administration. FNA lesions contain Kupffer cells, so many will retain radioisotope and appear as a hot spot on scan (Matthieu et al. 1986). Mattison and colleagues recently concluded that MRI can distinguish FNH from hepatocellular carcinoma in most instances, although they found some overlap between FNH and fibrolamellar hepatomas. Multiple tests are required to establish a radiologic diagnosis with any degree of certainty (Mattison, Glazer, and Quint 1987).

TREATMENT

Emergency surgery is rarely needed because focal nodular hyperplasia seldom bleeds. Patients who have pain as a primary symptom may require surgery. Operative management is usually reserved for individuals who are symptomatic or in whom there is diagnostic uncertainty. A nonoperative approach generally can be taken. FNH patients should not take oral contraceptives.

MALIGNANT LIVER TUMORS

HEPATOCELLULAR CARCINOMA

EPIDEMIOLOGY AND ETIOLOGY

The distribution of hepatocellular carcinoma (HCC) shows striking geographic variations. Globally, countries and populations are grouped according to incidence rates: (1) very high rates (20 or more per 100,000 males per year)—China, Southeast Asia, western and southern Africa, and Chinese populations in Singapore, Taiwan, and Hong Kong; (2) intermediate rates (6 to 19 per 100,000 males per year)—Japan, Bulgaria, Poland, France, Hungary, Yugoslavia, Czechoslovakia, Belgium, Austria, New Zealand Maoris, Hawaiians, and Chinese living in the United States; and (3) low rates (fewer than 5 cases per 100,000 males per year)—United Kingdom, United States, Canada, Australia, Israel, Scandinavia, Latin America, India, and New Zealand (International Union Against Cancer 1982).

Worldwide, hepatocellular carcinoma is more common in males both in high-incidence and low-incidence areas. In all populations the incidence rate increases with age, independent of risk until it eventually levels off in the elderly. High-incidence regions show a marked shift toward the younger age group; the average age in Africa is 40, and in Asia about 50. Studies have shown that individuals from high-incidence regions who emigrate to low-incidence regions retain their increased risk.

RISK FACTORS

Hepatocellular carcinoma occurs more commonly in the tropics, leading to suspicion of tropical nutritional disorders in causation. Epidemics of fatal liver disease in poultry during the 1960s were found to be related to commercial poultry feed contaminated by mycotoxin. Subsequent investigation showed the mycotoxin to be the result of *Aspergillus* fungi growing in cereals and other foods in hot, humid areas, particularly when harvested wet and stored improperly. Of the four major members of this group of mycotoxins, aflatoxin B_1 is the most toxic and carcinogenic. Aflatoxin-contaminated food has been reported to produce liver tumors in trout, rats, and rhesus monkeys fed aflatoxin B_1 over a long period of time (Adamson et al. 1976; Carnaghan 1967; Wogan 1977). Despite good correlations experimentally between the levels of injected aflatoxin and the frequency of cancer, direct evidence for chemical carcinogenesis in the human has not been proved.

The association of viral hepatitis and HCC in high-risk areas of West Africa has been known for more than 20 years. Blumberg's identification of the hepatitis B antigen in 1965 permitted sophisticated study of the relationship between hepatitis B and hepatocellular carcinoma (Blumberg, Alter, and Visnich 1965). There is a positive correlation between the geographic pattern of hepatitis B surface antigen (HBsAG) and the distribution of HCC into areas of high, intermediate, and low incidence. In high-incidence regions, hepatitis virus appears to be transmitted either in the prenatal period by carrier mothers or by contact with children who have been infected by carrier mothers. Molecular biological studies have shown integrated hepatitis B virus DNA in the livers of patients with chronic hepatitis as well as hepatocellular carcinoma. Prospective studies in Taiwan, Japan, and a number of other countries are providing strong evidence that the hepatitis B virus is probably a direct cause of HCC (Beasley 1982).

In the Western world, hepatocellular carcinoma has a low incidence, is more frequent in males, and generally occurs on a background of cirrhosis. In this setting, 80% to 90% of cases are related to ethanol-induced cirrhosis. Alcoholics with cirrhosis have a risk of hepatocellular carcinoma that increases with time, but alcoholics without cirrhosis seem not to have an increased risk for HCC (Anthony 1979; Lee 1966). Table 17.2 lists agents associated with the development of HCC.

HCC occurs in two gross patterns, a diffuse form and a nodular form. The diffuse or multicentric variety may evolve from a unicentric lesion (Peters 1976). In a

Table 17.2
ETIOLOGICAL AGENTS IN HEPATOCELLULAR CARCINOMA

Hepatitis B
Chronic liver disease
Iron
Mycotoxins
Irradiation
Androgens
Estrogens
Vinyl chloride
Arsenic
Parasitic infestation
Chronic venous obstruction

comparison study with HCC autopsy material from Los Angeles County Hospital, Pretoria University Hospital, and Japan, Okuda (1975) observed encapsulated margins commonly found in the tumors in Japan compared with infiltrative margins usually found in the tumors occurring in South Africa. He also reported more cirrhosis associated with the Japanese HCC, whereas in South Africa cirrhosis was less advanced and the HCCs grew faster, as judged by their poor prognosis (Primack, Vogel, and Kyalwazi 1975). In Japan, the duration of survival appeared to be longer, suggesting that HCC grows more slowly in cirrhotic liver (Okuda et al. 1984).

Of the numerous histologic patterns of HCC, only the fibrolamellar variant is of particular importance in treatment and clinical behavior. This lesion is more frequent in females, occurs at an earlier age, is not associated with cirrhosis, and tends to be solitary and thus more amenable to surgical resection (Nagorney, Adson, and Weiland 1985).

These tumors are usually AFP negative, have high serum binding of vitamin B_{12}, and produce neurotensin as a specific tumor marker (Collier et al. 1984; Paradinas et al. 1982). Eosinophilic, polygonal-shaped cells separated by lamellar fibrosis characterize fibrolamellar carcinomas histologically. These tumors may have a better prognosis than the usual HCC (Berman, Libbey, and Foster 1980).

Careful evaluation of resected HCC specimens will demonstrate invasion of the portal vein. Okuda and colleagues found this vein invasion in 14% of specimens when the lesion was less than 2.0 cm, and in 71% of liver specimens with lesions greater than 5.1 cm. These thrombi may involve the hepatic vein, vena cava, and portal vein and are believed to be a major source of metastases (Okuda, Ryu, and Takayoshi 1987).

DIAGNOSIS

The most common presenting features of HCC are abdominal pain, right upper quadrant mass, anorexia, weight loss, and ascites; however, about one-third of the patients are asymptomatic. Signs of cirrhosis such as spider angioma and gynecomastia are common. Fever of unknown origin, gastrointestinal bleeding, coma secondary to hepatic failure, hypercalcemia, or intraabdominal hemorrhage when the tumor bleeds are less common. A number of paraneoplastic syndromes have been reported in association with HCC (table 17.3).

Biochemical changes of HCC are similar to those of cirrhosis; increased alkaline phosphatase, elevated transaminase, and elevated bilirubin are present in about 50% of patients and usually predict a short survival (Chun, Cheng, and Geller 1984).

Tumor markers associated with HCC include AFP, an alpha-1-globulin normally detected in the human fetus after six weeks and disappearing a few weeks after birth. While AFP is also elevated in germ cell tumors and pregnancy, the immunoassay will detect between 70% and 90% of all HCC. A small percentage of patients with metastatic disease to the liver from the

Table 17.3
PARANEOPLASTIC SYNDROMES ASSOCIATED WITH HEPATIC CELL CARCINOMA

Hypercalcemia
Hypoglycemia
Cushing's syndrome (ACTH)
Precocious puberty (HCG)
Hyperlipidemia
Polycythemia
Microangiopathic hemolytic anemia
Leukocytosis
Disseminated intravascular coagulation

pancreas and stomach as well as some with primary liver disease will be AFP positive.

Reports have associated preoperative high levels of AFP (greater than 10,000 ng/mL) with median survivals half that of patients with levels less than 10,000 ng/mL, and normal levels with improved survival. Postresection AFP levels are useful in monitoring clinical progress (Idhde et al. 1985). Carcinoembryonic antigen (CEA) has been reported to be elevated in 39% to 70% of patients (MacNab, Urbanowitz, and Kew 1978)

Liebman and colleagues have described an abnormal prothrombin, des-y-carboxy prothrombin, detectable in 91% of patients with confirmed HCC. Low levels of the abnormal prothrombin were found in patients with chronic active hepatitis or metastatic carcinoma and no detectable levels in normal subjects. The test's place in clinical management has not yet been fully evaluated (Liebman et al. 1984).

DIAGNOSTIC TESTS

A variety of isotopes may successfully produce hepatic imaging, but technetium-99m sulfur colloid is the most frequent radioactive tracer. Most primary and metastatic tumors produce focal defects on liver scan when they reach 2 cm to 3 cm in size. Scans fail to distinguish between liver tumors and liver cysts or other space-occupying lesions, and this lack of specificity limits their role in detection.

Ultrasonography is both inexpensive and noninvasive, but it is operator dependent. The hyperechoic appearance of HCC may lead to confusion with benign as well as metastatic tumors.

The HCC has two forms: focal and diffuse. The focal form of HCC appears as a rounded or lobular mass lesion, often multiple, with high- and low-level echoes. Ultrasound may show both hepatic veins and portal veins and occasionally demonstrate intravascular tumor. The diffuse form is more difficult to diagnose with US study. The changes may be subtle and indistinguishable from diffuse changes seen with cirrhosis and chronic active hepatitis.

Hepatocellular carcinomas are best visualized on CT scans before and after administration of intravenous contrast media (Hosoki, Chatani, and Mori 1982). Hosoki has described three patterns associated with HCC on CT scanning. A lesion may appear as a low attenuation structure with less contrast than that of the normal liver parenchyma. Vascular tumors containing more central necrosis display a rapid increase in density during the arterial phase, which persists through the venous phase. In addition to demonstrating primary lesions greater than 1 cm, this process may identify compression or invasion of the portal or hepatic veins, as well as extrahepatic metastatic disease, particularly to the hepatoduodenal ligament and lungs.

Magnetic resonance imaging (MRI) has not as yet been demonstrated to be more useful in the liver than CT scanning. MRI studies, while hampered by technical problems related to respiratory motion that result in blurring of the image, are evolving rapidly with technical improvements and should soon play a significant role in the management of liver lesions.

HCCs are frequently multifocal and occur on a background of pre-existing cirrhosis, so they may be difficult to detect angiographically. Solitary lesions are generally hypervascular and may present with bizarre pathologic circulatory patterns, may increase in size, and may invade or obtain a blood supply from nearby structures such as the diaphragm or kidneys. A growing tumor may compress, obstruct, or invade the portal vein. Occasionally AV shunting occurs (Okuda 1975). Angiography is also important in demonstrating the vascular anatomy and in planning resection. This is especially important in the fibrolamellar variant of hepatocellular carcinoma, which is one of the more resectable tumors (Soreide, Czerniak, and Blumgart 1985)

Laparoscopy is more invasive than angiography but it provides direct visualization of the liver, peritoneal cavity, and viscera and allows for a percutaneous needle biopsy under direct vision. Laparoscopy may detect lesions on the liver surface and on the peritoneum that other studies have not identified. It may result in more accurate staging and in some cases the avoidance of unnecessary laparotomy. About 6% of laparoscopies produce complications, generally related to bleeding from the abdominal puncture wound (Korula and Reynold 1988).

The exact nature of a solid hepatic tumor cannot be determined without microscopic evaluation of a tissue sample. Percutaneous biopsy techniques include those of fine needle aspiration cytology (FNA) or core needle biopsy. Needle biopsy may be performed directed by US or CT, blindly into a palpable mass, or under direct vision using the laparoscope.

Routine biopsies of highly vascular lesions prone to hemorrhage or solid lesions that appear resectable should not be performed; the potential for tumor spillage and intraperitoneal spread outweighs the advantage obtained in knowing the diagnosis preoperatively. On the other hand, unresectable lesions or lesions arising in a background of other liver pathology should be biopsied in order to plan the best therapeutic regimen.

SURGERY

Surgery for malignant hepatic tumors, chiefly HCC, depends mainly on tumor size and location and the condition of the uninvolved liver. Patients with diffuse HCC and those with advanced cirrhosis are generally considered unresectable. Because many patients will have cirrhosis, it is important to preserve as much functioning liver tissue as possible to avoid postoperative liver failure (Tsuzuki, Ogata, Iida 1984).

For small lesions, subsegmental or segmental resections are preferable, especially if cirrhosis is present. Real time intraoperative US may assist technically in performing minimal resections by allowing exact localization and ligation of segmental portal and hepatic veins. This minimizes devitalized hepatic tissue and thus reduces the occurrence of abscess and bleeding.

Larger lesions require major resections of multiple liver segments (fig. 17.1). The resectability rate for primary HCC is about 10% but may be higher in the fibrolamellar tumors (Nagorney, Adson, and Weiland 1985). Operative mortality increases with the extent of resection and inversely with the degree of function of the remaining liver tissue. Operative mortality in the world's literature varies from 5% to 33% (Adson 1988; Bengmark et al. 1982; Inouye and Whelan 1979; Iwatsuki, Shaw, and Starzl 1983; Lee, Wong, and Ong 1982). The type and extent of tumor and coexistence of cirrhosis and hepatitis determines the long-term survival. One-year survival rates are reported at about 80% (Foster, Adson, and Schwartz 1982), while 5-year survival rates range from 30% to 46%. Many patients with primary hepatic cancer have undergone liver transplantation. Ideally, the patients selected for transplantation should have slowly growing lesions, fibrolamellar carcinomas, or lesions occurring in a setting of significant cirrhosis. Although the short-term results are encouraging, tumor metastases result in a steady decline in survival to about 25% at three years (Starzl, Iwatsuki, and Shaw 1988).

CHEMOTHERAPY

Chemotherapy for HCC has not been extensively evaluated; fluorouracil (5-FU) is probably the most studied drug. Unfortunately, there are little data to support its therapeutic effectiveness either as a single agent or in combination with other agents. Various delivery methods and regimens of 5-FU demonstrate response rates of 0% to 75% with a median survival of one to 17 months (Ong and Chan 1974). The difficulties in monitoring any type of study in this disease are: (1) the relative infrequency of HCC in the Western world; (2) the heterogeneity of patients: age, stage of disease, with and without cirrhosis, hepatitis, functional status, etc.; and (3) the heterogeneity of the tumor: multiple vs. solitary, slow-growing lesions, fibrolamellar tumors, or lesions occurring in a setting of significant cirrhosis.

Idhde and colleagues evaluated prognostic factors in HCC patients receiving systemic chemotherapy and concluded that two groups had prospects for prolonged survival. One group, Caucasians under the age of 25, fully ambulatory, having fibrolamellar tumors, lacking evidence of jaundice, hepatitis B markers, or cirrhosis and with a normal AFP had long-term survival even in the presence of extrahepatic metastases. Patients in the second group were older, not jaundiced, had tumors confined to the liver, and were fully ambulatory. Patients in these groups lived for 14 to 37 months. The remainder of patients died within five months of the initiation of therapy (Idhde et al. 1985).

The major blood supply to HCC is derived from the hepatic artery. This observation has fostered a variety of palliative treatments related to intra-arterial chemotherapy and hepatic artery embolization (HAE). A number of investigators have employed combination chemotherapy with intra-arterial embolization by Gelfoam. The addition of hepatic arterial chemoembolization using ethiodized oil (Lipiodol), chemotherapy, and Gelfoam has been utilized with some success. Recently Lin and colleagues (1988) demonstrated in a prospective randomized trial a 42% survival (at 22 months) for patients who received HAE compared to 13% for a group who received systemic 5-FU.

RADIATION THERAPY
External-beam radiation alone or in combination with chemotherapy has a role in the palliative management of HCC. Unfortunately, the limiting factor is the total organ dose tolerance of radiation therapy. Dosages of 3 Gy to 30 Gy may result in radiation hepatitis, subsequent fibrosis, and the development of a syndrome similar to the Budd-Chiari syndrome. Shrinking field techniques allow the delivery of higher doses of radiation therapy to solitary lesions.

A new radiation therapy technique is the use of radiation-labeled antibodies to ferritin. Ferritin is a normal tissue protein present in the heart, muscles, spleen, and bone marrow that is also synthesized and secreted by HCC. In the tumor neovasculature, high-tumor concentrations of ferritin and more static tumor blood flow allow normal tissue sparing and intratumoral concentration of labeled antiferritin antibody. Phase I and II studies of ^{131}I antiferritin have shown a 48% remission rate. The longest partial remission was six years and a complete remission of four years was recorded (Order et al. 1985).

Recently the production of ^{90}Y antiferritin has offered the advantages of a pure beta emitter with a high energy of 0.9 MeV, greater potential tumor dosage, and no need to isolate the patient during treatment. Phase I and Phase II studies have been favorable and more extensive therapeutic trials are planned (Order et al. 1986).

PREVENTION
Improved agricultural and grain storage techniques have reduced the contamination of grain by aflatoxin. However, such advances have been made chiefly in developed countries and not in developing ones. Vaccination is a secondary prevention method that has received a great deal of attention. Vaccination programs against hepatitis B could possibly reduce the HCC incidence significantly. Several authors have demonstrated transmission of hepatitis B virus in newborn infants (Beasley et al. 1983; Wong et al. 1984). With

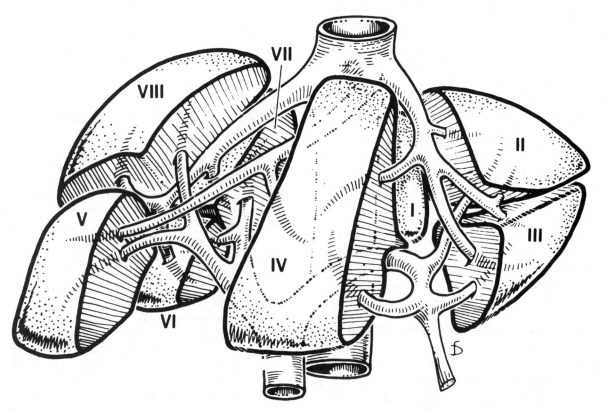

Fig. 17.1. Functional anatomy of the liver according to Couinaud's nomenclature. (Courtesy: Bismuth [1988].)

sufficient financial resources, immunization against hepatitis B virus to protect high-risk newborns is within reach (Zuckerman 1984). Mass vaccination programs in high-risk regions may significantly reduce morbidity and mortality from both liver disease and hepatocellular carcinoma.

CHOLANGIOCARCINOMA

Intrahepatic cholangiocarcinoma is an adenocarcinoma arising from bile ducts. In most instances it is associated with mucin production, a characteristic that permits distinction from HCC, and with dense fibrous tissue reaction.

Studies have documented an association between cholangiocarcinoma and chronic liver infections with *Opisthorchis viverrini*, particularly in Southeast Asia (Kurathong et al. 1985). A six-fold increase in death rate from hepatobiliary cancer has been observed in chronic typhoid carriers (Welton, Marr, and Friedman 1979). Peripherally occurring cholangiocarcinomas have been reported in patients taking oral contraceptives or high doses of anabolic steroids (Littlewood et al. 1980; Stromeyer, Smith, and Ishak 1979)

The clinical presentation of patients with cholangiocarcinoma parallels that of patients with hilar cholangiocarcinomas, i.e., fever, jaundice, and pain. Clinical studies are compatible with obstructive jaundice with a solitary mass lesion or, more likely, multiple lesions noted on a CT scan of the liver. These patients are not often resectable because the disease is multicentric, but intubational procedures might provide short-term palliation in some individuals. There are no good studies of radiation therapy or chemotherapy in the control of this lesion.

ANGIOSARCOMA

Angiosarcoma is an unusual liver neoplasm consisting of proliferating variably differentiated, endothelial cells associated with fibrosis. Multicentric tumors are very common.

While the cause is unknown, certain studies have shown a strong association with chemical exposure. Chronic arsenic exposure in vineyard workers (Roth 1957), arsenical medications for psoriasis (Regelson et al. 1968), thorium dioxide (Thorotrast) exposure (Visfeldt and Poulsen 1972), and idiopathic hemochromatosis have all been associated with the development of angiosarcoma of the liver (Sussman, Nydick, and Gray 1974). Creech and Johnson (1974) reported an association of angiosarcoma with vinyl chloride exposure. A year later, vinyl chloride was shown to induce angiosarcoma in rats (Maltoni and Lefemine 1975).

The most common symptoms are abdominal pain with weakness, weight loss, anorexia, and abdominal swelling. The liver may become quite large and frequently the patient has jaundice and ascites. Interestingly, factor VIII is usually present within the tumor cells and may be a helpful diagnostic determinant. Arteriography is probably the most useful diagnostic

study; CT scan follows. These tumors are usually large, multicentric, and clinically advanced. Frequently, little can be done for the patient; survival is usually a matter of a few months. Experience with chemotherapy or radiation therapy has been too limited to comment on. Death usually results from hepatic failure, gastrointestinal bleeding, and/or renal failure.

REFERENCES

Adam, Y.G.; Huvos, A.G.; and Fortner, J.G. 1970. Giant hemangiomas of the liver. *Ann. Surg.* 172:239-45.

Adamson, R.C.; Correa, P.; and Sieber S.M. et al. 1976. Carcinogenicity of aflatoxin B$_1$ in rhesus monkeys: two additional cases of primary liver cancer. *J. Natl. Cancer Inst.* 57:67-78.

Adson, M.A. 1988. Primary hepatocellular cancers: Western experience. In Blumgart, L.H. *Surgery of the liver and biliary tract.* p. 1155. Edinburgh, London, Melbourne, New York: Churchill-Livingstone.

Anthony, P.P. 1979. Precancerous changes in the human liver. In Lapis, K., and Johannessen, J.V. eds. *Liver carcinogenesis.* pp. 131-41. Washington, D.C.: Hemisphere.

Beasley, R.P. 1982. Hepatitis B virus as the etiologic agent in hepatocellular carcinoma: epidemiologic considerations. *Hepatology* 2:521-26.

Beasley, R.P.; Hwang, L.Y.; and Lee, G.C.Y. et al. 1983. Prevention of perinatally transmitted hepatitis B virus infections with hepatitis B immune globulin and hepatitis B vaccine. *Lancet* II:1099-1102.

Bengmark, S.; Hafstrom, L.; and Jeppsson, B. et al. 1982. Primary carcinoma of the liver: improvement in sight? *World J. Surg.* 6:54-60.

Berman, M.N.; Libbey, W.P.; and Foster, J.H. 1980. Hepatocellular carcinoma: polygonal cell type with fibrous stroma in atypical variant with a favorable prognosis. *Cancer* 46:1448-55.

Bismuth, H. 1988. Surgical anatomy and anatomical surgery of the liver. In Blumgart, L.H. ed. *Surgery of the liver and biliary tract.* pp. 3-9. Edinburgh, London, Melbourne, New York: Churchill-Livingstone.

Blumberg, B.S.; Alter, H.M.; and Visnich, S. 1965. A "new" antigen in leukemia. *JAMA* 191:541.

Carnaghan, R.B. 1967. Hepatic tumours and other chronic liver changes in rats following a single oral administration of aflatoxin. *Br. J. Cancer* 21:811-14.

Christopherson, W.M., and Mays, E.T. 1987. Risk factors, pathology, and pathogenesis of selected benign and malignant liver neoplasms. In Wanebo, J.H. ed. *Hepatic and biliary cancer.* pp. 23. New York: Marcel Dekker.

Chun, H.; Cheng, E.; and Geller, N. 1984. Hepatocellular carcinoma (HC): statistical analysis of 78 consecutive patients (PTS). *Proc. ASCCO*:C23.

Collier, N.A.; Bloom, S.R.; and Lee, Y.C. et al. 1984. Neurotensin secretion by fibrolamellar carcinoma of the liver. *Lancet* I:538-40.

Creech, J.L. Jr., and Johnson, M.N. 1974. Angiosarcoma of the liver in the manufacture of polyvinylchloride. *J. Occup. Med.* 16:150-51.

Foster, J.H.; Adson, M.A.; and Schwartz, S.I. et al. 1982. Symposium: benign liver tumors. *Contemp. Surg.* 21:67-102.

Foster, J.H. 1988. Benign liver tumours. In Blumgart, L.H. ed. *Surgery of the liver and biliary tract.* pp. 1115-27. Edinburgh, London, Melbourne, New York: Churchill-Livingstone.

Glazer, G.M.; Aisen, A.N.; and Francis, I.R. et al. 1985. Hepatic cavernous hemangioma: magnetic resonance imaging. *Radiology* 155:417-20.

Grieco, M.B., and Miscall, B.G. 1978. Giant hemangiomas of the liver. *Surg. Gynecol. Obstet.* 147:783-87.

Hosoki, T.; Chatani, M.; and Mori, S. 1982. Dynamic computerized tomography of hepatocellular carcinoma. *AJR* 139:1099-1106.

Idhde, D.C.; Matthews, M.T.; and Makuch, R.W. et al. 1985. Prognostic factors in patients with hepatocellular carcinoma receiving systemic chemotherapy: identification of two groups of patients with prospects for prolonged survival. *Am. J. Medicine* 78:399-406.

Inouye, A.A.; and Whelan, T.J. Jr. 1979. Primary liver cancer: a review of 205 cases in Hawaii. *Am. J. Surg.* 138:53-61.

International Union Against Cancer. 1982. Workshop on Biology of Human Cancer. Rep. 17: *Hepatocellular carcinoma.* Geneva.

Issa, P. 1968. Cavernous haemangioma of the liver: the role of radiotherapy. *Br. J. Radiol.* 41:26-32.

Iwatsuki, S.; Shaw, B.W. Jr.; and Starzl, T.E. 1983. Experience with 150 liver resections. *Ann. Surg.* 197:247-53.

Kurathong, S.; Lerverasirikul, P.; and Wongpaitoon, V. et al. 1985. *Opisthorchis viverrini* infection in cholangiocarcinoma: a perspective: case-controlled study. *Gastroenterology* 89:151-56.

Korula, J., and Reynold, T.B. 1988. Laparoscopy. In Blumgart, L.H. ed. *Surgery of the liver and biliary tract.* pp. 313-25. Edinburgh, London, Melbourne, New York: Churchill Livingstone.

Lee, F.I. 1966. Cirrhosis and hepatoma in alcoholics. *Gut* 7:77-85.

Lee, N.W.; Wong, J.; and Ong, G.B. 1982. Surgical management of primary carcinoma of the liver. *World J. Surg.* 6:66-75.

Liebman, H.A.; Furie, B.C.; and Tong, M.J. et al. 1984. Des-gamma-Carboxy (abnormal) prothrombin as a serum marker of primary hepatocellular carcinoma. *N. Engl. J. Med.* 310:1427-31.

Lin, D.Y.; Liaw, Y.F.; and Lee, T.Y. et al. 1988. Hepatic arterial embolization in patients with unresectable hepatocellular carcinoma: a randomized controlled trial. *Gastroenterology* 94:453-56.

Littlewood, E.R.; Barrison, I.G.; and Murray-Lyon, I.M. et al. 1980. Cholangiocarcinoma and oral contraceptives (letter). *Lancet* I:310.

MacNab, G.M.; Urbanowitz, J.M.; and Kew, M.C. 1978. Carcinoembryonic antigen in hepatocellular cancer. *Br. J. Cancer* 38:51-54.

Maltoni, C., and Lefemine, G. 1975. Carcinogenicity bioassays of vinyl chloride: current results. *Ann. N.Y. Acad. Sci.* 246:195-218.

Matthieu, D.; Breneton, J.N.; and Drouillard, J. et al. 1986. Hepatic adenomas in focal nodular hyperplasia: dynamic CT study. *Radiology* 160:53-58.

Mattison, G.R.; Glazer, G.M.; and Quint, L.E. et al. 1987. MR imaging of focal nodular hyperplasia: characterization and distinction from primary malignant hepatic tumors. *AJR* 148:711-5.

Nagorney, D.M.; Adson, M.A.; and Weiland, L.H. 1985. Fibrolamellar hepatoma. *Am. J. Surg.* 149:113-19.

Okuda, K. 1975. Demonstration of growing casts of hepatocellular carcinoma in the portal vein by celiac angiography: the thread and streak sign. *Radiology* 117:303.

Okuda, K.; Obata, H.; and Nakajima, Y. et al. 1984. Prognosis of primary hepatocellular carcinoma. *Hepatology* 4:3S-6S.

Okuda, K.; Ryu, M.; and Takayoshi, T. 1987. Surgical management of hepatoma: the Japanese experience. In Wanebo, J.H.

ed. *Hepatic and biliary surgery.* pp. 219-38. New York: Marcel Dekker.

Ong, G.B., and Chan, P.K. 1974. Primary carcinoma of the liver. *Surg. Gynecol. Obstet.* 143:855-63.

Order, S.E.; Klein, J.L.; and Leichner, P.K. et al. 1986. 90 yttrium antiferritin: new therapeutic radio-labeled antibody. *Int. J. Radiat. Oncol. Biol. Phys.* 12:277-81.

Order, S.E.; Stillwagon, G.B.; and Klein, J.L. et al. 1985. Iodine 131 antiferritin: new treatment modality in hepatoma. Radiation Therapy Oncology Group. *J. Clin. Oncol.* 3:1573-82.

Paradinas, F.J.; Melia, W.M.; and Williamson, M.L. et al. 1982. High serum vitamin B_{12} binding capacity as a marker of fibrolamellar variant of hepatocellular carcinoma. *Br. Med. J.* 285:840-42.

Peters, R.L. 1976. Pathology of hepatocellular carcinoma. In Okuda, K., and Peters, R.L. eds. *Hepatocellular carcinoma.* pp. 107-168. New York: John Wiley & Sons.

Primack, A.; Vogel, C.L.; and Kyalwazi, S.K. 1975. A staging system for hepatocellular carcinoma: prognostic factors in Ugandan patients. *Cancer* 35:1357-64.

Regelson, W.; Kim, U.; and Ospina, J. et al. 1968. Haemangioendothelial sarcoma of liver from chronic arsenic intoxication by Fowler's solution. *Cancer* 21:514-22.

Roth, F. 1957. Arsen leber tumoren (hamangioendotheliom). *Zeitschrift Fur Krebsforschung.* 61:468-503.

Sewell, J.H., and Weiss, K. 1961. Spontaneous rupture of hemangioma of the liver: review of literature and presentation of illustrative case. *Arch. Surg.* 83:729-33.

Soreide, O.; Czerniak, A.; and Blumgart, L.H. 1985. Large hepatocellular cancers: hepatic resection or liver transplantation. *Br. Med. J.* 291:853-57.

Starzl, T.L.; Iwatsuki, B.W.; and Shaw, B.W. 1988. Techniques of liver transplantation. In Blumgart, L.H. ed. *Surgery of the liver and biliary tract.* p. 1551. Edinburgh, London, Melbourne, New York: Churchill-Livingstone.

Stromeyer, F.W.; Smith, D.H.; and Ishak, K.J. 1979. Anabolic steroid therapy and intrahepatic cholangiocarcinoma. *Cancer* 43:440-43.

Sussman, E.B.; Nydick, I; and Gray, F.G. 1974. Hemangioendothelial sarcoma of the liver and hemochromatosis. *Arch. Pathol.* 97:39-42.

Tsuzuki, T; Ogata, Y.; and Iida, S. et al. 1984. Hepatic resection in 125 patients. *Arch. Surg.* 119:1025-32.

Visfeldt, J., and Poulsen H. 1972. On the histopathology of liver and liver tumors and thorium dioxide patients. *Acta. Pathol. Microbiol. Scand (A). Pathology* 80:97-108.

Welch, T.J.; Sheedy, P.F. II; and Johnson, C.M. et al. 1985. Focal nodular hyperplasia and hepatic adenoma: comparison of angiography, CT, US, and scintigraphy. *Radiology* 156:593-95.

Welton, J.C.; Marr, J.S.; and Friedman, S.M. 1979. Association between heptobiliary cancer and typhoid carrier state. *Lancet* I:791-94.

Wogan, G.N. 1977. Mycotoxins and other naturally occurring carcinogens. In Kraybill, H.F., and Mehlman, M.A. eds. *Environmental cancer: advances in modern toxicology.* vol. 3. pp. 263-90. New York: John Wiley & Sons.

Wong, V.C.W.; Ip, H.M.; and Reesink, H.W. et al. 1984. Prevention of HBsAG carrier state in newborn infants of mothers who are chronic carriers of HBsAg by administration of hepatitis B vaccine and hepatitis-B immunoglobulin: double-blind randomized placebo-controlled study. *Lancet* I:921-26.

World Health Organization. 1983. Prevention of liver cancer. *WHO Tech. Rep. SCR* p. 691.

Zukerman, A.J. 1984. Perinatal transmission of hepatitis B. *Arch. Disease Child.* 59:10007-10009.

Chapter 18

GASTRIC NEOPLASMS

Walter Lawrence, Jr., M.D.

Walter Lawrence, Jr., M.D.
Professor, Division of Surgical Oncology
Director Emeritus, Massey Cancer Center
Medical College of Virginia
Richmond, Virginia

INTRODUCTION

Clinically significant gastric neoplasms include both benign and malignant lesions. Several varieties of malignant neoplasms arise from the stomach, but the overwhelming preponderance are primary carcinomas arising from the mucosal glands. Until now, these cancers, as well as other lesions considered in the differential diagnosis, were primarily of surgical interest. However, the generally poor prognosis of gastric cancer after surgical therapy naturally leads to the current interest in potential benefits from other treatment modalities.

A primary purpose of this chapter is to provide information on the clinical presentation and natural history of gastric cancer, as well as state of the art management approaches. However, the hope is that future clinical developments will alter the poor prognosis. Possibly, today's student will change this discouraging baseline information by understanding the current status of this disease and developing new ideas about its prevention or management.

DIFFERENTIAL DIAGNOSIS

Benign gastric lesions include benign neoplasms and non-neoplastic processes, which all present in such a way that a malignant neoplasm must be considered as a possible diagnosis. Benign clinical problems are important in terms of the differential diagnosis and management of gastric lesions. The more common benign lesions in descending order of significance are gastric ulcers, leiomyomas, and gastric polyps. Another benign lesion of concern is pseudolymphoma, which simulates the less-common primary gastric lymphoma, which is malignant. The categorization of benign and malignant gastric lesions is shown in table 18.1.

PATHOLOGY OF GASTRIC CANCER

The first classification of gastric cancer and its gross pathology was constructed by Borrmann in 1926 and is summarized as follows:

Type I —Polypoid carcinoma: clearly demarcated; may be ulcerated; late metastasis; relatively good prognosis.

Type II —Ulcerating carcinoma ("ulcero-cancer"): sharply defined margins; difficult to differentiate from benign ulcer on gross examination; requires biopsy; relatively good prognosis.

Type III — Ulcerating and infiltrating: lacks clear-cut margins; extensive submucosal infiltration and usually extends to the serosa; most common type of gastric cancer; relatively poor prognosis.

Type IV — Diffuse infiltration: early metastasis, includes linitis plastica ("leather bottle stomach"), has poorest prognosis of all gastric cancers.
(Both types I and II appear to be decreasing in incidence in the United States, in contrast to types III and IV.)

Additional gross classifications include superficial spreading carcinoma (large, ulcerating and irregular lesions, confined to the mucosa and submucosa) and early gastric cancer (small, very early lesions that do not infiltrate beyond the submucosa). The early cancers constitute up to 30% of some series in Japan, but are quite rare in the United States.

HISTOLOGIC CATEGORIES

The original histologic classification for gastric cancer was developed by Broder, who described four grades (I-IV) based on the degree of differentiation present. A more recent, commonly used histological classification was described by Lauren (1965). He discussed two types: the *intestinal*, a well-differentiated lesion; and the

Table 18.1
DIFFERENTIAL DIAGNOSIS OF GASTRIC LESIONS

Benign
    Gastric (peptic) ulcer
    Leiomyoma
    Polyps (adenomatous, hyperplastic)
    Pseudolymphoma (often associated with gastric ulcer)

Malignant
    Adenocarcinoma (90%)
    Primary lymphoma (6%-8%)
    Leiomyosarcoma (1%-3%)
    Carcinoid, metastatic cancer, etc. (rare)

diffuse, or undifferentiated carcinoma. Epidemiologists prefer this differentiation because it enables them to demonstrate that the association of atrophic gastric cancer in certain countries and age groups may be entirely the result of increased numbers of the intestinal variety. These findings suggest that the intestinal and the diffuse types of lesions may have different etiologies. However, none of the less-common histologic classifications has as much effect on prognosis as the gross classification described by Borrmann.

LOCATION IN STOMACH

Most adenocarcinomas are found in the distal stomach on the lesser curvature; this is the same trend as in benign gastric ulcers. In one large series, 45% of all lesions were primarily in the distal third of the stomach, 33% in the pars media, and 22% in the proximal third. Each location has operative implications as well as an impact on prognosis; proximal lesions have the worst prognosis.

ROUTES OF SPREAD

Gastric carcinomas can spread in a number of ways (fig. 18.1). They can spread through the gastric wall and directly invade contiguous anatomic structures. By this mechanism gastric carcinomas can involve the pancreas,

spleen, esophagus, colon, duodenum, gallbladder, liver, or the adjacent mesenteries. Gastric carcinomas also spread via lymphatics and do so in approximately two-thirds of patients. The regional lymphatics involved are determined somewhat by the location of the primary lesion in the stomach. More distant lymphatic spread, particularly that detected in the left supraclavicular nodes, is a classic sign of inoperability (Virchow's node). Gastric carcinomas may also spread via the bloodstream to the liver, and less often to other sites. In addition, they can spread directly to the peritoneum where peritoneal implants, a rectal shelf, or ascites may be a manifestation of diffuse metastases.

CANCERS OTHER THAN ADENOCARCINOMAS

Adenocarcinoma is by far the most common stomach cancer, but several other types of malignant lesion are seen. Malignant lymphoma is the second most common stomach cancer and accounts for up to 8% of all cancers of this organ. Although this tumor presenting in the stomach may just be a manifestation of a systemic process, lymphoma will often have its primary and only site in the stomach. When this is the case, it may present as a discrete polypoid lesion, an ulcerated mass, or as giant rugal folds. Histologic differentiation must be made from pseudolymphoma, an unusual inflammatory

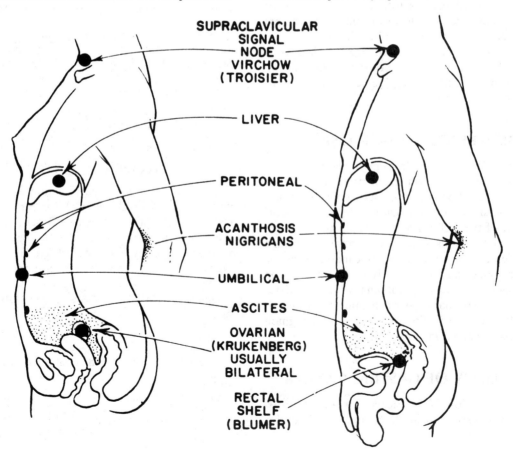

SUPRACLAVICULAR
SIGNAL
NODE
VIRCHOW
(TROISIER)

LIVER

PERITONEAL

ACANTHOSIS
NIGRICANS

UMBILICAL

ASCITES

OVARIAN
(KRUKENBERG)
USUALLY
BILATERAL

RECTAL
SHELF
(BLUMER)

Fig. 18.1. Diagram of gastric cancer routes of spread.

process that is sometimes associated with benign gastric ulcer (Orr, Lininger, and Lawrence 1984). Extranodal lymphomas arising as primary cancers of the stomach may or may not show regional lymph node metastasis.

The second most common cancer of mesodermal origin in the stomach is leiomyosarcoma, making up 1% to 3% of all gastric cancers (Appelman and Helwig 1977). Benign leiomyomas, however, occur much more frequently than leiomyosarcomas. The differentiation of sarcoma from a benign leiomyoma is often made on the basis of the frequency of mitotic figures in a histologic section. Other sarcomas are more clearly infiltrative on gross examination. Less frequent sarcomas arising in the stomach are liposarcoma, fibrosarcoma, carcinosarcoma, or malignant soft tissue tumors of vascular origin.

Other, rare types of malignant gastric tumors are carcinoids, plasmacytomas, and metastatic cancers. Carcinoids are generally small, firm, yellow, well-circumscribed submucosal lesions, as they are in other locations. Carcinoid tumors are argentaffin-positive on histologic staining. Some cancers that may rarely metastasize to the stomach arise in the lung, pancreas, prostate, breast, ovary, cervix, liver, and on the skin (malignant melanoma).

EPIDEMIOLOGY

To understand the etiology of any cancer in humans, it is necessary to know various features of the disease's natural history as well as demographic observations that might be clues to the etiology.

Two unusual observations have been made about the epidemiology of gastric cancer. The first is that the incidence of gastric cancer has been decreasing in the United States for more than 50 years (fig. 18.2), even though no major advances in diagnosis or treatment have been made during this period. Second, a wide variation in mortality rates from gastric cancer occurs from country to country. Gastric cancer is a relatively common cause of death in Japan, Chile, and Iceland, with the death rate being approximately five times that in the United States (Silverberg and Lubera 1988; Correa 1985). Much study still needs to be done to delineate those factors that contribute to these major differences.

Despite the continued decrease in incidence of gastric cancer in the United States, it was estimated that there would be 23,000 new cases in 1990 and approximately 14,000 deaths. This represents 2.3% of all new cancer cases. Within the gastrointestinal tract, gastric cancer is more common than cancers of the esophagus, small intestines, biliary tract, or liver but slightly less frequent than pancreatic cancer.

Gastric cancer is found more commonly in people between 50 and 70 years of age. It is predominantly a disease of men worldwide in a ratio of about two men to one woman. For no apparent reason, the incidence is greater in countries farther from the equator. Also, in

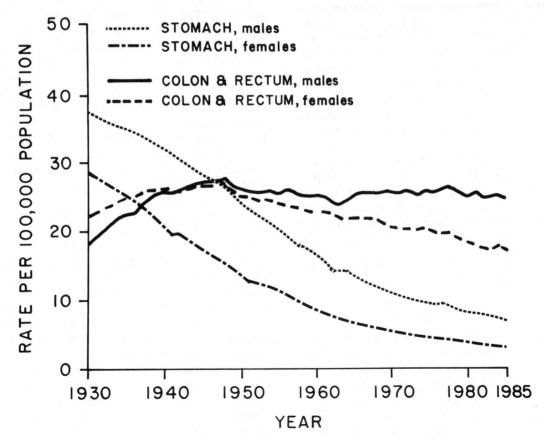

Fig. 18.2. Changing death rates for gastric cancer in the United States compared with trends for colon and rectal cancer.

most countries people in lower socioeconomic classes tend to develop gastric cancer much more frequently. There is no rural-urban or occupational difference in the incidence.

GENETICS

A small increased incidence has been noted in the direct relatives of people who had gastric cancer. Napoleon Bonaparte's family is the best-known example of the few families reported in which the incidence of gastric cancer is remarkably high. A study of Japanese immigrants, however, has detracted from suggestions of genetic influence on the incidence of gastric cancer (Haenszel and Kurihara 1968). Japanese emigrants to the United States maintain nearly the same incidence of gastric cancer as seen in the region where they spent their first 20 years. In contrast, their offspring have an incidence of gastric cancer that is almost comparable to that of Caucasians living nearby. These findings suggest that there are probably exposures in early life, rather than a genetic influence, that are the major causative factors in gastric cancer.

ASSOCIATED PATHOLOGY

Patients who have pernicious anemia, hypochlorhydria, or achlorhydria seem to develop gastric cancer more frequently. There have been reports of a 15% to 20% increased incidence in persons with blood group A. More recently, atrophic gastritis and intestinal metaplasia have been thought to be major precursor lesions (Correa, Cuello, and Duque et al. 1976; Stout 1945). Adenomatous polyps are not considered major precursor lesions for gastric cancer, but patients with adenomatous polyps do have an increased incidence of gastric cancer (Tomasulo 1971). In contrast to their occurrence in the colon, however, adenomatous polyps are uncommon in the stomach and are probably less common than cancer.

The exact relationship of benign gastric ulcer to gastric cancer is often debated. Observations have been made of carcinoma developing at the margins of pre-existing apparently benign ulcers, but others feel strongly that there is no etiological relationship between benign gastric ulcer and cancer. There are data that suggest patients with a prior gastrectomy and Billroth II anastomosis for benign disease have a higher incidence of stomach cancer, particularly after a 20-year interval (Caygill et al. 1986).

DIET

Much study has been done in attempting to delineate dietary causes for gastric cancer and many items have been incriminated (Risch, Jain, and Choi et al. 1985). It is believed that specific diets may contain carcinogens or some protective agent that is added during food preparation. An increased incidence of atrophic gastritis has been observed in many countries where gastric cancer flourishes. Also, Siurula and associates have observed progression of the disease from atrophic gastritis to

gastric cancer by repeated biopsies in a select group of patients (Siurula, Varis, and Wilijasala 1966).

What is the stimulus for this chain of pathological events when it does occur? Studies have shown that nitrosamines can produce gastric cancer in experimental animals (Magee and Barnes 1967). It is believed that they may be etiologic in man as well. Ruddell and associates have shown that nitrosamines can be produced in the stomach from nitrates (Ruddell, Bone, and Hill 1976). The intermediate in the synthesis of nitrosamines from nitrates is nitrites. Nitrites can be produced from nitrates by bacteria in the stomach, but the bacteria with enzymes capable of performing this reaction are killed by the acid present in a normal stomach. This might explain why gastric cancer develops more frequently in patients with atrophic gastritis and hypochlorhydria. Once nitrites are formed they quickly combine with amines that are naturally present in gastric juices to form nitrosamines. Although there is increasing evidence that nitrates and nitrosamines are, at least to some extent, involved in the etiology of gastric cancer, no definitive proof of this has yet been obtained.

DIAGNOSIS

Detection and diagnosis are the first steps in the management of patients with gastric cancer. Unfortunately, gastric cancer is difficult to diagnose at an early stage because there are no truly identifying signs or symptoms. The vast majority of patients present with nonspecific gastrointestinal complaints, such as vague epigastric discomfort or indigestion, occasional vomiting, belching, or postprandial fullness. Five percent to 10% of gastric cancer patients may have complaints similar to those of patients with classic peptic ulcer disease. Another 10% have nonspecific symptoms of chronic disease, such as anemia, weakness, and weight loss. A small number of patients are first seen with an acute intra-abdominal problem, such as massive upper gastrointestinal bleeding, acute obstruction of the esophagus or pylorus, and gastric perforation, often requiring emergency surgery.

There are no physical findings specifically associated with gastric cancer except where the disease is advanced. The only observation that may lead to an early diagnosis of gastric cancer is a positive stool occult blood test. Other physical signs that suggest more advanced disease include palpable ovarian mass, hepatomegaly, abdominal mass, ascites, jaundice, and cachexia. Although a palpable gastric cancer may be suitable for curative resection, this finding is often associated with a poor prognosis.

With no truly diagnostic symptoms or signs of gastric cancer, the physician must completely evaluate any patient (particularly in the over-40 age group) with an upper gastrointestinal disorder. The two oldest methods of evaluation are upper GI radiographic studies and gastric juice aspiration for cytology; the latter has been replaced by endoscopic approaches using either biopsy and/or brush cytology. Endoscopy is particularly useful to differentiate an ulcerated cancer from a benign gastric ulcer. The Japanese have identified a higher proportion of very superficial cancers using this approach. In most series, the combined use of cytologic examination from endoscopic brushings and pathologic examination of endoscopic biopsy specimens has produced the largest number of positive diagnoses of gastric cancer.

One way to increase early detection might be to screen a population that is at high risk. Early attempts at radiologic screening of asymptomatic populations in the United States showed a low rate of detection. The Japanese have been radiologically and endoscopically screening for gastric cancer more extensively, due to that country's increased mortality from gastric cancer. One demonstrated advantage of this screening approach in one study was that more than 40% of the cancers discovered were early and had a 5-year post-treatment survival rate of more than 90% (Kaneko, Nakamura, and Umeda et al. 1977).

STAGING

Clinical staging of the gastric cancer patient is based on the extent of the disease as shown by both physical examination and by radiologic and endoscopic studies (clinicodiagnostic stage). However, a more accurate staging classification for end result reporting after surgical treatment is based on the extent of the disease found at the time of surgical exploration of the abdomen, and the histological study of the excised surgical specimen when the cancer can be resected (clinico-pathologic stage).

The finding of cervical lymph node, liver, or peritoneal metastasis, or metastatic lesions to less frequent sites, establishes the clinical stage as stage IV, a category suitable for palliative treatment only. Such adverse

findings are often not apparent until celiotomy is performed, although pretreatment evaluations may allow proper categorization. At the time of celiotomy, the operative findings may reveal completely resectable disease and the tumor-nodes-metastasis (TNM) stage can then be determined from pathologic study of the resected specimen (table 18.2).

The principal factor affecting the TNM classification (American Joint Committee on Cancer 1983) from the standpoint of the primary tumor is the degree of penetration of the gastric wall by the carcinoma. The size or the location of the primary tumor is of less significance in assigning "T" for estimation of prognosis. Nodal involvement is a significant prognostic factor in the staging process, and the level of this ranges from either no metastasis to lymph nodes (N0), to lymphatic spread to immediately adjacent nodes (N1), to nodes in the perigastric area on both the lesser and greater curvatures (N2), to more distant nodes (N3). Distant metastases to the peritoneal surfaces, the liver, or other sites detected at operation are categorized as M1, a uniformly poor prognostic sign.

TREATMENT

Surgery is the only effective curative method in the primary treatment of gastric cancer and is the major approach for palliation as well. Despite improvements over the years in both operative and postoperative management, overall survival rates are still quite low.

SURGERY

All patients with gastric cancer, except those with evidence of peritoneal metastasis (ascites containing malignant cells or rectal shelf), documented liver metastasis, or other proven distant metastases (usually cervical lymph nodes), should be subjected to exploratory

Table 18.2
GASTRIC CANCER STAGING

AMERICAN JOINT COMMITTEE ON CANCER STAGING AND END RESULTS REPORTING (3rd ed.)

Tumor, Nodes, Metastasis Definitions

Stage 0	T_{is}	N0	M0	T_{is}-Limited to mucosa
Stage IA	T1	N0	M0	T1-Limited to mucosa and submucosa
Stage IB	T1	N1	M0	
	T2	N0	M0	
Stage II	T1	N2	M0	T2-To but not through serosa
	T2	N1	M0	T3-Through serosa but not adjacent structures
	T3	N0	M0	
Stage IIIA	T2	N2	M0	T4a-Through serosa and involves adjacent structures
	T3	N1	M0	T4b-Involves liver, diaphragm, pancreas, abdominal wall, retroperitoneum, small bowel, or duodenum via serosa
Stage IIIB	T3	N2	M0	N1-Perigastric nodes within 3 cm of tumor
	T4	N1	M0	N2-Perigastric nodes more than 3 cm from tumor (within celiac group)
Stage IV	T4	N2	M0	N3-Other intra-abdominal nodes (retroperitoneal, mesenteric, etc.)
	Any T	Any N	M1	M1-Distant metastasis

celiotomy to select both potentially curable patients and those who might benefit from palliative resection. If the cancer is regionally localized at exploration, adequate resection of the primary tumor, as well as actual and potential regional lymphatic extensions, is performed. Unfortunately, fewer than 40% of patients so explored are able to undergo a resection with some hope of cure on the basis of the findings at operation.

LYMPHATIC SPREAD

In designing a radical gastrectomy for patients with curable gastric cancer, the removal of potential regional lymphatic extensions must be considered (fig. 18.3). Although the incidence of regional lymphatic spread varies with different gross and histologic types of cancer, the overall incidence of lymphatic spread from carcinoma of the stomach is high—about 60%. In addition, gross observations often do not reveal whether lymph node metastases are present. Potential areas of lymphatic spread must always be considered in the design of radical gastrectomy, since the status of the regional lymphatics can be determined with confidence only after the resection has been completed. Unfortunately, removal of histologically involved lymph nodes is often not effective in terms of long-term cancer control, although about 15% of the patients with limited lymphatic spread do have long-term survival.

CHOICE OF OPERATION

The major options for surgical resection are distal subtotal gastric resection, proximal subtotal resection, or total gastrectomy (fig. 18.4). These procedures may include resection of adjacent organs involved with the

cancer by local extension, such as the body and tail of the pancreas, a portion of the liver, transverse colon, or perhaps the duodenum and head of the pancreas. Inclusion of extragastric organs in the resection is an infrequent consideration because, when these organs are involved, this is usually accompanied by other gross signs of incurability. This tends to discourage the surgeon from proceeding with a major resection, particularly when it includes the head of the pancreas.

Larger lesions of the pars media of the stomach and lesions of the proximal stomach are close to, or involve, the esophagogastric junction. This usually requires the proximal line of resection to be through the distal esophagus if an adequate margin around the cancer is to be removed. With either proximal or total gastrectomy for cancer in these sites, esophageal anastomosis is required. This has been associated with some increase in morbidity and mortality in the past, but less so in recent years.

The presence of microscopic spread around the gross margin of a gastric cancer is common, so removal of a generous margin of normal stomach around the carcinoma is a major principle of gastric resection for malignant lesions of all sites. In distal gastric lesions, generous resection of the adjacent first portion of the duodenum is required; in proximal lesions, the removal of a generous margin of distal esophagus is necessary. Frozen section examination of the site of transection is obtained at the time of operation in both situations. Failure to control a potentially curable cancer by not achieving an adequate gross margin around the primary tumor is a serious and avoidable error.

Although careful abdominal exploration is designed

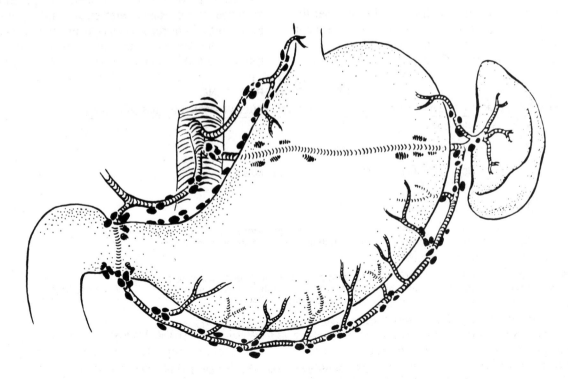

Fig. 18.3. Lymphatic drainage of the stomach.

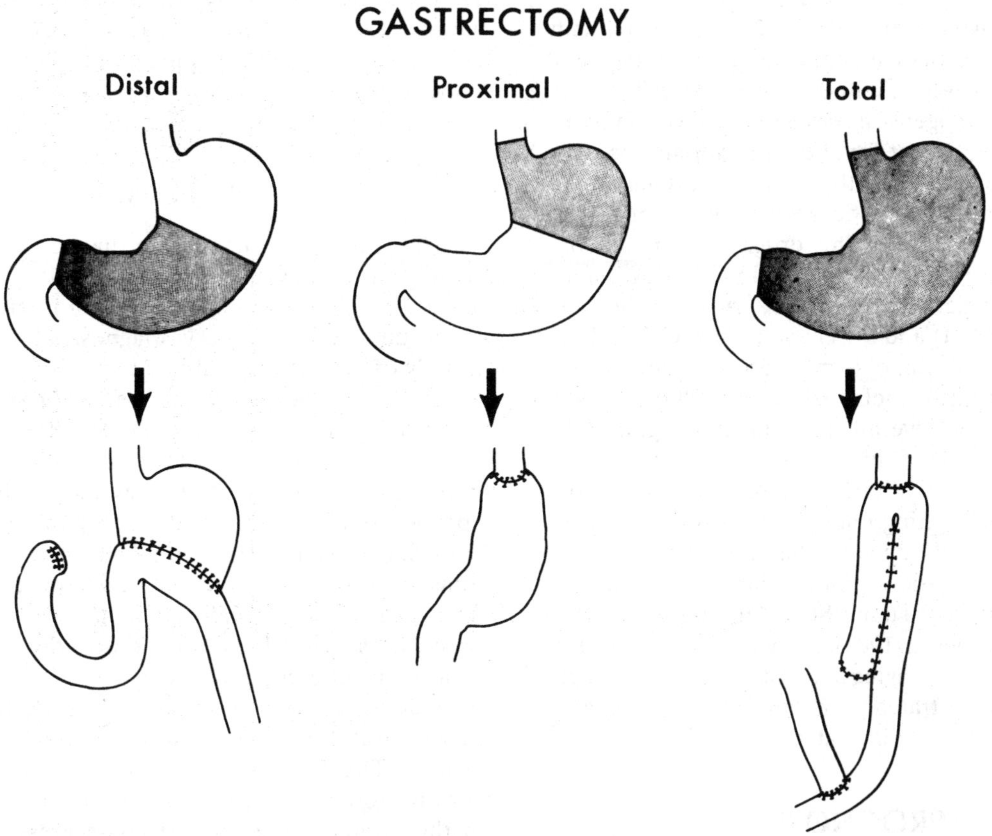

GASTRECTOMY

Distal   Proximal   Total

Fig. 18.4. Diagrams of operative resections employed for gastric cancer. Left to right: distal gastrectomy, proximal gastrectomy, total gastrectomy (method of reconstruction shown below each procedure).

to avoid radical surgery when cure is not possible, it is also important to confirm the diagnosis of cancer histologically if resection is not possible. If a resectable gastric cancer is observed grossly, it does not seem essential to obtain a positive biopsy prior to resection, particularly if the resectional procedure planned is less radical than a total gastrectomy.

PALLIATIVE OPERATIONS

A significant number of patients have unfavorable findings at the time of celiotomy, such as serosal implants, liver or ovarian metastasis, or metastatic disease in lymph nodes outside the range of a radical *en bloc* resection. This is the case in more than 60% of gastric cancer patients subjected to operation with the hope that curative resection is possible. A palliative procedure is then planned or the abdomen is closed without further operation, except for biopsy confirmation of the findings.

Palliative resection of gastric cancer is always preferred in these circumstances if the procedure can be accomplished without total gastrectomy, without transection of gross tumor at the site of planned anastomosis, and without a major hazard to the patient. If these conditions are met, palliative resection can significantly relieve symptoms in most patients and also appears to prolong survival. Palliative procedures such as gastrojejunostomy, gastrostomy, or jejunostomy rarely alleviate symptoms or prolong life expectancy. In

carefully selected patients, total gastrectomy can be used for palliation, particularly if the patient has obstruction as a major problem or if extensive lymphatic spread is the only finding preventing curative resection. These patients seem to have longer survival after palliative resection than those with liver or peritoneal metastasis. Considerable judgment is needed in making decisions about the choice of operative procedure when definite signs of incurability are detected at the exploration.

ROLE OF RADIATION THERAPY

Radiation therapy is rarely helpful for patients with gastric cancer that is unsuitable for curative resection, as the usual reason for nonresectability is the lack of localization of the cancer. Radiation therapy is sometimes useful, however, in relieving a localized area of obstruction, particularly in the region of the cardia, and for patients with chronically bleeding cancers that cannot be resected. This palliative tool is rarely indicated but may have benefit in highly selected cases. Some surgeons have recently been using intraoperative radiation therapy, but this adjuvant technique has not been used long enough to allow for a complete evaluation.

ROLE OF CHEMOTHERAPY

Many chemotherapeutic drugs have been tried as single agents for the palliation of gastric cancer, but the results have generally been disappointing. The antimetabolite

5-fluorouracil (5-FU) has been used most frequently. In one large review, approximately 22% of the patients treated with 5-FU had a limited degree of transient improvement and no definite increase in survival time. Many other single agents have been used with minimal palliative benefit, except for the drug Adriamycin.

There has been more enthusiasm for various combinations of chemotherapeutic agents for patients with advanced gastric cancer. The drugs in combinations include 5-FU, nitrosoureas, mitomycin-C, and Adriamycin. The combinations of 5-FU, Adriamycin, and mitomycin-C (FAM) and 5-FU and methyl CCNU have been associated with an objective response rate of 42% in prospective trials (MacDonald et al. 1980). It is still uncertain whether overall survival has significantly increased as a result of this palliative chemotherapy.

The overall results of operative resection for gastric cancer are disappointing enough to encourage aggressive clinical trials of adjuvant chemotherapy for all or selected groups of patients undergoing curative gastrectomy (Gastrointestinal Tumor Study Group 1982; Higgins et al. 1983; Fielding et al. 1983). Earlier results from one or two studies were encouraging but no clear-cut survival benefit has been demonstrated from these adjuvant programs. Further trials are clearly indicated.

PROGNOSIS

The prognosis for patients with gastric cancer remains poor because almost two-thirds of patients have either physical-examination or operative findings at the time of diagnosis that eliminate the possibility of surgical cure. No more than one-third of patients who are considered candidates for curative resection live five years or more after treatment (Lawrence and Terz 1977; Adashek, Sanger, and Longmire 1979). This overall success rate of 10% to 15% of all patients presenting with carcinoma of the stomach is discouraging. The majority of patients who develop regrowth of their cancers usually do so within three years of their primary surgical treatment, and in most series about 90% of the patients reaching the 5-year mark remain well.

Some prognostic factors somewhat modify these discouraging statistics and may be important in determining the prognosis for individual patients. Patients with a short history of symptoms tend to have a poorer prognosis than those with a longer history, and patients with the ulcer syndrome appear to do better than those presenting with the more common symptoms of indigestion. The gross pathologic type of lesion, the location of the cancer in the stomach, and the presence or absence of lymphatic metastases are more important indicators of prognosis than any specific features of the patient's history. The presence or absence of lymphatic metastasis is probably the most significant prognostic variable noted in all patients who have had curative gastric resection. Only a small proportion (15%) of patients with lymphatic metastasis enjoy long-term survival after radical resection that includes regional lymph nodes.

However, patients without lymphatic metastasis who are suitable for curative radical gastrectomy have a reasonably good prognosis; approximately 50% of these patients will have long-term survival.

THE FUTURE

The hope has been that earlier diagnosis would lead to significant improvement in the results of treatment. There are few examples, however, of improved survival based on attempts at early diagnosis. The explanation usually offered is the inability to achieve a diagnosis at an early *pathologic* stage of disease. Despite a lack of significant improvement in the result from operative treatment of gastric cancer in the United States, the improvement in long-term results in Japan would appear to demonstrate convincingly the importance of early diagnosis. In that country, alertness to early symptoms, more aggressive use of endoscopy, and the performance of high-quality air contrast radiographic procedures have all led to the detection of more superficial and more curable lesions. As a result, there has been a major overall improvement in Japan in the survival rates after resection for potentially curable lesions. The 5-year survival rate of about 50% after curative resection in Japan is almost twice that reported in the United States, where less-aggressive diagnostic approaches are employed. There may be other differences in gastric cancer between the two countries, but these treatment results should encourage efforts in early diagnosis, despite the relatively low incidence of gastric cancer in the United States.

As with all solid tumors treated primarily by surgery, there is the constant hope that overall treatment results may be improved by adjuvant chemotherapy. The results of controlled clinical trials have failed thus far to show significant benefit from chemotherapy given after gastric resection. Despite the lack of conclusive benefit, however, this adjuvant chemotherapeutic approach is still the major hope for the possible improvement in the survival of gastric cancer patients.

REFERENCES

Adashek, K.; Sanger, J.; and Longmire, W.P. Jr. 1979. Cancer of the stomach, a review of consecutive ten-year intervals. *Ann. Surg.* 189:6-10.

American Joint Committee on Cancer. 1988. *Manual for staging of cancer. 3rd ed.* Philadelphia: J.B. Lippincott.

Appelman, H.D., and Helwig, E.B. 1977. Sarcomas of the stomach. *Am. J. Clin. Pathol.* 67(1):2-10.

Caygill, C.P.J.; Hill, M.J.; and Kirkham, J.S. et al. 1986. Mortality from gastric cancer following gastric surgery for peptic ulcer. *Lancet* I:929-31.

Correa, P. 1985. Clinical implications of recent developments in gastric cancer pathology and epidemiology. *Semin. Oncol.* 12:2-10.

Correa, P.; Cuello, C.; and Duque, E. et al. 1976. Gastric

cancer in Colombia. III: natural history of precursor lesions. *J. Natl. Cancer Inst.* 57(5):1027-35.

Fielding, J.W.; Fagg, S.L.; and Jones, B.G. et al. 1983. An interim report of a prospective, randomized, controlled study of adjuvant chemotherapy in operable gastric cancer: British Stomach Cancer Group. *World J. Surg.* 7:390-99.

Gastrointestinal Tumor Study Group. 1982. Controlled trial of adjuvant chemotherapy following curative resection for gastric cancer. *Cancer* 49:1116-22.

Haenszel, W.M., and Kurihara, M. 1968. Studies of Japanese immigrants. I: mortality from cancer and other diseases in the United States. *J. Natl. Cancer Inst.* 40:43-68.

Higgins, G.A.; Amadeo, J.H.; and Smith, D.E. et al. 1983. Efficacy of prolonged intermittent therapy with combined 5-FU and methyl CCNU following resection for gastric carcinoma. *Cancer* 52:1105-12.

Kaneko, K.; Nakamura, T.; and Umeda, N. et al. 1977. Outcome of gastric carcinoma detected by gastric survey. *Gut* 18:626-30.

Lauren, P. 1965. The two histologic main types of gastric carcinoma: diffuse and so-called intestinal type carcinoma: an attempt at a histochemical classification. *Acta. Pathol. Microbiol. Scand.* 64:31-49.

Lawrence, W. Jr., and Terz, J.J. 1977. Management of gastrointestinal cancer. In Lawrence, W. Jr., and Terz, J.J. eds. *Cancer management.* pp. 202-19. New York: Grune & Stratton.

Magee, P.N. and Barnes, J.M. 1967. Carcinogenic nitroso compounds. *Adv. Cancer Res.* 10:163-246.

MacDonald, J.S.; Schein, P.S.; and Woolley, P.V. et al. 1980. 5-fluorouracil, doxorubicin, and mitomycin (FAM) combination chemotherapy for advanced gastric cancer. *Ann. Intern. Med.* 93:533-36.

Orr, R.; Lininger, J.R., and Lawrence, W. Jr. 1984. Gastric pseudolymphoma, a challenging clinical problem. *Ann. Surg.* 200:185-94.

Risch, H.A.; Jain, M.; and Choi, N.W. et al. 1985. Dietary factors and the incidence of cancer of the stomach. *Am. J. Epidemiol.* 122:947-59.

Ruddell, W.S.; Bone, E.S.; and Hill, M.J. 1976. Gastric juice nitrate, a risk factor for cancer in the hypochlorhydric stomach? *Lancet* II(7994):1037-39.

Silverberg, E. and Lubera, J. 1988. Cancer statistics, 1986. *CA* 38:5-22.

Siurula, M.; Varis, K.; and Wilijasala, M. 1966. Studies of patients with atrophic gastritis: a 10-15 year follow-up. *Scand. J. Gastroenterol.* 1:40-48.

Stout, A.P. 1945. Gastric mucosal atrophy and carcinoma of the stomach. *N.Y. J. Med.* 45:973-77.

Tomasulo, J. 1971. Gastric polyps. *Cancer* 27:1346-55.

Chapter 19

CANCER OF THE ESOPHAGUS

F. Henry Ellis, Jr., M.D., Ph.D.
Nathan Levitan, M.D.
Theodore C.M. Lo, M.D.

F. Henry Ellis, Jr., M.D., Ph.D.
Senior Consultant
Department of Thoracic and Cardiovascular Surgery
Lahey Clinic Medical Center
Burlington, Massachusetts

Nathan Levitan, M.D.
Section of Oncology
Lahey Clinic Medical Center
Burlington, Massachusetts

Theodore C.M. Lo, M.D.
Chairman
Department of Radiotherapy
Lahey Clinic Medical Center
Burlington, Massachusetts

INTRODUCTION

Carcinoma of the esophagus is relatively uncommon in the United States. Only an estimated 4% of all digestive tract cancers diagnosed during 1990 will arise in the esophagus (Silverberg, Boring, and Squires 1990). When carcinomas involving the esophagogastric junction (cardia) are included, the total cases are nearly doubled (fig. 19.1). The prognosis for patients with carcinoma of the esophagus, although poor, has improved. Untreated patients survive an average of four months after diagnosis. Even with modern forms of therapy, long-term survival is rare because, in many patients, the tumor has metastasized before the diagnosis has been made. On the other hand, patients with carcinoma of the esophagus are seeking medical care earlier. This fact, coupled with a more aggressive surgical approach that has increased operability and resectability rates and lowered hospital mortality rates, has led to an improvement in overall postoperative survival statistics. Furthermore, surgery today effectively relieves dysphagia, the disease's most common symptom.

Advances have also been made in the palliative treatment of patients with nonresectable carcinoma of the esophagus. Radiotherapeutic techniques including brachytherapy (Rowland and Pagliero 1985), laser therapy (*Lancet* 1987), photodynamic therapy (McCaughan, Williams, and Bethel 1985), and peroral intubation (Van den Brandt-Grädel, den Hartog Jager, and Tytgat 1987) provide effective palliation. However, none of these techniques has had an appreciable impact on life expectancy after initiation of treatment.

The role of chemotherapy remains undefined. Chemotherapeutic drugs with activity against this tumor

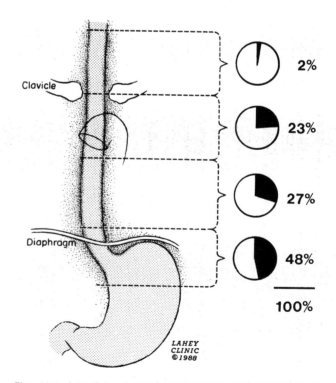

Fig. 19.1. Location of surgically treated carcinomas of the esophagus and cardia. (By permission of Lahey Clinic.)

include cisplatin, bleomycin, methotrexate, 5-fluorouracil, Adriamycin, vindesine, mitomycin C, and CCNU. Response rates to individual drugs range from 15% to 38% (Kelsen 1984). Considerably higher response rates have been reported (Vogl, Greenwald, and Kaplan 1981; Hellerstein et al. 1983; Gisselbrecht et al. 1983) with combinations of these drugs. Combination chemotherapy has been used experimentally in three ways: (1) preoperatively in an effort to shrink the tumor, increase resectability rates, and eliminate micrometastatic disease; (2) in combination with radiation therapy; and (3) alone as palliative therapy for patients with advanced unresectable or metastatic disease.

In our opinion, further improvement in long-term survival of patients with carcinoma of the esophagus will depend on improving diagnostic techniques to permit early diagnosis. The cost-effectiveness of screening methods to permit early diagnosis may not make these methods practical in the United States, but they have been successful in certain endemic areas in the world, particularly in Lin Xian County in the Henan Province of China (*Chin. Med. J.* 1976). On the other hand, use of these screening techniques seems eminently prudent for persons known to be at risk for the development of esophageal carcinoma, such as those with Barrett's esophagus. Improved survival may also follow the development of more effective systemic chemotherapy.

EPIDEMIOLOGY AND ETIOLOGY

EPIDEMIOLOGY
Carcinoma of the esophagus predominates in elderly men, the male-to-female ratio being approximately 3:1. Esophageal carcinoma usually develops in the seventh and eighth decades of life, although young adults and octogenarians are not exempt.

Prevalence varies widely in different parts of the world (table 19.1), varying from 7.6 per 100,000 in the United States where prevalence is considerably higher among black males than among white males (13.3 vs. 3.5) to 130 per 100,000 persons in endemic areas of China (Day 1975). An estimated 10,600 new cases of carcinoma of the esophagus will occur in the United States during 1990 (Silverberg, Boring, and Squires 1990).

Table 19.1
DEMOGRAPHIC FEATURES

Region	Prevalence per 100,000
Lin Xian County, China	130.0
North Iran	114.6
Transkei Region, South Africa	70.4
Turkmenia	51.1
Kazakhstan	47.8
Brittany	28.9
United States	
Black men	13.3
White men	3.5

ETIOLOGY
Surprisingly, these marked geographic differences in the incidence of carcinoma of the esophagus have not revealed more useful information on the cause of the disease. There is probably a variety of etiologic factors.

Nitrosamines and alcoholic beverages have been implicated in the high incidence of the disease among the Bantu in South Africa (McGlashan, Walters, and McLean 1968), and nitrosamines also have been implicated in the high incidence reported from Lin Xian County in China (Yang 1988). Low socioeconomic background, deficient diet, and exposure to opium tar have been implicated in northern Iran (Tuyns, Péquignot, and Jensen 1979). Alcohol and tobacco use have been implicated in northwest France and the United States (Wynder and Bross 1961).

Certain precancerous lesions have long been recognized. The incidence of esophageal carcinoma among patients with achalasia is approximately seven times that of normal individuals (Wychulis et al. 1971). The disease has been shown to occur with increasing frequency in the Paterson-Kelly (Plummer-Vinson) syndrome (Larsson, Sandstroom, and Westling 1975). When patients with caustic injury to the esophagus are observed for 24 years or more, the incidence has been reported to be 1,000 times greater than that of the normal individual (Kiviranta 1952). Of current interest is the association between adenocarcinoma of the esophagus and Barrett's esophagus, the prevalence varying from 8.6% (Naef, Savary, and Ozzello 1975) to nearly 50% (Skinner et al. 1983) depending on the patient population studied. The actual incidence of the disorder is more difficult to codify as it has been observed in anywhere from 1 per 81 (Sprung, Ellis, and Gibb 1984) to 1 per 441 patient-years of follow-up (Cameron, Ott, and Payne 1985). Clearly, more studies are required to identify the risk of carcinoma developing in the presence of Barrett's mucosa. Tylosis, an inherited condition characterized by epidermal thickening of the palms and soles, has a high association with esophageal carcinoma (Wynder and Bross 1961).

DETECTION AND DIAGNOSIS

CLINICAL DETECTION
Dysphagia is by far the most frequent complaint of patients with esophageal carcinoma. It is usually apparent first with ingestion of bulky foods, later with soft foods, and ultimately with liquids. Weight loss, regurgitation, and aspiration pneumonitis also may be present. In patients who do not experience dysphagia, the predominant symptoms are odynophagia (pain on swallowing) and gastroesophageal reflux symptoms, associated in some patients with minor degrees of blood loss.

Symptoms and signs suggesting advanced stages of the disease include cervical adenopathy; chronic cough, suggesting tracheal involvement; choking after eating, suggesting a fistula within the trachea; massive hemoptysis or hematemesis or both, suggesting perforation of the lesion into vascular structures; and hoarseness, suggesting recurrent laryngeal nerve paralysis. Pain is an unusual symptom and suggests local extension to adjacent structures.

DIAGNOSTIC PROCEDURES

Esophageal roentgenography is an essential part of the workup of any patient complaining of difficulty in swallowing. The characteristic finding of an irregular ragged mucosal pattern with luminal narrowing is typical of carcinoma of the esophagus. Unlike benign obstructive lesions, carcinoma is not usually associated with proximal dilation of the esophagus. Cinefluorography may also be useful in the diagnosis of problem cases. The exact role of computed tomography (CT) and magnetic resonance imaging (MRI) remains controversial, but it may be helpful in identifying invasion of tissues outside the confines of the esophagus. Computed tomography may be useful in preoperative staging, but it has not proved to be a reliable indicator of nonresectability.

Esophagoscopy is required to confirm the clinical suspicion of carcinoma. The use of fiberoptic instruments has simplified the performance of this study, which must be associated with biopsy to provide histologic material for evaluation.

Lesions involving the upper portion of the thoracic esophagus near the tracheal carina require bronchoscopy in addition to esophagoscopy to determine the presence or absence of involvement of the tracheobronchial tree.

As an aid to early diagnosis, use of supravital staining techniques with such agents as iodine (Lugol's solution), toluidine blue, indigo carmine, or sulfamycin may help identify potential biopsy sites during esophagoscopy. The addition of brush biopsy may provide useful material for cytologic study in patients at risk for the development of esophageal carcinoma. Another promising technique is the use of radioisotopes in tumor scanning. Materials preferentially picked up by squamous cancer cells, such as gallium-67 and cobalt-57-bleomycin (Blenoxane), may be useful in early diagnosis.

CLASSIFICATION

ANATOMIC STAGING

The definition of tumor and node (T and N) categories for carcinoma of the esophagus according to the American Joint Committee for Cancer staging (AJCC) (American Joint Committee on Cancer 1988) is summarized in table 19.2. The postsurgical staging is summarized in table 19.3. The AJCC also recognizes clinical, surgical, and recurrent staging categories.

HISTOPATHOLOGY

Squamous cell carcinoma accounts for approximately two-thirds of esophageal carcinomas. It arises from the

Table 19.2
POSTSURGICAL TUMOR (T) NODE (N) CLASSIFICATION*

Primary tumor

T_{IS}	Carcinoma *in situ*
T_1	Invasion of lamina propria or submucosa
T_2	Invasion of muscularis propria
T_3	Invasion of muscle to adventitia
T_4	Invasion of extraesophageal structures

Lymph nodes

N_x	Nodes cannot be assessed
N_0	No regional node metastasis
N_1	Regional node metastasis

*(Modified from: American Joint Committee on Cancer [1988].)

surface epithelium and is found equally in the upper and lower esophagus.

Adenocarcinoma is encountered more frequently today than in the past and is the second most common type. It usually arises in Barrett's esophagus. Tumors similar in microscopic appearance to those arising in salivary glands account for most of the remaining glandular tumors of the esophagus. They are considered to arise from the ducts of the esophageal submucous glands. Occasionally, an adenocarcinoma may occur in which squamous differentiation is histologically evident, and the term adenosquamous carcinoma is applied to them.

Carcinosarcoma and pseudosarcoma are less common lesions usually presenting as bulky intraluminal polypoid growths. Both are slow-growing tumors that warrant aggressive surgery.

Sarcomas represent less than 1% of all malignant esophageal tumors and include such histologic diagnoses as fibrosarcoma, leiomyosarcoma, and rhabdomyosarcoma. Primary melanoma is more commonly encountered among rare tumors. Verrucous squamous cell carcinoma is another rare tumor whose indolent biologic behavior makes it susceptible to cure. Finally, oat cell carcinoma of the esophagus has been reported and is considered a true apudoma arising from the argyrophilic Kulchitsky cells in the surface epithelium (see table 19.4).

STAGING WORKUP

Staging of esophageal carcinoma depends on the primary tumor's size and degree of penetration as well as the presence or absence of nodal involvement and

Table 19.3
POSTSURGICAL STAGE GROUPING*

Stage 0	T_{IS}	N_0	M_0
Stage I	T_1	N_0	M_0
Stage IIA	T_2	N_0	M_0
	T_3	N_0	M_0
Stage IIB	T_1	N_1	M_0
	T_2	N_1	M_0
Stage III	T_3	N_1	M_0
	T_4	Any N	M_0
Stage IV	Any T	Any N	M_1

*(Modified from: American Joint Committee on Cancer [1988].)

Table 19.4
HISTOPATHOLOGIC CLASSIFICATIONS

Squamous cell carcinoma
Adenocarcinoma
Adenoid cystic carcinoma
Mucoepidermoid carcinoma
Adenosquamous carcinoma
Carcinosarcoma and pseudosarcoma
Miscellaneous
  Sarcoma
  Melanoma
  Plasmacytoma
  Verrucous carcinoma
  Oat cell carcinoma

metastatic disease. Because relief of dysphagia is a primary treatment goal, therapy should be undertaken regardless of the disease stage. Accordingly, extensive screening for metastases seems unjustified in the absence of clinical and/or laboratory evidence.

RECOMMENDED PROCEDURES

Esophagography assesses the tumor's location, length, and degree of circumferential extent. *Laboratory tests* include complete blood cell count and chemistries with attention to indicators of liver abnormalities, that is, alkaline phosphatase, serum glutamic-oxaloacetic transaminase (SGOT), and bilirubin. *Bronchoscopy* is restricted to lesions of the upper thoracic and cervical esophagus to exclude tracheobronchial involvement. *Computed tomog-*

raphy provides helpful information for staging the degree of penetration of the esophageal wall by tumor and its possible involvement of adjacent structures. However, it is not a reliable index of resectability.

Radioisotope scanning should not be part of the routine workup of patients with esophageal carcinoma unless either clinical or laboratory findings or both suggest metastatic lesions.

PRINCIPLES OF TREATMENT

Widespread pessimism regarding treatment of patients with esophageal carcinoma persists despite recent advances (Earlam and Cunha-Melo 1980). Although some of this negativism is justified, it should not lead to total despair. Several aggressive surgical techniques provide excellent palliation and, in early disease, a reasonable chance for cure. Radiation therapy offers excellent palliation, and chemotherapy has been used in combination with surgery, radiation, or both.

SURGERY

An aggressive surgical approach to carcinoma of the esophagus provides the patient with excellent palliation, longevity, and a chance for cure. A radical resective procedure seems to have no surgical advantage compared with standard resection. Although radical surgery

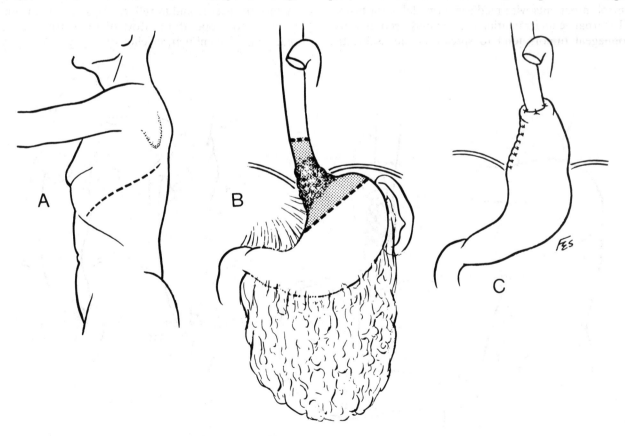

Fig. 19.2. Technique of esophagogastrectomy and esophagogastrostomy for carcinoma of the cardia. A = Site of incision; B = Extent of resection (shaded area); C = Completed esophagogastrostomy. (From Ellis, F.H. Jr., and Shahian, D.M. 1983. Tumors of the esophagus. In Glenn, W.W.L.; Baue, A.E.; Geha, A.S.; Hammond, G.L.; and Laks, H. eds. *Thoracic and cardiovascular surgery*. 4th ed. p. 566. Norwalk, Conn.: Appleton & Lange.)

is safer than in the past, it clearly adds to morbidity and mortality. Figs. 19.2 through 19.4 depict examples of standard techniques for esophagogastrectomy based on the location of the lesion. An esophagogastrectomy through the left chest is appropriate for most lesions in the lower esophagus (fig. 19.2), whereas for higher lesions (fig. 19.3) the combined laparotomy and right thoracotomy (Ivor Lewis) or a transhiatal approach (fig. 19.4) is preferred. For lesions at the thoracic inlet and cervical esophagus, a transhiatal approach (fig. 19.4), which has been applied to lesions at all locations of the esophagus, is preferred (Orringer 1984). The stomach is preferred as the esophageal replacement; colon interposition is reserved by most surgeons for patients in whom inadequate stomach remains after resection.

RADIATION THERAPY

Squamous cell carcinoma is radiosensitive, and local tumor control is frequently attainable. Radiation therapy is particularly useful for lesions above the aortic arch.

Radiation therapy is an excellent palliative modality for obstructive symptoms with a response rate reaching 75% (Hankins et al. 1972; Rider and Diaz Mendoza 1969; Wara, Mauch, and Thomas 1965). Added value may result when combined with dilation as needed. Radiation therapy is also a good treatment for pain control in patients with mediastinal nodal metastases.

External beam irradiation is commonly used. Because esophageal tumors tend to spread submucosally, the radiation treatment field should include if possible a 5 cm margin proximally and distally from the tumor volume as shown on barium swallow to ensure adequate tumor coverage. Patients usually are treated daily with fractionated radiation therapy of 9 Gy to 10 Gy per week. Because of normal lung and spinal cord tolerance, field modification is usually necessary at 45 Gy, and curative total tumor dose should be in the range of 60 Gy to 70 Gy. Split-course treatment is tolerated better by the patient but may compromise overall radiation effect (Levitt, Frazier, and James 1970). The pros and cons of multiple fraction per day schemes are being explored (DePaoli et al. 1988). Endocurietherapy using intracavitary sources of radiation, such as iridium 192, as a supplement to increase the dose to selected tumor sites is being investigated; preliminary results are encouraging (George 1980). Endocurietherapy is particularly effective in palliation for obstruction. Other types of radioactive sources have also been used (Rowland and Pagliero 1985; Hishikawa et al. 1982).

Palliative radiation therapy to symptomatic metastatic sites, such as bone, is effective.

CHEMOTHERAPY

A number of trials have been conducted using preoperative chemotherapy to eliminate distant microscopic metastatic disease and to reduce the size of the primary tumor before operation. Most of these trials use cisplatin-based combination chemotherapy. Investigators

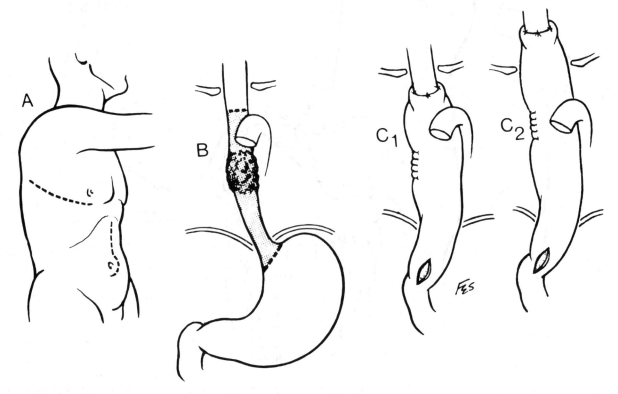

Fig. 19.3. A = Combined abdominal incision and right thoracotomy for lesions of the upper thoracic esophagus; B = Extent of resection (shaded area); C₁ = Esophagogastrostomy can be performed in the chest; C₂ = If submucosal spread is great, a cervical anastomosis through a third incision can be performed. (From Ellis, F.H. Jr. 1980. Esophagogastrectomy for carcinoma: technical considerations based on anatomic location of lesion. *Surg. Clin. North Am.* **60:273.)**

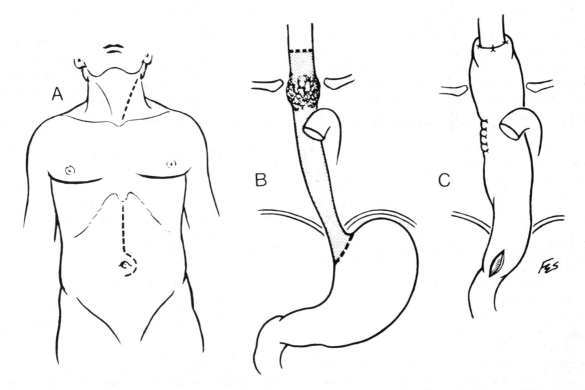

Fig. 19.4. For esophagectomy without thoracotomy, the patient is in the supine position. A = Upper midline and left cervical incisions (broken lines) are made; B = Extent of resection (shaded area) is shown; C = Completed anastomosis. (From Ellis, F.H. Jr. 1980. Esophagogastrectomy for carcinoma: technical considerations based on anatomic location of lesion. *Surg. Clin. North Am.* 60:275.)

(Kelsen et al. 1983) have reported major tumor regression in more than 60% of patients. No evidence exists that this combined treatment is associated with an improvement in survival.

COMBINATION CHEMOTHERAPY, RADIATION THERAPY, AND SURGERY

To improve local control further while destroying distant micrometastatic disease, concurrent preoperative chemotherapy and radiation therapy have been used (Fujimaki et al. 1975; Leichman et al. 1984). When a cisplatin-based combination chemotherapy regimen plus radiation therapy was given before operation, 18% of patients had no pathologic evidence of residual tumor at the time of surgery. Unfortunately, the mortality rate associated with this triple-modality therapy is unacceptably high. Prolonged survival has been observed in the small group of patients who had no pathologic evidence of residual tumor at the time of surgery, but no overall survival advantage has been demonstrated for patients treated in this fashion (Poplion et al. 1987).

CHEMOTHERAPY AND RADIATION THERAPY WITHOUT SURGERY

The efficacy of radiation therapy plus chemotherapy in reducing tumor bulk has led investigators to question whether patients would benefit from radiation therapy plus chemotherapy without surgery. One study (Coia, Engstrom, and Paul 1987) that used this approach revealed a median survival of 35 months in patients who had no clinical evidence of residual cancer after completion of therapy. Another study (Leichman et al. 1987) revealed a 1-year actuarial survival rate of 72% for patients treated in this fashion, and effective palliation of dysphagia was achieved. Surgery was reserved for patients whose disease failed to respond to chemotherapy or in whom persistent aspiration developed.

The use of chemotherapy in patients with esophageal carcinoma is investigational and should be reserved for patients who either refuse surgery or choose to participate in a research protocol. At present, surgical resection, radiation therapy, or both remain the standard treatments for patients with esophageal carcinoma.

SPECIAL CONSIDERATIONS OF TREATMENT

RADIATION COMPLICATIONS

Development of untoward reactions to irradiation depends on normal tissue tolerance and varies with the type of tissue, volume irradiated, total dose, and rate of administration. The type of complication depends on the structure involved.

Esophageal perforation or hemorrhage may occur as part of the natural history of the disease responding to therapy. Stricture could be a late effect.

Radiation fibrosis is an infrequent lung complication, dependent on the volume of pulmonary parenchyma exposed and radiation dose delivered. Transverse myelitis is reported after a total dose greater than 50 Gy has been delivered to the spinal cord, but this complication is avoidable with modern techniques. The radiation field rarely needs to cover the whole cardiac silhouette, but radiation cardiomyopathy can develop if the entire heart is treated with a total dose above 45 Gy. With supervoltage machines, significant radiation skin changes are no longer seen.

CHEMOTHERAPY COMPLICATIONS

Side effects of chemotherapy vary with the specific agents used. In general, myelosuppression, mucositis, and gastrointestinal toxicity develop. Many regimens use cisplatin, which can also cause nephrotoxicity, ototoxicity, and neurotoxicity.

SURGICAL COMPLICATIONS

Complications after surgery for carcinoma of the esophagus are much less common than in past years. Patients are coming for treatment earlier than before; this earlier treatment, coupled with advances in respiratory therapy, hyperalimentation, and anesthetic support during the operation, has decreased markedly the incidence of anastomotic leaks and respiratory failure.

Cardiovascular complications predominate as a cause of death among patients who failed to survive esophagogastrectomy. Myocardial infarction, cerebrovascular accident, and pulmonary embolus are the commonest offenders.

Problems with gastric emptying may follow esophagogastrostomy. Mechanical obstruction or decreased gastric tone, together with anastomotic strictures secondary to gastroesophageal reflux, or recurrent disease predominates in this category.

Anastomotic leakage is now uncommon. When it occurs, it is seen more often after colon interposition with a leaking esophagocolostomy. Cervical leaks are usually well managed conservatively with hyperalimentation.

RESULTS AND PROGNOSIS

SURGERY RESULTS

Current surgical results are far more encouraging than they were in past years. The hospital mortality rate has dropped appreciably, and a number of reports (Akiyama et al. 1981; Ellis, Gibb, and Watkins 1983; King et al. 1987; Mathisen et al. 1988) show rates under 5% with a low morbidity rate. In addition, operability and resectability rates are increasing so that more patients are candidates for long-term survival. In one series (Ellis 1989), this has led to a near quadrupling of the overall survival rate of all patients seen and admitted with carcinoma of the esophagus and cardia at two major United States clinics (from 4% to 15% over the past 40 years). Current 5-year survival figures are in the neighborhood of 20%, nearly reaching 40% for stage I and II lesions.

In contrast to earlier concepts, no appreciable difference in survival appears when location or cell type is considered. The only variant of prognostic importance is related to the stage of the disease, lending further credence to the concept that early diagnosis may be the ultimate key to long-term survival.

RADIATION THERAPY RESULTS

Pearson (1969) has reported a 5-year survival of 20% in patients treated with radiation therapy alone, but others have not been able to duplicate this record. An exhaustive review of the literature by Earlam and Cunha-Melo (1980) revealed only a 6% 5-year survival rate with radiation therapy alone.

CHEMOTHERAPY RESULTS

Chemotherapy alone is used only to provide palliation for patients with locally recurrent or metastatic disease. When chemotherapeutic agents are used individually, response rates range from 15% to 38% (Kelsen 1984). When combinations of these drugs are used, response rates as high as 80% have been reported (Gisselbrecht et al. 1983).

COMBINED THERAPY RESULTS

Earlier studies regarding combined use of preoperative radiation and surgery were encouraging, but subsequent prospective randomized studies of this combined form of treatment have failed to substantiate earlier enthusiasm. There is no statistically significant difference between the two modalities (Launois et al. 1981; Gignoux et al. 1987).

Cisplatin-based combination chemotherapy has been used preoperatively in experimental protocols with excellent response rates (Kelsen 1987; Hilgenberg et al. 1988).

Chemotherapy has been combined with radiation therapy preoperatively. Approximately 18% of patients treated in this fashion are found to be histologically free of tumor at the time of surgery (Fujimaki et al. 1975; Leichman et al. 1984; Poplion et al. 1987). Chemotherapy has been used in combination with radiation therapy in place of surgery, and effective palliation of dysphagia has been reported (Akiyama et al. 1981). Despite the ability of combination chemotherapy to reduce tumor size, prolonged survival has not been demonstrated.

REASONS FOR FAILURE

Symptoms occur late in the disease, usually after circumferential involvement of the esophagus, by which time the disease is often systemic rather than localized. Death usually is the result of metastases not evident when therapy is initiated. Early diagnosis is essential for good results to be achieved.

CLINICAL INVESTIGATIONS

Cost-effective methods permitting early diagnosis should be investigated, particularly for patients at risk for the development of cancer, such as persons with Barrett's esophagus.

Expansion of the role of radiation therapy should be encouraged, especially as it applies to the potential value of intracavitary radioactive sources.

Further studies of chemotherapeutic agents to eliminate metastatic disease are necessary if combined forms of therapy are to become more effective.

Protocols should be established to permit randomized prospective evaluation of the role of operation alone compared with operation and adjuvant forms of therapy, either radiation therapy or chemotherapy or both, in the management of this disease.

REFERENCES

Akiyama, H.; Tsurumaru, M.; and Kawamura, T. et al. 1981. Principles of surgical treatment for carcinoma of the esophagus: analysis of lymph node involvement. *Ann. Surg.* 194:438-46.

American Joint Committee on Cancer. 1988. *Manual for staging of cancer.* 3rd. ed. Philadelphia: J.B. Lippincott.

Cameron, A.J.; Ott, B.J.; and Payne, W.S. 1985. Incidence of adenocarcinoma in columnar-lined (Barrett's) esophagus. *N. Engl. J. Med.* 313:857-59.

Chin. Med. J. 1976. Early diagnosis and surgical treatment of esophageal cancer under rural conditions. *Chin. Med. J.* 2:113-16.

Coia, L.R.; Engstrom, P.F.; and Paul, A. 1987. Nonsurgical management of esophageal cancer: report of a study of combined radiotherapy and chemotherapy. *J. Clin. Oncol.* 5:1783-90.

Day, N.E. 1975. Some aspects of the epidemiology of esophageal cancer. *Cancer Res.* 35:3304-3307.

DePaoli, A.; Boz, G.; and Trovo, M.G. et al. 1988. Multiple fraction per day radiation therapy for inoperable esophageal cancer. *Int. J. Radiat. Oncol. Biol. Phys.* 14:855-60.

Earlam, R., and Cunha-Melo, J.R. 1980. Oesophageal squamous cell carcinoma. I: a critical review of surgery. *Br. J. Surg.* 67:381-90.

Earlam, R., and Cunha-Melo, J.R. 1980. Oesophageal squamous cell carcinoma. II: a critical review of radiotherapy. *Br. J. Surg.* 67:457-61.

Ellis, F.H. Jr. 1989. Surgery for cancer of the esophagus and cardia. *Mayo Clin. Proc.* 64:945-55.

Ellis, F.H. Jr.; Gibb, S.P.; and Watkins, E. Jr. 1983. Esophagogastrectomy: a safe, widely applicable and expeditious form of palliation for patients with carcinoma of the esophagus and cardia. *Ann. Surg.* 198:531-40.

Fujimaki, M.; Soga, J.; and Kawaguchi, M. et al. 1975. Role of preoperative administration of bleomycin and radiation in the treatment of esophageal cancer. *Jpn. J. Surg.* 5:48-55.

George, F.W. 3d. 1980. Radiation management in esophageal cancer: with a review of intraesophageal radioactive iridium treatment in 24 patients. *Am. J. Surg.* 139:795-804.

Gignoux, M.; Roussel, A.; and Paillot, B. et al. 1987. Value of preoperative radiotherapy in esophageal cancer: results of a study of the E.O.R.T.C. *World J. Surg.* 11:426-32.

Gisselbrecht, C.; Calvo, F.; and Mignot, L. et al. 1983. Fluorouracil (F), Adriamycin (A), and cisplatin (P) (FAP): combination chemotherapy of advanced esophageal carcinoma. *Cancer* 52:974-77.

Hankins, J.R.; Cole, F.N.; and Ward, A. et al. 1972. Carcinoma of the esophagus: philosophy for palliation. *Ann. Thorac. Surg.* 14:189-97.

Hellerstein, S.; Rosen, S.; and Kies, M. et al. 1983. Diamminedichloroplatinum and 5-fluorouracil combined chemotherapy of epidermoid esophageal cancer (Abstr C-497). *Proc. Am. Soc. Clin. Oncol.* 2:127.

Hilgenberg, A.D.; Carey, R.W.; and Wilkins, E.W. Jr. et al. 1988. Preoperative chemotherapy, surgical resection, and selective postoperative therapy for squamous cell carcinoma of the esophagus. *Ann. Thorac. Surg.* 45:357-63.

Hishikawa, Y.; Taniguchi, M.; and Kamikonya, N. et al. 1988. External beam radiotherapy alone or combined with high-dose-rate intracavitary irradiation in the treatment of cancer of the esophagus: autopsy findings in 35 cases. *Radiother. Oncol.* 11:223-27.

Kelsen, D. 1984. Chemotherapy of esophageal cancer. *Semin. Oncol.* 11:159-68.

Kelsen, D.; Hilaris, B.; and Coonley, C. et al. 1983. Cisplatin, vindesine, and bleomycin combination chemotherapy of local-regional and advanced esophageal carcinoma. *Am. J. Med.* 75:645-52.

Kelsen, D.P. 1987. Preoperative chemotherapy in esophageal carcinoma. *World J. Surg.* 11:433-38.

King, R.M.; Pairolero, P.C.; and Trastek, V.F. et al. 1987. Ivor Lewis esophagogastrectomy for carcinoma of the esophagus: early and late functional results. *Ann. Thorac. Surg.* 44:119-22.

Kiviranta, U.K. 1952. Corrosion carcinoma of the esophagus: 381 cases of corrosion and 9 cases of corrosion carcinoma. *Acta Otol.* 42:89-95.

Lancet. 1987. Endoscopic laser resection of inoperable tracheobronchial and oesophageal tumours (editorial). II:1126-27.

Larsson, L.G.; Sandstrom, A.; and Westling, P. 1975. Relationship of Plummer-Vinson disease to cancer of the upper alimentary tract in Sweden. *Cancer Res.* 35:3308-16.

Launois, B.; Delarue, D.; and Campion, J.P. et al. 1981. Preoperative radiotherapy for carcinoma of the esophagus. *Surg. Gynecol. Obstet.* 153:690-92.

Leichman, L.; Steiger, Z.; and Seydel, H.G. et al. 1984. Combined preoperative chemotherapy and radiation therapy for cancer of the esophagus: the Wayne State University, Southwest Oncology Group, and Radiation Therapy Oncology Group experience. *Semin. Oncol.* 11:178-85.

Leichman, L.; Herskovic, A.; and Leichman, C.G. et al. 1987. Nonoperative therapy for squamous-cell cancer of the esophagus. *J. Clin. Oncol.* 5:365-70.

Levitt, S.H.; Frazier, A.B.; and James, K.W. 1970. Split-course radiotherapy in the treatment of carcinoma of the esophagus. *Radiology* 94:433-35.

Mathisen, D.J.; Grillo, H.C.; and Wilkins, E.W. Jr. et al. 1988. Transthoracic esophagectomy: a safe approach to carcinoma of the esophagus. *Ann. Thorac. Surg.* 45:137-43.

McCaughan, J.S. Jr.; Williams, T.E. Jr.; and Bethel, B.H. 1985. Palliation of esophageal malignancy with photodynamic therapy. *Ann. Thorac. Surg.* 40:113-20.

McGlashan, N.D.; Walters, C.L.; and McLean, A.E. 1968. Nitrosamines in African alcoholic spirits and oesophageal cancer. *Lancet* II:1017.

Naef, A.P.; Savary, M.; and Ozzello, L. 1975. Columnar-lined lower esophagus: an acquired lesion with malignant predisposition. Report on 140 cases of Barrett's esophagus with 12 adenocarcinomas. *J. Thorac. Cardiovasc. Surg.* 70:826-35.

Orringer, M.B. 1984. Transhiatal esophagectomy without thoracotomy for carcinoma of the thoracic esophagus. *Ann. Surg.* 200:282-88.

Pearson, J.G. 1969. The value of radiotherapy in the management of esophageal cancer. *AJR* 105:500-13.

Poplion, E.; Fleming, T.; and Leichman, L. et al. 1987. Combined therapies for squamous-cell carcinoma of the esophagus: a Southwest Oncology Group Study (SWOG-8037). *J. Clin. Oncol.* 5:622-28.

Rider, W.D., and Diaz Mendoza, R. 1969. Some opinions on treatment of cancer of the esophagus. *AJR* 105:514-17.

Rowland, C.G., and Pagliero, K.M. 1985. Intracavitary irradiation in palliation of carcinoma of the esophagus and cardia. *Lancet* II:981-83.

Silverberg, E.; Boring, C.C.; and Squires, T. 1990. Cancer statistics 1990. *CA* 40:7-24.

Skinner, D.B.; Walther, B.C.; and Riddell, R.H. et al. 1983. Barrett's esophagus: comparison of benign and malignant cases. *Ann. Surg.* 198:554-56.

Sprung, D.J.; Ellis, F.H. Jr.; and Gibb, S.P. 1984. Incidence of adenocarcinoma in Barrett's esophagus (Abstr). *Am. J. Gastroenterol.* 79:817.

Tuyns, A.J.; Péquignot, G.; and Jensen, D.M. 1979. Role of diet, alcohol, and tobacco in oesophageal cancer as illustrated by two contrasting high-incidence areas in the north of Iran and west of France. *Front. Gastrointest. Res.* 4:101-10.

Van den Brandt-Grädel, V.; den Hartog Jager, F.C.A.; and Tytgat, G.N.J. 1987. Palliative intubation of malignant esophagogastric obstruction. *J. Clin. Gastroenterol.* 9:290-97.

Vogl, S.E.; Greenwald, E.; and Kaplan, B.H. 1981. Effective chemotherapy for esophageal cancer with methotrexate, bleomycin, and cis-diamminedichloroplatinum II. *Cancer* 48:2555-58.

Wara, W.; Mauch, P.; and Thomas, A. 1965. Palliation for carcinoma of esophagus. *Radiology* 85:952-55.

Wychulis, A.R.; Woolam, G.L.; and Andersen, H.A. et al. 1971. Achalasia and carcinoma of the esophagus. *JAMA* 115:1638-41.

Wynder, E.L., and Bross, L.J. 1961. A study of etiological factors in cancer of the esophagus. *Cancer* 14:389-413.

Yang, C.S. 1988. Research on esophageal cancer in China: a review. *Cancer Res.* 40:2633-44.

Chapter 20

MALIGNANT MELANOMA

Sonja Eva Singletary, M.D.
Charles M. Balch, M.D.

Sonja Eva Singletary, M.D.
Assistant Professor of Surgery
Department of General Surgery
The University of Texas
M.D. Anderson Cancer Center
Houston, Texas

Charles M. Balch, M.D.
Head, Division of Surgery
Chairman, Department of General Surgery
The University of Texas
M.D. Anderson Cancer Center
Houston, Texas

INTRODUCTION

Melanomas develop from the malignant transformation of the melanocyte, a cell of neural crest origin that produces the pigment melanin. Although melanoma currently represents only 1% to 3% of all cancers in the United States, the incidence of melanoma has been increasing by an average of 5% per year. In 1990, an estimated 27,600 new cases of and 6,300 deaths from melanoma will occur in the United States (Silverberg, Boring, and Squires 1990). Melanoma is a potentially curable cancer if it is diagnosed and properly treated at an early stage (Balch et al. 1983). Increased awareness of suspicious skin lesions, by both physicians and the public, and a simple physical examination can change the natural history of this disease. A national survey of 4,545 melanoma patients treated during 1980 demonstrated that 87% had clinically localized disease. In 39% of these patients, the melanomas were less than 0.76 mm thick, a size associated with a 95% or greater cure rate (Balch et al. 1984).

RISK FACTORS

One of the most important risk factors for melanoma is a recent change in a mole (Milton, Balch, and Shaw 1985). A change in the mole's color, diameter, or borders is the most common sign, occurring in over 70% of thin and curable melanomas. Bleeding, ulceration, or tenderness are usually late changes that indicate a more advanced melanoma (Sober et al. 1983). Itching is a nonspecific symptom that may attract the patient's attention to a previously unnoticed lesion.

Melanoma is 80% more frequent among whites than nonwhites. Melanoma lesions in nonwhite races are often in unusual sites such as the palmar surface of the hand, plantar surface of the foot, and in the mucous membranes.

The incidence of melanoma rises with increasing age; it is unusual in infants and young children, with an annual risk of less than 1 per 1,000,000 population (Rhodes et al. 1987). The peak age of incidence is in the fourth decade, without a sex prevalence. A patient with melanoma has a 3% to 5% risk of developing a second primary melanoma (Tucker, Boice, and Hoffman 1985). A familial history of melanoma increases a relative's risk by two to eight times (Holman and Armstrong 1984; Duggleby et al. 1981).

Dysplastic moles are usually large (>5 mm diameter) lesions with irregular pigmentation and borders. The presence of dysplastic moles, particularly in a patient with a familial tendency to melanoma, has a seven-fold to 70-fold increased risk factor for melanoma (Kraemer et al. 1986).

Congenital moles are pigmented nevi that are present at birth. The relative lifetime risk for developing melanoma in very large congenital moles is estimated to be 6.3%. The melanoma risk associated with small congenital moles is controversial (Rhodes et al. 1981).

An increased incidence of melanoma has been reported in renal transplant recipients (Greene, Young, and Clark 1981) and in patients with leukemia and lymphoma. In these patients, incidence is probably related to immunosuppression (Tucker et al. 1985).

Men or women with fair complexions (especially those with red hair) and a tendency to sunburn after relatively brief exposure to bright sunlight have a two-fold to three-fold increased risk of developing melanoma (Beral et al. 1983).

An association between melanoma and early childhood

exposure to excessive sun has been suggested based on patterns of migration to high-risk geographic areas (Cooke and Fraser 1985).

GROWTH PATTERNS

The four major kinds of melanomas based on growth patterns are: superficial spreading melanomas, nodular melanomas, lentigo maligna melanomas, and acral lentiginous melanomas (McGovern and Murad 1985). Each has unique clinical features and specific histological appearances.

SUPERFICIAL SPREADING MELANOMAS

Superficial spreading melanomas generally arise in a pre-existing nevus and constitute approximately 70% of all melanomas (Clark et al. 1975). The typical clinical history is a slowly evolving change of the precursor lesion over several years, followed by a rapid growth phase. Superficial spreading melanomas are predominantly flat because of a radial (horizontal) growth pattern. With penetration of the deeper layers of the dermis (vertical growth), the melanoma's surface may become more elevated and irregular. The characteristic appearance is a deeply pigmented lesion with variegated colors ranging from black, brown, or reddish-pink to white patches of regression. The melanoma's periphery is often notched or indented due to the lesion's expansion.

NODULAR MELANOMAS

Nodular melanomas are more aggressive tumors that commonly arise without evidence of a pre-existing lesion. They occur in 15% to 30% of melanoma patients and are seen more often in men than women. Histologically, the growth is vertical into the dermis without a radial component. Nodular melanomas are usually blue-black in color but may lack any pigment (amelanotic). Lesions that are polypoid, with a stalk or cauliflower appearance, are particularly virulent (Manci et al. 1981).

LENTIGO MALIGNA MELANOMAS

Lentigo maligna melanomas make up only 4% to 10% of melanomas and are typically located on the face in older Caucasians (McGovern et al. 1980). They are generally larger than 3 cm, and are flat, tan-colored lesions that have been present for many years. The lesion's borders are usually indented with prominent notching. The histological diagnosis of lentigo maligna requires the concomitant presence of severe changes in both the epidermis and dermis from sun exposure.

ACRAL LENTIGINOUS MELANOMAS

Acral lentiginous melanomas occur on the palms of the hands, soles of the feet, or beneath the nailbeds. Although this growth pattern makes up only 2% to 8% of melanomas in Caucasians, it constitutes 35% to 60% of melanomas in dark-skinned patients (Krementz et al. 1982). Acral lentiginous melanomas resemble tan or brown flat stains with very irregular borders on the palms or soles.

Subungual melanomas appear as brown to black discolorations under the nailbed, usually that of the great toe or the thumb. Ulceration is common in neglected lesions and is often mistaken for a fungal infection.

DIAGNOSIS

Any lesion that changes in size, contour, configuration, or color should be considered a possible melanoma and be biopsied. The biopsy, either excisional or by a core-punch technique, must adequately represent the full tumor's thickness and level of invasion into the various skin layers. This histopathological feature of the melanoma is critically important in predicting the risk of subsequent metastases and in determining the appropriate clinical management. Shave biopsies or electrodesiccation of a suspected melanoma are to be condemned.

STAGING

After biopsy, the pathologist measures the melanoma's thickness (Breslow's microstaging) and determines the level of invasion (Clark's microstaging).

Breslow's system (Breslow 1970) is the quantitative assessment of the maximum tumor thickness in millimeters as measured by an ocular micrometer. This technique is more reproducible and has been shown to correlate accurately with the risk of metastatic disease and prognosis.

Clark's system (Clark et al. 1969) categorizes five levels of invasion that reflect increasing depth of penetration into the underlying dermis or subcutaneous tissue. In Clark's Level I, the melanoma is confined to the epidermis above the basement membrane. After adequate excision, a Level I lesion never metastasizes. Clark's Level II shows invasion through the basement membrane into the papillary dermis; Level III has tumor cells at the junction of the papillary and reticular dermis; Level IV lesions extend into the reticular dermis; and Level V has penetration through to the subcutaneous fat. Reported mortality figures are: Level II lesions 8.3%; Level III lesions 35%; Level IV lesions 46%; and Level V lesions 55%.

The new staging system adopted by the American Joint Committee on Cancer (table 20.1) is based on the tumor microstaging of the primary melanoma and the known pattern of metastases (Ketcham and Balch 1985). The most common first site of metastases is the regional lymphatic nodal basin. Melanoma cells may also become entrapped within dermal lymphatics near the primary tumor (satellites) or between the primary tumor and regional lymph nodes (intransits). In stages I

Table 20.1
STAGING OF MELANOMA
(AMERICAN JOINT COMMITTEE ON CANCER)

Stage	Criteria
IA	Localized melanoma <0.75 mm or Level II* (T_1, N_0, M_0)
IB	Localized melanoma 0.76 mm to 1.5 mm or Level III* (T_2, N_0, M_0)
IIA	Localized melanoma 1.5 mm to 4 mm or Level IV* (T_3, N_0, M_0)
IIB	Localized melanoma >4 mm or Level V* (T_4, N_0, M_0)
III	Limited nodal metastases involving only one regional lymph node basin or <5 in-transit metastases but without nodal metastases (any T, N_1, M_0)
IV	Advanced regional metastases (any T, N_2, M_0) or any patient with distant metastases (any T, any N, M_1 or M_2)

*When the thickness and level of invasion criteria do not coincide within a T classification, thickness of lesion should take precedence.

and II, patients have clinically localized disease subdivided into A and B according to microstaging (thickness and level). Stage III patients have nodal metastases in a single lymph node basin, whereas stage IV patients have one of the following: (1) distant metastases; (2) nodal metastases involving two or more lymph node basins; (3) >5 in-transit metastases; or (4) nodal metastases either >5 cm in diameter or fixed.

EVALUATION FOR METASTASES

The most important initial evaluation for metastases is a complete medical history and physical examination. Although melanoma can metastasize to virtually any organ or tissue, knowledge of the patterns of metastases will help focus on the site most likely to harbor disease. The regional lymph nodes are the most common site of metastases, followed by skin, subcutaneous tissue, and lung (Balch and Milton 1985). Other potential areas of spread are the liver, bone, and brain. In the absence of symptoms or signs of metastases, a minimum number of laboratory and radiological tests should be ordered because the diagnostic yield is low and not cost-effective. A preoperative metastatic survey should include the following:

1. Physical examination and biopsy of suspected subcutaneous or skin metastasis or a second primary melanoma;

2. Chest x-ray for possible asymptomatic lung metastases. If suggestive of spread, this should be confirmed by lung tomograms or computed tomography (CT) scan;

3. Serum alkaline phosphatase and lactic dehydrogenase levels to evaluate possible hepatic involvement. If elevated or if symptoms of weight loss, anorexia, and upper abdominal pain are present, a liver ultrasound (US) or abdominal CT scan should be obtained;

4. Complete medical history and physical examination for possible brain involvement (symptoms of headache, signs of numbness, motor weakness) followed by brain CT scan if clinically indicated; and

5. Serum alkaline phosphatase analysis and bone scan for localized bone pain.

Routine CT scans or magnetic resonance imaging (MRI) studies in asymptomatic early stage melanoma are not cost-effective and should be done only when clinical signs or symptoms of occult metastases are present. For example, if the complete blood cell (CBC) count suggests anemia then further evaluation to detect blood loss secondary to gastrointestinal metastases should be done.

Clinical follow-up after the treatment of melanoma is based on the same principle. The frequency of clinic visits is dictated by the tumor thickness. For thin melanomas (<1 mm), biannual examinations should be sufficient because the risk of metastases is low. For thicker melanomas (>1 mm), the patient should be examined more frequently: every three to four months during the first two years, every six months until five years, and then once a year throughout the patient's lifetime.

PRINCIPLES OF TREATMENT

The surgical management of melanoma is based on the knowledge of factors that predict the risk of local recurrence and metastatic disease and on the potential morbidity of the operation (table 20.2). In early stage melanoma, tumor thickness is the primary criterion in determining the surgical approach to the primary site and the regional nodes (Urist, Balch, and Milton 1985). For patients with clinical evidence of metastases in regional nodes or at solitary distant sites, surgery is still usually indicated for local disease control.

PRIMARY MELANOMA

Surgical treatment of any primary melanoma consists of a wide excision of the tumor or a previous biopsy site with a margin of normal-appearing skin. The surgical margins are determined by the tumor's thickness, which correlates with the biological risk of local recurrence. Although melanoma *in situ* (Clark's Level I or atypical melanocytic hyperplasia) is a noninvasive lesion, there is a risk of local recurrence; therefore, an excision with a 1 cm margin with primary skin closure is indicated. For melanoma of less than 1 mm thickness, a margin of 1 cm

Table 20.2
PRIMARY PROGNOSTIC PREDICTORS OF CLINICAL COURSE IN PATIENTS WITH MELANOMA

Clinical Stage	Unfavorable Predictors
Localized melanoma	
a) Tumor thickness	a) >1.5 mm
b) Ulceration	b) Present
c) Sex	c) Male
d) Location	d) Trunk
Regional metastases	
a) Number of metastatic nodes	a) >1
b) Ulceration of primary	b) Present
Distant metastases	
a) Location	a) Visceral
b) Number of sites	b) >1

to 2 cm of skin is adequate (Veronesi et al. 1988). For melanoma greater than 1 mm in thickness, a 3 cm to 4 cm margin of skin is removed to reduce the risk of local recurrence and satellitosis. Subungual melanomas beneath the fingernails or toenails are treated by amputation of the digit.

After adequate excision, the risk of local recurrence is very low (about 3%). Features of the primary melanoma that predict high risk of local recurrence are a thickness of at least 4 mm (13% incidence), ulceration (11%), or location on the foot, hand, or scalp (5% to 12%) (Urist et al. 1985).

CLINICALLY NORMAL REGIONAL LYMPH NODES

The efficacy of elective (immediate) prophylactic lymph-node dissection to remove suspected microscopic or clinically occult metastatic melanoma is still controversial (Balch et al. 1985). Because not all melanoma patients benefit from this surgical procedure, the question is whether a certain subset of patients can be identified that will have improved survival rates after elective lymph-node dissection compared to lymph-node dissection when nodal metastases have grown large enough to be palpated.

The thickness of the primary melanoma is a quantitative estimate of the risk for occult metastatic melanoma at regional and distant sites and may help in the selection of patients who might benefit from an elective node dissection. Melanomas less than 1 mm are usually localized and offer a 95% or greater 10-year survival rate. Therefore, an elective lymphadenectomy would not be of benefit. Melanomas of intermediate thickness (1 mm to 4 mm) present an increasing incidence (up to 60%) of occult regional metastases but a relatively low incidence (<20%) of distant metastases. Patients with these intermediate-thickness lesions may have improved survival after elective node dissection performed relatively early in the natural history of the nodal metastases, at the time when the tumor burden is generally less than several million cells. Patients with melanomas thicker than 4 mm have a high risk (>60%) of regional nodal micrometastases and also a high risk (>70%) of occult distant metastases. An elective node dissection in these patients would have little curative potential but may provide staging information for patients entering clinical trials of adjuvant therapy.

In addition to tumor thickness, other prognostic factors (presence or absence of ulceration, growth pattern of the lesion, patient's sex and age, anatomic location of the melanoma, operative risk) should be considered in determining whether an elective node dissection is indicated. Ulcerated melanomas have a higher rate of microscopic metastases and a 5-year survival of 55% compared to 80% for nonulcerated melanomas, even when matched for other predictive factors such as tumor thickness (Balch et al. 1980). A lentigo maligna melanoma has a low incidence of metastases and a patient with this type of growth pat-

tern would not benefit from an elective node dissection (Urist et al. 1984). Extremity melanomas in women have a more favorable outlook than equivalent-thickness melanomas of the extremities in men. Patients with melanomas on the trunk, head, and neck fare worse regardless of sex. Obese patients and older patients have an increased incidence of postoperative wound complications (Urist et al. 1983).

An elective node dissection can be of benefit for well-selected patients and can be performed with little morbidity and virtually no mortality if good surgical judgment and technique are used. An elective modified neck dissection spares the spinal accessory nerve and avoids limitation of shoulder function. Because it is difficult to define precisely the pathways of nodal drainage to various parts of the neck, a partial neck dissection is generally not performed. For primary melanomas located on the face, ear, or anterior scalp, the superficial portion of the parotid gland is also excised to remove the parotid lymph nodes. A standard radical axillary lymphadenectomy is performed for melanomas of the arm or upper trunk and has a postoperative morbidity of less than 5%. An inguinal node dissection for melanomas of the leg or lower trunk generally includes only the femoral nodes to minimize the risk of significant leg edema. If there are demonstrable metastases to the femoral nodes at the time of elective node dissection, extension of the surgery to remove the iliac and obturator nodes has been recommended. Because melanomas of the trunk have several nodal basins potentially at risk for harboring microscopic metastases, a radionuclide cutaneous scan is an accurate and reproducible method for determining the sites of lymphatic drainage (Logic and Balch 1985).

Several prospective but nonrandomized trials of elective node dissections for more than 2,000 stage I melanoma patients treated at the University of Alabama in Birmingham, the University of Sydney, Australia, and the Duke Medical Center in North Carolina have demonstrated an improved survival rate in patients with intermediate thickness (1 mm to 4 mm) melanomas (Balch et al. 1982; Reintgen et al. 1983). The results from the Alabama and Australia data show an increased survival rate for patients with intermediate thickness melanomas of the trunk, head, and neck. The benefit of elective node dissection was greater in men than in women with extremity melanomas.

Randomized prospective studies from the World Health Organization (WHO) and from the Mayo Clinic did not show any increased survival for patients with melanomas of the extremities who had elective node dissections compared with similar patients treated by wide excision alone (Veronesi et al. 1982; Sim et al. 1978). However, it has been suggested that a small subgroup of patients in the WHO Melanoma Group Study may have benefited from an elective node dissection (Balch et al. 1985). Because the results of these randomized trials have not been completely accepted due to the stratification criteria used, a new randomized prospective analysis of elective node dissection for intermediate-thickness melanomas at all sites is being done by cooperative cancer centers in the United States and Canada. The WHO Melanoma Group has also initiated a randomized prospective trial for melanomas of the trunk.

CLINICALLY ENLARGED REGIONAL LYMPH NODES

Radical excision of the regional lymph nodes is the treatment of choice for patients with suspected or proven nodal metastases (Balch et al. 1981; Ames and Singletary 1985). When possible, an in-continuity lymph node dissection should be performed by excising all the intervening lymphatics and soft tissue between the primary melanoma and the regional nodes to decrease the risk of satellite (in-transit) metastases. Patients with clinical nodal metastases have an 85% chance of having occult distant metastases and the survival rate at 10 years is only 25% to 30% (Singletary et al. 1988; Singletary et al. 1986).

To date, adjuvant therapy for melanoma has not been proven to be beneficial and remains a critical area of investigation (Balch and Hersey 1985). In randomized trials, chemotherapeutic agents with established activity against advanced melanomas, imidazole carboxamide (DTIC) and the nitrosoureas, have not increased survival either as single agents or in combination therapy (Hill et al. 1981; Qualiana et al. 1980; Banzet et al. 1978). Randomized studies of immunomodulatory agents like bacillus Calmette-Guérin (BCG), *Corynebacterium parvum*, levamisole, and transfer factor also showed no activity alone or with chemotherapy (Balch and Hersey 1985; Veronesi et al. 1982). Nonrandomized adjuvant trials with melanoma-specific tumor cell vaccines suggest encouraging results and are being investigated in phase III clinical trials (Cassel, Murray, and Phillips 1983; Hersey et al. 1986).

IN-TRANSIT METASTASES

In-transit or satellite metastases arise in the lymphatics or soft tissue between the primary site of the melanoma and the regional lymph nodes. The incidence of in-transit metastases is approximately 2% to 3%. Favorable prognostic factors include: patients who are women; the location of in-transit metastases within the skin rather than in the subcutaneous tissue; a small number of in-transit metastases; and the presence of regional nodal metastases (Singletary, Tucker, and Boddie 1988; Balch et al. 1985).

Isolated limb perfusion with chemotherapy and hyperthermia is probably the most effective treatment for extremity lesions (Krementz et al. 1985). Surgical excision may be used for one or only a few lesions. Radiation therapy may be used for multiple lesions involving the trunk, head, and neck. Intralesional immunotherapy with agents like BCG has had some success.

Systemic chemotherapy with DTIC alone or with other drugs has shown little effect in controlling the disease.

Although most patients with in-transit metastases later develop systemic metastases, with median survival rates ranging from 19 months to 42 months, an aggressive regional treatment of in-transit metastases may offer significant palliation and give the best long-term results for some patients.

DISTANT METASTASES

The treatment goals for distant metastases are symptomatic relief, prolongation of life, and clinical staging to determine subsequent treatment. The anticipated benefit of treatment should exceed the toxic effects and risk. Treatment options depend on the sites and number of metastases, growth rate, previous treatment, and the patient's age, overall condition, and desires (Balch and Milton 1985).

METHODS OF TREATMENT

SURGERY

Surgical excision of metastatic melanoma often provides the most effective and the longest-lasting palliation (Wornom et al. 1986). The obvious limitation of surgery is that it is a local form of treatment, and the patient could eventually succumb to metastatic disease elsewhere. Surgery should, therefore, be confined to lesions that are accessible and limited in number and to patients on whom the operation can be performed safely.

RADIATION THERAPY

Radiation therapy will relieve bone pain from metastases, usually within one week. Cranial and spinal cord irradiation combined with dexamethasone therapy often effectively palliates central nervous system metastases. High-energy radiation therapy may control superficial metastases in the skin or soft tissue. A high-dose, low-fraction radiation schedule (e.g., 6 Gy given twice a week for 3 weeks) is important (Overgaard et al. 1986).

CHEMOTHERAPY

DTIC is considered the standard single agent to be used, but response rates average only 15% to 20% in most series (Hill, Krementz, and Hill 1984). Responses are seen most frequently in patients with skin, subcutaneous tissue, lymph node, and lung metastases. Unfortunately, the mean duration of responses is only four to six months.

Combinations of drugs have not been superior to DTIC alone. Initial encouraging results using a combination of cisplatin, vinblastine, and bleomycin (PVB) were not confirmed in randomized studies that compared PVB with DTIC alone (Luikart, Kennealey, and Kirkwood 1984). The addition of immunomodulators such as BCG or levamisole to combination chemotherapy has also shown no advantage (Costanzi et al. 1982; Costanzi et al. 1984). Recently, phase II trials have reported high response rates with cisplatin combinations, particularly in patients with liver metastases (Legha et al. 1988). These results need to be confirmed in randomized controlled studies.

IMMUNOTHERAPY

The lack of effective chemotherapy for metastatic melanoma and the development of recombinant DNA technology have led to the investigation of a variety of immunological and biological agents. Recombinant alpha-interferon has produced response rates of 10% to 20%, with an occasional long-term complete response observed (Creagan et al. 1986). Clinical trials with interleukin-2 (IL-2) and adoptive immunotherapy have also demonstrated antitumor activity. The protocol of the National Cancer Institute that uses a combination of high-dose injections of IL-2 and lymphokine-activated killer (LAK) cells has produced objective responses, including two complete responses, in six of 23 melanoma patients (Rosenberg et al. 1985). Confirmatory studies with IL-2 and LAK cells had similar results in six of 32 patients (Dutcher et al. 1987). Preliminary studies with high-dose IL-2 alone have shown responses in five of 16 patients treated with bolus injection (Rosenberg et al. 1987) and in five of 10 patients treated with continuous infusion (West et al. 1987). The toxic effects from high-dose IL-2 can be severe; oliguria, confusion, hypotension, cardiac arrhythmia, and myocardial infarction can occur. Further studies are needed to evaluate the efficacy of treatment with IL-2 plus LAK cells compared to IL-2 alone and to design the optimal doses and treatment schedules.

Animal model studies have shown tumor regression with a type of adoptive immunotherapy that uses lymphocytes isolated from tumor sites (tumor-infiltrating lymphocytes, or TIL) which are then further activated and expanded by IL-2. Substantial antitumor activity by TIL cells with lower doses of IL-2 were attained as compared to the response in animals treated with high-dose IL-2 and LAK cells (Rosenberg, Spiess, and Lafreniere 1986). Phase I trials using this approach are in progress.

Another area of investigation is the development of monoclonal antibodies directed against the antigens expressed on the surface of melanoma cells. These antibodies may then be used alone to activate the host immune system against the melanoma, or can be conjugated to a cytotoxic agent with direct delivery of the agent to the tumor site. Preliminary trials of IgG$_3$ subclass of unconjugated monoclonal antibodies against melanoma antigens, GD3 ganglioside and GD2 ganglioside, have produced partial responses in six of 30 patients studied (Houghton et al. 1986; Cheung et al. 1987). Toxic reactions were usually mild to moderate but the maximum tolerated dose is still undefined.

Monoclonal antibodies conjugated to radioisotopes, such as ^{131}I, are being evaluated for use in the detection of regional and distant metastases. The primary dose-limiting toxicity is from marrow irradiation resulting in thrombocytopenia and neutropenia (Larson et al. 1983). Antibodies have also been conjugated to the toxin ricin, a natural product of castor beans from the plant *Ricinus communis* and a potent inhibitor of protein synthesis. A phase II study of ricin-conjugated antibody resulted in one complete and three partial responses in 46 patients with melanoma (Spitler et al. 1987). The toxicity was mild, with flu-like symptoms and hepatic enzyme elevations.

The major therapeutic limitation of antimelanoma antibodies is the induction of an immune response against the antibody itself because most monoclonal antibodies are derived from mice. Currently, antibodies derived from humans or chimeric antibodies genetically constructed with the mouse antigen-binding regions ligated to human immunoglobulin sequences are being explored to eliminate the human antimouse response.

SUMMARY

A full-thickness biopsy of any cutaneous lesion that changes in size, color, contour, or configuration should be performed to establish the diagnosis and microstaging (tumor thickness, level of invasion, and ulceration). A complete history and physical examination, a chest x-ray, and liver function tests constitute the most important evaluative tests for metastases. Additional tests are to be obtained only if there are signs or symptoms suggestive of metastases.

The dominant prognostic factors for patients with localized melanoma are gender, tumor thickness, ulceration, and the site of the primary lesion. The most predictive factors for patients with regional node metastases are the number of metastatic nodes and ulceration of the primary tumor. The number and site of metastases were the most predictive for distant disease.

The treatment of primary melanoma is surgical excision with a margin of 1 cm to 2 cm of normal skin for thin melanomas and a margin of 2 cm to 3 cm for intermediate and thick lesions. A regional lymph-node dissection is indicated for clinically involved nodes and may be of benefit in selected patients with clinically normal nodes who have intermediate thickness melanoma (1 mm to 4 mm). Surgical excision of isolated and accessible distant metastases provides effective palliation. Radiation therapy should be considered for bone, brain, skin, and soft-tissue metastases. Response rates are usually low and of short duration after chemotherapy. Recent clinical trials using immunotherapy, however, appear promising.

REFERENCES

Ames, F.C., and Singletary, S.E. 1985. Cutaneous malignancies of the trunk and lower extremities. In Johnson, D.E., and Ames, F.C. eds. *Atlas of groin dissection*. pp. 111-36. Chicago: Year Book Medical Publishers.

Balch, C.M.; Soong, S.-J.; and Milton, G.W. et al. 1983. Changing trends in cutaneous melanoma over a quarter century in Alabama, USA, and New South Wales, Australia. *Cancer* 52(9):1748-53.

Balch, C.M.; Karakousis, C.; and Mettlin, C. et al. 1984. Management of cutaneous melanoma in the United States. *Surg. Gynecol. Obstet.* 158(4):311-18.

Balch, C.M., and Milton, G.W. 1985. Treatment for advanced metastatic melanoma. In Balch, C.M., and Milton, G.W. eds. *Cutaneous melanoma: clinical management and treatment results worldwide.* pp. 251-73. Philadelphia: J.B. Lippincott.

Balch, C.M., and Milton, G.W. 1985. Diagnosis of metastatic melanoma at distant sites. In Balch, C.M., and Milton, G.W. eds. *Cutaneous melanoma: clinical management and treatment results worldwide.* pp. 221-50. Philadelphia: J.B. Lippincott.

Balch, C.M.; Soong, S.-J.; and Milton, G.W. et al. 1982. A comparison of prognostic factors and surgical results in 1,786 patients with localized (stage I) melanoma treated in Alabama, USA, and New South Wales, Australia. *Ann. Surg.* 196(6):677-84.

Balch, C.M.; Wilkerson; J.A.; and Murad, T.M. et al. 1980 The prognostic significance of ulceration of cutaneous melanoma. *Cancer* 45(12):3012-17.

Balch, C.M.; Cascinelli, N.; and Milton, G.W. et al. 1985. Elective lymph node dissection: pros and cons. In Balch, C.M., and Milton, G.W. eds. *Cutaneous melanoma: clinical management and treatment results worldwide.* pp 131-57. Philadelphia: J.B. Lippincott.

Balch, C.M.; Soong, S.-J.; and Murad, T.M.; et al. 1981. A multifactorial analysis of melanoma, III: prognostic factors in melanoma patients with lymph node metastases (stage II). *Ann. Surg.* 193:377-88.

Balch, C.M.; Urist, M.M.; and Maddox, W.A. et al. 1985. Management of regional metastatic melanoma. In Balch, C.M., and Milton, G.W. eds. *Cutaneous melanoma: clinical management and treatment results worldwide.* pp. 93-130. Philadelphia: J.B. Lippincott.

Balch, C.M., and Hersey, P. 1985. Current status of adjuvant therapy. In Balch, C.M., and Milton, G.W. eds. *Cutaneous melanoma: clinical management and treatment results worldwide.* pp 197-218. Philadelphia: J.B. Lippincott.

Banzet, P.; Jacquillat, C.; and Livatte, J. et al. 1978. Adjuvant chemotherapy in the management of primary malignant melanoma. *Cancer* 41:1240-48.

Beral, V.; Evans, S.; and Shaw, H. et al. 1983 Cutaneous factors related to the risk of malignant melanoma. *Br. J. Dermatol.* 109(2):165-72.

Breslow, A. 1970. Thickness, cross-sectional areas, and depth of invasion in the prognosis of cutaneous melanoma. *Ann. Surg.* 172:902-8.

Cassel, W.A.; Murray, D.R.; and Phillips, H.S. 1983. A phase II study on the postsurgical management of stage II malignant melanoma with a Newcastle disease virus oncolysate. *Cancer* 52:856-60.

Cheung, K.; Lazarus H.; and Miraldi, F.D. et al. 1987. Ganglioside GD2-specific monoclonal antibody 3F8: a phase I study in patients with neuroblastoma and malignant melanoma. *J. Clin. Oncol.* 5(9):1430-40.

Clark, W.H. Jr.; From, L.; and Bernardino, E.A. et al. 1969. The histogenesis and biologic behavior of primary human malignant melanomas of the skin. *Cancer Res.* 29:705-26.

Clark, W.H. Jr.; Ainsworth, A.M.; and Bernardino, E.A. et al. 1975. The developmental biology of primary human malignant melanoma. *Semin. Oncol.* 2:83-103.

Cooke, K.R., and Fraser, J. 1985. Migration and death from malignant melanoma. *Int. J. Cancer* 36:175-78.

Costanzi, J.J.; Fletcher, W.S.; and Balcerzak, S.P. et al. 1984. Combination chemotherapy plus levamisole in the treat-ment of disseminated malignant melanoma: a Southwest Oncology Group study. *Cancer* 53:833-36.

Costanzi, J.J.; Al-Sarrafg, M.; and Groppe, C. et al. 1982. Combination chemotherapy plus BCG in the treatment of disseminated malignant melanoma: a Southwest Oncology Group study. *Med. Pediatr. Oncol.* 10:251-58.

Creagan, E.T.; Ahman, D.L.; and Frytak, S. et al. 1986. Recombinant leukocyte A interferon (rIFN-Alpha A) in the treatment of disseminated malignant melanoma: anal-ysis of complete and long-term responding patients. *Cancer* 58:2576-78.

Duggleby, W.F.; Stoll, H.; and Priore, R.L. et al. 1981. A genetic analysis of melanoma: polygenetic inheritance as a threshold trait. *Am. J. Epidemiol.* 114:63-72.

Dutcher, J.P.; Creekmore, S.; and Weiss, G.R. et al. 1987. Phase II study of high-dose interleukin-2 and lymphokine-activated killer cells in patients with melanoma. *Proc. Am. Soc. Clin. Oncol.* 6:970.

Greene, M.H.; Young, T.I.; and Clark, W.H. Jr. 1981. Malig-nant melanoma in renal transplant recipients. *Lancet* I: 1196-99.

Hersey, P.; Edwards, A.; and Coates, A. et al. 1986. Evidence that treatment with vaccinia melanoma cell lysates (VMCL) may improve survival of patients with stage II melanoma. *Cancer Immunol. Immunother.* 25:257-65.

Hill, G.J. Jr.; Krementz, E.T.; and Hill, H.Z. 1984. Dimethyl-triazenoimidazole carboxamide and combination therapy for melanoma, IV: late results after complete response to chemotherapy. *Cancer* 53:1299-1305.

Hill, G.J.; Moss, S.E.; and Golomb, F.M. et al. 1981. DTIC and combination therapy for melanoma, III: DTIC (NSC 45388) surgical adjuvant study COG Protocol 7040. *Cancer* 47:2556-62.

Holman, C.D.J., and Armstrong, B.K. 1984. Pigmentary traits, ethnic origin, benign nevi, and familial history as risk factors for cutaneous malignant melanoma. *J. Natl. Cancer Inst.* 72:257-66.

Houghton, A.N.; Vadhan, S.; and Wong, G. et al. 1986. Clinical study of a mouse monoclonal antibody directed against GD3 ganglioside in patients with melanoma. *Proc. Am. Soc. Clin. Oncol.* 5:231.

Ketcham, A.S., and Balch, C.M. 1985. Classification and staging systems. In Balch, C.M., and Milton, G.W. eds. *Cutaneous melanoma: clinical management and treatment results worldwide.* pp. 55-62. Philadelphia: J.B. Lippincott.

Kraemer, K.H.; Tucker, M.; and Tarone, R. et al. 1986. Risk of cutaneous melanoma in dysplastic nevus syndrome types A and B. *N. Engl. J. Med.* 315:1615-16.

Krementz, E.T.; Reed, R.J.; and Coleman, W.P. et al. 1982. Acral lentiginous melanoma: a clinicopathologic entity. *Ann. Surg.* 195:632-45.

Krementz, E.T.; Ryan, R.F.; and Carter, R.D. et al. 1985. Hyperthermic regional perfusion for melanoma of the limbs. In Balch, C.M., and Milton, G.W. eds. *Cutaneous melanoma: clinical management and treatment results world-wide.* pp. 171-95. Philadelphia: J.B. Lippincott.

Larson, S.M.; Carrasquillo, J.A.; and Krohn, K.A. et al. 1983. Localization of ^{131}I-labeled p97-specific Fab fragments in human melanoma as a basis for radiotherapy. *J. Clin. Invest.* 72:2101-14.

Legha, S.; Ring, S.; and Plager, C. et al. 1988. Evaluation of a triple drug regime containing cisplatinum (C), vinblastine (V), and DTIC (D) in patients (PTS) with metastatic melanoma. *Proc. Am. Soc. Clin. Oncol.* 7:250.

Logic, J.R., and Balch, C.M. 1985. Defining lymphatic drain-age patterns with cutaneous lymphoscintigraphy. In Balch, C.M., and Milton, G.W. eds. *Cutaneous melanoma: clinical management and treatment results worldwide.* pp 159-70. Philadelphia: J.B. Lippincott.

Luikart, S.D.; Kennealey, G.T.; and Kirkwood, J.M. 1984. Randomized phase III trial of vinblastine, bleomycin, and cis-dichlorodiammine-platinum versus dacarbazine in malignant melanoma. *J. Clin. Oncol.* 2:164-68.

Manci, E.A.; Balch, C.M.; and Murad, T.M. et al. 1981. Polypoid melanoma, a virulent variant of the nodular growth pattern. *Am. J. Clin. Pathol.* 75:810-15.

McGovern, V.J.; Shaw, H.M.; and Milton, G.W. et al. 1980. Is malignant melanoma arising in a Hutchinson's melanotic freckle a separate entity? *Histopathology* 4:235-42.

McGovern, V.J., and Murad, T.M. 1985. Pathology of melanoma: an overview. In Balch, C.M., and Milton, G.W. eds. *Cutaneous melanoma: clinical management and treatment results worldwide.* pp. 29-53. Philadelphia: J.B. Lippincott.

Milton, G.W.; Balch, C.M.; Shaw, H.M. 1985. Clinical characteristics. In Balch, C.M., and Milton, G.W. eds. *Cutaneous melanoma: clinical management and treatment results worldwide.* pp. 13-28. Philadelphia: J.B. Lippincott.

Overgaard, J.; Overgaard, M.; and Hansen, V. et al. 1986. Some factors of importance in the radiation treatment of malignant melanoma. *Radiother. Oncol.* 5:183-92.

Qualiana, J.; Tranum, B.; and Neidhardt, J. et al. 1980. Adjuvant chemotherapy with BCNU, hydrea and DTIC (BHD) with or without immunotherapy (BCG) in high-risk melanoma patients. *Proc. Am. Assoc. Cancer Res.* 21:399.

Reintgen, D.S.; Cox, E.B.; and McCarty, K.S. Jr. et al. 1983. Efficacy of elective lymph node dissection in patients with intermediate thickness primary melanoma. *Ann. Surg.* 198(3):379-85.

Rhodes, A.R.; Wood, W.C.; and Sober, A.J. et al. 1981. Nonepidermal origin of malignant melanoma associated with a giant congenital nevocellular nevus. *Plast. Reconstr. Surg.* 67:782-90.

Rhodes, A.R.; Weinstock, M.A.; and Fitzpatrick, T.B. et al. 1987. Risk factors for cutaneous melanoma: a practical method of recognizing predisposed individuals. *JAMA* 258:3146-54.

Rosenberg, S.A.; Spiess, P.J.; and Lafreniere, R. 1986. A new approach to adoptive immunotherapy of cancer with tumor-infiltrating lymphocytes. *Science* 233:1318-21.

Rosenberg, S.A.; Lotze, M.T.; and Muul, L.M. et al. 1985. Special report: observations in the systemic administration of autologous lymphokine-activated killer cells and recombinant interleukin-2 to patients with metastatic cancer. *N. Engl. J. Med.* 313:1485-92.

Rosenberg, S.A.; Lotze, M.T.; and Muul, L.M. et al. 1987. A progress report on the treatment of 157 patients with advanced cancer using lymphokine-activated killer cells and interleukin-2 or high-dose interleukin-2 alone. *N. Engl. J. Med.* 316:889-97.

Silverberg, E.; Boring, C.C.; and Squires, T.S. 1990. Cancer statistics. *CA* 40:9.

Sim, F.H.; Taylor, W.F.; and Ivins, J.C. et al. 1978. A prospective randomized study of the efficacy of routine elective lymphadenectomy in management of malignant melanoma: preliminary results. *Cancer* 41(3):948-56.

Singletary, S.E.; Shallenberger, R.; and Guinee, V.F. et al. 1988. Melanoma with metastasis to regional axillary or inguinal lymph nodes: prognostic factors and results of surgical treatment in 714 patients. *South. Med. J.* 81:5-9.

Singletary, S.E.; Byers, R.M.; and Shallenberger, R. 1986. Prognostic factors in patients with regional cervical nodal metastases from cutaneous malignant melanoma. *Am. J. Surg.* 152:371-75.

Singletary, S.E.; Tucker, S.L.; and Boddie, A.W. Jr. 1988. Multivariate analysis of prognostic factors in regional cutaneous metastases of extremity melanoma. *Cancer* 61:1437-40.

Sober, A.J.; Day, C.L.; and Kopff, A.N. et al. 1983. Detection of "thin" primary melanoma. *Cancer* 33:160-63.

Spitler, L.E.; Del Rio, M.; and Khentigan, A. et al. 1987. Therapy of patients with malignant melanoma using a monoclonal antimelanoma antibody ricin A chain immunotoxin. *Cancer Res.* 47:1717-23.

Tucker, M.A.; Boice, J.D.; and Hoffman, D.A. 1985. Second cancer following cutaneous melanoma and cancers of the brain, thyroid, connective tissue, bone, and eye in Connecticut, 1935-1982. *NCI Monogr.* 68:161-89.

Tucker, M.A.; Misfeldt, D.; and Coleman, C.N. et al. 1985. Cutaneous malignant melanoma after Hodgkin's disease. *Ann. Intern. Med.* 102:37-41.

Urist, M.M.; Balch, C.M.; and Soong, S.-J. et al. 1984. Head and neck melanoma in 534 clinical stage I patients: a prognostic factors analysis and results of surgical treatment. *Ann. Surg.* 200(6):769-75.

Urist, M.M.; Balch, C.M.; and Milton, G.W. 1985. Surgical management of the primary melanoma. In Balch, C.M., and Milton, G.W. eds. *Cutaneous melanoma: clinical management and treatment results worldwide.* pp. 71-90. Philadelphia: J.B. Lippincott.

Urist, M.M.; Maddox, W.A.; and Kennedy, J.E. et al. 1983. Patient risk factors and surgical morbidity after regional lymphadenectomy in 204 melanoma patients. *Cancer* 51(11):2152-56.

Urist, M.M.; Balch, C.M.; and Soong, S.-J. et al. 1985. The influence of surgical margins and prognostic factors predicting the risk of local recurrence in 3,445 patients with primary cutaneous melanoma. *Cancer* 55(6):1398-1402.

Veronesi, U.; Adamus, J.; and Bandiera, D.C. et al. 1982. Delayed regional lymph node dissection for stage I melanoma of the skin of the lower extremities. *Cancer* 49(11):2420-30.

Veronesi, U.; Adamus, J.; and Aubert, C. et al. 1982. A randomized trial of adjuvant chemotherapy and immunotherapy in cutaneous melanoma. *N. Engl. J. Med.* 307:913-16.

Veronesi, U.; Cascinelli, N.; and Adamus, J. et al. 1988. Thin stage I primary cutaneous malignant melanoma: comparison of excision with margins of 1 or 3 cm. *N. Engl. J. Med.* 318:1159.

Wallack, M.K.; Bask, J.A.; and Leftheriotis, E. et al. 1986. The positive relationship of clinical and serologic responses to vaccinia melanoma oncolysates. *Cancer* 57:649-55.

West, W.H.; Tauer, K.W.; and Yannelli, J.R. et al. 1987. Constant infusion recombinant interleukin-2 adoptive immunotherapy of advanced cancer. *N. Engl. J. Med.* 316:898-905.

Wornom, I.L.; Smith, J.N.; and Soong, S.-J. et al. 1986. Surgery as palliative treatment for distant metastases of melanoma. *Ann. Surg.* 204:181-85.

Chapter 21

UROLOGIC AND MALE GENITAL CANCERS

Irwin N. Frank, M.D.
Sam D. Graham, Jr., M.D.
William L. Nabors, M.D.

Irwin N. Frank, M.D.
Professor of Urology
The University of Rochester School of Medicine and Dentistry
Rochester, New York

Sam D. Graham, Jr., M.D.
Chief of Urology
The Emory Clinic
Atlanta, Georgia

William L. Nabors, M.D.
Assistant Professor
Department of Urology
The Emory Clinic
Atlanta, Georgia

PERSPECTIVE

Neoplasms occurring in the urinary tract and in the male genital tract are among the most common malignancies. It is estimated that they will account for approximately 32% of new cancers (excluding nonmelanoma skin cancer) occurring in men during 1990 (Cancer Statistics 1990). All modes of cancer therapy, including hormone control and chemotherapy, are used in the care of patients with these neoplasms. A collaborative approach to diagnosis and therapy is essential for optimal care and maximum survival, goals best achieved by accurate pretreatment staging of tumors.

Important advances in diagnostic and therapeutic regimens used in urologic oncology are applicable to other sites. In general, the staging of urologic malignancies is widely accepted, as evidenced by the translation between the tumor, node, metastasis (TNM) system and the ABCD stages of the American Urologic System (American Joint Committee 1988; International Union Against Cancer 1987). Computed tomography (CT) scanning, ultrasound (US), and magnetic resonance imaging (MRI) have had a dramatic impact on diagnosis and staging of renal cancers and are in general use in bladder and prostate cancers. Spontaneous regression of renal cancer metastases has stimulated the search for immunologic therapy using tumor-specific antibodies. The treatment of Wilms' tumor remains the success story of all neoplasms and the model for the multimodal approach in other pediatric and adult tumors (American Cancer Society 1987; D'Angio et al. 1980; Farber 1966).

Improvement in survival due to decreases in local and regional failures has been most evident in bladder and prostate cancers. In the 1980s, the integration of preoperative irradiation and/or chemotherapy with cystectomy has been used and better end results are now appearing in the literature. However, the choice of radiation dosage or drug regimen remains an issue, i.e., whether to utilize low-to-moderate vs. high doses. The acceptance of modern supervoltage irradiation over selected surgery is best exemplified by the high degree of tumor response in prostate cancer and by the long-term survivors, many of whom retain their potency.

Perhaps the most gratifying advance in the treatment of urologic tumors is the increased survival being attained in men with testicular cancers. Drug combinations have led to a marked increase in cures approaching the high survival rates seen in seminomas for patients with nonseminomatous cancers. These chemotherapy programs are evolving into many different protocols, resulting from cooperative group efforts and national clinical trials (American Cancer Society 1987). The challenge remains in finding systemic agents for the disseminated renal, prostate, and bladder cancers that still take their toll each year (International Histological Classification of Tumours 1981; Javadpour

The authors gratefully acknowledge Henry M. Keys, M.D., and Craig S. McCune, M.D., coauthors of "Urologic and Male Genital Cancers" in *Clinical Oncology: A Multidisciplinary Approach* (New York: American Cancer Society, 1983).

1983; Murphy et al. 1987; Murphy 1972; American Cancer Society 1987; Resnick and Kursh 1987; Skinner and Lieskovsky 1988; Walsh et al. 1986).

ADULT KIDNEY TUMORS

EPIDEMIOLOGY

Approximately 10,300 people die each year from adult kidney cancer. An estimated 24,000 new cases are diagnosed annually, comprising 2% of all cancers. The average age at the time of diagnosis is between 55 and 60 years.

Renal cell carcinoma occurs in 80% of the cases, with approximately a 2:1 male predominance. Transitional cell or squamous cell carcinomas of the renal pelvis are present in about 15% of cases, with an equal incidence in males and females.

The increased usage of CT scans and US in medical practice has led to an increased incidence of unsuspected renal tumors.

ETIOLOGY

The etiology of renal cell carcinoma is obscure. Some renal pelvic tumors might occur as a result of chronic inflammation and irritation secondary to calculous disease. Epidemiologic studies have suggested a significant correlation between smoking and renal cell carcinoma (Bennington and Laubscher 1978). Patients with acquired cystic disease due to renal failure are also prone to renal cell carcinoma. The autosomal dominant hereditary Von Hippel-Lindau disease is frequently associated with renal carcinoma. In addition, experimental models have suggested hormones and radiation as possible etiologies.

DETECTION AND DIAGNOSIS

CLINICAL DIAGNOSIS

This usually is a "silent" tumor in the early stages and symptoms usually denote a more advanced tumor. Typical presenting signs and symptoms are hematuria (70%), pain (50%), palpable mass (20%), polycythemia (3%), and fever (16%). A reversible hepatorenal syndrome (Slauffer's syndrome) and other paraneoplastic syndromes such as hypercalcemia due to parathyroid hormone production and erythrocytosis due to increased erythroprotein production also have been described.

A prolonged period exists between the onset of signs and symptoms and the diagnosis of renal cancer. Metastases are present in approximately one-third of patients at the time of diagnosis.

Improvement in the quality of excretory urography and nephrotomography, abdominal CT, and other imaging modalities has significantly increased the early detection of clinically asymptomatic and unsuspected cases (American Cancer Society 1987).

DIAGNOSTIC PROCEDURES

Urinalysis might show red blood cells. Excretory urography (intravenous pyelogram [IVP]) might reveal evidence of a space-occupying mass with pelvocalyceal displacement and alteration of the renal contour or a filling defect in the pelvocalyceal system.

Nephrotomography helps to differentiate a cyst from a solid tumor in approximately 95% of patients. Retrograde pyelography might demonstrate a filling defect in the presence of a tumor of the renal pelvis or the calyceal system, but it is of little value for workup of primary parenchymal lesions. Ultrasound is helpful in differentiating cystic from solid lesions. Needle aspiration of avascular cystic masses, including cytologic examination of fluid and injection of contrast materials, is a useful adjunct.

Computed tomography scans are useful in both the diagnosis and staging. The density (whether cystic or solid), size of tumor, extent of local invasion, vena caval or renal vein involvement, or metastases to the lymph nodes, liver, or lung can all be seen on abdominal CT. Magnetic resonance imaging has recently been suggested to show superior selectivity to CT scanning for visualization of renal veins or vena caval involvement (American Cancer Society 1987).

Selective renal arteriography is diagnostic in 80% of hypernephromas, with characteristic findings of neovasculature. It provides evidence of the lesion's extent and defines the renal blood supply preoperatively. Venacavography helps to determine the extent of the lesion in the renal vein or vena cava. Angiography, in general, is being replaced by CT and MRI, due to its potential complications and the increased detail available on CT or MRI.

Cytology is useful for tumors of the pelvocalyceal system, but of little use in parenchymal cancers. Additionally, brush biopsies or ureteroscopy may be helpful in defining filling defects in the collecting system.

CLASSIFICATION

ANATOMIC STAGING

The TNM system favored by the American Joint Committee (1988) and the International Union Against Cancer (1987) is gradually being adopted, but it may be simplified if the T stages and alphabetic designations are matched.

T STAGE

Tumor stage grouping (table 21.1) are as follows: T1, tumor confined to the kidney and capsule; T2, tumor >2.5 cm limited to the kidney; T3, tumor extends into major veins or exhibits perinephric invasion; and T4, tumor invades beyond Gerota's fascia.

Table 21.1
TUMOR (T), NODE (N) CLASSIFICATION KIDNEY CANCER

T1	<2.5 cm, limited to kidney
T2	>2.5 cm, limited to kidney
T3	Into major veins or perinephric invasion
T4	Invades beyond Gerota's fascia
N1	Single <2 cm
N2	Single >2 cm <5 cm, multiple <5 cm
N3	>5 cm

(Modified from: UICC [1987].)

The regional lymph nodes (nodal involvement, N) are the para-aortic and paracaval nodes. The juxtaregional lymph nodes are the pelvic nodes and the mediastinal nodes. The presence of distant metastases is indicated by M.

HISTOPATHOLOGY

The two malignancies most commonly found in the kidney are parenchymal (usually renal cell carcinoma) and carcinoma of the renal pelvis, collecting system, or ureter, usually transitional cell carcinoma (Mostofi 1967).

The *parenchymal* tumor has been referred to as a hypernephroma, renal cell carcinoma, or clear cell cancer. It locally infiltrates into the capsule and is highly angioinvasive, spreading into the renal vein and vena cava, and results in widespread hematogenous and lymphatic metastases especially to the lung, liver, nodes, and bone. The tumor's pathology differs from most tumors in terms of metastases to unusual sites (testes, skin, etc.), spontaneous regression, and delayed metastases, more resembling melanoma.

The *pelvis cancer* variety is more typical of the urothelial cancer of the bladder. It spreads by parenchymal infiltration, lymphatic involvement, and by seeding along the ureters. It may also be multifocal in origin.

CLINICAL STAGING

Recommended procedures. The following is the recommended usual sequence for clinical staging:

1. Excretory urography with tomography reveals the primary lesion, the degree of local extension, evidence of nodal compression, and deviation of the ureter. Ultrasound may delineate a solid vs. cystic mass.
2. Abdominal CT scan demonstrates the solid nature of the primary renal tumor; evidence of local extension; nodal, renal vein, and vena caval involvement; and liver metastases. MRI is of use if the level of vena caval involvement is in doubt. Venous angiographies are useful if the MRI is not diagnostic (American Cancer Society 1987).
3. Radiologic metastatic survey includes chest x-ray and bone scans.
4. Laboratory tests include complete blood count (CBC) and sequential multiple analysis (SMA-12), particularly liver chemistries, and calcium levels.

Optional and investigative procedures. Lymphangiography is not reliable for high para-aortic and paracaval nodes. Angiography is usually used only if all other methods fail to give the information required for diagnosis or staging.

PRINCIPLES OF TREATMENT

SURGERY

Renal cell carcinoma. Radical nephrectomy, in which the kidney, perinephric fat, Gerota's capsule, and regional nodes are removed, is preferred for all resectable lesions in stages A to C (Robson, Churchill, and Anderson 1968). In advanced cases, palliative nephrectomy is indicated for intractable bleeding and pain control. Occasional cures are reported with nephrectomy and resection of a solitary metastasis (brain, liver, bone). The presence of tumor in the renal vein and/or vena cava does not preclude surgical resection for cure. For bilateral tumors, which occur in approximately 1% of cases, treatment consists of nephrectomy (larger lesion) and partial nephrectomy (smaller lesion), or bilateral partial nephrectomy, if feasible. Bench surgery may be required for these procedures, involving surgical excision of the involved kidney, tumorectomy, and autotransplantation of the residual kidney. Occasionally, bilateral nephrectomies are indicated. The patient is then placed on chronic hemodialysis or peritoneal dialysis with the expectation of renal transplantation after a prolonged period (i.e., two years) of observation (American Cancer Society 1987).

RADIOTHERAPY

Radiotherapy is of little use in treating the kidney, but may be of benefit in treating local recurrences or symptomatic bony tumor. The radiation therapy field is limited to the renal bed, including lymph node drainage up to the diaphragm. Postoperative irradiation of 45 Gy to 50 Gy is used for residual or recurrent carcinoma (Flocks and Kadesky 1958).

CHEMOTHERAPY

Occasional responses to progesterone occur, and this hormone produces no toxicity. The true response rate is probably no greater than 5% (Hahn et al. 1978; Hahn et al. 1979).

Single-agent and combination chemotherapy have been evaluated to a limited degree, and response rates have been low. Vinblastine has been most extensively studied. Thus far it appears that no single agent or combination gives a response greater than 10% (deKernion and Berry 1980; Hahn et al. 1978; Hahn et al. 1979; Kaufman and Mims 1966).

IMMUNOTHERAPY

Most standard treatments (chemotherapy, radiation therapy, and surgery) are not effective for advanced renal cell carcinoma. Also, the tumor chemically and experimentally appears to be under the control of the immune system, so some patients are treated with some form of immunotherapy (Graham 1989). There are some responses seen with vaccines and nonspecific immunomodulators. Better responses (up to 20% to 30%) are seen with lymphormones (interferon and IL-2). More recently, the use of autolymphocyte therapy with supernumerary lymphormones has shown promise (Oshand et al. 1990).

Renal pelvis carcinoma. If operable, tumors of the collecting system warrant nephroureterectomy. The ureter is removed because of the tendency for transitional cell pelvic tumors to seed down along the ureter and into the bladder, or to be multifocal (Droller 1980; Fraley 1978; Gittes 1979; Grabstald, Whitmore, and Melamed 1971; Grace, Taylor, and Taylor 1967; Lathan and Kau 1974; McDonald and Priestly 1944).

Bilateral tumors may be treated endoscopically, or with partial resection of the renal pelvis/kidney, or with topical or systemic chemotherapy. Advanced lesions are treated with cisplatin-based chemotherapy. Distal ureteral lesions are treated with partial ureterectomy.

SPECIAL CONSIDERATIONS FOR TREATMENT

Instances of spontaneous regression of renal cell carcinoma recorded in the literature have led to a policy of debulking advanced tumors in the hope of inducing regression of metastases. In view of the experience, however, such successful outcomes are rare (1% to 2%). The mechanisms are unknown, but immunologic and hormonal factors are cited (Rubin 1968).

RESULTS AND PROGNOSIS

SURVIVAL RATES FOR RENAL CELL CARCINOMA

For stages A and B, there is a 5-year survival of 30% to 50%, and 10-year survival of 15% to 30%. Stage C has an approximate 5-year survival of 10% (Priestley 1939), and 10-year survival is approximately 5% (Riches, Griffith, and Thackaray 1957).

The best results (5- and 10-year survival of 65%) are reported by Robson (Robson 1963; Robson, Churchill, and Anderson 1968) and are attributed to thoracoabdominal nephrectomy with node dissection, primary ligation of the renal pedicle before tumor manipulation, and removal of the kidney with the fibrofatty envelope. Crude survival curves are shown in fig. 21.1.

Improved survival may result from earlier diagnosis of incidental carcinomas found on excretory urograms and tomograms, US, abdominal CT scans, and other imaging techniques (American Cancer Society 1987).

Results of the Rotterdam study (Van der Werf-Messing 1973) showed that preoperative irradiation may decrease the tumor's size and reduce the extent of invasiveness but does not influence survival significantly.

Advanced disease usually carries a dismal prognosis. However, reports of 750 survivals at nearly two years have been reported with immunotherapy (Oshand et al. 1990).

SURVIVAL RATES FOR PELVOCALYCEAL CARCINOMA

Transitional cell carcinoma of the renal pelvis has the following 5-year survival rates (McDonald and Priestly 1944): papillary without invasion, 52%; papillary with parenchymal infiltration, 16.7%; nonpapillary with infiltration, 7.1%; and venous or lymphatic involvement, 4.3%.

Five-year survival is rare for squamous cell carcinoma (McDonald and Priestley 1944).

PATTERNS OF FAILURE

Renal cell carcinoma. The most common pathway of failure is widespread metastatic disease either via nodal spread to hilar, paracaval, para-aortic, and mediastinal sites, or via hematogenous spread to bone, lung, liver, brain, and virtually any visceral site. Local recurrence is not common unless the tumor is incompletely resected, tumor spillage has occurred, or the tumor has penetrated the renal capsule.

Transitional cell carcinoma. Local recurrence is more common than distant metastases.

CLINICAL INVESTIGATIONS

For localized stages, no studies are in progress. For advanced and metastatic stages, no consistently effective systemic chemotherapy for renal cell carcinoma has been found. The thrust of current clinical research is to search for an effective single agent.

Immunologic approaches have produced objective responses in renal cell carcinoma. This has been seen with injections of aggregated tumor antigens (Niedhart et al. 1980), irradiated autologous tumor cells (McCune, Schapira, and Henshaw 1981), and by infusions of interferons, or sensitized autologous lymphocytes (LAK-IL-2) (Steele et al. 1981; Oshand 1990).

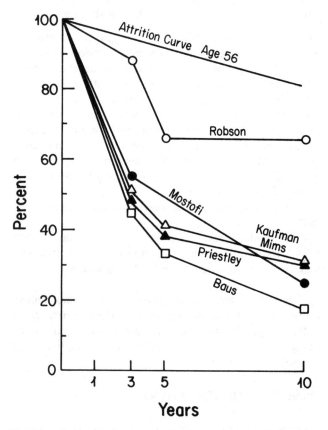

Fig. 21.1. Crude survival curves of several large series of renal carcinomas, treated surgically and followed-up for 10 years: Robson 1963; Kaufman and Mims 1966; Priestly 1939; Mostofi 1967; and the British Association of Urologic Surgeons (BAUS). (Courtesy: Kaufman and Mims [1966].)

EMBRYONAL KIDNEY TUMORS (WILMS' TUMOR)

EPIDEMIOLOGY

The origin of this large malignant tumor of childhood is mesodermal. Sixty-five percent occur before the third year and 75% occur before the fifth year. There is an equal incidence for both sexes, and bilateral involvement is present in approximately 7.2% of the patients.

DETECTION AND DIAGNOSIS

CLINICAL DETECTION

Typical presentation is a palpable abdominal mass in approximately 50% of patients. Other presenting signs are hematuria (approximately 20%), pain (approximately 30%), and hypertension (approximately 75%).

DIAGNOSTIC PROCEDURES

Excretory urogram with tomography is usually adequate for diagnosis. Ultrasound evaluation can rule out hydronephrosis or cystic disease; MRI may also be used before CT scan.

Computed tomography scan is useful for staging and evaluation of the other kidney. Aortography is useful, but rarely needed. Retrograde pyelography may be required when the excretory urogram is nondiagnostic, but it is seldom needed.

DIFFERENTIAL DIAGNOSIS

Wilms' tumor must be differentiated from hydronephrosis, neuroblastoma, multicystic disease of the kidney, and retroperitoneal sarcoma.

CLASSIFICATION

ANATOMIC STAGING

The National Wilms' Tumor Study (NWTS) classification is the most widely used system and is based upon surgical and pathologic findings (D'Angio et al. 1980).

In stage I, tumor is limited to kidney, confined within its intact capsule, and completely excised without evidence of tumor at its margin. In stage II, tumor extends beyond the kidney, but is completely excised grossly; tumor invades into perinephric fat; lymph nodes and veins must be resected with a clear margin. Stage II also applies if the tumor has been biopsied or if there is local spillage. Stage III is residual nonhematogenous tumor confined to abdomen, indicating tumor rupture at surgery; peritoneal implants; juxtaregional nodes in pelvis; or incomplete resection. Stage IV indicates hematogenous metastases beyond stage III.

HISTOLOGIC TYPES

Two general types are identifiable: favorable and unfavorable varieties (table 21.2). The latter type has focal and diffuse anaplasia and sarcomatous features associated with brain and skeletal metastases.

CLINICAL STAGING

Recommended procedures. The following is the sequence of recommended staging workup procedures:

1. Ultrasound of abdomen.
2. Excretory urography, including tomography.
3. CT scan, when possible, for staging and evaluation of the other kidney.
4. Chest films are necessary because the lungs are an important metastatic pathway. Suspicious lesions may require computed tomography (CT) for confirmation.
5. Laboratory survey includes CBC and SMA-12.
6. Laparotomy to determine primary and nodal extent and for definitive surgical treatment.

Optional and investigative procedures. Aortogram and renal arteriography may be difficult to perform in children. Retrograde pyelography can be helpful, but is seldom needed. Procedures *not* recommended include lymphangiography, and skeletal survey since bone metastases are very uncommon. Magnetic resonance imaging is still being evaluated and may be impossible to perform on small children (American Cancer Society 1987).

PRINCIPLES OF TREATMENT

SURGERY

Transperitoneal nephrectomy should be performed as soon as possible. Local lymphadenectomy is rarely required. The flank approach is contraindicated because neither the contralateral kidney nor the entire abdomen can be explored.

RADIOTHERAPY

In the past radiotherapy was given routinely, but its use has been declining. At present, low-dose radiotherapy is used in patients with stage III disease and is combined with chemotherapy. It is also used in a similar manner for stage IV.

Complications of radiotherapy include minimal scoliosis, radiation nephritis, and occasionally, temporary bone-marrow suppression.

Table 21.2
WILMS' TUMOR PROGNOSIS ACCORDING TO HISTOLOGIC TYPE 427 CASES REVIEWED

Histology	Number (%)	Number Relapse-free at 2 Years (%)	Number Alive at 2 Years (%)
FH*	378 (89)	305 (89)	338 (89)
UH**	49 (10)	14 (29)	19 (39)
Total	427	319	357

*FH = Favorable histology
**UH = Unfavorable histology
14 of the FH deaths and two of the UH deaths were not caused by tumor.
(Courtesy: D'Angio et al. [1980].)

CHEMOTHERAPY

Effective use of combination cyclic chemotherapy consisting of VACA (vincristine, actinomycin D, cyclophosphamide, and doxorubicin [Adriamycin]) is one of the most successful programs.

TREATMENT ACCORDING TO STAGES

For stage I, nephrectomy is indicated. Postoperative radiation therapy is not recommended except for large tumors (more than 300 g) and for older children (more than 2 years of age). Elective cyclic actinomycin D is utilized.

Nephrectomy and VACA are recommended for stages II and III.

For stage IV, nephrectomy, radiation therapy to the renal bed and lungs, and VACA are suggested.

RESULTS AND PROGNOSIS

HISTORICAL RESULTS WITHOUT CHEMOTHERAPY

Children under 2 years of age had a 73%, 2-year survival rate. Of those from 3 to 9 years of age, 18.5% had a 2-year survival rate. Doubling time as a prognostic criterion was accurate in 338 of 340 cases. This postulate states that the patient's period of risk for tumor recurrence is equal to the child's age at the time of diagnosis with a gestation period of nine months. This does not take the effect of chemotherapy into consideration (D'Angio et al. 1980).

RESULTS WITH CHEMOTHERAPY

In 1966, Farber, from the Boston Children's Hospital, reported that when actinomycin D was administered routinely at the time of nephrectomy and followed by local irradiation, metastases were prevented in almost all patients. The 2-year survival rate of 40% without drug therapy increased to 89% with actinomycin D.

Previously incurable, bilateral pulmonary metastases were treated with combined total lung irradiation and actinomycin D. They became curable in 58% of cases with some failure because of metastases elsewhere (D'Angio et al. 1980). Vincristine has shown similar tumoricidal activity.

The addition of doxorubicin has improved relapse-free survival for stage III of favorable histology from 80% to 90%, but late cardiotoxicity is a concern.

RESULTS WITH AND WITHOUT RADIOTHERAPY

There is no difference in outcome for stage I in patients under 2 years of age. The improvement in outcome with radiotherapy occurs for stage I children over 2 years of age.

HISTOLOGIC TYPE

Unfavorable histology occurs in 11% of all patients and is three times more lethal than the favorable histology (see table 21.2).

CANCER OF THE URETER

EPIDEMIOLOGY AND ETIOLOGY

Carcinoma of the ureter occurs predominately in males (2:1) in their 60s and 70s. The ureter is a relatively uncommon site for primary tumors; more than one-half are located in the lower third of the ureter. Carcinoma of the ureter is most commonly transitional cell carcinoma and is similar histologically to tumors of the bladder and the renal pelvis (Gittes 1979; Riches, Griffith, and Thackaray 1957). Since transitional cell carcinoma is frequently multifocal, tumors of the ureter may be found in 10% of patients with transitional cell carcinoma of the bladder, and a similar incidence is found in the bladder with primary ureteral tumors.

DETECTION AND DIAGNOSIS

CLINICAL DETECTION

Hematuria is the most common sign, occurring in 74% of the cases. Pain from obstruction, local extension, or metastases is the most common symptom and occurs in 50% of patients (Gittes 1979; Riches, Griffith, and Thackaray 1957).

DIAGNOSTIC PROCEDURES

Urine exam may show red blood cells (RBCs) that are ureteral casts. Urinary cytology is highly recommended. In addition to voided cytologies, it may be necessary to obtain selected cytologies from each ureter, as well as brush cytologies of any lesions seen on retrograde urograms. Excretory urography (IVP) may detect obstruction or a filling defect in the ureter. Cystoscopy may reveal blood from the involved ureter. Retrograde ureterography and pyelography are recommended, although brush biopsy and ureteroscopy are frequently necessary. Ultrasound and/or CT scan may help rule out uric acid calculi if a filling defect is seen (Gittes 1979; Riches, Griffith, and Thackaray 1957).

PRINCIPLES OF TREATMENT

Primary therapy for transitional cell carcinoma is nephroureterectomy if the lesion is resectable. Lesions of the distal ureter may be managed by distal ureterectomy with a cuff of bladder and reimplantation of the ureter. Local excision may be performed if the renal function is reduced, or for a solitary kidney.

Cisplatin-based chemotherapy is used for advanced cases with local extension or metastases.

RESULTS AND PROGNOSIS

Five-year survival is approximately 25%, with low-grade tumors having a better prognosis. This is primarily due to the fact that most tumors are advanced when first detected. Invasion of the thin ureteral wall is common, resulting in local extension which alters prognosis.

BLADDER CANCER

EPIDEMIOLOGY

Bladder carcinoma is the most frequent malignant tumor of the urinary tract, with estimations for 1990 at 49,000 new cases. Eighty-four percent occur on the lateral and posterior walls of the bladder and 40% on the trigone. This disease is most common in the 50- to 70-year age group, and accounts for 2% of all cancer deaths in the United States. It is estimated that 6,500 men and 3,200 women (a 2:1 ratio) will die from bladder cancer in 1990 (Cancer Statistics 1990).

ETIOLOGY

Aniline dye used in the textile, rubber, and cable industries is related to etiology. There is a long latent period (6 to 20 years) from exposure until tumor transformation in humans. Beta-naphthylamine, 4-amino diphenyl, and tobacco tar can cause tumors in animals. In humans, cigarette smoking is associated with a sixfold higher incidence of bladder tumors.

Chronic bladder infections and calculous disease or *Schistosoma haematobium* may be etiologic in squamous cell carcinoma. Adenocarcinoma may occur in exstrophy of the bladder or in a urachal remnant (Caldwell 1970; de-Kernion and Skinner 1978; Prout 1980; Rubin 1968; Whitmore et al. 1968; Whitmore and Marshall 1962).

DETECTION AND DIAGNOSIS

CLINICAL DETECTION

Typical presentations include gross hematuria, which is the most common clinical finding and the first sign in approximately 75% of patients. Microscopic hematuria is present in most cases. Frequency, bladder irritability, and dysuria occur in about one-third of patients and increase in the later stages of the disease.

Bleeding is characteristically intermittent. This delays diagnosis because the patient and the physician may defer workup if the urine clears.

For early diagnosis, the presence of unexplained gross or microscopic hematuria requires evaluation. Urine cytology is recommended in high-risk populations, such as workers exposed to carcinogens.

DIAGNOSTIC PROCEDURES

Urinalysis often shows microhematuria when urine is grossly clear. Excretory urogram (IVP) is used to evaluate the upper urinary tracts and bladder filling. Cystoscopy is usually diagnostic. DNA ploidy by cytology and flow cytometry is helpful in diagnosing and screening patients at higher risk, and for follow-up of therapy. The yield from this study can be increased by brisk lavage of the bladder with normal saline. Cytology may be of screening value in industry and may detect lesions at an early stage in follow-up.

Pelvic CT scan aids in staging. Other imaging techniques, such as MRI, are being evaluated. Flow cytometry of urine may be of value for diagnosis and prognosis.

CLASSIFICATION

Depth of tumor penetration into the bladder wall is the single most important factor in predicting the ultimate prognosis of a particular lesion; this factor forms the basis for staging of bladder cancer.

The presence of multiple tumors without invasion and the location of the lesion might be important factors in determining the mode of therapy. Tumors might seed downward from a renal pelvic or ureteral primary (deKernion and Skinner 1978; Jewett and Strong 1946; Prout 1980). Metastases occur by lymphatic and hematogenous routes. Common metastatic sites are regional lymph nodes (Smith and Whitmore 1981), liver, lung, and bones.

Bimanual assessment under anesthesia is reflected in clinical classification. Modification of staging by endoscopic biopsy depends on depth of biopsy in muscle.

Tables 21.3 and 21.4 outline the TNM classification systems for bladder cancer. There is concurrence between the AJC and the UICC classification (American Joint Committee 1988; International Union Against Cancer 1987). Translations of the TNM system (American Joint Committee 1988) into the ABCD American Urologic (Jewett-Marshall) staging system are possible (see table 21.5).

HISTOPATHOLOGY

Transitional cell carcinoma is the most common carcinoma of the bladder in the United States (85%), though squamous cell and adenocarcinoma may also occur. The tumor's histologic appearance (grade) may give some indication of its potential to infiltrate and spread. Most noninvasive tumors are low-grade (I-II), while invasive lesions are usually high-grade (grade III-IV). Carcinoma *in situ* is a flat (nonpapillary) grade III tumor with an especially ominous prognosis if associated with an otherwise noninvasive tumor. The grade of the tumor also correlates with exfoliation of the tumor cells that are picked up on cytology or flow cytometry.

Squamous cell carcinoma accounts for 5% of cases. Adenocarcinoma accounts for less than 1% of cases and may be of urachal or cystitis glandularis origin.

CLINICAL STAGING

Clinical staging of transitional cell carcinoma is necessary to plan treatment. Despite the elegant staging systems available, the treatment decisions are based on (1) superficial disease (confined to mucosa); (2) muscle invasive disease (confined to bladder); and (3) systemic disease.

Table 21.3
TUMOR (T), NODE (N) CLASSIFICATION BLADDER CANCER TNM

Urinary bladder	
Tis	*In situ:* flat tumor
Ta	Papillary noninvasive
T1	Subepithelial connective tissue
T2	Superficial muscle (inner half)
T3	Deep muscle or perivesical fat
T3a	Deep muscle (outer half)
T3b	Perivesical fat
T4	Prostate, uterus, vagina, pelvic wall, abdominal wall
N1	Single <2 cm
N2	Single >2 cm <5 cm, multiple <5 cm
N3	>5 cm

(Courtesy: UICC [1987].)

Table 21.4
TNM CLINICAL CLASSIFICATION

T = Primary Tumor
The suffix (m) should be added to the appropriate T category to indicate multiple tumors. The suffix "is" may be added to any T to indicate presence of associated carcinoma *in situ.*
TX   Primary tumor cannot be assessed
T0   No evidence of primary tumor
Tis   Carcinoma *in situ:* flat tumor
Ta   Noninvasive papillary carcinoma
T1   Tumor invades subepithelial connective tissue
T2   Tumor invades superficial muscle (inner half)
T3   Tumor invades deep muscle or perivesical fat
T3a   Tumor invades deep muscle (outer half)
T3b   Tumor invades perivesical fat
T4   Tumor invades any of the following: prostate, uterus, vagina, pelvic wall, abdominal wall

Note: If pathology report does not specify that tumor invades muscle, consider it as invasion of subepithelial connective tissue. If depth of muscle invasion is not specified by the surgeon, code as T2.
(Courtesy: UICC [1987].)

Recommended procedures. The following is the sequence of recommended staging workup procedures (see fig. 21.2):

1. Cystoscopy with biopsy or resection into muscle. In addition, biopsies of the bladder or prostatic urethra are usually indicated, especially if there is concern about multifocal disease. A barbotage specimen may be sent for cytology and flow cytometry.
2. Bimanual examination to stage the tumor.
3. Excretory urography or retrograde pyelogram to determine obstruction of the ureters and extension, lymph node involvement, or other tumors of the pelvocalyceal system or ureters.

If the tumor is invasive, then additional studies are required. These include:

4. Radiographic survey, which includes chest film and abdominal (pelvic) CT scan. Bone scan is useful only if bony metastases are clinically suspected.
5. Laboratory tests, including CBC and SMA-12 chemistries.

Optional and investigative procedures. Cystography, in the form of triple voiding cystogram, may show bladder wall infiltration, but has seldom been used since the advent of CT scanning or other imaging techniques.

Table 21.5
CLASSIFICATION AND STAGING OF BLADDER CANCER

TNM CLASSIFICATION*
1.   Primary tumor (0T): The suffix "m" should be added to the appropriate T category to indicate multiple lesions.
2.   Regional lymph nodes (N): The absence or presence and extent of regional lymph node metastasis.
STAGE GROUPING (AMERICAN)
0 -   Superficial tumor confined to mucosa and carcinoma *in situ*
A -   Superficial tumor confined to submucosa
B -   Muscle invasion
a.   B1 - Superficial
b.   B2 - Deep
C -   Extension through serosa and/or perivesical fat
D -   Metastatic
D1 - Lymph nodes, below the aortic bifurcation
D2 - Lymph nodes above the aortic bifurcation and/or distant metastases

(*American Joint Committee [1988]; UICC [1987].)

Laparotomy or pelvic exploration will evaluate the extent of the primary lymph nodes. Clips may be placed on positive nodes to locate them on radiographs when determining radiation treatment fields. Metal clips may interfere with subsequent CT scan interpretation, as well as MRI.

PRINCIPLES OF TREATMENT

GENERAL PRINCIPLES
The following factors must be considered before determining the mode and extent of therapy: anatomic and histologic classification (stage and grade); location of tumor; patient's general health; associated genitourinary problems (prostatism, urinary tract infection, ureteral obstruction, compromised renal function); patient's ability to tolerate and to care for any urinary diversion; history of tumor recurrence rate (an increased rate may

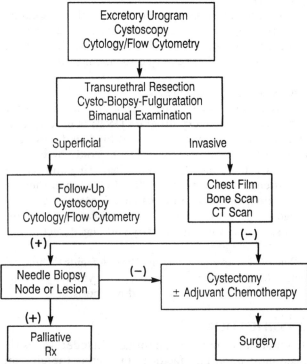

Fig. 21.2. Carcinoma of the bladder: clinical evaluation and treatment. This plan may be altered because of factors such as patient's age, general health, etc.

influence therapy plan); previous surgery or radiation therapy; and training, experience, and skill of the surgeon, medical oncologist, or radiation therapist.

SURGERY

Endoscopic resection and fulguration are usually used to diagnose and treat superficial lesions with a slow recurrence rate, and to control bleeding in patients who are poor operative risks or who have advanced disease. Treatment with a Nd:YAG laser is also a possibility for some patients. Segmental bladder resection is reserved for large single lesions at the bladder dome or the lateral wall in a patient who is too high a risk for total cystectomy, or for cases of adenocarcinoma. Recurrence rates of approximately 50% are seen in superficial tumors and may be treated with repeated endoscopic procedures or intravesical chemotherapy.

Total cystectomy requires a urinary diversion and includes resection of local pelvic nodes, prostate, seminal vesicles, and penile urethra if there is disease in the prostatic urethra. Cystectomy is indicated when the tumor is invasive, high-grade, superficial but not controllable with conservative modalities, and when the patient has a good life expectancy with no metastases outside the pelvic area. Common forms of diversion are ileal loop (ureteroileal-cutaneous), colon loop (ureterocolic-cutaneous), rectal bladder (ureteral-rectal with colostomy fecal diversion), or continent diversions which do not require external collection devices.

PREFERRED SURGICAL PROCEDURES
BY CLASSIFICATION

For superficial stage (0, A, B1), low-grade carcinoma (I,II): endoscopic resection and fulguration; segmental bladder resection in selected cases; and total cystectomy in patients who do not respond to conservative methods, or are at high risk for progression (carcinoma *in situ*); intravesicle instillation for some cases and for carcinoma *in situ*.

For deep stage (B2, C), high-grade carcinoma (III, IV): total cystectomy with urinary diversion; cystoprostatectomy-urethrectomy for lesions near or distal to the bladder neck; segmental bladder resection in a few selected cases.

For metastatic stage (D), high-grade carcinoma (III, IV): urinary diversion occasionally for palliation (Gittes 1979; Whitmore and Marshall 1962).

RADIOTHERAPY

Radiation therapy may be used as definitive therapy, adjuvant therapy, or in combination therapy. Definitive radiation therapy alone is seldom recommended due to the low response and survival rates (<20%), and the complications resulting from radiation damage to the detrusor muscle of the bladder. Radiation has been examined in the adjuvant setting with radical cystectomy, and except in occasional stage B2C (T3a, T3b) lesions, no additional benefit has been seen (Wallace and Bloom 1976). More recently, radiation has been used in combination with cisplatin (a radiopotentiator) with some reports of increased success. Clinical trials are currently evaluating this modality.

In metastatic stage (D), high-grade (III, IV), radiation may be used as a palliative measure in controlling pain and bleeding. In selected cases of an advanced stage bladder tumor limited to the pelvis with ureteral obstruction, diversionary procedures such as an ileal loop will allow delivery of an uninterrupted high-dose course. This may increase survival and decrease symptoms and blood loss (American Cancer Society 1987; Goodman et al. 1981; Miller and Johnson 1972; Van der Werf-Messing 1973; Van der Werf-Messing 1979; Whitmore et al. 1977; Whitmore et al. 1968).

CHEMOTHERAPY

There is no established systemic chemotherapeutic regimen for the treatment of metastatic bladder carcinoma. In recent years, the following drugs have been investigated and found to give response rates (partial regressions) in the range of 10% to 41%: methotrexate, doxorubicin (Adriamycin), 5-fluorouracil (5-FU), cyclophosphamide (Cytoxan), mitomycin C, and cisplatin (Goodman et al. 1981; Prout 1980; Yagoda 1980). The single agent with the best responses has been cisplatin. It is currently being utilized with vinblastine and methotrexate (with or without Adriamycin) in a variety of protocols (Yagoda 1985). More recently, to reduce the toxicity of the regimen, platinum analogs (i.e., carboplatinum) and VP-16 have been substituted in the MVAC (methotrexate, vinblastine, Adriamycin, cisplatin) regimen. MVAC has also been examined as a neoadjuvant regimen, though there is no data at this time to support its efficacy.

Intravesical instillations for superficial bladder cancer have been studied with at least several agents, and there is evidence that the recurrence rate can be significantly reduced by this approach. The agents most used are *bacillus Calmette-Guérin* (BCG), thiotepa, doxorubicin, and mitomycin C (American Cancer Society 1987; Soloway 1980). The most effective agent for carcinoma *in situ* is BCG, although mitomycin C also exhibits some effect.

RESULTS AND PROGNOSIS

Currently, patients with superficial disease have an excellent prognosis of up to 85% to 90% 5-year survival, and a 10% chance of progression overall. Factors such as size of

Table 21.6
COMPARATIVE SURVIVAL RESULTS OF
BLADDER CANCER AT 5 YEARS

Stage	Supervoltage Irradiation (%)	Total Cystectomy (%)
0,A,B	12 to 71	32 to 80
B2,C	7 to 28	8 to 36
D	0	0 to 12
Total	6 to 33	13 to 43

Note: The large range presented at each stage results from patient selection and associated medical diseases.
(Compiled from: Caldwell [1970].)

tumor, number of tumors, time of recurrence, grade, histologic stage, presence of carcinoma *in situ*, and detection of normal cell antigens, all have some bearing on prognosis. Disease invading muscle is currently treated by cystectomy with a 55% to 60% 5-year survival. Systemic disease has a grim prognosis (see table 21.6).

PATTERNS OF FAILURE
Patterns of failure after irradiation are different from patterns after surgery (Batata et al. 1980). Evaluation of the local failure rate after radiation therapy is complicated because recurrence of bladder cancer can result from a new lesion or relapse of the previous lesion. A similar pattern of recurrence is seen with conservative surgical procedures designed to preserve bladder function. In cystectomy, however, the most common site of relapse is distant metastases, and less than 15% will have local recurrence.

CLINICAL INVESTIGATIONS
Clinical investigations currently include the role of adjuvant chemotherapy prior to or after cystectomy and urinary diversion, and evaluation of chemotherapeutic or immunotherapeutic agents for local instillation in the bladder for superficial, low-grade tumors and carcinoma *in situ*. Additionally, modification of the surgical technique to preserve potency and continence and attempts to develop bladder sparing procedures are being investigated.

CANCER OF THE PROSTATE

EPIDEMIOLOGY
Prostate carcinoma is now the most common male cancer in the United States, accounting for 21% of all newly diagnosed cancers. With the graying of America, its frequency will continue to increase. The median age of incidence is 70 years; the incidence increases with each decade after age 50. The incidence rate is 89 per 100,000 for the male population, 87.7 per 100,000 white males, and 123.4 per 100,000 nonwhite males (Cancer Statistics Review 1973-1986 [1989]).

Approximately 106,000 new cases of prostate carcinoma are discovered each year, and approximately 30,000 deaths occur per year (Cancer Statistics 1990). The autopsy incidence of histologic prostate carcinoma (based on serial sections) is 14% to 46% of men over 50 years of age (Suen, Lau, and Yermakov 1974). The common histologic tumor is adenocarcinoma. Sarcoma is rarely seen; ductal, transitional cell carcinoma also occurs.

ETIOLOGY
The etiology is unknown, although there appears to be some hormonal relationship (Catalona and Scott 1986; Hutchinson 1981).

Environmental and familial factors may contribute to an increased incidence. An increased incidence has been shown in persons migrating to the United States from areas with a low incidence of prostate cancer. Significant clustering within families is documented. Certain industries

have an excess in mortality due to prostatic carcinoma; these include workers who are exposed to cadmium, workers in tire and rubber manufacturing, farmers, mechanics, and sheet metal workers (Carter et al. 1989).

PRESENTATION AND DIAGNOSIS

CLINICAL PRESENTATION
Approximately 60% of patients have localized cancer when first diagnosed (*CA* 1989). Most of these patients will be asymptomatic or have symptoms of lower urinary tract obstruction. Marked irritative symptoms, in the absence of infection, should prompt a search for this malignancy. Associated hematuria is rare.

Advanced presentation includes bladder outlet obstructive symptoms with urinary retention, ureteral obstruction with possible anuria, azotemia, uremia, anemia, and anorexia. Bone pain is the most frequent complaint of patients who present with metastatic disease.

DIAGNOSIS
Digital rectal examination remains the gold standard for detection of prostatic carcinoma. Fifty percent of palpable nodules will be found to be carcinomatous (Jewett et al. 1968). Fig. 21.3 outlines diagnostic procedures.

The use of transrectal ultrasonography (TRUS) for the early detection of prostatic carcinoma remains controversial. Though it is roughly twice as sensitive as a digital rectal examination, there is concern that clinically insignificant tumors may be detected, resulting in over-treatment (Chodak 1989). Most urologists use TRUS for the evaluation and directed biopsy of lesions within clinically abnormal glands.

Diagnosis is made by histologic or cytologic examination. Core needle biopsy is used in the United States. Fine needle aspiration is used more commonly in Europe; the technique was receiving increased use in the United States, only to be largely supplanted by the biopsy gun. This system utilizes a spring drive 18 gauge needle and delivers uniform cores with little displacement of the prostate gland and without the need for an anesthetic agent. Often, a patient undergoing prostatectomy for presumed benign disease will be found to have an unsuspected carcinoma.

Neither prostatic acid phosphatase (PAP) nor prostate-specific antigen (PSA) are useful in screening for prostatic carcinoma. Though PSA is more sensitive than PAP, 36% of patients with nonmalignant diseases will be found to have a moderately elevated PSA (Drago et al. 1989).

EARLY DETECTION
Men over 40 should receive a careful rectal exam during routine physical examinations. Studies are under way to test asymptomatic men older than 55 years to determine whether annual transrectal US plus PSA will detect early treatable cancers.

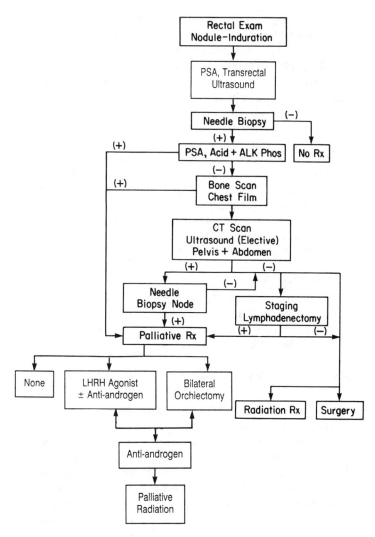

Fig. 21.3. Carcinoma of the prostate: clinical evaluation and treatment. This plan may be altered because of factors such as patient's age, general health, etc.

CLASSIFICATION

ANATOMIC STAGING

The American Urologic System consists of ABCD stages that have been translated into TNM categories by the American Joint Cancer Committee (1988) and the International Union Against Cancer (1987). The TNM classification for prostatic cancer is outlined in table 21.7.

STAGE GROUPING

Incidental finding by the pathologist and clinically unsuspected carcinoma is either stage A1 (three or fewer foci, well differentiated) or stage A2 (diffuse or more than three foci, poorly differentiated, and more extensive than A1).

Clinically palpable lesions in the prostate are stage B1 (<1.5 cm involving one lobe) and stage B2 (>1.5 cm diffusely involved).

Extension beyond the prostatic capsule without evidence of metastases is stage C.

Metastatic carcinoma is stage D1 (involvement of the pelvic lymph nodes below the aortic bifurcation) and

stage D2 (lymph node involvement above the aortic bifurcation and/or distant metastases to other sites).

HISTOPATHOLOGY

The vast majority of prostatic carcinomas are adenocarcinomas. Multiple grading systems are available, with the Gleason grading system becoming the most frequently utilized. It is based on both the tumor's glandular differentiation and growth pattern. Scores range from 2 to 10, and have been shown to be predictive of associated lymph node metastases (Paulson 1979).

CLINICAL STAGING

Clinical staging is generally accomplished using the following procedures. A CBC and SMAC are obtained in all patients. An elevated serum PAP is very suggestive of metastatic disease. The PSA is roughly proportional to prostatic volume. A PSA greater than 40 ng/mL to 50 ng/mL is usually associated with locally advanced or metastatic disease (Stamey 1987; Palken 1990).

Recommended procedures. A radioisotopic bone scan is more sensitive than a skeletal survery and is obtained to rule out metastatic disease. CT scan of the pelvis is recommended for detection of pelvic lymphadenopathy and TRUS may reveal local extension.

Optional and investigative procedures. Lymphangiography is rarely used, but it can determine extent of para-aortic and pelvic node involvement (Prando et al. 1979). Percutaneous fine-needle biopsy of enlarged lymph nodes found on the CT scan, MRI, or lymphangiogram (Prando et al. 1979) can be performed and is particularly useful in patients presenting with a high Gleason grade tumor. Scalene-node biopsy may demonstrate metastatic disease. Bone marrow aspiration and acid-phosphatase determination in search of metastatic disease is not very useful. Pelvic lymph nodes up to the aortic bifurcation can be explored.

PRINCIPLES OF TREATMENT

SURGERY

Radical prostatectomy is usually performed by the retropubic route. The prostate gland, seminal vesicles,

Table 21.7
TUMOR (T), NODE (N) CLASSIFICATION
PROSTATE CANCER SUMMARY

Prostate	
T1	Incidental
T1a	<3 foci
T1b	>3 foci
T2	Clinically or grossly, limited to gland
T2a	<1.5 cm
T2b	>1.5 cm/> one lobe
T3	Invades prostatic apex/beyond capsule/bladder neck/seminal vesical/ not fixed
T4	Fixed or invades other adjacent structures
N1	Single <2 cm
N2	Single >2 cm <5 cm, multiple <5 cm
N3	>5 cm

(Source: UICC [1987].)

and a narrow cuff of bladder neck are removed. Pelvic lymph nodes can be resected and sampled for staging. This is effective treatment for a localized lesion in a healthy male with an otherwise good prognosis for a 10-year survival. Patients with stages A2, B1, and B2 disease are considered to be candidates for surgical cure. Traditionally, patients with A1 disease were considered to generally have a benign course. Recently, up to 16% of these patients were found to have progressed (Epstein and Walsh 1987). The nerve sparing operation of Walsh, in which capsular and periprostatic nerves are spared, has preserved potency in a majority of patients. The immediate results show good cancer control and represent a major new advance (Walsh and Lepor 1987).

Pelvic lymphadenectomy has not been determined to be of therapeutic value (Catalona and Scott 1986; Jewett 1980), but it allows for more precise staging because pelvic nodes are generally the first site of metastatic spread.

RADIOTHERAPY

Locally invasive cancers, stages B and C, are treatable with supervoltage irradiation as are A2 and some A1 cancers; this applies to cancers within the capsule and those with extracapsular spread (Bagshaw 1974; Catalona and Scott 1986; Del Regato 1979; Meljenko, Perez, and Bauer 1980; Ray, Cassady and Bagshaw 1973; Van der Werf-Messing, Sourek-Zikova, and Blonk 1976). Highly focused modern techniques allow for delivery of 60 Gy to 70 Gy to the prostate cancer (Kiesling et al. 1980) with minimal morbidity.

The major issue of radiotherapy is the incorporation of pelvic and para-aortic lymph nodes. Most centers will treat pelvic lymph nodes. Extended fields for para-aortic irradiation are under study.

An alternate approach to prostate cancer management is to utilize iodine 125 seed implants at the time of pelvic lymphadenectomy, extending the dissection to the high common iliac nodes and lower para-aortic area (Batata et al. 1980; Guerriero, Carlton, and Hudgins 1980; Hilaris, Kim, and Tokita 1976; Hilaris et al. 1976).

Radiation therapy is effective in treating pain due to metastatic bone disease. Moderate doses often provide prompt pain relief. For extensive bone metastases, hemibody radiation in a single dose of 7 Gy to 8 Gy can provide dramatic pain relief in 70% to 80% of patients within 24 to 48 hours (Salazar et al. 1981).

Prior to estrogen therapy, pretreatment to the normal breasts with a modest dose (15 Gy) of radiation prevents nipple tenderness, but not necessarily gynecomastia.

HORMONAL THERAPY

The evaluation for metastatic prostate cancer has for almost 50 years centered around orchiectomy or the administration of estrogens. Both will remove 90% to 95% of circulating testosterone. Median survival is one to three years in ambulatory patients (DeVoogt et al. 1983). Estrogen administration may result in thromboembolic and cardiovascular complications.

Luteinizing hormone-releasing hormone agonists have been shown to be equivalent to orchiectomy or diethylstilbestrol (DES) (Leuprolide Study Group 1984; Geeling 1989). However, they are expensive and are associated with a flare phenomenon characterized by an increase in bone pain and outlet obstruction. Flutamide (Eulexin) is a nonsteroidal anti-androgen approved in the United States for use with a LHRH agonist; it blocks the uptake and/or nuclear binding of androgens in the target tissues. Combined androgen ablation using a LHRH agonist and flutamide has been shown to produce significantly better results, particularly in patients with minimal disease (Crawford 1989). Other drugs which can be used for ablation of both testicular and adrenal androgens include cyproterone acetate, megestrol acetate, aminoglutethamide, and ketoconozol.

CHEMOTHERAPY

No standard effective chemotherapy regimen exists for cases refractory to hormone therapy. Clinical investigation is in process in this area (American Cancer Society 1987; Paulson 1981; Schmitt et al. 1980).

RESULTS AND PROGNOSIS

RADICAL PROSTATECTOMY (FOR CURE)

Fifteen-year survival in patients with carcinoma clinically confined to the gland and treated with radical prostatectomy is equivalent to age or matched control population (*JAMA* 1987). Moreover, with the improvement in surgical technique brought about by Walsh, postoperative potency is 50% to 70%, while the incontinence rate has dropped to 1% to 2% (Badalament and Drago 1990).

RADIATION THERAPY (FOR CURE)

Supervoltage therapy. Of 661 patients with locally invasive cancer (stages B2 and C) who have been followed to 15 years, the 5-, 10-, and 15-year survival rates after supervoltage therapy are 70%, 50%, and 30%, respectively (Bagshaw et al. 1975). Additional advantages are maintenance of potency in approximately 75% of cases, and no incontinence (Batata et al. 1980).

Radioisotopic interstitial injection. This is a highly specialized approach. Two studies found iodine 125 preferable to radioisotopic gold delivery at doses of 180 Gy to 300 Gy to the prostate cancers (Hilaris, Kim, and Tokita 1976; Hilaris et al. 1976).

In the Rotterdam study (Van der Werf-Messing, Sourek-Zikova, and Blonk 1976), in comparable groups of stage C (T) patients, there was a 4-year survival of 82% with radiotherapy alone, a 65% survival with hormonal therapy, and 50% survival rate with combined radiation therapy and hormonal therapy. Van der Werf-Messing et al. (1976) note that with careful follow-up, progressive or recurrent disease occurring after either mode of therapy can be successfully salvaged by the other. They advocate sequential rather than concurrent use of irradiation and hormonal therapy.

The disparity in survival figures (55% to 70%) reported at five years in different series depends upon tumor grade for stage C lesions and the associated incidence of positive pelvic and para-aortic lymph nodes (50% to 70%) (Bagshaw et al. 1975; Hilaris et al. 1976; Lipsett, Cosgrave, and Green et al. 1976).

The use of radioisotopic techniques yields high local control. Hilaris and colleagues (1976) report slow and complete tumor regression starting at three months up to one year after iodine 125 implants, with local failure of 10% after doses of 180 Gy. Survival rates with this approach and pelvic lymph node dissections are close to 70% at five years for all stages. Bone metastases are much more common with high grade and stage tumors and positive lymph nodes (Bagshaw 1974; Bagshaw 1980; Bagshaw 1978; Batata et al. 1980; Cupps et al. 1980; Del Regato 1979; Miljenko, Perez, and Bauer 1980; Perez 1980; Ray, Cassady, and Bagshaw 1973).

PATTERNS OF FAILURE

Patients who die of metastatic prostate cancer often demonstrate excellent local control of the disease. Metastases to bones with bone marrow replacement may be the event that leads to death. Most other organs can be affected, but osseous metastases predominate.

It is difficult to compare results of series utilizing different modalities because comparable groups of patients are not being studied; that is, staging differs as does associated medical disease.

In a careful analysis of postirradiation failures, the local recurrence rate was dependent upon stage (Lipsett et al. 1976; Miljenko, Perez, and Bauer 1980). There may also be a correlation with irradiation dosage and survival rates.

TESTIS CANCER

EPIDEMIOLOGY AND ETIOLOGY

Testis cancer represents only about 1% of all cancer in males, but it is one of the most frequently occurring cancers in young adult men. The average patient age is about 32 years. The incidence among blacks is two-thirds less than that of whites (Devesa and Silverman 1978).

A significantly increased incidence of carcinoma is found developing in cryptorchid testes. Twenty-four percent of testis cancer patients with bilateral cryptorchidism developed carcinoma in the other testis, as compared with 1% of the patients with naturally descended testes in the scrotum.

Etiologic factors are unknown.

DETECTION AND DIAGNOSIS

CLINICAL DETECTION

Typically, there are no early symptoms. A testicular mass is the early finding, and approximately 96% of solid tumors of the testis are malignant. Most are painless, though patients may complain of a dull ache or sense of heaviness. Pain is associated with hemorrhage into the tumor.

Differential diagnosis includes epididymitis; spermatocele; hydrocele; benign tumor of testis, epididymis, or tunica albuginea (rare); orchitis; infarction; and trauma.

Early detection is accomplished best by self-palpation of the testis, and on physical examination.

Among metastatic symptoms and signs, para-aortic lymph node involvement can produce ureteral obstruction or can present as an abdominal mass, and pulmonary symptoms from metastases of unknown origin may be evident in a young patient.

DIAGNOSTIC PROCEDURES

The physician should palpate the testes and surrounding structures for a testicular mass, examine the breasts for signs of gynecomastia, transilluminate intrascrotal lesions, and perform an abdominal examination for a palpable mass.

Ultrasound of the scrotum will locate and delineate an intrascrotal lesion. Excretory urogram with lateral projections may show ureteral deviation from para-aortic or paracaval node involvement.

Radioimmunoassay (RIA) for serum alpha-fetoprotein (AFP) and a subunit human chorionic gonadotrophin (A-HCG) should be performed (Javadpour 1978; Javadpour 1980).

Other diagnostic procedures include abdominal CT scan for staging, and chest film and CT scan of lungs and/or lung tomograms for metastatic disease.

Pedal lymphangiography (Wallace 1969) may be performed, but to a large extent CT scans have replaced it for nonseminomatous testis tumor evaluation. Lymphangiography may be more valuable in the workup of the patient with a seminoma. A positive radiographic interpretation showed excellent correlation (95%) with surgical findings. A positive dissection was predicted by pedal lymphangiogram in 68% of patients (Wallace 1969; Anderson et al. 1979; Babain and Johnson 1980; Caldwell et al. 1980; Fraley et al. 1980; Javadpour 1979; Morse, and Whitmore 1986; Smith 1978).

CLASSIFICATION

ANATOMIC STAGING

Anatomic classification and expansion of histologic typing has occurred because both are important factors in determining the prognosis and treatment of testis cancer.

The UICC has published a TNM classification (International Union Against Cancer 1987).

The incidence of positive lymphadenectomy was 38% for testicular tumors other than seminomas (Maier et al. 1969).

The TNM classification of primary tumor (T), nodal involvement (N), and distant metastases (M) is outlined in table 21.8 (International Union Against Cancer 1987).

STAGE GROUPING

This is an older, alternative approach. In stage A, tumor is confined to the testis. Involvement of retroperitoneal lymph nodes is found in the following stages: stage B1, minimal (fewer than 6 positive nodes and no node >2

**Table 21.8
TUMOR (T), NODE (N) CLASSIFICATION
TESTIS CANCER TNM**

Testis	
pTis	Intratubular
pT1	Testis and rete testis
pT2	Beyond tunica albuginea or into epididymis
pT3	Spermatic cord
pT4	Scrotum
N1	Single <2 cm
N2	Single >2 cm <5 cm, multiple <5 cm
N3	>5 cm
pTNM	Pathological Classification
pT =	Primary Tumor
pTX	Primary tumor cannot be assessed (in the absence of radical orchiectomy TX is used)
pT0	Histological scar or no evidence of primary tumor
pTis	Intratubular tumor: preinvasive cancer
pT1	Tumor limited to testis, including rete testis
pT2	Tumor invades beyond tunica albuginea or into epididymis
pT3	Tumor invades spermatic cord
pT4	Tumor invades scrotum
pN =	Regional Lymph Nodes

The pN categories correspond to the N categories.

| pM = | Distant Metastasis |

The pM categories correspond to the M categories.

(Courtesy: UICC [1987].)

cm in diameter); stage B2, moderate (more than 6 positive nodes or any node >2 cm, but <5 cm in diameter); stage B3, massive, or nodal mass >5 cm; and stage C, metastatic tumor to nodes above the diaphragm or to distant sites (Smith 1978).

HISTOPATHOLOGY

There are two theories on the histogenesis of testicular tumors: the holistic or single germ cell origin theory (fig. 21.4) is favored over the dual origin theory, which hypothesizes a separate origin for seminomas and teratomatous cancers (Dixon and Moore 1953; Friedman 1978; Mostofi 1980; Smith 1978). A representation of the dual origin for the derivation of testicular tumors follows (Mostofi 1980):

Representative Distributions
1. Germinal Origin (97%)
   — Seminoma (pure)
     47.7% (Smith 1978)
     Typical (classical)
     Anaplastic
     Spermatocystic (atypical)
   — Embryonal carcinoma
     20% to 25%
   — Teratoma
     5% to 9%
   — Teratoma with malignant areas
     25% to 30%
     (Teratocarcinoma)
   — Choriocarcinoma
     1% to 3%
2. Nongerminal Origin (3%)
   — Interstitial cell tumors
   — Gonadal-stromal tumors

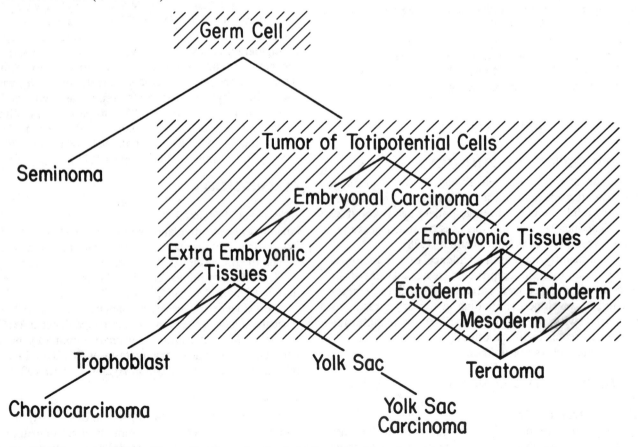

Fig. 21.4. A representation of the unified theory for the derivation of testicular tumors. (Courtesy: Mostofi [1980].)

This schema does not include consideration of so-called carcinoma *in situ,* a microscopic foci of cancer that is still undergoing definition and evaluation.

DIAGNOSIS AND CLINICAL STAGING

The following are recommended procedures for clinical staging:

1. Clinical evaluation, scrotal ultrasound, and histopathologic analysis of the testis and cord are used to determine penetration into the cord, epididymis, or scrotum.

2. Radiographic survey is usually limited to a chest film and CT scans.

3. Excretory urogram, including lateral film evaluation, determines the course of the ureters for evidence of lateral deviation, elevation, or obstruction due to adjacent lymph node involvement.

4. Laboratory survey includes CBC counts and SMA-12.

5. Human chorionic gonadotrophin (HCG) and alpha-fetoprotein (AFP) markers (radio-immunoassays) are recommended before surgery (Javadpour 1978; Javadpour 1980) and offer valuable information regarding staging and prognosis. They are also helpful in the follow-up period.

6. Pedal lymphangiogram may be a useful study for seminomas (Wallace 1969).

7. Venacavagram and isotope scans of liver, brain, and bones are optional procedures.

In patients in whom a testicular tumor is a possibility, inguinal exploration with high ligation of the cord followed by orchiectomy is carried out. Vascular control should be achieved prior to manipulation of the tumor. Open biopsy is usually contraindicated, as is scrotal exploration.

PRINCIPLES OF TREATMENT

SURGERY

If the pathology reveals embryonal carcinoma, teratocarcinoma, adult teratoma, or seminoma with an elevated AFP level, a bilateral retroperitoneal lymph node dissection is usually carried out. In the presence of bulky nodal involvement (B3) or metastatic disease above the diaphragm or to distant organs (C), chemotherapeutic-induced debulking should precede surgery. The surgical lymphadenectomy provides debulking and staging information needed for planning further therapy. For metastatic disease limited to the lungs or abdomen, after a complete response to chemotherapy, surgery is deferred and careful follow-up employed as part of a clinical trial. Early results for nonbulky disease are encouraging (American Cancer Society 1987; Donahue, Einhorn, and Williams 1980; Javadpour 1978; Maier et al. 1969; Skinner 1978).

RADIOTHERAPY

Seminomas. Irradiation of the retroperitoneal and homolateral iliac nodes to the level of the diaphragm is the usual form of treatment for stage A1, B1, and B2 tumors. Surveillance for stage I seminomas is experimental. Prophylactic mediastinal irradiation does not significantly improve survival, and may prevent the optimal use of subsequent chemotherapy (Thomas et al. 1982; Herman et al. 1983). The major thrust of current clinical investigations is to find out whether induction plus limited chemotherapy without maintenance can be successful for nonbulky disease limited to lung or abdomen alone. Careful follow-up is necessary and initial results are promising (American Cancer Society 1987; Caldwell et al. 1980; Maier, Sulak, and Mittmeyer 1968; Thomas, Rider, and Dembo 1982; Williams et al. 1980; Yagoda and Vugrin 1979).

Nonseminomas. Cytoreductive surgery and chemotherapy have largely replaced radiation therapy as the treatment of low stage (A, B1, B2) nonseminomatous testes tumors. Occasionally, radiation therapy may be helpful in the treatment of localized metastatic disease that cannot be excised and does not respond to chemotherapy.

CHEMOTHERAPY

Seminomas. Chemotherapy is useful in cases that fail to respond to radiation therapy and for bulky metastatic disease (Yagoda and Vurgin 1979). It appears that for advanced metastatic bulky disease, combined chemotherapy and cytoreductive surgery will be highly successful (American Cancer Society 1987).

Nonseminomas. Dramatic progress in combining chemotherapeutic agents has had a marked impact on patient survival with metastatic disease. Initially, the essential drugs were cisplatin, vinblastine, and bleomycin with actinomycin D and cyclophosphamide being added in some regimens. The chemotherapy was usually given over a period of three to six months. The side effects can be quite severe and many patients require hospitalization for some portion of the chemotherapy administration. While many patients will have a complete remission, others will have only partial remission, and will require surgery to remove residual tumor. Following chemotherapy, the residual masses removed at surgery will be found to be scar in 40%, teratoma in 40%, and cancer in 20% of cases (Donohue and Rowland 1984).

Should residual carcinoma be found, additional chemotherapy is indicated. Relapses usually occur within 18 months following the initiation of chemotherapy. Relapsing patients and those refractory to initial chemotherapy attempts can be treated with salvage chemotherapy. Prolonged complete remissions, probably representing cures, are frequent. Significant toxicity occurs with these chemotherapeutic regimens (Donahue, Einhorn, and Williams 1980; Einhorn and Stephens 1980; Skinner 1978; Williams et al. 1980).

RESULTS AND PROGNOSIS

The dramatic responses to single-agent and combination drug chemotherapy have made even more advanced cases of testis cancer potentially curable. Radiation therapy still has a curative role for seminomas, but has been almost replaced by chemotherapy for nonseminomatous tumors. Tumor markers (AFP and HCG) aid in the early diagnosis and are equally important in follow-up because they may be the earliest indication of recurrent tumors.

SEMINOMAS

Radiation therapy resulted in 2- to 5-year, disease-free survival rates of 91% (table 21.9) for 1,346 patients with stage A and stage B disease (Caldwell et al. 1980).

Chemotherapy is similar to that for nonseminomas (American Cancer Society 1987). Einhorn and Williams (1980) found a 63% complete response with a minimal follow-up of two years; 58% of patients had no evidence of disease (NED). Others have reported better results (American Cancer Society 1987; Javadpour 1979; Maier, Sulak, and Mittmeyer 1968; Thomas, Rider, and Demo 1982; Williams et al. 1980; Yagoda and Vugrin 1979).

NONSEMINOMAS

Complete remission can be obtained in 50% to 70% of patients with metastatic disease by chemotherapy alone, and another 10% to 15% of patients can be made disease-free by surgical removal of residual tumor. Relapses occur in 10% to 20% of patients who have achieved a complete remission. It appears that almost all relapses occur within 18 months following the initiation of chemotherapy. Relapsing patients and those refractory to initial chemotherapy attempts can be treated with salvage chemotherapy.

Einhorn and Williams (1980) report that all stage B patients who relapsed after surgery and who were detected with minimal disease had a 100% complete response (CR) if no prior chemotherapy or radiotherapy was given. This was also true for stage B2 or large abdominal mass presentations (B3).

A complete response rate depends upon the amount of metastatic disease: minimal disease, 90% complete response; advanced thoracic disease, 67%; advanced abdominal disease, 20%, using a vinblastine, actinomycin D, bleomycin (VAB-4) program (Einhorn and Williams 1980).

CLINICAL INVESTIGATIONS

The major thrust of current clinical investigations is to see if, for nonbulky disease limited to lungs or abdomen alone, whether induction plus limited chemotherapy without maintenance can be successful. Careful follow-up is necessary and initial results are promising (American Cancer Society 1987).

FOR LOCALIZED DISEASE

A search for other tumor markers is being carried out. A 15% false-negative tumor marker accuracy now exists. A reduction in the false-negative rate may lessen the need for retroperitoneal lymph node dissection for staging.

FOR ADVANCED AND METASTATIC STAGES

Randomized studies evaluating adjuvant chemotherapy are in progress. Much attention is being devoted to reducing the significant toxicity associated with combined drug chemotherapy. Alterations in drug doses and intervals of therapy, as well as drug combinations, are being evaluated. Prospective study regarding the need for maintenance chemotherapy following intensive induction chemotherapy is under way. The early results suggest that maintenance chemotherapy may not be required after adequate response to initial chemotherapy (Einhorn and Stephens 1980).

REFERENCES

American Joint Committee on Staging and End Results. 1988. *Reporting manual for staging of cancer.* Chicago: AJC, J.B. Lippincott.

American Cancer Society. 1987 National Conference on Urologic Cancer. *Cancer* 60(Suppl):437-718.

Table 21.9
2- TO 5-YEAR DISEASE-FREE SURVIVAL FOR PATIENTS WITH SEMINOMA

Researchers (years patients were studied)	Stage A	Stage B	Stage C (& D)*	Stage A & B (%)
Ytredal and Bradfield (1947-1971)	69/71	6/6	0/1	97
Maier and Sulak (1940-968)	274/284	31/34	3/18	96
Earle, Bagshaw, and Kaplan (1956-1971)	71/71	23/27	3/4	96
Culp, Boatman, and Wilson (1960-1970)	55/58	5/19	5/32	78
Peckham and McElwain (1963-1971)	77/78	25/27	3/5	97
Del Vecchio, Tawil, and Beland (1951-1969)	27/30	3/4	1/2	88
Doornsbos, Hussey, and Johnson (1944-1971)	74/79	37/48	3/14	87
Lindsey and Glenn (1959-1974)	33/41	7/8	3/4	82
van der Werf Messing (1950-1974)	145/153	58/74	13/30	89
Kademian, Bosch, and Caldwell (1959-1974)	35/36	10/11	1/3	96
Blandy (years not available)	91/98	25/35	2/17	87
Slawson (1957-1973)	32/33	15/21	–	87
Total	983/1032	245/314	37/130	
	95%	78%	28%	91

*In those series where a staging system of A-D is used, those patients with stage D disease are included.
(Courtesy of: Caldwell et al. [1980].)

Anderson, T.; Waldmann, T.A.; and Javadpour, N. et al. 1979. Testicular germ cell neoplasms: recent advances in diagnosis and therapy. *Ann. Intern. Med.* 90:373-85.

Babaian, R.J., and Johnson, D.E. 1980. Management of stages I and II nonseminomatous germ cell tumors of the testis. *Cancer* 45(Suppl):1775-91.

Bagshaw, M.A. 1980. Extended radiation therapy of cancer of the prostate. *Cancer* 45(Suppl):1912-21.

Bagshaw, N.A.; Ray, G.R.; and Pistenma, D.A. et al. 1975. External beam radiation therapy of primary carcinoma of the prostate. *Cancer* 36:723-28.

Bagshaw, M.A. 1978. Radiotherapy for cancer of the prostate. In deKernion, J.B., and Skinner, D.G. eds. *Genitourinary cancer.* pp. 213-31. Philadelphia: W.B. Saunders.

Bagshaw, M.A. 1974. Definitive radiotherapy in carcinoma of the prostate. In Rubin, P. ed. *Current concepts in cancer.* pp. 222-23. Chicago: American Medical Association.

Batata, M.A.; Hilaris, B.S.; and Chu, F.C.H. et al. 1980. Radiation therapy in adenocarcinoma of the prostate with pelvic lymph node involvement at lymphadenectomy. *Int. J. Radiat. Oncol. Biol. Phys.* 6:149-53.

Batata, M.A.; Whitmore, W.F.; and Chu, F.C.H. et al. 1980. Patterns of recurrence in bladder cancer after radiation therapy vs. drugs. *Int. J. Radiat. Oncol. Biol. Phys.* 6:155-60.

Bennington, J.R., and Laubscher, F.A. 1978. Epidemiologic studies on carcinoma of the kidney. 1: association of renal adenocarcinoma with smoking. *Cancer* 21:1069-71.

Byar, D.R. 1973. The Veterans Administration Cooperative Urological Research Group's studies of cancer of the prostate. *Cancer* 32:1126-30.

CA. 1989. 39(1):3-20.

Caldwell, W.; Kademian, M.T.; and Frias, Z. et al. 1980. The management of testicular seminomas, 1979. *Cancer* 45(Suppl):1769-74.

Caldwell, W.L. 1970. *Cancer of the urinary bladder with emphasis on treatment by irradiation.* pp. 1-116. St. Louis: Green.

Cancer Statistics 1990. *CA* 40(1):9-26.

Cancer Statistics Review 1973-1976. 1989. NIH Publ. No. 89-2789. Bethesda, Md.: National Cancer Institute.

Carter, B.S. et al. 1989. Epidemiologic evidence regarding predisposing factors to prostate cancer. *The Prostate* 16:187- 97.

Catalona, W.J., and Scott, W.W. 1986. Carcinoma of the prostate. In Walsh, P.C.; Gittes, R.F.; and Perlmutter, A.D. et al. eds. *Campbell's urology.* 5th ed. vol. 2. pp. 1463-1534. Philadelphia: W.B. Saunders.

Chodak, G.W. 1985. Early detection of prostate cancer. *Hormone Res.* 32(Suppl 1):35.

Cupps, R.E.; Utz, D.C.; and Flemming, T.R. et al. 1980. Definitive radiation therapy for prostatic carcinoma: Mayo Clinic experience. *J. Urol.* 124:855-59.

D'Angio, G.H.; Beckwith, J.B.; and Breslow, N.E. et al. 1980. Wilms' tumor: an update. *Cancer* 45(Suppl):1791-98.

deKernion, J.B., and Skinner, D.G. eds. *Genitourinary cancer.* pp. 213-31. Philadelphia: W.B. Saunders.

deKernion, J.B., and Skinner, D.G. 1978. Epidemiology, diagnosis, and staging of bladder cancer. In Skinner, D.G., and deKernion, J.B. eds. *Genitourinary cancer.* pp. 213-31. Philadelphia: W.B. Saunders.

deKernion, J.B., and Berry, D. 1980. The diagnosis and treatment of renal cancer. *Cancer* 45:1947-56.

Droller, M.J. 1980. Transitional cell carcinoma: an overview. In *Controversies in urologic oncology. Urol. Clin. North Am.* 7:519-21.

Del Regato, J.A. 1979. Long-term curative results of radiotherapy of patients with inoperable prostatic carcinoma. *Radiology* 131:291-97.

Denis, L.; Niijima, T.; and Prout, G. Jr. et al. eds. 1986. Developments in bladder cancer. In *Progress in clinical and biological research.* vol. 221. New York: Alan R. Liss.

Dixon, F.J. Jr., and Moore, R.A. 1953. Testicular tumors: a clinicopathological study. *Cancer* 6:427-54.

Donahue, J.P.; Einhorn, L.H.; and Williams, S.D. 1980. Cytoreductive surgery for metastatic testis cancer: considerations of timing and extent. *J. Urol.* 123:876-80.

Drago, S.R. et al. 1989. *Urology* 34(4):187-92.

Einhorn, L.H., and Williams, S.D. 1980. Chemotherapy of disseminated seminoma. *Cancer Clin. Trials* 3:307-13.

Einhorn, L.H., and Stephens, D.W. 1980. Chemotherapy of disseminated testicular cancer: a random prospective study. *Cancer* 46:1339-44.

Farber, S. 1966. Chemotherapy in leukemia and Wilms' tumor. *JAMA* 198:826-36.

Flocks, R.H., and Kadesky, M.C. 1958. Malignant neoplasms of the kidney: an analysis of 353 patients followed 5 years or more. *J. Urol.* 79:196-201.

Foti, A.G.; Cooper, J.F.; and Herschman, H. et al. 1977. Detection of prostatic cancer by solid-phase radioimmunoassay of serum prostatic acid phosphatase. *N. Engl. J. Med.* 297:1357-61.

Fraley, E.E. 1978. Cancer of the renal pelvis. In Skinner, D.H., and deKernion, J.B. eds. *Genitourinary cancer* pp. 134-49. Philadelphia: W.B. Saunders.

Fraley, E.E.; Lange, P.; and Williams, R. et al. 1980. Staging of early nonseminomatous germ cell testicular cancer. *Cancer* 45(Suppl):1762-67.

Fraley, E.E.; Lange, P.H.; and Kennedy, B.J. 1979. Germ cell testicular cancer in adults. *N. Engl. J. Med.* 301:1370-77.

Friedman, N.E. 1978. Pathology of testicular tumors. In Skinner, D.G., and deKernion, J.E. eds. *Genitourinary cancer.* pp. 430-47. Philadelphia: W.B. Saunders.

Gittes, R.F. 1979. Tumors of the bladder. In Harrison, J.H.; Gittes, R.F.; and Perlmutter, A.D. et al. eds. *Campbell's urology.* 4th ed. pp. 1033-70. Philadelphia: W.B. Saunders.

Gittes, R.F. 1979. Tumors of the ureter and renal pelvis. In Harrison, J.H.; Gittes, R.H.; and Perlmutter, A.D. et al. eds. *Campbell's urology.* vol. 2. pp. 1010-32. Philadelphia: W.B. Saunders.

Gleason, D.F. 1966. Classification of prostatic carcinoma. *Cancer Chemother. Rep.* 50:125-28.

Gleason, D.F., and Mellinger, G.T. 1974. The Veterans Administration Cooperative Urological Research Group: prediction of prognosis for prostatic adenocarcinoma by combined histological grading and clinical staging. *J. Urol.* 111:58-64.

Goodman, G.B.; Hislop, T.G.; and Elwood, J.M. et al. 1981. Conservation of bladder function in patients with invasive bladder cancer treated by definitive irradiation and selective cystectomy. *Int. J. Radiat. Oncol. Biol. Phys.* 7:469-573.

Grabstald, H.; Whitmore, W.F.; and Melamed, M. 1971. Renal pelvic tumors. *JAMA* 218:845-54.

Grace, D.A.; Taylor, W.N.; and Taylor, J.N. 1967. Carcinoma of the renal pelvis: a 15-year review. *J. Urol.* 98:566-69.

Green, N.; Broth, E.; and George, F.W. et al. 1979. Prostate carcinoma: therapeutic considerations in the management of gross lymph node metastases. *Int. J. Radiat. Oncol. Biol. Phys.* 5:891-97.

Guerriero, W.G.; Carlton, E.C. Jr; and Hudgins, P.T. 1980. Combined interstitial and external radiotherapy in the definitive management of carcinoma of the prostate. *Cancer* 45(Suppl):1922-28.

Hahn, R.G. 1979. Bladder cancer treatment considerations for metastatic disease. *Semin. Oncol.* 6:236-39.

Hahn, R.G.; Bauer, M.; and Creech, W.J. et al. 1978. Phase II study of vinblastine, methyl-CCNU, and medroxyprogesterone in advanced renal cell cancer. *Cancer Treat. Rep.* 62:1093-95.

Hahn, R.G.; Bauer, M.; and Walter, J. et al. 1979. Phase II study of single-agent therapy with megestrol acetate, VP-16-213, cyclophosphamide, and dianhydrogalactiol in advanced renal cell carcinoma. *Cancer Treat. Rep.* 63:513-15.

Helmstein, K. 1972. Treatment of bladder carcinoma by a hydrostatic pressure technique: report on 43 cases. *Br. J. Urol.* 44:434-50.

Hilaris, B.S.; Whitmore, W.F.; and Batata, M. et al. 1976. Behavioral patterns of prostate adenocarcinoma following iodine 125 implants and pelvic nodes dissections (abstr). *Int. J. Radiat. Oncol. Biol. Phys.* 1(Suppl):90.

Hilaris, B.S.; Kim, J.H.; and Tokita, N. 1976. Low-energy radionuclides for permanent interstitial implantation. *Am. J. Roentgenol.* 126:171-78.

Huggins, C., and Hodges, C.V. 1941. Studies on prostatic cancer: effect of castration, of estrogen, and of androgen injection on serum phosphatase in metastatic carcinoma of the prostate. *Cancer Res.* 1:293-97.

Hutchinson, G.B. 1981. Incidence and etiology of prostate cancer. *Urology* 17(Suppl):4-10.

International histological classification of tumours, nos. 1-25. vols. 1, 2. Geneva: World Health Organization.

International Union Against Cancer (UICC). 1973. Commission of Clinical Oncology. *TNM classification of malignant tumors.* Geneva: UICC.

International Union Against Cancer (UICC). 1987: *TNM classification of malignant tumours.* 4th, fully rev. ed. New York: Springer-Verlag.

Javadpour, N. 1980. The role of biological tumor markers in testicular cancer. *Cancer* 45(Suppl):1755-61.

Javadpour, N. 1978. Biologic tumor markers in management of testicular and bladder cancer. *Urology* 12:177-83.

Javadpour, N. ed. 1983. *Principles and management of urologic cancer.* Baltimore: Williams & Wilkins.

Javadpour, N. 1979. Testicular germ cell tumors. In *Principles and management of urologic cancer.* pp. 419-44. Baltimore: Williams & Wilkins.

Javadpour, N. The National Cancer Institute experience with testicular cancer. *J. Urol.* 102:651-59.

Jewett, H.J. 1980. Radical perineal prostatectomy for palpable, clinically localized nonobstructive cancer: experience at the Johns Hopkins Hospital 1909-1963. *J. Urol.* 124:492-94.

Jewett, H.J.; Bridge, R.W.; and Gray, G.F. et al. 1968. The palpable nodule of prostatic cancer: results 15 years after radical surgery. *JAMA* 203:403-406.

Jewett, H.J., and Strong, G.H. 1946. Infiltrating carcinoma of the bladder: relation of depth of penetration of the bladder wall to incidence of local extension and metastases. *J. Urol.* 55:366-72.

Kaufman, J.J., and Mims, M. 1966. Tumors of the kidney. In Ravitch, M.M.; Ellison, E.H.; and Julian, O.C. et al. eds. *Current problems in surgery.* pp. 1-44. Chicago: Year Book Medical Publishers.

Kiesling, V.J.; McAninch, J.W.; and Goebel, J.L. et al. 1980. External beam radiotherapy for adenocarcinoma of the prostate: a clinical follow-up. *J. Urol.* 124:851-54.

Lathan, H.S., and Kau, S. 1974. Malignant tumors of the renal pelvis. *Surg. Gynecol. Obstet.* 138:613-22.

Lindberg, B. 1972. Treatment of rapidly progressing prostatic carcinoma with Estracyt. *J. Urol.* 108:303-306.

Lipsett, J.A.; Cosgrove, M.S.; and Green, M.D. et al. 1976. Factors influencing prognosis in the radiotherapeutic management of carcinoma of the prostate. *Int. J. Radiat. Oncol. Biol. Phys.* 1:1049-58.

Maier, J.G.; Sulak, M.H.; and Mittemeyer, E.T. 1968. Seminoma of the testis: analysis of treatment, success, and failure. *Am. J. Roentgenol.* 102:596-602.

Maier, J.G.; VanBuskirk, K.E.; and Sulak, M.E. et al. 1969. An evaluation of lymphadenectomy in treatment of malignant testicular germ cell neoplasm. *J. Urol.* 101:356-59.

McCune, C.S.; Schapira, D.V.; and Henshaw, E.C. 1981. Specific immunotherapy of advanced renal carcinoma: evidence for the polyclonality of metastases. *Cancer* 47:1984-87.

McDonald, J.R., and Priestly, J.T. 1944. Carcinoma of the renal pelvis: histologic study of 75 cases with special reference to prognosis. *J. Urol.* 51:245-58.

Miljenko, V.P.; Perez, C.A.; and Bauer, W. 1980. Prognostic parameters in radiotherapeutic management of localized carcinoma of the prostate. *J. Urol.* 124:485-87.

Miller, L.S. 1980. T3 bladder cancer: the case for higher radiation dosage. *Cancer* 45(Suppl):1875-1978.

Miller, L.S., and Johnson, D.E. 1972. Megavoltage irradiation for bladder cancer alone: postoperative or preoperative? *Proceedings of the 7th National Cancer Conference, Sept. 27-29, 1972.* pp. 771-82. Philadelphia: J.B. Lippincott.

Morse, M.J., and Whitmore, W.F. 1986. Neoplasms of the testis. In Walsh, P.C.; Gittes, R.F.; and Perlmutter, A.D. et al. eds. *Campbell's urology.* 5th ed. vol. 2. pp. 1532-82. Philadelphia: W.B. Saunders.

Mostofi, F.K. 1967. Pathology and spread of renal cell carcinoma. In King, J.S. Jr. ed. *Renal neoplasia.* pp. 45-85. Boston: Little, Brown and Company.

Mostofi, F.K. 1975. Grading of prostate cancer. *Cancer Chemother. Rep.* 59:111-17.

Mostofi, F.K. 1980. Pathology of germ cell tumors of testis: a progress report. *Cancer* 45(Suppl):1735-54.

Murphy, L.J. 1972. *The history of urology.* p. 127. Springfield: Charles C. Thomas.

Murphy, G.P.; Khoury, S.; and Kuss, R. et al. eds. 1987. *Prostate cancer, parts A and B.* New York: Alan R. Liss.

Murphy, G.P. 1981. Current status of classification and staging of prostate cancer. *Cancer* 45:1889-96.

Neidhart, J.A.; Murphy, S.G.; and Henrich, L.A. et al. 1980. Active specific immunotherapy of stage IV renal carcinoma with aggregated tumor antigen adjuvant. *Cancer* 46:1128-34.

Paulson, D.F. 1979. Uro-oncology research group. *J. Urol.* 121:300-302.

Paulson, D.F. 1981. Multimodal therapy of prostate cancer. *Urology* 17(Suppl):53-56.

Perez, C.A. 1980. Irradiation of cancer of the prostate localized to pelvis: analysis of tumor response and prognosis. *Int. J. Radiat. Oncol. Biol. Phys.* 6:555-63.

Prando, A.; Wallace, S.; and Von Eschenbach, A.C. et al. 1979. Lymphangiography in staging of carcinoma of the prostate: the potential value of percutaneous lymph node biopsy. *Radiology* 131:641-45.

Priestley, J.T. 1939 Survival following removal of renal neoplasms. *JAMA* 113:902-906.

Prout, G.R. Jr. 1980. Classifying and staging bladder cancer. *Cancer* 45(Suppl):1832-41.

Prout, G.R. Jr.; Slack, N.H.; and Bross, I.D. 1970. Irradiation and 5-fluorouracil and adjuvants in the management of invasive bladder carcinoma: a cooperative group report after 4 years. *J. Urol.* 104:116-29.

Ray, G.R.; Cassady, J.R.; and Bagshaw, M.A. 1973. Definitive radiation therapy of carcinoma of the prostate: report of 15 years of experience. *Radiology* 106:407-18.

Resnick, M.I., and Kursh, E. eds. 1987. *Current therapy in genitourinary surgery.* Toronto: B.C. Decker, Inc.

Riches, E.W.; Griffith, I.H.; and Thackaray, A.C. 1957. New growths of the kidney and ureter. *Br. J. Urol.* 23:297-356.

Robson, C.J.; Churchill, B.M.; and Anderson, W. 1968. Results of radical nephrectomy for renal cell carcinoma. *Trans. Am. Assoc. Genitourin. Surg.* 60:122-29.

Robson, C.J. 1963. Radical nephrectomy for renal cell carcinoma. *J. Urol.* 89:37-42.

Rubin, P. ed. 1974. Cancer of the urogenital tract. In *Current concepts in cancer.* parts IV-XX. pp. 117-254. Chicago: American Medical Association.

Rubin, P. 1968. Introduction and comment: conservatism vs. radicalism in treatment. *JAMA* 206:2719-28.

Rubin, P. 1968. Cancer of the urogenital tract: bladder cancer incidence, frequency, etiological factors. *JAMA* 206:1761-76.

Rubin, P. ed. 1968. Cancer of the urogenital tract: kidney, part X. *JAMA* 204:603-13.

Steele, G.; Wang, B.S.; and Richie, J.P. et al. 1981. Results of xenogeneic I-RNA therapy in patients with metastatic renal cell carcinoma. *Cancer* 47:1286-88.

Salazar, O.M.; Rubin, P.; and Hendrickson, F.R. et al. 1981. Single half-body irradiation for the palliation of multiple bone metastases from solid tumors: a preliminary report. *Int. J. Radiat. Oncol. Biol. Phys.* 7:773-81.

Schmitt, J.D.; Scott, W.W.; and Gibbons, R. et al. Chemotherapy programs of the National Prostatic Cancer Project (NPCP). *Cancer* 45:1937-46.

Scott, W.W.; Menon, M.; and Walsh, P.C. 1980. Hormonal therapy of prostate cancer. *Cancer* 45:1929-36.

Skinner, D.G. 1978. Management of nonseminomatous tumors of the testis. In Skinner, D.G., and deKernion, J.B. eds. *Genitourinary cancer.* pp. 470-93. Philadelphia: W.B. Saunders.

Skinner, D.G., and Lieskovsky, G. eds. 1988. *Diagnosis and management of genitourinary cancer.* Philadelphia: W.B. Saunders.

Smith, J.A., and Whitmore, W.F. 1981. Regional lymph node metastasis from bladder cancer. *J. Urol.* 125:591-93.

Smith, R.B. 1978. Diagnosis and staging of testicular tumors. In Skinner, D.G., and deKernion, J.B. eds. *Genitourinary cancer.* pp. 448-69. Philadelphia: W.B. Saunders.

Soloway, M.S. 1980. The management of superficial bladder cancer. *Cancer* 45:1856-65.

Suen, K.C.; Lau, L.L.; and Yermakov, V. 1974. Cancer and old age: an autopsy study of 3,535 patients over 65 years old. *Cancer* 33:1164-68.

Thomas, G.M.; Rider, W.D.; and Dembo, A.J. 1982. Seminoma of the testis: results of treatment and patterns of failure after radiation therapy. *Int. J. Radiat. Oncol. Biol. Phys.* 8:165-74.

Van der Werf-Messing, B. 1973. Carcinoma of the bladder treated by preoperative irradiation followed by cystectomy: second report. *Cancer* 32:1084-88.

Van der Werf-Messing, B. 1979. Preoperative radiation therapy followed by cystectomy to treat carcinoma of the urinary bladder, category T3, NX, 0-4 M0. *Int. J. Radiat. Oncol. Biol. Phys.* 5:395-401.

Van der Werf-Messing, B. 1973. Carcinoma of the kidney. *Cancer* 32:1056-61.

Van der Werf-Messing, B.; Sourek-Zikova, V.; and Blonk, D.I. 1976. Localized advanced carcinoma of the prostate: radiation therapy vs. therapy. *Int. J. Radiat. Oncol. Biol. Phys.* 1:1043-48.

Van der Werf-Messing, B. 1981. Cancer of the bladder (T1, NX, M0) radiation only vs. TUR. *Int. J. Radiat. Oncol. Biol. Phys.* 7:299-303.

Van der Werf-Messing, B.; Friedell, G.H.; and Menon, R.S. et al. 1981. Carcinoma of the urinary bladder (T3, NX, M0) treated by preoperative irradiation followed by simple cystectomy. *Int. J. Radiat. Oncol. Biol. Phys.* 8:1849-55.

Wallace, N. 1969. Lymphography in the management of testicular tumors. *Clin. Radiol.* 20:453-58.

Wallace, D.M., and Bloom, H.J.G. 1976. The management of deeply infiltrating (T3) bladder carcinoma: controlled trial of radical radiotherapy vs. postoperative radiotherapy and radical cystectomy (first report). *Br. J. Urol.* 48:587-97.

Walsh, P.C.; Gittes, R.F.; and Perlmutter, A.D. et al. eds. 1986. *Campbell's urology.* 5th ed. vol. 2. sec. IX, XII. Philadelphia: W.B. Saunders.

Walsh, P.C., and Lepor, H. 1987. The role of radical prostatectomy in the management of prostatic cancer. *Cancer* 60(Suppl):526-37.

Whitmore, W.F. Jr.; Grabstald, H.; and Mackenzie, A.R. et al. 1968. Preoperative irradiation with cystectomy in the management of bladder cancer. *Am. J. Roentgenol.* 102:570-76.

Whitmore, W.F. Jr.; Batata, M.A.; and Hilaris, B.S. et al. 1977. A comparative study of 2 preoperative radiation regimens with cystectomy for bladder cancer. *Cancer* 40:1077-86.

Whitmore, W.F. Jr., and Marshall, V.F. 1962. Radical total cystectomy for cancer of the bladder: 230 consecutive cases 5 years later. *J. Urol.* 87:853-68.

Williams, S.D.; Einhorn, L.E.; and Greco, F.A. et al. 1980. V0-16-213 salvage therapy for refractory germinal neoplasms. *Cancer* 46:2154-58.

Yagoda, A. 1980. Chemotherapy of metastatic bladder cancer. *Cancer* 45:1879-88. Yagoda, A., and Vugrin, D. 1979. Theoretical considerations in the treatment of seminoma. *Semin. Oncol.* 6:74-81.

Chapter 22

SKIN CANCER: BASAL CELL AND SQUAMOUS CELL CARCINOMA

Robert J. Friedman, M.D.
Darrell S. Rigel, M.D.
Diane S. Berson, M.D.
Jason Rivers, M.D., F.R.C.P.(C.)

Robert J. Friedman, M.D.
Clinical Assistant Professor
Department of Dermatology
New York University Medical Center
New York, New York

Darrell S. Rigel, M.D.
Clinical Assistant Professor
Department of Dermatology
New York University Medical Center
New York, New York

Diane S. Berson, M.D.
Clinical Instructor
Department of Dermatology
New York University Medical Center
New York, New York

Jason Rivers, M.D., F.R.C.P.(C.)
Past Melanoma Fellow
Department of Dermatology
New York University Medical Center
New York, New York

BASAL CELL CARCINOMA

DEFINITION

Basal cell carcinoma (basal cell epithelioma) is a malignant neoplasm of the skin that arises from the basal cells of the epidermis and its appendages (figs. 22.1-22.4). It is characterized by slow local growth capable of causing extensive tissue destruction. It is the most prevalent cancer in humans. Although metastases are rare, these tumors can lead to death if left untreated.

EPIDEMIOLOGY

Basal cell carcinoma (BCC) will account for most of the estimated 600,000 new cases of nonmelanoma skin cancers in the United States in 1990 (ACS 1990). BCC occurs predominantly on skin exposed to ultraviolet radiation, a fact which has been recognized for many years (Fitzpatrick et al. 1982). It rarely develops in very dark-skinned persons, but when it does, the neoplasm primarily occurs on sun-exposed areas of the head and neck (Brody 1970). Men are affected more often than women, but this sex difference is becoming less noticeable, presumably because of changes in lifestyle and sun exposure habits of women. Once infrequent before the age of 40, current trends of increased sun exposure have made BCCs more common in people still in their 20s. The incidence rate rises annually, perhaps compounded by the depletion of the ozone layer, which prevents much of the carcinogenic radiation in ultraviolet light (UVL) from reaching the earth (Fitzpatrick et al. 1982).

PATHOGENESIS

Ultraviolet light (UVL) is the factor most frequently implicated in the pathogenesis of skin cancer. People who live close to the equator have an increased likelihood of developing skin cancer (Fears, Scotto, and Schneiderman 1977; Scotto, Kopf, and Urbach 1979; Swanbeck 1971; Urbach 1971), as do individuals with outdoor professions and those who tend to burn and not tan. The risk is substantially decreased in people who tan easily and in those who are naturally dark-skinned

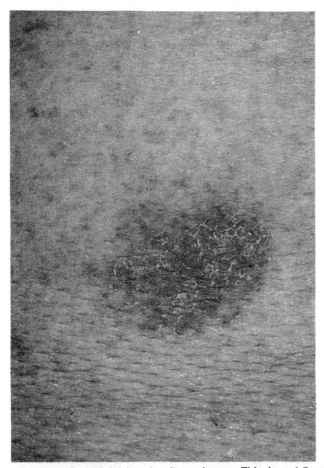

Fig. 22.1. Superficial basal cell carcinoma. This is a 1.5-cm erythematous plaque with a rolled telangiectatic pearly border.

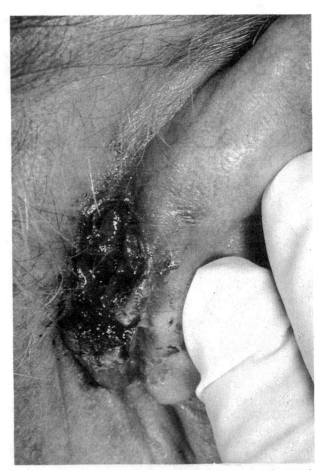

Fig. 22.2. Ulcerated basal cell carcinoma. This 1.4-cm ulcerated nodule has the typical pearly borders seen in this neoplasm.

(Brody 1970; Urbach 1971; Marshall 1968; Ten Seldam 1963; Vitaliano and Urbach 1980).

Cumulative exposure to UVL over many years is necessary for the development of skin cancer (Fears, Scotto, and Schneiderman 1977; Vitaliano and Urbach 1980), which explains its infrequency in children. The predominant spectrum for photocarcinogenesis lies between 290 nm and 320 nm (UVL) (Black and Chan 1977; Johnson 1973). In mice the use of UVL-absorbing sunscreens suppresses the development of cutaneous neoplasia (Kligman, Akin, and Kligman 1980).

Ionizing radiation may also induce BCC (Ridley and Spittle 1974; Martin, Strong, and Spiro 1970; Good, Diaz, and Bowerman 1980; Madison 1980; Traenkle 1963) after a long latency period (Ridley and Spittle 1974; Martin, Strong, and Spiro 1970; Good, Diaz, and Bowerman 1980; Madison 1980; Modan et al. 1974). As with carcinomas caused by UVL, DNA damage probably plays a critical role (Cleaver 1968; Cleaver 1969; Lehmann et al. 1977; Kraemer 1981). Chemicals such as arsenic (Wagner et al. 1979) and topically applied nitrogen mustard (Lee et al. 1982) have also been associated with the development of BCC.

The immune system may contribute to the pathogenesis of skin tumors. Squamous cell carcinoma appears at an increased rate in immune-compromised patients with lymphoma and leukemia (Cohen 1980; Weimar, Ceilley, and Goeken 1979; Manusow and Weinerman 1975; Harville and Aaron 1973; Turner and Callen 1981), in renal transplant patients, and in nontransplant patients on immunosuppressive medication (Halgrimson et al. 1973; Hoxtell et al. 1977; Marshall 1974; Walden, Robertson, and Jeremy 1971; Mullen, Silverberg, and Penn 1976; Smith and Brysk 1981). Whether immune suppression *per se* affects the biology of BCC is currently unclear. The development of BCCs in patients infected with human immunodeficiency virus (HIV) has recently been reported (Fisher and Warner 1987; Slazinski, Stall, and Mathew 1984; Ruocco and Satriano 1986; Sitz, Koppen, and Johnson 1987); in one of these patients the BCC metastasized (Sitz, Koppen, and Johnson 1987).

BIOLOGIC ACTIVITY

The stroma is critical for both initiating and maintaining the development of BCC. Transplantation of basal cell carcinomas devoid of stroma often is not successful (Van Scott and Reinertson 1961; Lyles, Freeman, and Knox 1960; Gerstein 1963; Pawlowski and Haberman 1979), which may account for the infrequency with which BCCs metastasize. A sufficient blood supply is also required for maintenance. As expected, these tumors can elicit an angiogenic factor (Wolf and Hubler 1975), accounting for the telangiectatic vessels characteristically seen on the tumor's surface. BCCs generally

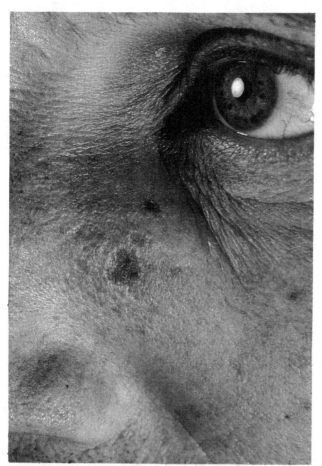

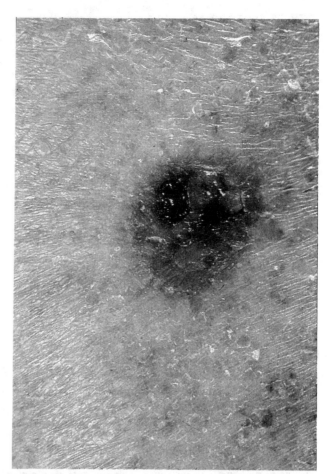

Fig. 22.3. Pigmented basal cell carcinoma. This 8-mm pigmented nodule with rolled pearly borders is present on the left cheek of this young patient. The classical rolled border allows the differentiation of this lesion from a melanocytic neoplasm.

Fig. 22.4. Pigmented basal cell carcinoma. This 1-cm ulcerated pigmented nodule could not be clinically distinguished from an ulcerated malignant melanoma. Only a biopsy allowed for the proper diagnosis.

have a slow growth rate, owing to the opposing forces of growth and tumor regression. The dominant phase dictates the rate at which the tumor enlarges (Franchimont et al. 1982). Many studies indicate that collagenase may contribute to the spread of BCC (Bauer et al. 1977; Hashimoto, Yamanishi, and Dabbous 1972; Montandon, Kocher, and Gabbiani 1982; Barsky, Grossman, and Bhuta 1987).

Metastasis for BCC is infrequent; incidence ranges from 0.0028% to 0.1% (Mikail et al. 1977; Von Domarus and Steven 1984). It occurs most commonly via lymphatic spread to regional nodes and hematogenous spread to long bones and lungs. When metastases are present, the primary lesion is usually located in the head and neck area and has been long standing. BCC may invade both the vasculature and perineurium. Although the adenoid and basosquamous (metatypical) variants of BCC metastasize most often, all of the histologic subtypes have the potential to do so.

In contrast to their low metastatic rate, BCCs are locally invasive and destructive. Basal cell carcinoma always follows the path of least resistance, explaining why invasion of bone, cartilage, and muscle is a late event. If the tumor does reach these areas it will migrate along the perichondrium (Robinson, Pollack, and Robins 1980; Levine and Ballin 1980; Ceilly, Bumsted, and

Smith 1979; Bailin et al. 1980; Mora and Robins 1978), periosteum (Levine and Bailin 1980; Bailin et al. 1980), or fascial plane (Mora and Robins 1978). This in part explains the high recurrence rates encountered in the eyelid region (Mora and Robins 1978; Ceilly and Anderson 1978; Rosen 1987), nose (Mora and Robins 1978; Roenigk et al. 1986), and scalp (Gormley and Hirsch 1978; Binstock, Stegman, and Tromovitch 1981).

Embryonic fusion planes are vulnerable to the deep invasion of BCC, where higher than expected rates of recurrence are seen following therapy. These areas include the inner canthus, philtrum, mid-lower chin, nasolabial groove, preauricular area, and the retroauricular sulcus (Levine and Bailin 1980; Ceilly, Bumsted, and Smith 1979; Bailin et al. 1980; Mora and Robins 1978; Gullane 1986; Granstrom, Aldenburg, and Jeppsson 1986).

Basal cell carcinomas usually do not penetrate into the subcutis because of its insufficient vascular supply. They may spread perineurally (Mark 1972; Ballantyne, McCarter, and Ibanez 1963; Hanke et al. 1983) but this is uncommon and usually seen with recurrent aggressive lesions (Mark 1972; Hanke et al. 1983). The patient may feel numbness, tingling, or pain, and experience motor weakness or paralysis (Mark 1972; Ballantyne, McCarter, and Ibanez 1963; Hanke et al. 1983).

CLINICAL MANIFESTATIONS

Nodular (or nodulo-ulcerative) BCC is the most common type of primary BCC. The lesion usually presents as a flesh-colored or pink translucent nodule with superimposed telangiectasis. Ulceration may accompany growth of the tumor. The occasional presence of melanin accounts for the variable amount of visible pigment and may make the lesion appear black, resembling a melanocytic neoplasm. Over many years these tumors can grow and invade deeply, destroying an eyelid, nose, or ear. The destruction may be so extensive that the ulcer's primary etiology is not easily discernible. Close inspection of the ulcer's periphery, however, often reveals a pearly telangiectatic rolled border.

The superficial multicentric variant of BCC is most often found on the trunk and extremities, although it may also occur in the head and neck region. The lesion is usually an erythematous, slightly scaly patch that typically has a rolled translucent border. Atrophy and pigmentary alterations appear in areas in which regression has occurred. Lesions vary in size and may be single or multiple. Their appearance may be similar to that of various benign inflammatory processes such as nummular dermatitis and psoriasis. Early radial growth of these tumors is responsible for their large size; however, they can also penetrate vertically, forming nodules and ulceration. A high recurrence rate following surgical removal is caused by persistent subclinical centrifugal extension of the lesions.

The morpheaform type of BCC presents as an indurated sclerotic plaque of varying size with occasional telangiectases, resembling a lesion of morphea. It can also clinically and histologically mimic metastatic carcinoma. Morpheaform BCCs infiltrate aggressively and subclinically, tending to recur after seemingly adequate treatment. Cystic BCCs are characterized by clear bluish cystic lesions containing a clear fluid that can be expressed with manipulation. When present on the face they resemble hidrocystomas. Occasionally the cystic changes that can be seen histologically are quite subtle clinically, thus giving the tumor the appearance of a common nodular BCC.

BCC with squamous metaplasia (basosquamous or metatypical carcinoma) is a histologic classification, although it is clinically more aggressive than other BCCs. Some believe it has characteristics more like that of a squamous cell carcinoma (SCC), with an increased incidence of metastases and postoperative recurrences (Borel 1973; Farmer and Helwig 1980; Fidler 1978; Lund 1957; Montgomery 1967; Murphy 1975; Schuller et al. 1979; Stellmack, Rehrmann, and Koch 1971; Thomas 1968). Metastatic lesions may histologically reveal a poorly differentiated SCC (Borel 1973; Farmer and Helwig 1980); the primary tumor in such cases is probably composed of relatively more squamoid cells. The estimated incidence of metastasis for this type of BCC is 9.7% (Borel 1973).

There are conflicting opinions about the role of irradiation in the induction of this tumor (Montgomery 1967; Schuller et al. 1979; Conley 1966). Some believe that the metatypical histologic features gradually evolve with each successive recurrence of BCC (Borel 1973; Farmer and Helwig 1980; Murphy 1975; Stellmack, Rehrmann, and Koch 1971; Conley 1966).

The fibroepithelioma of Pinkus is a rare variant of BCC usually found on the lower back, although it can appear elsewhere. The lesion, a firm smooth nodule classically pedunculated, resembles a fibroma.

TREATMENT OVERVIEW

The most important goal in the management of a patient with BCC is complete elimination of the lesion. Also important are the need for conservation of normal structure and function and an optimal cosmetic result. Although often stressed, the latter should not take precedence over total removal of the lesion, since in the long run the cosmetic defect would be even larger if more procedures were required. One study revealed a high incidence of recurrent BCCs in young women for whom cosmetic outcome was given priority over adequate treatment (Robins and Albom 1975).

Although BCCs enlarge slowly and seldom metastasize, their potential for aggressive local growth should not be underestimated when determining a treatment. The decision to repeatedly desiccate and curette a recurrent BCC rather than to surgically remove it, if its depth had not been appreciated, could eventually result in extensive tissue destruction. There are many treatment options for this tumor; the clinician should use the one with which he or she has the most experience.

The anatomic location and the type of tumor should also be considered. A clinician inexperienced in performing the optimal procedure for a given patient should make a referral to an appropriately skilled expert.

Prevention is significant in the management of skin cancer patients, who should be informed about the potential hazards of excessive sun exposure and the importance of regular sunscreen use.

CURETTAGE AND ELECTRODESICCATION

This method is the one dermatologists most commonly use in the treatment of BCCs. Some authors contend that the procedure should be repeated a fixed number of times (Knox, Freeman, and Heaton 1962; Kopf et al. 1977; Tromovitch 1965); however, treating deeper than is required to eradicate the tumor will only contribute to poor cosmesis. Some investigators have excluded the electrodesiccation in order to optimize the cosmetic result, achieving cure rates only slightly lower than with the combination of curettage and electrodesiccation (Reymann 1975; McDaniel 1978; Reymann 1971; McDaniel 1983). Although this modification decreases the incidence of hypertrophic scarring, it does not prevent postinflammatory pigmentary alterations (McDaniel 1978; McDaniel 1983).

Cure rates using curettage and electrodesiccation have been reported as high (Spiller and Spiller 1984;

Knox et al. 1960; Salasche 1983; Edens et al. 1983; Kopf et al. 1977; Tromovitch 1965; McDaniel 1978; McDaniel 1983; Salasche 1984), but only certain lesions are amenable to this form of therapy. BCCs arising in areas that are characterized by a high rate of recurrence (i.e., eyelids, nose, lips, ears, scalp, temple, and embryonic fusion planes) should not be treated this way because there is no definitive proof that a tumor has been destroyed. Lesions greater than 1 cm in diameter and those without well-defined clinical borders should also be considered for alternative forms of treatment (Salasche 1984).

EXCISION

Surgical excision provides a specimen that can be histologically evaluated. If performed skillfully, it can produce a cosmetically good result and heal quickly. Theoretically, excision is appropriate for most BCCs but it takes more time and requires more experience than desiccation and curettage. It may also sacrifice normal tissue in the process. The cure rates are inferior to those for Mohs surgery in the treatment of recurrent BCCs (Menn et al. 1971), morpheaform BCCs (Salasche and Ammonette 1981; Burg et al. 1975), some large superficial multicentric BCCs (Sloane 1974), and BCCs in high-risk (anatomic site and type) areas (Bart et al. 1978; Dubin and Kopf 1983).

Wolf and Zitelli (1987) have shown that for non-morpheaform BCCs with a distinct border that are 2 cm or less in diameter, 4 mm clear margins were necessary to eliminate 98% of the lesions. They reported that the subclinical extension of the tumors was not uniform in all directions; in tumors larger than 2 cm in diameter, subclinical spread was so irregular that they could not offer advice regarding an appropriate margin.

The question as to the proper depth of excision remains unanswered. For small primary BCCs, excision into fat is generally appropriate since spread into the subcutis is rare. However, large, recurrent, or high-risk BCCs may infiltrate into the subcutaneous tissue.

MOHS MICROGRAPHIC SURGERY

This modality permits the best histologic verification of complete removal and allows maximum conservation of tissue (Robins 1981; Mohs 1978). It is the preferred treatment for large penetrating tumors; for morpheaform, recurrent, poorly delineated, high-risk, and incompletely removed BCCs; and for those sites in which tissue conservation is imperative (Hanke et al. 1983; Menn et al. 1971; Salasche and Ammonette 1981; Burg et al. 1975; Robins 1981; Mohs 1978; Robinson 1987; Tromovitch and Stegman 1978).

Mohs surgery is more time-consuming than routine surgery and is not always easily accessible. Although this technique was developed to manage the most aggressive BCCs, other surgical specialists may need to be consulted for help either in removing deeply invasive tumors or in repairing the surgical defect (Baker, Swanson, and Grekin 1987; Riefkohl, Pollack, and Gerogiade 1985).

RADIATION THERAPY

Radiation therapy is helpful in the treatment of some BCCs. Its major advantage that it spares normal tissue, obviating the need for complicated surgical procedures. It is often preferred for BCCs of the nose, ear, and near the eyes since reconstructive surgery is not required and functional integrity (e.g., lacrimal duct) is preserved (Braun-Falco, Lukacs, and Goldschmidt 1976; Gladstein, Kopf, and Bart 1978; Chahbaziam and Brown 1980; Chahbaziam and Brown 1984). Its use offers elderly patients an alternative to a surgical procedure they may not be willing to undergo (Gladstein, Kopf, and Bart 1978). Radiation therapy has also been used for palliation in inoperable BCC and can provide the patient with a better quality of life (Hunter 1987). However, it should not be used in younger patients because of potential late radiation sequelae (Braun-Falco, Lukacs, and Goldschmidt 1976; Gladstein, Kopf, and Bart 1978; Hunter 1987).

The 5-year cure rates for primary BCCs treated with radiation is 90% to 95% (Dubin and Kopf 1983; Braun-Falco, Lukacs, and Goldschmidt 1976; Gladstein, Kopf, and Bart 1978; Chahbaziam and Brown 1980; Chahbaziam and Brown 1984; Brady, Binnick, and Fitzpatrick 1987). Although one dose of x-ray can adequately treat a small BCC of 1 cm or less in size, appropriate treatment usually consists of fractionated doses given over several sessions to maximize cure and cosmesis (Braun-Falco, Lukacs, and Goldschmidt 1976; Gladstein, Kopf, and Bart 1978; Chahbaziam and Brown 1980; Chahbaziam and Brown 1984; Brady, Binnick, and Fitzpatrick 1987). The skin of the head and neck endures the effects of radiation therapy better than that of the trunk and extremities. Cure rates for recurrent BCC are poorer than for primary lesions (Gladstein, Kopf, and Bart 1978), probably due to the tumor's subclinical spread.

Complications of radiation therapy include scarring (Brady, Binnick, and Fitzpatrick 1987; Goldschmidt and Sherwin 1983), cutaneous necrosis (Gladstein, Kopf, and Bart 1978; Hunter 1987; Brady, Binnick, and Fitzpatrick 1987), and chronic radiation dermatitis (Braun-Falco, Lukacs, and Goldschmidt 1976). Whereas surgical scars improve with time, cosmesis deteriorates after radiation therapy. At nine to 12 years, only 50% of patients have a good cosmetic result (Gladstein, Kopf, and Bart 1978; Brady, Binnick, and Fitzpatrick 1987).

CRYOSURGERY

Cryosurgery has become an accepted treatment for certain BCCs. Treatment of a BCC with cryosurgery requires use of a liquid nitrogen spray unit; cotton-tipped swabs in liquid nitrogen are not acceptable. A double freeze-thaw cycle to a tissue temperature of $-50°C$ is required to sufficiently destroy the tumor. A margin of normal-appearing skin should also be frozen to ensure eradication of subclinical disease (Zacarian 1985; McLean et al. 1978).

Cryosurgery is not advised for BCCs of the scalp. Lesions on the lower legs treated with cryosurgery heal slowly and often yield poor cosmetic results. Cryosurgery is recommended for BCCs of the eyelids because the procedure preserves normal tissue and obviates the need for reconstructive surgery (Zacarian 1985; Frauenfelder 1985; Kuflik 1985). Potential complications include loss of the eyelashes, scarring, hypopigmentation, and increased eyelid thickness (Frauenfelder 1985; Kuflik 1985). In this anatomic area cure rates as high as 97% have been reported for BCCs smaller than 1 cm in diameter (Frauenfelder 1985); the cure rate decreases with larger and recurrent lesions (Frauenfelder 1985; Kuflik 1985). Cure rates for cryosurgery of BCCs in other areas are excellent (97% to 98%) for tumors less than 2 cm in diameter. Larger tumors and morpheaform, recurrent, and high-risk BCCs are more likely to recur after therapy (Zacarian 1985; Spiller and Spiller 1985).

Cryosurgery is not advised for BCCs attached to periosteum and for patients who have blood dyscrasias, dysglobulinemia, cold intolerance, autoimmune disease, or who are receiving immunosuppressive therapy or renal dialysis (Zacarian 1985). Complications include tissue depression, hypertrophic scarring, and postinflammatory pigmentary changes (Zacarian 1985; Zacarian 1985). The occurrence of pain at first during the freeze and later during the thaw can be avoided by preoperative infiltration of the treatment area with epinephrine-free xylocaine. Blistering, crusting, and swelling can also develop, but these effects usually resolve within a few weeks.

LASERS

The carbon dioxide (CO_2) laser has been used in the management of BCC and has several advantages over conventional surgery. Its sealing of small blood vessels and nerves provides a relatively bloodless surgical field and reduced postoperative pain (Bailin, Ratz, and Lutz-Nagey 1981; Sacchini et al. 1984). It can be used in the focused cutting mode to excise the tumor or in the defocused vaporizing mode in combination with curettage to treat large or multiple superficial multicentric BCCs (SMBCCs).

INTERFERON

Greenway et al. (1986) have successfully treated eight BCC patients with intralesional human recombinant alpha-2 interferon (IFN); 1.5×10^6 IU were injected into the lesions three times a week for three weeks. Microscopic studies of the treated areas revealed no residual tumor. Side effects of IFN therapy include fever, malaise, myalgias, chills, transient leukopenia, discomfort, and itching at the injection site. Further investigation of interferon therapy should provide some insight into its effectiveness.

RETINOIDS

Experience with the use of retinoids for BCC is limited. Its use most often has been for patients with the basal cell nevus syndrome (Hodak et al. 1987; Crestofollini et

al. 1984). Partial regression of BCC has resulted from the use of 4.5 mg/kg/day of isotretinoin and 1 mg/kg/day of etretinate. High-dose isotretinoin (1.5 mg/kg/day) has a preventive effect (Crestofollini et al. 1984; Peck 1986), However, side effects limit the use of these agents for long periods, and discontinuation of therapy can lead to relapse (Crestofollini et al. 1984; Peck 1986).

CHEMOTHERAPY

Chemotherapy is appropriate for locally aggressive or metastatic tumors. Disseminated disease is otherwise associated with a poor prognosis, with an average survival of 10 to 20 months (Mikhail et al. 1977; Farmer and Helwig 1980; Safao and Good 1977). A complete systemic workup is required when evaluating a patient for metastases. This includes a thorough medical history, physical examination, complete blood counts, liver profile, chest x-ray, bone and liver scans, and CT scans, when appropriate.

For metastatic disease limited to the regional nodes, surgery with or without radiation is indicated (Coker et al. 1983; Hartman, Hartman, and Green 1986; Wieman, Shiveley, and Woodcock 1983). Systemic chemotherapy, occasionally in combination with radiation, should be used in cases with more extensive metastases including those involving bone. Cisplatin, bleomycin, cyclophosphamide, 5-fluorouracil, and vinblastine have been studied; cisplatin has been the most effective and is associated with the longest remission (Coker et al. 1983; Hartman, Hartman, and Green 1986; Wieman, Shiveley, and Woodcock 1983). Cisplatin, doxorubicin, and radiation therapy can achieve palliation in widely disseminated or inoperable BCC.

FOLLOW-UP

It is imperative to examine regularly patients with BCC. Although most recurrences appear within five years, many can develop later (Grover 1973). Subsequent new primary BCCs can also appear; 20% to 30% do so within one year of treatment of the original lesion (Bergstresser and Halprin 1975; Spoor 1972; Epstein 1987; Robinson 1987.

Finally, it is important to advise patients to avoid excessive sun exposure and to regularly apply a sunscreen with a sun protective factor (SPF) of 15 or greater whenever they are exposed to direct or reflected sunlight.

SQUAMOUS CELL CARCINOMA

DEFINITION

Squamous cell carcinoma (SCC) is a malignant tumor of the keratinizing cells of the epidermis (figs. 22.5-22.7). Unlike basal cell carcinoma, SCC has the propensity to metastasize to regional lymph nodes and distant sites.

EPIDEMIOLOGY

Squamous cell carcinoma is the second most common skin cancer in humans. It is a disease of older people,

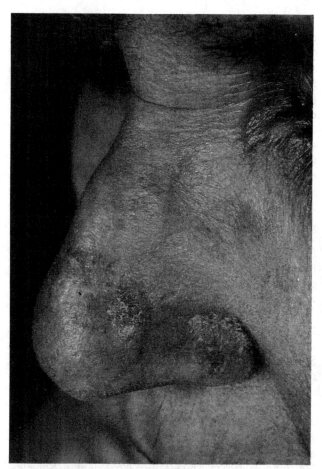

Fig. 22.5. Actinic keratosis. Multiple scaly erythematous plaques are seen on the latter aspect of the nose.

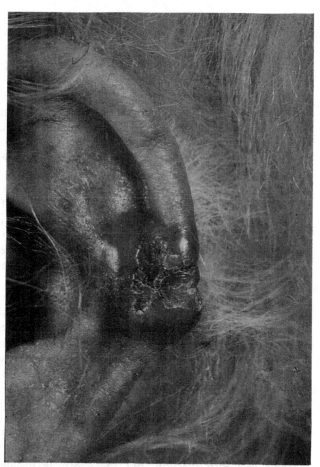

Fig. 22.6. Squamous cell carcinoma. This erythematous ulcerated nodule was slowly growing on the helix of this elderly patient. The lack of a pearly border helps distinguish this lesion from a basal cell carcinoma.

with men outnumbering women 2:1 (Scotto, Fears, and Fraumeni 1983). In one large retrospective study, the mean age at diagnosis for SCC was 68.1 years in men and 72.7 years in women (Aubry and Mac Gibbon 1985). In one report, 2.6% of patients with SCC were between the ages of 30 and 39 years (Katz, Urbach, and Lilienfeld 1957).

Evidence suggests that most human SCCs are related to the total accumulated lifetime dose of solar radiation (Kripke, Urbach, and Witkop 1983). It is also clear that skin pigmentation protects against the induction of skin cancer. People of Celtic descent, with fair complexions, poor tanning ability, and a predisposition to sunburn, are at increased risk for developing SCC (Blum 1948). Evidence links ultraviolet B (UVB) to the development of SCC: (a) SCC appears on parts of the body most often exposed to sunlight (Silverstone and Gordon 1966); (b) SCC is more prevalent in outdoor workers (Stoll and Schwartz 1987) and in those who have spent the longest periods outdoors (Urbach, Rose, and Bonnem 1972); (c) the incidence of SCC increases with a decrease in latitude (Bauer et al. 1977; Blum 1948; Auerbach 1961); and (d) experiments have produced SCC on the skin of mice by repeated exposure to ultraviolet wavelengths between 280 nm and 320 nm (UVB) (Kripke, Urbach, and Witkop).

Recently it has been suggested that the use of oral psoralen and ultraviolet A (UVA) radiation for the treatment of psoriasis may be associated with the development of SCC in these patients (Stern et al. 1979; Stern et al. 1984). In the past few years commercial tanning booths, designed for year-round maintenance of a "beautiful tan", have proliferated. The lamps in most tanning booths emit primarily in the UVA spectrum (Rivers et al. 1990; Devgun, Johnson, and Patterson 1982; Deffey 1986). There is no direct evidence that these devices cause skin cancer, but they do induce alterations in the immune system (Rivers et al. 1990; Hersey et al. 1983). Because UVA can augment the carcinogenic effect of UVB in mice (Staberg et al. 1983), it remains to be seen if the incidence of SCC in tanning-booth patrons will increase. Other predisposing factors are exposure to chemical carcinogens (arsenic and organic hydrocarbons) and ionizing radiation (Aubry and Mac Gibbon 1985).

PATHOGENESIS

SCC is thought to arise from the same factors that initiate or promote the development of BCC. The evidence for a relationship between sunlight (UVL) and SCC is even stronger than that for BCC (Scotto, Kopf, and Urbach 1979; Urbach 1971; Auerbach 1961; Diffey,

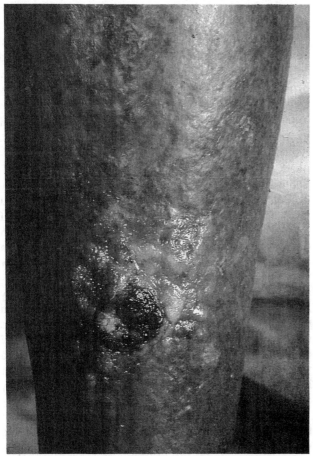

Fig. 22.7. Squamous cell carcinoma. This large ulcerated nodule had been present on the anterior lower leg of this patient for several years.

Tate, and Davis 1979). The rate at which solar keratoses undergo malignant transformation has been estimated as up to 20% (Bendl and Graham 1971). However, Marks et al. (1988) have recently demonstrated that the risk of malignant transformation of a solar keratosis to SCC within one year was less than 1 in 1,000. Heritable conditions associated with SCC include xeroderma pigmentosum and oculocutaneous albinism (Mohl and Nickoloff 1986). In addition, SCC may develop in areas of chronic inflammation, such as lesions of discoid lupus erythematosus (Sehgal et al. 1983); chronic osteomyelitis (Sedlin and Fleming 1963); acne conglobata (Camisa 1984); lupus vulgaris (Hekele and Seyss 1951); hidradenitis suppurativa (Humphrey, Playforth, and Leavell 1969); pilonidal sinus (Sagi et al. 1984); thermal burns (Muhlemann, Geiffiths, and Briggs 1982; Horton, Crawford, and Love 1957); and leg ulcers (Stoll and Schwartz 1987).

Immune suppression may also play a role in the pathogenesis of SCC. Patients receiving immunosuppressive therapy (Marshall 1974; Walden, Robertson, and Jeremy 1971; Westburg and Stone 1973) and renal transplant patients (Halgrimson et al. 1973; Hoxtell et al. 1977; Mullen, Silverberg, and Penn 1976) are prone to SCC. Skin cancers in these patients appear primarily on sun-exposed skin (Halgrimson et al. 1973; Hoxtell et al. 1977; Marshall 1974; Walden, Robertson, and Jer-

emy 1971; Mullen, Silverberg, and Penn 1976; Lutzner 1984). This correlation suggests that immune suppression and UVL act as cofactors in the development of SCC.

An animal model has been developed in which UVB can induce a selective state of immunosuppression that allows tumors to persist (Kripke 1982; Kripke 1983; Kripke 1981; Kripke 1977; Kripke 1977; Kripke 1981; Kripke 1974; Roberts, Schmitt, and Daynes 1979; Daynes et al. 1981). The UVL exposure appears to interfere with antigen processing by Langerhans cells, which in turn gives rise to T suppressor cells that lead to a state of immune tolerance (Kripke 1983; DeMorgas, Winkelmann, and Jordon 1970; Gurish et al. 1981; Nordlund 1983; Zelickson and Mottaz 1970; Loews, Bergstresser, and Strelein 1980; Schwartz et al. 1981; Gilchrest et al. 1983).

Finally, recent research has focused on the role the human papilloma virus (HPV), specifically HPV-5, HPV-16, and HPV-18, plays in the development of SCC (Syrjanen 1987; Stone et al. 1987; Loning et al. 1987; Pfister 1987).

BIOLOGIC ACTIVITY

The biologic behavior of SCC is determined by a number of variables. Immerman et al. observed a 20% incidence of recurrence in 86 patients with invasive SCC. Determining depth of penetration of the lesions revealed that only those tumors that penetrated to the reticular dermis and subcutis recurred. Patients with moderately or poorly differentiated tumors had a greater degree of recurrence (Immerman et al. 1983).

Dzubow et al. (1982) found that in both sexes, SCC of the lower extremities was the most likely site of recurrence after Mohs' surgery.

The tendency for regional lymph node metastasis is also variable. Tumors arising in areas of chronic inflammation, Bowen's disease, discoid lupus erythematosus, lichen sclerosus et atrophicus, chronic osteomyelitis, radiation dermatitis, chronic draining sinuses, and ulcers have a high rate of metastases, ranging from 10% to 30% (Moller, Reymann, and Hou-Jensen 1979). Although tumors that are actinically induced behave in a more biologically benign fashion than de novo SCCs, all lesions have the potential to become invasive both locally and to metastasize to draining lymph nodes (Freeman, Knox, and Heaton 1964).

Actinic keratoses can become metastatic SCC (Fukamizu et al. 1985). Friedman et al. (1985) have demonstrated that all trunk and extremity primary SCCs that later developed local or nodal recurrence were at least 4 mm deep and penetrated into the reticular dermis or subcutis. Every fatal lesion was at least 10 mm deep and invaded the subcutis.

The extent of cellular differentiation also determines a given SCC's metastatic potential. Tumors that invade the regional lymph nodes tend to be more anaplastic than those that have not metastasized (Lund 1965; Shiu, Chu, and Fortner 1980).

SCCs arising in nonglabrous mucocutaneous sites (lip, vulva, penis, perianal area) are more likely to metastasize than those involving other glabrous hair-bearing areas of the skin (Moller, Reymann, and Hou-Jensen 1979). The incidence of metastases for SCC of the skin has varied, from 3% for patients with primary cutaneous SCC (Moller, Reymann, and Hou-Jensen 1979) to 11% for patients with mucocutaneous labial lesions, and 10% to 40% of those with SCC developing in a pre-existing inflammatory condition. This increased incidence has been demonstrated in SCCs developing at sites of inflammation caused by different processes. Carcinomas developing at burn scar sites reportedly have a metastatic rate of 18% (Arons et al. 1965); those with chronic osteomyelitis a rate of 31% (Sedlin and Fleming 1963); those induced by radiation a 20% rate (Martin, Strong, and Spiro 1970); and those arising in discoid lupus erythematosus a 30% metastatic rate (Moller, Reymann, and Hou-Jensen 1979). Tumors are more likely to disseminate to regional lymph nodes than to organs (Mohl and Nickoloff 1986), although intravascular metastases to viscera have appeared in as many as 5% to 10% of all metastatic cases (Epstein et al. 1968).

Distant metastases may also occur via perineural involvement. In one study, 14% of SCCs showed perineural spread (Goepfert et al. 1984), while others have found rates as high as 36% (Carter et al. 1983). Regional lymph node and distant metastases were increased in the patients with perineural involvement. SCC of the head and neck usually spreads to cervical nodes and distantly to the central nervous system, the latter either hematogenously or via the perineural space, which directly connects to the subarachnoid space. Areas that tend to have nerve involvement include the midface, lip, and the mandibular branch of the trigeminal nerve (Goepfert et al. 1984). Although these patients are asymptomatic they show a lower 10-year survival (23% vs. 88%) and a higher local recurrence rate (47% vs. 7.3%) than those without neural involvement (Goepfert et al. 1984). Despite a poor prognosis, Mohs micrographic surgery can occasionally achieve successful treatment (Cottell 1982).

CLINICAL MANIFESTATIONS

SCC occurs within, and may be confined to, the epidermis. Intraepidermal, or *in situ,* squamous-cell carcinoma may occur in a pre-existing thermal keratosis, hydrocarbon keratosis, actinic keratosis, arsenical keratosis, and also in morphologic entities like Bowen's disease, Bowenoid papulosis, and erythroplasia of Queyrat (Stoll and Schwartz 1987). Intraepidermal SCC remains within the epidermis for a variable period to time but may breach the dermoepidermal junction and become an invasive SCC with the propensity to metastasize.

An intraepidermal carcinoma or a premalignant lesion usually precedes invasive squamous cell carcinoma clinically. SCC, other than that arising from an *in situ* tumor, is rarely seen on skin that appears normal (Stoll and Schwartz 1987). Although there are no specific characteristics to make a definitive diagnosis of SCC, most lesions consist of plaques that may be covered with scale, crust, or ulceration. They usually lack the pearly rolled border and superficial telangiectases found in BCCs. Although most are reddish, SCCs that are hyperkeratotic or that occur on mucocutaneous surfaces may be white. The clinical differential diagnosis includes other tumors (BCC, keratoacanthoma, adnexal neoplasm); precancerous lesions (actinic keratosis, Bowen's disease); and some inflammatory diseases (psoriasis, infections, pseudoepitheliomatous hyperplasia).

Squamous cell carcinoma of the nose was studied by Binder et al., who found that 21 of 114 patients had involvement of underlying cartilage and bone. In 77% of these 21 individuals, lesions were greater than 3 cm in diameter and symptoms had been present for more than a year. The incidence of nodal metastases in this study was 8% (Binder, Cady, and Catlin 1968), while previously it had been reported as high as 21% (Conley 1966). Every patient in Binder's study who developed metastases had involvement of the cervical lymph nodes (ipsilateral in six cases, bilateral in two cases, and contralateral in one case), had symptoms for at least a year, and showed involvement of cartilage or bone; most had a primary lesion larger than 3 cm in diameter. Only one patient developed distant metastases.

The majority of SCCs developing on the lip arise from the lower lip in an area of chronic actinic cheilitis. The reported risk of metastasis from SCC of the lip has ranged between 5% and 37% (Stoll and Schwartz 1987).

SCC can also occur on the nail bed, nail folds, and matrix; more than 100 cases had been reported by 1984 (Mikhail 1984). The patient usually has symptoms of swelling, redness, and discomfort. If the nail matrix is affected, atrophy or loss of the nail plate can result. The differential diagnosis of these lesions includes paronychia, pyogenic granuloma, verrucae, nail dystrophies, and tumors such as glomus, keratoacanthoma, and melanoma. There have been two reports of metastases to regional lymph nodes from subungual SCC, while the incidence is 30% for hand tumors that have extended to bone or tendon (Mikhail 1984).

Small SCCs appearing on the trunk and extremities are easily treated, although advanced lesions are aggressive. In a recent review of 106 patients the causes of the SCC included previous exposure to radiation (notably on hands of radiologists and dentists), burn scars, chronic inflammatory dermatoses, ulcers, osteomyelitis, and arsenic ingestion (Shiu, Chu, and Fortner 1980). Factors associated with a poor prognosis included a low degree of histologic differentiation, location on the sacrum or perineum, and degree of lymphatic metastases. SCCs of the trunk and extremities usually spread to the axillary and inguinal lymph nodes, whereas hand and foot tumors metastasize to epitrochlear and popliteal nodes, respectively. Cutaneous and subcutaneous metastatic nodules were found in transit between the primary lesion and the draining lymph nodes in 11 patients. Fourteen patients showed evidence of visceral metastases. These were curable surgically if no bone or lymph node involvement was present. There was no therapeutic advantage to prophylactic node dissection.

SCC of the penis is rare; its incidence for all cancers in males is less than 1% (Hoppman and Fraley 1978; Skinner, Leadbetter, and Kelley 1972). The incidence is greater in Uganda, Mexico, China, India, and Puerto Rico. The patient is invariably uncircumcised and often has phimosis and poor hygiene. SCC of the penis may develop within lesions of leukoplakia, erythroplasia of Queyrat, and balanitis xerotica obliterans. Verrucous carcinoma of the penis (Buschke-Lowenstein tumor) is histologically well-differentiated with features of a wart, but it clinically behaves like an aggressive SCC. Radiation therapy of such lesions is contraindicated; it may induce malignant transformation of the tumor and development of metastases.

Penile SCC usually occurs between the ages of 40 and 60. It may present with a penile nodule, ulceration, discharge, edema, or inguinal adenopathy. The most common site of involvement is the glans; however, it can develop anywhere along the shaft. Metastasis to the inguinal lymph nodes from carcinoma of the penis has been reported in 33% to 50% of patients at the time of the first examination (Stoll and Schwartz 1987).

Verrucous carcinoma is a subtype of low-grade SCC that can affect cutaneous and mucosal surfaces (Ackerman 1948; Andreasson et al. 1983; Biller, Ogura, and Bauer 1971; Japaze, Van Dinh, and Woodruff 1982; Jones, Levin, and Ballard 1981; Lowe and McKee 1983; Powley 1964; Stafford and Frootko 1986; Brownstein and Shapiro 1976; Kao, Graham, and Helwig 1982; Sanchez-Yus, Velasco, and Robledo 1986). This tumor occurs most often in middle-aged and elderly men (Brownstein and Shapiro 1976; Aird et al. 1954; Melo, Melo, and Souza 1981; Mohs and Sahl 1979; Rheingold and Roth 1978; Thompson 1968). The tumor is characterized by a warty exophytic neoplasm containing sinuses with a greasy, malodorous discharge. The cutaneous lesions are found most often on the plantar surface of the foot (McKee et al. 1981). Mucosal lesions of the oral cavity present as white fungating plaque.

The course of verrucous carcinoma is usually indolent although it can cause severe local tissue destruction (Aird et al. 1954; Mohs and Sahl 1979; McKee et al. 1981; Mallatt, Ceilley, and Dryer 1980; Mora 1983). Distant metastases have been described only after radiation therapy to mucosal lesions (Perez et al. 1966; Proffitt, Spooner, and Kosek 1970). In a study of 46 patients with cutaneous verrucous carcinoma, only one developed inguinal metastases, and no patient had disseminated or fatal disease after a 19-year follow-up period (Kao, Graham, and Helwig 1982).

TREATMENT OVERVIEW

Many of the same treatments for BCC are appropriate for SCC. The type of therapy should be selected on the basis of size of the lesion, anatomic location, depth of invasion, degree of cellular differentiation, and history of previous treatment.

CURETTAGE AND ELECTRODESICCATION

Squamous cell carcinomas less than 2 cm in diameter are amenable to this form of therapy. Honeycutt and Jansen (1973) had a 99% cure rate of 281 SCCs after a 4-year follow-up. Two recurrences were noted in lesions over 2 cm in diameter. However, in a separate study involving 29 cases of SCC from the lower lip, there were three recurrences, all in lesions less than 2 cm in diameter. Others have reported 5-year cures ranging from 97% to 98.8% in selected cases (Freeman, Knox, and Heaton 1964; Chernosky 1978).

EXCISION

Surgical excision can remove almost any carcinoma. Freeman et al. (1964) reported a 91% 5-year cure rate for a high-risk group of 91 patients with SCC not amenable to curettage and electrodesiccation. Lesions greater than 3 cm in diameter of the scalp, forehead, and distal extremities are best treated by excision because of the poor healing qualities of thin layers of subcutaneous tissue overlying bone (Stoll and Schwartz 1987). Carcinomas of the eyelid and lip commissures are usually excised because function and cosmesis can be better preserved. Carcinomas of the penis, vulva, and anus are usually treated by excision because of the frequent need for lymph node dissection and because of the poor tolerance of these areas to irradiation (Stoll and Schwartz 1987). Surgical excision is the treatment of choice for verrucous carcinoma (Flynn and Wiemer 1978; Johnson et al. 1985; Tornes et al. 1985).

MOHS MICROGRAPHIC SURGERY

Mohs surgery is useful for carcinomas that fall into one of the following groups: (1) residual carcinoma following previous therapy; (2) recurrent carcinoma; (3) clinically ill-defined carcinoma; (4) carcinoma invading bone and cartilage; (5) carcinoma arising in late radiation dermatitis; and (6) carcinoma arising in areas at high risk for recurrence.

Mohs accomplished a 94.8% 5-year cure rate using his microscopically controlled procedure for primary cutaneous SCC (Mohs 1980). The cure rate varied with the degree of histologic differentiation (98.9% for grade I to 45.2% for grade IV) and lesion size (99.5% for lesions smaller than 1 cm to 58.9% for lesions larger than 3 cm in diameter). Successful treatment also depended on anatomic location: forehead 84.3%, leg 85.6%, foot and toes 71.4%. Dzubow et al. (1982) reported on 414 cases of primary cutaneous SCC and found a 5-year mortality-table-adjusted cure rate of 93.3%. Only the number of surgical stages correlated significantly with recurrence rate. This modality is especially useful where the preservation of the maximum amount of tissue for function and cosmesis is necessary (Mohs and Sahl 1979; Mallatt, Ceilley, and Dryer 1980; Mora 1983; Swanson and Taylor 1980).

RADIATION THERAPY

As with BCC, radiation therapy is excellent for elderly patients with SCC who are unwilling to undergo surgery. It is especially suitable for lesions of the nose, lip, eyelid, and the region of the canthus. Radiation therapy in a fractionated dose schedule has a better cosmetic result and probably an enhanced therapeutic effect.

The use of radiation therapy for verrucous carcinoma has been controversial because of the potential for anaplastic transformation or a higher rate of metastases (Kraus and Perez-Mesa 1966; Smith, Kuhajda, and Harris 1985; Van Nostrand and Olofsson 1972).

OTHER MODALITIES

Cryotherapy of SCC is useful in selected patients (Zacarian 1979). New or experimental treatments include the Nd:YAG laser (Brunner et al. 1985); CO_2 laser (Brunner et al. 1985); photodynamic therapy (Meyskens et al. 1982); retinoids (Meyskens et al. 1982; Kingston, Gaskell, and Marks 1983; Lippman and Meyskens 1987); and 5-fluorouracil given either topically or systemically (Odom 1987; Andrews et al. 1979).

FOLLOW-UP

Invasive squamous cell carcinoma is potentially fatal and warrants close follow-up. The association between solar radiation and the development of SCC is firmly established and it is important to advise patients to avoid excessive exposure to the sun and to always use a sun block with a high sun-protective factor (SPF).

REFERENCES

Ackerman, L.V. 1948. Verrucous carcinoma of the oral cavity. *Surgery* 23:670-78.

Aird, I.; Johnson, H.D.; and Lennox, B. et al. 1954. Epithelioma cuniculatum: a variety of squamous cell carcinoma peculiar to the foot. *Br. J. Surg.* 42:245-50.

American Cancer Society. *Cancer facts and figures 1990.*

Andreasson, B.; Bock, J.E.; and Strom, K.V. et al. 1983. Verrucous carcinoma of the vulval region. *Acta Obstet. Gynecol. Scand.* 62:183-86.

Andrews, J.M. et al. 1979. Extensive malignancies of facial skin treated by perfusion with 5-fluorouracil and conservative excision. *Br. J. Plast. Surg.* 32:253.

Arons, M.S.; Lynch, J.B.; and Lewis, S.N. et al. 1965. Scar tissue carcinoma. I: a clinical study with special reference to burn scar carcinoma. *Ann. Surg.* 161:170-88.

Aubry, F., and Mac Gibbon, B. 1985. Risk factors of squamous cell carcinoma of the skin. *Cancer* 55:907-11.

Auerbach, H. 1961. Geographic variation in incidence of skin cancer in the United States. *Public Health Rep.* 76:345-48.

Bailin, P.L.; Levine, H.L.; and Wood, B.G. et al. 1980. Cutaneous carcinoma of the auricular and periauricular region. *Arch. Otolaryngol.* 106:692.

Bailin, P.L.; Ratz, J.L.; and Lutz-Nagey, L. 1981. CO_2 laser modification of Mohs surgery. *J. Dermatol. Surg. Oncol.* 7:621.

Baker, S.R.; Swanson, N.A.; and Grekin, R.C. 1987. An interdisciplinary approach to the management of basal cell carcinoma of the head and neck. *J. Dermatol. Surg. Oncol.* 13:1095.

Ballantyne, A.J.; McCarter, A.B.; and Ibanez, M.L. 1963. The extension of cancer of the head and neck through peripheral nerves. *Am. J. Surg.* 106:651.

Barsky, S.H.; Grossman, D.A.; and Bhuta, S. 1987. Desmoplastic basal carcinomas possess unique basement membrane-degrading properties. *J. Invest. Dermatol.* 88:324.

Bart, R.S.; Schrager, D.; and Kopf, A.W. et al. 1978. Scalpel excision of basal cell carcinomas. *Arch. Dermatol.* 114:739.

Bauer, E.A.; Gordon, J.M.; and Reddick, M.E. et al. 1977. Quantitation and immunocytochemical localization of human skin collagenase in basal cell carcinoma. *J. Invest. Dermatol.* 69:363-67.

Bendl, B.J., and Graham, J.H. 1971. New concepts on the origin of squamous cell carcinomas of the skin: solar (senile) keratosis with squamous cell carcinoma—a clinico-pathologic and histochemical study. *Proc. Natl. Cancer Conf.* 6:471-88.

Bergstresser, P.R., and Halprin, K.M. 1975. Multiple sequential skin cancers: the risk of skin cancer in patients with previous skin cancer. *Arch. Dermatol.* 111:995.

Biller, H.F.; Ogura, J.H.; and Bauer, W.C. 1971. Verrucous carcinoma of the larynx. *Laryngoscope* 81:1323-29.

Binder, S.C.; Cady, B.; and Catlin, D. 1968. Epidermoid carcinoma of the skin of the nose. *Am. J. Surg.* 116:506-12.

Binstock, J.H.; Stegman, S.J.; and Tromovitch, T.A. 1981. Large aggressive basal cell carcinomas of the scalp. *J. Dermatol. Surg. Oncol.* 7:565.

Black, H.S., and Chan, J.T. 1977. Experimental ultraviolet light carcinogenesis. *Photochem. Photobiol.* 26:183-99.

Blum, H.F. 1948. Sunlight as a causal factor in cancer of the skin of man. *J. Natl. Cancer Inst.* 9:247-58.

Borel, D.M. 1973. Cutaneous basosquamous carcinoma: review of the literature and report of 35 cases. *Arch. Pathol.* 95:293-97.

Brady, L.W.; Binnick, S.A.; and Fitzpatrick, P.J. 1987. Skin cancer. In Perez, C.A. and Brady, L.W. eds. *Principles and practice of radiation oncology.* p. 377. Philadelphia: J.B. Lippincott.

Braun-Falco, O.; Lukacs, S.; and Goldschmidt, H. 1976. In *Dermatologic radiotherapy.* p. 69. New York: Springer-Verlag.

Brody, I. 1970. Contributions to the histogenesis of basal cell carcinoma. *J. Ultrastruct. Res.* 33:60-79.

Brownstein, M.H., and Shapiro, L. 1976. Verrucous carcinoma of skin: epithelioma acuniculatum plantare. *Cancer* 38:1710-16.

Brunner, R.; Landthaler, M.; and Haina, D. et al. 1985. Treatment of benign, semimalignant and malignant skin tumors with the ND:YAG laser. *Lasers Surg. Med.* 5:105-10.

Burg, G.; Hirsch, R.D.; and Konz, B. et al. 1975. Histographic surgery: accuracy of visual assessment of the margins of basal-cell epithelioma. *J. Dermatol. Surg.* 1:21.

Camisa, C. 1984. Squamous cell carcinoma arising in acne conglobata. *Cutis* 33:185-88.

Carter, R.L.; Foster, C.S.; and Dinsdale, E.A. et al. 1983. Perineural spread by squamous cell carcinomas of the head and neck: a morphological study using antiaxonal and antimyelin monoclonal antibodies. *J. Clin. Pathol.* 36:269-75.

Ceilly, R.I., and Anderson, R.L. 1978. Microscopically controlled excision of malignant neoplasms on and around eyelids followed by immediate surgical reconstruction. *J. Dermatol. Surg. Oncol.* 4:55.

Ceilly, R.I.; Bumsted, R.M.; and Smith, W.H. 1979. Malignancies on the external ear: methods of ablation and reconstruction of defects. *J. Dermatol. Surg. Oncol.* 5:762.

Chahbaziam, C.M., and Brown, G.S. 1980. Radiation therapy for carcinoma of the skin of the face and neck: special considerations. *JAMA* 244:1135.

Chahbaziam, C.M., and Brown, G.S. 1984. In Gilbert, H.A. ed. *Skin cancer in modern radiation oncology classic literature and current management.* p. 158. Philadelphia: Harper & Row.

Chernosky, M.E. 1978. Squamous cell and basal cell carcinomas: preliminary study of 3,818 primary skin cancers. *South Med. J.* 71:802-803.

Cleaver, J.E. 1968. Defective repair replication of DNA in xeroderma pigmentosum. *Nature* 218:652-56.

Cleaver, J.E. 1969. Xeroderma pigmentosum: a human disease in which an initial stage of DNA repair is defective. *Proc. Natl. Acad. Sci. USA* 63:428-35.

Cohen, C. 1980. Multiple cutaneous carcinomas and lymphomas of the skin. *Arch. Dermatol.* 116:687-89.

Coker, D.D.; Elias, E.G.; Viravathana, T. et al. 1983. Chemotherapy for metastatic basal cell carcinoma. *Arch. Dermatol.* 119:44.

Conley, J. 1966. Cancer of the skin of the nose. *Arch. Otolaryngol.* 84:55-60.

Cottell, W.L. 1982. Perineural invasion by squamous cell carcinoma: *J. Dermatol. Surg. Oncol.* 8:589-600.

Crestofollini, M.; Zumiani, G.; and Scappini, P. et al. 1984. Aromatic retinoid in the chemoprevention of nevoid basal cell carcinoma syndrome. *J. Dermatol. Surg. Oncol.* 10:778.

Daynes, R.A.; Bernhard, E.J.; and Gurish, M.F. et al. 1981. Experimental photoimmunology: immunologic ramifications of UV-induced carcinogenesis. *J. Invest. Dermatol.* 77:7-85.

Deffey, B.L. 1986. Use of UV-A sunbeds for cosmetic tanning. *Br. J. Dermatol.* 115:67-76.

DeMorgas, J.M.; Winkelmann, R.K.; and Jordon, R.E. 1970. Immunofluorescence of epithelial skin tumors. I. patterns of intercellular substance. *Cancer* 25:1399-1403.

Devgun, M.S.; Johnson, B.E.; and Paterson, C.R. 1982. Tanning, protection against sunburn and vitamin D formation with a UV-A "sunbed." *Br. J. Dermatol.* 107:275-84.

Diffey, B.L.; Tate, T.J.; and Davis, A. 1979. Solar dosimetry of the face: relationship of natural ultraviolet radiation exposure to basal cell carcinoma localization. *Phys. Med. Biol.* 24:931-39.

Dubin, N., and Kopf, A.W. 1983. Multivariate risk score for recurrent cutaneous basal cell carcinomas. *Arch. Dermatol.* 119:373.

Dzubow, L.M.; Rigel, D.S.; and Robins, P. 1982. Risk factors for local recurrence of primary cutaneous squamous cell carcinomas. *Arch. Dermatol.* 118:900-902.

Edens, B.L.; Bartlow, G.A.; and Haghighi, P. et al. 1983. Effectiveness of curettage and electrodesiccation in the removal of basal cell carcinoma. *J. Am. Acad. Dermatol.* 9:383.

Epstein, E.; Epstein, N.; and Bragg, K. et al. 1968. Metastases from squamous cell carcinoma of the skin. *Arch. Dermatol.* 97:245-51.

Epstein, E. 1987. Value of follow-up after treatment of basal cell carcinoma. *Arch. Dermatol.* 108:798.

Farmer, E.R., and Helwig, E.B. 1980. Metastatic basal cell carcinoma: a clinicopathologic study of 17 cases. *Cancer* 46:748-57.

Fears, T.R.; Scotto, J.; and Schneiderman, M.A. 1977. Mathematical models of age and ultraviolet effects of the incidence of skin cancer among whites in the United States. *Am. J. Epidemiol.* 105:420-27.

Fidler, I.J. 1978. Tumor heterogeneity and the biology of cancer invasion and metastases. *Cancer Res.* 38:2651-60.

Fisher, B.K., and Warner, L.C. 1987. Cutaneous manifestations of the acquired immunodeficiency syndrome: update 1987. *Int. J. Dermatol.* 26:615.

Fitzpatrick, T.B.; Parrish, J.A.; and Hayanes, H.A. et al. 1982. Ozone depletion and skin cancer. *Dermatol. Caps. Comm.* 4:10.

Flynn, K.J., and Wiemer, D.R. 1978. Treatment of an epithelioma cuniculatum plantare by local excision and a plantar skin flap. *J. Dermatol. Surg. Oncol.* 4:773-75.

Franchimont, C.; Pierard, G.E.; and Cauwenberge, D.V. et al. 1982. Episodic progression and regression of basal cell carcinoma. *Br. J. Dermatol.* 106:305.

Frauenfelder, F.T. 1985. Cryosurgery of eyelid, conjunctival, and intraocular tumors. In Zacarian, S.A. ed. *Cryosurgery for skin cancer and cutaneous disorders.* p. 259. St. Louis: C.V. Mosby.

Freeman, R.G.; Knox, J.M.; and Heaton, C.L. 1964. The treatment of skin cancer: a statistical study of 1,341 skin tumors comparing results obtained with irradiation, surgery, and curettage followed by electrodesiccation. *Cancer* 17:535-38.

Friedman, H.I.; Cooper, P.H.; and Wanebo, H.J. 1985. Prognostic and therapeutic use of microstaging of cutaneous squamous cell carcinoma of the trunk and extremities. *Cancer* 56:1099-1105.

Fukamizu, H.; Inoue, K.; Matsumoto, K.; and Okayama, H. et al. 1985. Metastatic squamous cell carcinomas derived from solar keratosis. *J. Dermatol. Surg. Oncol.* 11:518-22.

Gerstein, W. 1963. Transplantation of basal cell epithelioma to the rabbit. *Arch. Dermatol.* 88:834-36; 113:436-38.

Gilchrest, B.; Szabo, G.; and Flynn, E. et al. 1983. Chronologic and actinically induced aging in human facial skin. *J. Invest. Dermatol.* 80:815-55.

Gladstein, A.H.; Kopf, A.W.; and Bart, R.S. 1978. Radiotherapy of cutaneous malignancies. In Goldschmidt, H. ed. *Physical modalities in dermatologic therapy: radiotherapy, electrosurgery, phototherapy, cryosurgery.* p. 95. New York: Springer-Verlag.

Goepfert, H.; Dichtel, W.J.; Medina, J.E. et al. 1984. Perineural invasion in squamous cell skin carcinoma of the head and neck. *Am. J. Surg.* 148: 542-47.

Goldschmidt, H., and Sherwin, W.K. 1983. Office radiotherapy of cutaneous carcinomas. I. radiation techniques, dose schedules, and radiation protection. *J. Dermatol. Surg. Oncol.* 9:31-46.

Good, A.E.; Diaz, L.A.; and Bowerman, R.A. 1980. Basal cell carcinomas following roentgen therapy of ankylosing spondylitis. *Arthritis Rheum.* 23:1065-67.

Gormley, D.E., and Hirsch, P. 1978. Aggressive basal cell carcinoma of the scalp. *Arch. Dermatol.* 114:782.

Granstrom, G.; Aldenburg, F.; and Jeppsson, P.H. 1986. Influence of embryonal fusion lines for recurrence of basal cell carcinoma in the head and neck. *Otolaryngol. Head Neck Surg.* 95:76.

Greenway, H.T.; Cornell, R.C.; and Tanner, D.J. et al. 1986. Treatment of basal cell carcinoma with intralesional interferon. *J. Am. Acad. Dermatol.* 15:437.

Gregory, R.O., and Goldman, L. 1986. Application of photodynamic therapy in plastic surgery. *Lasers Surg. Med.* 6:62-66.

Grover, R.W. 1973. Basal cell carcinoma. *Arch. Dermatol.* 107:138.

Gullane, P.G. 1986. Extensive facial malignancies: concepts and management. *J. Otolaryngol.* 15:44.

Gurish, M.F.; Roberts, L.K.; and Krueger, G.G. et al. 1981. The effect of various sunscreen agents on skin damage and the induction of tumor susceptibility in mice subjected to ultraviolet irradiation. *J. Invest. Dermatol.* 76:246-51.

Halgrimson, C.G.; Penn, I.; and Booth, A. et al. 1973. Eight-to-ten year follow-up in early cases of renal homotransplantation. *Transplant Proc.* 5:787-91.

Hanke, C.W.; Wolf, R.L.; Hochman, S.A. et al. 1983. Perineural spread of basal cell carcinoma. *J. Dermatol. Surg. Oncol.* 9:742.

Hartman, R.; Hartman, S.; and Green, N. 1986. Long-term survival following bony metastases from basal cell carcinoma: report of a case. *Arch. Dermatol.* 122:912.

Harville, D., and Aaron, J. 1973. Cutaneous oncogenesis and immunosuppression. *Cutis* 11:188-91.

Hashimoto, K.; Yamanishi, Y.; and Dabbous, M.K. 1972. Electron microscopic observations of collagenolytic activity of basal cell epithelioma of the skin *in vivo* and *in vitro.* *Cancer Res.* 32:2561-67.

Hekele, K., and Seyss, R. 1951. Die malignen Tumoren in lupo vulgari. *Hautarzt* 2:349.

Hersey, P.; Hasic, E.; and Edwards, A. et al. 1983. Immunological effects of solarium exposure. *Lancet* I:545-48.

Hodak, E.; Ginzburg, K.A.; and David, M. et al. 1987. Etretinate treatment of nevoid basal cell carcinoma syndrome: therapeutic and chemopreventive effect. *Int. J. Dermatol.* 26:606-609.

Hoppmann, H.J., and Fraley, E.E. 1978. Squamous cell carcinoma of the penis. *J. Urol.* 120:393-98.

Honeycutt, W.M., and Jansen, G.T. 1973. Treatment of squamous cell carcinoma of the skin. *Arch. Dermatol.* 108:670-72.

Horton, C.E.; Crawford, H.H.; and Love, H.G. 1957. The malignant potential of burn scar. *Plast. Reconstr. Surg.* 22:348-352.

Humphrey, L.J.; Playforth, H.; and Leavell, V.W. 1969. Squamous cell carcinoma arising in hidradenitis suppurativum. *Arch. Dermatol.* 100:59-62.

Hunter, R.D.; Easson, E.C.; and Pointon, R.C.S. eds. 1987. *Skin in the radiotherapy of malignant disease.* p. 135. New York: Springer-Verlag.

Immerman, S.C.; Scanlon, E.F.; and Christ, M. et al. 1983. Recurrent squamous cell carcinoma of the skin. *Cancer* 51:1537-40.

Japaze, H.; Van Dinh, T.; and Woodruff, J.D. 1982. Verrucous carcinoma of the vulva: study of 24 cases. *Obstet. Gynecol.* 60:462-66.

Johnson, D.E.; Lo, R.K.; Srigley, J.; and Ayala, A.G. 1985. Verrucous carcinoma of the penis. *J. Urol.* 133:216-18.

Johnson, B.E. 1973. Solar radiation and skin cancer. *Br. J. Cancer* 28:91.

Jones, M.J.; Levin, H.S.; and Ballard, L.A. Jr. 1981. Verrucous squamous carcinoma of the vagina: report of a case and review of the literature. *Cleve. Clin. Quart.* 48:305-13.

Kao, G.F.; Graham, J.H.; and Helwig, E.B. 1982. Carcinoma cuniculatum (verrucous carcinoma of the skin): a clinicopathologic study of 46 cases with ultrastructural observations. *Cancer* 49:2395-2403.

Katz, A.D.; Urbach, F.; and Lilienfeld, A.M. 1957. Frequency and risk of metastases in squamous cell carcinoma of the skin. *Cancer* 10:1162-66.

Kingston, T.; Gaskell, S.; and Marks, R. 1983. The effects of a novel potent oral retinoid (Ro 13-6298) in the treatment of multiple solar keratoses and squamous cell epithelioma. *Eur. J. Cancer. Clin. Oncol.* 19:1201-1205.

Kligman, L.H.; Akin, F.J.; and Kligman, A.M. 1980. Sunscreens prevent ultraviolet photocarcinogenesis. *J. Am. Acad. Dermatol.* 3:30-35.

Knox, J.; Lyles, T.W.; Shapiro, E.M. et al. 1960. Curettage and electrodesiccation in the treatment of skin cancer. *Arch. Dermatol.* 82:197.

Knox, J.M.; Freeman, R.G.; and Heaton, C.L. 1962. Curettage and electrodesiccation in the treatment of skin cancer. *South. Med. J.* 55:1212.

Kopf, A.W.; Bart, R.S.; and Schrager, D. et al. 1977. Curettage-electrodesiccation treatment of basal cell carcinomas. *Arch. Dermatol.* 113:439.

Kraemer, K.H. 1981. Cancer prone genodermatoses and DNA repair. *Prog. Dermatol.* 15:1-6.

Kraus, F.T., and Perez-Mesa, C. 1966. Verrucous carcinoma: clinical and pathologic study of 105 cases involving oral cavity, larynx and genitalia. *Cancer* 19:26-38.

Kripke, M.L. 1974. Antigenicity of murine skin tumors induced by ultraviolet light. *J. Natl. Cancer Inst.* 53:1333-1336.

Kripke, M.L. 1977. Latency, histology and antigenicity of tumor induced by ultraviolet light in three inbred mouse strains. *Cancer Res.* 37:1395-1400.

Kripke, M.L. 1977. Ultraviolet radiation and tumor immunity. *J. Reticuloendothelial Soc.* 22:217-22.

Kripke, M.L. 1981. Immunologic mechanisms in UV radiation carcinogenesis. *Adv. Cancer Res.* 34:69-106.

Kripke, M.L.; Morison, W.L.; and Parrish, J.A. 1981. Differences in the immunologic reactivity of mice treated with UVB or methoxsalen plus UVA radiation. *J. Invest. Dermatol.* 76:445-48.

Kripke, M.L. 1982. Role of UVL-induced immunosuppression in experimental photocarcinogenesis. *Prog. Dermatol.* 16:1-6.

Kripke, M.L. 1983. In Parrish, J.A. ed. *Immunobiology of photocarcinogenesis: the effect of ultraviolet radiation on the immune system, a scientific round table.* pp. 87-106. Englewood, N.J.: Johnson & Johnson Baby Products.

Kripke, M.; Urbach, F.; and Witkop, C. 1983. Ultraviolet radiation carcinogenesis. In *Biology of skin cancer (excluding melanomas): a series of workshops on the biology of human cancer.* Report No. 15.

Kuflik, E.G. 1985. Cryosurgery for carcinoma of the eyelids: a 12-year experience. *J. Dermatol. Surg. Oncol.* 11:243.

Lee, L.A.; Fritz, K.A.; and Golitz, L. et al. 1982. Second cutaneous malignancies in patients with mycosis fungoides treated with topical nitrogen mustard. *J. Am. Acad. Dermatol.* 7:590-98.

Lehmann, A.R.; Kirk-Bell, S.; and Corlett, C.F. et al. 1977. Repair of ultraviolet light damage in a variety of human fibroblast cell strains. *Cancer Res.* 37:904-10.

Levine, H.L., and Bailin, P.L. 1980. Basal cell carcinoma of the head and neck: identification of the high-risk patient. *Laryngoscope* 90:955.

Lippman, S.M., and Meyskens, F.L. 1987. Treatment of advanced squamous-cell carcinoma of the skin with isotretinoin. *Ann. Intern. Med.* 107:499-502.

Loews, G.B.; Bergstresser, P.R.; and Strelein, J.W. 1980. Epidermal Langerhans cell density determines whether contact hypersensitivity or unresponsiveness follows skin painting with DNFB. *J. Immunol.* 124:445-53.

Loning, T.; Meichsner, M.; and Milde-Langosch, K. et al. 1987. HPV DNA detection in tumours of the head and neck: a comparative light microscopy and DNA hybridization study. *ORL J. Otorhinolaryngol. Relat. Spec.* 49:259-69.

Lowe, D., and McKee, P.H. 1983. Verrucous carcinoma of the penis (Buschke-Lowenstein tumour): a clinicopathological study. *Br. J. Urol.* 55:427-29.

Lund, H.Z. 1957. *Tumors of the skin.* Fascicle 2, Sec 1. pp. 205-235. Washington, D.C.: AFIP.

Lund, H.Z. 1965. How often does squamous cell carcinoma of the skin metastasize? *Arch. Dermatol.* 92:635-37.

Lutzner, M.A. 1984. Skin cancer in immunosuppressed organ transplant recipients. *J. Am. Acad. Dermatol.* 11:891-93.

Lyles, T.W.; Freeman, R.G.; and Knox, J.M. 1960. Transplantation of basal cell epitheliomas. *J. Invest. Dermatol.* 34:353.

Madison, J.F. 1980. Basal cell epitheliomas after repeat fluoroscopic examinations of the chest. *Arch. Dermatol.* 116:323-24.

Mallatt, B.D.; Ceilley, R.I.; and Dryer, R.F. 1980. Chemosurgical reports: management of verrucous carcinoma on a foot by a combination of chemosurgery and plastic repair, report of a case. *J. Dermatol. Surg. Oncol.* 6:532-34.

Manusow, D., and Weinerman, B.H. 1975. Subsequent neoplasia in chronic lymphocyte leukemia. *JAMA* 232:267-71.

Mark, G. 1972. Basal cell carcinoma with intraneural invasion. *Cancer* 40:2181.

Marks, R.; Rennie, G.; and Selwood, T.S. 1988. Malignant transformation of solar keratosis to squamous cell carcinoma. *Lancet* I:795-96.

Marshall, D.R. 1968. The clinical and pathological effects of prolonged solar exposure. II: association with basal cell carcinoma. *Aust. N.Z. J. Surg.* 38:89-97.

Marshall, V. 1974. Premalignant and malignant skin tumors in immunosuppressed patients. *Transplant* 17:272-75.

Martin, H.; Strong, E.; and Spiro, R.H. 1970. Radiation induced skin cancer of the head and neck. *Cancer* 25:61-71.

McDaniel, W.E. 1978. Surgical therapy for basal cell epitheliomas by curettage only. *Arch. Dermatol.* 114:1491.

McDaniel, W.E. 1983. Therapy for basal cell epitheliomas by curettage only: further study. *Arch. Dermatol.* 119:901.

McKee, P.H.; Wilkinson, J.D.; and Black, M.M. et al. 1981. Carcinoma (epithelioma) cuniculatum: a clinicopathological study of 19 cases and review of the literature. *Histopath* 5:425-36.

McLean, D.I.; Haynes, H.A.; and McCarthy, P.L. et al. 1978. Cryotherapy of basal cell carcinoma by a simple method of standardized freeze-thaw cycles. *J. Dermatol. Surg. Oncol.* 4:175.

Menn, H.; Robins, P.; and Kopf, A.W. et al. 1971. The recurrent basal cell epithelioma: a study of 100 cases of recurrent re-treated basal epitheliomas. *Arch. Dermatol.* 103:628.

Melo, C.R.; Melo, I.S.; and Souza, L.P. 1981. Epithelioma cuniculatum, a verrucous carcinoma of the foot. *Dermatologica* 163:338-42.

Meyskens, F.L. Jr.; Gilmartin, E.; and Alberts, D.S. et al. 1982. Activity of isotretinoin against squamous cell cancers and preneoplastic lesions. *Cancer Treat. Rep.* 66:1318-19.

Mikhail, G.R. 1984. Subungual epidermoid carcinoma. *J. Am. Acad. Dermatol.* 11:291-98.

Mikhail, G.R.; Nims, L.P.; and Kelly, A.P. Jr. et al. 1977. Metastatic basal cell carcinoma: review pathogenesis and report of two cases. *Arch. Dermatol.* 113:1261.

Modan, B.; Hannah, M.; and Baidatz, D. et al. 1974. Radiation induced head and neck tumors. *Lancet* I:277-79.

Mohl, J., and Nickoloff, B.J. 1986. Fatal cutaneous squamous cell carcinoma in a forty-three-year-old male. *J. Dermatol. Surg. Oncol.* 112:276-79.

Mohs, F.E. 1978. In *Chemosurgery: microscopically controlled surgery for skin cancer.* Springfield, Ill.: Charles C. Thomas.

Mohs, F.E. 1978. Carcinoma of the skin: a summary of results in chemosurgery. In *Chemosurgery: microscopically controlled surgery for skin cancer.* p. 153. Springfield, Ill.: Charles C. Thomas.

Mohs F.E., and Sahl, W.J. 1979. Chemosurgery for verrucous carcinoma. *J. Dermatol Surg. Oncol.* 5:302-306.

Moller, R.; Reymann, F.; and Hou-Jensen, K. 1979. Metastases in dermatological patients with squamous cell carcinoma. *Arch. Dermatol.* 115:703-705.

Montandon, D.; Kocher, O.; and Gabbiani, G. 1982. Cancer invasiveness: immunofluorescent and ultrastructure methods of assessment. *Plast. Reconstr. Surg.* 69:365-71.

Montgomery, H. 1967. Epithelial neoplasms: basal and squamous cell neoplasms and keratoacanthoma. In *Dermatopathology.* vol. 2. pp. 934-40. New York: Harper & Row.

Mora, R.G., and Robins, P. 1978. Basal cell carcinoma in the center of the face: special diagnostic, prognostic and therapeutic considerations. *J. Dermatol. Surg. Oncol.* 4:315.

Mora, R.G. 1983. Microscopically controlled surgery (Mohs' chemosurgery) for treatment of verrucous squamous cell carcinoma of the foot (epithelioma cuniculatum). *J. Amer. Acad. Dermatol.* 8:354-62.

Muhlemann, M.F.; Geiffiths, R.W.; and Briggs, J.C. 1982. Malignant melanoma and squamous cell carcinoma in a burn scar. *Br. J. Plast. Surg.* 35:474-77.

Mullen, D.L.; Silverberg, S.G.; and Penn, I. 1976. Squamous cell carcinoma of the skin and lip in renal homograft recipients. *Cancer* 37:729-34.

Murphy, K.J. 1975. Metastatic basal cell carcinoma with squamous appearances in the nevoid basal cell carcinoma syndrome. *Br. J. Plast. Surg.* 28:331-34.

Nordlund, J.J. 1983. Chemical agents which mimic the effects of ultraviolet radiation on the epidermis: a possible role for oxidation of arachidonic acid in expression of surface markers on epidermal cells. In Parrish, J.A. ed. *The effect of ultraviolet radiation on the immune system: a scientific round table.* pp. 161-180. Englewood, N.J.: Johnson & Johnson Baby Products.

Odom, R.B. 1987. Fluorouracil. In Epstein, E., and Epstein, N. eds. *Skin surgery.* p. 396. Philadelphia: W.B. Saunders.

Pawlowski, A., and Haberman, H.F. 1979. Heterotransplantation of human basal cell carcinomas in "nude" mice. *J. Invest. Dermatol.* 72:310-13.

Peck, G.L. 1986. Topical tretinoin in actinic keratoses and basal cell carcinoma. *J. Am. Acad. Dermatol.* 15:829.

Perez, C.A.; Kraus, F.T.; Evans, J.C.; and Powers, W.E. 1966. Anaplastic transformation in verrucous carcinoma of the oral cavity after radiation therapy. *Radiology* 86:108-15.

Pfister, H. 1987. Human papillomaviruses and impaired immunity vs. epidermodysplasia verruciformis. *Arch. Dermatol.* 123:1469-70.

Powley, J.M. 1964. Buschke-Lowenstein tumour of the penis. *Br. J. Surg.* 51:76-77.

Proffitt, S.D.; Spooner, T.R.; and Kosek, J.C. 1970. Origin of undifferentiated neoplasm from verrucous epidermal carcinoma of oral cavity following irradiation. *Cancer* 26:389-93.

Reymann, F. 1975. Multiple basal cell carcinomas of the skin: treatment with curettage. *Arch. Dermatol.* 111:877.

Reymann, F. 1971. Treatment of basal cell carcinoma of the skin with curettage. *Arch. Dermatol.* 103:623.

Rheingold, L.M., and Roth, L.M. 1978. Carcinoma of the skin of the foot exhibiting some verrucous features. *Plast. Reconstr. Surg.* 61:605-609.

Ridley, C.M., and Spittle, M.F. 1974. Epitheliomas of the scalp after irradiation. *Lancet* I:509.

Riefkohl, R.; Pollack, S.; and Gerogiade, G.S. 1985. A rationale for the treatment of difficult basal cell and squamous cell carcinoma of the skin. *Ann. Plast. Surg.* 15:99.

Rivers, J.K.; Norris, P.G.; and Murphy, G.M. et al. 1990. UVA sunbeds: tanning, photoprotection, immunological changes and acute adverse effects. *Br. J. Dermatol.*

Roberts, L.K.; Schmitt, M.; and Daynes, R.A. 1979. Tumor susceptibility generated in mice treated with sulcarcinogenic doses of 8-methoxypsoralen and long-wave ultraviolet light. *J. Invest. Dermatol.* 73:306-309.

Robins, P., and Albom, M.J. 1975. Recurrent basal cell carcinoma in young women. *J. Dermatol. Surg.* 1:49.

Robins, P. 1981. Chemosurgery: my 15 years of experience. *J. Dermatol. Surg. Oncol.* 7:779.

Robinson, J.K.; Pollack, S.V.; and Robins, P. 1980. Invasion of cartilage by basal cell carcinoma. *J. Am. Acad. Dermatol.* 2:499.

Robinson, J.K. 1987. What are adequate treatment and following care for nonmelanoma cutaneous cancer? *Arch. Dermatol.* 123:331.

Robinson, J.K. 1987. Risk of developing another basal cell carcinoma: a five-year prospective study. *Cancer* 60:118.

Roenigk, R.K.; Ratz, J.L.; and Bailin, P.L. et al. 1986. Trends in the presentation and treatment of basal cell carcinomas. *J. Dermatol. Surg. Oncol.* 12:860, 986.

Rosen, H.M. 1987. Periorbital basal cell carcinoma requiring ablative craniofacial surgery. *Arch. Dermatol.* 123:376.

Ruocco, V.; and Satriano, R.A. 1986. Basal cell cancer and classic Kaposi's sarcoma in a locally immunocompromised patient. *Int. J. Dermatol.* 25:594.

Sacchini, V.; Lovo, G.F.; and Avioli, N. et al. 1984. Carbon dioxide laser in scalp tumor surgery. *Laser Surg. Med.* 4:261.

Safao, B., and Good, R.A. 1977. Basal cell carcinoma with metastases: review of literature. *Arch. Pathol. Lab. Med.* 101:327.

Sagi, A.; Rosenberg, L.; Greiff, M.; and Mahler, D. 1984. Squamous cell carcinoma arising in a pilonidal sinus: a case report and review of the literature. *J. Dermatol. Surg. Oncol.* 10:210-12.

Salasche, S.J., and Ammonette, R.A. 1981. Morpheaform basal cell epitheliomas: a study of subclinical extensions in a series of 51 cases. *J. Dermatol. Surg. Oncol.* 7:3878-79

Salasche, S.J. 1983. Curettage and electrodesiccation in the treatment of midfacial basal cell epithelioma. *J. Am. Acad. Dermatol.* 8:496.

Salasche, S.J. 1984. Status of curettage and desiccation in the treatment of primary basal cell carcinoma. *J. Am. Acad. Dermatol.* 10:285.

Sanchez-Yus, E.; Velasco, E.; and Robledo, A. 1986. Verrucous carcinoma of the back. *J. Am. Acad. Dermatol.* 14:947-50.

Schuller, D.E.; Berg, J.W.; and Sherman, G. et al. 1979. Cutaneous basosquamous carcinomas of the head and neck: a comparative analysis. *Otolaryngol. Head Neck Surg.* 87:420-27.

Schwartz, J.; Solt, D.B.; and Pappo, J. et al. 1981. Distribution of Langerhans cells in normal and carcinogen-treated mucosa of buccal punches of hamsters. *J. Dermatol. Surg. Oncol.* 7:1005-10.

Scotto, J.; Kopf, A.W.; and Urbach, F. 1979. Nonmelanoma skin cancer among Caucasians in four areas of the United States. *Cancer* 34:1333-38.

Scotto, J.; Fears, T.R.; and Fraumeni, J.F. 1983. *Incidence of nonmelanoma skin cancer in the United States.* USDHS, NIH Publication No. 83-2433.

Sedlin, E.D., and Fleming, J.L. 1963. Epidermal carcinoma arising in chronic osteomyelitis foci. *J. Bone Joint Surg.* 45:827-37.

Sehgal, V.N.; Reddy, B.S.N.; and Koranne, R.V. et al. 1983. Squamous cell carcinoma complicating chronic discoid lupus erythematosus. *J. Dermatol.* 10:81-84.

Shiu, M.H.; Chu, F.; and Fortner, J.G. 1980. Treatment of regionally advanced epidermoid carcinoma of the extremity and trunk. *Surg. Gyn. Obstet.* 150:558-62.

Silverstone, H., and Gordon, D. 1966. Regional studies in skin cancer, 2nd report: wet tropical and sub-tropical coast of Queensland. *Med. J. Aust.* 2:733-40.

Sitz, K.V.; Koppen, M.; and Johnson, D.F. 1987. Metastatic basal cell carcinoma in acquired immunodeficiency syndrome-related complex. *JAMA* 257:340.

Skinner, D.G.; Leadbetter, W.F.; and Kelley, S.B. 1972. Surgical management of squamous cell carcinoma of the penis. *J. Urol.* 107:273-77.

Slazinski, L.; Stall, J.R.; and Mathew, C.R. 1984. Basal cell carcinoma in a man with acquired immunodeficiency syndrome. *J. Am. Acad. Dermatol.* 11:140.

Sloane, J.P. 1974. The value of typing basal cell carcinomas in predicting recurrence after surgical excision. *Br. J. Dermatol.* 96:127-32.

Smith, E.B., and Brysk, M.M. 1981. Immunity and skin cancer. *South. Med. J.* 74:44-46.

Smith, R.R.L.; Kuhajda, F.P.; and Harris, A.E. 1985. Anaplastic transformation of verrucous carcinoma following radiotherapy. *Am. J. Otolaryngol.* 6:448-52.

Spiller, W.F., and Spiller, R.F. 1984. Treatment of basal cell epithelioma by curettage and electrodesiccation. *J. Am. Acad. Dermatol.* 11:808.

Spiller, W.F., and Spiller, R.F. 1985. Cryosurgery and adjuvant surgical techniques for cutaneous carcinomas. In Zacarian, S.A. ed. *Cryosurgery for skin cancer and cutaneous disorders.* p. 187. St. Louis: C.V. Mosby.

Spoor, H.J. 1972. Skin cancer: relationship to topically applied hormones. *Cutis* 9:335.

Staberg, B.; Wulf, H.C.; and Poulsen, T. et al. 1983. Carcinogenic effect of sequential artificial sunlight and UV-A irradiation in hairless mice: consequences for solarium "therapy". *Arch. Dermatol.* 119:641-43.

Stafford, N.D., and Frootko, N.J. 1986. Verrucous carcinoma in the external auditory canal. *Am. J. Otolaryngol.* 7:443-45.

Stellmack, R.K.; Rehrmann, A.; and Koch, H. 1971. Malignant degeneration of basal cell carcinomas of the face;

basal-squamous carcinoma. *Plast. Reconstr. Surg.* 48:471-73.

Stern, R.S.; Thibodeau, L.A.; and Kleinerman, R.A. et al. 1979. Risk of cutaneous carcinoma in patients treated with oral methoxalen photochemotherapy for psoriasis. *N. Engl. J. Med.* 300:809-13.

Stern, R.S.; Laird, N.; Melski, J.; and Parrish, J.A. et al. 1984. Cutaneous squamous cell carcinoma in patients treated with PUVA. *N. Engl. J. Med.* 310:1156-61.

Stoll, H.L., and Schwartz, R.A. 1987. Squamous cell carcinoma. In Fitzpatrick, T.B.; Eisen, A.Z.; Wolff, K.; Freedberg, I.M.; and Austen, K.F. eds. *Dermatology in general medicine.* 3rd ed. pp. 746-758. New York: McGraw-Hill.

Stone, M.S.; Noonan, C.A.; Tschen, J.; and Bruce, S. 1987. Bowen's disease of the feet: presence of human papillomavirus 16 DNA in tumor tissue. *Arch. Dermatol.* 123:1517-20.

Swanbeck, G. 1971. Aetiological factors in squamous cell skin cancer. *Br. J. Dermatol.* 85:394-96.

Swanson, N.A., and Taylor, W.B. 1980. Plantar verrucous carcinoma. *Arch. Dermatol.* 116:794-97.

Syrjanen, K.J. 1987. Human papillomavirus (HPV) infections and their associations with squamous cell neoplasia. *Arch. Geschwulstforsch* 57(6):417-44.

Ten Seldam, R.E.J. 1963. Skin cancer in Australia. *Natl. Cancer Inst. Monogr.* 10:153-79.

Thomas, C.C. 1968. Basal cell carcinoma of the left leg with metastases to the left inguinal lymph nodes, multiple skin metastases and involvement of the bone marrow. *Arch. Dermatol.* 97:596-98.

Thompson, S.G. 1968. Epithelioma cuniculatum: an unusual tumour of the foot. *Br. J. Plast. Surg.* 18:214-17.

Tornes, K.; Bang, G.; and Koppang, H.S. et al. 1985. Oral verrucous carcinoma. *Int. J. Oral Surg.* 14:485-92.

Traenkle, H.L. 1963. X-ray induced skin cancer in man. *Natl. Cancer Inst. Monogr.* 10:423-32.

Tromovitch, T.A. 1965. Skin cancer treatment by curettage and desiccation. *Calif. Med.* 103:107.

Tromovitch, T.A., and Stegman, S.J. 1978. Microscopic-controlled excision of cutaneous tumors: chemosurgery fresh tissue technique. *Cancer* 41:653.

Turner, J.E., and Callen, J.B. 1981. Aggressive behavior of squamous cell carcinoma in a patient with preceding lymphocytic lymphoma. *J. Am. Acad. Dermatol.* 4:446-50.

Urbach, F. 1971. Geographic distribution of skin cancer. *J. Surg. Oncol.* 3:219-34.

Urbach, F.; Rose, D.B.; and Bonnem, N. 1972. Genetic and environmental interactions in skin carcinogenesis. In *Environment and cancer.* pp. 335-71. Baltimore: Williams & Wilkins.

Van Nostrand, A.W.P., and Olofsson, J. 1972. Verrucous carcinoma of the larynx. *Cancer* 30:691-702.

Van Scott, E.J., and Reinertson, R.P. 1961. Modulating influence of stromal environment on epithelial cells studied in human autotransplants. *J. Invest. Dermatol.* 36:109-31.

Vitaliano, P.P., and Urbach, F. 1980. Relative importance of risk factors in nonmelanoma carcinoma. *Arch. Dermatol.* 116:454-56.

Von Domarus, H., and Steven, P.J. 1984. Metastatic basal cell carcinoma: report of five cases and review of 170 cases in the literature. *J. Am. Acad. Dermatol.* 10:1043.

Wagner, S.L.; Maliner, J.S.; and Morton, W.E. et al. 1979. Skin cancer and arsenical intoxication from well water. *Arch. Dermatol.* 115:1205-1207.

Walden, B.K.; Robertson, M.R.; and Jeremy, D. 1971. Skin cancer and immunosuppression. *Lancet* II:1282-83.

Weimar, V.M.; Ceilley, R.I.; and Goeken, J.A. 1979. Aggressive biologic behavior of basal and squamous cell cancers in patient with chronic lymphocytic leukemia or chronic lymphocytic lymphoma. *J. Dermatol. Surg. Oncol.* 5:609-14.

Westburg, S.P., and Stone, O.J. 1973. Multiple cutaneous squamous cell carcinomas during immunosuppressive therapy. *Arch. Dermatol.* 107:893-95.

Wieman, T.J.; Shiveley, E.H.; and Woodcock, T.M. 1983. Responsiveness of metastatic basal cell carcinoma to chemotherapy: a case report. *Cancer* 52:1583.

Wolf, J.E., and Hubler, W.R. 1975. Tumor angiogenic factor and human skin tumors. *Arch. Dermatol.* 111:321-27.

Wolf, D.J., and Zitelli, J.A. 1987. Surgical margins for basal cell carcinoma. *Arch. Dermatol.* 123:340-44.

Zacarian, S.A. 1979. Cryosurgery of malignant lesions and selection of patients. *Dermatology* 2:39.

Zacarian, S.A. 1985. Cryosurgery for cancer of the skin. In Zacarian, S.A. ed. *Cryosurgery for skin cancer and cutaneous disorders.* p. 96. St. Louis: C.V. Mosby.

Zacarian, S.A. 1985. Complications, indications, and contraindications. In Zacarian, S.A. ed. *Cryosurgery for skin cancer and cutaneous disorders.* p. 283. St. Louis: C.V. Mosby.

Zelickson, A.S., and Mottaz, J. 1970. The effect of sunlight on human epidermis: a quantitative electron microscopic study of dendritic cells. *Arch. Dermatol.* 101:312-15.

Chapter 23

HEAD, NECK, AND THYROID CANCER

Charles M. Norris, Jr., M.D., F.A.C.S.

Blake Cady, M.D.

Charles M. Norris, Jr., M.D., F.A.C.S.
Assistant Clinical Professor of Otolaryngology
Harvard Medical School
New England Deaconess Hospital
Boston, Massachusetts

Blake Cady, M.D.
New England Deaconess Hospital
Boston, Massachusetts

PART I: HEAD AND NECK CANCER

INTRODUCTION

A practical discussion of head and neck cancer concerns squamous cell (or epidermoid) carcinoma of the upper aerodigestive tract. Head and neck oncology increasingly and appropriately involves the participation and judgment of multiple medical disciplines—medical oncology, radiation therapy, head and neck surgery, dentistry, maxillofacial prosthodontics, nutrition, speech therapy, social work, nursing, and hospice care. The patient, even when successfully treated, often faces functional and social problems that can have great psychological impact. While they are a small portion of all cancers, head and neck malignancies are a visible and significant threat to life and lifestyle. Multiple relevant variables dictate an individualized approach to treatment decisions. Treatment and mortality parameters cannot be universally applied, as the natural history and consequent clinical expectations vary from site to site. Survival should not concern only statistics, but quality of life as well. Rather than impart to the reader a series of clinical observations, facts, and numerical data, this chapter provides insight into the philosophy of patient management in a more global oncologic sense.

EPIDEMIOLOGY

Squamous cell carcinoma of the upper aerodigestive tract mucosa generally is a disease afflicting males in their fifth and sixth decades, accounting for roughly 8.5% of all malignancies in this group (Cann, Fried, and Rothman 1985). The proportion of females with these lesions has always been less by a factor of 2 to 4, depending on the site. This disparity is declining, especially in laryngeal carcinoma, as more women, who have been smoking for longer periods of time, attain the traditional age group of risk. Overall, approximately 43,000 new cases of head and neck cancer will have been diagnosed in the United States in 1990 (Silverberg, Boring, and Squires 1990).

ETIOLOGY

The multivariate etiology of head and neck cancer is understandable, given the number of environmental agents that can come into contact with the breathing and swallowing passages. Tobacco (whether inhaled or chewed), ethyl alcohol, and the combination of tobacco and alcohol, are the best established and most significant carcinogens of mucosal malignancy in the oral cavity, oropharynx, hypopharynx, and larynx. However, these are neither invariable nor exclusive in a given patient (see table 23.1) (Suen and Myers 1981). Since the effect of multiple etiologic factors can be synergistic, the elimination of even a single factor can greatly influence overall risk.

Nutritional deficiency and suboptimal orodental health are also generally implicated in a number of patients, and are frequent social concomitants of alcoholism. Viral and genetic observations have provided additional insight into cancer pathogenesis, but are not as readily eliminated as the environmental factors. The lack of identifiable carcinogens in a given individual does not preclude the occurrence of head and neck cancer. While multiple risk factors may coexist in a patient, they should not be weighed so heavily that they detract from other possible clinical considerations.

NATURAL HISTORY

PRIMARY SITE

Squamous cell head and neck cancer generally originates on the surface of the mucosal lining of the upper aerodigestive tract. True or apparent submucosal lesions occur when the tumors start within epithelial invaginations, such as the tonsils or tongue base, or from the ducts of minor salivary glands. Recurrent cancer after previous treatment is often submucosal and elusive, invisible

Table 23.1
CARCINOGENS IN HEAD AND NECK CANCER

SITE	CARCINOGEN FACTORS	OTHER FACTORS
Nasal cavity Paranasal sinuses	Wood dust (furniture) Leather manufacturing Textile industry Nickel refining Thorotrast (radiochemical) Mustard gas	? chronic sinusitis ? cigarette smoke
Nasopharynx	Nitrosamines	Epstein-Barr virus Genetics: Chinese
Oral cavity	Cigarettes Ethyl alcohol Snuff, chewing tobacco Textile industry Leather manufacturing	Syphilis Vitamin deficiencies
Hypopharynx Larynx	Cigarettes Asbestos (ship builders) Mustard gas Ethyl alcohol Wood exposure	Nutrition deficiencies
Esophagus	Ethyl alcohol Cigarettes	Nutrition deficiencies Race: Eskimos, blacks
Salivary gland	Radiation	Genetics: Eskimos

(Adapted from: Suen and Myers eds. [1981].)

to the eye, but possibly palpable. The so-called typical mucosal carcinoma appears as an ulceration, roughening, thickening, outcropping, or cauliflower-like fungation, or combinations of these. Early lesions are either reddish (erythroplastic) or whitish (leukoplakic) in color. Surface infection, necrosis, or bleeding may evolve as a tumor grows. Progressive infiltration into underlying muscles results in their dysfunction. Centripetal mucosal expansion, as well as invasion along tissue planes (including perichondrium or periosteum) or nerves, occurs. Direct invasion into bone is a late development, though tumors may extend into bony structures through pre-existent anatomic openings, such as a nerve canal or dental extraction site. Extension along nerves, or within lymphatics or small vessels, can facilitate the spread of malignant cells beyond the area discernible by examination techniques.

Inflammation, mass or pressure effect, nerve impingement, or muscle dysfunction cause primary site symptoms. However, symptoms may be lacking altogether. Tumors in certain sites (tongue base, pyriform sinus, nasopharynx, paranasal sinuses) tend to become noticeable to the patient only when in advanced stages. Symptom trends and patterns of tumor spread vary from site to site, but are neither unique nor exclusive.

LYMPHATIC SPREAD
Epidermoid cancer in the head and neck spreads both locally (at and around the primary site of origin) and regionally, via lymphatic channels through which tumor implantation into lymph nodes occurs. Enlarged cervical nodes, in the presence of a known head and neck

malignancy, reflect this implantation and may be an initial symptom or sign. Different sites and histologic subtypes have varying propensities for occult or overt lymphatic spread. Progressive lymphatic spread of head and neck malignancies also tends to occur in recognizable anatomic patterns that may be altered after previous surgery or radiation treatment. The sequestration of persisting tumor cells can lead to elusive manifestations of tumor recurrence in spite of diligent observation.

DISTANT SITES
The invasion of malignant cells into the venous circulation allows dissemination throughout the body. Not all seeds will grow, and the tendency for any tumor cell to establish itself and propagate in a distant site depends on a number of factors. These include the cancer cell's own biology, its ability to pass through the recipient tissue's capillary wall, its resistance to local and systemic immune surveillance and to any active medical therapy, and the receptiveness of the host tissue. The incidence of distant metastasis differs according to the location of the primary lesion. Generally, there is a dose-response phenomenon: the larger the primary tumor or more extensive the nodal deposits, the greater the risk of distant dissemination. The lungs are the most common location for distant metastasis from head and neck cancer. Bone, liver, and brain sites are much less likely.

A tumor's natural history affects its recurrence after treatment. Thus, particular patterns of spread are also reflected in associated patterns of failure. Tumors that tend to spread early into either lymphatics or the bloodstream, but are themselves responsive to treatment at the primary site, tend to recur at either the nodal or distant site, or both. Tumor site, histology, and extent of a tumor have patterns of spread that are reflected in its natural history, and also in the patient's course. This somewhat predictable biologic behavior must be considered when determining the type and extent of treatment, and plans for follow-up.

CLASSIFICATION AND STAGING
Classification and staging of cancers are necessary in order to clinically compare patient groups within and among treating institutions, communicate data in the same language, provide treatment guidelines, and evaluate treatment response. The ideal staging system is simple enough to recall from memory in daily use. It must be relevant to the natural history of the disease process in question and complete enough to allow a statistical inquiry into the most significant aspects of the disease, as well as into those variables that can reasonably and practically be evaluated routinely during a patient's evaluation and course of treatment. Most importantly, there should be a correlation between the extent of disease at the time of treatment (stage), the treatment rendered, and the outcome, expressed both in quantity and quality of life.

Reflecting the patterns of spread observed in head and neck cancer, a version of the "TNM" system of tumor classification has developed (table 23.2) (Beahrs, Henson,

Table 23.2
CLASSIFICATION OF HEAD AND NECK CANCERS

CLASSIFICATION

PRIMARY TUMOR (T)
general — for all sites
TX   no available information on primary tumor
T0   no evidence of primary tumor
TIS   carcinoma *in situ*

ORAL CAVITY, OROPHARYNX
T1   greatest diameter of primary tumor < or = 2 cm
T2   > 2 cm or = 4 cm
T3   > 4 cm
T4   massive tumor, with deep invasion into maxilla, mandible, pteygoid muscles, deep tongue muscle, skin, soft tissues of neck

HYPOPHARYNX
T1   tumor confined to region of origin
T2   extension into adjacent region or site, without fixation of hemilarynx
T3   extension into adjacent region or site, with fixation of hemilarynx
T4   massive tumor, invading bone or soft tissues of neck

NASOPHARYNX
T1   tumor confined to one site, or identified on biopsy only (no tumor visible)
T2   involvement of two sites within nasopharynx
T3   extension into nasal cavity or oropharynx
T4   invasion into skull and/or cranial nerve involvement

LARYNX
Glottic
T1   confined to true vocal cords; normal mobility; includes anterior or posterior commissure
T2   supra- or subglottic extension; normal or impaired mobility
T3   confined to larynx proper; cord fixation
T4   cartilage destruction and/or extension out of larynx
Supraglottic
T1   confined to site of origin; normal mobility
T2   extension to glottis or adjacent supraglottic site; normal or impaired mobility
T3   confined to larynx proper; cord fixation and/or extension into hypopharynx or pre-epiglottic space
T4   massive tumor; cartilage destruction and/or extension out of larynx
Subglottic
T1   confined to subglottic region
T2   glottic extension; normal or impaired mobility
T3   confined to larynx proper; cord fixation
T4   massive tumor; cartilage destruction and/or extension out of larynx

NODAL METASTASIS (N)
NX   nodes cannot be assessed
N0   no clinically positive nodes
N1   single, clinically positive, ipsilateral node; < or = 3 cm
N2A   single, clinically positive, ipsilateral node; > 3 or = 6 cm
N2B   multiple, clinically positive, ipsilateral nodes; all < or = 6 cm
N3A   clinically positive, ipsilateral node(s); one > 6 cm
N3B   bilateral, clinically positive nodes (each side subclassified)
N3C   contralateral, clinically positive node(s), only

DISTANT METASTASIS (M)
MX   not assessed
M0   no distant metastases identified
M1   distant metastasis present
specify site:
            PUL - pulmonary
            OSS - osseous
            BRA - brain
            LYM - lymph nodes (noncervical)
            MAR - bone marrow
            PLE - pleura
            SKI - skin
            OTH - other

STAGE GROUPINGS
Stage I   T1 N0 M0
Stage II   T2 N0 M0
Stage III   T3 N0 M0 T1, T2, or T3 N1 M0
Stage IV   T4 N0 or N1 M0
             Any T N2 or N3 M0
             Any T Any N M1

and Hutter et al. 1988). The designation T, for tumor, classifies the primary origin of the malignancy according to several variables, which vary from site to site. These include tumor size or extension into adjacent anatomic structures. Assigning a T-value depends on accurately locating and measuring the tumor, either by inspection, palpation, endoscopic exam, or other modality such as imaging study. For a given anatomic subdivision in the upper aerodigestive tract, advancing T-stage correlates with disease severity and prognosis, but a comparison between sites of like T-stages is not at all valid, due to site differences in tumor natural history. Although it has some impact on prognosis, the present system does not include histologic grading as a parameter for T-staging. (Other classification schemes proposed have included this variable, particularly in Europe.)

The N classification, for nodal, seeks to group the number, size, and laterality of lymphatic metastases. Assigning an N-level is generally more consistent, with good correlation between pretreatment N-stage and outcome. Clinically false-positive nodes are rare.

M, for metastasis, designates the systemic dissemination of cancer cells to other organs of the body. The term M0 communicates only that at a point in time, usually prior to treatment, the modalities employed for examination detected no *identifiable* metastases. Because it is rare, even in the presence of massive primary and nodal disease, for pulmonary or other sites of blood-borne spread to be evident at initial presentation, evaluation is often limited to a chest x-ray. Any suggestive symptoms outside the head and neck area are considered and worked up accordingly. M1, qualified by a location, designates metastasis to that location.

Interestingly, when a distant metastasis is identified the patient is not curable and treatment should maximize subjective well-being. The effects of uncontrolled head and neck cancer tend to be slow but extremely debilitating in terms of physical appearance, airway effects, swallowing, and pain; therefore such treatment may well be equivalent to the original recommendation. The prognosis of an advanced head and neck cancer may be worse than that of an early pulmonary lesion, in which case the former would be treated as planned, and workup of the latter deferred.

No classification and staging system alone will provide clear-cut, unvarying instructions for patient management. As Sisson points out, the "shortcomings [of the TNM system] are as much a reflection of the complexity of the disease itself as a condemnation of the staging system" (Sisson and Pelzer 1985). The classification scheme does, however, represent a common denominator for comparison in a constantly changing discipline.

APPROACH TO PATIENT

DIAGNOSIS AND EVALUATION

In contrast to many other regions of the body, most of the areas involved with head and neck cancer are accessible to examination. Medical comorbidity is common in patients with head and neck cancer, particularly that due to liver disease and chronic obstructive pulmonary disease, reflecting alcohol and tobacco use, respectively. Any prior history of malignant or premalignant disease of the upper aerodigestive tract, lung, or esophagus, and the evaluations and treatment rendered, is critical. A history of other malignancy may modify life expectancy and thereby influence future treatment considerations. Cardiac, neurologic, renal, hematologic, and otologic disease, and diabetes mellitus can limit surgical or chemotherapeutic treatment options, and may even constitute a greater life threat than an early head and neck cancer. Family history, with rare exception, is generally more indicative of a patient's social milieu than his cancer risk. Previous experience with a family member who had cancer, however, may substantially affect a patient's perception and possible misconception of his own disease and its treatment.

The so-called symptoms of head and neck cancer, as expressed by the patient, may not be symptoms at all, but the patient's own observation of a "lump" in the neck, or a "growth," or a slowly healing "sore" in the mouth. Unilateral pain, dysarthria, hoarseness or *any form of voice change,* dysphagia, stridor, positional dyspnea, aspiration symptoms such as choking, odynophagia, and any kind of bleeding are manifestations that alone or in combination may indicate a lesion in the upper aerodigestive tract. They reflect a loss of mucosal integrity, mass effect, or dysfunction of a portion of the involved anatomy. More localizing, but still with other potential explanations, are unilateral nasal obstruction or bleeding, facial pain, serous otitis media (due to eustachian tube compromise), and orbital or ocular symptoms, indicating a possible lesion in the nose, paranasal sinuses, or nasopharynx.

Otalgia is a significant concomitant of head and neck neoplasms. It may be due to referred pain from any of the nerves innervating the oral cavity, oropharynx, mandible, maxilla, hypopharynx, or larynx; it signifies deep invasion of the tumor. Persistent otalgia without explanation and with an unremarkable head and neck exam should be further evaluated. Lesions of the tongue base, pyriform sinus, and cervical esophagus can be particularly elusive to office physical examination.

Although the manifestations of a neck mass may suggest a benign nature, any neck mass in an adult should be viewed as malignant and probably metastatic until proven otherwise (Norris and Miller 1985). Concomitant sources of regional infection, fluctuation in size, tenderness and pain, a high jugular or midline location, oval shape, mobility, soft or cystic consistency, and bilaterality all suggest, but do not guarantee, a benign cervical lymph node. A complete mucosal exam and symptom review are advisable. It is important to determine whether a solitary mass is a lymph node, another cervical structure, or a mass within a major salivary gland or the thyroid gland, all of which can be sources of neoplasia, but with vastly differing natural histories.

Almost all primary head and neck malignancies are discernible through complete office examination. A systematic approach is recommended, with good illumination, a reasonably comfortable patient, and the practiced use of equipment. A general evaluation of face and neck symmetry, eyes, skin lesions, respiratory status, and various stigmata of systemic disease is important. Otoscopic ear exam and nasal cavity exam via nasal speculum should be followed by detailed visualization and palpation of all accessible mucosal surfaces of the nasopharynx, oral cavity, oropharynx, hypopharynx, and larynx. A tongue retractor and various mirrors are generally used, coupled with coaxial illumination from either a direct or indirect source. An array of rigid and flexible fiberoptic telescopes for insertion into the nose or oral cavity facilitates the exam of areas not otherwise well visualized. The importance of digital and bimanual palpation of the oral cavity and oropharynx cannot be overemphasized.

Palpation of the neck, noting both normal landmarks and abnormal contours or masses, requires practice. Benign adenopathy is common. Worrisome lymph nodes can be anywhere, and will tend to be firm or hard, round, 2 cm or greater in size, possibly immobile or partially immobile, and often single and unilateral. "Normal" nodes are unusual in the supraclavicular or posterior triangle portions of the neck. The location and tissue of origin of any mass must be questioned. Distinguishing a high jugular lymph node from a mass in the *tail of the parotid,* for example, can be difficult. Auscultation of the neck is useful to pick up evidence of carotid artery compression, intrinsic occlusive disease, or possibly the bruit associated with some unusual vascular tumors or malformations. Subtle subglottic or tracheal airway compromise may be detected via stethoscope.

Further evaluation of a patient already diagnosed with head and neck cancer focuses on the lesion's histologic type, local extent, and metastatic spread. Biopsy for histologic review of lesions in some locations can be accomplished in an office setting, as can the cytologic evaluation of a needle aspirate (fine needle biopsy) from a neck mass. Generally, however, an examination under anesthesia is both necessary and more informative. In addition to palpation of the oral cavity and neck, direct laryngoscopy (of the oropharynx, hypopharynx, and larynx), rigid esophagoscopy, nasopharyngoscopy, and bronchoscopy (including the trachea and subglottic airway) are carried out in some combination appropriate for the lesion. This "triple" endoscopy, or "quad-scoping," is important for assessing a suspect lesion in greater detail and identifying any other coincident abnormalities, including second primary mucosal lesions of the upper aerodigestive tract or lung (Shaha et al. 1988; Atkins et al. 1984; Shikhani et al. 1986). A very accurate description of pretreatment tumor location and extent is essential to specify optimal treatment, assess response, and observe the treated patient in follow-up.

Blood work is performed as a baseline assessment of the patient's general medical condition, and includes routine tests reflecting liver, renal, and hematologic function. Nutritional indicators, arterial blood gases, pulmonary function testing, and creatinine clearance are all considered. Various serologic markers, including carcinoembryonic antigen (CEA) and Epstein-Barr virus (EBV) antibody titers, can be useful in follow-up.

Finally, imaging studies are an important, and sometimes critical, adjunct to clinical evaluations. A chest x-ray is routine, to evaluate cardiopulmonary health and rule out parenchymal lesions. Barium swallow examination of the hypopharynx/esophagus is relevant and useful, but rarely, if ever, supplants a good endoscopic examination. Anteroposterior tomography of the larynx or sinuses may delineate tumor extension in these areas, perhaps below the vocal cords or into the facial bones, respectively. Mandible x-rays may identify bone invasion from an oral cavity or oropharyngeal tumor. They may not, however, reveal a tumor within the jaw due to extension through intrinsic foramina or tooth extraction sockets. A radionuclear bone scan of the jaw, when correlated with the patient's symptoms and physical findings, may suggest periosteal involvement or subclinical cortical bone erosion. Total body, brain, or liver scanning have a very low incidental yield in identifying distant metastases, and are performed only if indicated by specific symptoms or other findings.

Axial and coronal CT scanning of the head and neck is essentially the imaging study of choice for most advanced head and neck lesions. Cross-sectional images facilitate an anatomic evaluation of unexplained symptomatology associated with less advanced lesions, and allow a noninvasive exploration of areas not otherwise examinable, such as the paranasal sinuses, parapharyngeal and pterygomaxillary spaces, orbits, and anterior skull base. The role of magnetic resonance imaging (MRI) will be similar to that of CT scanning. Although its nonradiation technology and high resolution are desirable, MRI is limited by its lack of universal ability and interpretive experience in the head and neck area. Soft tissue resolution including that of the tumor-tissue interface is occasionally superb, but bone delineation is poor. At present, MRI is most useful for representing the soft tissue extent of tumors that have transgressed the skull base, or which involve the parapharyngeal spaces. The areas in which it is superior to CT scanning are currently becoming established (MRI Report 1988).

Arteriography, either by formal angiography or by digital subtraction technique, is used very selectively in squamous cell carcinoma, primarily to discern carotid artery involvement. Arteriography is particularly useful in cases of rare, nonepidermoid tumors of the head and neck, such as chemodectomas, angiofibromas, large or malignant hemangiomas, and some others. In these cases, angiography may be diagnostic and also provide a means of preoperative therapeutic embolization in order to lessen bleeding.

TREATMENT FUNDAMENTALS

Surgery and radiation, alone or in combination, are the cornerstones of curative treatment in head and neck cancer. Conventional resectional surgery, endoscopic surgery, laser surgery, cryotherapy, and electrocautery are surgical treatment modalities. Radiation may be delivered by external beam, interstitial implantation, or surface-contact. Chemotherapy by itself, in spite of its demonstrated ability to reduce or eradicate clinically detectable squamous cell cancer, is not curative. Currently, chemotherapy is undergoing vigorous assessment as an adjunct to surgery and radiation.

Other research in the treatment of head and neck cancer centers around ways of improving the efficacy, or decreasing the morbidity, of existing therapies. While the combination of radiation and surgery is well established as more effective against some advanced lesions, the optimum manner and sequence in which these are administered for a given cancer type, stage, and site is a controversial area subject to continued review.

Conservation surgery, the achievement of adequate tumor resection with less radical tissue removal or functional impairment, is a frequent topic of report, as are further refined techniques in the reconstruction of tumor defects or the rehabilitation of functional deficits. Radiation sensitizers are pharmacologic agents capable of increasing the effect of ionizing radiation on hypoxic tumor cell masses, while maintaining or decreasing the normal tissue side effects. Treatment with hyperbaric oxygen has a similar rationale. Technologic improvements in the power and type of radiation have made possible the use of electron and neutron beam therapies. An area of active investigation concerns the twice-daily format for external beam therapy, in which either the conventional or higher doses are delivered through an increased number of fractions administered more rapidly over compressed time periods (hyperfractionation, and accelerated fractionation). The correlation of such clinical research inquiries with investigations into the basic science of tumor carcinogenesis, biology, evolution, and natural history is critical to the perspective of an active practitioner in this field today, whether as a surgeon, radiation therapist, or medical oncologist.

The goals of *cancer treatment* are to eliminate the known tumor, deter its recurrence, and prevent the emergence of occult cancer cells. These objectives must be integrated into the goals of *patient management,* which are to meet the goals of cancer treatment with the maintenance of satisfactory physiologic function, reasonable appearance, and social interaction, and to rehabilitate the patient for a lifestyle compatible with his or her own priorities and standards. Needless to say, physicians have no control over some of these goals and little influence over some others. The art becomes one of exercising well-informed, accurately communicated judgment as to the best compromises to make.

The natural history of head and neck cancers indicates there is an expected pattern of spread for each type, site, and stage. Consequently, definitive therapy must be directed at the identifiable disease, and prophylactic, or elective, therapy must be aimed at areas of possible cancer cell dispersal, based on the likelihood of this occurrence. The amount and combination of therapy is further tem-

pered with a probability contrast between treatment morbidity, likelihood of efficacy, and the preservation of future options. The physiologic morbidity of either surgery or radiation in the head and neck area influences life-sustaining and socially necessary function and appearance, with secondary psychological, domestic, and occupational consequences. Table 23.3 identifies areas of potential physical impairment.

It can be difficult to accurately convey to patients the effects of treatment on their future. Assessing patients' motivation and powers of rehabilitation, both physical and emotional, compounds the task. And yet, the patients' informed desires regarding treatment must be considered among the many factors influencing treatment planning.

SURGERY

In contrast to radiation, the operative eradication of a tumor and its areas of potential spread is a more expeditious treatment that avoids both the immediate and long-term side effects of radiation. The treated tissue volume is less and is available for pathologic analysis, allowing the surgeon to determine treatment adequacy and to confirm pretreatment staging classification. Furthermore, surgery preserves radiation as a future treatment option, and avoids the higher complication rate of postradiation surgery.

While a number of standard procedures are described for dealing with tumors of different locations and sizes, treatment is individualized for each patient. Although creating a wide margin around the primary tumor is desirable, the efficacy of this is limited by the functional or cosmetic importance of the adjacent tissue, as well as the feasibility of surgically or prosthetically reconstructing the resulting defect. The relative importance and efficacy of any surgical procedure must also be seen in relation to overall cancer control. For example, it may be worthwhile to remove a small tumor of the lateral tongue, while the same lesion in the midline base of the tongue would require a very extensive procedure with the same, or less, effectiveness than radiation. Reconstruction, both cosmetic and functional, is an integral component of surgical management, and may involve more technically sophisticated procedures than tumor site ablation.

Table 23.3
AREAS OF POTENTIAL PHYSICAL IMPAIRMENT

Speech:	
phonation	larynx
articulation	tongue, teeth, palate, lips
chewing	jaw, teeth, salivary lubrication, relevant musculature
Swallowing:	
deglutition	tongue, palate, pharynx, esophagus, salivary lubrication
airway protection	larynx, esophagus; coordinated reflexes and sensation
Breathing	larynx, trachea
Senses	taste, smell, sight, hearing

Secondary effects of above on nutrition, chronic pulmonary health

Appearance

RADIATION

Radiation avoids the small, but definite, risk of perioperative mortality that remains in judiciously selected and carefully managed surgical patients. No tissue is removed, so the cosmetic effect can be minimal. Functional side effects do occur, but they generally are much less dramatic than those of surgery. These side effects are caused by the loss of mucosal lubrication (due to radiation effect on salivary gland function) and taste; by chronic mucosal inflammation and fragility; and by scarring, fibrosis, and edema around the treated area. These radiation reactions extend to all exposed tissues, not just the mucosa. Fibrosis of various muscles can cause dysfunction (e.g., trismus, or vocal cord fixation). Chronic edema, adding to the swallowing discomfort caused by salivary insufficiency, can also result in chronic dysphagia, dysphonia, and airway obstruction. The risk of soft tissue, cartilage, or bone necrosis is small with present management and technical practice, but must be weighed in the decision.

The logistics of radiation therapy involve daily treatments for five to eight weeks, which is a disadvantage. An advantage is the ability of radiation to treat multiple regions simultaneously, as in the case of coexistent multiple primary mucosal lesions. As elective treatment for occult lymphatic disease, either independently or in conjunction with surgery, radiotherapy carries relatively little morbidity and is effective.

The dose of radiation is determined by the site and volume of tumor, its proclivity for spread, and the intent of treatment (curative or palliative). Palliative doses are likely to be lower, with smaller field sizes, in order to minimize side effects. Larger (T3 or T4) tumors tend to need higher doses, (>70 Gy), while smaller ones (T1 or T2) may be cured with 60 Gy to 70 Gy. The clinically negative neck (N0) is traditionally treated with doses of 50 Gy to 55 Gy. Doses much higher than 70 Gy, if delivered externally, increase complications substantially. Usually, several different focus angles of the beam onto the tumor are used in order to lessen the deleterious effects of radiation on the interposed normal tissues. The fields (or portals) of delivery for external radiotherapy are simulated by computer to ensure accurate dosing in the area of tumor, and to allow the consistent daily administration of the beam. Regions needing additional treatment (a radiation boost) use smaller field sizes to administer treatment (a shrinking field technique).

Higher doses can also be delivered through the insertion or implantation of radioactive materials such as gold or iridium via seeds, needles, removable catheters, or surface contact. The interstitial technique (brachytherapy) is particularly useful in the tongue base, tonsil fossa, and oral cavity. Surface exposure is occasionally used to deliver additional radiation to the nasopharynx or to a maxillectomy cavity.

COMBINATION THERAPY

As a rule, surgical salvage (indicating the successful retreatment of a recurrent or persistent cancer after previous treatment) for radiation failure is more likely than radiation salvage after previous surgery. According to Million and Cassisi a recurrence after radiation is more likely to be at the epicenter of the original lesion, rather than at its periphery. Therefore, a surgical procedure, albeit with functional and operative sequelae, is more likely to anatomically encompass the recurrence with a reasonable margin. Recurrence at the primary site after surgery, by contrast, will more likely develop submucosally at the periphery of the original tumor, in the margin of resection. The difficulty in discerning recurrent tumor from postoperative fibrosis is formidable, and often results in diagnostic delay. Even if recurrence is suspected, obtaining and histologically confirming tissue from a previously operated site can be problematic. Such a tumor recurrence, in a scarred, distorted, and relatively avascular tissue field, is likely to have multiple areas of sequestration and hypoxia. These features probably account for the tumor's resistance to radiation salvage in this setting.

Radiation and surgery are frequently employed together. As a very general guideline, in the absence of clinically identifiable lymphatic spread, small lesions (T1 or T2) are equally well served by either radiation or surgery, and the choice is based on relative morbidity for the site. Additional weight is given to radiation if the patient has a high risk of occult nodal disease. Surgical alternatives including neck dissection are possible. For large primary tumors (T3 or T4) or clinically evident nodal disease (N1, N2, or N3), combined treatment with radiation and surgery is indicated, with sequence and sites of emphasis determined by the staging and site of tumor, perceived effectiveness, combined morbidity, and individual preference.

CHEMOTHERAPY

A number of antineoplastic drugs are effective against epidermoid cancer of the head and neck. While chemotherapy does not have the capacity to cure this family of malignancies, it can bring about a considerable reduction in tumor cell population, volume, and density. Systemic therapy would allow the possible eradication of tumor cells dispersed hematogenously or early tumor colonies in distant organs. By lessening the tumor volume at the primary and nodal sites, a subsequent curative therapy such as radiation may work better. Surgery, by encompassing a smaller tumor mass, could have greater latitude for larger margins of resection. Alternatively, a lower tumor density at the margin may result in a decrease in tumor viability (Norris et al. 1986). An actively investigated offshoot of these mechanisms may be that pretreatment with chemotherapy (induction chemotherapy) would lessen the extent of subsequent treatment needed, or even eliminate one of the combined modalities presently performed for advanced head and neck cancer (Ervin et al. 1987; Dreyfuss et al. 1990). A more traditional but very important use for chemotherapy has been in the palliation of incurable patients.

Methotrexate, bleomycin, and particularly cisplatin and 5-fluorouracil (5-FU), are the best-established agents used in chemotherapy trials today. The principles of induction chemotherapy are to administer combinations of established drugs with differing mechanisms of antineoplastic action and nonoverlapping major toxicities in a dose and timing sequence that takes advantage of each agent's action on the tumor cell cycle.

As an independent variable, adjuvant chemotherapy in head and neck cancer has not yet been conclusively shown to improve survival. While the degree of response to chemotherapy does correlate with survival, it is not clear that this trend is due to the chemotherapy itself or to the fortuitous biology of an individual tumor that renders it sensitive to both traditional treatment and chemotherapy. Well-designed, randomized, prospective clinical trials with long-term follow-up will help to determine the role for chemotherapy in the treatment of advanced head and neck cancer patients. A practical role in early lesions is not envisioned.

ORAL CAVITY/OROPHARYNX

The oral cavity is bordered by the vermillion border of the lips anteriorly, and the hard-soft palate junction, anterior tonsillar pillar, and circumvallate papillae posteriorly. Included are the mobile tongue, floor of mouth, gingiva, hard palate, buccal mucosa, and retromolar trigone. Though relatively accessible to self-exam, dental evaluation, and routine physical examination, there are often delays in the diagnosis of oral cavity cancer because of a lack of unique symptomatology, or confusion with traumatic, inflammatory, or infectious lesions (Crissman, Gluckman, and Whitely et al. 1980). The oropharynx extends from the rear border of the oral cavity to the base of tongue and pharyngeal walls, inferiorly, to the level of the vallecula. Included are the tonsillar pillars, fossae, and tonsils (if present), soft palate, tongue base, and both the lateral and posterior pharyngeal walls to the level of the pyriform sinus introitus and base of epiglottis, inferiorly. In general, the morbidity of treatment increases and the prognosis worsens as one progresses backward from the lips to the oropharynx, and from there to the hypopharynx.

After the larynx, the oral cavity and oropharynx are the most common sites for squamous cell carcinoma of the head and neck (MacComb, Fletcher, and Healey 1967). The patients tend to be males in their 50s and 60s, but the number of females affected is growing (Wey, Lotz, and Triedman 1987; Cusumano and Persky 1988). There is also a downward trend in the age group most affected. Tobacco use of any kind and alcohol consumption are etiologically significant. Oral cancers are commonly associated with poor dentition, chronic oral infection, and local trauma of any cause. As with skin cancer, sun exposure is implicated in carcinomas of the exposed vermillion, an area that also comes in contact with cigarettes, pipes, or cigars.

The histology of oral cavity and oropharyngeal malignancy is almost always squamous cell carcinoma. Minor salivary gland adenocarcinomas may occur; these would tend to be nonulcerated or submucosally infiltrative, but these features are not exclusive and biopsy is required to establish the diagnosis. The oropharynx includes the lymphoid tissue of the palatal and lingual tonsils and can be the site of lymphoma.

Lesions in the oral cavity and oropharynx tend to be poorly delineated, often spread submucosally, and are not confined by the anatomic midline. Deep muscle involvement of the tongue or pterygoid musculature is a particularly ominous finding. The invasion of bony structures (mandible, palate, maxilla, maxillary sinus, spine) is serious in terms of both prognosis and treatment morbidity. Extension of the primary tumor across the midline is particularly distressing, as this renders surgical treatment much more debilitating.

Nodal metastases are relatively uncommon with lesions in the oral cavity, but are more frequent when the site of the primary lesion is further into the oropharynx, or when the lesion's size increases. This feature, along with the higher incidence of poorly differentiated lesions, accounts, in part, for the worse prognosis of oropharyngeal lesions compared with oral cavity cancers. Bilateral nodal spread is likely with oropharyngeal primaries, at least microscopically. In the evaluation of oral cavity and oropharyngeal cancers, palpation of both primary and nodal areas is of paramount importance, as well as inquiry into signs or symptoms reflecting deep (i.e., T4) involvement. Mandible x-rays and/or bone scan are required for assessing bone involvement, and CT scan is required to assess parapharyngeal, spine, carotid, or pterygoid muscle involvement. Endoscopy and examination under anesthesia are essential to fully evaluate primary site extent and to explore the possibility of synchronous second primaries (Shibuya, Hisamitsu, and Shioiri et al. 1988).

Few other fields of oncology have so many variables to consider in formulating a treatment recommendation, particularly for advanced head and neck cancer. Education of patients is measured not as a function of the time spent talking with them or the number of consultants to whom they are exposed, but rather in their achieving a true perspective in terms with which they can identify. Decisions concerning the quantity and quality of future life must be accorded the patient, particularly when the most effective treatment may also be the most threatening to physical and psychological integrity.

TREATMENT/OUTCOME

In general, the treatment of *early* stage primary lesions of the oral cavity/oropharynx is based on the perceived side effects and morbidity. Radiation techniques and surgery are both equally effective. To a certain extent, as the site of the tumor moves posteriorly, the morbidity of surgery increases. Most patients tend to underestimate the degree and duration of radiation side effects and overestimate those of early stage surgery, many of which are transient or reasonably accommodated.

Advanced lesions generally require combined treatment, traditionally by both radiation and surgery, in various patterns and sequences. The role for adjunctive chemotherapy, either as initial treatment and/or as final treatment, remains controversial. Surgical exposure can be difficult, especially for posterior lesions, which compounds morbidity and reconstructive aspects. The complex anatomy of the floor of the mouth and the difficulty of administering radiation when lesions are close to bony structures are modifying factors. Posterior lesions, even early ones, have an increased likelihood of *occult* nodal metastasis. Among the lymphatic drainage pathways are nodes inaccessible to standard surgical techniques (i.e., retro- and parapharyngeal), or for which contralateral surgical treatment would be considered excessive. Even aggressive radical surgery for early stage lesions of the oropharynx may not remove all gross and subclinical disease, and consequently, radiation would be appropriate.

Clinically overt nodal metastasis, with either oral cavity or oropharyngeal primaries, confers an advanced staging and generally requires combined treatment. However, this does not necessarily entail combined treatment of *both* primary and nodal disease. For example, a small oropharyngeal primary with ipsilateral nodal disease may be treated with radiation and implant to cure the primary lesion and sterilize the contralateral neck, and with surgery (neck dissection) to control the known nodal disease. More advanced primaries will require surgery as well in order to achieve maximum cure potential.

Extremely advanced disease may be determined to represent an incurable situation, for which aggressive, potentially debilitating treatment may not be appropriate in preserving the quality of a patient's existence for the limited time he or she may have. As such, nonsurgical techniques for palliation may be recommended, in an effort to minimize morbidity and preserve some control of tumor for a period of time.

Surgery (primary site). Surgery on anteriorly located structures may be attempted transorally. Primary closure, especially of the mobile tongue following partial glossectomy but also of the buccal mucosa or mouth floor, is often possible. If not, split thickness or dermal skin grafting is feasible. A variety of local, intraoral flaps allow the transfer of tissue from one area of the oral cavity to another. For larger or less accessible anterior (oral cavity) lesions, and for most posterior (oropharyngeal) lesions, intraoral surgery is limiting, and a transcervical approach for exposure, with or without mandible or lip splitting procedures, will be required. Reconstruction can require elaborate means, including the transfer of distant tissue such as a pectoralis major myocutaneous (muscle-skin pedicle) flap, bone graft, or artificial prosthesis (jaw plate). The reconstructive endeavors may be as formidable a procedure as the tumor extirpation itself.

The preoperative assessment of resectability can be difficult, and in some cases impossible. Margins are limited by the confined anatomy of the oral cavity and oropharynx. Increasing the boundaries of resection,

even if anatomically feasible, usually results in significant increases in patient morbidity. Frozen section analysis of the margins taken during surgery, appropriately oriented and related to the tumor-patient defect, are essential but still do not give absolute assurance of the adequacy of resection. Postoperative radiation, advocated by some as reasonable back-up for an area of incompletely excised tumor, should not readily be relied upon. The tongue base and lower pharynx are particularly treacherous areas and may require adjunctive total laryngectomy in order to avoid postoperative aspiration problems. Some surgeons consider this inappropriately excessive initial treatment. However, for the palliation of recurrent disease, total laryngectomy may provide relief from pain and aspiration, and allow oral intake to resume.

Surgery (nodal metastasis). The surgical treatment of known nodal disease is generally via radical neck dissection, possibly with preservation of the spinal accessory nerve (modified radical neck dissection). Such surgery entails the removal of all of the nodal groups in the accessible cervical region, obligating coincident removal of the internal jugular vein, sternocleidomastoid muscle, and cervical sensory nerves. Other forms of less radical neck dissection are occasionally appropriate. Radiation is often used to treat clinically uninvolved nodal areas.

Radiation. Radiation, if chosen for primary site treatment, can be delivered by either external beam technique, or by combined external/interstitial implant methods. Treatment of nodal disease, either occult or evident, is incorporated into the plan. Generally a minimum of 60 Gy to 70 Gy must be delivered to ensure the 80% to 85% cure rate of T1-T2 oral cavity/oropharyngeal lesions. Nodal disease prophylaxis requires 45 Gy to 55 Gy, although areas within the primary site field will get more. Areas of known nodal disease will often be treated with postradiation neck dissection. If this is not planned, neck doses will have to be higher, at least 60 Gy, with a resultant increase in side effects. In general, nodal prophylaxis by radiation should at least be considered for all but the smallest oral cavity lesions and for most oropharyngeal lesions. A substantial boost of radiation dose to the primary site can be delivered without additional exposure of uninvolved external structures via the interstitial implant of radioactive material directly into the tumor.

Combined therapy. Combined therapy is generally the rule for oral cavity/oropharyngeal lesions in the following circumstances (S = surgery, XRT = radiation therapy, CHEMO = chemotherapy):

- Large 1° OC/CP **>>>** S first on 1° ± neck; w/clinically negative neck **>>>** XRT second, to neck + 1°

- Small 1° OC/OP **>>>** XRT first, to 1° + neck; w/clinically positive neck **>>>** S second, on neck, ± radiation implant to 1°

- Major 1º + neck disease >>> S + XRT, w/XRT first if resectability in question; OR >>> CHEMO + S + XRT

- Recurrent disease >>> S or XRT, for "salvage" of either location after previous Tx failure w/other modality, unless palliative only; +/or CHEMO

As with most sites in the head and neck, early lesions (T1 and T2 disease of the oral cavity and T1 cancers of the oropharynx, without nodal involvement) have a good chance for cure. Second primary lesions are especially a problem in oral cavity malignancy. The addition of either nodal disease, an advanced primary, or a recurrence after previous treatment, is a significant determinant in decreasing survival and incorporates a substantial risk of distant (usually pulmonary) metastasis. Overall 5-year survival for oral cavity tumors is in the 50% range; oropharyngeal lesions fare worse, at about 35%. Tumors at the base of the tongue and pharyngeal walls, and any tumor involving bone, are particularly deadly. The treatment of advanced tumors in either site leaves survivors with major, possibly life-threatening morbidity.

LARYNX

The larynx is the most frequent site of carcinoma in the adult upper aerodigestive tract. Anatomically, physiologically, and pathogenetically, the larynx has three distinct subdivisions: glottic, supraglottic, and subglottic.

The glottic region encompasses the true vocal cords, excluding the arytenoid cartilage. The glottic larynx measures only 4 mm to 6 mm in vertical dimension. Its primary functions are phonation, airway protection during swallowing, and coughing, an important pulmonary cleaning mechanism. Because symptoms of cancers in the glottic portion of the larynx occur early, there is an opportunity for earlier diagnosis. Lymphatics are sparse, so nodal metastasis is clinically rare, occurs late, and usually only with long-standing advanced local disease. The relative prognosis of glottic carcinoma is correspondingly better, both overall and stage for stage. Limitation of vocal cord mobility, due to deep muscle invasion, and thyroid cartilage invasion represent poor prognostic features with direct treatment implications.

The supraglottic area encompasses the false vocal cords, arytenoid area, epiglottis, and aryepiglottic folds. This portion of the larynx interfaces superiorly with the oropharynx and laterally and posteriorly with the hypopharynx. The supraglottic larynx functions as an air passage, but mainly as a shield and sphincter to protect the airway. Malignancies in this anatomic subdivision, as in the hypopharynx, can be silent, and therefore generally present at a more advanced stage. There is a much higher likelihood of occult or palpable nodal metastasis in supraglottic lesions, and fewer barriers to primary site extension. These features account for the worsening prognosis as tumor location shifts away from the true vocal cords.

The subglottic portion is the airway below the true vocal cords and above the first tracheal ring, basically representing the mucosa within the cricoid cartilage. Carcinomas arising in the subglottic larynx are rare. Most often, subglottic involvement is through extension of a glottic or supraglottic tumor. Because the subglottis is mainly an air conduit, symptoms from tumor involvement include stridor. The region's rich lymphatic network drains into the paratracheal and superior mediastinal nodes, rendering surgical treatment considerably less feasible.

While phonation is the most obvious concern, it is less important physiologically than airflow or pulmonary protection during swallowing. Chronic aspiration can be lethal in both the short and long term. Research and treatment techniques for laryngeal cancer seek to achieve more result with less therapy, or at least the same result with fewer side effects. Consequently, surgery which spares portions of the functional laryngeal anatomy ("conservation" laryngeal surgery) is a constantly refined, and requested, treatment modality. Hyperfraction radiation and induction chemotherapy may also facilitate effective nonsurgical cure.

Squamous cell carcinoma of the larynx is the classic smoker's cancer of the head and neck and generally occurs after many decades of cigarette use. Its occurrence in nonsmokers is extremely unusual. The glottic portion is most commonly involved. Alcohol is not a significant independent or synergistic etiologic cofactor, as it is in the oral cavity or hypopharynx. Hoarseness and other vocal complaints are common symptoms.

Squamous cell carcinoma is by far the predominant histology encountered. Like the oral cavity, the true vocal cords are subject to considerable functional trauma and environmental insult. They are often the site of various inflammatory and premalignant changes. Carcinoma in situ may exist either independently or in association with invasive carcinoma. Because of the wide spectrum of hyperplasia, metaplasia, dysplasia, and other atypia seen in the mucosa of laryngeal biopsies, the diagnosis of carcinoma in situ or even invasive carcinoma may be deceptive. Variant epidermoid carcinomas are also found in the larynx and oral cavity. These include verrucous carcinoma, carcinosarcoma, pseudosarcoma, and others (Lundgren, Van Nostrand, and Harwood et al. 1986; Giordano, Ewing, and Adams et al. 1983). The distinction of verrucous carcinoma is important because, while nodal spread is rare and a T1 or T2 presentation is the rule, treatment with radiation is not as effective as with conventional squamous cell carcinoma, and surgical techniques must be given greater weight. Small-cell carcinoma and adenocarcinomas of minor salivary gland origin are reported, but are a very small proportion of laryngeal malignancies (Batsakis, Rice, and Solomon 1980; Baugh et al. 1986). The rare primary subglottic carcinoma is treated similarly to glottic lesions; its prognosis is worse.

Endoscopy in laryngeal malignancy is mandatory (Pillsbury and Kirchner 1979); CT scanning (Katsantonis et al. 1986; Isaacs et al. 1988; Hirano et al. 1988) may identify occult extension, particularly into or through the thyroid cartilage or pre-epiglottic space. Anteroposterior laryngeal tomography can also be useful in assessing subglottic extension prior to endoscopy, and may facilitate airway management. Pulmonary function testing is needed if conservation surgery is contemplated. Chest x-ray is necessary to review any associated pulmonary functional disease, or to identify a possible coexistent lung cancer.

TREATMENT

The treatment of early lesions (generally T1 and some T2), in the absence of overt nodal disease (N0) is generally successful and equally effected by either surgery or radiation alone. Consequently, the choice of treatment is dictated largely by morbidity anticipated in the glottic area. Given the minimal likelihood of occult nodal disease, limited surgery may be preferable, provided that the multifunctional integrity of the larynx can be maintained. Radiation would then be reserved for recurrent disease or second primaries. Small glottic lesions confined to the tendonous part of the vocal cord can be excised using endoscopic carbon dioxide laser technique. Larger (but still T1 or T2) glottic lesions, those involving the anterior commissure, or lesions with any trace of limited cord mobility would be better treated with either an external surgical approach, i.e., partial laryngectomy, or radiation. At least 60 Gy is considered necessary. This dose generally will be tolerated because the treatment field is so small (confined to the glottic larynx).

Partial laryngectomy procedures include: supraglottic laryngectomy; epiglottidectomy; cordectomy; anterior commissure resection; vertical hemilaryngectomy; frontolateral and extended frontolateral partial laryngectomy; and near-total laryngectomy. Accurate, pretreatment clinical staging is critical. An underestimate of local disease extension could result in inappropriate treatment if a patient has been prepared for partial laryngectomy and intraoperative findings mandate more extensive surgery. By contrast, clinical overstaging is relatively unlikely to occur.

Early supraglottic lesions are anatomically amenable to conservative surgical techniques, but the likelihood of occult local extension and/or nodal metastasis requires treatment encompassing both the primary site and the neck. This will often be by external radiation to both, including at least 66 Gy to the primary. Supraglottic laryngectomy alone is less frequently performed at this time. Most commonly, this procedure would be envisioned for a more extensive T2 lesion, in which case planned postoperative radiotherapy would be appropriate. Neck dissection would be incorporated in the presence of nodal disease.

Advanced (T3 or T4) lesions of either the glottic or supraglottic larynx generally require total laryngectomy and postoperative radiation to both the neck and larynx fields. Positive nodal metastases, whether identified pre- or intraoperatively, require neck dissection. Radiation is the treatment of choice for suspect, but unconfirmed, nodal metastases (based on primary site location and extent). Present clinical research in laryngeal cancer surrounds nonsurgical therapy for T3 lesions. Hyperfractionation radiotherapy in some hands (Parsons, Cassisi, and Million 1984; Wang, Blitzer, and Suit 1985) would appear to offer a reasonable cure potential, but its use remains controversial because the associated morbidity may not always differ substantially from that of surgery. Induction chemotherapy eliciting a histologically confirmed complete response, followed by definitive radiation to the larynx and neck, is another nonsurgical means of treatment. Such a combined sequence is presently undergoing prospective evaluation (Dimery, Kramer, and Choksi et al. 1989). Although T4 lesions at either site have limited curability, the chances of cure reside in at least radical surgery and postoperative radiation.

Traditionally, the treatment of recurrent disease following previous radiotherapy, whether glottic or supraglottic, has required total laryngectomy with ipsilateral neck dissection. In the supraglottic larynx, there is generally little argument. Nonetheless, the role of partial laryngectomy after radiation failure in glottic carcinoma has become controversial. In selected cases with unilateral endolaryngeal involvement, conservation surgery may be possible. The obstacles are formidable, however, and include the substantial difficulty of preoperatively determining disease extent. Other pitfalls include postradiation healing complications and persistent edema or fibrosis that compromises laryngeal function and future recurrence monitoring.

OUTCOME

The fate of a patient with glottic carcinoma is most significantly affected by the presence of vocal cord fixation, which almost halves the 95% cure rate achievable in T1, and 80% to 85% achievable in T2, glottic lesions. The addition of clinically perceptible nodal metastases has the same effect. Advanced (T3 or T4) lesions with nodal metastases entail a less than 30% 5-year survival rate. Supraglottic laryngeal cancer is generally more lethal, stage for stage, for both early and more advanced lesions, with or without positive adenopathy. Survival rates are generally 10% to 25% worse than the corresponding glottic lesion. The prognosis in primary subglottic cancer is generally poor.

HYPOPHARYNX/CERVICAL ESOPHAGUS

The segregating of the hypopharynx and cervical esophagus is somewhat artifactual due to considerable overlap and similarity in the anatomic, physiologic, and treatment considerations for tumors in these areas. Tumor extension from one anatomic region into another is a common factor in determining the extent of surgical treatment. However, tumors of the hypopharynx/ esophagus are distinctive for their often surreptitious evolution to advanced stages with relatively modest symptomatology.

The hypopharynx extends from the inferior border of the oropharynx to just above the cricopharyngeus muscle portion of the upper alimentary tract. Included are the pyriform sinuses, the posterior pharyngeal wall, and the postcricoid portion of the larynx. The hypopharynx basically surrounds the larynx, whose aryepiglottic folds and epiglottis separate it anatomically from the pyriforms (hypopharynx) and tongue base (oropharynx). Tumors will frequently straddle boundaries, making it difficult to name and classify lesions. Generally, a visual estimation of the tumor's epicenter is taken as the site of origin, though such basis for designation may be tempered by observations on the tumor's clinical behavior. The cervical esophagus borders on and includes the cricopharyngeus muscle region, which comprises the functional upper esophageal sphincter. This area represents a substantial narrowing of the hypopharyngeal lumen, so that tumors which impinge on the cricopharyngeus vicinity will require pharyngoesophageal reconstruction during surgery, in order to reinstate alimentary integrity. The lower border of the cervical esophagus is generally considered to be the thoracic inlet.

Epithelial malignancies of the hypopharynx and cervical esophagus are generally similar clinically, and, with the possible exception of some salivary gland histologies and melanoma, are the deadliest group of head and neck tumors. As with other head and neck mucosal sites, they are often the result of the prolonged and excessive use of alcohol and inhaled tobacco products.

In the preliminary patient evaluation, a barium swallow is often performed although this study can vastly underestimate the extent of disease and does not replace the need for direct evaluation. Endoscopy must determine at least the mucosal margins of the lesion, direct involvement of the larynx or trachea, and a need for esophageal reconstruction. Flexible endoscopy of the hypopharynx has significant limitations and should not be substituted for a rigid endoscopic examination under anesthesia. CT scanning can suggest tracheal or prevertebral fascia involvement and mediastinal or nodal disease. In the event that distal endoscopy is not possible due to obstructing or friable disease (risking perforation), a CT scan can help delineate the inferior margin of tumor.

TREATMENT/OUTCOME

Early tumors (T1 and some T2 primaries) are rare; they are generally treated with external radiation to the primary, areas of anticipated spread, and to the cervical and upper mediastinal node regions. Occasionally a small lesion confined to the lateral wall of the pyriform sinus or pharynx may lend itself to complete excision by lateral pharyngectomy, with primary or flap reconstruction. The likelihood of metastatic nodal disease dictates some form of nodal treatment, usually at least elective doses of radiation.

More advanced stages of primary site disease generally require combined treatment, involving radical pharyngolaryngectomy or laryngoesophagectomy with appropriate reconstruction. Advanced disease of the hypopharynx/cervical esophagus carries such a high probability of at least occult nodal disease that radical

or modified radical neck dissections should also be performed at the time of surgery. Postoperative external radiation to an approximate dose of 60 Gy would be the general rule, optimally to begin three to six weeks following surgery. The patient's ability to heal, recuperate, start rehabilitation, and get on with radiation is critical to the success of combined treatment rendered in this sequence. If the patient's surgical tolerance status or tumor resectability is questionable, preoperative radiation with associated hyperalimentation measures can be considered, allowing for staged surgical procedures subsequently. By virtue of cytoreduction and gross tumor shrinkage, unresectable tumors may become resectable during chemotherapy, thereby permitting surgery on an as yet unirradiated patient.

Overall survival in this group of tumor patients is generally less than 30%. The rare early stage lesion without involved adenopathy may be cured 60% to 70% of the time. Even the apparently successful control of local (primary site plus or minus extension) and regional (nodal) disease for a period of time may result in survival failure due to blood-borne metastases. Delayed distant metastasis along with second sites of primary cancer are a possibility in any patient with head and neck malignancy. The former represents an invariably incurable situation and is particularly common with advanced nodal involvement. As local and regional control has improved due to combined therapies, the proportion of patients succumbing to delayed distant disease has increased. This fact, in part, accounts for the desirability for some form of systemic (whole body) therapy, like chemotherapy.

A patient's motivation to avoid the loss of laryngeal function is understandably great. The rationale to avoid surgery while maintaining a proportionate level of cure is presently being explored through the use of hyperfractionated radiation schedules and/or induction chemotherapy. It is paradoxically true that a patient may be better off, both objectively and subjectively, following radical surgery, even if only for palliation. The elimination of pain or obstruction to breathing and swallowing may not be achieved by radiation alone, and surgical salvage after full-dose radiation entails a substantially increased complication rate. Based on personal standards and philosophy, a patient may want a traditionally less effective or experimental treatment plan in order to modify what he or she views as unacceptable morbidity.

NASOPHARYNX

Along with the tongue base and pyriform sinus, the nasopharynx is a classic occult site for upper aerodigestive tract malignancy. Nasopharyngeal carcinoma (NPCa) (Batsakis, Solomon, and Rice 1981) entails a different epidemiologic and etiologic spectrum, unassociated with tobacco use, and is relatively uncommon among Caucasians (Henderson, Louie, and Soo Hoo Jing et al. 1976). The symptoms are varied and poorly localized, and the patients tend to be younger. The result of these factors is that NPCa is not always considered, and therefore not found (Dickson 1981).

The limits of the nasopharynx extend anteriorly to the plane of the choanae, which demarcate the nasal cavity. The lateral walls incorporate the eustachian tube orifices and a part of the pharyngeal walls, with inferior limits at the level of the palate. Superiorly, the nasopharynx includes the mucosa overlying the skull base and sphenoid rostrum. Examination of the nasopharynx should be a part of any head and neck evaluation, particularly in an adult patient with a neck mass or unilateral ear complaints.

NPCa is endemic in parts of China, where it is the most common malignancy of the head and neck and also accounts for a significant proportion of all cancers (Hsu, Huang, and Lynn et al. 1982; Ho 1978). This observation has prompted one of the more fascinating epidemiologic investigations in medicine. The evidence has favored environmental factors, as opposed to a genetic susceptibility, and particularly the Epstein-Barr virus is implicated. Antibody titers to EBV are elevated in a significant number of patients, Asian or Caucasian, with NPCa.

The most common local symptom of NPCa is no symptom at all. Frequently, the patient will present with a self-identified neck mass, indicative of the early tendency of this lesion to spread into the lymphatic system. Ear symptoms, including fullness, pain, or otitis media, and nasal symptoms, such as obstruction or bleeding, may be elicited. More extensive disease may result in throat pain, neurologic or ocular symptoms— headache, proptosis, facial pain, diplopia, hoarseness, and dysphagia. The latter four reflect cranial nerve involvement in and around the skull base (Neel 1985).

The diagnostic procedure of choice is CT scanning, in both the axial and coronal planes. Triple endoscopy is not routinely necessary, though examination under anesthesia may be advisable to visualize the lesion and safely obtain sufficient biopsy material. Cranial nerve examination is mandatory.

The histology of NPCa is usually squamous cell carcinoma, or a variant thereof. Salivary gland tumors and lymphomas occur, but are quite rare. Lymphoepithelioma, or nonkeratinizing (undifferentiated) squamous cell carcinomas are encountered more often than the usual keratinizing type. This fact has contributed to some confusion in the past with regard to both histologic interpretation and classification. A typical example would involve a patient presenting with an otherwise asymptomatic neck mass. Premature removal of the mass for diagnosis may indeed reveal an undifferentiated carcinoma, for which a primary site cannot clearly be determined. The differential diagnosis by routine light microscopy alone includes lymphoma and metastatic cancer from a variety of sites, above and below the clavicles. Modern awareness and histologic techniques, particularly the advent of immunohistochemistry, have considerably refined the approach to the differential diagnosis of undifferentiated carcinoma. Lymphocyte markers and antibody labels to a variety of tissue types permit the "fingerprinting" of a biopsy specimen. An appropriate treatment plan depends on knowing whether a lesion is a lymphoma, a nasopharyngeal carcinoma, or a metastatic malignancy because the staging and therapy for each are very different. An examination of the nasopharynx in many instances can quickly lead to the likely diagnosis.

TREATMENT/OUTCOME

Treatment factors are somewhat unique in nasopharyngeal carcinoma, because operations on the primary site of origin are only very rarely considered. The anatomy of the area is complex and relatively inaccessible by surgery; it includes the multiple neurovascular foramina of the skull base, and the neighboring cranial nerves, great vessels, and extensive networks of lymphatics. Radiation techniques are employed to treat the primary site and nodal areas (Dickson 1981; Hoppe, Goffinet, and Bagshaw 1976). A wide field encompassing the entire nasopharynx and extending from the skull base to the supraclavicular region is necessary; doses are generally 65 Gy to 70 Gy. During treatment, as the nasopharyngeal tumor involutes, the radiation portals may be narrowed to lessen the dose on the bony structures of the skull base and spine, and on the spinal cord itself (shrinking field technique). The local dose may be augmented in selected cases through the use of transnasal surface contact irradiation.

Because of the well-known tendency for NPCa to develop extensive, bilateral nodal metastases, treatment of all cervical nodal areas is mandatory. Over half the patients will initially present with clinically identifiable nodal disease. The apparent volume of node metastases may far exceed that which might be expected from a relatively small primary lesion. The role of neck dissection in NPCa is indefinite, but as a general rule, radical neck dissection would be reserved for that patient with residual, palpable nodal disease several weeks after completing radiation therapy, and for recurrent nodal disease in the absence of distant metastases or a nasopharyngeal recurrence. Patients with massive nodal disease at presentation are also considered for neck dissection, though the benefit has not been established.

Rarely, a patient will have limited recurrent disease localized in the nasopharynx that can be treated surgically by a complex approach to the lateral skull base. This surgery is practiced at relatively few major hospital centers and is not established treatment. The greatest experience is in Europe, where results suggest a benefit in a small, highly selected group of patients.

The delayed appearance of disseminated distant metastases is a significant problem in NPCa, and is responsible for more deaths than uncontrolled local or regional disease. Induction chemotherapy to reduce the population and density of malignant cells in NPCa is attractive in theory, because of both the distant metastatic problem and the extensive nodal tumor burden with which many patients present. Tumor response to chemotherapy in NPCa is generally better than in other areas, allowing patients to enter the subsequent radiation phase of treatment with smaller volumes of disease. As with other sites of epidermoid cancer in the head and neck, however, a benefit in survival due to the inclusion of chemotherapy is not yet established.

Survival in NPCa is directly related to the pretreatment volume of disease (T and N stage of the primary site and nodes) and the histology. The rare T1 keratinizing lesion without palpable adenopathy may have an 80% 5-year survival; patients with advanced local (T3 or T4) or regional (N2 or N3) disease will have only a 10% to 20% likelihood of being alive at five years. Lymphoepithelioma entails a modestly more favorable prognosis.

NASAL CAVITY/PARANASAL SINUSES

Primary malignancy of the nasal cavity is very rare. Most often the nasal cavity is secondarily involved by sinus malignancies, which tend to extend surreptitiously from region to region within this multicompartmented but interconnected anatomic network. Symptoms are not exclusive and diagnostic delay is common. Sinus malignancy is also quite rare, and the practitioner who claims to have never heard of a case is not unusual. As usual, squamous cell carcinoma is the predominate histology, although minor salivary glands abound in the nose and sinuses and adenocarcinomas are seen (Goepfert et al. 1983; Batsakis 1980; Batsakis 1980; Duncavage, Campbell, and Hanson et al. 1983; Rejowski, Campanella, and Block 1982). Esthesioneuroblastoma (Levine, McLean, and Cantrell 1986) is an unusual neuroendocrine malignancy that arises high in the roof of the nasal cavity in association with the olfactory groove. Malignant melanoma also may arise in the nasal cavity or sinus mucosa (Trapp, Fu, and Calcaterra 1987).

Sinus cancer is not clearly related to smoking. An association has been identified with components of solvents used in furniture finishing, and possibly with nickel (Roush 1979; Halperin, Goodman, and Stayner et al. 1983). Chronic sinusitis may precede the diagnosis, particularly of maxillary sinus cancer, and chronic sinusitis is felt to be of some etiologic significance. The maxillary is by far the most common paranasal sinus involved with cancer. The rudiments of treatment are similar for other sinuses, but the surgical details are varied and a full discussion of ethmoid, frontal, and sphenoid cancers would be out of proportion to their clinical relevance. In these other sinuses, the diagnosis of malignancy is usually not made until some effect on the nose, orbit, skull, cranial nerves, or frontal lobe has been realized, reflecting advanced disease. The fortuitous identification of a tumor within the nasal cavity of an otherwise asymptomatic individual is unlikely, emphasizing the insidious way in which sinus malignancies can spread from any site of origin.

Classification schema for each sinus and the nasal cavity are not established. For the maxillary sinus, however, primary site staging is relatively well worked out, and accurately reflects prognosis. Nodal metastatic disease is rare and as a rule reflects a far-advanced, long-standing local cancer. Distant metastasis occurs in

conjunction with recurrent, extensive local tumor. The latter is more often the cause of death. Ohngren's line is an historically useful anatomic reference point within the maxillary sinus. It represents an oblique plane through the maxillary sinus (from the medial canthus to the angle of the mandible) dividing the sinus into an anteroinferior portion and a posterosuperior portion. Anteroinferior lesions will tend to extend through the wall of the sinus into the gingivobuccal sulcus, or inferiorly into the palate or dental structures. Medial extension into the anterior inferior nasal cavity may permit an earlier diagnosis and imply a more favorable prognosis than for lesions above Ohngren's line. This is the basis for the distinction between the T2 and T3 classifications. Posterosuperior lesions will extend into the orbit, infraorbital rim and nerve, or into the ethmoid sinuses and possibly through the anterior cranial fossa. Posterior erosion into the pterygomaxillary fossa and skull base has abysmal prognostic implications (table 23.4).

A lesion in one sinus or the nasal cavity requires a thorough investigation of all nasal and paranasal compartments. Physical examination is of limited usefulness in assessing the limits of tumor extension or resectability, so CT scanning in both the axial and coronal planes is critical. As in other sites where surgical treatment for cure involves considerable morbidity, a chest x-ray and other studies to rule out distant metastasis should be considered.

TREATMENT/OUTCOME

Sinus cancer is a disease in which the likelihood of cure without surgery as a part of the treatment plan, for any stage, is small. The rare, fortuitously identified T1 lesion could be cured with surgery alone, but for the most part combined therapy with surgery, either preceded or followed by radiation, is the standard.

If a given tumor seems clearly resectable, some physicians prefer surgery to be followed with radiation, thereby minimizing problems with healing or with closed-space drainage during radiation. A higher radiation dose delivered to a more precisely delineated field may then be administered. Field boosts by either electron beam or surface mold techniques are possible. Borderline or unresectable disease might be considered for presurgical treatment with radiation, or even chemotherapy, in order to provide initial tumor shrinkage and permit more effective surgery. The amount of wide-field radiation is limited by bone tolerance and the risk of osteoradionecrosis of the maxilla, orbit, or skull

Table 23.4
MAXILLARY SINUS CLASSIFICATION

T1 —	tumor confined to infrastructure mucosa (below Ohngren's line); no bone erosion
T2 —	tumor confined to suprastructure mucosa (above Ohngren's line); no bone erosion or infrastructure with erosion of medial or inferior walls only
T3 —	tumor invading orbit, pterygoid muscles, skin of cheek, anterior ethmoid sinuses
T4 —	extensive tumor invading cribriform plate, posterior ethmoid, sphenoid, nasopharynx, pterygoid plates, or skull base

base. Historically, a substantial number of patients who survived for more than two years after treatment died of treatment complications, if not of recurrent disease.

The surgery for cancer of the maxillary sinus is one of several variously modified maxillectomy procedures. An inferior partial maxillectomy may suffice for a very early anteroinferior lesion, or a medial maxillectomy via lateral rhinotomy for a limited nasal cavity lesion. Most often, a radical total maxillectomy, with or without orbital exenteration, is called for. Skin and soft tissue reconstruction of the exposed bony surfaces is necessary. The palate defect is handled with an obturator prosthesis, resembling a denture, which must be fashioned prior to surgery and be available for intraoperative insertion. The extension of surgical resection through the anterior skull base is feasible in selected cases, using what is referred to as a craniofacial procedure, in which the head and neck surgeon collaborates with a neurosurgeon. The approach is a combined one via both conventional midface access (lateral rhinotomy) and by a subfrontal craniotomy. Most often, this form of radical surgery would be used in lesions involving the ethmoid sinus, either as the primary site or by invasion; cribriform plate (esthesioneuroblastoma); or orbital roof.

The overall prognosis in maxillary sinus cancer is abysmal. In spite of aggressive treatment, lesions recur in the surgical cavity and lead to death by intracranial invasion and ensuing complications. Patients may not live long enough to manifest distant metastasis. The rare, early, unifocal, T1 or T2 primary nasal cavity carcinoma does carry a better prognosis. The chances in other sinus cavity primaries are difficult to predict, due to their relative rarity.

SALIVARY GLAND

The salivary gland diseases include an eclectic mix of benign and malignant tumors. The histologies are as varied as the biological behavior of the lesions and run the gamut from innocent to deadly. Some of the malignancies display a rather long natural history, but are ultimately lethal. The sites of origin are diverse, and include the major salivary glands (parotid, submandibular, and sublingual) as well as the multiple, small minor salivary glands located immediately below the mucosa diffusely throughout the entire upper aerodigestive tract. For all neoplasms of salivary gland origin, generally the larger the gland, the greater the likelihood of benign disease. Hence, most parotid tumors are benign, and most minor salivary gland tumors are malignant.

The parotid gland is the most common site for either benign or malignant lesions. In spite of the tendency for parotid tumors to be benign in 75% to 80% of cases, the remaining malignancies occur several times more frequently than cancers of the submandibular, sublingual, or minor salivary glands. The average age of patients is in the fourth to fifth decade, considerably younger than those with squamous cell carcinoma of the upper aerodigestive tract. Radiation has been implicated as a

Table 23.5
HISTOLOGY OF SALIVARY GLAND MALIGNANCY

Mucoepidermoid — low grade, high grade
Adenoid cystic (cylindroma)
Acinic cell
Malignant mixed
Adenocarcinoma — various degrees of differentiation
Squamous cell carcinoma
Other miscellaneous and unusual

potential cause of both benign and malignant tumors (Batsakis and Spitz 1984). A classification of salivary gland cancers is not in widespread use, because stage and prognosis are not as well-correlated as in other head and neck malignancies. Whereas treatment is more often dictated by histology (table 23.5) than stage, classification criteria are relatively impractical.

Mucoepidermoid (Nascimento, Amaral, and Prado et al. 1986) lesions predominate within the parotid gland, while adenoid cystic carcinomas predominate elsewhere. Other tumor types are uncommon, and are extremely rare outside the parotid gland. Squamous cell and high-grade mucoepidermoid carcinomas are particularly lethal. Low-grade mucoepidermoid carcinoma, on the other hand, behaves essentially in a benign fashion, with recurrences rare after simple complete removal. Intermediate in behavior is adenoid cystic carcinoma, which will often result in patient mortality, but only after a prolonged clinical course punctuated by late recurrences (five to 15 years after initial treatment) of pulmonary metastases. Either of these manifestations may evolve quite slowly, remaining asymptomatic and untreated for many months.

The biological natural history typified by adenoid cystic carcinoma (Nascimento, Amaral, and Prado et al. 1986) emphasizes the true nature and philosophy of palliative treatment. The best therapy for a palpable mass, or for multiple nodular shadows on chest x-ray, when these represent incurable disease, may well be no treatment at all. If curable, treat the patient's tumor; when incurable, treat patients themselves and their symptoms. Consequently, in an incurable situation, if the endpoint morbidity of a particular treatment, be it chemotherapy, hormonal manipulation, radical radiation, or surgery, is worse than the patients' symptoms or consequences anticipated in their near future, then leaving them alone, except for periodic reassessment and support, is the most humane course of action. The focus of palliative management should be on the quality of life as patients see it, not on statistical longevity. Some symptoms are more readily controlled than others, through different means. For example, pain from a bone metastasis could always be ameliorated through pharmacology, yet a brief course of focal radiation may work better with fewer side effects. Dyspnea due to multiple pulmonary metastases may respond to hormonal or chemotherapy therapy; the former is less toxic and should generally be tried first. While curing and rehabilitating patients is paramount, it is both important and rewarding to be able to manage the terminal and preterminal care of the patients for whom cure is not possible.

Parotid tumors tend to occur almost exclusively in the lateral, or superficial lobe of the gland. Benign tumors are generally discrete and mobile, reflecting their encapsulation and focal nature. Malignancies may appear grossly encapsulated, but tend to infiltrate the gland stroma. The most common presenting symptom is that of a lump. Pain, rapid expansion, poor mobility, or facial nerve weakness are other symptoms associated with malignancy. Adenoid cystic lesions have a proclivity for perineural invasion and spread. Submandibular and minor salivary gland tumors also tend to present as painless, submucosal masses. Hematogenous metastasis is as much, if not a greater problem than the lymphatic spread of salivary gland malignancies. Either or both, however, can occur with any histology, but much less predictably than with epidermoid cancer of the upper aerodigestive tract.

Fine needle aspiration cytology is performed with increasing frequency for masses of the major salivary glands, in an effort to suggest the diagnosis of malignancy prior to open surgical exploration. Incisional biopsy, lest it spread tumor or injure the facial nerve, is rarely indicated except in massive lesions or questionable operative candidates, for whom nonsurgical initial treatment will be most appropriate. Needle aspiration, however, is not always diagnostic and even in experienced hands will result in a certain number of false-positive and false-negative interpretations. CT scans can be useful in determining the deep extent of disease, bony involvement, or occult metastasis.

Submandibular masses (Batsakis 1986) are generally explored and completely excised along with the gland and the submandibular triangle contents, followed by intraoperative frozen section analysis. Depending on the diagnostic certainty and extent of treatment implied, further surgery may then be carried out. A similar approach to diagnosis, entailing superficial parotid lobectomy and facial nerve dissection, is necessary if needle aspiration biopsy fails to suggest a pretreatment diagnosis. In either event, histologic confirmation must be obtained before excessive surgery is carried out, especially if facial nerve resection is a possibility. Such confirmation may require permanent histologic staining techniques and thereby force the postponement and subsequent staging of definitive surgical therapy. Minor salivary tumors can generally be biopsied in a standard fashion, utilizing general anesthesia and endoscopic technique.

TREATMENT/OUTCOME

Salivary gland malignancy is a surgical disease, with radiation playing an adjuvant role and chemotherapy a palliative one. Investigation of chemotherapy as initial treatment for far-advanced or unresectable disease is of interest, but not nearly as promising as induction chemotherapy for epidermoid head and neck cancer. Salivary tumors are hormone responsive, but to a variable and unpredictable extent. Palliative treatment with sex hormones is feasible, but has no parallel role in initial curative treatment.

Surgical exploration of the gland and proximate nodal lymphatics is the approach of choice, with removal of the entire gland (total parotidectomy) and contained tumor. Enlarged lymph nodes are handled with neck dissection, with or without preliminary frozen section sampling. Elective ipsilateral neck dissection is warranted for high-grade mucoepidermoid and squamous cell lesions, and probably for larger malignant mixed and adenoid cystic tumors. The approach to the facial nerve remains controversial, but the trend is toward preserving it, even if this requires the blunt peeling of tumor off of a major branch. Gross nerve trunk or branch invasion, or preoperative facial paralysis in the presence of a high-grade or adenoid cystic lesion, generally would require nerve sacrifice. Various means of reconstituting the nerve are available, including interposition grafting (from the sural nerve, or other expendable peripheral nerve) or nerve transfer from the hypoglossal or spinal accessory. Some surgeons feel, in the absence of pre-existent paralysis, that the facial nerve should always be preserved, even at the expense of leaving gross or microscopic tumor behind. Postoperative radiation therapy is then relied upon to eradicate residual disease. Given all the facts, a patient may have particularly strong feelings about the surgical philosophy, which must be reconciled with those of the surgeon. Minor salivary gland cancers are approached with an operation appropriate for the involved anatomic area, much in keeping with epidermoid lesions in the same location.

Historically, salivary malignancies were not considered to be curable by radiation, or even to be very radioresponsive. This is true when gross disease is treated, although there is usually some palliative benefit in unresectable lesions or in inoperable patients. However, postoperative radiation is valuable as an adjunct for the treatment of theoretical or actual microscopic disease, or minute amounts of gross disease residue. Whether this reflects improved utilization, better technology, or a more open-minded treatment approach is unclear. Local and regional control of salivary gland malignancies is improved with a combined approach. The use of postoperative radiation has helped foster the trend toward facial nerve preservation, thus reducing the morbidity of aggressive treatment. In general, radiation should be planned in all patients with adenoid cystic or high-grade carcinomas, and in those of any histology with residual disease after surgery. Recurrent local or regional disease is similarly handled: surgery if feasible, followed by radiation if not previously given.

Composite 5-year survival for high-grade mucoepidermoid malignancies is approximately 40%. The prognosis for malignant mixed tumors is somewhat better, and for squamous cell carcinoma of the parotid somewhat worse. By contrast, adenoid cystic carcinoma fares comparatively well during the first five years, with survival rates in the 70% to 80% range. However, cancer-related mortality continues for years, in keeping with the prolonged natural history and tendency toward delayed and slowly evolving metastasis. Survival, excluding deaths due to unrelated causes, has been shown to drop to 40% at 10 years and 22% at 20 years.

NECK

Thus far, discussion of the neck (Norris and Miller 1985) as a site of cancer has largely concerned nodal metastases from primary tumors of the upper aerodigestive tract. In fact, 70% of neck masses in an adult population will be malignant. Of these, three-quarters will be metastatic and one-quarter will be primary cancers arising in various neck structures. Metastatic lesions will represent spread from primary cancer sites in the mucosa of the upper aerodigestive tract.

Excluding skin, thyroid, and major salivary gland neoplasms, primary malignancy from one of the many structures of the cervical anatomy are uncommon. Lymphoma, arising in a cervical lymph node, is the best known. Among other sources and histologies are skeletal muscle (rhabdomyosarcoma); adipose tissue (liposarcoma); fibrous tissue (fibrosarcoma); vascular (angiosarcoma, leiomyosarcoma); neuroendocrine (malignant Schwannoma, carotid body tumors); and bone (osteogenic sarcoma). These will all generally require some form of open surgical procedure for diagnosis. However, in an adult the likelihood is high that a mass represents metastasis from a mucosal site and the initial investigation should evaluate this possibility. While historically controversial, it is generally considered harmful to incise the normal tissue planes of the neck in the presence of nodal metastasis, lest this cause scarring, vascular and lymphatic disruption, and possible tumor spread.

A careful history may elicit symptomatology attracting attention to one area of the mouth or throat, and promoting accessory examinations. A thorough office examination of the head and neck skin, oral cavity, nasopharynx, hypopharynx, and larynx will often identify the so-called unknown primary tumor. Traditionally, in patients referred for evaluation because of a neck mass, whether suspected or biopsy-proven metastatic squamous cell carcinoma, the site of the primary cancer will usually be in the nasopharynx, pyriform sinus, base of tongue, or tonsil fossa. The location of the node can help implicate the source. For example, a high posterior triangle nodal metastasis is likely to have emanated from the nasopharynx, while a solitary low jugular nodal metastasis is very unlikely to reflect nasopharyngeal cancer. Occasionally, all that is needed is a tongue retractor and illumination, but the physician should be prepared to perform, or refer the patient for, a complete head and neck examination.

Even such efforts occasionally will fail to identify the primary lesion. At that point, either a formal endoscopic examination under anesthesia or fine-needle aspiration biopsy should be performed. The results of needle aspiration can be misleading and should not be the sole determinant of how to manage a patient. Negative cytology (implying benign disease) should not be overly reassuring. While most epidermoid carcinoma and thyroid histologies are relatively reliably determined, lymphomas and poorly differentiated or undifferentiated squamous cell carcinomas can be diagnostically elusive. If physical examination, accessory testing (imaging and blood studies), needle aspiration, and endoscopy are all inconclusive, then open biopsy will be necessary. Preparation to perform definitive surgical therapy, if appropriate for the diagnosis encountered, is considered, discussed preoperatively, and based on reliable intraoperative frozen section evaluation. Tissue handling at the time of biopsy should allow the pathologist to perform all necessary testing, including electron microscopy, immunocytochemistry, and lymphoma markers.

Some patients will have a clinical profile less suspicious for upper aerodigestive tract cancer — patients who are younger, who do not smoke, or who have adenopathy in multiple body locations. Early fine-needle aspiration will help focus subsequent investigations. As in all areas of medicine, however, the less invasive, lower morbidity, nonirrevocable procedures should be considered first, even if they are somewhat less likely to yield the diagnosis. Definitive treatment options and their urgency must also be factored into the judgment schema. Adenocarcinoma metastatic to cervical nodes may have arisen from an occult thyroid or parotid gland tumor source. Metastatic nodal disease in the neck from a source below the clavicles is very rare and represents, with rare exception, incurable disease from the lung, breast, gastrointestinal tract, genitourinary tract, or other organ system.

In spite of all diagnostic efforts, an occasional patient will have metastatic epidermoid carcinoma to the cervical nodes from an unidentifiable, very small, submucosal, and asymptomatic upper aerodigestive tract source. One-third of these patients will be cured by neck dissection alone; that is, without definitive primary site treatment. Various systemic and local-regional immunologic mechanisms have been proposed to explain this phenomenon. Some centers have advocated simple total excisional biopsy of the metastatic node, avoiding formal neck dissection or radical neck dissection where possible. Definitive external radiation is thereafter administered to the nodal fields and most, or all, mucosal sites of the upper aerodigestive tract from nasopharynx to cervical esophagus in order to treat the presumptive primary and occult lymphatic disease. A third treatment alternative, also dual-modality, entails multilevel radiation therapy, either followed by or preceded by neck dissection. Immediate neck dissection would be envisioned in a case of metastatic squamous cell carcinoma in which open biopsy has become necessary. Preliminary neck dissection would also permit the histologic confirmation of needle aspiration cytology results and eliminate the risk of inappropriate treatment. A patient referred after simple open biopsy would undergo preliminary radiation followed by neck dissection, assuming the primary site remained elusive.

Elaborating upon the clinical features and treatment

of primary malignancies of the cervical soft tissue structures is beyond the scope of this chapter. Lymphomas are nonsurgical systemic diseases, for which surgery is of diagnostic and staging importance only. Some head and neck sarcomas will require surgical removal, but not invariably as the first or even most definitive step. As a rule, and increasingly so in all areas of oncology, head and neck neoplasia is a multidisciplinary field.

PART II: THYROID CANCER

INTRODUCTION

Cancers of the thyroid gland have elicited far more concern than their incidence might indicate. They frequently afflict the young adult, and occasionally teenagers; their clinical behavior varies widely from the nearly uniformly fatal anaplastic cancer to the nearly benign-behaving papillary carcinomas of the young. Both these cancers are derived from the same follicular cell. Recent advances in rapid and simple diagnosis, and case selection through needle biopsy, have been accompanied by much earlier clinical presentation and the virtual disappearance of the giant and spindle-cell anaplastic varieties (Cady et al. 1985). Thus, the management and results of this disease in recent years has been another chapter in the story of improving results in cancer treatment, although the major gains can be attributed to earlier diagnosis.

Another reason for continued interest and controversies about therapy has been the current recognition that two vastly different outcomes of therapy are based largely on age at diagnosis, with further outcome alterations based on size and extent of disease in older patients (Cady and Rossi 1988). It has been difficult for physicians, surgeons, and endocrinologists to accept the fact that a human cancer of identical pathological appearance microscopically could have huge differences in outcome, based largely on age; and that traditional correlation with outcomes such as size, node metastases, and extent of primary cancer do not relate at all to outcome in younger patients but do strongly correlate to survival in older patients. Because of the seemingly incomprehensible correlations or lack of correlations, much of this section will deal with empirical biological information, with less emphasis placed on those highly controversial details of therapeutic management.

ETIOLOGY AND EPIDEMIOLOGY

The only specific epidemiological association in thyroid cancer is with childhood radiation therapy. Differentiated thyroid carcinoma develops with some frequency after even very small doses of radiation exposure in infants and children, though not in adults. A formula of population incidence suggests that about 2.5 cases/rad/year/million people may be a reasonable estimate of risk of thyroid cancer (Foster 1975). No series of differentiated thyroid cancers, however, have displayed a history of such radiation in more than a small number

of cases, usually 10% to 15%. If a large group of children who received radiation is followed years later, however, a high percentage (about 10%) will develop papillary cancers, although usually only a microscopic focus or a very small primary cancer will be found (Favus et al. 1976). The incidence of benign abnormalities detected by either palpation or radioactive scan in such patients is substantial. Inhabitants of the Marshall Islands exposed to radioactive fallout from atomic explosions frequently have palpable thyroid irregularities or nodules. More important than mere incidence, however, is the benign biologic nature of these radiation-associated thyroid cancers, and the vast number of thyroid cancers detected on studies of routine autopsies. This benign behavior highlights the greatest puzzle in understanding thyroid cancer; that is, the enormous discrepancy between the frequent microscopic or small foci, the infrequent clinical thyroid cancer, and the rarity of death when analyzing country-wide statistics.

In autopsy studies from Finland, Japan, the United States, Poland, Canada, and Colombia, the incidence of microscopic foci of thyroid cancer has been reported as high as 36%, 28%, 13%, 9%, and 6% respectively when thyroid glands are subjected to whole organ step sectioning (Harach, Franssila, and Wasenius 1985). Even in randomly sampled glands removed for Grave's disease or other benign conditions in the United States, as many as 6% of glands will contain microscopic foci of differentiated carcinoma. Thus, a conservative estimate of the number of such cancers is 25 million (at a 10% incidence) or only 2.5 million (at a 1% incidence). Only about 12,000 clinical thyroid cancers and 1,025 deaths were estimated for 1990 by the American Cancer Society (Silverberg, Boring, and Squires 1990). Such wide discrepancies between microscopic foci and clinical cancer seems to be a characteristic of some endocrine organ cancers (i.e., prostate, breast), but only in thyroid cancers are such a small number of deaths associated with such a large number of microscopic foci. This discrepancy remains the major hurdle in understanding the etiology and epidemiology of this cancer.

One variation in the proportion of the major subtypes or differentiated cancers depends on the amount of dietary iodine and the incidence of endemic goiter, with areas of iodine deficiency and high incidence of goiter having greater proportions of follicular carcinoma and a higher incidence of clinical cancer (Williams et al. 1977). The proportion of follicular carcinomas has steadily declined in the United States; for the past 50 years papillary carcinomas have constituted the overwhelming majority of thyroid cancers in people with adequate dietary iodine. This is not true in parts of Europe, however, where salt is still not iodized. Precise biochemical explanation for this variation in incidence and type is unknown, but it has been postulated that it is related to chronic elevation of thyroid stimulating hormone (TSH) and follicular cell stimulation. Differentiated thyroid carcinoma incidence resulting from abnormalities of the TSH-thyroid hormone axis are produced in animal models indicating that high TSH levels may be associated with a higher incidence of differentiated thyroid cancer. It is speculative and unclear whether the implications of such an animal model actually relate to the human condition.

Follicular thyroid carcinoma is probably the result of progressive growth of benign follicular adenomas, but whether follicular carcinomas also arise *de novo* is unclear: DNA analysis of nuclear protein of follicular lesions does not help to resolve this uncertainty because of the equally high incidence of aneuploidy in all follicular lesions, regardless of size or vascular invasion.

CLINICAL PRESENTATION

The usual clinical presentation is a palpable nodule discovered on physical examination. Currently in the United States, the majority of cancers are less than 2 cm in diameter, and fewer than 10% are over 5 cm in diameter (Cady et al. 1985). This is due to a high level of general public awareness of health issues, heightened concern about masses, physician sophistication regarding physical examination, a realization that solitary nodules have a high incidence of neoplasia, and the infrequency of goiter in the general population, in contrast to two generations ago.

Prominent or dominant nodules in multinodular glands, nodules that are increasing in size, and nodules in general in men, convey a greater risk of being diagnosed as cancer. Another common presentation is an unexpected microscopic or small (less than 1 cm) focus discovered when a gland is removed for another reason, such as Grave's disease, adenomatous goiter, or Hashimoto's thyroiditis.

Cancers in 25% of young patients and 10% of adults over age 50 are first detected because of a palpable lymph node metastasis in the neck (Cady et al. 1976). Before 1940, such node metastases were known as "lateral aberrant thyroids" and were assumed to be an embryological phenomena, because rarely did such patients become ill or die. These lymph node metastases are usually large (>2 cm), frequently multiple, occasionally bilateral, and may accompany either a palpable, or frequently a nonpalpable, primary papillary cancer in the thyroid gland. Such large node metastases do not convey a poor prognosis, but may require distinct therapeutic strategies.

Diffuse enlargement and rapid growth may suggest an anaplastic spindle and giant cell carcinoma, particularly when developing from a long-standing nodule of stable size, or a thyroid lymphoma, an uncommon but not rare disease. Physical-examination diagnostic features of thyroid cancer include hardness, fixation, vocal cord paralysis, and displacement or narrowing of trachea or esophagus. Examination of the vocal cords should be considered if any vocal changes have occurred.

DIAGNOSTIC TESTS

Usually patients have blood tests of thyroid function after presentation with a palpable thyroid abnormality,

but functional tests are seldom of value in evaluating nodules in the absence of clinical evidence of abnormal thyroid function. The nodule that is a cancer suspect is not the goiter or nodule that elicits concern about hypothyroidism. Antithyroid antibodies indicative of immune thyroiditis (Hashimoto's disease) may suggest a benign etiology of the thyroid nodule, but both differentiated thyroid carcinomas and thyroid lymphomas may be associated with Hashimoto's disease; therefore, the presence of antithyroid antibodies in no way rules out the diagnosis of malignancy.

Radioactive iodine (RAI) scans of the thyroid help define whether nodules are functional, or "hot" (autonomous with suppression of surrounding thyroid), or nonfunctional, or "cold" (hypofunctional compared to the remainder of the glands). Hot or functional nodules are seldom cancer and this finding decreases, but does not eliminate, the possibility of cancer. Ultrasonic examination of the thyroid gland can diagnose a cyst; however, many mixed cystic and solid lesions, and even occasional cysts detected by ultrasonography, may be papillary carcinomas. Therefore, all palpable cysts deserve at least a needle aspiration. Solid lesions convey a higher-than-average risk of neoplasm and indicate the need for further diagnostic studies, needle sampling, or biopsy.

Needle biopsy of the thyroid, whether by means of a large core-cutting or needle-aspiration technique, has had an enormous impact on the management of thyroid nodules in the past decade. By directly sampling cells from the palpable nodule, the general risk of the lesion being a neoplasm can usually be ascertained; however, a specific diagnosis cannot usually be obtained and should not be expected. Pathological examination of aspirated cells provides either the indication for surgical removal or the assumption that the palpable nodule is a part of an adenomatous goiter. Thyroid cancers of the follicular variety are not diagnosed by histologic criteria, but by evidence of glandular cells in abnormal locations such as lymph nodes, blood vessels, and compressed pseudocapsule. Any needle biopsy showing neoplastic cells or a hypercellular or microfollicular pattern indicates that surgical removal is necessary. Many papillary cancers, however, can be diagnosed specifically by needle biopsies. The clinician should note the aspirates that are clearly benign and nonneoplastic (i.e., adenomatous goiter), which select out those patients that do not require surgery. However, factors such as large size, pain or discomfort, fullness, compression of the trachea or esophagus, or unsightly appearance may clearly indicate the need for surgery, even if the needle aspirate is innocuous.

PATHOLOGY

Differentiated thyroid cancers are either of papillary or follicular types (Cady et al. 1976; Zampi, Carcangui, and Rosai 1985). Papillary varieties may have varying proportions of follicular features, even predominantly follicular features. They are characterized as mixed papillary and follicular cancer, defined by having some papillary elements. In contrast, follicular carcinoma is purely follicular, and usually has a tumor pseudocapsule of compressed, normal, surrounding thyroid tissue. Follicular carcinoma displays major or minor invasion of this tumor pseudocapsule or blood vessels. Obviously, random sectioning of the tumor pseudocapsule has sampling limitations, so that occasionally metastases are apparently associated with follicular adenoma. More extensive sampling of the original tumor pseudocapsule may reveal involvement characteristic of follicular carcinoma, however.

Anaplastic carcinomas usually display giant or spindle cells. Remnants or papillary carcinoma near such aggressive cancers suggest that anaplastic carcinomas occasionally (fewer than 1%) arise from long-standing untreated tumors. Areas of anaplastic or undifferentiated cells may occur in differentiated thyroid cancers and are associated with poor outlook, unless these areas are very small. Very poorly differentiated follicular carcinomas also carry a poor prognosis (Zampi, Carcangiu, and Rosai 1985).

Thyroid lymphoma is usually of the histiocytic type but may involve other types. Extensive histochemical and electron microscopy should be done routinely, and this requires close cooperation with the pathologist.

Rare forms of thyroid cancer, such as squamous cell, occur, but metastases usually from lung, breast, or melanoma to the thyroid gland are not uncommon. Direct involvement by extension from adjacent head and neck squamous cell carcinomas also occurs.

STAGING

Because of the overwhelming importance of age on prognosis, traditional anatomic staging criteria are modified. Prognostic categories may seem incongruous, but reflect a lack of correlation between local tumor extent and outcome in young patients (Beahrs and Myers 1983). For instance, many reports indicate the infrequency of a fatal outcome in children, despite frequent extensive disease and even pulmonary metastases at presentation (Buckwalter, Gurll, and Thomas 1981).

Because extension of the primary cancer can be best evaluated by physical examination prior to surgery, as can node metastases, other evaluative tests are not usually required. However, if advanced local disease is suspected, a CT examination of the thyroid area may provide useful information.

Distant metastases are uncommon with the early clinical nature of the disease, and rarely occur in sites other than lung at the time of presentation. Routine tests other than a chest x-ray are not useful. Bone scans and liver scans are to be avoided. In children under age 17, pulmonary metastases are more common (about 5% of cases) but are adequately diagnosed preoperatively by chest x-ray. Computed tomography scans or radioactive iodine (RAI) scans of the lungs need not be done prior to operation.

THERAPY

Surgery should be performed to remove all suspicious nodules. Total thyroid lobectomy should be the minimum operation on clinically significant differentiated thyroid cancers, but subtotal lobectomy is adequate for occult, microscopic, or small nodules of the anterior or exterior surface of the thyroid or isthmus. Since 90% of differentiated cancers are at very low risk of recurrence or death (Cady and Rossi 1988), conservative resections are adequate, particularly because thyroid-bed recurrence is not reduced by performing more than a total lobectomy. When clinical factors indicate a higher risk of recurrence or metastases, such as extraglandular extension, large size, or age over 50, a total ipsilateral lobectomy should be accompanied by removal of at least some of the opposite lobe in order to facilitate the use of radioactive iodine for diagnosis and therapy of possible metastases. However, it is not necessary to perform a total thyroidectomy or contralateral total lobectomy, particularly because of the marked increase in hypoparathyroidism that results from this operation.

PROGNOSIS

Prognosis is related to the age of patients and the extent of primary disease in older patients. All patients under 40, and women under 50 years of age, will seldom die of the disease, and even pulmonary metastases are cured in the vast majority of such young patients. Prognosis worsens with each age decade over 50, however, so that elderly patients have a poor outlook, as do older patients with large primary cancers.

POSTOPERATIVE MANAGEMENT

Thyroid hormone given in doses sufficient to reduce TSH levels to undetectable is the standard practice, but minimal cancers with virtual 100% cure rates treated by hemithyroidectomy can probably be spared such lifetime medication.

Radioactive iodine (RAI) ablation of residual thyroid tissue and its use for treatment of metastases is highly successful for the minority of patients whose metastases actually take up the RAI (Ruegemer et al. 1988), as the cellular dose of radioactivity is enormous (Maxon et al. 1983). Unfortunately, most patients with metastases do not concentrate RAI (Ruegemer et al. 1988). External radiotherapy and chemotherapy may offer palliation.

REFERENCES

Atkins, J.P. Jr.; Keane, W.M.; and Young, K.A. et al. 1984. Value of panendoscopy in determination of second primary cancer. *Arch. Otolaryngol.* 110:533-34.

Barton, R.T. 1980. Management of carcinoma arising in the lateral nasal wall. *Arch. Otolaryngol.* 106:685-87.

Batsakis, J.G. 1986. Carcinomas of the submandibular and sublingual glands. *Ann. Otolaryngol. Rhinol. Laryngol.* 95: 211-12.

Batsakis, J.G. 1980. The pathology of head and neck tumors:

nasal cavity and paranasal sinuses, part 5. *Head Neck Surg.* 2:410-19.

Batsakis, J.G.; Rice, D.H.; and Soloman, A.R. 1980. The pathology of head and neck tumors: squamous and mucous-gland carcinomas of the nasal cavity, paranasal sinuses, and larynx, part 6. *Head Neck Surg.* 2:497-508.

Batsakis, J.G., and Spitz, M.R. 1984. Major salivary gland carcinoma. *Arch. Otolaryngol.* 110:45-49.

Batsakis, J.G.; Rice, D.H.; and Soloman, A.R. 1980. The pathology of head and neck tumors: squamous and mucous-gland carcinomas of the nasal cavity, paranasal sinuses, and larynx. *Head Neck Surg.* 2:497-508.

Batsakis, J.G.; Solomon, A.R.; and Rice, D.H. 1981. The pathology of head and neck tumors: carcinoma of the nasopharynx. *Head Neck Surg.* 3:511-21.

Baugh, R.F.; Wolf, G.T.; and Beals, T.F. et al. 1986. Small cell carcinoma of the larynx: results of therapy. *Laryngoscope* 96:1283-90.

Beahrs, O.H.; Henson, D.E.; and Hutter, R.V.P. et al. 1988. *Manual for staging of cancer.* 3rd ed. Philadelphia: J.B. Lippincott.

Beahrs, O.H., and Myers, M.H. eds. 1983. *Manual for staging of cancer.* 2nd ed. pp. 55-57. Philadelphia: J.B. Lippincott.

Bradfield, J.S., and Scruggs, R.P. 1983. Carcinoma of the mobile tongue: incidence of cervical metastases in early lesions related to method of primary treatment. *Laryngoscope* 93:1332-36.

Buckwalter, J.; Gurll, N.J.; and Thomas, C. 1981. Cancer of the thyroid in youth. *World J. Surg.* 5:15-25.

Cady, B.; Rossi, R.; and Silverman, M. et al. 1985. Further evidence of the validity of risk group definition in differentiated thyroid carcinoma. *Surgery* 98:1171-78.

Cady, B; Sedgwick, C.E.; and Meissner, W.A. et al. 1976. Changing clinical, pathologic, therapeutic, and survival patterns in differentiated thyroid carcinoma. *Ann. Surg.* 184:541-53.

Cady, B., and Rossi, R. 1988. An expanded view of risk group definitions in differentiated thyroid carcinoma. *Surgery* 104(6): 947-53.

Callery, C.D.; Spiro, R.H.; and Strong, E.W. 1984. Changing trends in the management of squamous carcinoma of the tongue. *Am. J. Surg.* 148:449-54.

Cann, C.I.; Fried, M.P.; and Rothman, K.J. 1985. Epidemiology of squamous cell cancer of the head and neck. *Otolaryngol. Clin. North Am.* 18:367-88.

Chretien, P.B.; Johns, M.E.; and Shedd, D.P. et al. 1985. *Head and neck cancer.* vol. 1. Philadelphia: B.C. Decker, Inc.

Collin, C.F., and Spiro, R.H. 1984. Carcinoma of the cervical esophagus: changing therapeutic trends. *Am. J. Surg.* 460-66.

Council on Scientific Affairs. 1988. Magnetic resonance imaging of the head and neck region: present status and future potential. Report of the Panel on Magnetic Resonance Imaging. *JAMA* 260:3313-26.

Crissman, J.D.; Gluckman, J.; and Witeley, J. et al. 1980. Squamous-cell carcinoma of the floor of the mouth. *Head Neck Surg.* 3:2-7.

Cunningham, J.J.; Johnson, J.T.; and Myers, E.N. et al. 1986. Cervical lymph node metastasis after local excision of early squamous cell carcinoma of the oral cavity. *Am. J. Surg.* 152:361-66.

Cusumano, R.J., and Persky, M.S. 1988. Squamous cell carcinoma of the oral cavity and oropharynx in young adults. *Head Neck Surg.* 10:229-34.

Davis, R.K.; Shapshay, S.M.; and Strong, M.S. et al. 1983. Transoral partial supraglottic resection using CO_2 laser. *Laryngoscope* 93:429-32.

DeSanto, L.W. 1985. Cancer of the supraglottic larynx: a review of 260 patients. *Otolaryngol. Head Neck Surg.* 93: 705-11.

DeSanto, L.W.; Pearson, B.W.; and Olsen, K.D. 1989. Utility of near-total laryngectomy for supraglottic, pharyngeal, base-of-tongue, and other cancers. *Ann. Otolaryngol. Rhinol. Laryngol.* 98:2-17.

DeVita, V.T. Jr.; Hellman, S.; and Rosenberg, S.A. *Cancer: principles and practice of oncology.* 3rd ed. Philadelphia: J.B. Lippincott.

Dickson, R.I. 1981. Nasopharyngeal carcinoma: an evaluation of 209 patients. *Laryngoscope* 91:333-54.

Dimery, I.W.; Kramer, A.M.; and Choksi, A.J. et al. 1989. Neoadjuvant chemotherapy and radiotherapy in larynx preservation (clinical conference). *Am. J. Clin. Oncol.* 12: 173-77.

Donegan, J.O.; Gluckman, J.L.; and Crissman, J.D. 1982. The role of suprahyoid neck dissection in the management of cancer of the tongue and floor of mouth. *Head Neck Surg.* 4:209-12.

Dreyfuss, A.I.; Clark, J.R.; and Wright, J.E. et al. 1990. Continuous infusion high-dose leucovorin with 5-fluorouracil and cisplatin for untreated stage IV carcinoma of the head and neck. *Ann. Intern. Med.* 112:167-172.

Dumich, P.S.; Pearson, B.W.; and Weiland, L.H. 1984. Suitability of near-total laryngopharyngectomy in pyriform carcinoma. *Arch. Otolaryngol.* 110:664-69.

Duncavage, J.A.; Campbell, B.H.; and Hanson, G.A. 1983. Diagnosis of malignant lymphomas of the nasal cavity, paranasal sinues and nasopharynx. *Laryngoscope* 93:1276-80.

Eapen, L.J.; Gerig, L.G.; and Catton, G.E. et al. 1988. Impact of local radiation in the management of salivary gland carcinomas. *Head Neck Surg.* 10:239-45.

Ervin, T.J.; Clark, J.R.; and Weichselbaum, R.R. 1987. An analysis of induction and adjuvant chemotherapy in the multidisciplinary treatment of squamous cell carcinoma of the head and neck. *J. Clin. Oncol.* 5:10-20.

Favus, M.J.; Schneider, A.B.; and Stachura, M.E. et al. 1976. Thyroid cancer occurring as a late consequence of head and neck irradiation: evaluation of 1,056 patients. *N. Engl. J. Med.* 294:1020-25.

Fee, W.E. Jr.; Goepfert, H.; and Johns, M.E. 1990. *Head and neck cancer.* vol. 2. Philadelphia: B.C. Decker, Inc.

Fogel, T.D.; Harrison, L.B.; and Son, Y.H. 1985. Subsequent upper aerodigestive malignancies following treatment of esophageal cancer. *Cancer* 55:1882-85.

Foster, R. 1975. Thyroid irradiation and carcinogenesis: review with assessment of clinical implications. *Am. J. Surg.* 130:608-11.

Gilbert, R.W.; Birt, D.; and Shulman, H. et al. 1987. Correlation of tumor volume with local control in laryngeal carcinoma treated by radiotherapy. *Ann. Otolaryngol. Rhinol. Laryngol.* 96:514-18.

Giordano, A.M.; Ewing, S.; and Adams, G. et al. 1983. Laryngeal pseudoscarcoma. *Laryngoscope* 93:735-40.

Goepfert, H.; Luna, M.A.; and Lindberg, R.D. et al. 1983. Malignant salivary gland tumors of the paranasal sinuses and nasal cavity. *Arch. Otolaryngol.* 109:662-68.

Halperin, W.E.; Goodman, M.; and Stayner, L. et al. 1983. Nasal cancer in a worker exposed to formaldehyde. *JAMA* 249:510-12.

Harach, H.R.; Franssila, K.O.; and Wesenius, V. 1985. Occult papillary carcinoma of the thyroid: a normal finding in Finland. A systematic autopsy study. *Cancer* 56:531-38.

Henderson, B.E.; Louie, E.; and SooHoo Jing, J. et al. 1976. Risk factors associated with nasopharyngeal carcinoma. *N. Engl. J. Med.* 292:1101-1106.

Hirano, M.; Kurita, S.; and Cho, J.S. 1988. Computed tomography in determining laryngeal involvement of hypopharyngeal carcinoma. *Ann. Otolaryngol. Rhinol. Laryngol.* 97: 476-82.

Ho, J.H. 1978. An epidemiologic and clinical study of nasopharyngeal carcinoma. *Int. J. Radiat. Oncol. Biol. Phys.* 4:182-98.

Hoppe, R.T.; Goffinet, D.R.; and Bagshaw, M.A. 1976. Carcinoma of the nasopharynx: eighteen years' experience with megavoltage radiation therapy. *Cancer* 37:2605-12.

Hsu, M.M.; Huang, S.C.; and Lynn, T.C. et al. 1982. The survival of patients with nasopharyngeal carcinoma. *Otolaryngol. Head Neck Surg.* 90:289-95.

Isaacs, J.H. Jr.; Mancuso, A.A.; and Mendenhall, W.M. et al. 1988. Deep spread patterns in CT staging of T2-4 squamous cell laryngeal carcinoma. *Otolaryngol. Head Neck Surg.* 99:455-64.

Kaiser, T.N.; Sessions, D.G.; and Harvey, J.E. 1989. Natural history of treated T1N0 squamous cell carcinoma of the glottis. *Ann. Otolaryngol. Rhinol. Laryngol.* 98:217-19.

Katsantonis, G.P.; Archer, C.R.; and Rosenblum, B.N. et al. 1986. The degree to which accuracy of preoperative staging of laryngeal carcinoma has been enhanced by computed tomography. *Otolaryngol. Head Neck Surg.* 95:52-62.

Kirchner, J.A. 1984. Pathways and pitfalls in partial laryngectomy. *Ann. Otolaryngol. Rhinol. Laryngol.* 93:301-305.

Knegt, P.P.; De Jong, P.C.; and Van Andel, J.G. et al. 1985. Carcinoma of the paranasal sinuses. *Cancer* 56:57-65.

Langer, M.; Choi, N.C.; and Orlow, E. et al. 1986. Radiation therapy alone or in combination with surgery in the treatment of carcinoma of the esophagus. *Cancer* 58:1208-13.

Leipzig, B.; Cummings, C.W.; and Chung, C.T. et al. 1982. Carcinoma of the anterior tongue. *Ann. Otolaryngol.* 91: 94-97.

Levine, P.A.; McLean, W.C.; and Cantrell, R.W. 1986. Esthesioneuroblastoma: the University of Virginia experience 1960-1985. *Laryngoscope* 96:742-46.

Lore, J.M. Jr. 1988. *An atlas of head and neck surgery.* 3rd ed. Philadelphia: W.B. Saunders.

Lundgren, J.A.V.; Van Nostrand, P.; and Harwood, A.R. et al. 1986. Verrucous carcinoma (Ackerman's tumor) of the larynx: diagnostic and therapeutic considerations. *Head Neck Surg.* 9:19-26.

MacComb, W.S.; Fletcher, G.H.; and Healey, J.E. Jr. 1967. Intraoral cavity. In MacComb, W.S., and Fletcher, G.H. eds. *Cancer of the head and neck.* pp. 89-151. Baltimore: Williams & Wilkins.

Maceri, D.R.; Lampe, H.B.; and Makielski, K.H. et al. 1985. Conservation laryngeal surgery: a critical analysis. *Arch. Otolaryngol.* 111:362-65.

Marks, J.E.; Breaux, S.; and Smith, P.G. et al. 1985. The need for elective irradiation of occult lymphatic metastases from cancers of the larynx and pyriform sinus. *Head Neck Surg.* 8:3-8.

Marks, J.E.; Lee, F.; and Freeman, R.B. et al. 1981. Carcinoma of the oral tongue: a study of patient selection and treatment results. *Laryngoscope* 91:1548-59.

Marks, J.E.; Smith, P.G.; and Sessions, D.G. 1985. Pharyngeal wall cancer. *Arch. Otolaryngol.* 11:79-85.

Maxon, H.R.; Thomas, S.R.; and Hertzberg, V.S. et al. 1983. Relation between effective radiation dose and outcome of radioiodine therapy for thyroid cancer. *N. Engl. J. Med.* 309:937-41.

Mendelson, B.C.; Woods, J.E.; and Bearhs, O.H. 1976. Neck dissection in the treatment of carcinoma of the anterior two-thirds of the tongue. *Surg. Gynecol. Obstet.* 143:75-80.

Mendenhall, N.P.; Parsons, J.T.; and Cassisi, N.J. et al. 1987. Carcinoma of the nasal vestibule treated with radiation therapy. *Laryngoscope* 97:626-32.

Mendenhall, W.M.; Parsons, J.T.; and Vogel, S.B. et al. 1988. Carcinoma of the cervical esophagus treated with radiation therapy. *Laryngoscope* 98:769-71.

Mendenhall, W.M.; Parsons, J.T.; and Devine, J.W. et al. 1987. Squamous cell carcinoma of the pyriform sinus treated with surgery and/or radiotherapy. *Head Neck Surg.* 10:88-92.

Million, R.R., and Cassisi, N.J. 1984. *Management of head and neck cancer.* Philadelphia: J.B. Lippincott.

Myers, E.N., and Suen, J.Y. 1989. *Cancer of the head and neck.* 2nd ed. New York: Churchill Livingstone.

Nascimento, A.G.; Amaral, A.L.P.; and Prado, L.A.F. et al. 1986. Adenoid cystic carcinoma of salivary glands. *Cancer* 57:312-19.

Nascimento, A.G.; Amaral, A.L.P.; and Prado, L.A.F. et al. 1986. Mucoepidermoid carcinoma of salivary glands: a clinicopathologic study of 46 cases. *Head Neck Surg.* 8: 409-17.

Neel, H.B. III. 1985. Nasopharyngeal carcinoma: clinical presentation, diagnosis, treatment, and prognosis. *Otolaryngol. Clin. North Am.* 18:479-90.

Norris, C.M. Jr., and Miller, D. 1985. The neck mass. In English, G.M. ed. *Otolaryngology.* Philadelphia: Harper & Row.

Norris, C.M. Jr.; Clark, J.R.; and Frei, E. III et al. 1986. Pathology of surgery after induction chemotherapy: an analysis of resectability and locoregional control. *Laryngoscope* 96:292-302.

O'Brien, C.J.; Soong, S-J.; and Herrera, G.A. et al. 1986. Malignant salivary tumors: analysis of prognostic factors and survival. *Head Neck Surg.* 9:82-92.

Ossoff, R.H.; Sisson, G.A.; and Shapshay, S.M. 1985. Endoscopic management of selected early vocal cord carcinoma. *Ann. Otolaryngol. Rhinol. Laryngol.* 94:560-64.

Parsons, J.T.; Cassisi, N.J.; and Million, R.R. 1984. Results of twice-a-day irradiation on squamous cell carcinomas of the head and neck. *Int. J. Radiat. Oncol. Biol. Phys.* 10:2041-51.

Pillsbury, H.R.C., and Kirchner, J.A. 1979. Clinical vs. histopathologic staging in laryngeal cancer. *Arch. Otolaryngol.* 105:157-59.

Pingree, T.F.; Davis, R.K.; and Reichman, O. et al. 1987. Treatment of hypopharyngeal carcinoma: a 10-year review of 1,362 cases. *Laryngoscope* 97:901-904.

Rejowski, J.E.; Campanella, R.S.; and Block, L.J. 1982. Small cell carcinoma of the nose and paranasal sinuses. *Otolaryngol. Head Neck Surg.* 90:516-17.

Riley, R.W.; Fee W.E. Jr.; and Goffinet, D. et al. 1983. Squamous cell carcinoma of the base of the tongue. *Ann. Otolaryngol. Rhinol. Laryngol.* 91:143-50.

Robbins, K.T.; Davidson, W.; and Peters, L.J. et al. 1988. Conservation surgery for T2 and T3 carcinomas of the supraglottic larynx. *Arch. Otolaryngol. Head Neck Surg.* 114:421-26.

Rousch, G.C. 1979. Epidemiology of cancer of the nose and paranasal sinuses: current concepts. *Head Neck Surg.* 2: 3-11.

Ruegemer, J.J.; Hay, I.D.; and Bergstralh, E.J. et al. 1988. Distant metastases in differentiated thyroid carcinoma: a multivariate analysis of prognostic variables. *J. Endo. Metabol.* 67(3):501-508.

Seiden, A.M.; Mantravadi, R.P.; and Haas, R.B. et al. 1984. Advanced supraglottic carcinoma: a comparative study of sequential treatment policies. *Head Neck Surg.* 7:22-27.

Shaha, A.R.; Hoover, E.L.; and Mitranim, M. et al. 1988. Synchronicity, multicentricity, and metachronicity of head and neck cancer. *Head Neck Surg.* 10:225-28.

Shaha, A.R.; Spiro, R.H.; and Shah, J.P. 1984. Squamous carcinoma of the floor of mouth. *Am. J. Surg.* 148:455-59.

Shemen, L.J.; Huvos, A.G.; and Spiro, R.H. 1987. Squamous cell carcinoma of salivary gland origin. *Head Neck Surg.* 9:235-40.

Shibuya, H.; Hisamitsu, S.; and Shioiri, S. et al. 1987. Multiple primary cancer risk in patients with squamous cell carcinoma of the oral cavity. *Cancer* 60:3083-86.

Shikhani, A.H.; Matonoski, G.M.; and Jones, M.M. et al. 1986. Multiple primary malignancies in head and neck cancer. *Arch. Otolaryngol. Head Neck Surg.* 112:1172-79.

Shindia, H.; Hartsough, A.B.; and Weisberger, E. et al. 1987. Epithelial carcinoma of the nasal fossa. *Laryngoscope* 97: 717-23.

Silverberg, E.; Boring, C.C.; and Squires, T.S. 1990. Cancer statistics 1990. *CA* 40:9-26.

Sisson, G.A.; and Pelzer, H.J. 1985. Staging system by sites: problems and refinements. *Otolaryngol. Clin. North Am.* 18:397-402.

Spaulding, C.A.; Krochak, R.J.; and Hahn, S.S. et al. 1986. Radiotherapeutic management of cancer of the supraglottis. *Cancer* 57:1292-98.

Spiro, R.H. 1986. Salivary neoplasms: overview of a 35-year experience with 2,807 patients. *Head Neck Surg.* 8:177-84.

St-Pierre, S., and Baker, S.R. 1983. Squamous cell carcinoma of the maxillary sinus: analysis of 66 cases. *Head Neck Surg.* 5:508-13.

Suen, J.Y., and Myers, E.N. eds. 1981. *Cancer of the head and neck.* p. 3. New York: Churchill Livingstone.

Teichgraeber, J.F., and Clairmont, A.A. 1984. The incidence of occult metastases for cancer of the oral tongue and floor of the mouth: treatment rationale. *Head Neck Surg.* 7:15-21.

Thawley, S.E.; Simpson, J.R.; and Marks, J.E. 1983. Preoperative irradiation and surgery for carcinoma of the base of the tongue. *Ann. Otolaryngol. Rhinol. Laryngol.* 92:485-90.

Trapp, T.K.; Fu, Y-S., and Calcaterra, T.C. 1987. Melanoma of the nasal and paranasal sinus mucosa. *Arch. Otolaryngol. Head Neck Surg.* 113:1086-89.

Tsujii, H.; Kamada, T.; and Arimoto, T. et al. 1986. The role of radiotherapy in the management of maxillary sinus carcinoma. *Cancer* 57:2261-66.

Wang, C.C.; Blitzer, P.H.; and Suit, H.D. 1985. Twice-a-day radiation therapy for cancer of the head and neck. *Cancer* 55:2100-2104.

Wang, C.C. 1983. *Radiation therapy for head and neck neoplasms.* Boston: John Wright.

Weber, A.L., and Stanton, A.C. 1984. Malignant tumors of the paranasal sinuses: radiologic, clinical, and histopathologic evaluation of 200 cases. *Head Neck Surg.* 6:761-76.

Wey, P.D.; Lotz, M.J.; and Triedman, L.J. 1987. Oral cancer in women nonusers of tobacco and alcohol. *Cancer* 60:1644-50.

Williams, E.D.; Doniach, I.; and Bjarnason, O. et al. 1977. Thyroid cancer in an iodine-rich area: a histopathological study. *Cancer* 39:215-22.

Yuen, A.; Medina, J.E.; and Goepfert, H. et al. 1984. Management of stage T3 and T4 glottic carcinomas. *Am. J. Surg.* 148:467-72.

Zampi, C.; Carcangui; and Rosai, J. 1985. Thyroid tumor pathology. *Sem. Diag. Pathol.* 2:87-136.

Chapter 24

CANCER OF THE CENTRAL NERVOUS SYSTEM AND PITUITARY

Joseph Ransohoff, M.D.
Maxim Koslow, M.D.
Paul R. Cooper, M.D.

Joseph Ransohoff, M.D.
Professor and Chief of Neurosurgery
Department of Neurosurgery
New York University Medical Center
New York University School of Medicine
New York, New York

Maxim Koslow, M.D.
Research Associate Professor of Neurosurgery
Department of Neurosurgery
New York University Medical Center
New York University School of Medicine
New York, New York

Paul R. Cooper, M.D.
Associate Professor of Neurosurgery
Department of Neurosurgery
New York University Medical Center
New York University School of Medicine
New York, New York

PART I: CANCER OF THE CENTRAL NERVOUS SYSTEM

INTRODUCTION

Central nervous system (CNS) tumors logically fall into subgroups that include both brain and spinal cord tumors; primary and secondary tumors; and benign and malignant tumors. The benign tumors, such as meningiomas, neurinomas, and hemangioblastomas, present little oncologic challenge, although they may represent difficult surgical management problems. However, primary CNS gliomas constitute the majority of brain tumors and spinal cord tumors and are of great oncological interest. While primary CNS tumors are all basically malignant, some are considered to be benign depending upon their growth rate and their response to therapy. Also, primary CNS tumors, such as craniopharyngiomas and choroid plexus papillomas, do not fall into the classification of the broad group of gliomas.

Secondary or metastatic tumors to the CNS are major therapeutic problems. They bridge the gap between neuro-oncology and general oncology and, in certain institutions, represent the majority of patients with CNS neoplasms.

INCIDENCE

A variety of factors make it difficult to accurately estimate the incidence of various brain tumors; incidence varies greatly among institutions and areas. An estimated 15,600 new cases of primary brain and central nervous system tumors will occur in 1990 (Silverberg, Boring, and Squires 1990). There appears to be an increase in the incidence of supratentorial gliomas, although it is difficult to confirm this in view of the increased sophistication of the newer neurodiagnostic techniques. Estimates of new cases of total CNS tumors for 1987 were 12,000; an estimated 11,100 deaths were projected from these neoplasms in 1990 (Silverberg, Boring, and Squires 1990). All patients with primary central nervous system tumors of the glioma series will eventually die of their tumors unless they succumb to other diseases. The incidence of primary brain tumors in the United States is increasing, particularly among individuals age 75 or older (Greig, Ries, and Yancik et al. 1990). Many patients with systemic cancer, particularly those with melanoma and lung cancer, die of metastases to the CNS. In childhood, primary CNS tumors are the second leading cause of death from cancer; leukemia is first.

CENTRAL NERVOUS SYSTEM GLIOMAS

Comparatively little is known regarding the etiology, development, and growth regulatory mechanisms of gliomas. These tumors are characterized by a striking heterogeneity that can be observed macroscopically at surgery, microscopically, and genotypically by cytogenetic analysis (Seminars in Oncology 1986).

Although heterogeneity is a significant stumbling block to understanding the basic biology of glial neoplasms, the recent application of recombinant DNA technology to the study of these solid tumors has provided some insights (Seminars in Oncology 1986; Cusimano 1989).

In spite of the dearth of basic data, these neoplasms have certain characteristics that make them ideal tumors for clinical investigations. Central nervous system gliomas rarely metastasize outside of the nervous system unless seeded to extracranial sites secondary to surgical intervention. Medulloblastomas, for example, are well known to seed through ventricular shunts, and once distributed, grow rapidly in extracerebral tissues. Seeding within the CNS via cerebrospinal fluid (CSF) pathways is a more common mode of spread, and multicentric gliomas frequently occur in the latter stages of the disease. There is a group of patients who will eventually succumb to their CNS malignancies but who are otherwise relatively healthy and can tolerate vigorous therapy including surgery, radiation therapy, chemotherapy, and the developing field of CNS immunotherapy.

CLASSIFICATION OF GLIOMAS

The current tendency is to simplify these classifications of gliomas into benign astrocytomas, anaplastic astrocytomas, and glioblastomas. There is no hard line of separation among these three groups, which represent a continuum from the most benign to the highly malignant. Subgroups are determined by the cellular atypism, the presence of mitotic figures, the incidence of endothelial hyperplasia, and the presence of necrotic areas. Newer techniques of molecular biology in the study of gliomas may lead to a more sophisticated subclassification and, hence, to a more logical program of therapy.

DIAGNOSIS

Gliomas in adults generally present symptomatically as seizures. The incidence depends upon the tumor's proximity to the areas of the brain that subserve seizure activity. These include the temporal lobe, which produces psychomotor and petit mal seizures, and the sensory motor area, which produces focal motor or sensory seizures and/or grand mal epilepsy. Gliomas arising in the occipital and posterior temporal areas may produce visual field defects; central gliomas involving the corpus callosum may present with progressive intellectual deterioration without focal neurological signs. Depending upon the tumor's proximity to the ventricular system, patients may have increased intracranial pressure without focal neurological deficits. The

increased use of computed tomography (CT) scans and magnetic resonance imaging (MRI) scans has resulted in fewer patients presenting with severe papilledema and the increased intracranial pressure syndrome, including nausea and vomiting. The exception to this is when midline tumors produce acute obstruction of the ventricular system.

Diagnostically, a high index of suspicion is essential with a symptomatic patient. The use of CT scan with and without contrast material and, more recently, MRI scan with and without gadolinium enhancement, are the mainstays of early diagnosis of CNS gliomas. Cerebral angiography may be of value in planning for surgical intervention, but it rapidly is losing importance in establishing a definitive diagnosis. Lumbar puncture is rarely indicated; pneumoencephalography and ventriculography are obsolete, and electroencephalography alone is of little diagnostic value.

PROGNOSIS

In terms of prognosis, it is well established on the basis of a large series of randomized studies by the Brain Tumor Cooperative Group (Seminars in Oncology 1986) that the three most important factors are: age, with survival being far better in younger patients; the patient's functional neurologic status (Karnofsky score); and the size of residual tumor after surgical excision. These prognostic factors are superimposed upon the tumor's grade (i.e., degree of anaplasia) found by histologic examination. The subclassifications of gliomas, including astrocytomas (the most common), oligodendrogliomas, ependymomas, and gangliogliomas, do not basically alter prognosis.

TREATMENT

SURGERY

The surgical management of brain and spinal cord gliomas serves the dual function of reducing the tumor burden and establishing a definite pathological diagnosis. Radical reduction of tumor burden while maintaining a high quality of postoperative neurological status is clearly indicated in all but the very elderly and debilitated patients. The upper brain stem and pons are not amenable either to direct surgical approach and debulking or stereotactic biopsy, as an alternative. Stereotactic biopsy is a simple and safe diagnostic procedure. In small tumors located in the region of the thalamus and midline corpus callosum it may be the surgical procedure of choice (Seminars in Oncology 1986; Kornblith, Walker, and Cassady 1987).

The use of radiation therapy without a definite pathological diagnosis is rarely justified, as the long-term effects of megavolt therapy to the CNS have been shown to produce significant changes in mental functioning, which is most severe in childhood (Leibel and Sheline 1987). Deficits include deterioration of short-term memory; disturbing changes in personality with severe flattening of affect; and, in children, significant retardation of cognitive development. Anatomically, progressive cerebral atrophy has been well documented by CT scan studies (Leibel and Sheline 1987).

RADIATION

Radiation therapy is indicated once the pathological diagnosis has been established and maximal surgical intervention carried out. It is very rare to find the patient who does not respond to radiation therapy and yet who responds to chemotherapy, immunotherapy, or one of the other treatment modalities. Radiation therapy is generally delivered via external beam using the linear accelerator. The current trend is to reduce the amount of whole brain radiation by coning down on the area of residual tumor or the site of tumor excision. This is based on the fact that the great majority of gliomas, whether benign or malignant, recur within a few centimeters of the original tumor site (Kornblith, Walker, and Cassady 1987; Leibel and Sheline 1987). The use of agents designed to increase the tumor's radiosensitivity has been disappointing. Such drugs as the misonidazoles and 5-bromodeoxyuridine (BUDR) have been used in a number of patients, randomized and nonrandomized. The potential role of radiosensitization should continue to be an area for clinical and laboratory investigation.

Interstitial radiation therapy has received a good deal of attention in the last few years. There appears to be good evidence that stereotactically placed interstitial radiation therapy in small gliomas, particularly in those that have recurred following standard therapy, can significantly prolong survival time. However, cure has not been achieved. Recurrence is common, generally just beyond the irradiated fields (Gutin 1987).

CHEMOTHERAPY

Many chemotherapeutic agents have been used orally, intravenously, and by direct carotid perfusion to treat malignant astrocytomas. BCNU (carmustine) has been the drug of choice for a number of years. The Brain Tumor Cooperative Group demonstrated that BCNU statistically increased median survival time compared to radiation therapy alone; a median survival of about 35 weeks was increased to 50 weeks (Seminars in Oncology 1986). The results were better in the anaplastic astrocytoma than in the full-blown glioblastoma. Intracarotid BCNU, however, produced severe white-matter damage due to the perfusion and was discontinued. Intracarotid cisplatin appears to be effective, and intravenous PCNU, a derivative of BCNU, appears also to have a beneficial effect. However, neither of these drugs nor the other agents which have been used are more effective than intravenous BCNU. Nitrosoureas have limited value because of dose-related renal and pulmonary fibrosis.

There has not been enough experience with the other agents to establish the long-term complications other than the expected effects on the hematopoietic system. There is considerable interest in the development of new experimental drugs, using tissue-culture techniques as well as experimental animal models.

Most cytotoxic agents used in the treatment of CNS neoplasms have been adapted from the armamentarium of drugs used in the treatment of other cancers. The drugs were chosen because they meet the particular need for CNS therapy: They cross the blood-brain barrier. Spiromustine, a drug specifically designed for brain tumor therapy, is a conjugate of nitrogen mustard and hydantoin (Dilantin). The technique of opening the blood-brain barrier by the administration of intracarotid mannitol and then using selected drugs is being investigated as a means of improving delivery. The most recent promising area for improved delivery of cytotoxic agents is the use of biodegradable anhydrous wafers impregnated with chemotherapeutic agents that can be placed in the bed of the tumor resection at the time of surgery. The anhydrous wafers can be constructed to deliver the selected chemotherapeutic agents on a slow-release basis over a period of many months. Theoretically, this technique would combine constant perfusion with chemotherapy during the period of radiation therapy and thereafter. Because most of these tumors recur locally, it is an attractive concept that has yet to be proven in a clinical trial.

OTHER INVESTIGATIONAL MODALITIES

The use of monoclonal antibodies as carriers of either chemotherapeutic agents or radioactive materials is another area of investigation. Of central importance in the development of monoclonal conjugates is the identification of specific tumor antigens. The considerable research effort has not as yet been especially fruitful. However, it serves as an example of how knowledge gleaned from basic research can be applied to the development of clinical treatment strategies. Molecular biologic techniques have shown that a significant percentage of high-grade gliomas have increased expression of epidermal growth factor (EGF). This has led to a clinical trial of an EGF antibody conjugated with ^{131}I administered by the intracarotid route. It is too early to evaluate the efficacy of this approach.

Recent interest has been focused on the use of biological response modifiers (BRMs). Unlike cytotoxic agents that act directly on tumor cells, BRMs exert their effect or effects through the mediation of host responses. Clinical trials of BRMs have become possible due to the availability of large quantities of such molecules developed by recombinant DNA technology. For CNS tumors, clinical trials evaluating BRMs are in progress. There is particular interest in systemically administered beta-interferon and local administration of interleukin-2 (IL-2) in combination with autologous lymphokine activated killer cells (LAK cells). While anecdotal claims for efficacy in some individual cases have been made, further evaluation is needed.

Many therapeutic strategies are being evaluated in the treatment of these highly malignant tumors, whose response to various modes of therapy can be well documented by neurological examination and CT and MRI imaging. These tumors kill in a consistent fashion and, therefore, lend themselves to well-designed randomized clinical trials for phase III studies in the management of recurrent gliomas.

Management of intramedullary spinal cord tumors does not differ significantly compared to intracerebral gliomas. Successful surgery can be done using the operating microscope, ultrasound (US) localization, and the laser and US aspirator with reasonably successful clinical recovery. The intramedullary ependymomas can often be cured surgically and patients with lower-grade astrocytomas may survive for many years, particularly in childhood, with or without postoperative radiation therapy. The higher-grade tumors, particularly the glioblastomas occurring in the spinal cord, are uniformly rapidly fatal, generally due to widespread CSF seeding. This phenomenon is not frequently seen with the intracranial gliomas, including those which freely communicate with the CSF pathways due to surgical intervention.

CHILDHOOD CNS TUMORS

In childhood, the need for aggressive and appropriate adjunctive therapy is even more evident than in adults. An increase in survival of several years in adults is not a significant achievement, but in childhood life expectancy is significantly longer. On the other hand, the effects of radiation therapy on the developing brain are more disastrous than for an adult. A well-documented significant drop in I.Q. is common after whole brain irradiation (Leibel and Sheline 1987). Therefore, many children are observed clinically and radiographically after excision of lower-grade astrocytomas, with radiation therapy withheld until recurrence appears. There are also many well-developed protocols for adjunctive chemotherapy for children using multiple drugs which, at times, show documented significant responses.

The medulloblastoma or primary neuroectodermal tumor is a special subgroup of pediatric tumors. When these tumors are localized in the cerebellar hemisphere and radical surgery is done followed by radiation therapy, there is a significant 5-year disease-free survival. It has been clearly established that entire neuraxis irradiation must be administered. When CSF seeding can be documented, and there is residual tumor after surgery, the results are not nearly as satisfactory in spite of neuraxis irradiation.

Pineal tumors seen in children and young adults are a major clinical challenge. The surgical approach to these tumors can be quite successful, and radical excision of the lower-grade pineal tumors often results in long-term survivals as well as cures. Radiation therapy and many chemotherapeutic agents have been used to manage the more malignant tumors that occur in the pineal gland region. CSF markers can often confirm the presence of the more malignant tumors. Stereotactic biopsy is also readily achievable at a relatively low risk. A number of clinicians, however, still use more conservative measures including ventricular shunting (tumors

in this region frequently cause obstructive hydrocephalus) and a trial of radiation therapy before either stereotactic biopsy or surgery. Pineal tumors include gliomas and a variety of teratomas, pineoblastomas, and/or germ cell tumors (germinoma, embryonal carcinoma, choriocarcinoma). With the exception of gliomas, pineal tumors have a high incidence of diffuse dissemination throughout the CNS via the CSF pathways. The teratomas and germ cell tumors may yield CSF markers including alpha-fetoprotein (embryonal carcinoma component) and chorionic gonadotrophic hormone (choriocarcinoma component). These markers may be used to follow therapeutic response and recurrence. Patients with germ cell tumors frequently present with symptoms of diabetes insipidus due to tumor involvement of the pituitary stalk/hypothalamus. Unfortunately, with the exception of the pure germinoma which carries an excellent prognosis after radiation therapy, these tumors are highly malignant and have a poor long-term outcome in spite of adjuvant chemotherapy.

The optic pathway gliomas are rare in adults but common in childhood. These tumors are usually very low grade and may arise within the optic nerves or chiasm directly, or present as anterior third ventricle astrocytomas invading the optic pathways. The latter group may be successfully debulked, although surgery is not curative. By and large, radiation therapy is the main treatment modality. In view of the indolent nature of these tumors, radiation therapy can be withheld until there is clear evidence of progression demonstrated by decreasing visual function or increasing size of the neoplasm as seen on MRI scan.

Craniopharyngiomas are histologically benign tumors. However, if they are not successfully treated, they lead to loss of vision, disturbed hypothalamic function, and ventricular obstruction as they enlarge and obliterate the anterior third ventricle and foramen of Monro. In children and young adults, these tumors can be successfully removed, sometimes *in toto*, with preservation of good visual function. At times, the pituitary stalk can be preserved and neuroendocrine activity will return to normal. Total excision that disrupts the pituitary stalk is often justified in children because adequate neuroendocrine replacement is available. In adults, it is rarely possible to achieve total removal. Subtotal removal followed by radiation therapy is effective in retarding the tumor's growth. Total excision in adults is often followed by disastrous changes in personality and short-term memory secondary to the tumor's adherence to the anterior third ventricle region and the septal area.

MENINGIOMAS

Meningiomas are benign tumors and logically do not fall into the area of neuro-oncology. These tumors can be cured by total excision including a widespread removal of the dural attachment, but there is a 20% recurrence rate even when excellent surgery has presumably completely removed the tumor. The recurrence rate is far higher with meningiomas arising from the base of the skull where total excision of the dural attachment is not possible. The recent advent of laser techniques to fulgurate the dural origin of these tumors may prove more effective in preventing recurrence.

Of greater interest are the so-called atypical meningiomas and the frankly malignant meningiomas. Also, the hemangiopericytoma, which some physicians consider a variant of the meningioma, has a higher recurrence rate than the usual benign meningioma. This tumor has a high incidence of metastases to sites outside the CNS and is classified by many pathologists as an entity distinct from meningiomas. It is believed to arise from pericytes of blood vessels.

Radiation therapy has been effective in the control of meningioma regrowth when residual tumor was clearly present at the completion of surgery. At times, small meningiomas at the base of the skull involving the superior orbital fissure, optic pathways, and similar regions can be treated with radiation therapy primarily. This has resulted in well-documented recovery of neural function and documented long-term follow-up of a reduction in tumor growth (Kupersmith, Warren, and Newall et al. 1987). The use of selective cerebral angiography with embolization of the extracranial blood supply to these tumors using inert particles or, at times, absolute alcohol is another technique used to reduce tumor growth. It also serves as important adjunctive therapy prior to surgery of hypervascular meningiomas.

METASTASES TO CNS

The management of metastases to the brain is highly controversial. Radiation therapy without surgery is sometimes recommended; other clinicians feel strongly that total removal of a single metastatic intracranial nodule followed by prophylactic whole-brain radiation is a technique of choice (Kornblith, Walker, and Cassady 1987). These differing opinions can be better resolved when the patient is considered in terms of management of the intracranial lesion. On one hand, the intracranial tumor is found during the evaluation of a patient with known systemic cancer. The patient with widespread cancer who is simultaneously harboring an intracranial mass is not suitable for surgical intervention and rarely for radiation therapy. However, the patient who has an intracranial metastatic tumor and no evidence of other systemic cancer has a far better prognosis. The presumption in the latter situation is that the primary tumor has been suppressed by the patient's immunological defense mechanisms, whereas this spontaneous mode of tumor control is not available when lesions are present in the CNS. In the middle is the patient whose primary tumor has been removed and is potentially under good control. With a reasonable life expectancy based on the primary disease and a single intracranial lesion as demonstrated on MRI scan in a resectable area, surgery followed by radiation therapy may be clearly indicated.

Metastatic cancer to the spinal column with secondary spinal cord compression is equally controversial in terms of management. The majority of these tumors have spread to the vertebral body or bodies and cause anterior compression of the spinal cord. The results of posterior laminectomy followed by radiation therapy are probably no better and are potentially worse than the control of spinal cord edema with corticosteroids and radiation therapy alone.

However, more recent neurosurgical and orthopedic developments enable surgeons to do an anterior approach to the spinal column and totally excise the involved vertebra, decompress the spinal cord, and orthopedically stabilize the area. This can offer dramatic long-term protection from paraplegia. In such cases the patient's prognosis depends on the stage of the primary disease process.

PART II: CANCER OF THE PITUITARY

CLASSIFICATION

Benign adenomas of the pituitary gland are relatively common in neurosurgical practice and are the most frequently encountered neoplastic lesion seen in the sellar and parasellar regions. These tumors form glandular structures that are morphologically similar in appearance to their tissue of origin. The cell borders are distinct, the cells themselves demonstrate little or no pleomorphism, nucleoli are inconspicuous, and mitotic activity is infrequently seen.

Malignant lesions originating from the pituitary gland are rare and make up only 1% to 2% of all pituitary tumors in most large series; their very existence has been questioned by some authorities (Zulch 1965). There is also disagreement and uncertainty over the criteria that are necessary to classify a lesion as a pituitary malignancy.

There are a number of reasons for the confusion. A high percentage of benign pituitary adenomas demonstrate microscopic evidence of invasion of the dura of the sella. Although these tumors are clinically and histologically benign, the presence of dural invasion suggests that the tumor may not be completely removable by operative means and that local recurrence may take place from residual tumor attached to or invading the dura.

Another group of pituitary adenomas with a benign histological appearance act aggressively and invade the cavernous sinus or extend into the anterior and middle cranial fossae. Some authorities (Bailey and Cutler 1940; Jefferson 1940) consider these lesions to be malignant, while others (Russell and Rubenstein 1977) do not consider local invasion to be a sufficient criterion for the classification of a tumor as malignant. U and Johnson (1984) felt that benign tumors compressed adjacent structures, whereas malignant ones were characterized by a tendency to local invasion.

Jefferson (1940), in his classic monograph, believed that 4% to 5% of pituitary tumors invaded the cavernous sinus. Computerized axial tomography (CT) scanning and magnetic resonance imaging (MRI) have allowed more accurate definition of cavernous sinus invasion; it is likely that this figure is three to four times greater than Jefferson's estimate. He referred to locally invasive tumors as "malignant adenomas." The term seems oxymoronic; these tumors are probably best referred to as invasive or aggressive adenomas. In spite of their biologic behavior, Landolt (1975) in an electron microscopic study could discern no difference in appearance between invasive tumors and noninvasive adenomas.

Histologically benign pituitary adenomas can metastasize within the CNS or to distant sites (Madonick et al. 1963; Ogilvy and Jakubowski 1973). The term "metastasizing adenoma" is perhaps most appropriate for these lesions.

There is little controversy about the last group of lesions in this continuum: the pituitary carcinomas. These tumors originate from pituitary cells and have the characteristic histological features of an epithelial malignancy: The nuclei show marked pleomorphism, multinucleated giant cells are sometimes seen, mitotic figures are frequent, nucleoli are prominent, cytoplasm is scanty, the cell borders are ill-defined, and the tumor lacks an acinar or sinusoidal pattern (Bailey and Cutler 1940; Feiring, Davidoff, and Zimmerman 1953; Nudleman, Choi, and Kusske 1985; Ogilvy and Jakubowski 1973; U and Johnson 1984; Zulch 1965). Their growth patterns are characterized by local invasion and metastasis within the CNS or systemically, or a combination of these.

Any classification of malignant pituitary tumors must take into account their biological as well as their histological appearance. These tumors may exhibit discrepancies between the lesion's histological appearance and its expected behavior (Luzi et al. 1987; Madonick et al. 1963; Martin, Hales, and Wilson 1981; Ogilvy and Jakubowski 1973). Table 24.1 (Zafar, Mellinger, and Chason 1984) classifies pituitary tumors according to both their clinical behavior and histological appearance.

HISTOPATHOLOGY OF PITUITARY CARCINOMA

Feiring and coworkers required that cellular pleomorphism, numerous mitotic figures, and multinucleated giant cells be present before a tumor could be labeled a

Table 24.1
CLASSIFICATION OF PITUITARY TUMORS

Histologically Benign Adenomas
  1. Encapsulated pituitary adenoma
  2. Locally invasive adenoma
  3. Diffusely invasive adenoma
  4. Metastasizing adenoma
Pituitary Carcinoma
  1. Locally invasive carcinoma
  2. Diffusely invasive carcinoma
  3. Metastatic carcinoma

(Modified from: Zafar, Mellinger, and Chason [1984].)

pituitary carcinoma. Increased cellularity and loss of acinar pattern may also be present. However, benign, noninvasive pituitary adenomas may also show cellular pleomorphism and increased mitotic activity (Martin, Hales, and Wilson 1981). In deciding when to label a pituitary tumor malignant, the degree of cellular pleomorphism and mitotic activity is helpful. However, there is no single objective point when a benign pituitary adenoma becomes a pituitary carcinoma; the progression of histologic changes may form a continuum and lead to the labeling of one tumor a histologically aggressive adenoma and another a carcinoma. Some clinicians will not consider a pituitary tumor to be malignant regardless of its histological pattern unless there is evidence of metastasis.

Systemic carcinoma metastatic to the pituitary gland must be excluded before a tumor can be labeled a primary pituitary malignancy (Nudleman, Choi, and Kusske 1985). Tumors that can metastasize to the pituitary include those originating in the breast, lung, kidney, and colon. Features that are helpful in characterizing a tumor as one of pituitary origin include the presence of secretary granules on electron microscopy, a light microscopic appearance bearing some resemblance to the normal pituitary gland, and the absence of a primary malignant tumor of epithelial origin elsewhere in the body.

Immunohistochemical staining may be helpful in establishing the identity of a metastatic pituitary tumor. The epithelial nature of a tumor may be confirmed by the presence of cytokeratin on immunohistochemical staining (Luzi et al. 1987). Prolactin-specific staining is incontrovertible evidence of a tumor's pituitary origin (Martin, Hales, and Wilson 1981). Although ACTH can be produced by systemic tumors, the presence of ACTH granules in a metastatic lesion and in a histologically similar lesion within the sella is strong evidence of pituitary origin (Zafar, Mellinger, and Chason 1984). Pituitary tumors producing a clinical picture of acromegaly can also metastasize. Myles and coresearchers (Myles, Johns, and Curry 1984) confirmed the pituitary origin of a metastatic growth hormone-secreting tumor through the use of immunohistochemical studies, although the patient had no symptoms or signs of acromegaly prior to her death.

CLINICAL MANIFESTATIONS

The clinical manifestations of pituitary tumors result from direct extension from an intraseller tumor; subarachnoid seeding and growth of tumor in the subarachnoid space within the CNS; distant metastases outside the nervous system; and production of ACTH, growth hormone, or prolactin.

The clinical picture of malignant pituitary tumors that extend in contiguity from the sella may be identical to those produced by benign adenomas: a typical pattern of bitemporal loss of visual fields and decrease in visual acuity (Feiring, Davidoff, and Zimmerman 1953). Unlike the benign adenomas, the patient's history tends to be short and symptoms progress rapidly (Bailey and Cutler 1940). Benign tumors rarely produce the rapid onset and progression of visual loss or cranial nerve dysfunction that results from intratumoral hemorrhage or necrosis. However, signs of cranial nerve dysfunction are seen relatively frequently with malignant tumors and result from invasion of structures adjacent to the sella. It is common to see extraocular muscle palsies (Myles, Johns, and Curry 1984; Nudleman, Choi, and Kusske 1985; St. E. D'Abrera et al. 1973) due to involvement of the third, fourth, or sixth cranial nerves. Third-nerve involvement will also produce ptosis and pupillary dilatation. Facial sensory loss may occur from involvement of the trigeminal nerve in the cavernous sinus or superior orbital fissure (Fleischer, Reagan, and Ransohoff 1972; Myles, Johns, and Curry 1984; Nudleman, Choi, and Kusske 1985).

A prior history of a pituitary adenoma is no assurance that recurrent symptoms of involvement of parasellar structures is due to a benign process. Residual pituitary adenomas that were histologically and clinically benign at the time of initial treatment may undergo malignant transformation and recur (Ogilvy and Jakubowski 1973; Symon, Logue, and Mohanty 1982; U and Johnson 1984).

Hormonal production from pituitary tumors is frequently, but not invariably, seen. Abnormally high levels of ACTH have been reported in one-half of patients with metastatic pituitary malignancies (Nudleman, Choi, and Kusske 1985). Bilateral adrenalectomy in patients with Cushing's disease from ACTH-producing pituitary tumors removes the end-organ hormonal inhibition. Frequently, this results in increased growth and aggressiveness of the pituitary tumor with hyperpigmentation as a result of the melanocyte-stimulating effect of high levels of ACTH (Nelson's syndrome). Less frequently, prolactin (Martin, Hales, and Wilson 1981; U and Johnson 1984) or growth hormone (Feiring, Davidoff, and Zimmerman 1953; Ogilvy and Jakubowski 1973) are produced by malignant pituitary tumors with amenorrhea and galactorrhea in the former, and signs and symptoms of acromegaly in the latter.

Malignant pituitary tumors may also spread through the CNS via the subarachnoid space or cerebral ventricles (St. E. D'Abrera et al. 1973). Tumor cells gain access to the subarachnoid space at the time of operation or spontaneously through invasion. Tumor cells float in the cerebrospinal fluid (CSF) and grow in the subarachnoid space. They may then form tumor masses in the subarachnoid cisterns at the base of the brain; invade the cerebral parenchyma (Fleischer, Reagan, and Ransohoff 1972; Martin, Hales, and Wilson 1981; U and Johnson 1984); or infiltrate the cranial nerves (Myles, Johns, and Curry 1984; Nudleman, Choi, and Kusske 1985), cauda equina (Epstein et al. 1964), and spinal cord (Zafar, Mellinger, and Chason 1984).

Extraneural metastases of CNS neoplasms are exceedingly rare, as is systemic spread of pituitary tumors. Landolt (1975) found only 25 pituitary tumors with distant metastases in a review of the literature. The mechanism by which pituitary tumors metastasize to distant sites is uncertain. Because there are no lymphatics within the CNS, hematogenous spread is most likely due to invasion of the walls of the surrounding venous plexuses or the cavernous sinus (Ogilvy and Jakubowski 1973). The most common site of metastasis is the liver (Landolt 1975; Queiroz et al. 1975) but spread to lymph nodes (Luzi et al. 1987; Scholz, Gastineau, and Harrison 1962; St. E. D'Abrera, Burke, and Bleasel 1973), kidney, lung (Nudleman, Choi, and Kusske 1985), and bone (Myles, Johns, and Curry 1984) have been reported.

DIAGNOSTIC EVALUATION

DIFFERENTIAL DIAGNOSIS

Plain films are a cost-effective screening study to rule out enlargement of the sella or destruction of bone at the base of the skull in patients who are suspected of having a pituitary lesion. However, MRI is now the diagnostic modality of choice for the evaluation of sellar and parasellar lesions. Scanning should be performed in the coronal and sagittal planes to accurately define the tumor's extent. Because bone is inadequately visualized by MRI, CT scanning should also be performed if a destructive lesion in the region of the sella is suspected.

Enlargement of the sella turcica is essential to the diagnosis of a pituitary tumor. While an incompetent diaphragma sella may result in a disproportionate amount of suprasellar tumor compared to intrasellar tumor, the sella will be enlarged if a pituitary tumor 1 cm or larger in size is present. Bone destruction at the base of the skull may occur with aggressive pituitary adenomas but its presence should suggest a meningioma, metastatic malignancy, chordoma, or malignant pituitary tumor. Bony destruction with a normal-sized sella is unlikely to be due to a pituitary lesion. Craniopharyngiomas are frequently cystic with areas of calcification and can be located within or above the sella, but their characteristic appearance should cause little difficulty in distinguishing them from lesions of pituitary origin. Hyperostosis of the base of the skull, an irregularly shaped lesion, and minimal sellar enlargement should suggest a meningioma. If necessary, cerebral angiography may be utilized to show a characteristic vascular pattern that will enable a meningioma to be distinguished from a pituitary tumor or a malignant lesion.

Most tumors originating from the pituitary gland can be readily distinguished from lesions of nonpituitary origin, but there is no absolutely reliable means of separating benign and malignant pituitary lesions on imaging studies alone. While the presence of severe bony destruction may be suggestive of malignancy, histological confirmation of malignancy and observation for continued aggressive growth will usually be necessary for a definitive diagnosis.

Nonradiographic information may also be useful in the differential diagnosis of seller and parasellar lesions. Diabetes insipidus is rarely seen with pituitary adenomas, but is common with craniopharyngiomas and metastatic lesions to the pituitary or hypothalamus. An elevated level of growth hormone or ACTH is *prima facie* evidence of a pituitary tumor. Hyperprolactinemia below 100 ng/mL may be caused by a prolactin-secreting tumor or inhibition of prolactin inhibitory factor from a parasellar lesion. However, a level greater than 100 ng/mL strongly suggests the presence of a prolactin-secreting pituitary tumor. The presence of a primary systemic malignancy should arouse suspicion of a metastasis to the CNS, as should multiple lesions seen on MRI or a CT scan.

Cytological examination of CSF obtained at lumbar puncture may show the presence of malignant cells if a pituitary carcinoma or other malignancy is present. It is unlikely, however, that cytopathological examination will be able to differentiate among the various types of epithelial malignancies.

TREATMENT

Treatment of benign or malignant pituitary tumors begins with surgical removal. For the most part, the transsphenoidal approach is the preferred technique if: (1) the sella turcica is enlarged; (2) diagnostic studies leave little doubt that the tumor is of pituitary origin; and (3) the intracranial extension of the tumor is basically in the midline above the sella without significant lateral extension. Treatment via craniotomy is less frequently used to remove pituitary tumors since the optic nerves and chiasm are located between the surgeon and tumor, placing the visual apparatus at more risk for injury than with the transsphenoidal approach. However, if there is uncertainty about the diagnosis or if the tumor extends far laterally, posteriorly, or anteriorly, craniotomy is the preferred operative approach.

Regardless of the operative technique, the goal is to remove as much tumor as possible. Total removal of a malignant pituitary tumor by craniotomy or a transsphenoidal approach is rarely, if ever, possible and adjunctive therapy should be considered in the postoperative period. Radiation therapy is clearly effective in retarding the growth of residual benign pituitary adenomas. Although the number of patients with malignant pituitary lesions treated with radiation is small, most authorities believe it to be efficacious in the treatment of both the primary tumor and metastatic foci (Bailey and Cutler 1940; Epstein et al. 1964; Martin, Hales, and Wilson 1981; Myles, Johns, and Curry 1984; Zafar, Mellinger, and Chason 1984). Others, however, have noted no beneficial effect (Feiring, Davidoff, and Zimmerman 1953).

Bromocriptine, a dopamine agonist, reduces the size and prolactin production of most benign prolactin-secreting pituitary adenomas. Experience with the use of this agent in the management of malignant tumors is small and less encouraging. Martin et al. (1981) reported a patient with a malignant prolactin-secreting tumor who developed a cerebellar metastasis in spite of bromocriptine therapy. Malignant prolactin-producing tumors are so rare that no definitive statement can be made regarding the efficacy of bromocriptine. However, a trial of bromocriptine as primary treatment or adjunct to operation is indicated if a tumor produces prolactin.

Unfortunately, chemotherapy has not been effective in reducing the size of nonsecreting tumors or those that produce ACTH. Clinical trials are being held to determine the efficacy of a somatostatin analogue that reduces growth hormone production from benign tumors in patients with acromegaly. While this agent appears to be effective in lowering growth hormone levels in most patients with benign growth hormone secreting tumors and in reducing the size of some tumors, there has been no experience in its use in patients with malignant tumors.

SUMMARY AND CONCLUSIONS

Malignant tumors of the pituitary gland are rare. Their existence has been questioned, but numerous well-documented reports have appeared in the literature and there now seems little doubt that they do occur. Histopathological characteristics do not consistently predict the behavior of pituitary tumors and any classification that depends solely on their microscopic appearance without taking into account their clinical behavior is inadequate. It is also appropriate to classify benign-appearing lesions that metastasize as malignant, in addition to those which are histologically anaplastic.

Because malignant pituitary tumors are so rare, suggestions for their management are tentative. Treatment beginning with operative removal of the primary lesion, generally via a transsphenoidal approach, seems most appropriate to decompress the visual apparatus and to establish a diagnosis. Postoperative radiation therapy of the primary and metastatic lesions is effective in delaying or preventing tumor regrowth. Data on the efficacy of bromocriptine therapy for prolactin-secreting tumors and somatostatin analogues for growth-hormone-secreting tumors are lacking, but their use would seem to be reasonable.

Unfortunately once metastasis has occurred the clinical course is short, therapy is palliative at best, and most patients are dead within three years from the onset of symptoms (Zafar, Mellinger, and Chason 1984).

REFERENCES

Bailey, O.T., and Cutler, E.C. 1940. Malignant adenomas of the chromophobe cells of the pituitary body. *Arch. Pathol.* 29:368-99.

Cusimano, M.D. 1989. An update on the cellular and molecular biology of brain tumors. *Can. J. Neurol. Sci.* 16:22-27.

Epstein, J.A.; Epstein, B.S.; and Molbo, L. et al. 1964. Carcinoma of the pituitary gland with metastases to the spinal cord and roots of the cauda equina. *J. Neurosurg.* 21:846-53.

Feiring, E.H.; Davidoff, L.M.; and Zimmerman, H.M. 1953. Primary carcinoma of the pituitary. *J. Neuropath. Exper. Neurol.* 12:205-23.

Fleischer, A.A.; Reagan, T.; and Ransohoff, J. 1972. Primary carcinoma of the pituitary with metastasis to the brain stem. *J. Neurosurg.* 36:781-84.

Greig, N.H.; Ries, L.G.; and Yancik, R. et al. 1990. Increasing annual incidence of primary malignant brain tumors in the elderly. *Proc. Am. Assoc. Cancer Res.* 31:229.

Gutin, P.H. et al. 1987. Recurrent malignant gliomas: survival following interstitial brachytherapy with high-activity iodine 125 sources. *J. Neurosurg.* 67:864-73.

Jefferson, G. 1940. Extrasellar extension of pituitary adenomas. *Proc. Royal Soc. Med.* 33:433-58.

Kornblith, P.L.; Walker, M.D.; and Cassady, J.R. eds. 1987. *Neurologic oncology.* Philadelphia: J.B. Lippincott.

Landolt, A.M. 1975. Ultrastructure of human sella tumors. *Acta Neurochir. Suppl.* 22:94-103.

Leibel, S.A., and Sheline, G.E. 1987. Radiation therapy for neoplasms of the brain. *J. Neurosurg.* 66:1-22.

Luzi, P.: Miracco, C.; and Lio, R. et. al. 1987. Endocrine inactive pituitary carcinoma metastasizing to cervical lymph nodes: a case report. *Hum. Pathol.* 18:90-92.

Madonick, M.J.; Rubinstein, L.J.; and Rona Dasco, M. et al. 1963. Chromophobe adenoma of pituitary gland with subarachnoid metastases. *Neurology* 13:836-40.

Martin, N.; Hales, M.; and Wilson, C.B. 1981. Cerebellar metastasis from a prolactinoma during treatment with bromocriptine. *J. Neurosurg.* 55:615-19.

Myles, S.T.; Johns, R.D.; and Curry, B. 1984. Clinicopathological conference: carcinoma of the pituitary gland with metastases to bone. *Can. J. Neurol. Sci.* 11:310-17.

Nudleman, K.L.; Choi, B.; and Kuspke, J.A. 1985. Primary pituitary carcinoma: a clinicopathological study. *Neurosurgery* 16:90-95.

Ogilvy, K.M., and Jakubowski, J. 1973. Intracranial dissemination of pituitary adenomas. *J. Neurol. Neurosurg. Psychiatry* 36:199-205.

Queiroz, L.; Facure, N.O.; and Facure, J.J. et al. 1975. Pituitary carcinoma with liver metastases and Cushing's syndrome: report of a case. *Arch. Pathol.* 99:32-35.

Russell, D.S., and Rubenstein, L.J. 1977. *Pathology of tumours of the nervous system.* 2nd ed. London: Edward Arnold.

Rose, F.C., and Fields, W.S. eds. 1985. Neuro-oncology. In *Progress in experimental tumor research.* vol. 29. Basel: Karger.

Rosenblum, M.L., and Wilson, C.B. eds. 1984. Brain tumor therapy. In *Progress in experimental tumor research.* vol. 28. Basel: Karger.

Schmidek, H.H. 1987. The molecular genetics of nervous system tumors. *J. Neurosurgery* 67:1-16.

Scholz, D.A.; Gastineau, C.F.; and Harrison, E.G. Jr. 1962. Cushing's syndrome with malignant chromophobe tumor of the pituitary and extracranial metastasis. *Mayo Clin. Proc.* 37:31-42.

Seminars in Oncology. 1986. *Brain tumors* 13(1).

Seminars in Oncology. 1986. *Biological response modifiers* 13(2).

Silverberg, E.S.; Boring, C.C.; and Squires, S.S. 1990. Cancer statistics 1990. *CA* 40:9-26.

St. E. D'Abrera, V.; Burke, W.J.; and Bleasel, K.F. et al. 1973. Carcinoma of the pituitary gland. *J. Pathol.* 109:335-43.

Symon, L.; Logue, V.; and Mohanty, S. 1982. Recurrence of pituitary adenomas after transcranial operation. *J. Neurol. Neurosurg. Psychiatry* 45:780-85.

U, H.S., and Johnson, C. 1984. Metastatic prolactin-secreting pituitary adenoma. *Hum. Pathol.* 15:94-96.

Zafar, M.S.; Mellinger, R.C.; and Chason, J.L. 1984. Cushing's disease due to pituitary carcinoma. *Henry Ford Med. J.* 32:61-66.

Zulch, K.J. 1965. *Brain tumors: their biology and pathology.* New York: Springer-Verlag.

Chapter 25

TUMORS OF THE EYE AND OCULAR ADNEXA

Frederick A. Jakobiec, M.D.
I Rand Rodgers, M.D.

Frederick A. Jakobiec, M.D.
Chief, Ophthalmology Service
Massachusetts Eye and Ear Infirmary
Chairman, Department of Ophthalmology
Harvard Medical School
Boston, Massachusetts

I Rand Rodgers, M.D.
Ophthalmic Plastic and Reconstructive Surgery; Ophthalmic Oncology
North Shore University Hospital — Cornell University Medical College
Manhasset, New York and
Mount Sinai Medical Center
New York, New York

OVERVIEW

Between 5% and 9% of all skin cancers arise on the eyelid. Basal cell carcinomas make up 90% of malignant eyelid neoplasms, followed by squamous cell carcinomas and sebaceous cell carcinomas. Included in a differential diagnosis are inflammatory, viral, and benign tumors. Treatment is directed toward establishing a diagnosis. In cases of eyelid malignancies, the usual principle of cancer surgery—to excise the tumor with wide margins of normal tissue—is complicated by the possibility of compromising ocular function. Attention must be directed not only upon tumor excision but also upon the cosmetic appearance, tear and lid function, and the overall effect on the eye itself.

The conjunctiva may be involved with benign and malignant processes. Pigmented conjunctival lesions pose the greatest diagnostic dilemmas. The patient's age and the lesion's clinical appearance determine whether a biopsy is indicated. A pathologist with expertise in either ophthalmic pathology or pigmented lesions is exceedingly helpful.

Intraocular neoplasms are exceedingly rare. Approximately 250 to 400 new cases of retinoblastoma and 1,500 cases of uveal tract malignant melanomas are diagnosed each year in the United States. Retinoblastoma is the eighth most common cancer among children 15 years and younger; because of its hereditary predisposition, hereditary retinoblastoma serves as a prototype of hereditary human cancer. The diagnosis of choroidal melanoma was fraught with difficulty 20 years ago because up to 20% of eyes with suspected melanomas were found to have other diseases on pathologic examina-

tion. With improved diagnostic techniques as well as the establishment of ocular oncology centers, the controversies regarding malignant melanoma have shifted from diagnostic accuracy to management decisions.

Orbital lesions pose complex diagnostic and therapeutic problems for the ophthalmologist. Almost every soft tissue neoplasm, both benign and malignant, can occur within the orbit. In addition, complex malformations, infections, and noninfectious inflammatory responses as well as systemic diseases may involve the orbit.

EYELID LESIONS

INFLAMMATORY DISEASES AND "PSEUDOTUMORS"

The chalazion is the most frequent lipogranulomatous reaction of the eyelid (Apple and Rabb 1985; Aurora and Blodi 1970; Font 1985). It typically arises spontaneously from noninfectious obstruction of sebaceous gland ducts. It is painless, evolves slowly, and presents as localized tarsal thickening. Inflammation of the surrounding lid or conjunctiva is minimal. In histopathological terms, there is a confluent series of focal granulomas with small microabscesses each centered on a lipid globule. The differential diagnosis includes less frequently occurring granulomatous conditions such as sarcoid, tuberculosis, leprosy, or fungal diseases, and the masquerade syndrome of sebaceous gland carcinoma. Treatment of chalazia includes application of warm compresses, incision and curettage, and steroid injection (Pizzarello et al. 1978).

338

Molluscum contagiosum ("Henderson-Patterson" bodies) is a member of the poxvirus group (Middlekamp and Munger 1967). Multiple dome-shaped, tan-colored nodules characterize it clinically. The lesions have umbilici and contain yellowish thickened material. When the nodules appear on the lid margin, viral particles often travel into the conjunctival cul-de-sac and produce a follicular conjunctivitis. In histopathologic terms, the epidermis has invasive acanthosis with invaginated pear-shaped lobules. The infected epidermal cells degenerate to create the umbilicated appearance. The molluscum virus intracytoplasmic inclusion bodies are round to oval eosinophilic structures and involve the malpighian layer. Treatment includes excision, curettage, or cauterization. Molluscum contagiosum of the palpebral conjunctiva has recently been associated with the acquired immunodeficiency syndrome (Charles 1989).

BENIGN EYELID TUMORS

Squamous cell papillomas are the most frequent benign eyelid lesions (Apple and Rabb 1985; Aurora and Blodi 1970; Font 1985). Their morphology determines subclassifications. Squamous papillomas may be flat, sessile, or polypoid and they may form a cutaneous horn or have a corrugated surface. Papillomas are often multiple; their coloration is similar to adjacent skin, and they tend to involve the lid margin. Squamous papillomas may have a number of origins: viral, solar-radiation, or idiopathic. All squamous papillomas display acanthosis, hyperkeratosis, and parakeratosis. Finger-like projections of vascularized connective tissue covered by papillae make up the lesion. Excision is adequate treatment except in cases of viral papillomas, where cryotherapy is required to minimize recurrence of the lesion.

Pseudoepitheliomatous hyperplasia (PEH) is clinically and histologically confused with carcinoma (Aurora and Blodi 1970; Font 1985). Typically, PEH is associated with a chronic inflammatory process secondary to infectious processes, medications, radiation therapy, burns, and insect bites. Malignant lymphoma and granular cell myoblastoma may also evoke a pseudocarcinomatous response in the overlying epidermis. The vast majority of these lesions, however, have an undetermined etiology. Histopathologically, an inflammatory cell infiltrate underlies invasive acanthosis. Atypical mitoses, nuclear hyperchromatism, and alterations in nuclear-to-cytoplasmic ratio are not present. Keratoacanthoma and inverted follicular keratosis are two specific examples of PEH.

In the past, keratoacanthomas were often misdiagnosed as squamous cell carcinomas (Boniuk and Zimmerman 1967). Because these lesions often spontaneously regress, they have been dubbed "self-healing" carcinomas. These lesions are now widely recognized as benign. A viral etiology has been suggested, but a virus has not been documented by cultures and electron microscopic studies. These benign tumors appear clinically as dome shaped and contain a large, central keratotic plug projecting from the center of the mass. Microscopic examination reveals a cup-shaped nodular elevation with epidermal thickening surrounding a central keratin mass. There is usually an inflammatory cell response at the base.

Inverted follicular keratosis is a second example of pseudoepitheliomatous hyperplasia (Boniuk and Zimmerman 1963). It has been referred to as a baso-squamous cell acanthoma. This lesion presents as a nodular or wart-like keratotic mass. The lesions are benign, but tend to recur if excision is incomplete.

Seborrheic keratosis (basal cell papilloma, senile verruca) is a common benign lesion found on the eyelids and faces of older individuals (Apple and Rabb 1985; Aurora and Blodi 1970; Font 1985). Classically, these lesions have a greasy appearance and hyperpigmentation. They are also slightly raised and friable. Histologically, the acanthotic epidermis contains keratin-filled cysts. Occasionally, because of an increase in melanin pigment granules, seborrheic keratoses can be confused with a pigmented basal cell carcinoma or a malignant melanoma. Seborrheic keratoses are not premalignant lesions, so they do not evolve into squamous or basal cell carcinomas.

Xanthelasmas are localized, reactive lesions composed of foamy histiocytes. Approximately two-thirds of patients with xanthelasmas are normolipenic, but the remainder suffer from essential hyperlipidemia (Fredrickson, Levy, and Lees 1967). Xanthelasmas are generally bilateral, yellow-tan in color, and flat. Most lesions are excised for cosmetic reasons.

Benign tumors of sebaceous gland origin include sebaceous hyperplasia and sebaceous adenoma. Clinically, these lesions are small, soft, yellow nodules. Histologically, sebaceous hyperplasia has well-demarcated lobules of mature sebaceous glands. The admixture of normal-appearing sebaceous elements with lobules of cells closely resembling immature sebaceous cells characterizes sebaceous adenoma. Muir-Torre syndrome is of clinical importance. It presents a curious association between sebaceous gland adenomas and visceral neoplasms, particularly proximal adenocarcinomas of the colon (Torre 1968). All patients with biopsy-proven sebaceous adenoma should be carefully evaluated for malignancy.

Benign vascular eyelid lesions include capillary hemangiomas and cavernous hemangiomas. Capillary hemangiomas are the most common, occurring in 1 of every 200 live births (Walsh and Tompkins 1956). The soft, reddish-purple lesions generally appear within the first two weeks of life. Many rapidly enlarge during the next six months. By age 7 years, 75% to 90% have totally regressed. This tumor consists of lobules of capillaries interspersed with sparse fibrous septa. Lesions causing functional impairment or serious cosmetic deformity may require therapy. Intralesional steroid injection is the preferred treatment modality (Kusher 1981; Hiles and Pilchard 1971).

Cavernous hemangiomas typically arise in the second to fourth decades of life and are slowly progressive (Apple and Rabb 1985). The superficial lesions change the overlying skin to a dark blue color, while the deep ones cause no color change. Blood circulating within the vascular channels is typically stagnant, and this stagnation results in secondary thrombosis and phlebolith formation. Cavernous hemangiomas are composed of large, dilated, blood-filled vascular spaces lined by a flat layer of endothelium. Electron microscopy reveals smooth muscle cells comprising the walls of the cavernous hemangioma, a feature which capillary hemangiomas do not share (Iwamoto and Jakobiec 1979). Extensive cavernous hemangiomas may be associated with thrombocytopenic purpura, or Kasabach-Merritt syndrome (Kasabach and Merritt 1940); gastrointestinal hemangiomas, or blue rubber bleb syndrome (Bean 1958b); and enchondromas and exostoses of the hand, or Maffucci's syndrome (Bean 1958a).

Nevi are benign melanocytic lesions. Their clinical appearance varies considerably. They frequently occur on the eyelid or lid margin surface. They may increase in size and pigmentation over time. Histologically, nevi are of three types: junctional, compound, and intradermal. Junctional nevi arise from the deep layers of the epidermis and do not involve the underlying dermis. Compound nevi exhibit junctional activity and extend deep into the dermis. An intact layer of collagen separates dermal nevi from the overlying dermis. Unlike junctional and compound nevi, intradermal nevi do not become malignant (Apple and Rabb 1985; Aurora and Blodi 1970; Font 1985).

MALIGNANT EYELID TUMORS

Basal cell carcinoma is the most frequent primary malignant epithelial tumor of the eyelid (Aurora and Blodi 1970). It typically afflicts fair-skinned adults, and involves the lower eyelid and inner canthus. Actinic exposure is a predisposing factor. Basal cell carcinomas may be associated with rhinophymas, nevus sebaceous of Jadassohn, and the nevoid basal cell carcinoma syndrome (Acker and Helwig 1967; Gorlin and Goltz 1960; Lever and Schaumburg-Lever 1975).

Based upon their clinical appearance, basal cell carcinomas are classified as nodulo-ulcerative, pigmented, morphea (sclerosing), and superficial (Lever and Schaumburg-Lever 1975). The nodulo-ulcerative form is the classic raised, firm, pearly nodule containing telangiectatic vessels. The lesion is called a rodent ulcer when the nodule undergoes central necrosis. Pigmented basal cell carcinomas frequently are diagnosed as malignant melanomas (Hornblass and Stevano 1981). The pigmentation is due to either melanin pigment within the tumor cells or collection of melanophages within epithelial lobules. Pigmented basal cell carcinomas are otherwise similar to their nodulo-ulcerative counterparts. The morphea or sclerosing basal cell carcinoma is a pale, indurated plaque. Elongated strands of basaloid cells embedded in a dense, fibrous stroma characterize

it histologically. The morphea basal cell epithelioma is aggressive, and infiltrates into the adjacent dermis and subcutis. It may erode into the paranasal sinuses and invade orbital structures. The superficial forms typically appear on the trunk and only rarely on the eyelid. The lesions are erythematous scaling patches with fine, pearly borders.

Basal cell carcinomas rarely metastasize. Doxanas and Green (1979) reviewed 507 basal cell carcinomas of the eyelid and found six tumor deaths, all resulting from orbital and intracranial tumor extension. Farmer and Helwig (1980) studied 17 cases of metastatic basal cell carcinoma. Thirteen of the 17 primary tumors were located in the head, and one involved the lower eyelid and infraorbital region. The mean survival was 1.6 years, with lung, bone, lymph nodes, liver, spleen, and adrenal glands as the more common sites of metastasis.

Treatments of primary basal cell carcinomas include surgical excision, irradiation, and cryotherapy (Fraunfelder et al. 1980; Gladstein 1978; Mohs 1976; Robins 1981).

Squamous cell carcinoma may arise *de novo* or from premalignant lesions such as actinic keratosis or xeroderma pigmentosum (Gaasterland, Rodrigues, and Moshell 1982). It may also arise as a complication of radiation therapy. The ratio of squamous cell carcinoma to basal cell carcinoma is 1:39 (Kwitko, Boniuk, and Zimmerman 1963). In clinical terms, squamous cell carcinoma presents as an elevated, indurated plaque with irregular borders and focal regions of ulceration. Histologic features include pleomorphism, hyperchromatic nuclei, atypical mitotic figures, hyperkeratosis, and deep invasion of tumor cells into the dermis. Early lesions of squamous carcinoma have an excellent prognosis; wide, local surgical excision is curative. Advanced and neglected tumors often metastasize to lymph nodes of the head and neck.

Sebaceous gland carcinoma is a rare adenocarcinoma that affects older individuals (Boniuk and Zimmerman 1968; Rao et al. 1982). The median age at diagnosis is 65. Several cases of sebaceous gland carcinoma have occurred before age 40 in patients who underwent radiation therapy for either retinoblastoma (Boniuk and Zimmerman 1968) or cavernous hemangioma of the face (Schlernitzauer and Font 1976). Sebaceous gland carcinoma arises almost exclusively in the skin of the eyelids from the meibomian glands and zeis glands; rarely, it arises from sebaceous glands in the caruncle or brow. Sebaceous gland carcinoma is more common in the upper eyelid because there are more meibomian glands in the upper tarsus. These tumors frequently mimic other neoplastic or inflammatory conditions; they may appear as atypical or recurring chalazia. The neoplastic cells may invade the overlying epithelium to form scattered nests, or may completely replace the entire epithelium and create the clinical impression of a persistent, unilateral conjunctivitis or blepharoconjunctivitis. Histologic exam documents pleomorphic cells with hyperchromatic nuclei containing a finely vacuolated cytoplasm. These tumors spread in an intraepithelial manner, similar to that of ductal carcinoma of the breast. They may also spread by direct extension into adjacent structures, including lymphatics. Rao, McLean and Zimmerman (1978) studied 95 patients, 22 of whom developed preauricular and cervical lymphadenopathy.

An important feature of sebaceous carcinoma is the tumor's multicentric origin. Independent foci with upper and lower eyelid involvement is seen in 6% to 10% of cases (Rao et al. 1982). Consequently, this tumor is difficult to completely excise.

If the tumor has extended into the orbit, exenteration is the treatment of choice. Involvement of the eyelid requires full-thickness wide excision with map biopsy of the bulbar conjunctiva. If the bulbar conjunctiva contains tumor cells, cryotherapy may help (Lisman, Jakobiec, and Small 1989). Scrutinous follow-up examinations are essential, and, if necessary, map biopsies must be repeated. This tumor is rare except in the eyelid, so an experienced ocular pathologist is of benefit in making a diagnosis.

METASTATIC EYELID TUMORS

Metastatic tumors to the eyelid are uncommon (Apple and Rabb 1985; Aurora and Blodi 1970; Font 1985). Primary cancers that have been known to metastasize to the eyelid include breast, cutaneous melanoma, lung, gastric, colon, thyroid, parotid, and kidney.

TUMORS OF THE CONJUNCTIVA

CONGENITAL TUMORS
Dermoids are benign solid tumors of the conjunctiva and are commonly located at the temporal limbus. They are white in color and may be finely vascularized. On histologic exam, the overlying epithelium is often irregular and keratinized; the substantia propria may contain hairs and sebaceous glands, cartilage, nerve fiber bundles, or smooth muscle. Dermoids in combination with auricular appendages constitute Goldenhar's syndrome (Goldenhar 1952). Dermoids are excised if they are cosmetically disfiguring or if they interfere with motility.

Dermatolipomas are dermoids composed primarily of fatty tissue and lack hairs and sebaceous glands.

BENIGN TUMORS
Benign hereditary intraepithelial dyskeratosis is a rare, autosomal-dominant, inherited condition occurring in certain triracial families in North Carolina (Von Sallman and Paton 1960). Clinically, the nasal and temporal bulbar conjunctiva contains dyskeratotic plaques. Similar leukoplakic lesions of the oral mucosa exist. The tumors are benign and have no malignant potential.

Conjunctival papillomas can grow in either sessile or pedunculated form. The human papilloma virus usually causes the latter (Lass, Grove, and Papale 1983). Viral papillomas generally occur in younger patients, are multiple, and recur if incompletely excised. Viral papillomas eventually regress if untreated. For cosmetically disfiguring, irritating, or recurring lesions, excision with adjuvant cryotherapy is recommended.

The nonviral papillomas are sessile and represent squamous hyperplasia, dysplasia, or carcinomas growing in a papillomatous pattern. They occur in older patients, are solitary, and may involve the cornea.

PREMALIGNANT AND MALIGNANT EPITHELIAL CONJUNCTIVAL TUMORS
The classification of epithelial neoplasms of the conjunctiva (formerly referred to as Bowen's disease) is similar to those of the cervix (McGavic 1942). The designation CIN in ophthalmology refers to conjunctival/corneal intraepithelial neoplasia. The disease spectrum may be divided into: (1) benign; (2) dysplastic; (3) carcinoma *in situ;* and (4) squamous cell carcinoma. The designation CIN no longer applies after invasion beyond the epithelium; such extension denotes squamous carcinoma (Spencer and Zimmerman 1985).

Chronic irritation, such as from exposure to sunlight, is a presumed causative factor (Blodi 1973).

The more-benign lesions are believed to gradually transform into more-malignant ones, but this process may take years.

A gelatinous, pearly white appearance characterizes the relatively benign carcinoma *in situ.* The tumor begins in the limbus and spreads to involve adjacent conjunctiva and cornea; a fine vascularized papillomatous pattern may be present. Carcinoma *in situ* is histologically characterized by severe dysplasia and anaplasia involving the entire thickness of the epithelium but not extending beyond it (Pizzarello and Jakobiec 1978). Excisional biopsy and cryotherapy is the recommended treatment (Kaufman 1988). Corneal involvement is treated by gently scraping away the abnormal cells from the underlying Bowman's layer. Cryotherapy to the adjacent conjunctiva destroys abnormal cells that may remain, and thus decreases the recurrence rate.

Squamous cell carcinoma is carcinoma *in situ* that has invaded beyond the epithelial basement membrane. Metastases are rare and deaths due to the tumors are exceedingly uncommon. Local invasion of subepithelial tissues is much more common than metastases; squamous carcinoma may invade the interior of the eye and grow vigorously (Iliff, Marback, and Green 1975). Extensive invasion may necessitate exenteration.

PIGMENTED CONJUNCTIVAL LESIONS
Congenital melanosis oculi is a congenital blue nevus of the episclera and sclera in association with increased iris and choroidal pigmentation. It appears clinically as multiple, slate-gray patches of the episclera and sclera. It does not involve the conjunctiva. Periocular unilateral pigment (nevus of Ota) is commonly associated. The term oculodermal melanocytosis refers to the combination of ocular and cutaneous pigmentation (Helmick and Pringle 1956). Malignant transformation is rare, but may involve the skin, uveal tract, orbit, and meninges (Reese 1976).

Conjunctival nevi may be pigmented or amelanotic (Abramson 1988). They nearly always begin in childhood and involve the interpalpebral zone. These nevi contain goblet cells within inclusion cysts. The secretion of mucus by goblet cells can lead to an increase in lesion size and produce the false impression of malignant degeneration. Conjunctival nevi may, on occasion, become malignant (Henkind 1978).

Primary acquired melanosis (PAM) is flat, conjunctival pigmentation (Abramson 1988). Unlike congenital melanosis oculi, acquired pigmented conjunctival lesions move within the conjunctiva and are brown or black. Primary acquired melanosis differs from secondary acquired melanosis (due to Addison's disease, radiation, pregnancy, or medications) and from acquired racial melanosis, characterized by a perilimbal ring of pigmentation developing after birth in black patients (Spencer and Zimmerman 1985).

There are two types of PAM (Folberg, McLean, and Zimmerman 1984; Folberg, McLean, and Zimmerman 1985a). The diagnosis of PAM without atypia is made if there is either overproduction of melanin without melanocytic hyperplasia, or melanocytic hyperplasia is present but the melanocytes lack atypia. Primary acquired melanosis with atypia is diagnosed if atypical melanocytes are present within the epithelium. This histologic distinction has important clinical implications: PAM without atypia rarely progresses to melanoma, but PAM with atypia does; atypical lesions composed of epitheliod cells or exhibiting intraepithelial pagetoid extension have, respectively, a 75% or 90% chance of becoming invasive melanoma (Folberg, McLean, and Zimmerman 1985b; Jakobiec, Folberg, and Iwamoto 1989).

Conjunctival malignant melanomas are uncommon ocular neoplasms occurring one-fortieth as often as choroidal melanomas. Conjunctival melanomas may arise in any portion of the conjunctiva but most commonly at the limbus. The degree of pigmentation is variable and the tumors are usually heavily vascularized. Melanomas may arise from pre-existing nevi (40%), *de novo* (30%), or from PAM (30%) (Abramson 1988). If a malignant conjunctival melanoma is suspected, an otolaryngology consultation to rule out localized head and neck metastases may be beneficial. Recommended treatment is surgical excision with adjuvant cryotherapy. A 5% recurrence rate is reported for this treatment modality (Jakobiec et al. 1988).

INTRAOCULAR TUMORS

RETINOBLASTOMA

EPIDEMIOLOGY
An estimated 250 to 400 new cases of retinoblastoma are diagnosed each year in the United States (Abramson 1982; Weichselbaum et al. 1979).

Retinoblastoma is the most common intraocular malignancy of childhood. It follows malignant melanoma as the most common primary intraocular neoplasm (Zimmerman). Retinoblastoma accounts for 1% of all tumor deaths in the pediatric age group.

The increasing frequency of occurrence is leading some investigators to suspect an environmental oncogenic factor as an etiology (Sang and Albert 1977; Schappert-Kimmijser, Hemmes, Nijland 1966).

Retinoblastoma is typically diagnosed between 12 and 18 months of age, with 90% of cases diagnosed prior to age 3 years. Spontaneous regression occurs in 1% of all cases (Parks and Zimmerman 1960).

ETIOLOGY
Retinoblastoma occurs both in hereditary and nonhereditary forms. Approximately 30% to 40% of patients with retinoblastoma have a hereditary predisposition to the tumor, as well as to other neoplasia including osteosarcoma. Only one-quarter of patients with hereditary retinoblastoma have a family history; the remaining three-quarters are caused by new mutations of the germ cells. The hereditary form of the disease is an autosomal dominant trait but with incomplete penetrance and variable expressability. Table 25.1 summarizes the transmission patterns for retinoblastoma.

The Knudson hypothesis states that two mutations are necessary for the emergence of a retinoblastoma tumor (Knudson, Hethcote, and Brown 1975). Children who have hereditary retinoblastoma inherit the first mutation, which is present in all cells of their body. Because of this germinal mutation these patients can pass the gene to offspring and their so-called secondary tumors. In hereditary retinoblastomas, the first inherited germinal mutation predisposes to the second acquired somatic mutation, which is necessary for tumorigenesis. In the nonhereditary retinoblastomas, both

Table 25.1
TRANSMISSION PATTERNS FOR RETINOBLASTOMA*

What is the chance that my child will inherit retinoblastoma?	UNILATERAL CASE		BILATERAL CASE	
	Positive Family History	Negative Family History	Positive Family History	Negative Family History
If the inquirer is:				
Parent of affected patient	40%	1%	40%	6%
Affected patient	40%	8%	40%	40%
Sibling of affected patient	7%	1%	7%	1%

*Assumes a penetrance rate of 80%

mutations are acquired and somatic. The tumor is, therefore, unilateral with no tendency for secondary tumors, and no transmission of the disease to the affected's offspring.

In the 1970s investigators noted a chromosomal deletion in a subpopulation of patients with retinoblastoma (Weichselbaum et al. 1979). High resolution chromosome banding placed the deletion side within the q14 band of chromosome 13. Subsequent studies discovered the gene for the enzyme esterase D to be located on chromosome 13 in close linkage to the retinoblastoma gene. Assays for esterase D have been used in identifying carriers for the retinoblastoma gene (Benedict et al. 1983). In 1986 the gene for retinoblastoma was identified and cloned (Friend et al. 1986; Lee et al. 1987). The gene spans 200 kilobases on chromosome 13 at band q14 and is associated with a 4.7 kilobase RNA transcript. The gene product is a nuclear phosphoprotein with DNA binding activity (Whyte et al. 1988). This gene functions as a dominant suppressor of tumor formation or anti-oncogene (Huang, Lee, and Shew 1988). Although retinoblastoma has an autosomal dominant inheritance pattern at the clinical level, alteration or inactivation of both of the two homologous alleles is necessary for the disease to occur, and thus at the molecular level the gene is recessive. Such information supports the Knudson two-hit hypothesis. The first abnormal gene is inherited and present in all cells of patients with hereditary retinoblastoma, while a somatic mutation occurs within a single retinal cell in nonhereditary disease. In all cases of retinoblastoma the second mutation occurs in the retinal cells, which then gives rise to the tumor.

Prenatal diagnosis may be possible if there is a strong family history of retinoblastoma. Amniocentesis has been reported on five families predisposed to retinoblastoma using restriction length and isozymic alleles of loci on chromosome 13 (Cavenee, Murphree, and Shull 1986). The calculated predictive accuracy was greater than 94% in cases with informative loci flanking the retinoblastoma loci. Several researchers emphasize that the possibility of recombination reduces the accuracy of prenatal diagnosis as individual chromosome specific markers are linked to, but distinct from, the retinoblastoma locus (Gilbert 1986). Furthermore, one must study two generations, which must include both a parent and a child with retinoblastoma. Thus, prenatal diagnosis of sporadic cases, which are the majority, is virtually impossible (Cavenee, Murphree, and Schull 1986).

CLINICAL DIAGNOSIS

The presenting signs and symptoms of retinoblastoma are determined by the tumor's size, location, and biologic behavior. Leukocoria and strabismus are the most common signs (Ellsworth 1969). Other presenting signs include visual disturbances, heterochromia, spontaneous hyphema, and uveitis.

A complete ocular examination in the office can lead a physician to suspect the diagnosis of retinoblastoma. The examination should include assessment of visual function, slit lamp biomicroscopy of the anterior segment and vitreous, and indirect ophthalmoscopy.

Examination under anesthesia permits a more detailed study of the disease process. Intraocular pressures and corneal diameters can also be evaluated. Ultrasound, MR, and CT scanning may be helpful in making the diagnosis. Other ancillary tests are listed in table 25.2.

The differential diagnosis includes Coat's disease, nematode endophthalmitis, persistent hyperplastic primary vitreous, retrolental fibroplasia, uveal coloboma, retinal dysplasia, and congenital cataract (Abramson 1982; Ellsworth 1969).

A patient in whom retinoblastoma is strongly suspected should undergo a complete general history and physical examination supplemented by bone scan, bone marrow aspiration, lumbar puncture for cerebrospinal fluid analysis, and karyotype analysis. Family members must be examined to look for ophthalmoscopic evidence of a regressed retinoblastoma.

PATHOLOGY

The retinoblastoma eye contains a chalky white to gray tumor that usually contains calcium deposits. Zimmerman (1985) has described three growth patterns of retinoblastoma. Endophytic growth occurs when the tumor grows from the retina inward toward the vitreous cavity. In these cases the patient may have clinical signs of a cellular infiltration of the vitreous resembling an endogenous endophthalmitis. An exophytic growth pattern occurs when the tumor grows from the retina outward toward the subretinal space. These eyes typically have a total retinal detachment and a subretinal yellow-white material resembling the exudative detachment of advanced Coat's disease. The third pattern is the multicentric infiltration of tumor cells throughout the entire retina. This pattern is seen in older patients

Table 25.2
ANCILLARY TESTS FOR RETINOBLASTOMA

I. Frequently performed
    1) CT scan (Roentgenograms)
    2) Ultrasound
II. Occasionally performed
    1) Paracentesis
    2) Cytology
    3) Enzymes
III. Rarely performed
    1) Needle biopsy
    2) Serum ELISA (Toxocara)
IV. New tests: reliability unknown
    1) MRI
    2) Chromosomes (RLFPs)
    3) Immune complexes
V. Tests of uncertain value
    1) Transillumination
    2) Serum alpha-fetoprotein
    3) AD antigens (Hanganutzin-Deicher antigen)
    4) $P32$ test
    5) CEA
    6) Fluorescein angiography
    7) Urine catecholamines
    8) Lymphocyte cytoxicity test
    9) Serum haptoglobin

with retinoblastoma (Morgan 1971; Nicholson and Norton 1980).

Histological appearance is that of small, rounded cells with large hyperchromatic nuclei and scant cytoplasm. Most retinoblastomas have zones of viable tumor alternating with areas of necrosis, where the tumor has outgrown its blood supply. The tumor may become so necrotic as to destroy itself entirely, giving rise to spontaneous regression (Burnier, McLean, and Zimmerman 1990). Zones of calcification may be present.

Higher magnification may show several types of rosettes. The Flexner-Wintersteiner rosette (Flexner 1891; Wintersteiner 1897) consists of differentiated tumor cells arranged around a patent central space. The rim of the central space is analogous to the terminal bars of the photoreceptors (Tso, Fine, and Zimmerman 1969; Tso, Fine, and Zimmerman 1970). The Flexner-Wintersteiner rosette is virtually pathognomonic for retinoblastoma. Fleurettes demonstrate bulbous cellular extension representing differentiation along the lines of outer photoreceptor segments. The Homer-Wright rosette is found in several tumors besides retinoblastomas. Unlike the Flexner-Wintersteiner rosette, there is no central lumen.

PRINCIPLES OF TREATMENT

Surgery. Surgery (Abramson and Ellsworth 1980; Abramson, Ellsworth, and Rozakis 1982; Abramson et al. 1981; Shields 1983; Shields and Augsburger 1981) to remove the affected eye is the treatment of choice for most children with retinoblastoma. Treatment of the second eye in bilateral cases depends on the size and extent of the tumor.

When enucleation is performed, it is important to excise as much of the optic nerve as possible along with the globe. A histological examination of the cut end of the optic nerve is necessary.

Photocoagulation. Photocoagulation (Meyer-Schwickerath 1961) of retinoblastomas is rarely undertaken. Its only possible indication is for exceedingly small retinoblastomas located posterior to the equator and confined to the retina.

Cryotherapy. Cryotherapy (Abramson, Ellsworth, and Rozakis 1982) is effective for small- to medium-sized tumors located anterior to the equator. Bruch's membrane and the internal limiting membrane of the retina are preserved with no specific complications. Lesions greater than 7 disc diameters are not suitable for cryotherapy.

Radiotherapy. Radiotherapy (Abramson et al. 1981; Balmer and Gaillard 1983; Shields 1983; Shields and Augsburger 1981) can be used to treat retinoblastoma, which is sensitive to relatively moderate doses of irradiation that the tumor-free retina can withstand. More differentiated retinoblastomas may be somewhat more radioresistant.

For bilateral advanced cases of retinoblastoma, external beam radiotherapy is usually the preferred treatment. The goal is to preserve at least one eye with some useful vision. External beam radiation therapy is also common for less-advanced cases in which the tumor has invaded the macula, optic disc, or vitreous.

The total dose of radiation, retraction of treatment, fractionation schedule, and method of shielding depend on the extent of disease. Radiation oncologists and ophthalmologists must jointly determine these parameters.

The lens of the eye is quite sensitive to radiation damage and, despite attempts at shielding, a radiation cataract may develop. This cataract may be removed later.

In infants, a frequent complication of radiotherapy is radiation therapy's growth-retarding effect on bones of the orbital region. Marked facial asymmetry is often the sequela of radiotherapy administered to patients under age 2 years.

Radiation therapy may also be responsible for the late appearance of orbital osteogenic sarcoma and rhabdomyosarcoma. These and other tumors may also arise outside of radiation sites (Jensen and Miller 1971; Schipper 1980).

Radioactive plaque therapy. Radioactive plaques may be useful in those eyes in which external beam radiation therapy has failed to destroy all viable tumor (Stallard 1964). Rarely, it is used as the primary treatment for patients with small- to medium-sized tumors.

Chemotherapy. Chemotherapy alone as treatment for primary retinoblastoma is not of value.

Adjuvant chemotherapy is used in some children following enucleation for advanced retinoblastoma, but the risk-benefit ratio has not been determined completely.

Chemotherapy (vincristine-cyclophosphamide-doxorubicin) is being used for treatment of metastatic disease.

RESULTS AND PROGNOSIS

The Reese-Ellsworth classification (Sang and Albert 1977) groups retinoblastomas according to probability that some form of treatment can eradicate the tumor and preserve useful vision. The Reese-Ellsworth classification (table 25.3) takes into account the number, size, and location of tumors and the presence or absence of vitreous seeding. According to this classification, retinoblastomas are grouped from very favorable (group I) to very unfavorable (group V) probabilities of eye preservation with useful vision.

Treatment results depend heavily upon the stage at which the tumor is first diagnosed. In addition, the degree of cellular differentiation, the presence or absence of optic nerve involvement, and the presence or absence of choroidal involvement correlate with long-term prognosis. Patients with well-differentiated tumors have a higher survival rate than patients with poorly

Table 25.3
CRITERIA OF SUITABILITY FOR TREATMENT IN RETINOBLASTOMA PATIENTS

Group I Very Favorable	Group II Favorable	Group III Doubtful	Group IV Unfavorable	Group V Very Unfavorable
Solitary tumor, less than 4 DD* in size, at or behind equator	Solitary lesion 4-10 DD in size, at or behind equator	Any lesion, anterior to equator	Multiple tumors, some larger than 10 DD	Massive tumors, involving over half the retina
Multiple tumors, none over 4 DD in size, all at or behind equator	Multiple tumors, 4-10 DD in size, behind equator	Solitary tumors, larger than 10 DD, behind equator	Any lesion, extending anteriorly to ora serrata	Vitreous seeding

*DD = disc diameter

differentiated tumors. Children with gross invasion of tumor beyond the line of optic nerve transection have a much poorer prognosis than do those with no invasion of the optic nerve. Although there is some suggestion that massive choroidal involvement by retinoblastoma may worsen the prognosis, the predictive value of this factor is not as well established as that of the other two features.

Long-term survivors of irradiation have a 1.5% chance of developing second primary cancer; the most common is osteosarcoma. Nonradiogenic neoplasms have also been reported. Pineal tumors may occur at the time of retinoblastoma diagnosis or many years after successful treatment (Jakobiec et al. 1977). Histologically, the tumor is composed of Flexner-Wintersteiner rosettes and fleurettes (Stefanko and Manschot 1979). Bader has proposed the term trilateral retinoblastoma to signify such solitary midline lesions.

CLINICAL INVESTIGATIONS

Work is presently under way at fully sequencing the retinoblastoma gene. Given the limitations of genetic analysis with restriction fragment length polymorphisms, investigators are attempting to directly identify the disease-causing mutation in the retinoblastoma gene (Yandell, Campbell, and Dayton 1989). Tumors are screened exon by exon using specific polymerase chain amplification and direct sequence analysis to identify variations in DNA sequence that differ from those in normal tissue (Yandell and Dryja 1989). If the initial mutation can be identified, new germinal mutations leading to the hereditary form of retinoblastoma can be quickly distinguished from the nonhereditary mutations. Prenatal diagnosis of hereditary retinoblastoma would be more accurate.

MALIGNANT MELANOMA OF THE CHOROID

EPIDEMIOLOGY

Malignant melanoma of the choroid is an uncommon neoplasm (Strickland and Lee 1981). Only an estimated 1,500 cases of uveal melanoma are diagnosed each year in the United States, or about 0.5 cases per 100,000 people per year.

The average age of patients with choroidal melanoma is 50 years (Paul, Parnell, and Fraker 1962); however, the incidence continues to rise until age 70 before

declining. Less than 4% of patients with choroidal melanomas are under 30 years of age (Barr, McLean, and Zimmerman 1981).

Choroidal melanomas occur much more frequently in whites than blacks (Scotto, Fraumeni, and Lee 1976). Women in the reproductive years and perimenopausal period are more likely to present with choroidal melanoma than men of similar age.

Growth of melanomas in women who are pregnant or on birth control pills or estrogen supplements has been documented (Frenkel and Klein 1966). Attempts at finding estrogen receptors have been fruitless.

ETIOLOGY

The etiology of choroidal melanomas is poorly understood. Inheritance may occur on rare occasion (Oosterhuis, Went, and Lynch 1982), particularly in the B-K mole syndrome (Bellet et al. 1980). Choroidal melanomas may derive from some combination of environmental factors and areas of increased pigmentation.

The role of environmental carcinogens has been difficult to document, but choroidal melanoma may ultimately be linked to cigarette smoking (Keeney, Waddell, and Perrayt 1982). N-nitrosonornicotine, a potent carcinogen in cigarette smoke, is concentrated in the choroid. In animal experiments, the carcinogen passes the placenta and localizes in the choroid of the fetus. The lower 5-year survival rate of smokers with choroidal melanoma lends credence to this hypothesis.

Patients with the nevus of Ota syndrome and ocular melanocytosis have an increased risk of developing malignant melanomas at sites of increased pigmentation (Nik, Glew, and Zimmerman 1982).

Many researchers believe that the majority of choroidal melanomas arise in a pre-existent nevus. The presence of bland nevoid cells at the base of the tumor against the sclera or at the margin or periphery of choroidal melanomas supports this hypothesis (Yanoff and Zimmerman 1967).

DETECTION

The clinical presentation of choroidal melanoma varies greatly (Shields 1983). Posterior pole lesions most commonly present with signs of increasing hyperopia. Melanomas that arise in the comparatively silent anterior choroid or ciliary body region may be asymptomatic until they reach an advanced state. At that time, they may cause pigmentation of tissue in the chamber angel, focal shallowing of the anterior chamber, episcleral nodules, episcleral dilated sentinel vessels, sector cataract, and lens subluxation or tilting. Scotomas, floaters, photopsia, and pain are other signs and symptoms of choroidal melanomas. Pain is a particularly ominous symptom and is often associated with glaucoma.

Both hyperopia and metamorphopsia are associated with serous detachments caused by choroidal tumors. Vitreous hemorrhage is generally a very late complication.

Melanoma should always be suspected in phthisical or blind, painful eyes (Shields et al. 1977).

DIAGNOSIS

Misdiagnosis of choroidal malignant melanoma has decreased markedly since the 1950s (Davidorf et al. 1983), due to improved diagnostic techniques and careful following of sequential steps in the differential diagnosis of choroidal melanoma.

Indirect ophthalmoscopy is the most important diagnostic test for choroidal melanoma. The shape of the lesion often resembles a mushroom or collar button; the latter appearance often results from rupture of the tumor through Bruch's membrane. Patchy areas of retinal pigment epithelial (RPE) atrophy, hyperplasia, or fibrous metaplasia over the lesion's surface often give it a mottled appearance.

The degree of the lesion's pigmentation often adds little diagnostic information; many tumors are amelanotic. An orange to golden-brown pigment consisting of macrophages filled with lipofuscin and melanin granules may lie over the tumor.

Drusen may be present, but are much more common in nevi than in melanomas.

Serous retinal detachment is common. Diffuse lesions with large base diameters frequently cause extensive detachment.

Ultrasound is exceedingly valuable in diagnosing these tumors (Ossoinig and Blodi 1974; Ossoinig and Till 1969). Ultrasound views lesions in eyes with opaque media and can calculate tumor thickness in the anteroposterior dimension. Any lesion measuring less than 2 mm in thickness is most likely a nevus. Tumor heights of 2 mm to 3 mm, 3 mm to 5 mm, and greater than 5 mm represent small, medium, and large lesions, respectively (Ossoinig and Till 1989). On A-scan, a melanoma is characterized by a sharply rising surface signal, spontaneous vascular movements, low to medium internal reflectivity, and a regular internal structure. On B-scan, a melanoma is solid with acoustic shadow-casting along the posterior surface of the mass resembling choroidal excavation. Extrascleral extension may be determined on ultrasound.

At present, CT scanning and MR imaging provide limited information. One important observation that these modalities may provide, however, is whether or not there is extrascleral or epibulbar extension.

Transillumination is one of the most underutilized diagnostic aids (Jakobiec and Levinson 1985). To perform it, the physician observes either the blockage of light through the pupil as the light source is moved behind the lesion, or the shadow of the tumor that is projected on the sclera when the light source is on the opposite side of the globe. Both methods provide an accurate assessment of the size, extent, and solidity of the lesion. Transillumination is helpful in differentiating retinoschisis, retinal detachments, and choroidal effusions from a melanoma, as these all transilluminate well.

Fluorescein angiography is a common diagnostic aid (Gass 1977), although there is no diagnostically useful or distinct fluorangiographic pattern of a melanoma. However, melanomas tend to display patchy hyperfluoresence due to retinal pigment epithelial changes and late staining.

Ultrasound-directed needle biopsy is a technique for obtaining cellular aspirates for histologic analysis (Jakobiec, Coleman, and Chattock 1979). Because of the intricate technique and potential risks, it is reserved for situations in which the diagnosis is uncertain and enucleation is planned.

The $^P32$ test cannot differentiate nevi from melanomas, nor can it distinguish low-grade from high-grade melanomas (Minckler, Font, and Shields 1978; Zakov, Smith, and Albert 1978). Many false positive results are possible. The $^P32$ test may also traumatize the lesion. Visual field and electroculogram (EOG) testing is of no value.

DIFFERENTIAL DIAGNOSIS

Table 25.4 lists the lesions that mimic choroidal and ciliary body melanomas (Ferry 1964). The first and foremost distinction is whether the lesion represents a large nevus or a small melanoma. Lesions measuring less than 2 mm thick, even those with a large base, can be diagnosed as nevi, provided there is no centrifugal growth through the choroid. In patients with lesions greater than 2 mm thick, this distinction cannot be made on a single examination. Only sequential examinations documenting the absence of growth would lend credence to the diagnosis of a nevus. Nevi, like melanomas, may have multiple drusen on the surface. Nevi may cause subretinal neovascular nets, and even exudative detachments (Gass 1977).

The melanocytoma is a variant of the choroidal nevus (Shields and Font 1972). Although melanocytomas have a predilection for the nerve, these benign tumors may occur in the ciliary body or in the choroid. Melanocytomas can increase in size and can cause subretinal neovascularization.

Hemorrhagic complications of non-neoplastic conditions are included in the differential diagnosis (Shields and Zimmerman 1973). Neovascularization beneath the retinal pigment epithelium may result in subretinal heme, which is easily confused with an elevated pigmented mass.

Astrocytomas are whitish, richly vascularized lesions. Astrocytomas may be associated with tuberous sclerosis,

Table 25.4
LESIONS THAT MIMIC CHOROIDAL AND CILIARY BODY MELANOMAS

RETINAL
- Preretinal hemorrhage
- Macroaneurysm
- Metastasis (extremely rare)
- Astrocytic tumors (including mixed vascular-glial lesions)
- Massive gliosis of retina filling vitreous cavity
- Exophytic peripapillary hemangioblastoma (von Hippel lesion)
- Macular and ectopic disciform lesions with hemorrhage

RETINAL PIGMENT EPITHELIUM (RPE)
- RPE hypertrophy and hyperplasia
- RPE adenomas and carcinomas (non-metastasizing)
- Sub-RPE neovascularization with hemorrhage
- Sub-RPE mounds of reticulum cell sarcoma
- Complex RPE-retinal vascular hamartoma

CHOROID
- Amelanotic nevus, large pigmented nevus and melanocytoma
- Bilateral diffuse choroidal nevi with retinal detachment (associated with malignancy)
- Cavernous hemangioma
- Osseous choristoma
- Reactive lymphoid hyperplasia
- Solid vascular and peripheral nerve tumors (extremely rare)
- Metastatic carcinoma

OTHER SITES
- Scleritis
- Melanocytoma of ciliary body
- Conventional and mesectodermal leiomyomas and peripheral nerve tumors of ciliary body (extremely rare)
- Adenomas and carcinomas of pigmented and nonpigmented ciliary epithelium

but more frequently are isolated retinal lesions; they may have associated retinal exudates.

Hypertrophy and hyperplasia of the retinal pigment epithelium results in oval-shaped, jet-black, perhaps multiple lesions.

Retinal pigment epithelial adenomas and adenocarcinomas are rare. These lesions are always intensely pigmented and block fluorescence from the underlying choroid. They do not invade the choroid (Tso and Albert 1972).

The most common nonmelanocytic choroidal tumor is the cavernous hemangioma, an intensely red-orange lesion that has a predilection for the posterior pole. It may be elevated and associated with cystoid macular edema, subretinal exudate, and metaplasia of the pigment epithelium to bone. Ultrasound will reveal vascular pulsations, and the lesion will blanch when pressure is applied to the globe.

Osseous choristoma is a salmon- or cream-colored lesion occurring most commonly in young women. It is typically located in the posterior pole or peripapillary zone. Fluorescein angiography discloses widespread areas of retinal pigment atrophy. Ultrasound and CT reveal the presence of bone within the choroid.

The choroid is the most frequent ocular site of a nonocular carcinoma metastasis (Albert, Rubinstein, and Scheie 1967; Bullock and Yanes 1980). Metastatic lesions are generally flatter than primary intraocular melanomas, appear nonpigmented and creamy, grow rapidly, are multiple in number, and cause coarse clumping of the pigment epithelium. Ultrasound indicates a higher internal reflectivity in a metastatic lesion because of the associated fibrosis.

METASTATIC WORKUP

Prior to therapy for a suspected choroidal melanoma, the patient should undergo a metastatic workup. Liver enzymes should be assayed, including gamma-glutamyl transpeptidase (Zimmerman 1983). Liver-spleen scan, chest x-ray, and a complete physical examination are mandatory.

Fewer than 1% to 2% of patients presenting with choroidal melanoma have had clinical evidence of distant metastases at the time of clinical diagnosis.

CLASSIFICATION

Table 25.5 lists the pretreatment clinical staging of uveal melanomas (Beahrs and Myers 1983).

CELLULAR CLASSIFICATION

Callender's initial classification of spindle A, spindle B, and epithelioid cell lesions has undergone a major revision (Callender 1931).

Spindle A cells contain a longitudinal fold in the nuclear membrane. The cells have a small, slender nucleus with ill-defined or absent nuclei. Spindle A cells are now recognized as benign (McLean, Zimmerman, and Evans 1978).

Spindle B cells have a larger, plumper nucleus containing coarse chromatin and a deeply stained, small, round nucleolus.

Epithelioid cells are larger, more pleomorphic polygonal cells than spindle A or B. They may contain multiple nucleoli.

Mixed tumors contain a mixture of epithelioid and spindle B cells. To be classified as a mixed tumor, at least 5% of the cells must be epithelioid.

PRINCIPLES OF TREATMENT

Ionizing radiation is the most promising noninvasive therapeutic modality available. Brachytherapy is being used in most treatment centers. With this technique, plaques containing gamma-emitting isotopes are affixed to the globe for a set period and deliver a fixed dosage to the tumor (Packer et al. 1980; Rotman et al. 1977; Stallard 1966). The dosage is calculated to deliver a maximum of 80 Gy to 100 Gy to the tumor's apex. Both iodine 125 and cobalt 60 are used. Iodine 125 has a more favorable isodose fall-off curve which limits the amount of radiation reaching nontarget tissues. Iodine 125 seeds are affixed within gold mounts that provide much greater protection to both the surgeon and nontarget orbital tissues than does cobalt, which is impregnated into lead shields molded to fit the scleral surface.

Approximately 50% of patients receiving cobalt 60 plaques have developed radiation-induced complications including retinopathy, vitreous hemorrhage, optic nerve necrosis, and cataracts. Most centers now use iodine 125 plaques instead of cobalt 60. Even though iodine 125 has no greater tumoricidal property than cobalt 60, it induces fewer ocular complications.

Proton beam radiation is gaining favor as a treatment for choroidal melanomas (Char et al. 1982; Gragoudas et al. 1982). Linear accelerators deliver radiation in the form of heavily charged particles, either protons or helium ions. Such teletherapy is available only in Boston and San Francisco. The area of the choroidal melanoma to be treated is generally marked with transillumination and tantalum clips. Radiation is given over several sessions. The Bragg effect describes the significant advantage of these particles over gamma radiation. Namely, when these charged particles penetrate tumor tissue, their energy is not transferred gradually as with gamma rays; instead, they release sudden large bursts of energy on impact with the tumor. As long as the nontarget tissue is shielded, the immediate release of energy theoretically limits the effects of the particles to the tumor itself. Cataracts are the most common post-treatment complication.

Photocoagulation is of limited efficacy in the treatment of choroidal melanoma (Lund 1966). Several studies have proven that incident light does not penetrate deeply enough into the tumor to destroy it. Additionally, preretinal membranes and macular degeneration may occur.

Hyperthermia induced by either microwave or ultrasound may damage tumor cells (Finger et al. 1984). In combination with radiation, there appears to be a synergistic effect.

Photosensitive hematoporphyrin derivatives injected prior to laser photoirradiation have never been documented to totally arrest a choroidal melanoma. Because hematoporphyrin derivatives are distributed throughout the entire body, patients cannot be exposed to the sun for at least four to six weeks after each treatment.

Eye wall resections of small choroidal melanomas are technically feasible but exceedingly difficult (Peyman and Raichand 1978). Cytologically proven melanomas have been completely excised by this method. Ciliary body melanomas, if small, may be removed via an iridocyclectomy. Such local surgery is often associated with significant postoperative visual morbidity from induced astigmatism, cataract formation, and retinal dysfunction secondary to vitreous loss.

Enucleation is generally reserved for large melanomas that do not respond to radiation therapy, or for melanoma arising in a blind eye. Enucleation should be carried out with as little trauma as possible to avoid dislodging tumor cells into the blood stream. Some centers administer 20 Gy of external-beam radiation to the diseased eye prior to enucleation.

Exenteration is reserved for cases of large extraocular extension of melanoma (Kersten et al. 1985). If there are only small focal episcleral extensions of tumor, exenteration can be avoided by suturing Tenon's capsule and adjacent orbital soft tissue over the nodule. For small anterior episcleral extensions beneath the conjunctiva, the conjunctiva surrounding the nodule is removed with the globe.

Chemotherapy is reserved for cases of metastatic melanoma.

RESULTS AND PROGNOSIS

McLean and coworkers evaluated 16 different risk factors and found that seven correlated with outcome (McLean, Foster, and Zimmerman 1977; McLean, Foster, and Zimmerman 1982). These factors are cell type, pigmentation, largest dimension, degree of scleral invasion, mitotic activity, location of anterior margin of the tumor (the farther anterior, the worse the prognosis), and optic nerve invasion.

Traditionally, enucleation has been the procedure of choice for treating choroidal melanoma. Zimmerman (Zimmerman and McLean 1979), however, has hypothesized that enucleation may push malignant melanoma cells into large tumor-associated vascular lumen and into the systemic bloodstream. Two findings support this argument: the general absence of metastases in patients at the time of diagnosis and the development of distant metastases in many patients 18 to 24 months after enucleation. Niederkorn (1984), with the aid of a mouse ocular melanoma model, has identified other factors possibly involved in the establishment of metastases. His studies show that ocular manipulations and traumatic enucleations increase the numbers of metastases in animals with suppressed natural killer cells and T-lymphocytes. Although immunosurveillant cells may not completely suppress primary tumor growth, they may prevent micrometastases. It is hypothesized that natural killer cells and T-lymphocytes become sensitized to the primary tumor and, after having gained access to the systemic circulation, suppress metastatic spread. Enucleation is thought to lead to suppressed sensitization of these cells and a drop in their levels, which allows the establishment of metastases.

Randomized case control studies are under way to assess the optimal treatment of choroidal melanomas. The Collaborative Ocular Melanoma Study (COMS), under the support of the National Eye Institute, is a multicenter controlled study (Straatsma et al. 1988). The study consists of two randomized trials and one prospective observational study. The first trial studies patients with choroidal melanomas 3 mm to 8 mm in height and up to 16 mm in largest basal diameter. These patients are randomly assigned to treatment by ^{125}I plaque irradiation or enucleation. The second randomized trial is for patients with tumors greater than 8 mm in height or 16 mm in largest basal diameter. These patients are randomly assigned to treatment by enucleation or enucleation preceded by 20 Gy of external beam radiation in five divided doses. The prospective study is for choroidal melanomas 1 mm to 3 mm in height and at least 5 mm in largest basal diameter. These patients are being treated according to the preferences of the treating ophthalmologist and the patient.

ORBITAL TUMORS

LACRIMAL GLAND

Benign and malignant lacrimal gland tumors constitute between 10% and 15% of biopsied orbital lesions (Henderson and Farrow 1980). Inflammatory lesions and lymphoid tumors are equally as common as epithelial tumors.

The clinical history (duration and symptoms), the presence or absence of radiographically demonstrable bone changes, and the contour of the lesion constitute the three most important factors in evaluating lacrimal tumors.

EPITHELIAL TUMORS

Benign mixed tumors account for 50% of epithelial lacrimal gland tumors (Font and Gamel 1978). The classic history is of a painless, slowly developing lacrimal gland mass (Stewart, Krohel, and Wright 1979). It is generally well-tolerated and rarely produces diplopia or visual deterioration. The globe is generally proptotic and displaced downward and inward. The lateral aspect of the lid is full and may be slightly ptotic. Palpation of the supertemporal orbit reveals a firm, smooth mass; CT scan reveals a rounded, ovoid lesion. Longstanding cases may cause bone erosion of the supertemporal orbit.

The gross pathology of the benign mixed tumor is of an encapsulated tumor containing bosselations. Histology reveals a mixture of epithelial and mesenchymal elements. The epithelioid units are organized into ducts. The surrounding stroma results from metaplasia of epithelial cells into myxoid tissue, cartilage, and, rarely, bone. Management is surgical excision of the entire lesion within its capsule via a lateral orbitotomy. Excision through the lid or rupture of the capsule and piecemeal delivery entail a high recurrence rate. Malignant degeneration of recurrent tumors may occur, although the survival rate at 15 years follow-up is almost 100%.

Adenoid cystic carcinoma arising *de novo* makes up 25% to 30% of epithelial lacrimal gland tumors (Font and Gamel 1980; Lee et al. 1985). In contrast to benign mixed tumors, this disease affects women somewhat more frequently than men. The average age at diagnosis is 39 years, but it may occur within the first two decades and even in the seventh decade of life. Patients complain of numbness, pain, and headaches. Ptosis, proptosis, and diplopia develop a short time after the onset of pain; CT scanning reveals a globular, rounded lesion with more irregular and serrated edges than a benign mixed lesion (Jakobiec et al. 1982). The bone changes are destructive or sclerotic and contrast with the rather regular, corticated pressure indentations found in benign mixed tumors. This highly aggressive tumor has a propensity to infiltrate nerve and muscle. In suspected cases, a biopsy through the lid is recommended (Jakobiec 1980). Once definite diagnosis is made on permanent sections, radical surgery is recommended. Because of poor results with exenteration [20% survival at 10 years (Gamel and Font 1982)], radical exenteration or

orbitectomy is recommended in which the lateral and superior walls of the orbit are removed to dura with the orbital soft tissues. Such surgery requires the collaboration of a head and neck surgeon and neurosurgeon due to exposure of the brain and necessity for large skin flaps. Adjuvant radiotherapy is recommended by some clinicians. No data are available on long-term survival rates of radical orbitectomy.

Malignant mixed tumors account for 13% of epithelial tumors (Font and Gamel 1978). A malignant mixed tumor is a benign mixed tumor that has undergone malignant degeneration. The average age of patients with adenoid cystic carcinoma developing in a benign mixed is only slightly older than of those with a pure benign mixed (43 vs. 39 years), but is older in those with adenocarcinoma (52). If malignant degeneration occurs within a recurrent benign mixed tumor, the patient usually becomes symptomatic within six months of the prior debulking. In all cases of suspected malignant mixed tumor, the preauricular and cervical lymph nodes should be palpated to rule out regional metastases. Once the diagnosis is made, radical orbitectomy with parotid and cervical lymph node dissection is the treatment of choice (Jakobiec 1982). If, however, the patient has regional metastases, localized radiotherapy after a debulking procedure is all that can be recommended. Once a malignant degeneration occurs, the long-term outlook is extremely poor, with death usually ensuing within three years. Malignant mixed tumors have a poorer prognosis than adenoid cystic types because of the former's tendency for lymphogenous dissemination and pulmonary metastases.

Less than 10% of epithelial lacrimal gland lesions are adenocarcinomas arising *de novo* (Font and Gamel 1978). The median age at diagnosis is 56 years, but the ages range from 18 to 80. The clinical and radiologic findings are similar to those with adenoid cystic carcinoma. On rare occasions, sebaceous differentiation may occur. For patients free of metastatic disease, radical orbitectomy with regional lymph node dissection may offer the best prognosis, but as yet no studies substantiate this claim.

LYMPHOID TUMORS

As many as one-fourth to one-third of orbital lymphoid tumors arise within the lacrimal gland (Jakobiec, McLean, and Font 1979). Patients are symptomatic for an average of six months or less. They present with painless swelling of the lateral eyelid and displacement of the globe (Knowles and Jakobiec 1980). CT scan reveals oblong molding of the lesion to sclera and bone (Yeo et al. 1982). The tumors frequently involve the palpebral lobe of the lacrimal gland. Biopsy and tissue marker studies are recommended.

VASCULAR TUMORS

Cavernous hemangioma is a benign, well-encapsulated orbital lesion (Harris and Jakobiec 1978). The average

age of onset is 42 years, with a range of 18 to 67 years. Females predominate over males. The typical history is slowly progressive proptosis, and minimal decrease in visual acuity. The tumor is generally well-tolerated; even with high degrees of proptosis, the cornea is not exposed because of the ability of the lids to stretch. Fundus examination may reveal optic nerve head swelling and choroidal striae. Visual field examination may reveal enlargement of the blind spot or field compression. The tumor grows rapidly during pregnancy. CT scan reveals a well-circumscribed lesion, usually within the muscle cone. The tumor enhances with contrast about 20 minutes following infusion. Surgery is recommended when the lesion impairs vision or disturbs motility, or when cosmesis concerns the patient. At surgery, an intensely violet-colored tumor is found. The surgeon must be particularly careful when excising apical lesions because of potential damage to the optic nerve, orbital nerves, and ocular muscles.

Hemangiopericytomas differ from cavernous hemangiomas in several ways (Jakobiec, Howard, Jones 1974), with a shorter duration of symptoms, greater evidence of orbital and conjunctival vascular congestion, and a lack of lid accommodation. The most frequent complaints are proptosis, pain, diplopia, and decreased visual acuity (Croxatto and Font 1982). On CT scan, hemangiopericytomas appear as well-encapsulated tumors displaying dramatic enhancement. On MR the tumors are hyperintense to brain on T2 weighted images. Surgery is indicated when the tumor is suspected because the lesion is potentially malignant. At surgery, hemangiopericytomas are dark blue to violet. Complete local excision of the tumor within its pseudocapsule offers the best management. When the tumor is incompletely excised, most clinicians will follow the patient, provided he or she retains ocular function. If the lesion has caused visual compromise, whether recurrent or incompletely excised at the first surgery, an exenteration should be performed. Local recurrent lesions are capable of invading the brain.

A varix is a benign orbital tumor characterized by intermittency of proptosis, variation of proptosis depending upon head position, and worsening of proptosis during Valsalva (Krohel and Wright 1979). A thrombosis may develop within a varix and spontaneous orbital hemorrhage may occur if the variceal wall ruptures. Venography demonstrates an enlarged ophthalmic vein (Handa and Mori 1968). Conservative management is recommended for low grades of proptosis because these lesions bleed profusely at surgery if their origins are not ligated.

Other vascular lesions include venous angiomas, vascular leiomyoma, and arteriovenous malformations.

MESENCHYMAL TUMORS

Rhabdomyosarcoma is the most common primary orbital malignancy of childhood (Ashton and Morgan 1965; Kirk and Zimmerman 1969; Porterfield and Zimmerman 1962). This tumor affects children with an average age at presen-

tation of 7 years; it affects boys more commonly than girls and often presents with a fulminant proptosis. Rhabdomyosarcomas have been diagnosed soon after birth. In addition to proptosis of rapid onset, the eyelids may be swollen and the conjunctiva chemotic. CT scan documents a well-defined, circumscribed mass which enhances with contrast. Bone destruction and invasion of the brain or adjacent sinuses may occur.

Once the clinical suspicion is high, a biopsy should be performed without delay (Knowles, Jakobiec, and Potter 1976). For anterior lesions, a percutaneous biopsy through the lid is performed. Once a definitive diagnosis is made, radiotherapy of 50 Gy to 60 Gy is delivered through combined lateral and anterior portals. Adjuvant chemotherapy using vincristine and Actinomycin D is administered. A metastatic workup is also undertaken.

Fibrous histiocytoma presents with signs and symptoms similar to hemangiopericytomas (Jakobiec and Howard et al. 1974). On the average patients suffer from a 2.5-year history of proptosis, orbital congestion, conjunctival chemosis, and visual acuity defects. The patients range in age from 4 to 85 years, with a median of 43 (Font and Hidayat 1982). A CT scan will reveal a well-circumscribed tumor, most frequently located in the superior orbit. Complete surgical excision is the recommended treatment for fibrous histiocytomas. If the first surgery incompletely excises the tumor and ocular function remains intact, it is best to follow the patient; if a recurrence develops, exenteration should be performed. For those rare cases of malignant fibrous histiocytoma discovered at the first surgery (Rodrigues, Furgiuele, and Weinreb 1977), exenteration should be performed provided there is no widespread tumor dissemination. Radiotherapy is not effective in this disease.

NERVE SHEATH TUMORS

Approximately 4% of orbital tumors are of peripheral nerve sheath origin (Jakobiec and Jones 1979). Plexiform neurofibromas account for one-half of all nerve sheath tumors, Schwannomas one-quarter, and isolated neurofibromas one-quarter.

Most peripheral nerve tumors arise from sensory nerves, which accounts for the associated pain.

Plexiform neurofibromas are pathognomonic of von Recklinghausen's disease. This tumor arises in childhood and is associated with *cafe au lait* spots, melanomas, meningiomas, optic nerve gliomas, and thyroid carcinomas. Von Recklinghausen's disease is inherited in an autosomal dominant pattern. Patients typically present with redundancy of the upper eyelid, enlarged corneal nerves, iris nodules, and an enlarged orbit (Woog et al. 1982). The sphenoid bone may be absent, causing pulsatile exophthalmos. The globe is proptotic, motility may be disturbed, and the patient may complain of pain. Orbital neurofibromas should be excised if vision or motility is impaired. The CO_2 laser may be useful in such an operation. Radiation therapy plays no role in this disease. Malignant degeneration of this tumor is extremely rare (Jakobiec, Font, and Zimmerman 1985), although von Recklinghausen patients are at a greater risk of developing malignant nerve sheath tumors than the general population (Harkin and Reed 1969).

Schwannomas present as slowly progressive, well-tolerated proptosis (Rootman, Goldberg, and Robertson 1982), often with concurrent motility disturbance and pain. Optic nerve dysfunction may occur if the lesion approximates the optic nerve. A well-circumscribed lesion is revealed by CT scan; MR imaging shows a lesion hypointensive to brain on T1 weighted images and hyperintensive on T2 weighted images. Surgery is recommended if vision is impaired or motility disturbed. Schwannomas are readily removed from the orbit, but may recur if incompletely excised. Schwannomas almost never undergo malignant degeneration (Schatz 1971).

Lymphoid tumors of the orbit typically afflict individuals in their late 50s or 60s (Jakobiec 1982; Jakobiec, McLean, and Font 1979; Knowles et al. 1976). Patients present with painless, progressive proptosis, motility disturbances, and, rarely, visual deterioration. Inflammatory signs such as erythema or chemosis are not present. Examination may reveal fullness of the lids and orbit; the lesions feels firm and rubbery, but not rock-hard. A CT scan documents a lesion typically involving the superior orbit, which is molded to contiguous structures. Biopsy is the recommended intervention. At surgery, the lesions are typically salmon-colored. Histologically, they are classified as either benign reactive hyperplasia, atypical hyperplasia, or malignant (Jakobiec and Font 1986).

All patients with orbital lymphoid tumors should undergo a systemic workup. A thorough physical examination, chest x-ray, CBC count, serum protein electrophoresis (SPEP), bone and liver scan, and bone marrow biopsy are recommended. Patients with benign reactive hyperplasia have a 20% incidence of concomitant or systemic disease within five years, those with atypical lymphoid hyperplasias have a 40% incidence, and those with malignant a 60% incidence (Jakobiec, McLean, and Font 1979).

If the systemic workup is unremarkable, local orbital radiotherapy with shielding of the eyeball is recommended (Jereb et al. 1984; Kennerdell, Johnson, and Deutsch 1979; Kim and Fayos 1976; Sergott, Glaser, and Charyulu 1981). The recommended dose is 15 Gy to 20 Gy administered to benign tumors and 20 Gy to 30 Gy to malignant tumors. Systemic chemotherapy is not administered. If systemic lymphoma is diagnosed, chemotherapy alone is given.

REFERENCES

Abramson, D.H. 1982. Retinoblastoma: diagnosis and management. *Cancer* 32:130-40.

Abramson, D.H. 1988. The diagnosis of retinoblastoma. *Bull. N.Y. Acad. Med.* 64:283-17.

Abramson, D.H., and Ellsworth, R.M. 1980. The surgical management of retinoblastoma. *Ophthalmol. Surg.* 11:596-98.

Abramson, D.H.; Ellsworth, R.M.; and Rozakis, G.W. 1982. Cryotherapy for retinoblastoma. *Arch. Ophthalmol.* 100: 1253-56.

Abramson, D.H.; Jereb, B.; and Ellsworth, R.M. et al. 1981. External beam radiation for retinoblastoma. *Bull. N.Y. Acad. Med.* 57:787-803.

Acker, D.W., and Helwig, E.B. 1967. Rhinophyma with carcinoma. *Arch. Dermatol.* 95:250-54.

Albert, D.M.; Rubinstein, R.A.; and Scheie, H.G. 1967. Tumor metastasis to the eye I: incidence in 213 adult patients with generalized malignancy. *Am. J. Ophthalmol.* 63:723-26.

Apple, D.J., and Rabb, M.F. 1985. *Ocular pathology: clinical applications and self-assessment.* 3rd ed. pp. 444-86. St. Louis: C.V. Mosby.

Ashton, N., and Morgan, G. 1965. Embryonal sarcoma and embryonal rhabdomyosarcoma of the orbit. *J. Clin. Pathol.* 18:699-714.

Aurora, A.L., and Blodi, F.C. 1970. Lesions of the eyelids: a clinicopathologic study. *Surv. Ophthalmol.* 15:94-104.

Balmer, A., and Gaillard, C. 1983. *Retinoblastoma: diagnosis and treatment in turning points in cataract formation syndromes and retinoblastoma.* pp. 36-96. Basel: Karger.

Barr, C.C.; McLean, I.W.; and Zimmerman, L.E. 1981. Uveal melanoma in children and adolescents. *Arch. Ophthalmol.* 99:2133-36.

Beahrs, O.H.; and Myers, M.H. 1983. *Manual for staging of cancer.* 3rd ed. pp. 197-202. Philadelphia: J.B. Lippincott.

Bean, W.B. 1958a. Dyschondroplasia and hemangiomata (Maffucci's syndrome). *Arch. Intern. Med.* 102:544-50.

Bean, W.B. 1958b. *Vascular spiders and related lesions of the skin.* Springfield: Charles C. Thomas.

Bellet, R.E.; Shields, J.A.; and Soll, D.B. et al. 1980. Primary choroidal and cutaneous melanomas occurring in a patient with the B-K mole syndrome phenotype. *Am. J. Ophthalmol.* 89:567-70.

Benedict, W.F.; Murphree, A.L.; and Banerjee, A. et al. 1983. Patient with chromosome deletion: evidence that the retinoblastoma gene is a recessive cancer gene. *Science* 219: 973-75.

Blodi, F. 1973. Squamous cell carcinoma of conjunctiva. *Doc. Ophthalmol.* 34:93-108.

Boniuk, M., and Zimmerman, L.E. 1963. Eyelid tumors with reference to lesions confused with squamous cell carcinoma II: inverted follicular keratosis. *Arch. Ophthalmol.* 69:698-707.

Boniuk, M., and Zimmerman, L.E. 1968. Sebaceous gland carcinoma of the eyelid, eyebrow, caruncle, and orbit. *Trans. Am. Acad. Ophthalmol. Otolaryngol.* 72:619-42.

Boniuk, M., and Zimmerman, L.E. 1967. Eyelid tumors with reference to lesions confused with squamous cell carcinoma III: keratoacanthoma. *Arch. Ophthalmol.* 77:29-40.

Bullock, J.D., and Yanes, B. 1980. Ophthalmic manifestations of metastatic breast cancer. *Ophthalmology* 87:961-73.

Burnier, M. Jr.; McLean, I.W.; and Zimmerman, L.E. et al. 1990. Retinoblastoma: the relationship of proliferating cells to blood vessels. *Invest. Ophthalmol. Vis. Sci.* 31:2037-40.

Cavenee, W.K.; Murphree, A.L.; and Shull, M.M. 1986. Prediction of familial predisposition to retinoblastoma. *N. Engl. J. Med.* 19:1201-1207.

Callender, G.R. 1931. Malignant melanotic tumors of the eye: a study of histologic types in 111 cases. *Trans. Am. Acad. Ophthalmol. Otolaryngol.* 36:131-42.

Char, D.H. et al. 1982. Helium ion therapy for choroidal melanoma. *Arch. Ophthalmol.* 100:935-40.

Charles, N. 1989. Personal correspondence.

Croxatto, J.O., and Font, R.L. 1982. Hemangiopericytoma of the orbit: a clinicopathologic study of 30 cases. *Hum. Pathol.* 13:210-18.

Davidorf, F.H.; Letson, A.D.; and Weiss, E.T. et al. 1983. Incidence of misdiagnosed and unsuspected choroidal melanomas: a 50-year experience. *Arch. Ophthalmol.* 101:410-12.

Doxanas, M.T., and Green, W.R. 1979. Adult lid lesions: basal cell carcinoma. Presented at the 38th meeting of the Wilmer Residents' Association. Baltimore, Md. April 1979.

Ellsworth, R.M. 1969. The practical management of retinoblastoma. *Trans. Am. Ophthalmol. Soc.* 67:462-34.

Farmer, E.R., and Helwig, E.B. 1980. Metastatic basal cell carcinoma: a clinicopathologic study of seventeen cases. *Cancer* 46:748-57.

Ferry, A.P. 1964. Lesions mistaken for malignant melanoma of the posterior uvea: a clinicopathologic analysis of 100 cases with ophthalmoscopically visible lesions. *Arch. Ophthalmol.* 72:463-69.

Fine, B.S., and Yanoff, M. 1979. *Ocular pathology: a text and atlas.* 2nd ed. Philadelphia: Harper & Row.

Finger, P.T.; Packer, S.; and Svitra, P.P. et al. 1984. Hyperthermic treatment of intraocular tumors. *Arch. Ophthalmol.* 102:1477-81.

Flexner, S. 1891. A peculiar glioma (neuroepithelioma?) of the retina. *Bull. Johns Hopkins Hosp.* 2:115

Folberg, R.; McLean, I.W.; and Zimmerman, L.E. 1985. Primary acquired melanosis of the conjunctiva. *Hum. Pathol.* 16:129-35.

Folberg, R.; McLean, I.W.; and Zimmerman L.E. 1984. Conjunctival melanosis and melanoma. *Ophthalmology* 91:673-78.

Folberg, R.; McLean, I.W.; and Zimmerman, L.E. 1985. Malignant melanoma of the conjunctiva. *Hum. Pathol.* 16:136-43.

Font, R.L., and Hidayat, A.A. 1982. Fibrous histiocytoma of the orbit: a clinicopathologic study of 150 cases. *Hum. Pathol.* 13:199-209.

Font, R.L. 1985. Eyelids and lacrimal drainage system. In Spencer, W.H. ed. *Ophthalmic pathology: an atlas and textbook.* vol 3. pp. 2141-2336. Philadelphia: W.B. Saunders.

Font, R.L., and Gamel, J.W. 1980. Adenoid cystic carcinoma of the lacrimal gland: a clinicopathologic study of 79 cases. In Nicholson, D.H. ed. *Ocular pathology update.* pp. 277-83. New York: Masson Publishing.

Font, R.L., and Gamel, J.W. 1978. Epithelial tumors of the lacrimal gland: an analysis of 265 cases. In Jakobiec, F.A. ed. *Ocular and adnexal tumors.* pp. 787-805. Birmingham: Aesculapius Publishing Co.

Fraunfelder, F.T. et al. 1980. Cryosurgery for the malignancies of the eyelid. *Ophthalmology* 87:461-65.

Fraunfelder, F.T., and Roy, F.H. 1980. *Current ocular therapy.* Philadelphia: W.B. Saunders.

Fredrickson, D.S.; Levy, R.I.; and Lees, R.S. 1967. Fat transport in lipoproteins: an integrated approach to mechanisms and disorders. *N. Engl. J. Med.* 276:34-44.

Frenkel, M., and Klein, H.Z. 1966. Malignant melanoma of the choroid in pregnancy. *Am. J. Ophthalmol.* 62:910-13.

Friend, S.H.; Bernards, R.; and Rogelj, S. et al. 1986. A human DNA segment with properties of the gene that predisposes to retinoblastoma and osteosarcoma. *Nature* 323:643-46.

Gaasterland, D.E.; Rodrigues, M.M.; and Moshell, A.N. 1982. Ocular involvement in xeroderma pigmentosa. *Ophthalmology* 89:980-86.

Gamel, J.W., and Font, R.L. 1982. Adenoid cystic carcinoma of the lacrimal gland: the clinical significance of a basaloid histologic pattern. *Hum. Pathol.* 13:219-25.

Gass, J.D.M. 1977. Problems in the differential diagnosis of choroidal nevi and malignant melanomas: The XXXIII Edward Jackson Memorial Lecture. *Am. J. Ophthalmol.* 83:299-323.

Gass, J.D.M. 1972. Fluorescein angiography: an aid in the differential diagnosis of intraocular tumors. *Int. Ophthalmol. Clin.* 12:85.

Gilbert, F. 1986. Retinoblastoma and cancer genetics. *N. Engl. J. Med.* 314:1248-50.

Gladstein, A.H. 1978. Efficacy, simplicity, and safety of x-ray therapy of basal cell carcinomas on periocular skin. *J. Dermatol. Surg. Oncol.* 4:586-93.

Goldenhar, M. 1952. Associations malformatives de l'oeil et de l'orielle, en particulier le syndrome epibulbaire — appendices auriculaires — fistula auris congenita et ses relations avec la dysostose mandibulofaciale. *J. Genet. Hum.* 1:243-82.

Gorlin, R.J., and Goltz, R.W. 1960. Multiple nevoid basal cell epithelioma, jaw cysts, and bifid rib: a syndrome. *N. Engl. J. Med.* 262:908-12.

Gragoudas, E.S.; Goitin, M.; and Verhey, L. et al. 1982. Proton-beam irradiation of uveal melanomas: results of 5 1/2-year study. *Arch. Ophthalmol.* 100:928-34.

Handa, H., and Mori, K. 1968. Large varix of the superior ophthalmic vein: demonstration by angular phlebography and removal by electrically induced thrombosis — case report. *J. Neurosurg.* 29:202-205.

Harkin, J., and Reed, R. 1969. Tumors of the peripheral nervous system. In *Atlas of tumor pathology.* ser. 2, fas. 3. Washington, DC: Armed Forces Institute of Pathology.

Harris, G.J., and Jakobiec, F.A. 1978. Cavernous hemangioma of the orbit: a clinicopathologic analysis of sixty-six cases. In Jakobiec, F.A. ed. *Ocular and adnexal tumors.* pp. 741-81. Birmingham: Aesculapius Publishing Co.

Helmick, E., and Pringle, R. 1956. Oculocutaneous melanosis or nevus of Ota. *Arch. Ophthalmol.* 56:833-38.

Henderson, J.W., and Farrow, G.M. 1980. Primary malignant mixed tumors of the lacrimal gland. *Ophthalmology* 87:466-75.

Henkind, P. 1978. Conjunctival melanocytic lesions: natural history. In Jakobiec, F.A. ed. *Ocular and adnexal tumors.* pp. 572-82. Birmingham: Aesculapius Publishing Co.

Hiles, D.A., and Pilchard, W.A. 1971. Corticosteroid control of neonatal hemangiomas of the orbit and ocular adnexa. *Am. J. Ophthalmol.* 71:1003-1008.

Hornblass, A., and Stevano, J.A. 1981. Pigmented basal cell carcinomas of the eyelids. *Am. J. Ophthalmol.* 92:193-97.

Huang, H. J-S.; Lee J-K.; and Shew J-Y. et al. 1988. Suppression of the neoplastic phenotype by replacement of the RB gene in human cancer cells. *Science* 242:1563-66.

Iliff, W.; Marback, R.; and Green, R. 1975. Invasive squamous cell carcinoma of the conjunctiva. *Arch. Ophthalmol.* 93:119-22.

Iwamoto, T., and Jakobiec, F.A. 1979. Ultrastructural comparison of capillary and cavernous hemangioma of the orbit. *Arch. Ophthalmol.* 97:1144-53.

Jakobiec, F.A.; Coleman, D.J.; and Chattock, A. 1979. Ultrasonically guided needle biopsy and cytologic diagnosis of solid intraocular tumors. *Ophthalmology* 86:1662-78.

Jakobiec, F.A., and Levinson, A.W. 1985. Choroidal melanoma: etiology and diagnosis. *Am. Acad. Ophthalmol.* vol. 3, mod. 5.

Jakobiec, F.A. 1982. Orbital inflammations and lymphoid tumors. pp. 52-85. In *Proc. N. Orleans Acad. Med.*

Jakobiec, F.A. 1980. Lacrimal gland tumors. In Fraunfelder, F. ed. *Current ocular therapy.* pp. 492-94. St. Louis: C.V. Mosby.

Jakobiec, F.A. 1982. Tumors of the lacrimal gland and lacrimal sac. In *Symposium on Diseases and Surgery of the Lids, Lacrimal Apparatus, and Orbit: transactions of the New Orleans Academy of Ophthalmology.* pp. 190-202. St. Louis: C.V. Mosby.

Jakobiec, F.A.; Folberg, R.; and Iwamoto, T. 1989. Clinicopathologic characteristics of premalignant and malignant melanocytic lesions of the conjunctiva. *Ophthalmology* 96: 147-66.

Jakobiec, F.A.; Font, R.L.; and Zimmerman, L.E. 1985. Malignant peripheral nerve sheath tumors of the orbit: a clinicopathologic study of eight cases. *Trans. Am. Ophthalmol. Soc.* 83:17-35.

Jakobiec, F.A., and Jones, I.S. 1979. Neurogenic tumors. In Jones, I.S., and Jakobiec, F.A. eds. *Diseases of the orbit.* pp. 371-416. Hagerstown: Harper & Row.

Jakobiec, F.A.; Howard, G.; and Jones, I.S. et al. 1974a. Fibrous histiocytoma of the orbit. *Am. J. Ophthalmol.* 77:333-45.

Jakobiec, F.A.; Howard, G.; and Jones, I.S. et al. 1974b. Hemangiopericytoma of the orbit. *Am. J. Ophthalmol.* 78:816-34.

Jakobiec, F.A.; Yeo, J.H.; and Trokel, S.L. et al. 1982. Combined clinical and computed tomographic diagnosis of lacrimal fossa lesions. *Am. J. Ophthalmol.* 94:785-807.

Jakobiec, F.A.; McLean, I.; and Font, R. 1979. Clinicopathologic characteristics of orbital lymphoid hyperplasia. *Ophthalmology* 86:948-66.

Jakobiec, F.A. et al. 1988: Cryotherapy for conjunctival PAM and melanoma. *Ophthalmology* 95:1058-69.

Jakobiec, F.A., and Font, R.L. 1986. Orbital diseases. In Spencer, W. ed. *Ophthalmic pathology: an atlas and textbook.* pp. 2663-2711. Philadelphia: W.B. Saunders.

Jakobiec, F.A.; Tso, M.O.M.; and Zimmerman, L.E. et al. 1977. Retinoblastoma and intracranial malignancy. *Cancer* 39:2048-58.

Jakobiec, F.A. ed. 1978. *Ocular and adnexal tumors.* Birmingham: Aesculapius Publishing Co.

Jensen, R.D., and Miller, R.W. 1971. Retinoblastoma: epidemiologic characteristics. *N. Engl. J. Med.* 285:307-11.

Jereb, B.; Lee, H.; Jakobiec, F.A. et al. 1984. Radiation treatment of conjunctival and orbital lymphoid tumors. *Int. J. Radiat. Oncol. Biol. Phys.* 10:1013-19.

Kasabach, H.H., and Merritt, K.K. 1940. Capillary hemangioma with extensive purpura: report of a case. *Am. J. Dis. Child.* 59:1063-70.

Kaufman, H.E. 1988. *The cornea.* New York: Churchill Livingston.

Keeney, A.H.; Waddell, W.J.; and Perrayt, T.C. 1982. Carcinogenesis and nicotine in malignant melanoma of the choroid. *Trans. Am. Ophthalmol. Soc.* 80:131-42.

Kennerdell, J.S.; Johnson, B.L.; and Deutsch, M. 1979. Radiation treatment of orbital lymphoid hyperplasia. *Ophthalmology* 86:942-47.

Kersten, R.C.; Tse, D.; and Anderson, R.L. et al. 1985. Role of orbital exenteration in malignant melanoma with extrascleral extension. *Ophthalmology* 92:436-43.

Kim, Y.H., and Fayos, J.V. 1976. Primary orbital lymphoma: a radiotherapeutic experience. *Int. J. Radiat. Oncol. Biol. Phys.* 1:1099-1105.

Kirk, R.C., and Zimmerman, L.E. 1969. Rhabdomyosarcoma of the orbit. *Arch. Ophthalmol.* 81:559-64.

Knowles, D.M., and Jakobiec, F.A. 1980. Orbital lymphoid neoplasms: a clinicopathologic study of 60 cases. *Cancer* 46:576-89.

Knowles, D.M.; Jakobiec, F.A.; and Potter, G. et al. 1976. Ophthalmic striated muscle neoplasms: a clinicopathologic review. *Surv. Ophthalmol.* 21:219-61.

Knudson, A.G. Jr.; Hethcote, H.W.; and Brown, B.W. 1975. Mutation and childhood cancer: a probabilistic model for the incidence of retinoblastoma. *Proc. Natl. Acad. Sci. USA* 71:5116-20.

Krohel, G.B., and Wright, J.E. 1979. Orbital hemorrhage. *Am. J. Ophthalmol.* 88:254-58.

Kushner, B.J. 1981. Intralesional corticosteroid injection for infantile adnexal hemangioma. *Am. J. Ophthalmol.* 93:496-508.

Kwitko, M.L.; Boniuk, M.; and Zimmerman, L.E. 1963. Eyelid tumors with reference to lesions confused with squamous cell carcinoma I: incidence and errors in diagnosis. *Arch. Ophthalmol.* 69:693-97.

Lass, J.H.; Grove, A.S.; and Papale, J.J. et al. 1983. Detection of human papillomavirus DNA sequences in conjunctival papilloma. *Am. J. Ophthalmol.* 96:670-74.

Lee, D.A.; Campbell, R.J.; and Waller, R.R. et al. 1985. A clinicopathologic study of primary adenoid cystic carcinoma of the lacrimal gland. *Ophthalmology* 92:128-34.

Lee, W-H.; Bookstein, R.; and Hong, F., et al. 1987. Human retinoblastoma susceptibility gene: cloning, identification, and sequence. *Science* 235:1394-99.

Lever, W.F., and Schaumburg-Lever, G. 1975. *Histopathology of the skin.* 5th ed. Philadelphia: J.B. Lippincott.

Lisman, R.P.; Jakobiec, F.A.; and Small, P. 1989. Sebaceous carcinoma of the eyelids: the role of adjunctive cryotherapy in the management of conjunctival pagetoid spread. *Ophthalmology* 96:1021-26.

Lund, O. 1966. Changes in choroidal tumors after light coagulation (and diathermy coagulation): a histopathological investigation of 43 cases. *Arch. Ophthalmol.* 75:458-66.

Margileth, A.M., and Museles, M. 1965. Current concepts in diagnosis and management of congenital cutaneous hemangiomas. *Pediatrics* 36:410-16.

McGavic, J. 1942. Intraepithelial epithelioma of cornea and conjunctiva (Bowen's disease). *Am. J. Ophthalmol.* 25:167-76.

McLean, I.W.; Foster, W.D.; and Zimmerman, L.E. 1977. Prognostic factors in small malignant melanomas of choroid and ciliary body. *Arch. Ophthalmol.* 95:48-58.

McLean, I.W.; Foster, W.D.; and Zimmerman, L.E. 1982. Uveal melanoma: location, size, cell type, and enucleation as risk factors in metastasis. *Hum. Pathol.* 13:123-32.

McLean, I.W.; Zimmerman, L.E.; and Evans, R.M. 1978. Reappraisal of Callender's spindle A type of malignant melanoma of the choroid and ciliary body. *Am. J. Ophthalmol.* 86:557-64.

Meyer-Schwickerath, G. 1961. The preservation of vision by treatment of intraocular tumors with light coagulation. *Arch. Ophthalmol.* 66:458-66.

Middlekamp, J.N., and Munger, B.L. 1967. Ultrastructure and histogenesis of molluscum contagiosum. *J. Pediatr.* 64:888-905.

Minckler, D.; Font, R.L.; and Shields, J.A. 1978. Nonmelanoma ocular lesions with positive ^{32}P tests. In Jakobiec, F.A. ed. *Ocular and adnexal tumors.* pp. 245-56. Birmingham: Aesculapius Publishing Co.

Mohs, F.E. 1976. Chemosurgery for skin cancer: fixed tissue and fresh tissue techniques. *Arch. Dermatol.* 112:211-15.

Morgan, G. 1971. Diffuse infiltrating retinoblastoma. *Br. J. Ophthalmol.* 55:600-606.

Nicholson, D.H., and Norton, E.W. 1980. Diffuse infiltrating retinoblastoma. *Trans. Am. Ophthalmol. Soc.* 78:265-89.

Niederkorn, J.Y. 1984. Enucleation-induced metastasis of intraocular melanomas in mice. *Ophthalmology* 91:692-700.

Nik, N.D.; Glew, W.B.; and Zimmerman, L.E. 1982. Malignant melanoma of the choroid in the nevus of Ota of a black patient. *Arch. Ophthalmol.* 100:1641-43.

Oosterhuis, J.A.; Went, L.N.; and Lynch, H.T. 1982. Primary choroidal and cutaneous melanomas, bilateral choroidal melanomas, and familial occurrence of melanomas. *Br. J. Ophthalmol.* 66:230-33.

Ossoinig, K.C., and Blodi, F.C. 1974. Preoperative differential diagnosis of tumors with echography III: diagnosis of intraocular tumors. In Blodi, F.C. ed. *Current concepts in ophthalmology.* vol. 4. St Louis: C.V. Mosby.

Ossoinig, K.C., and Till, P. 1969. Methods and results of ultrasonography in diagnosing intraocular tumors. In Gitter, K.A.; Keeney, A.H.; and Sarin, L.K. et al. eds. *Ophthalmic ultrasound.* St Louis: C.V. Mosby.

Packer, S.; Rotman, M.; and Fairchild, R.G. et al. 1980. Irradiation of choroidal melanoma with iodine 125 ophthalmic plaque. *Arch. Ophthalmol.* 98:1453-57.

Parks, M.M., and Zimmerman, L.E. 1960. Retinoblastoma. *Clin. Proc. Child. Hosp. (Wash.)* 16:77-84.

Paul, E.V.; Parnell, B.L.; and Fraker, M. 1962. Prognosis of malignant melanomas of the choroid and ciliary body. *Int. Ophthalmol. Clin.* 2:387.

Peyman, G.A., and Raichand, M. 1978. Resection of choroidal melanoma. In Jakobiec, F.A. ed. *Ocular and adnexal tumors.* pp. 61-69. Birmingham: Aesculapius Publishing Co.

Pizzarello, L.D.; Jakobiec, F.A.; and Hofeldt, A.J. et al. 1978. Intralesional corticosteroid therapy of chalazia. *Am. J. Ophthalmol.* 85:818-21.

Pizzarello, L.D., and Jakobiec, F.A. 1978. Bowen's disease of the conjunctiva: a misnomer. In Jakobiec, F.A. ed. *Ocular and adnexal tumors.* chap. 39. Birmingham: Aesculapius Publishing Co.

Porterfield, J.F., and Zimmerman, L.E. 1962. Rhabdomyosarcoma of the orbit: a clinicopathologic study of 55 cases. *Virchows Arch.* 335(abstr):329-44.

Rao, N.A.; McLean, I.W.; and Zimmerman, L.E. 1978. Sebaceous carcinoma of the eyelid and caruncle: correlation of clinical pathologic features with prognosis. In Jakobiec, F.A. ed. *Ocular and adnexal tumors.* p. 461. Birmingham: Aesculapius Publishing Co.

Rao, N.A.; Hidayat, A.A.; and McLean, I.W. et al. 1982. Sebaceous gland carcinoma of the ocular adnexa: a clinicopathologic study of 104 cases with 5-year follow-up data. *Hum. Pathol.* 13:113-22.

Reese, A.B., and Ellsworth, R.M. 1963. The evaluations and current concept of retinoblastoma therapy. *Trans. Am. Acad. Ophthalmol. Otolaryngol.* 67:164-72.

Reese, A.B. 1976. *Tumors of the eye.* 3rd ed. New York: Harper & Row.

Robins, P. 1981. Chemosurgery: my 15 years experience. *J. Dermatol. Surg. Oncol.* 7:779-89.

Rodrigues, M.M.; Furgiuele, F.P.; and Weinreb, S. 1977. Malignant fibrous histiocytoma of the orbit. *Arch. Ophthalmol.* 95:2025-28.

Rootman, J. 1988. *Diseases of the orbit.* Philadelphia: J.B. Lippincott.

Rootman, J.; Goldberg, C.; and Robertson, W. 1982. Primary orbital Schwannomas. *Br. J. Ophthalmol.* 66:194-204.

Rotman, M.; Long, R.S.; and Packer, S. et al. 1977. Radiation therapy of choroidal melanoma. *Trans. Ophthalmol. Soc. UK* 97:431-35.

Sang, D.N., and Albert, D.M. 1977. Recent advances in the study of retinoblastoma. In Peyman G.A.; Apple, D.J.; and Sanders, D.R. eds. *Intraocular tumors.* pp. 285-329. New York: Appleton-Century-Crofts.

Schappert-Kimmijser, J.; Hemmes, G.D.; and Nijland, R. 1966. The heredity of retinoblastoma. *Ophthalmologica* 152:197-213.

Schatz, H. 1971. Benign orbital neurilemmoma: sarcomatous transformation in von Recklinghausen's disease. *Arch. Ophthalmol.* 86:268-74.

Schipper, J. 1980. Retinoblastoma: a medical and experimental study. Thesis, University of Utrecht. p. 144. April 29, 1980.

Schlernitzauer, D.A., and Font, R.L. 1976. Sebaceous gland carcinoma of the eyelid following radiation therapy for cavernous hemangioma of the face. *Arch. Ophthalmol.* 94:1523-25.

Scotto, J.; Fraumeni, J.F.; and Lee, J.A. 1976. Melanoma of the eye and other noncutaneous sites. *J. Natl. Cancer Inst.* 56:489-91.

Sergott, R.C.; Glaser, J.S.; and Charyulu, K. 1981. Radiotherapy for idiopathic inflammatory orbital pseudotumor. *Arch. Ophthalmol.* 99:853-56.

Shields, J.A., and Font, R.L. 1972. Melanocytoma of the choroid clinically simulating a malignant melanoma. *Arch. Ophthalmol.* 87:396-400.

Shields, J.A. 1983. *Diagnosis and management of intraocular tumors.* St. Louis: C.V. Mosby.

Shields, J.A.; McDonald, P.R.; and Leonard, B.C. et al. 1977. The diagnosis of uveal malignant melanomas in eyes with opaque media. *Am. J. Ophthalmol.* 83:95-105.

Shields, J.A. 1983. *Diagnosis and management of intraocular tumors.* pp. 151-254. St Louis: C.V. Mosby.

Shields, J.A., and Zimmerman, L.E. 1973. Lesions stimulating malignant melanoma of the posterior uvea. *Arch. Ophthalmol.* 89:466-71.

Shields, J.A., and Augsburger, J.J. 1981. Current approaches to the diagnosis and management of retinoblastoma. *Surv. Ophthalmol.* 25:347-72.

Shields, J.A. 1983. *Diagnosis and management of intraocular tumors.* pp. 497-532. St. Louis: C.V. Mosby.

Spencer, W.H., and Zimmerman, L.E. 1985. Conjunctiva. In Spencer, W.H. ed. *Ophthalmic pathology: an atlas and textbook.* pp. 107-228. Philadelphia: W.B. Saunders.

Spencer, W.H. ed. 1985. *Ophthalmic pathology: an atlas and textbook.* vols. 1-3. 3rd ed. Philadelphia: W.B. Saunders.

Stallard, H.B. 1964. The conservative treatment of retinoblastoma. In Boniuk, M. ed. *Ocular and adnexal tumors.* St Louis: C.V. Mosby.

Stallard, H. 1966. Radiotherapy for malignant melanoma of the choroid. *Br. J. Ophthalmol.* 50:147-55.

Stefanko, S.Z., and Manschot, W.A. 1979. Pinealoblastoma with retinoblastomatous differentiation. *Brain* 102:321-32.

Stewart, W.B.; Krohel, G.B.; and Wright, J.E. 1979. Lacrimal gland and fossa lesions: an approach to diagnosis and management. *Ophthalmology* 86:886-95.

Straatsma, B.R.; Fine, S.L.; and Earle, J.D. et al. 1988. Enucleation vs. plaque irradiation for choroidal melanoma. *Ophthalmology* 95:1000-1004.

Strickland, D., and Lee, J.A.H. 1981. Melanomas of eye: stability of rates. *Am. J. Epidemiol.* 113:700-702.

Tarkkanen, A., and Tuovinen, E. 1971. Retinoblastoma in Finland 1912-1964. *Arch. Ophthalmol.* 49:293-300.

Torre, D. 1968. Multiple sebaceous tumors. *Arch. Dermatol.* 98:549-51.

Tso, M.O.M.; Fine, B.S.; and Zimmerman, L.E. 1970. The nature of retinoblastoma II: photoreceptor differentiation—an electron microscopic study. *Am. J. Ophthalmol.* 69:350-59.

Tso, M.O.M.; Fine, B.S.; and Zimmerman, L.E. 1969. The Flexner-Wintersteiner rosettes in retinoblastoma. *Arch. Pathol.* 88:665-671.

Tso, M.O.M., and Albert, D.M. 1972. Pathologic conditions of the retinal pigment epithelium: neoplasms and nodular non-neoplastic lesions. *Arch. Ophthalmol.* 88:27-38.

Von Sallman, L., and Paton, D. 1960. Hereditary benign intraepithelial dyskeratosis I: ocular manifestations. *Arch. Ophthalmol.* 63:421-29.

Walsh, T.S., and Tompkins, V.N. 1956. Some observations on the strawberry nevus of infants. *Cancer* 9:869-904.

Weichselbaum, R.R.; Zakov, Z.N.; and Albert, D.M. et al. 1979. New findings in the chromosome 13 long-arm deletion syndrome and retinoblastoma. *Ophthalmology* 86:1191-98.

Whyte, P.; Buchkovich, K.J.; and Horowitz, J.M. et al. 1988. Association between an oncogene and anti-oncogene: the adenovirus EIA proteins bind to the retinoblastoma gene product. *Nature* 334:124-29.

Wintersteiner, H. 1897. *Das Neuroepithelioma Retinae: Eine anatomische und klinische Studie.* Leipzig: Franz Deuticke.

Woog, J.J.; Albert, D.M.; Solt, L.C. et al. 1982. Neurofibromatosis of the eyeball and orbit. *Int. Ophthalmol. Clin.* 22:157-87.

Yandell, D.W.; Campbell, T.A.; and Dayton, S.H. 1989. Oncogenic point mutations in the human retinoblastoma gene: their application to genetic counseling. *N. Engl. J. Med.* 321:1689-95.

Yandell, D.W., and Dryja, T.P. 1989. Detection of DNA sequence polymorphisms by enzymatic amplification and direct genomic sequencing. *Am. J. Hum. Genet.* 45:547-55.

Yanoff, M., and Zimmerman, L.E. 1967. Histogenesis of malignant melanomas of the uvea II: relationship of uveal nevi to malignant melanomas. *Cancer* 20:493-507.

Yeo, J.H.; Jakobiec, F.A.; and Abbott, G.F. et al. 1982. Combined clinical and computed tomographic diagnosis of orbital lymphoid tumors. *Am. J. Ophthalmol.* 94:235-45.

Zakov, Z.N.; Smith, T.R.; and Albert, D.M. 1978. False-positive P32 uptake tests. *Arch. Ophthalmol.* 96:2240-43.

Zimmerman, L.E., and McLean, I.W. 1979. An evaluation of enucleation in the management of uveal melanomas. *Am. J. Ophthalmol.* 87:741-60.

Zimmerman, L.E. 1983. Gamma-glutamyl transpeptidase in the prognosis of patients with uveal melanoma. *Am. J. Ophthalmol.* 96:409-10.

Zimmerman, L.E. 1978. The histogenesis of conjunctival melanomas: the first Algernon B. Reese lecture. In Jakobiec, F.A. ed. *Ocular and adnexal tumors.* pp. 600-30. Birmingham: Aesculapius Publishing Co.

Zimmerman, L.E. 1985. Retinoblastoma and retinocytoma. In Spencer, W.H. ed. *Ophthalmic pathology: an atlas and textbook.* vol. 2. pp. 1292-1351. Philadelphia: W.B. Saunders.

Chapter 26

MALIGNANT TUMORS OF BONE

Henry J. Mankin, M.D.
Christopher G. Willett, M.D.
David C. Harmon, M.D.

Henry J. Mankin, M.D.
Chief of the Orthopaedic Service
Massachusetts General Hospital
Boston, Massachusetts

Christopher G. Willett, M.D.
Radiation Medicine Service
Massachusetts General Hospital
Boston, Massachusetts

David C. Harmon, M.D.
Department of Hematology/Oncology
Massachusetts General Hospital
Harvard Medical School
Boston, Massachusetts

INTRODUCTION

In an overview of neoplastic disorders that affect the population, it is quite apparent that malignant primary bone tumors do not constitute a major health hazard. Virtually unknown in infancy, rare prior to 10 years of age, and at highest peak in the teens, only about 4,000 new cases of bone cancer occur annually in the United States. When compared to the risk for metastatic carcinoma to the skeleton, the numbers vary with age but are at least two orders of magnitude greater than for primary lesions.

Nevertheless, bone tumors fascinate clinicians and scientists and are important parts of the domains of radiation therapists, medical oncologists, radiologists, pathologists, and orthopaedic surgeons. The first reason for this extraordinary status is that the tumors represent a diagnostic challenge because they have a vast array of presentations and considerable variations in biological behavior. Since they recapitulate the development and structure of the skeletal system, the connective tissue biologist finds these lesions fascinating; they are often a rich and convenient source of important chemical constituents of the skeletal system.

To the clinician, the presentation of these lesions is so striking and the problems so devastating to the patient (often a child) and his or her family that patients with neoplasms such as Ewing's sarcoma and osteosarcoma become the central focus of considerable effort and concern on the part of the caretaking team.

Finally, and perhaps most importantly, an extraordinary amount of productive research has been done in recent years on the clinical and basic aspects of these diseases. As a result, there has been a marked improvement in outlook for patients with lesions that only a few decades ago were thought to be virtually incurable.

The commonest malignant tumors of the bone include osteosarcoma, Ewing's sarcoma, lymphoma, chondrosarcoma, and parosteal osteosarcoma.

OSTEOSARCOMA

Central osteosarcoma of the bone is the most common malignant primary bone tumor in childhood, and of all age groups if myeloma is excluded. The lesion occurs with the highest frequency in males in their teen years (ages 10-22). A second, smaller peak in incidence occurs considerably later in life with the development of Paget's sarcoma, thought to be a variant of the central osteosarcoma of childhood. In children and young adults, the tumors are most frequently found in the distal femur and proximal tibia; they are usually metaphyseal, or less commonly diaphyseo-metaphyseal, in location. Pathologically, the tumors seem to arise from primitive mesenchymal cells that produce a primarily osseous, fibrous, cartilaginous, or telangiectatic pattern. By definition, all osteosarcomas contain malignant osteoblasts that synthesize usually thin, wispy, and purposeless fragments of trabecular bone. The tumors are often eccentrically placed in the bone. By the time the patient is seen by the physician, the tumor is usually of substantial size and has broken out of the bone to involve first the periosteum and subsequently the adjacent soft tissues. Tumors arising in the elderly patient, often with Paget's disease, are more common in the humerus, pelvis, and proximal femur and may show a more varied histological pattern.

The usual presenting findings in patients with osteosarcoma are pain, local tenderness, enlargement of the part, and limitation of movement of the adjacent joint; occasionally there is a pathological fracture. Biochemical studies most commonly show only a modest to moderate elevation of the serum alkaline phosphatase. Only occasionally or in neglected cases does the patient present with systemic symptoms and findings. Imaging studies of an osteosarcoma show a highly characteristic pattern on routine radiographs, angiography, bone scan, CT, and MRI; rarely are there significant problems in suspecting the diagnosis. The principal findings are those of a productive lesion with simultaneous bone production and destruction, usually with marked cortical disruption and a large soft-tissue component at the time of discovery. The bone scan routinely shows a marked increase in activity at the tumor site.

The natural history of osteosarcoma is one of rapid enlargement of the primary tumor with an almost equal propensity for distant metastases usually to the lung, but sometimes to other bones, lymph nodes, or rarely, soft tissues and viscera. About 5% to 10% of patients with osteosarcoma present with pulmonary metastases at the outset. If untreated, the tumor is probably universally and rapidly fatal; death occurs with extensive metastases manifesting in less than one year. If the primary disease is eradicated by amputation or resection alone, the results are better but over time are almost as dismal; statistics show only a 5% to 20% 5-year survival.

The introduction of multidrug adjuvant chemotherapy protocols and, more recently, neoadjuvant therapy (both pre- and postoperative treatment) have remarkably influenced survival data. The most recent trends suggest a complete reversal of the figures for the untreated patients (i.e., 80% to over 90% survival). A randomized controlled trial has proven this dramatic benefit from adjuvant chemotherapy with high-dose methotrexate, doxorubicin, cisplatin, bleomycin, cyclophosphamide, and actinomycin. Most of the advantage comes from controlling distant micrometastases, but the local failure rate is also reduced, perhaps helping the surgeon to spare limbs. Current regimens employ a year's worth of intensive therapy requiring hospitalization and much emotional as well as medical attention.

Even metastatic osteosarcoma can be cured if limited numbers of metastases are amenable to surgical resection plus chemotherapy. Long-term survivals of 20% to 40% have been reported (Han, Telander, and Pairolero et al. 1981). More intensive regimens including ifosfamide are being tested in hopes of boosting these figures.

Irradiation has been used only for those osteosarcomas whose lesions were not resectable with good margins, such as osteosarcomas arising in the mandible, the maxilla, or the pelvis.

EWING'S SARCOMA AND OTHER ROUND-CELL LESIONS

The second most frequent tumor in the teenage group is Ewing's sarcoma. Originally thought by Ewing and a number of early investigators to be an endothelioma of bone, the current thinking is even more confusing and there is still doubt as to the cell of origin (Spjit, Dorfman, and Ackerman et al. 1971). The tumor consists of sheets and cords of monotonously similar small, round cells with prominent dark staining nuclei and very scant cytoplasm. Almost every field contains foci of necrotic cells, and special stains for glycogen show that material in a high percentage of cases. Even with immunohistochemistry and electron microscopy, differentiation of the lesion from lymphoma, myeloma, metastatic neuroblastoma, and other neuroectodermal tumors may be difficult.

Most Ewing's tumors arise in the shaft of a long bone or a portion of the pelvis. Males are predisposed, but less noticeably than for osteosarcoma. The peak age is similar to that for osteosarcoma although the lesion is more frequent than osteosarcoma in preteens. Also, the upper cutoff is much sharper, with cases rarely occurring in patients over age 25. The femur, tibia, fibula, and humerus are the most prevalent appendicular skeletal sites. Patients with Ewing's sarcoma are often ill with their disease and frequently present with anorexia, weight loss, chills, fever, and malaise. The local part may show enlargement, tenderness, and signs of inflammation suggestive of an infection; a blood study is often at least in part confirmatory because the sedimentation rate, white blood count, alkaline phosphatase, and LDH may be elevated. Radiographic and other imaging studies usually demonstrate, even at the earliest discovery, the classical permeative (moth-eaten) pattern to the cortex and medullary cavity often with periosteal layering (onion skin). Usually at the time of outset, the tumor extends from the medullary cavity through the cortex and results in a large soft-tissue mass. The lesion is very destructive and may result in a pathological fracture.

Untreated Ewing's tumors have an even more baleful prognosis than osteosarcoma. Fortunately, just as in all round-cell tumors, Ewing's tumor is radiosensitive and patients can obtain a remission and local control by such therapy. However, resecting or radiating the primary tumor did not materially alter the very dismal outlook for these patients (Pritchard, Dahlin, and Dauphine et al. 1975). Fully 15% of the patients presented with metastases to lungs at the time of discovery, and subsequent spread to other bones and viscera was common. In most of the series that were reviewed prior to the introduction of multidrug adjuvant chemotherapy, 5-year survival was less than 5% to 10% (Glaubiger, Makuch, and Schwarz 1981).

The modern era of chemotherapy associated with radiation or appropriate resective surgery has altered these statistics. Ewing's sarcoma often responds dramatically to combination chemotherapy which may include cyclophosphamide, doxorubicin, vincristine, actinomycin, etoposide, ifosfamide, and sometimes bleomycin, DTIC, methotrexate, carmustine, cisplatin, or 5-fluorouracil. Thus, immediate chemotherapy is the essential first component of therapy and should be continued, typically, for one year. Though treatment is toxic and demands close supervision and sometimes transfusions, multimodality therapy can cure even metastatic disease in perhaps 25% of cases. Increasing the intensity of treatment with total body radiation and autologous marrow transplantation with growth factors may improve the odds.

LYMPHOMA

Primary lymphoma of bone is less common than Ewing's sarcoma and occurs in an older age group. The tumors are equally divided between the sexes and occur principally in patients over the age of 25, with a peak occurring at around age 40. The femur is the most frequent site but the tumors can occur almost anywhere. Primary lymphoma of bone may be a misnomer because some of the cases may represent disseminated (stage IV) lymphoma that presents as a bony lesion. Thus, attempts should be made to search for the presence of bone-marrow deposits, enlarged abdominal and other lymph nodes, splenomegaly, and so forth. Most of the primary lymphomas of bone are non-Hodgkin's in type, present a wide range of cell types, and have variable prognoses. Immunohistochemical studies are essential to establish the cell type of the lymphoma and to rule out Ewing's sarcoma, since the treatment protocols for the two diseases are considerably different.

These patients are far less ill at presentation than are patients with Ewing's sarcoma. It is rare to see an individual with a primary lymphoma of bone with a significant systemic response. The radiographic and imaging patterns may be very similar to those seen in Ewing's sarcoma, but there is often less destruction. In some cases of lymphoma, the soft-tissue extension so characteristic of Ewing's sarcoma may not be evident.

In general, the prognosis for patients with primary lymphoma of bone is far better than that for patients with Ewing's sarcoma. Treatment is with intensive multidrug, multicycle chemotherapy (usually a variant of cyclophosphamide, doxorubicin, vincristine, and prednisone [CHOP]) combined with radiation directed to the affected bone. Radiation treatment to 50 Gy is regularly successful in achieving local control of primary lymphoma of bone. The local tumor, regional lymph nodes, or mediastinal and abdominal masses respond well to the lymphoma drug regimen. Well over 70% of the patients have sustained remissions, and in fact seem to be cured (Mindenhall, Jones, and Kramer 1987).

CHONDROSARCOMA

Chondrosarcoma is rare in childhood but becomes more prevalent with advancing age. At age 50 and above it may be the most prevalent form of primary tumor of bone (excluding myeloma). Certain genetic disorders that affect the bones and involve fetal cartilage remnants materially enhance the likelihood of developing a chondrosarcoma. These include the enchondromatoses which consist of Ollier's disease or Mafucci's syndrome (enchondromatosis and multiple venous malformations). Of less concern are the hereditary multiple osteocartilaginous exostoses that may also undergo malignant degeneration, but which are far less likely to do so and those that do rarely achieve the high-grade status of the enostotic lesions. Even less frequently seen are patients with juxtacortical chondrosarcomas arising in the periosteum of the shaft of the humerus or femur. Such tumors seem to be akin to the periosteal osteosarcoma and are considered to be low-grade malignancies.

Malignant cartilage lesions are often lytic in appearance on imaging studies and, depending on the nature of the tumor, display varying amounts of expansion of the cortex, thickening of the cortical shadow, destruction of bone, and a soft-tissue mass. All cartilage tumors (both benign and malignant) may show rounded or punctate calcification both in the primary centrally placed lesion and in the soft-tissue extension outside the bone. Diagnosis and grading of cartilage tumors on the basis of histology is very difficult. Furthermore, sampling is a problem since tumors may have areas of high-grade (differentiated chondrosarcoma) adjacent to regions of low-grade or even benign tumor. Flow cytometry has been somewhat helpful in this area but it still remains a major problem.

The prognosis for chondrosarcoma is much better than for lesions of osseous origin, Ewing's tumor, or lymphoma. Although many of the tumors are high-grade, they are considerably slower to metastasize and for the most part surgery is the treatment of choice. Where margins are expected to be close, surgical resection should be combined with radiation. Patients with chondrosarcoma need not be treated with adjuvant chemotherapy unless metastasis has occurred, but even in such circumstances the drug treatment is thought to add little.

PAROSTEAL OSTEOSARCOMA

The peak age of incidence for these uncommon, low-grade malignant tumors occurs in the late-teens to 40-year age group. The tumors occur slightly more frequently in males. The planum popliteum is the most common site, with the femoral shaft the second most common. The tumors are much more mature histologically than the central osteosarcoma and frequently have an appearance that is difficult to distinguish from myositis ossificans or a benign osteoma. Imaging studies show the lesion to be arising from the cortex and demonstrating a closely applied mass of seemingly mature bone. The peripheral-most portion is likely to demonstrate a soft-tissue component in even the most ossified lesions. Less frequently, particularly early in their course, the tumors may invade the cortex and extend into the medullary cavity. Most experts agree that patients with this condition have a considerably poorer outlook and their treatment should be similar to that for patients with central osteosarcomas.

A patient with a parosteal osteosarcoma is usually asymptomatic or has minimal pain at the site. The principal complaints are of a very slowly enlarging bony mass and limitation of motion of the adjacent joint (usually the knee). The treatment of these lesions is usually surgical and most commonly requires a wide resection (sometimes with allograft replacement or arthrodesis of the knee). Most patients with a successful resection need not have chemotherapy and are unlikely to develop pulmonary metastases.

Another category of lesion, the periosteal osteosarcoma, is more frequently noted in the tibia and occurs more often in young women. The lesion shows more cartilage in its substance, and in fact may be a juxtacortical chondrosarcoma. It has a slightly poorer prognosis than the parosteal tumor (Ritts, Pritchard, and Unni et al. 1987).

REFERENCES

Alho, A.; Connor, J.F.; and Mankin, H.J. et al. 1983. Assessment of malignancy of cartilage tumors using flow cytometry: a preliminary report. *J. Bone Joint Surg.* [Am] 65(6):779-85.

Bacci, G.; Springfield, D.; and Capanna, R. et al. 1987. Neoadjuvant chemotherapy for osteosarcoma of the extremity. *Clin. Orthop.* 224:268-76.

Bacci, G.; Avella, M.; and Picci, P. et al. 1988. Metastatic patterns in osteosarcoma (review). *Tumori* 74(4):421-27.

Cohen, E.K.; Kressel, H.Y.; and Frank, T.S. et al. 1988. Hyaline cartilage-origin bone and soft-tissue neoplasms: MR appearance and histologic correlation. *Radiology* 167(2):477-81.

Donaldson, S.S. 1985. The value of adjuvant chemotherapy in the management of sarcoma in children (review). *Cancer* 55(Suppl 9):2184-97.

Dosoretz, D.E.; Murphy, G.F.; and Raymond, A.K. et al. 1983. Radiation therapy for primary lymphoma of bone. *Cancer* 51(1):44-46.

Eilber, F.R., and Rosen, G. 1989. Adjuvant chemotherapy for osteosarcoma (review). *Semin. Oncol.* 16(4):312-22.

Evans, R.; Nesbit, M.; and Askin, F. et al. 1985. Local recurrence, rate and sites of metastases, and time to relapse as a function of treatment regimen, size of primary, and surgical history in 62 patients presenting with nonmetastatic Ewing's sarcoma of the pelvic bones. *Int. J. Radiat. Oncol. Biol. Phys.* 11(1):129-36.

Frie, E., III. 1985. Curative cancer chemotherapy (review). *Cancer Res.* 45(12 Pt. 1):6523-37.

Furman, W.L.; Fitch, S.; and Hustu, H.O. et al. 1989. Primary lymphoma of bone in children. *J. Clin. Oncol.* 7(9):1275-80.

Glasser, D.B.; Lane, J.M.; and Muschler, G. 1990. Osteosarcoma. In Evarts, C.M. ed. *Surgery of the musculoskeletal system.* pp. 4851-82. New York: Churchill Livingstone.

Glaubiger, D.L.; Mackuch, R.W.; and Schwarz, J. 1981. Influence of prognostic factors on survival in Ewing's sarcoma. *Natl. Cancer Inst. Monogr.* 56:285-88.

Hall, R.B.; Robinson, L.H.; and Malawar, M.M. et al. 1985. Periosteal osteosarcoma. *Cancer* 55(1):165-71.

Han, M.T.; Telander, R.L.; and Pairolero, P.C. et al. 1981. Aggressive thoracotomy for pulmonary metastatic osteogenic sarcoma in children and young adolescents. *J. Pediatr. Surg.* 16:928-33.

Jaffe, N. 1989. Chemotherapy for malignant bone tumors (review). *Orthop. Clin. North Am.* 20(3):487-503.

Jurgens, H.; Treuner, J.; and Winkler, K. et al. 1989. Ifosfamide in pediatric malignancies (review). *Semin. Oncol.* 16(1 Suppl 3):46-50.

Klein, M.J.; Kenan, S.; and Lewis, M.M. 1989. Osteosarcoma: clinical and pathological considerations (review). *Orthop. Clin. North Am.* 20(3):327-45.

Kreicbergs, A.; Silfversward, C.; and Tribukait, B. 1984. Flow DNA analysis of primary bone tumors: relationship between cellular DNA content and histopathologic classification. *Cancer* 53(1):129-36.

Leeson, M.C.; Makely, J.T.; and Carter, J.R. et al. 1989. The use of radioisotope scans in the evaluation of primary lymphoma of bone (review). *Orthop. Rev.* 18(4):410-16.

Lindell, M.M. Jr.; Shirkhoda, A.; and Raymond, A.K. et al. 1987. Parosteal osteosarcoma: radiologic-pathologic correlation with emphasis on CT. *AJR* 148(2):323-28.

Link, M.; Goorin, A.; and Mises, A. et al. 1986. The effect of adjuvant chemotherapy on relapse-free survival in patients with osteosarcoma of the extremity. *N. Engl. J. Med.* 314:1600-1606.

Mankin, H.J., and Gebhardt, M.C. 1985. Advances in the management of bone tumors (review). *Clin. Orthop.* 200:73-84.

Mankin, H.J.; Connor, J.F.; and Schiller, A.L. et al. 1985. Grading of bone tumors by analysis of nuclear DNA content using flow cytometry. *J. Bone Joint Surg.* [Am] 67(3):404-13.

Mankin, H.J.; Gebhart, M.C.; and Springfield, D.S. et al. 1990. Chondrosarcoma. In Evarts, C.M. ed. *Surgery of the musculoskeletal system.* pp. 4895-4928. New York: Churchill Livingstone.

McLean, R.G.; Choy, D.; and Hoschl, R. et al. 1985. Role of radionuclide imaging in the diagnosis of chondrosarcoma. *Med. Pediatr. Oncol.* 13(1):32-6.

Mendenhall, N.P.; Joneg, J.J.; and Kramer, B.S. et al. 1987. The management of primary lymphoma of bone. *Radiother. Oncol.* 9(2):137-45.

Meyers, P.A. 1987. Malignant bone tumors in children: Ewing's sarcoma (review). *Hematol. Oncol. Clin. North Am.* 1(4):667-73.

Miser, J.; Kinsella, T.; and Triche, T. et al. 1988. Preliminary results of treatment of Ewing's sarcoma of bone in children and young adults: six months of intensive combined modality therapy without maintenance. *J. Clin. Oncol.* 6:484-90.

Pritchard, D.J. 1990. Small round-cell tumors. In Evarts, C.M. ed. *Surgery of the musculoskeletal system.* pp. 4853-93. New York: Churchill Livingstone.

Pritchard, D.J.; Dahlin, D.C.; and Dauphine, R.T. et al. 1975. Ewing's sarcoma: a clinical-pathological and statistical analysis of patients surviving five years or longer. *J. Bone Joint Surg.* 57A:10-16.

Ritts, G.D.; Pritchard, D.J.; and Unni, K.K. et al. 1987. Periosteal osteosarcoma. *Clin. Orthop.* 219:299-307.

Rosen, G. 1986. Neoadjuvant chemotherapy for osteogenic sarcoma: a model for the treatment of other highly malignant neoplasms. *Rec. Results Cancer Res.* 103:148-57.

Sailer, S.L.; Harmon, D.C.; and Mankin, H.J. et al. 1988. Ewing's sarcoma: surgical resection as a prognosis factor. *Int. J. Radiat. Oncol. Biol. Phys.* 15:43-52.

Schajowicz, F.; McGuire, M.H.; and Santini-Araujo, E. et al. 1988. Osteosarcomas arising on the surfaces of long bones. *J. Bone Joint Surg.* [Am] 70(4):555-64.

Spjit, H.A.; Dorfman, H.D.; and Fedner, R.E. et al. 1971. *Atlas of tumor pathology fascicle 5: tumors of bone and cartilage.* pp. 216-28. Washington, D.C.: Armed Forces Institute of Pathology.

Sundaram, M.; McGuire, M.H.; and Herbold, D.R. et al. 1986. Magnetic resonance imaging in planning limb-salvage surgery for primary malignant tumors of bone. *J. Bone Joint Surg.* [Am] 68(6):809-19.

Xiang, J.H.; Spanier, S.S.; and Benson, N.A. et al. 1987. Flow cytometric analysis of DNA in bone and soft-tissue tumors using nuclear suspensions. *Cancer* 59(11):1951-58.

Chapter 27

SOFT TISSUE SARCOMAS

Mitchell C. Posner, M.D.
Murray F. Brennan, M.D.

Mitchell C. Posner, M.D.*
Surgical Fellow
Department of Surgery
Memorial Sloan-Kettering Cancer Center
New York, New York

Murray F. Brennan, M.D.
Chairman, Department of Surgery
Memorial Sloan-Kettering Cancer Center
New York, New York

INTRODUCTION

Sarcomas of the soft tissues, although derived from a common anlage, comprise a wide variety of solid neoplasms with diverse anatomic and morphologic characteristics. Although they occur infrequently, this group of solid tumors has generated renewed interest in recent years. Soft tissue sarcomas are a model for an organized multimodality approach to the therapy of malignant disease. While success with such regimens is seen in childhood sarcomas, their benefit has been less dramatic among adults. Enthusiasm continues, however, as clinical trials designed to evaluate multimodality therapy determine its efficacy.

INCIDENCE AND DEMOGRAPHICS

Soft tissue sarcomas are relatively rare neoplasms. An estimated 5,700 new cases were diagnosed in the United States in 1990 (Silverberg et al. 1990). However, this figure does not include a large number of soft tissue sarcomas coded to specific sites. The incidence is similar to that of testicular tumors (5,900) and carcinoma of the tongue (6,100), and is slightly less frequent than Hodgkin's disease (7,400). Approximately 3,100 die of the disease annually. Soft tissue sarcomas show no predilection for any particular age group, nor is there any clear sex predominance. These findings were confirmed in a retrospective analysis of 423 patients with localized extremity lesions at our institution between 1968 and 1978 (Collin et al. 1986; Collin et al. 1987; Collin et al. 1987).

A further attempt to define demographics and presentation characteristics led to the development of a prospective data base. From July 1, 1982, through December 31, 1987, 1,091 patients with histologically confirmed diagnoses

*Present Address:
    Assistant Professor of Surgery
    University of Pittsburgh School of Medicine
    Department of Surgery
    Montefiore Hospital
    Pittsburgh, Pennsylvania

of soft tissue sarcoma were admitted to Memorial Sloan-Kettering Cancer Center. The median age at presentation was 50 years (range 16-89). Tumors were slightly more common in males (54%) than in females (46%). Ninety percent were white, 6% black, and the remaining patients were distributed among other races.

The most common sites of initial presentation (fig. 27.1) were the extremities (49.8%). Lower extremity lesions (38.9%) predominated over upper limb tumors (10.9%), with most located in the proximal thigh. Other primary sites included retroperitoneum/intra-abdominal (15.2%), trunk (12.9%), genitourinary (7.2%), visceral (5.4%), and head and neck (4.8%).

Histopathological examination revealed the following predominant subtypes in decreasing order of frequency: liposarcoma, leiomyosarcoma, malignant fibrous histiocytoma, and fibrosarcoma (fig. 27.2). The primary presentation site has been shown to correlate with the relative frequency of particular histological types. Liposarcomas, malignant fibrous histiocytomas, tendosynovial sarcomas, and fibrosarcomas predominate in the extremity and head and neck regions. In the retroperitoneal and visceral sites, leiomyosarcomas and liposarcomas are most common (fig. 27.3).

Of the 1,091 patients admitted, 22% presented with metastases. Multiple factors are associated with the development of metastatic disease. Histologically, leiomyosarcoma was the most common type in those patients with metastases, while fibrosarcomas infrequently metastasized (fig. 27.4). Retroperitoneal and visceral sarcomas were more likely to be associated with metastases than extremity lesions (fig. 27.5). Most patients initially present with high-grade lesions; in those with metastatic disease, 76% had high-grade tumors (fig. 27.6). Most patients at first presentation have large tumors; those greater than 5 cm are more likely to have associated metastases than smaller lesions (fig. 27.7).

ETIOLOGY

Although genetic, environmental, and iatrogenic factors have been implicated as etiologic agents of soft tissue sarcoma, no conclusive evidence exists to substantiate such claims. Familial syndromes, particularly neurofibromatosis (Von Recklinghausen's disease) have been suggested as predisposing factors. Patients with malignant peripheral nerve tumors, schwannomas, or neurofibrosarcomas with prior neurofibromatosis have been identified. Neurofibrosarcomas arise in 2% to 3% of all patients with hereditary neurofibromatosis (Crowe, Schull, and Neel 1956; D'Agostino, Soule, and Miller 1963).

SOFT TISSUE SARCOMAS SITE

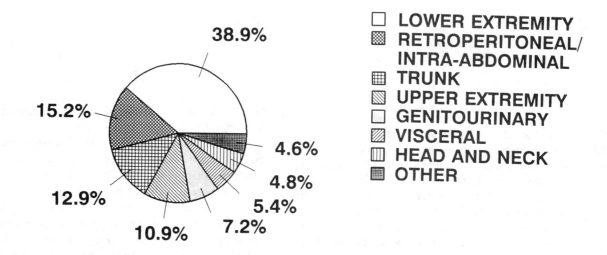

Fig. 27.1. Primary sites of initial presentation, MSKCC, 7/82-12/87, n = 1,091.

SOFT TISSUE SARCOMAS HISTOLOGIC TYPE

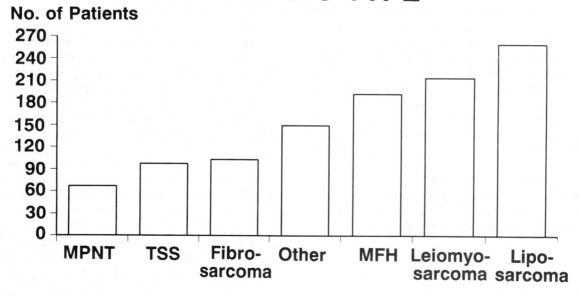

Fig. 27.2. Histopathological subtypes, MSKCC, 7/82-12/87, MPNT = Malignant Peripheral Nerve Tumor; TSS = Tendosynovial Sarcoma; MFH = Malignant Fibrous Histiocytoma, n = 1,091.

PREDOMINANT HISTOLOGIC TYPE BY SITE

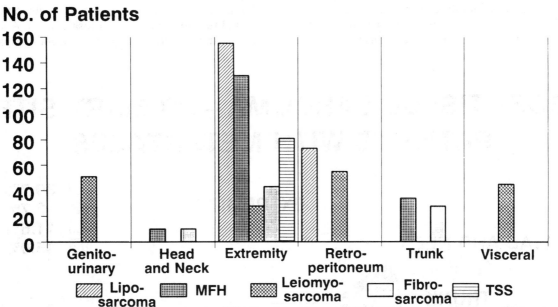

Fig. 27.3. Predominant histologic type by site, MSKCC, 7/82-12/87, n = 1,088. MFH = Malignant Fibrous Histiocytoma; TSS = Tendosynovial Sarcoma.

SOFT TISSUE SARCOMA—HISTOLOGIC TYPE PATIENTS WITH METASTASES

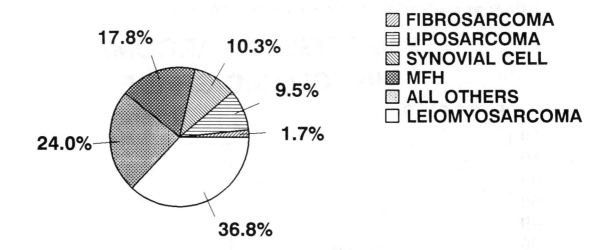

Fig. 27.4. Histologic type: Patients with metastases, MSKCC, 7/82-12/87, n = 242. MFH = Malignant Fibrous Histiocytoma.

Prior therapeutic radiation exposure is frequently suggested as a causative factor and numerous cases of sarcomas, both bone and soft tissue, arising in previously irradiated fields have been reported. Breast cancer and Hodgkin's disease are first malignancies in which radiation-induced sarcomas most often arise (Davidson, Westbury, and Harmer 1986; Souba et al. 1986). The true incidence may be obscure because of the long latency period (5 to 28 years) and failure to recognize this entity (Souba et al. 1986).

Lymphangiosarcoma is most often identified in the chronic lymphedematous extremity. Lymphadenectomy in association with mastectomy is the most common cause of persistent lymphedema. The role of radiotherapy as a contributing factor in this setting has been raised, although lymphangiosarcoma frequently arises outside the irradiated field and has been observed in lymphedematous extremities without prior radiation exposure (Borel Rinkes and de Jongste 1986; Sordillo et al. 1981). Lymphedema-related lymphangiosarcoma has been described in traumatic, idiopathic, congenital, and chronic filarial lymphedema (Muller, Hajdu, and Brennan 1987). By increasing the risk of developing lymphedema postmastectomy, radiotherapy may be a contributing factor.

Trauma is often mentioned as a possible etiology of desmoid tumors (low-grade fibrosarcomas). Abdominal wall desmoids originating in previous laparotomy

SOFT TISSUE SARCOMA – PRIMARY SITE PATIENTS WITH METASTASES

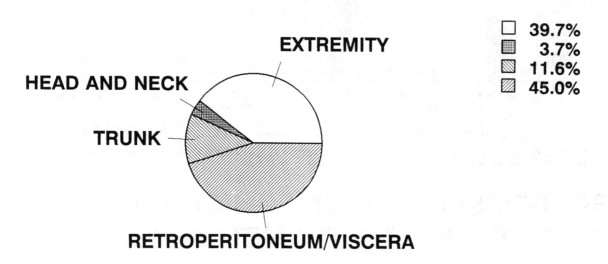

☐ 39.7%
▦ 3.7%
▨ 11.6%
▧ 45.0%

Fig. 27.5. Primary site: Patients with metastases, MSKCC 7/82-12/87, n = 242.

SOFT TISSUE SARCOMA HISTOLOGIC GRADE

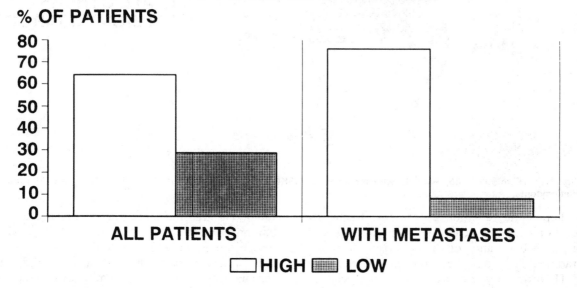

Fig. 27.6. Histologic grade. In patients with metastatic disease, 76% are found to have high-grade tumors. MSKCC 7/82-12/87.

SOFT TISSUE SARCOMA
TUMOR SIZE

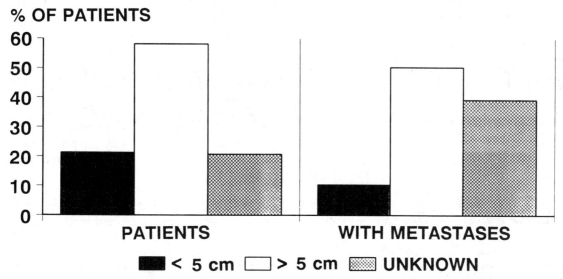

Fig. 27.7. Tumor size. Patients with tumors >5 cm are more likely to present with associated disease. MSKCC 7/82-12/87.

incisions, as well as an apparent causal association in the postpartum female, support this hypothesis (Hayry et al. 1982). In a recent review, eight of 12 abdominal wall desmoid tumors had antecedent history of trauma or recent pregnancy (Posner et al. 1989).

The possible association of toxic chemical exposure with the development of soft tissue sarcoma causes great concern in the United States. Individuals exposed to phenoxyherbicides (phenoxyacetic acid and chlorophenols) may be at high risk of developing soft tissue sarcomas. Agent Orange, the herbicide used extensively during the Vietnam War, contained dioxin, an extremely toxic chemical with teratogenic and carcinogenic potential. A more recent study revealed that Vietnam veterans in general did not have an increased risk of soft tissue sarcoma compared to controls (Kang et al. 1987). However, subgroups of ground troops, who were estimated to have increased exposure to the defoliant, were at higher risk than other soldiers.

HISTOPATHOLOGY

Proper recognition of specific cellular subtypes provides essential information regarding tumor behavior and for instituting protocol management. Major advances, especially in immunohistochemical techniques and electron microscopy, have contributed to precise identification. Detection of intermediate filament proteins (i.e., vimentin) is an accurate screening method for sarcomas vs. epithelial tumors. Tissue-specific markers help differentiate tumors of myogenic, neurogenic, or endothelial origin. Nonspecific markers such as S-100 or Actin further elucidate cellular origin (Roholl et al. 1985).

Once the histologic type of neoplasm is confirmed, histologic grading becomes paramount. Tumor grade is the single best prognostic indicator for the development of metastases and eventual outcome. Grading is based on criteria that include degree of differentiation, cellularity, amount of stroma, necrosis, vascularity, and number of mitoses (table 27.1). The lack of uniformity among various grading systems has led to confusion and misinterpretation in analyzing interinstitutional data. The MSKCC's system distinguishes only between high- and low-grade lesions (Hajdu 1985). This simplified approach readily enables the evaluation of both the recurrence potential (local or distant) and results of various treatment modalities, with minimal ambiguity. Even so, sampling error during pathologic examination can lead to biased results.

STAGING

The staging system proposed by the American Joint Committee for Cancer (AJCC) is based on four variables: histologic grade, tumor size, regional lymph node involvement, and presence of distant metastases

Table 27.1
GUIDELINES TO HISTOLOGIC GRADING OF SARCOMAS

LOW-GRADE SARCOMAS	HIGH-GRADE SARCOMAS
Good differentiation	Poor differentiation
Hypocellular	Hypercellular
Much stroma	Minimal stroma
Hypovascular	Hypervascular
Minimal necrosis	Much necrosis
<5 mitosis per 10 HPF	>5 mitosis per 10 HPF

Table 27.2
FACTORS INFLUENCING PROGNOSIS OF SARCOMAS

	FAVORABLE PROGNOSTIC SIGNS	UNFAVORABLE PROGNOSTIC SIGNS
Size	Small	Large
Site	Superficial	Deep
Histologic grade	Low	High

CORRELATION BETWEEN PROGNOSTIC SIGNS AND STAGE

PROGNOSTIC SIGNS	STAGE OF SARCOMA
3 favorable signs	Stage 0
2 favorable signs and 1 unfavorable sign	Stage I
1 favorable sign and 2 unfavorable signs	Stage II
3 unfavorable signs	Stage III
Evidence of metastasis	Stage IV

(Russell et al. 1977). For localized tumors, grade is the primary determinant of advancing stage (I-III). Stage IV lesions are either locally invasive or disseminated. An alternative staging system also recognizes the importance of size, site, and whether the tumor is superficial or deep to the muscular fascia (table 27.2). Each parameter's relative impact on outcome has been determined from a large retrospective analysis. Advancing tumor stage in this system represents the additive effects of poor prognostic variables, if present. The advantages of this type of staging system over the one currently in use are being evaluated.

EXTREMITY SITE SOFT TISSUE SARCOMAS

DIAGNOSIS

An effective management plan requires precise preoperative evaluation, incorporating all pertinent diagnostic methods to assess both the primary and possible metastatic disease. Most patients present with an asymptomatic mass (Collin et al. 1988). However, the majority of tumors are large and involvement of surrounding muscle and adjacent neurovascular structures may produce symptoms. Meticulous physical examination should be directed at determining location, approximate size, and depth and assessing direct invasion of underlying bone or neurovascular structures.

The presence of metastatic disease is then determined. The lung is the most frequent site of metastatic involvement. Initially anteroposterior and lateral radiographs of the chest are all that is necessary until histologic diagnosis is confirmed. Examination of regional lymph node basin is mandatory. Regional lymphadenopathy in general is uncommon but certain histopathologic types are associated with a higher incidence of lymph node involvement (Weingrad and Rosenberg 1978). These include epithelioid synovial cell sarcoma, in which 30% of patients develop lymph node metastases; rhabdomyosarcoma; and leiomyosarcoma.

Because histologic diagnosis determines further diagnostic measures, and no physical, biochemical, or radiologic information reliably predicts malignancy, tissue biopsy is the next logical step. The method of obtaining tissue is crucial. Fine needle aspiration rarely establishes the diagnosis of malignancy and is grossly inadequate for histopathological subtyping. Tru-Cut biopsy, which yields a core of tissue, has been shown to be highly sensitive in the diagnosis of sarcoma, but lacking in specificity (Kissin et al. 1986). Frequently the pathologist cannot determine grade or cell of origin from the specimen. Open biopsy remains the diagnostic procedure of choice. Excisional biopsy, or enucleation, is only indicated for small superficial lesions. For larger lesions, this technique invariably disrupts the pseudocapsule and may compromise the subsequent definitive *en block* resection. Incisional biopsy, in a plane longitudinal to the extremity's long axis, is most appropriate for all other lesions.

The specimen should be prepared so the pathologist receives fresh and fixed tissue. Surface markers and electron microscopic examination thus can be performed in addition to conventional light microscopy. Once the diagnosis of sarcoma is confirmed and both grade and histogenesis is determined, systematic use of more precise radiological techniques is in order to further define the primary and possible metastasis.

Computed tomography (CT) has been considered the optimal imaging modality for staging localized extremity lesions, but magnetic resonance imaging (MRI) now appears to have surpassed CT as the imaging device best able to delineate these lesions (fig. 27.8). Two recent reports (Demas et al. 1988; Chang et al. 1987) underscore the advantages of MRI and demonstrate its superior sensitivity and specificity in tumor resolution. Computed tomography continues to be the optimal imaging tool when evaluating lung metastases (fig. 27.9) and all patients with high-grade lesions should have a CT evaluation of the chest. Often, sarcomas previously described as localized will be disseminated on CT, while those with metastases on plain radiographs of the chest will have a higher yield of ipsilateral nodules and unsuspected contralateral lesions with CT (Chang et al. 1979).

With the advent of these sophisticated noninvasive imaging modalities, angiography rarely provides any valuable additional information and is not recommended. Likewise, bone scanning has been shown to be of limited value as a diagnostic tool (Walker, Healey, and Brennan, unpublished data). Poor specificity and sensitivity in delineating bone invasion makes this an unreliable staging device.

PROGNOSTIC FACTORS FOR LOCAL RECURRENCE AND SURVIVAL

In order to properly evaluate the efficacy of various management regimens on patient outcome, the definition of specific factors that influence both local recurrence and survival is essential. Prospective randomized trials designed to evaluate adjuvant therapy can only be implemented and properly analyzed once study groups

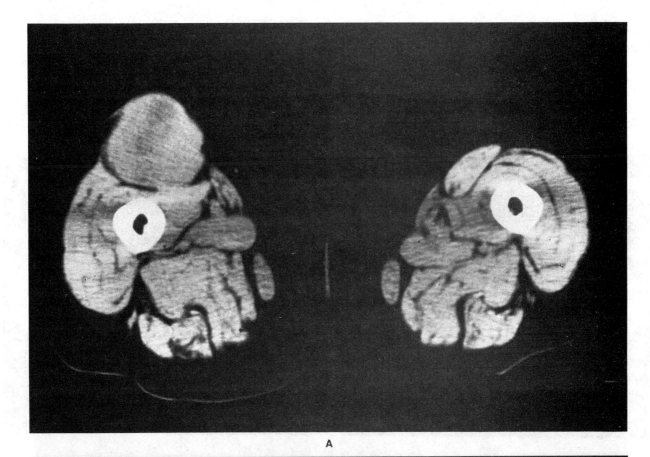

A

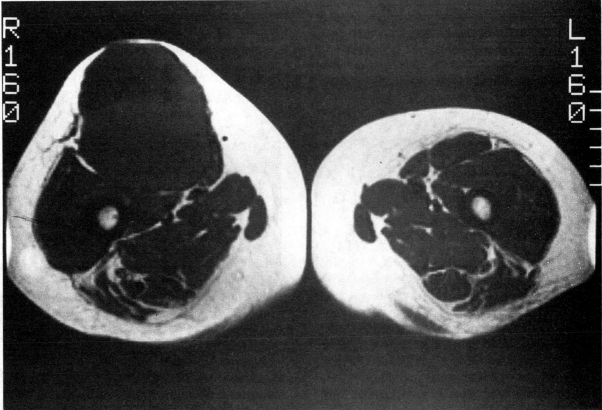

B

Fig. 27.8. Large, high-grade liposarcoma of the thigh in a 65-year-old patient. Preoperative evaluation by (A) computed tomography (CT) and (B) magnetic resonance imaging (MRI).

are stratified with respect to these variables. Patient subgroups identified as either at minimal risk for treatment failure or doomed to failure are not candidates for these studies, which strengthens the subsequent analysis.

Within this framework we instituted a detailed retrospective analysis of 423 patients with localized extremity lesions treated at MSKCC during the years 1968 to 1978

(Collin et al. 1986; Collin et al. 1987; Collin et al. 1987). This sample had 315 lower-extremity and 108 upper-extremity sarcomas. Males and females were equally represented. In all, 278 (66%) presented with their primary untouched, while 145 presented with locally recurrent disease. Tumors were proximal (above the knee or elbow) in 273 patients (65%), superficial to the

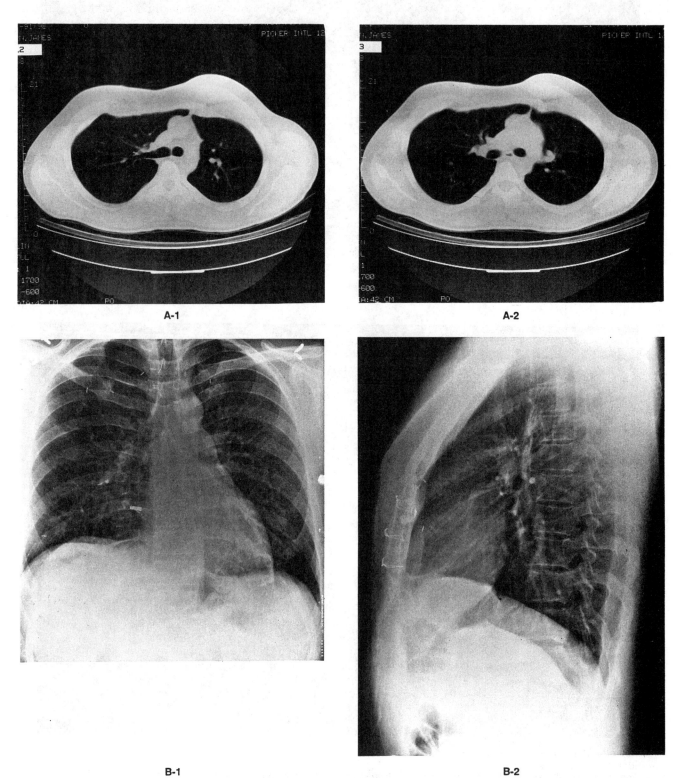

Fig. 27.9. Computed tomography (A1-A2) demonstrating lung metastases in patient with previously resected malignant fibrous histiocytoma of the chest wall. Standard radiographs (B1-B2) did not reveal metastases.

fascia in 206 of 393 evaluable cases, and greater than 10 cm in 120 of 252 patients (48%) for whom tumor size was available. Tumors were classified as high-grade in 256 cases (61%).

Univariate analysis of patient, tumor, and treatment factors demonstrated select variables that influenced local disease-free interval (LDFI) and survival (table 27.3). Patient-related variables predictive of subsequent local recurrence were age greater than 53 and presentation with locally recurrent disease. Tumors that were classified high grade and tumors associated with regional lymph node involvement were more likely to recur locally. Invasion of bone or neurovascular structures was a significant predictor of local recurrence in those patients undergoing limb sparing surgery (LSS), but was only of borderline significance in the group as a

Table 27.3
FACTORS AFFECTING LOCAL RECURRENCE AND SURVIVAL BY UNIVARIATE ANALYSIS

		Median LDFI		Median Survival	
	n	Months	p Values	Months	p Values
Patient Factors:					
Age >53	182	189[1]	.0009	74	.0004
≤53	241	196+		196+	
Presentation					NS[a]
Primary	278	194+	<.0001		
Recurrent	145	57			
Tumor Factors:					
Symptoms			NS		
Painful				63	.003
Painless				167	
Site			NS		
Proximal				91	
Distal				191+	.01
Depth			NS		
Superficial				194+	.003
Deep				80	
Size (Excised)			NS		
<5.0 cm				148	
5.0-9.9 cm				79	.001*
≥10.0 cm				41	
Grade[2]					
High	256	194+	.03	52	<.0001
Low	154	196+		196+	
Nodes					
Positive	17	8	.002	7	<.0001
Negative	150	194+		79	
Treatment Factors:					
Invasion (all patients)					
Yes	130	172+	.08	46	<.0001
No	282	196+		196+	
Invasion (LSS only)					NS[a]
Yes	63	71	.02		
No	213	193+			
Operation[3]					
Amputation	138	196+	.005	30	<.00001
LSS	276	194+		194+	
Margins (LSS only)					
Adequate	160	194+		194+	
Marginal	72	169+	.000001*	169+	.00002*
Inadequate	44	119+		64	
Margins (all patients)					
Adequate	288	196+		144	
Marginal	78	169+	<.001*	192+	.0003*
Inadequate	48	20		49	
Biopsy					
Immediate surgery	23	189+		79	
Delayed surgery	196	194+	.04*	193+	.0007*
No biopsy	195	194+		80	
Local Treatment					
Failure	52	-		149	.0001
vs. no failure[4]	225	-		196+	
Local only					
Failure	46	-		149	.00003
vs. no failure	225	-		196+	

[a] NS = Not significant
[1] + indicates median survival not reached
[2] Excludes 13 patients in whom grade could not be determined
[3] Excludes 9 patients treated nonsurgically
[4] Two-year landmark; all patients censored prior to the landmark are excluded from the analysis
*Log-rank test comparing all categories. If p <.05, one or more of the categories is significantly different from the others
(Modified from: Collin, Friedrich, and Godbold et al. [1988].)

whole. Local recurrence was less frequent following amputation vs. limb sparing surgery. If an adequate margin was obtained, regardless of the extent of procedure, it favorably influenced LDFI.

Multivariate analysis was used to define variables that independently correlated with an increased risk of local recurrence (table 27.4). These factors included age greater than 53, presentation with local recurrence, inadequate surgical margins, limb sparing surgery, and high-grade lesions. Specific histological subtypes (embryonal rhabdomyosarcoma, malignant peripheral nerve tumor, and angiosarcoma) also were associated with decreased LDFI.

Factors that affect survival were analyzed (see table 27.3) (Collin et al. 1987). Variables that adversely affect survival included increased age, painful mass, proximal site, location deep to the fascia, invasion of bone or neurovascular structures, and large tumor size. High grade and regional lymph node involvement were also poor prognosticators. Several histologic types including fibrosarcoma, liposarcoma, and malignant fibrous histiocytoma were associated with survival benefit. Need for amputation or the absence of adequate surgical margins portended a poor outcome as did local failure.

When subjected to multivariate analysis, the following variables were independent predictors of decreased survival: painful mass, age greater than 53, proximal site, size greater than 10 cm, high grade, lymph node involvement, need for amputation, and inadequate surgical margins (see table 27.4).

The log-hazard ratio allows stratification of patients into high-, intermediate-, and low-risk groups. This prognostic index can be applied broadly in the design of trials that examine therapeutic benefit of adjuvant regimens, and to confirm the validity of various staging systems.

Table 27.4
FACTORS PREDICTIVE OF LOCAL RECURRENCE BY MULTIVARIATE ANALYSIS

Age >53 years
Presentation with recurrent disease
High tumor grade
Histopathology of:
    Embryonal rhabdomyosarcoma
    Angiosarcoma
    Malignant peripheral nerve tumor
    Limb sparing operation
    Inadequate margins

FACTORS PREDICTIVE OF DECREASED SURVIVAL BY MULTIVARIATE ANALYSIS

Age >53 years
High tumor grade
Painful mass at presentation
Proximal site
Size ≥10 cm
Positive regional nodes
Amputation
Inadequate margins

(Modified from: Collin, Friedrich, and Godbold et al. [1988].)

TREATMENT

Management of extremity soft tissue sarcomas has evolved considerably over the past decade. Aggressive resection remains the primary method of local control, but limb sparing procedures are now clearly the goal of surgical therapy. While amputation was frequently employed early on to obtain clear margins, function-saving procedures now predominate. Limb sparing surgery must, when feasible, be wide margin in scope. However, in order to preserve neurovascular and/or bony structures, 2 cm to 3 cm of uninvolved surrounding tissue may not be feasible in certain extremity locations. Consequently, the use of radiation therapy as an adjunct to surgery has been critically examined.

The early work of Lindberg et al. (Lindberg 1983) and Suit et al. (Suit, Russell, and Martin 1973; Suit, Russell, and Martin 1975; Suit and Russell 1975; Suit et al. 1981), substantiated the premise that high dose radiation therapy can control residual microscopic foci of soft tissue sarcoma. The group at the National Cancer Institute evaluated the role of adjuvant external beam radiation therapy following limb sparing surgery vs. amputation in a prospective randomized trial (Rosenberg et al. 1982). Although the rate of local recurrence in the limb sparing group approached statistical significance (4 of 27 vs. 0 of 16), disease-free survival and overall survival were comparable to the amputation group.

Brachytherapy, the placement of radioactive sources directly into tumor or at the extirpation site, has been extensively explored at MSKCC as an alternative to conventional methods of radiation delivery (Shiu et al. 1984; Shiu et al. 1986; Brennan et al. 1987). For direct application of residual gross disease, iodine 125 seeds are used as a permanent implant. Tumor bed treatment involves the temporary implantation of iridium 192 on postoperative day five or six via percutaneous catheters that are removed following four to five days of treatment. In this manner, delivery of 45 Gy over this time is equivalent to 60 Gy of external beam radiation therapy (Shiu et al. 1988). Radiation effects on wound healing are considerable regardless of the route of delivery, but wound complications can be minimized by postponing delivery of radiation therapy until the fifth or sixth postoperative day as demonstrated by a recent prospective randomized trial at Memorial Hospital (Arbeit, Hilaris, and Brennan 1987; Ormsby et al. 1989). However, despite the enthusiasm and encouraging results of adjuvant radiation treatment, its optimal application has yet to be elucidated. Thus, it should not be used as an alternative to aggressive and adequate resection of local disease.

ADJUVANT CHEMOTHERAPY

The value of chemotherapy for soft tissue sarcomas is controversial. Absence of treatment groups comparably stratified for important prognostic criteria in numerous chemotherapeutic trials, in addition to administration of multimodality therapy in various combinations with

Table 27.5
ACTIVITY OF DOXORUBICIN IN SOFT TISSUE SARCOMA

	Year	Author	Dose mg/m^2	No. of patients	Response rate (%)
Southwest Oncology Group	1973	O'Bryan, R.M.	60-75	41	29
Baltimore Cancer Research Center	1973	Benjamin, R.S.	60	21	38
CTEP/NCI Summary	1975	Blum, R.H.	varied	151	26
Southwest Oncology Group	1977	O'Bryan, R.M.	25-75	82	28
Mayo Clinic	1977	Creagan, E.T.	60-75	15	7
Eastern Coop. Oncology Group	1982	Schoenfeld, D.A.	70	54	30
Gynecologic Oncology Group	1983	Omura, G.A.	60	80	16
Gynecologic Oncology Group	1985	Muss, H.B.	60	26	19
Eastern Coop. Oncology Group	1987	Borden, E.C.	70	94	17

surgery and radiation, make evaluation difficult. Adriamycin (doxorubicin) is the common denominator in all these chemotherapeutic regimens, since it is the most effective agent in disseminated soft tissue sarcoma (table 27.5). Its value as an adjuvant has been studied in multiple prospective randomized trials summarized in table 27.6. Despite conflicting evidence regarding its efficacy, it appears that patients at increased risk for an unfavorable outcome benefit from adjuvant chemotherapy. In patients with high-grade extremity lesions, two studies clearly demonstrate increased survival (Rosenberg et al. 1982; Gherlinzoni et al. 1986), while one study shows no difference (Antman et al. 1984). The other trials are not conclusive but suggest improved outcome; most, including negative trials, demonstrate a quantitative decrease in pulmonary metastases (Alvegard 1986; Edmondson et al. 1984; Bramwell et al. 1985).

METASTATIC DISEASE

The lung is the most common site for dissemination. Pulmonary metastases are frequently the first site of recurrence in patients with high-grade extremity lesions and are seen in 15% to 20% of patients with low-grade histology (Donohue et al. 1988). Long-term survival following complete resection of all metastatic disease is not uncommon, with 20% to 25% of patients alive and disease-free at five years (Putnam et al. 1984; McCormick and Martini 1979). The major determinants of favorable outcome include tumor doubling time greater than 20 days, disease-free interval greater than 12

months, and the presence of fewer than four nodules on linear tomograms (Putnam et al. 1984). The surgical approach to lung metastasis is controversial. Median sternotomy has gained favor in recent years over staged lateral thoracotomy. Advantages of bilateral exploration include the detection of occult metastases in a significant percentage of patients, and avoidance of a second thoracotomy without increasing pulmonary complications (Roth et al. 1986). Preoperative radiological evaluation is necessary to determine if the early detection of occult disease translates into a survival benefit.

RESULTS

The role of adjuvant radiation therapy in preventing local failure following excision of extremity or superficial trunk sarcoma is being examined at our institution in a prospective randomized trial. Since July 1982, all patients who undergo complete tumor extirpation are randomized to receive or not to receive radiation therapy with the brachytherapy technique. This involves afterloading of ^{192}I on the fifth or sixth postoperative day to deliver a dose of 45 Gy over four to five days. The patients are stratified according to prognostic criteria of histologic grade, size, proximal location, and presentation as recurrent disease.

An update on recently published data (Brennan et al. 1987) with median follow-up of 20 months (fig. 27.10) demonstrates a statistically significant reduction in local recurrence using brachytherapy. This benefit appears to result from the effects of radiation therapy in patients

Table 27.6
ADJUVANT CHEMOTHERAPY FOR SOFT TISSUE SARCOMA

Author	Year	Grade	Site	n	Chemo.	Survival
Rosenberg	1982	High Int.	Ext.	65	ADR 550 CYCL	Treated 84% Controls 57% Overall 5-yr. survival: p=0.01
Gherlinzoni*	1986	High	Ext.	59	ADR 450	Improved DFS, less pulm. mets. p = <0.05
Antman	1984	High Int.	All Ext.	42 25	ADR 450	No difference DFS or OS, less pulm. mets.
Alvegard	1986	High	Ext.	146	ADR 540	No difference
Edmonson	1984		All	61	ADR 550	less pulm. mets.
Bramwell	1985		All Ext.	247 48	CYVADIC	No difference less pulm. mets. survival: p=0.078

OS = overall survival; DFS = disease-free survival; ADR = Adriamycin as mg/m^2; CYCL = cyclophosphamide; CYVADIC = Cytoxan, vincristine, Adriamycin, dacarbazine
*Some patients received preoperative chemotherapy.

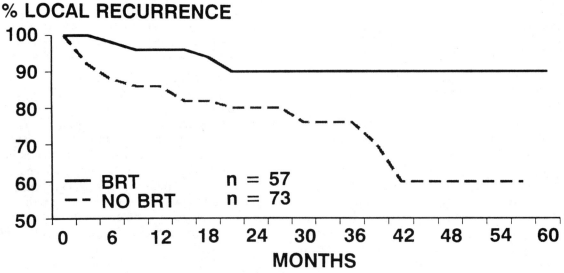

**SOFT TISSUE SARCOMA
TIME TO ANY LOCAL RECURRENCE**

Fig. 27.10. Local recurrence in soft tissue sarcoma; MSKCC 7/82-12/87. With median follow-up of 20 months, there is a statistically significant reduction in the brachytherapy (BRT) arm (p=.03).

with high-grade tumors. No difference in survival was detected and the study continues as longer follow up is obtained.

An effort to diminish the cardiac toxicity associated with bolus intravenous injection of Adriamycin led to a prospective randomized trial to examine the toxicity and efficacy of continuous intravenous administration of the agent (Brennan et al. 1987). Patients with locally controlled high-grade extremity lesions were randomized to receive chemotherapy by bolus or continuous infusion up to a total dose of 540 mg/m². As measured by radionuclide cardiac angiography, cardiac toxicity was diminished by continuous administration (table 27.7). There was no difference in survival between the two groups. Longer follow-up is necessary.

A group of patients with resectable extremity lesions who have a greatly diminished 5-year survival has been identified. These patients present with large, (>10 cm), proximal, and high-grade tumors. The outlook is dismal for patients with large, high-grade retroperitoneal, visceral, or trunk lesions. A preoperative chemotherapy regimen is under investigation for these patients in an effort to improve ease of resectability and long-term survival.

RETROPERITONEAL SITE SOFT TISSUE SARCOMAS

The anatomic location and local invasiveness of soft tissue sarcomas of the retroperitoneum continue to be a therapeutic challenge. There is not enough evaluable data regarding these lesions to make valid conclusions regarding efficacy of various treatment alternatives. There is a clear need to define prognostic variables and assess adjuvant therapeutic modalities in a prospective randomized forum.

Retroperitoneal sarcomas are rare, comprising less than 15% of soft tissue sarcomas (Cody et al. 1981). During the period 1982 to 1987, 150 patients were explored for retroperitoneal sarcomas at Memorial Hospital (table 27.8). As with all sarcomas, there was no age or sex predilection. Sixty-seven patients presented with primary (45%) and 49 (33%) with recurrent disease. The remaining patients had metastases at presentation. Because of their location, most tumors are larger than 10 cm on presentation. Low- and high-grade histology are equally represented, while leiomyosarcoma and liposarcoma types predominate.

Table 27.7
POST-TREATMENT LEFT VENTRICULAR EJECTION FRACTION FOR PATIENTS RECEIVING >300 MG/M² DOXORUBICIN

		Dose (mg/m²)		LVEF	
	n	Median	Range	Rest abnormal %	Exercise abnormal %
Bolus	21	431	300-500	48*	52*
Continuous	25	540	300-540	16	20

*p = 0.03 Fischer's Exact Test
(From: Brennan, Friedrich, and Almadrones et al. [1987].)

Table 27.8
RETROPERITONEAL SARCOMAS MEMORIAL HOSPITAL 1982-1987

	Primary	Recurrent	With Metastases
Biopsy only	4	3	4
LSS	56	41	16
Explored only	1	1	—
No surgery	6	5	13
Total	67(45%)	50(33%)	33(22%)

DIAGNOSIS

Invariably, retroperitoneal sarcomas present once the tumor size is considerable. Nonspecific symptoms during the growth phase result in a prolonged duration at presentation. An abdominal mass is palpable in approximately 75% of patients; another 15% are identified incidentally during physical examination for other purposes (Cody et al. 1981). In a retrospective analysis at Memorial Hospital, during the years 1971 to 1982, diffuse back pain was present in 50% of the patients and 25% had symptoms suggestive of peripheral nerve or nerve root compression. Gastrointestinal symptomatology was surprisingly infrequent, with only 5% developing small bowel obstruction (Jaques et al. 1989).

Diagnostic radiology is a valuable tool for delineating precise tumor location, relationship to adjacent retroperitoneal and intra-abdominal structures, and the presence of liver or intraperitoneal dissemination. Computed tomography has been the procedure of choice for evaluation of the primary (size, consistency, and anatomic relationships), defining residual tumor, and in detecting recurrent disease (fig. 27.11). Magnetic

resonance imaging may prove to be invaluable for assessing tumors in this location (fig. 27.12). The better soft tissue resolution and enhanced distinction between normal and abnormal tissue, demonstrated in a recent report (Demas et al. 1988), is encouraging. Tumor depiction without ionizing radiation and intravenous contrast clearly favors MRI.

Angiography should be used sparingly to define vascular supply of the lesion or provide a road map for resection of hepatic metastases, when indicated. Assessment of vascular involvement by tumor is unreliable and is better served by MRI.

Percutaneous needle aspiration or core biopsy have limited ability to provide reliable preoperative information. Instances in which resectability is questioned or an alternative diagnosis is suspected require open biopsy.

Preoperative search for metastatic disease should be directed at likely sites of involvement, such as the liver and lungs. Routine chest x-ray will usually identify the patient with pulmonary involvement. Chest CT is reserved for abnormalities detected on plain radiographs. Assessment of the hepatic parenchyma would be necessarily accomplished during standard CT or MRI evaluation of the primary tumor.

PROGNOSTIC FACTORS

The predictive variables for local recurrence and survival are ill-defined for retroperitoneal lesions. Histologic grade is an important prognosticator but histologic type is not a reliable predictor of survival. Although size

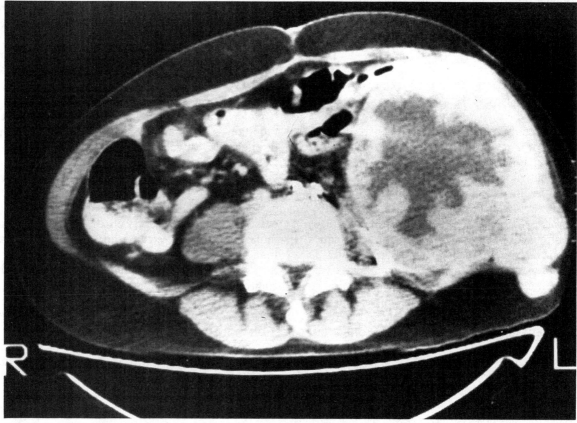

Fig. 27.11. CT of retroperitoneal sarcoma in 43-year-old patient. Note large size and central necrosis.

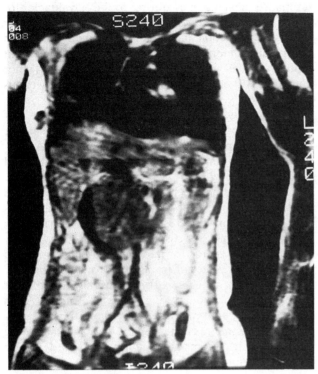

Fig. 27.12. MRI of retroperitoneal sarcoma. Note involvement of inferior vena cava.

and neurovascular involvement are addressed by the present AJCC staging system (Russell et al. 1977), invasion of adjacent organs or contiguous structures is not. Therefore, resectability, which has been shown to be a primary determinant of both local failure and survival, is overlooked. Critical analyses of variables predictive of outcome are necessary to confirm the reliability of the present staging system and appropriately stratify patients when evaluating multimodality regimens.

TREATMENT

Aggressive resection of all gross disease with an adequate margin of uninvolved tissue is the primary goal in treating these neoplasms. Their location makes tumor invasion of contiguous structures frequent. Proper exposure is best achieved transperitoneally by either a midline or bilateral subcostal approach. Organs frequently involved are the kidney, adrenal gland, colon, pancreas, stomach, small bowel, and diaphragm (Jaques et al. 1989). One or more of these viscera should be removed, when appropriate, to ensure a tumor-free margin. Neither the number of organs involved nor the lesion's size should dictate unresectability. Only the

surgeon's ability to remove all gross disease determines resectability. In a recent review of the Memorial experience, 80% of patients required resection of at least one adjacent organ to obtain clean margins. Complete resection could only be achieved in select patients by partial resection of major vessels (IVC, iliac artery/vein, superior mesenteric artery, etc.) and appropriate vascular reconstruction.

If complete excision is not feasible, partial resection of greater than 95% of tumor is the aim, in conjunction with interstitial radioactive implantation of gross residual disease when possible. This has improved the resectability rate over recent years. Of 56 patients referred for primary treatment of their tumor at Memorial Hospital between 1971 and 1982, 27 (48%) were completely resected and 22 (39%) partially resected. Ninety percent who presented with local failure were either completely or partially resected (table 27.9). Although morbidity (23%) and mortality (6%) are substantial, both have decreased dramatically in recent years. A similar approach should be taken for local recurrence. Lung or liver metastases should be resected aggressively if control of the primary tumor is feasible.

RADIATION AND CHEMOTHERAPY

Despite aggressive surgery, only 40% of patients are rendered disease-free by this single modality, and 5-year survival rates are approximately 40% following complete resection (Cody et al. 1981). Radiation therapy may be an attractive alternative or adjunctive approach, but the effective dose necessary to elicit a response is difficult to deliver. This is due not only to size and location of the tumor, but also to the radiation tolerance of intestine and other intra-abdominal organs. Primary radiation therapy rarely results in long-term survival and only in those with favorable histology (Kinne et al. 1973; Wist et al. 1985; Harrison et al. 1986). The Memorial experience and selected others are summarized in table 27.10. Brachytherapy and intraoperative radiation are techniques designed to limit toxicity and are being investigated. At this time, radiation therapy following adequate tumor resection is not considered standard practice. Clinical studies addressing the issue of adjuvant radiation are ongoing.

The role of chemotherapy in retroperitoneal sarcomas has yet to be elucidated. In patients who do not undergo curative resection, the single agent Adriamycin induces a partial or complete response in a select number of patients. No combination regimen has been shown to be more effective than Adriamycin, and all are invariably more toxic (Greenall et al. 1986). Likewise,

Table 27.9
RESECTABILITY RATE OF RETROPERITONEAL SOFT TISSUE SARCOMAS IN THE 1971-1982 MSKCC SERIES

Prior Treatment	Completely Resected	Partially Resected	Unresectable
No prior surgery	27 (48%)	22 (39%)	7 (13%)
Prior complete resection	15 (50%)	12 (40%)	3 (10%)

(From: Jaques, Coit, and Brennan [1989].)

Table 27.10
PUBLISHED RESULTS OF RADIATION THERAPY AS PRIMARY TREATMENT FOR UNRESECTABLE RETROPERITONEAL SOFT TISSUE SARCOMAS

Series	Year	No. of Patients	Tumor Dose (Gy)	Survival (%)	
				1-yr.	5-yr.
Kinne	1973	8*	20-50	25%	25%
Wist	1985	11	mean 39	55%	10%
Harrison	1986	10	7-49 mean 35	40%	10%

*All liposarcomas
(From: Jaques, Coit, and Brennan [1989].

the role of adjuvant chemotherapy needs further investigation. In a study from the National Cancer Institute, all patients had curative attempts at resection plus radiation therapy with or without combination chemotherapy (Adriamycin, Cytoxan, methotrexate). No benefit was demonstrated in the adjuvant chemotherapy arm and the chemotherapy administered was associated with significant morbidity (Glenn et al. 1985). Our institution is examining the efficacy of neoadjuvant combination chemotherapy in high-risk sarcoma patients.

OUTCOME

A retrospective analysis of the 1971-1982 data base identified 86 patients who underwent exploration for retroperitoneal sarcomas at Memorial Hospital. Fifty-four presented with their primary unresected, while 32 had recurrent disease. Overall survival was 63% at two years, and 37% at five years (table 27.11). Survival benefit is evident in those patients undergoing either complete or partial resection. No difference in 5-year survival is demonstrated between patients completely resected and the partial resection group, presumably due in part to the effect of radiation therapy. In patients presenting for their first definitive operation, complete resection affords the best survival (table 27.12). Local recurrence, with or without distant metastases, following complete tumor extirpation occurred in 42% of patients. The median disease-free interval was 15 months, necessitating careful and frequent follow-up (every two to three months), accompanied by CT scan every four to six months for two to three years. Despite poor outcome, local recurrence warrants aggressive attempts at resection, as all nonresected patients are dead at two years post recurrence (table 27.12). Site of distant metastases was equally distributed between lung and liver.

OTHER SITES

VISCERAL

Visceral sarcomas comprised approximately 5% of all soft tissue tumors seen at Memorial Hospital between 1982 and 1987. The majority (56%) were located in the stomach or small intestine. Other common sites included the rectum, colon, and liver. The predominant histopathological type was leiomyosarcoma. Symptoms associated with visceral sarcomas include gastrointestinal bleeding, intestinal obstruction, abdominal pain, and/or mass. Although nonspecific, these symptoms often precipitate radiologic and endoscopic procedures that provide valuable preoperative information. Upper or lower barium studies may identify an intramural or extramural lesion (Shiu et al. 1982), but have largely been supplanted by endoscopic examination, which can also provide a tissue diagnosis. In previous reviews from MSKCC (Shiu et al. 1982; Shiu et al. 1983), three clinicopathologic factors were associated with an unfavorable outcome: large tumor size, invasion of adjacent organs or contiguous structures, and high histopathologic grade.

Surgical treatment should be tailored to the lesion's size, extent, and location. Small gastric tumors can be excised by wedge resection with a variable margin of uninvolved tissue. Similar lesions of the small intestine or colon are adequately treated by segmental resection of the bowel and a portion of its mesentery. Small rectal tumors can be treated by simple excision via a number of sphincter-saving approaches. Larger tumors or tumors that invade adjacent organs or structures require more extensive resections encompassing all involved viscera when feasible. Pancreaticoduodenectomy, abdominoperineal resection, and pelvic exenteration should be considered in some cases since surgical extirpation holds the only chance for cure. The

Table 27.11
SURVIVAL OF PATIENTS WITH RETROPERITONEAL SARCOMA AFTER SURGICAL TREATMENT 1971-1982 SERIES*

	All Patients	Completely Resected	Partially Resected	Unresectable
2-yr survival	63%	76%	56%	30%
5-yr survival	37%	43%	45%	10%

*Eighty-six patients underwent operation at Memorial Hospital, 54 for initial surgical therapy and 32 for treatment of recurrent sarcoma.
(From: Jaques, Coit, and Brennan [1989].)

**Table 27.12
COMPARISON OF SURVIVAL AFTER SURGICAL
TREATMENT OF PRIMARY VERSUS RECURRENT
RETROPERITONEAL SOFT TISSUE SARCOMA**

	Survival (%)	
Resection type	2-year	5-year
Complete resection:		
Primary	85	56
Recurrence	60	20
Partial resection:		
Primary	63	45
Recurrence	42	25
Unresectable:		
Primary	43	14
Recurrence	0	0

(From: Jaques, Coit, and Brennan [1989].)

value of radiotherapy, as with retroperitoneal tumors, is limited by the radiation-tolerance of surrounding tissues. Radiation therapy may palliate in select instances. The role of chemotherapy has not been systematically examined or defined.

GENITOURINARY

The uterus (55%) is the most common site of presentation for sarcomas of the genitourinary tract. The most frequent histological types identified are leiomyosarcoma and mixed Müllerian sarcoma; the latter portends an unfavorable outcome. Prognosis is determined by tumor extent in addition to histopathology (Wen et al. 1987). Local tumor control is improved by the combination of aggressive resection and radiotherapy (Badib et al. 1969; Salazar et al. 1978), without change in survival. In an effort to improve survival, adjuvant chemotherapy has been examined in a number of trials with mixed results (Buchsbaum, Lifshitz, and Blythe 1979; Omura and Blessing 1978; Hannigan et al. 1983), mostly negative.

HEAD AND NECK

Sarcomas of the head and neck region are uncommon, accounting for 52 (5%) of 1,091 sarcoma patients admitted to our institution in the past five years. In adults, the predominant subtypes are malignant fibrous histiocytoma, fibrosarcoma, and embryonal rhabdomyosarcoma. In a recent review (Weber et al. 1986) histologic type, size, and treatment were factors that had prognostic value. The presence of malignant fibrous histiocytoma or rhabdomyosarcoma on histologic examination predicted poor survival while fibrosarcoma had improved survival at five years. Patients with large tumors (>5 cm) had reduced survival rates. Adequate resection with negative surgical margins improved disease-free survival, but the ability to widely excise tumor in this anatomic location is restricted. Radiotherapy has value for patients in whom adequate resection is not feasible. Chemotherapy is not considered standard treatment outside of investigational protocols. A prospective randomized trial of adjuvant chemotherapy following resection plus radiotherapy showed no survival benefit for the treatment arm (Rosenberg et al. 1981).

REFERENCES

Alvegard, T.A., for the Scandinavian Sarcoma Group. 1986. Adjuvant chemotherapy with Adriamycin in high grade malignant soft tissue sarcoma. *Proc. ASCO* 5(abstr):485.

Antman, K.; Suit, H.; and Amato, D. et al. 1984. Preliminary results of a randomized trial of adjuvant doxorubicin for sarcomas: lack of apparent difference between treatment groups. *J. Clin. Oncol.* 2:602-608.

Arbeit, J.M.; Hilaris, B.S.; and Brennan, M.F. 1987. Wound complications in the multimodality treatment of extremity and superficial truncal sarcomas. *J. Clin. Oncol.* 5:480-88.

Badib, A.O.; Vongtama, V.; and Kurohara, S.S. et al. 1969. Radiotherapy in the treatment of the sarcoma of the corpus uteri. *Cancer* 24:724-29.

Benjamin, R.S.; Wiernik, P.H.; and Bachur, N.R. 1974. Adriamycin chemotherapy: efficacy, safety and pharmacologic basis of an intermittent single high-dose schedule. *Cancer* 33:19-27.

Blum, R.H. 1975. Overview of studies with Adriamycin (NSC-123127) in the United States. *Cancer Chemother. Rep.* 6:247-51.

Borden, E.C.; Amato, D.A.; and Rosenbaum, C. et al. 1987. Randomized comparison of three Adriamycin regimens for metastatic soft tissue sarcomas. *J. Clin. Oncol.* 5:840-50.

Borel Rinkes, I.H.M., and de Jongste, A.B. 1986. Lymphangiosarcoma in chronic lymphedema. *Acta. Chir. Scand.* 152:227-30.

Bramwell, V.H.C.; Rouesse, J.; and Santoro, A. et al. 1985. European experience of adjuvant chemotherapy for soft tissue sarcoma: preliminary report of randomized trial of cyclophosphamide, vincristine, doxorubicin and dacarbazine. *Cancer Treat. Symp.* 3:99-107.

Brennan, M.F.; Friedrich, C.; and Almadrones, L. et al. 1987. Prospective randomized trial examining the cardiac toxicity of adjuvant doxorubicin in high grade extremity sarcomas. In *Adjuvant therapy of cancer V.* Orlando, Fla.: Grune & Stratton.

Brennan, M.F.; Hilaris, B.; and Shiu, M.H. et al. 1987. Local recurrence in adult soft tissue sarcoma: randomized trial of brachytherapy. *Arch. Surg.* 122:1289-93.

Buchsbaum, H.J.; Lifshitz, S.; and Blythe, J.G. 1979. Prophylactic chemotherapy in stage I and II uterine sarcoma. *Gynecol. Oncol.* 8:346-48.

Chang, A.E.; Schaner, E.G.; and Conkle, D.M. et al. 1979. Evaluation of computed tomography in detection of pulmonary metastases: prospective study. *Cancer* 43:913-16.

Chang, A.E.; Matory, Y.L.; and Dwyer, A.J. et al. 1987. Magnetic resonance imaging vs. computed tomography in the evaluation of soft tissue sarcomas of the extremities. *Ann. Surg.* 205:340-48.

Cody, H.S. III; Turnbull, A.O.; and Fortner, J.G. et al. 1981. Continuing challenge of retroperitoneal sarcomas. *Cancer* 47:2147-52.

Collin, C.; Hajdu, S.I.; and Godbold, J. et al. 1986. Localized, operable soft tissue sarcoma of the lower extremity. *Arch. Surg.* 121:1425-33.

Collin, C.; Hajdu, S.I.; and Godbold, J. et al. 1987. Localized, operable soft tissue sarcoma of the upper extremity. *Ann. Surg.* 205:331-39.

Collin, C.; Godbold, J.; and Hajdu, S. et al. 1987. Localized extremity soft tissue sarcoma: analysis of factors affecting survival. *J. Clin. Oncol.* 5:601-12.

Collin, C.; Friedrich, C.; and Godbold, J. et al. 1988. Prognostic factors for local recurrence and survival in patients with localized extremity soft-tissue sarcoma. *Semin. Surg. Oncol.* 4:30-37.

Creagan, E.T.; Hahn, R.G.; and Ahmann, D.L. et al. 1977. Clinical trial of Adriamycin (NSC-123127) in advanced sarcomas. *Oncology* 34:90-91.

Crowe, F.W.; Schull, W.J.; and Neel, J.V. 1956. *A clinical, pathological and genetic study of multiple neurofibromatosis.* Springfield, Ill.: Charles C. Thomas.

D'Agostino, A.N.; Soule, E.H.; and Miller, R.H. 1963. Sarcomas of the peripheral nerves and somatic soft tissues associated with multiple neurofibromatosis (von Recklinghausen's disease). *Cancer* 16:1015-27.

Davidson, T.; Westbury, G.; and Harmer, C.L. 1986. Radiation-induced soft tissue sarcoma. *Br. J. Surg.* 73: 308-309.

Demas, B.E.; Heelan, R.T.; and Lane, J. et al. 1988. Soft tissue sarcoma of the extremities: prospective comparison of MRI and CT in determination of anatomic extent of disease. *AJR* 150:615-20.

Donohue, J.H.; Collin, C.; and Friedrich, C. et al. 1988. Low-grade soft tissue sarcomas of the extremities: analysis of risk factors for metastasis. *Cancer* 62:184-93.

Edmondson, J.H.; Fleming, T.R.; and Ivins, J.C. et al. 1984. Randomized study of systemic chemotherapy following complete excision of nonosseous sarcomas. *J. Clin. Oncol.* 2:1390-96.

Gherlinzoni, F.; Bacaci, G.; and Pippi, P. et al. 1986. Randomized trial for the treatment of high grade soft tissue sarcoma of the extremities: preliminary observations. *J. Clin. Oncol.* 4:552-58.

Glenn, J.; Sindelar, W.F.; and Kinsella, T. et al. 1985. Results of multimodality therapy of resectable soft-tissue sarcomas of the retroperitoneum. *Surgery* 97:316-25.

Greenall, M.J.; Magill, G.B.; and DeCosse, J.J. et al 1986. Chemotherapy for soft tissue sarcoma. *Surg. Gynecol. Obstet.* 162:193-98.

Hajdu, S.I. 1985. *Differential diagnosis of soft tissue and bone tumors.* Philadelphia: Lea and Febiger.

Hannigan, E.V.; Freedman, R.S.; and Elder, K.W. et al. 1983. Treatment of advanced uterine sarcoma with Adriamycin. *Gynecol. Oncol.* 16:101-104.

Harrison, L.B.; Gutierrez, E.; and Fischer, J.J. 1986. Retroperitoneal sarcomas: Yale experience and review of the literature. *J. Surg. Oncol.* 32:159-64.

Hayry, P.; Reitamo, J.J.; and Totterman, S. et al. 1982. The desmoid tumor II: analysis of factors possibly contributing to the etiology and growth behavior. *Am. J. Clin. Pathol.* 77:674-80.

Jaques, D.P.; Coit, D.G.; and Brennan, M.F. 1989. Soft tissue sarcoma of the retroperitoneum. In Shiu, M.H., and Brennan, M.F. eds. *Surgical management of soft tissue sarcoma.* pp. 170-88. Philadelphia: Lea and Febiger.

Kang, H.; Enziger, F.; and Breslin, P. et al. 1987. Soft tissue sarcoma and military service in Vietnam: case-control study. *J. Natl. Cancer Inst.* 79:693-99.

Kinne, D.W.; Chu, F.C.H.; and Huvos, A.G. et al. 1973. Treatment of primary and recurrent retroperitoneal liposarcoma: twenty-five-year experience at Memorial Hospital. *Cancer* 31:53-64.

Kissin, M.W.; Fisher, C.; and Carter, R.L. et al. 1986. Value of Tru-Cut biopsy in the diagnosis of soft tissue sarcomas. *Br. J. Surg.* 73:742-44.

Lindberg, R.D. 1983. Role of radiotherapy. In Baker L.H. ed. *Soft tissue sarcomas.* Boston: Martinus Nijhoff.

McCormick, P.M.; and Martini, N. 1979. Changing role of surgery for pulmonary metastases. *Ann. Thorac. Surg.* 28: 139-45.

Muller, R.; Hajdu, S.I.; and Brennan, M.F. 1987. Lymphangiosarcoma associated with chronic filarial lymphedema. *Cancer* 59:179-83.

Muss, H.B.; Bundy, B.; and DiSaia, P.J. et al. 1985. Treatment of recurrent or advanced uterine sarcoma: randomized trial of doxorubicin vs. doxorubicin and cyclophosphamide (a Phase III trial of the Gynecologic Oncology Group). *Cancer* 55:1648-53.

O'Bryan, R.M.; Luce, J.K.; and Talley, R.W. et al. 1973. Phase II evaluation of Adriamycin in human neoplasia. *Cancer* 32:1-8.

O'Bryan, R.M.; Baker, L.H.; and Gottlieb, J.E. et al. 1977. Dose response evaluation of Adriamycin in human neoplasia. *Cancer* 39:1940-48.

Omura, G.A.; Major, F.J.; and Blessing, J.A. et al. 1983. Randomized study of Adriamycin with and without dimethyl triazenoimidazole carboximide in advanced uterine sarcomas. *Cancer* 52:626-32.

Omura, G.A.; and Blessing, J.A. 1978. Chemotherapy of stage III, IV and uterine sarcomas: randomized trial of Adriamycin vs. AD + DTIC. *Proc. ACR and ASCO* (abstr 103).

Ormsby, M.V.; Hilaris, B.S.; and Nori, D. et al. 1989. Wound complications of adjuvant radiation therapy in patients with soft-tissue sarcomas. *Ann. Surg.* 210:93-99.

Posner, M.L.; Shiu, M.A.; and Newsome, J. et al. 1989. The desmoid tumor–not a benign disease. *Arch. Surg.* 124: 191-96.

Putnam, J.B. Jr.; Roth, J.A.; and Wesley, M.N. et al. 1984. Analysis of prognostic factors in patients undergoing resection of pulmonary metastases from soft tissue sarcoma. *J. Thorac. Cardiovasc. Surg.* 87:260-68.

Roholl, P.J.M.; DeJong, A.S.H.; and Ramaekers, F.C.S. 1985. Application of markers in the diagnosis of soft tissue tumors. *Histopathology* 9:1019-35.

Rosenberg, S.A.; Tepper, J.; and Glatstein, E. et al. 1981. Adjuvant chemotherapy for patients with soft tissue sarcomas. *Surg. Clin. North Am.* 61:1415-23.

Rosenberg, S.A.; Tepper, J.; and Glatstein, E. et al. 1982. Treatment of soft tissue sarcomas of the extremities: prospective randomized evaluations of (1) limb-sparing surgery plus radiation therapy compared with amputation and (2) the role of adjuvant chemotherapy. *Ann. Surg.* 196:305-15.

Rosenberg, S.A.; Tepper, J.; and Glatstein, E. et al. 1982. Treatment of soft tissue sarcomas of the extremities. *Ann. Surg.* 196:305-15.

Roth, J.A.; Pass, H.I.; and Wesley, M.N. et al. 1986. Comparison of median sternotomy and thoracotomy for resection of pulmonary metastases in patients with adult soft-tissue sarcomas. *Ann. Thorac. Surg.* 42:134-38.

Russell, W.O.; Cohen, J.; and Enzinger, F.M.; et al. 1977. Clinical and pathological staging system for soft tissue sarcomas. *Cancer* 40:1562-70.

Salazar, O.M.; Bonfiglio, T.A.; and Patten, S.F. et al. 1978. Uterine sarcomas: natural history, treatment and prognosis. *Cancer* 42:1152-60.

Schoenfeld, D.A.; Rosenbaum, C.; and Horton, J. et al. 1982. Comparison of Adriamycin vs. vincristine and Adriamycin vs. vincristine, Actinomycin D, and cyclophosphamide for advanced sarcoma. *Cancer* 50:2757-62.

Shiu, M.H.; Farr, G.H.; and Papachristou, D.N. et al. 1982. Myosarcomas of the stomach: natural history, prognostic factors and management. *Cancer* 49:177-87.

Shiu, M.H.; Farr, G.H.; and Egeli, R.A. et al. 1983. Myosarcomas of the small and large intestine: clinicopathologic study. *J. Surg. Oncol.* 24:67-72.

Shiu, M.H.; Turnbull, A.D.; and Nori, D. et al. 1984. Control of locally advanced extremity soft tissue sarcomas by function-saving resection and brachytherapy. *Cancer* 53: 1385-92.

Shiu, M.H.; Collin, C.; and Hilaris, B. et al. 1986. Limb preservation and tumor control in the treatment of popliteal and antecubital soft tissue sarcomas. *Cancer* 57:1632-39.

Shiu, M.H.; Hilaris, B.; and Brennan, M.F. 1988. Brachytherapy and limb sparing resection in the management of soft tissue sarcoma. In Ryan, J.R. and Baker, L.O. eds. *Recent concepts in sarcoma treatment.* pp. 104-14. London: Kluwer Academie.

Silverberg, E.; Boring, C.; and Squires, T. 1990. Cancer statistics. *CA* 40:7-24.

Sordillo, P.P.; Chapman, R.; and Hajdu, S.I. et al. 1981. Lymphangiosarcoma. *Cancer* 48:1674-79.

Souba, W.W.; McKenna, R.J.; and Meis, J. et al. 1986. Radiation-induced sarcomas of the chest wall. *Cancer* 57:610-15.

Suit, H.D.; Russell, W.O.; and Martin, R.G. 1973. Management of patients with sarcoma of soft tissue in an extremity. *Cancer* 31:1247-55.

Suit, H.D.; Russell, W.O.; and Martin, R.G. 1975. Sarcoma of soft tissue: clinical and histopathologic parameters and response to treatment. *Cancer* 35:1478-83.

Suit, H.D.; and Russell, W.O. 1975. Radiation therapy of soft tissue sarcomas. *Cancer* 36:759-64.

Suit, H.D.; Proppe, K.H.; and Mankin, H.J. et al. 1981. Preoperative radiation therapy for sarcoma of soft tissue. *Cancer* 47:2269-74.

Weber, R.S.; Benjamin, R.S.; and Peters, L.J. et al. 1986. Soft tissue sarcomas of the head and neck in adolescents and adults. *Am. J. Surg.* 152:386-92.

Weingrad, D.W.; and Rosenberg, S.A. 1978. Early lymphatic spread of osteogenic and soft tissue sarcoma. *Surgery* 84:231-40.

Wen, B.C.; Tewfik, F.A.; and Tewfik, H.H. et al. 1987. Uterine sarcoma: retrospective study. *J. Surg. Oncol.* 34:104-108.

Wist, E.; Solheim, O.P.; and Jacobsen, A.B. et al. 1985. Primary retroperitoneal sarcomas. *Acta Radiol.* 24:305-10.

Chapter 28

HODGKIN'S DISEASE AND NON-HODGKIN'S LYMPHOMAS

Harmon J. Eyre, M.D.
Max L. Farver, M.D.

Harmon J. Eyre, M.D.
Professor of Medicine
Director of Clinical Research
Utah Cancer Center
University of Utah School of Medicine
Salt Lake City, Utah

Max L. Farver, M.D.
Assistant Professor of Internal Medicine
Department of Internal Medicine
University of South Dakota
Yankton, South Dakota

INTRODUCTION

The malignant lymphomas—Hodgkin's disease and non-Hodgkin's lymphomas—constitute a heterogeneous group of cancers that arise from the lymphoreticular system. They are the seventh most common cancer in the United States, but because of the younger average age of the lymphoma population, they account for more years of potential life lost than many of the more common adult cancers (Silverberg, Boring, and Squires 1990; Devesa et al. 1987). The cell of origin of Hodgkin's disease is still not completely defined, but it appears to be from the monocyte-histiocyte series (Pinkus, Thomas, and Said 1985). The origin of the malignant cell in non-Hodgkin's lymphomas is most commonly from B lymphocytes, and less frequently from T lymphocytes (Foon, Schroff, and Gale 1982).

Malignant lymphomas are among the most-studied human tumors and are among the most curable of all cancers. They are being extensively evaluated with immunophenotypes, gene rearrangements, cytogenetic abnormalities, and oncogene activation being determined. New therapeutic approaches are using combination chemotherapy, chemotherapy combined with radiotherapy, and high-dose chemotherapy with autologous marrow rescue in patients with refractory disease (DeVita, Jaffe, and Hellman 1985; Rosenberg and Kaplan 1982). The next few years will continue to bring rapid advances in understanding the pathogenesis and therapy of lymphomas; even higher cure rates should result.

HODGKIN'S DISEASE

EPIDEMIOLOGY

Hodgkin's disease (HD) accounts for approximately 14% of all malignant lymphomas. For 1990, it was estimated that 7,400 new cases (4,200 male, 3,200 female), and 1,600 deaths would occur (Silverberg, Boring, and Squires 1990). It occurs in a bimodal age-incidence distribution: the incidence rates rise sharply after age 10, peak in the late 20s, and then decline until age 45. After 45 the incidence again increases steadily with age. The histologic pattern and anatomic distribution vary with age. The nodular sclerosis form of the disease predominates in young adults and the mixed cellularity form is most common in the older age group. Twenty-five percent of elderly patients have only subdiaphragmatic disease at diagnosis, compared with fewer than 5% of young adult patients. More than half of the young patients have mediastinal involvement, compared with less than 25% of the elderly patients (DeVita, Jaffe, and Hellman 1985; Rosenberg and Kaplan 1982; National Cancer Institute 1988; Cutler and Young 1975).

ETIOLOGY

The clinical manifestations of fever, chills, and leukocytosis, and the histologic similarity to a granulomatous process, have suggested an infectious etiology. The epidemiology of Hodgkin's disease implies that the childhood social environment influences risk of the disease in young adulthood. The risk of acquiring the disease is associated with factors that diminish or delay exposure to infectious agents, such as higher social class, more education, small family size, and early birth-order position (Paffenbarger, Wing, and Hyde 1977; Grufferman et al. 1977; Vianna and Polan 1978).

Epstein-Barr virus (EBV) is a possible etiologic agent, a suggestion supported by the virus' ability to transform lymphocytes, and by the presence of Reed-Sternberg-like cells in lymphoid tissue of patients with infectious mononucleosis. This hypothesis, although supported by an early report of a 3.6-fold increase in the incidence of Hodgkin's disease among persons with histories of infectious mononucleosis, is not supported by other reports that show a weak association between EBV and HD (Diehl et al. 1984). The proportion of patients with antibodies to EBV viral capsid antigen is similar to that of controls, but the HD patients consistently have higher titers. These antibody titers have been shown to increase with progressive loss of cell-mediated immunity, as well as after splenectomy and treatment (Hesse et al. 1977). Hodgkin's disease is associated with some of the prodromal manifestations seen in acquired immune deficiency syndrome (AIDS) when it presents in advanced stages with a higher incidence of marrow involvement.

An increased incidence in persons with close personal contact with known cases of Hodgkin's disease has been used to support the hypothesis that it is contagious. However, subsequent studies have not shown an excess incidence among students who attended school with a student who had the disease (Grufferman, Cole, and Levitan 1979). There is no increased risk among physicians and nurses who are exposed to patients with the disease (Grufferman, Doung, and Cole 1976). However, there is a 7-fold increased risk for Hodgkin's disease in siblings of known cases, and a 3-fold risk for other first-degree relatives (Grufferman et al. 1977). In one family, all four siblings were affected and found to have one human leukocyte antigen (HLA) in common, suggesting the important role of genetic factors in the etiology of Hodgkin's disease (Robertson et al. 1987).

Although the question of neoplastic cell lineage remains unclear, current evidence suggests that the Reed-Sternberg (R-S) cell is derived from the monocyte-macrophage cell line. These cells possess Fc and complement receptors and lectin receptors, and express a granulocyte-related differentiation antigen, Leu-M1 (Pinkus, Thomas, and Said 1985). Reed-Sternberg cells have been shown to have polyclonal immunoglobulins in their cytoplasm, which supports the theory that they retain the phagocytic processes of monocyte-macrophage cell lines (Kadin et al. 1978). The giant cells cultured *in vitro* have also been shown to secrete the monokine interleukin-1 into the culture media (Ford et al. 1982). This monokine causes proliferation of T lymphocytes and fibroblasts and acts as an endogenous pyrogen (Oppenheim et al. 1982); both are common histologic and clinical features of Hodgkin's disease.

Multiple host defense mechanisms are adversely affected by Hodgkin's disease. Abnormalities in cellular immunity were demonstrated in batteries of skin tests (Young et al. 1972). Lymphocyte depletion (<1500/mcl of blood) is seen in 40% to 50% of patients and is more common in advanced disease. These lymphocytes proliferate poorly when stimulated. Macrophages adhere poorly to foreign surfaces and have abnormal antigen processing (Case et al. 1976). The clinical importance of these immune defects, combined with the effects of immunosuppressive therapy and splenectomy, is seen in the increased incidence of infectious complications. About 75% of the serious infections are caused by common bacterial pathogens and 25% are due to unusual pathogens such as *Pneumocystis carinii, Nocardia, Listeria, Aspergillus,* and *Candida*. Herpes zoster infections are common and may be the presenting symptoms (Kaplan 1980a).

CLINICAL PRESENTATION AND DETECTION

The typical presentation is characterized by painless lymphadenopathy in a young adult, although there may be associated constitutional symptoms of malaise, fever, night sweats, pruritus, and weight loss. The enlarged lymph node is usually (90%) supradiaphragmatic, and is frequently (60% to 80%) in the cervical region (Moran and Ultmann 1974). Axillary or mediastinal lymphadenopathy is less common. Massive mediastinal lymph nodes may result in symptoms of cough, wheezing, dyspnea, or superior vena cava syndrome. Subdiaphragmatic presentations are uncommon (10%) in young patients, but represent the only site of disease in 25% of the elderly patients. Involvement of retroperitoneal nodes, liver, spleen, and bone marrow usually occurs after the disease becomes generalized. Mesenteric lymph nodes are rarely involved, although in advanced cases any organ can be involved (Stein 1981).

A number of diagnostic procedures are used. They are:

Lymph node biopsy. The largest, most central node in an involved group should be removed with the capsule intact. Cervical nodes are preferable to axillary and inguinal nodes since the latter can frequently exhibit reactive changes and not be diagnostic. Needle biopsies yield limited amounts of tissue and are often not helpful for diagnosis. The pathologist should be notified prior to the surgical procedure in order to prepare fresh tissue for the various marker and cytogenetic studies prior to freezing or fixing the tissue in buffered formalin or Zenker solution.

Hematologic findings. Mild normochromic, normocytic anemia and a neutrophilic leukocytosis are common. Lymphopenia is present in approximately 50% of the cases at presentation and is more common in advanced stages. Eosinophilia may occur. Hemolytic anemia has been reported, usually in advanced disease, and is frequently Coombs' negative (Bjorkholm, Hol, and Merk 1982). Elevated erythrocyte sedimentation rates are common and have been correlated with exacerbations and advanced disease (Moran and Ultmann 1974).

Blood chemistries. Elevated serum alkaline phosphatase suggests liver or bone involvement, but may be nonspecific in younger patients. Hypergammaglobulinemia is common in early disease, but Ig levels may become low in advanced disease or during treatment. Elevated serum copper and ceruloplasm have been reported in active disease (Stein 1981).

Radiologic studies. Radiologic studies are important in both diagnosis and staging and may be the technique to initially detect lymphadenopathy or organ involvement.

PATHOLOGIC AND CLINICAL STAGING

HISTOPATHOLOGY

Hodgkin's disease is distinguished from other lymphomas by the presence of Reed-Sternberg cells (R-S cells) which are large, binucleate cells with vesicular nuclei and prominent eosinophilic nucleoli. The R-S cells are essential for the diagnosis of Hodgkin's disease, but they have been reported in benign conditions such as hyperplastic or inflammatory nodes, mononucleosis, some viral infections, and phenytoin therapy. Lymph nodes containing Hodgkin's disease show disruption of their normal nodal architecture by a diffuse and frequently mixed infiltration of neutrophils and a variable number of R-S cells. In 1966, Lukes and Butler proposed a histologic classification that appeared to correlate well with clinical stage and aggressiveness of disease (Lukes, Butler, and Hicks 1966). This scheme was later simplified into the Rye classification (table 28.1), which is widely used by pathologists and clinicians to subclassify the histology into four groups. These histologic features are illustrated in fig. 28.1.

Lymphocyte predominant. This group accounts for about 5% to 10% of patients with Hodgkin's disease. Abundant mature lymphocytes diffusely infiltrate the abnormal lymph nodes; R-S cells are few in number and difficult to find. The prognosis is excellent for patients with this subtype, with a 5-year survival rate of approximately 90%.

Nodular sclerosis. This is the most common subtype (30% to 60%). Interlacing bands of collagen that divide the cellular infiltrate into discrete island produce the lymph node's nodular appearance. Also present is a variant of the classic R-S cell, referred to as a lacunar

Table 28.1
HISTOPATHOLOGIC CLASSIFICATION OF HODGKIN'S DISEASE (RYE CLASSIFICATION)

Histology	Relative Frequency
Lymphocyte predominant	5% to 10%
Nodular sclerosis	30% to 60%
Mixed cellularity	20% to 40%
Lymphocyte depleted	5% to 10%

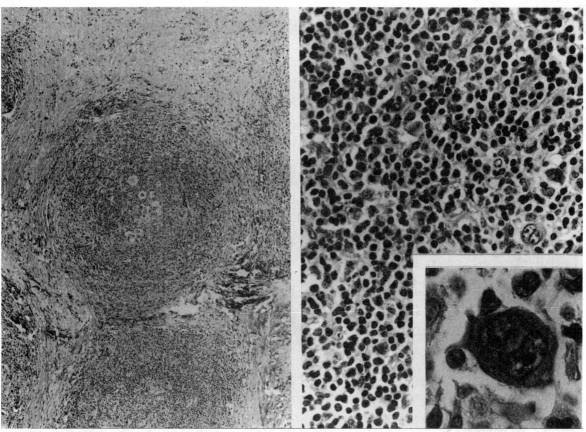

Fig. 28.1. (Left) nodular sclerosis Hodgkin's disease, low-power view. (Right) mixed cellularity Hodgkin's disease, medium-power view. (Inset) Reed-Sternberg cell, high-power view.

R-S cell because of its very faint staining cytoplasm that appears to be an empty space, or lacunae. Prognosis is good, with a high 5-year survival. This disease pattern is most frequently seen in young female adults. At diagnosis it is most often localized in the cervical nodes and mediastinum.

Mixed cellularity. This histologic group is the second most common, making up about 33% of the total. The nodes contain a pleomorphic infiltrate of eosinophils, normal lymphocytes, and readily identifiable R-S cells. Prognosis is slightly less favorable than the first two categories, with a 5-year survival of all stages of 50% to 60%.

Lymphocyte depleted. This is the least common subgroup of Hodgkin's disease reported. The R-S cell predominates and mature lymphocytes are virtually absent in affected lymph nodes. This pattern occurs primarily in older patients and is associated with B symptoms and an advanced stage at presentation. It has the least favorable prognosis of all the histologic types of HD with a 5-year survival rate of less than 50%.

ANATOMICAL STAGING

The 1971 Ann Arbor Symposium on staging in Hodgkin's disease recommended the following system using clinical staging (CS) and pathologic staging (PS) (Carbone et al. 1971). Clinical stage is determined by performing a thorough history and physical examination, blood counts and chemistries, chest x-ray, abdominal CT scan, and bipedal lymphangiography. Pathologic stage is based on the CS and information gained by the histologic review of tissue obtained by bone marrow biopsy, laparotomy, or from other sites. (Staging is illustrated in fig. 28.2 and described in table 28.2).

The following are the stages of the Ann Arbor staging system. Stage I is involvement of a single lymph-node region (I) or of a single extranodal site (I_E). Stage II is involvement of two or more lymph-node regions on the same side of the diaphragm (II) or localized involvement of an extranodal site and one or more lymph-node regions on the same side of the diaphragm (II_E).

Stage III is involvement of lymph-node regions on both sides of the diaphragm (III), and may include a single extranodal site (III_E), the spleen (III_S), or both (III_{SE}). Stage III has more recently been subdivided into lymphatic involvement of the upper abdomen in the spleen, splenic, celiac, and portal nodes (III_1), and the lower abdomen nodes in the periaortic, mesenteric, and iliac regions (III_2) (Desser et al. 1977).

Stage IV is diffuse or disseminated disease of one or more extralymphatic organs or tissues with or without associated lymph-node involvement. The pathologically proven extranodal site of disease should be identified by the following symbols: H = hepatic; L = lung; P = pleura; M = marrow; D = dermal; O = osseous.

As diagnostic imaging studies have improved, more staging is performed by computed tomography (CT), magnetic resonance imaging (MRI), isotope scanning, and ultrasonography. These techniques are frequently combined with directed needle biopsies and in many cases staging can be accurately completed without extensive surgery. These newer approaches have led to recommended changes in the Ann Arbor staging classification (Lister et al. 1989).

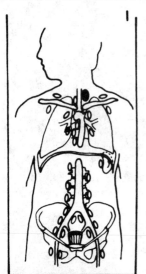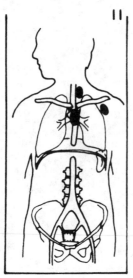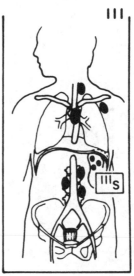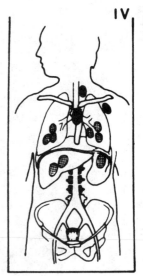

● INVOLVED NODE

⊗ INVOVED ORGAN

S INVOLVED SPLEEN

Fig. 28.2. Ann Arbor staging of the lymphomas. Stage I—single node region; stage II—two or more node regions on the same side of the diaphragm; stage III—lymph nodes or spleen involved on both sides of the diaphragm; stage IV—multiple or disseminated involvement of organs. Contiguous extralymphatic organ involvement can occur with stages I-III designated by I_E, II_E, III_E.

Table 28.2
STAGE/SUBSTAGE CLASSIFICATION
HODGKIN'S DISEASE
(ANN ARBOR STAGING SYSTEM)

Stage		Substage
Stage I	Single node region	I
	Single extralymphatic; organ/site	I (E)
Stage II	Two or more node regions on same side of diaphragm	II
	Single node region + localized single extralymphatic; organ/site	II (E)
Stage III	Node regions on both sides of diaphragm	III
	+ localized single extralymphatic	III (E)
	organ/site; spleen, both	III (S)
		III (ES)
Stage IV	Diffuse involvement extralymphatic organ/site node regions	IV
All stages	Without weight loss/fever/sweats	A
divided	With weight loss/fever/sweats	B

E = Extranodal
S = Spleen involved
(Compiled from: Carbone et al. [1971].)

A or B symptoms. A refers to patient without certain general symptoms; B refers to those with certain general symptoms. B symptoms include: unexplained fever with oral temperatures above 38°C, night sweats, and unexplained weight loss of more than 10% of body weight during the previous six months. Unexplained pruritus and alcohol-induced pain do not qualify as B symptoms. The presence of unexplained anemia has been demonstrated to be detrimental to outcome and perhaps should be considered a B symptom.

The value of the Ann Arbor staging system has been clearly demonstrated (Kaplan 1980a) by allowing clinicians to determine treatment and prognosis and compare patients enrolled in different treatment protocols. Despite the explicit staging definitions and their ability to be reproduced, there is some controversy in separating patients with E lesions from those with stage IV disease (Connors and Klimo 1984).

STAGING PROCEDURES

A careful, complete staging workup is essential to determine the extent of disease before proper treatment can be selected. Required procedures (Jones 1980; *Cancer Treat. Rep.* 1982) include an adequate surgical biopsy to be examined by an experienced pathologist and a detailed history including information about the presence of fever, sweating, weight loss, pruritus, and infections.

A thorough physical examination should be conducted, with special attention paid to all node-bearing areas, Waldeyer's ring, liver and spleen size, and a pelvic examination for women. Laboratory procedures with complete blood counts (CBCs), and blood chemistries should be performed. CBCs should include a differential white blood count (WBC), platelet count, reticulocyte count, and an erythrocyte sedimentation rate (ESR). A peripheral blood smear should be reviewed. Blood chemistries should include serum alkaline phosphatase and liver and kidney function tests.

Radiologic studies with PA and lateral chest x-ray are required and should be followed up with a chest CT scan if findings are suspicious or abnormal (Redman et al. 1977). Bipedal lymphangiography (LAG) is important for guiding biopsies during laparotomy and designing radiation ports. It can also be used to follow abnormal nodes with serial abdominal plain films. LAG is 95% sensitive (Clouse et al. 1985) with rare false positives in the grossly abnormal lymph nodes. The limitations of LAG are that high celiac, splenic hilar, portal, and mesenteric nodes are not visualized.

Abdominal CT scans are complementary to LAG and can detect suspicious (1 cm diameter) and enlarged (2 cm diameter) nodes in the regions not seen by LAG. Scans can provide information about the urinary tract and the structure and size of the liver and spleen (Strijk, Wagener, and Bogman 1985). The administration of oral and IV contrast produce optimal test results. However, the CT scan does not replace LAG because it is less sensitive (80%), has more false positives, is more costly, and does not demonstrate the abnormal, foamy node architecture of Hodgkin's disease (Redman et al. 1977; Clouse et al. 1985).

Procedures that are required under certain circumstances include bone marrow biopsy, which is recommended for most patients, particularly those with locally advanced disease, systemic symptoms, suspected bone involvement, and unexplained cytopenia (Weiss, Brunning, and Kennedy 1975). The biopsies are frequently bilateral and are usually taken from the posterior iliac crest with a Jamshidi needle. The sensitivity of the procedure is directly related to the quantity of tissue available for study; larger specimens may be obtained at the time of laparotomy.

Staging laparotomy with splenectomy should be performed when the information gained by the procedure will influence therapeutic decisions (Kaplan 1980a). The procedure includes an abdominal exploration with attention to both nodal and possible extranodal sites of disease, biopsy of both lobes of the liver, splenectomy, LAG-directed abdominal lymph-node biopsies, iliac crest bone marrow biopsy, and oophoropexy in selected cases.

Surgical staging is important in CS I, II, and IIIA patients due to the inaccuracy of clinical staging. After laparotomy, treatment plans were changed for 35% of patients; of these 25% to 35% were upstaged and about 10% were downstaged (Taylor, Kaplan, and Nelsen 1985). Clinically negative spleens were pathologically involved in one-third of the cases. Splenectomy may also have the therapeutic benefit of improving tolerance to chemotherapy (Kaplan 1980a). Laparotomy and splenectomy are associated with a 10% postoperative morbidity and less than 0.5% mortality. Splenectomized patients are at risk for increased infections, especially *Streptococcus pneumoniae* and *Hemophilus influenzae*, and should be given polyvalent pneumococcal vaccine before splenectomy.

In addition, intravenous pyelography, abdominal ultrasound, or inferior vena cavagram can be helpful if LAG or CT scan is equivocal or unsatisfactory. Skeletal x-rays should be obtained for areas of bone tenderness or pain. Percutaneous liver biopsy has a low sensitivity, while laparoscopic-directed liver biopsy is comparable to open surgical biopsy.

Optional or investigational procedures are radioisotope bone scans in patients with bone pain and equivocal x-rays; radioisotope liver or spleen scans; and gallium-67 scans, which may be useful in detecting recurrent disease in nodes above the diaphragm. Tests for delayed hypersensitivity with PPD, *Candida*, or *Trichophyton* can be normal even in advanced disease, but anergy in a patient with apparent localized disease may indicate dissemination.

PRINCIPLES OF TREATMENT

MULTIDISCIPLINARY TREATMENT APPROACH
The initial treatment plan is critical in determining the eventual outcome because the overwhelming majority of patients, even with the most advanced stages of disease, are potentially curable if optimal therapy is employed. Every aspect of staging and treatment planning should be thoroughly discussed by the patient's management team: medical and radiation oncologists, surgeon, pathologist, and radiologist. If competent physicians in each of these areas are not available, then the patient should be referred to a center where many patients with Hodgkin's disease are treated.

SURGERY
The primary roles of surgery in HD are to obtain diagnostic tissue and to perform a laparotomy when indicated. An experienced surgical team will decrease operative morbidity and mortality while increasing diagnostic yield.

Therapeutic excision of enlarged nodes in early stage disease is not indicated. Removal of stable residual bulky masses following therapy usually reveals fibrosis (Chen, Osborne, and Butler 1987).

Therapeutic splenectomy for hypersplenism, to increase tolerance to chemotherapy, or to reduce radiation field size may be indicated in selected cases (Schreiber et al. 1985).

RADIATION THERAPY
Irradiation is curative in most patients with limited Hodgkin's disease, i.e., stages I, II, and some IIIA (Cornbleet et al. 1985; Leslie, Mauch, and Hellman 1985; Prosnitz et al. 1978). The addition of chemotherapy to radiation may be indicated in patients with adverse prognostic factors such as B symptoms, bulky disease, and stage III_2 (Kaplan 1980a; Desser et al. 1977; Farber et al. 1980). Some basic concepts apply to curative radiation therapy for HD: use of megavoltage radiation (linear accelerators); treatment by opposed fields; tumoricidal doses; careful field simulation and verification; and close follow-up of all patients. Treatment should only be administered by a qualified radiation oncologist with full physics and dosimetric facilities. The general techniques of radiation therapy are illustrated in fig. 28.3.

The use of extended fields to include the adjacent, clinically negative nodal sites is essential for high cure rates (Kaplan 1980b). Extended field irradiation is based on the contiguity theory of Kaplan and Rosenberg (1966), which suggests that the disease is a monoclonal, unicentric neoplasm that predictably spreads by lymphatics to contiguous node groups. Total nodal irradiation (TNI) sequentially treats a mantle field above the diaphragm. Subtotal nodal irradiation (STNI) refers to a mantle field followed by irradiation to the pera-aortic

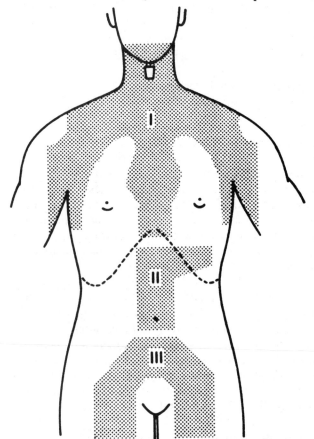

Fig. 28.3. Radiation fields (shaded areas) commonly employed in Hodgkin's disease. I = mantle; II = para-aortic-splenic pedicle; III = pelvic. I + II = subtotal nodal irradiation (STNI). I + II + III = total nodal irradiation (TNI).

Table 28.3
REPRESENTATIVE RESULTS OF RADIATION THERAPY IN LAPAROTOMY-STAGED HODGKIN'S DISEASE

Stage	Number of Patients in Series	5-year Freedom from Disease (%)	5-year Survival (%)	Reference
PS IA, IIA	111	85	95	(Mauch, Goodman, and Hellman 1978)
PS IA, IIA	98	77	90	(Zagars and Rubin 1985)
PS IA, IIA	131	77	95	(Prosnitz et al. 1980)
PS IB, IIB	53	75	86	(Hoppe 1980)
PS IIIA	86	66	86	(Rosenberg et al. 1982a)

PS = Pathologic stage

nodes and splenic pedicle. In PS I and IIA disease, STNI has become standard therapy and has the advantage of sparing the pelvic bone marrow and reducing exposure of the gonads. Carefully constructed field shapes and blocks (shielding) are used to protect the lungs, heart, spinal cord, larynx, kidneys, gonads, and iliac crests.

The tumoricidal dose level in HD is approximately 40 Gy to 45 Gy, delivered at the rate of 10 Gy per week (Kaplan 1980b). Clinically negative adjacent nodal regions can adequately be treated with 35 Gy. The necessary dose of radiation when used in combination with chemotherapy may be less.

The most efficient treatment of deep-lying tissues uses an opposed field technique that provides a homogenous dose distribution throughout the treatment volume and minimizes the chance of radiation damage to adjacent structures such as the heart and liver. All the standard treatment fields employed in treating Hodgkin's disease use an opposed field, usually anterior and posterior, technique.

Consolidation irradiation applies to the lower doses (15 Gy to 20 Gy) given to areas of known disease in advanced stages (IIIB or IV) after a complete response to chemotherapy (table 28.3) (Farber et al. 1980).

CHEMOTHERAPY

Multiagent chemotherapy of advanced HD (stages IIIB and IV) produces a complete remission and a 5-year disease-free survival in the majority of patients (DeVita et al. 1980; Longo et al. 1986; Bonadonna et al. 1975). The development of multiple drug combinations in the treatment of Hodgkin's disease has provided much of the foundation of modern medical oncology. Several single agents had been shown to have antitumor activity by inducing short-lived complete remissions. DeVita and coworkers at the National Cancer Institute were the first to combine four active agents and give them in a cycle to minimize toxicity and produce a synergistic antitumor effect. This concept is now used in the treatment of a wide variety of solid tumors and hematologic malignancies.

Single chemotherapeutic agents. Single chemotherapeutic agents (table 28.4) can produce complete and partial responses (CR + PR) in 50% to 70% of patients with HD, although the remissions last only a few months

Table 28.4
CHEMOTHERAPEUTIC AGENTS USEFUL IN LYMPHOMAS

Alkylating agents	Nitrogen mustard (mechlorethamine) Chlorambucil Cyclophosphamide Carmustine (BCNU) Lomustine (CCNU)
Vinca alkaloids	Vincristine (Oncovin) Vinblastine
Antibiotics	Doxorubicin (Adriamycin) Bleomycin
Other	Prednisone Procarbazine Methotrexate Dimethyl triazeno imidazole carboxamide (DTIC)

and complete responses (10% to 15%) are unusual (Coltman 1980). Single agents can be useful in palliating advanced disease in elderly patients or patients who are heavily pretreated and due to severe myelosuppression will not tolerate combined therapy.

Combination chemotherapy. The MOPP regimen (table 28.5) — nitrogen mustard (mechlorethamine), vincristine (Oncovin), procarbazine, and prednisone — first used by DeVita et al. resulted in a high complete response rate and a confirmed durable remissions (DeVita et al. 1980; Longo et al. 1986). The CR rate for the 188 patients was 84%, with 66% remaining disease-free for more than 10 years. Patients with no B symptoms and those receiving higher doses of vincristine had a higher CR rate and longer survival. Patients entering

Table 28.5
MOPP* REGIMEN

Agent	Dose/Administration Route	Day		
		1	8	14
Mechlorethamine	6 mg/m² IV	X	X	
Vincristine	1.4 mg/m² IV	X	X	
Procarbazine	100 mg/m² PO	XXXXXXXX		
Prednisone (1st and 4th cycles only)	40 mg/m² PO	XXXXXXXX		

Repeat cycle beginning on day 29

*MOPP = Nitrogen mustard, vincristine (Oncovin), procarbazine, prednisone complete remission in five cycles or less had significantly longer remissions than those requiring six or more cycles. Since the introduction of MOPP, investigators have added or substituted other drugs in an effort to reduce toxicity and improve results. These MOPP variants will require further studies to prove their superiority.

Bonadonna et al. demonstrated with the ABVD regimen (table 28.6) that a drug combination differing from MOPP in the component pharmacologies and mechanisms of action could result in a CR rate similar to that achieved with MOPP (Bonadonna et al. 1975). This regimen has proven to be noncross-resistant with MOPP due to its ability to salvage MOPP failures (59% CR, 13% PR) (Santoro, Bonfante, and Bonadonna 1982). ABVD—doxorubicin (Adriamycin), bleomycin, vinblastine, and dimethyl triazeno imadazole carboxamide (DTIC)—is often considered a second-line regimen because of potential cardiac and pulmonary toxicity. However, a recent report comparing MOPP and radiation therapy vs. ABVD and radiation therapy suggested that the ABVD group had no increased cardiopulmonary toxicity and had less risk of secondary leukemia (Santoro et al. 1987). Numerous single-institution studies have been reported with other second-line salvage therapies (Buzaid, Lippman, and Miller 1987). Most regimens incorporate a nitrosourea and doxorubicin; none appears clearly superior to or less toxic than ABVD.

Table 28.6
ABVD* REGIMEN

Agent	Dose/Administration Route	Day 1	15
Doxorubicin	25 mg/m² IV	X	X
Bleomycin	10 mg/m² IV	X	X
Vinblastine	6 mg/m² IV	X	X
DTIC	375 mg/m² IV	X	X

Repeat cycle beginning on day 29

*ABVD = Doxorubicin (Adriamycin), bleomycin, vinblastine, dimethyl triazeno imidazole carboxamide (DTIC)

COMBINED CHEMOTHERAPY AND RADIATION THERAPY

Refinements in treatment have led to the identification of specific subsets of patients who appear to benefit from irradiation and chemotherapy combination therapy. These include patients showing localized disease with masses exceeding one-third the diameter of the thoracic cavity (stages I or II with so-called massive mediastinum) (Hoppe 1985a); patients with stage IIIA disease with bulky sites (Henkelmann, Hagemester, and Fuller 1988); patients with stages IIIB or IV disease who achieve only a partial remission with chemotherapy that are converted to complete remission with added radiation therapy; and children where the use of combination chemotherapy may allow for reduced doses of irradiation, which spares bone growth (Behrendt, Von Bunnigen, and Van Leeuwen 1987).

The guidelines for treatment selection in HD are shown in table 28.7. These suggestions have to be modified depending on the careful evaluation of each individual. Results of therapy have been exciting, with a steady increase in the 5-year relative survival rate (fig. 28.4) and a corresponding drop in the mortality rate (fig. 28.5).

COMPLICATIONS OF TREATMENT

The side effects of radiation include temporary bone-marrow suppression, radiation pneumonitis (10%), pericarditis (<5%), and laboratory evidence of hypothyroidism (>30%). Transverse myelitis can occur if the spinal cord is overdosed by poor technique.

Chemotherapy with alkylating drugs increases the risk for secondary malignancies, particularly acute leukemia. The Stanford group found a 17.6% cumulative risk (6-fold excess risk) of secondary cancers (Tucker, Coleman, and Cox 1988). The risk of secondary leukemia is greatest in patients over 40 (20.7% actuarial risk at 7 years) (Coltman and Dixon 1982). Patients surviving more than 11 years after treatment appear to be at no increased risk of developing acute leukemia. Non-Hodgkin's lymphomas are also seen in increased numbers as a complication of treatment.

Table 28.7
GUIDELINES FOR TREATMENT OF HODGKIN'S DISEASE

Stage	Recommended Therapy	Alternative Therapy
I, II (A or B, negative laparotomy)	Subtotal lymphoid irradiation	Irradiation to involved field with combination chemotherapy
I, II (A or B, with mediastinal mass >1/3 diameter of the chest)	Combination chemotherapy followed by irradiation to involved field	Subtotal lymphoid irradiation followed by chemotherapy
IIIA₁, (minimal abdominal disease)	Total lymphoid irradiation	Combination chemotherapy with irradiation to involved sites
IIIA₂ (extensive abdominal disease)	Combination chemotherapy with irradiation to involved sites	Total lymphoid irradiation or combination chemotherapy alone
IIIB	Combination chemotherapy	Combination chemotherapy with irradiation to involved sites
IV (A or B)	Combination chemotherapy	Combination chemotherapy with irradiation to involved sites

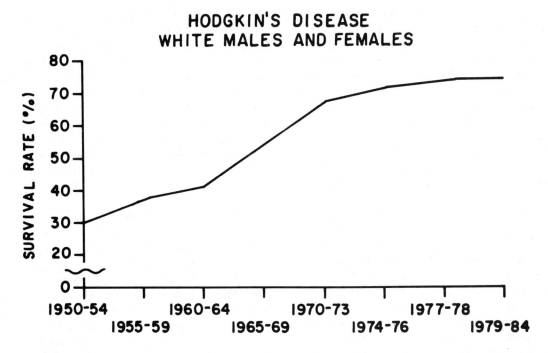

Fig. 28.4. Improvements in the 5-year relative survival rates in the United States from 1950 to 1984: 30% to 74%.

FUTURE DIRECTIONS

Ongoing studies include noncross-resistant alternating regimens, integrating chemotherapy and radiation therapy, biologic response modifiers, and high-dose chemotherapy with bone marrow transplantation (Canellos, Nadler and Takvorian 1988; Jones et al. 1990). Further studies are necessary to demonstrate the efficacy and toxicity of these modalities.

NON-HODGKIN'S LYMPHOMAS

EPIDEMIOLOGY

The American Cancer Society estimated that 35,600 new patients with non-Hodgkin's lymphoma would be detected in 1990, including 18,600 males and 17,000 females. It is estimated that 18,200 deaths would occur (Silverberg, Boring, and Squires 1990). The incidence rates have increased 123% since 1950, and although the mortality rates have increased as well, they have not risen as fast. Higher age-adjusted incidence rates are due primarily to increases among older persons. Lower-magnitude increases occur in the 35-to-64-year age group, while rates among young adults have not changed substantially (Devesa et al. 1987). Much of the increase in incidence in the older age group is attributed to a rising incidence of diffuse large-cell lymphoma histologic subtype.

ETIOLOGY

A viral etiology has been implicated in the pathogenesis of some types of non-Hodgkin's lymphoma (NHL). Burkitt's lymphoma, Mediterranean lymphoma, and T-cell leukemia/lymphoma have been shown by epidemiologic, electron microscopy, cell culture, and immunologic studies to have features implicating viral etiologies. Serologic studies have demonstrated an association between HTLV-I and T-cell leukemia/lymphoma. This virus has been isolated from T

Fig. 28.5. Incidence rates (2.8-3.4 per 100,000) age adjusted to 1970 for Hodgkin's disease have remained relatively stable. Mortality rates have declined by 61%, from 1.7 to 0.7 per 100,000.

lymphocytes of patients with T-cell lymphoma/leukemia in Japan and from some apparently healthy family members of NHL patients. In regions in Japan, 12% to 15% of the population have antibodies to HTLV-I (Sarin and Gallo 1984). Studies also have demonstrated an association between HTLV-I, and HTLV-II in other areas including the Caribbean and the Southeastern United States (Blayney et al. 1983).

Non-Hodgkin's lymphomas are seen with increased frequency in patients with acquired immune deficiency syndrome (AIDS), and in patients who are immunosuppressed following kidney and heart transplants. Notable in the latter diseases is the increased incidence of central nervous system non-Hodgkin's lymphoma. Increased risk of lymphomas are also seen in Wiskott-Aldrich syndrome, X-linked immunodeficiency, ataxia telangiectasia, and possibly Sjøgren's syndrome (Rosenberg and Kaplan 1982).

Cytogenetic abnormalities in almost all NHLs are seen when the cells are examined carefully (Rowley and Ultmann 1983). In Burkitt's lymphoma, there is frequently translocation between chromosome 8 and chromosome 14, which results in the c-*myc* oncogene being placed into the normal location for the immunoglobulin heavy-chain locus. Less common are translocations between chromosomes 8 and 2, as well as chromosomes 8 and 22, which also are associated with the c-*myc* oncogene being moved to the light-chain loci, for kappa and lambda respectively. The translocation of the c-*myc* oncogene to these locations perhaps brings it under the influence of the promoter region for the immunoglobulin synthesis, thus promoting the c-*myc* oncogene expression. Other chromosome translocations that appear to involve other growth-regulation loci have been observed.

Advances in immunology, particularly in the development of monoclonal antibody technology, have led to the characterization of non-Hodgkin's lymphomas as neoplasms of the immune system. Subclasses of lymphoma are now showing similarities in immunologic phenotype to stages in the normal differentiation of T and B lymphocytes (Foon, Schroff, and Gale 1982). Molecular genetic analysis has shown that loci involved in the monoclonal cell population for many B-cell lymphomas involve these areas, other specific sites on chromosome 11, and chromosome 18. The T-cell receptor alpha-chain gene locus on chromosome 14 and the T-cell receptor beta-chain locus on chromosome 7 have been involved in translocations. Studies have predicted that specific cytogenetic abnormalities in lymphoma will result in useful prognostic information (Rodriguez et al. 1987).

CLINICAL PRESENTATION

CLINICAL DETECTION
Most NHL patients are asymptomatic, although 20% may have some constitutional or B symptoms. Often, patients will give a history of "waxing and waning" adenopathy over several months before diagnosis. In

non-Hodgkin's lymphoma, early involvement of the oropharyngeal lymphoid tissue, skin, gastrointestinal tract, and bone is more common than with Hodgkin's disease (DeVita, Jaffe, and Hellman 1985; Rosenberg and Kaplan 1982). In both adults and children, initial intra-abdominal manifestations are also much more common. Tumor involvement in the mesenteric lymph nodes and GI tract is common. Leukemic transformation of NHL occurs in 10% to 15% of patients (Rosenberg et al. 1961). Coombs' positive autoimmune hemolytic anemia occurs more commonly in NHL than in HD.

INITIAL DIAGNOSTIC PROCEDURES
Lymph node biopsy. Central to the diagnosis of all lymphomas is the recognition of lymphadenopathy and the careful histologic evaluation of a lymph node biopsy. Because NHLs occur more commonly in extranodal sites than in HD, needle biopsies are more diagnostically helpful. This is true of both organ and marrow involvement. Careful coordination with the pathologist is necessary in order to obtain adequate samples for diagnosis.

Hematology and chemistry. As with HD, additional initial laboratory evaluations include CBC counts, with differential and platelet count, and blood chemistries evaluating liver and kidney function. Hypogammaglobulinemia is more frequent in NHL than in HD.

Radiologic studies. Radiological studies are essential in the evaluation and staging of patients with non-Hodgkin's lymphoma, as they are with Hodgkin's disease.

PATHOLOGIC AND CLINICAL STAGING

HISTOPATHOLOGY
Histologic classifications proposed for non-Hodgkin's lymphomas have included those of Rappaport, Lukes and Collins, Kiel, and Lennert. The most widely reported is Rappaport's, on which most of the literature in the United States to the mid-1980s is based. In 1982, a conference held to resolve these differences resulted in the working formulation histologic classification (Rosenberg et al. 1982b). The Rappaport classification and working formulation classification are seen in table 28.8. The low-grade lymphomas are predominately B-cell tumors; intermediate-grade lymphomas include B-cell and some T-cell lymphomas; immunoblastic lymphomas are predominately B-cell tumors; and the lymphoblastic group usually is composed of T-cell tumors. Burkitt's and non-Burkitt's small noncleaved cell tumors are predominately B-cell tumors. The histiocytic lymphomas are from the monocyte macrophage line. Mycosis fungoides is from T-cell origin.

Tumors with a good prognosis include all the low-grade NHLs, and some of the intermediate-grade tumors with long natural histories. Tumors with a poor prognosis include the rapidly progressive high-grade tumors, and some from the intermediate-grade group, particularly diffuse large-cell tumors. Most B-cell tumors are monoclonal

Table 28.8
HISTOPATHOLOGIC CLASSIFICATION OF NON-HODGKIN'S LYMPHOMAS

Grade	Working Formulation	Study Code	Rappaport Classification
	Favorable		
Low Grade	Small lymphocytic (SL)	A	Diffuse, lymphocytic, well differentiated
	Follicular, predominantly small cleaved-cell (FSC)	B	Nodular, lymphocytic, poorly differentiated
	Follicular, mixed small cleaved, large-cell (FM)	C	Nodular, mixed, lymphocytic and histiocytic
	Unfavorable		
Intermediate Grade	Follicular, predominantly large	D	Nodular, histiocytic
	Diffuse, small cleaved-cell (DSC)	E	Diffuse, lymphocytic
	Diffuse, mixed small- and large-cell (DM)	F	Diffuse, mixed, lympho- and histiocytic
	Diffuse, large-cell (DL): Cleaved or noncleaved-cell	G	Diffuse, histiocytic
	Unfavorable		
High Grade	Immunoblastic (IBL)	H	Diffuse, histiocytic
	Lymphoblastic (LL): Convoluted- or nonconvoluted-cell	I	Diffuse, lymphoblastic
	Small noncleaved-cell (SNC): Burkitt's or non-Burkitt's	J	Diffuse, undifferentiated
Miscellaneous Histiocytic			
	Mycosis fungoides		
	Extramedullary plasmacytoma		
	Composite		
	Unclassifiable		

and produce either a kappa or lambda light-chain immunoglobulin (usually IgM) cell associated molecule.

The histologic features of the four most common subgroups of NHLs are illustrated in fig. 28.6.

Follicular small-cleaved cell lymphoma. The vast majority of the neoplastic cells are small indented lymphocytes with only occasional large cells. Mitotic figures are few. Monoclonal populations of these lymphocytes are frequently found in the peripheral blood of many patients with follicular lymphomas who do not otherwise have evidence of leukemic changes or elevated lymphocyte counts. The significance of these circulating cells is not yet clear. This is the most common histologic subtype, accounting for approximately 40% of NHL patients. In this subgroup, patients predominately present with stages III and IV disease and have a high incidence of bone marrow involvement.

Follicular mixed small-cleaved and large-cell lymphomas. The large cells are more abundant and, in some cases, appear to be mixed with equal numbers of the smaller cells. As with the other follicular lymphomas, the lymph node architecture shows distinct nodules usually present throughout the lymph node. However, in the mixed cellular lymphomas, more frequent areas of diffuse infiltrate are common. This histologic subgroup accounts for the second most common group of non-Hodgkin's lymphomas, representing 20% to 40% of patients. Again, marrow involvement is frequent and most patients have stages III and IV disease at diagnosis.

Diffuse large-cell lymphomas. This subgroup has large lymphocytes with nuclear diameters much greater than a normal lymphocyte. The cells have cytologic

features of large noncleaved or large cleaved follicular cells. The cells contain nucleoli and abundant cytoplasm that is slightly amphophilic. Mitoses are more commonly identified in this subgroup. These tumors tend to present frequently in extranodal as well as nodal sites, tend to disseminate rapidly, and involve unusual areas such as the CNS, bone, and GI tract.

Immunoblastic lymphomas. These constitute high-grade neoplasms composed of cells commonly exhibiting a high mitotic rate. Subtypes including plasmacytoid, clear cell, and polymorphic categories have been proposed. The correlation between the morphologic appearance and immunologic subtype is less predictable in this group of high-grade lymphomas.

ANATOMIC STAGING
The same Ann Arbor staging symposium recommendations used in staging Hodgkin's disease (see table 28.2; fig. 28.2) are used for the staging of non-Hodgkin's lymphoma (Carbone et al. 1971).

The pattern of dissemination in non-Hodgkin's lymphomas is less frequently orderly; there are numerous illustrations of patients with early organ involvement with minimal adenopathy, and, more commonly, extranodal sites. The prognosis is influenced more by the histologic subtype rather than by the anatomic extent of disease, as in HD (Ultmann and Jacobs 1985).

STAGING PROCEDURES
A careful, complete staging workup is essential to determine the extent of disease before proper treatment can be selected (Chabner et al. 1980).

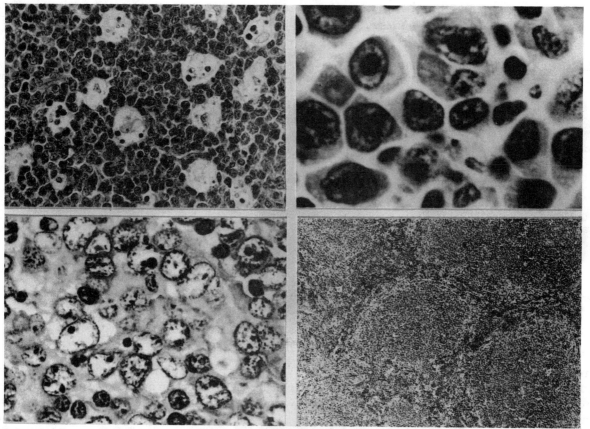

Fig. 28.6. (Top left) follicular small-cleaved cell lymphoma, low-power view. (Top right) diffuse large cell lymphoma, high-power view. (Bottom left) immunoblastic lymphoma, high-power view. (Bottom right) Burkitt's lymphoma "starry sky" pattern, low-power view.

Required procedures include an adequate surgical biopsy examined by an experienced lymphoma pathologist confirming the diagnosis and a complete history and physical examination with particular emphasis on all lymphoid tissue including Waldeyer's ring, lymph nodes, and liver and spleen size.

Also required are CBC counts including differential, white blood cell count, platelet count, reticulocyte count, and erythrocyte sedimentation rate; and blood chemistries including liver and kidney function tests, uric acid, and quantitative immunoglobulins.

Bone marrow biopsy should be done because of the high frequency of bone marrow involvement in NHL. The yield is proportional to the quantity of marrow obtained; bilateral bone marrow biopsies usually have a greater yield than do unilateral biopsies.

Required radiographic studies include PA and lateral chest x-rays, followed by CT scan if abnormalities or suggestions of disease are shown. Abdominal CT scans are particularly useful in detecting upper retroperitoneal and mesenteric nodes, as well as liver and spleen involvement. The CT scan is displacing the need for lymphangiography in many NHL patients. Bipedal lymphangiography (LAG) can be used to evaluate borderline lymphadenopathy on the abdominal CT scan. The internal nodal architecture is more clearly defined with the lymphangiogram than with the CT scan.

Optional procedures include staging laparotomy, although surgical evaluation of the abdomen is rarely justified in the management of patients with non-Hodgkin's lymphoma. The procedure should be done only if it clearly makes a major difference in the selection of treatment. The patients are generally older and frequently have more complications than those with Hodgkin's disease; thus the risks versus benefits should be clearly weighed. Laparotomy-staged series reveal an increased incidence of hepatic, mesenteric, and gastrointestinal involvement in NHL in contrast to HD (Goffinet et al. 1977).

In patients with extensive GI involvement, staging laparotomy should include resection of the involved gastrointestinal lymphoma, if feasible, to reduce the frequency of perforation and/or bleeding complications (Weingard et al. 1982).

In non-Hodgkin's lymphomas, involvement of the liver frequently can be demonstrated by peritoneoscopy with directed biopsies. Should liver involvement change the plan of therapy, this procedure may be useful. In patients with bone pain or equivocal x-rays, radioisotope bone scans may demonstrate bone involvement. The gallium-67 scans are of little use in non-Hodgkin's lymphoma, but occasionally they may be helpful in differentiating tumors from other masses in the supra-diaphragmatic region.

The clinical characteristics of many of the 1,014 patients with NHL evaluated by the working formula tion study group to determine histology are summarized in table 28.9. There was a high incidence of marrow involvement in stage III and stage IV disease in the low-grade lymphomas and the equal distribution of stages I and II versus stages III and IV with less marrow involvement in the intermediate- and high-grade groups. The survival curve (fig. 28.7) demonstrates the value of histologic subclassification of non-Hodgkin's lymphomas and is helpful with treatment planning.

PRINCIPLES OF TREATMENT

MULTIDISCIPLINARY TREATMENT APPROACH

As with Hodgkin's disease, the non-Hodgkin's lymphomas frequently demand multidisciplinary treatment planning in order to achieve the most optimal cure rates. Because the non-Hodgkin's lymphomas disseminate widely by hematogenous routes rather than through orderly, contiguous node extension as in Hodgkin's disease (Rosenberg and Kaplan 1982; Vokes et al. 1985), radiation therapy is usually used as an adjunct to chemotherapy rather than as primary treatment. However, radiation therapy has a role in the management of localized disease (stages I, I_E, and early stage II disease defined as nonbulky or with limited stage II involvement).

SURGERY

The primary role of surgery is in establishing the diagnosis and contributing to the anatomic staging, although staging laparotomies are utilized much less often in NHL. In a few circumstances surgery is a

Table 28.9
THE RELATIONSHIP BETWEEN HISTOLOGY, PATHOLOGIC STAGE, AND BONE MARROW INVOLVEMENT AT DIAGNOSIS

Histology	Stages (%)			Bone Marrow Involved
	I	II	III	
Small lymphocytic	3	8	89	71
Follicular, small cleaved-cell	8	10	82	51
Diffuse, small cleaved-cell	9	19	72	32
Diffuse large-cell	16	30	54	10
Large-cell, immunoblastic	23	29	58	12

beneficial part of the disease management. The first is in resection of extranodal gastrointestinal involvement. Gastrointestinal non-Hodgkin's lymphomas, when treated with chemotherapy or radiation therapy, have a significant risk of perforation and/or bleeding that can be fatal. To prevent this complication, it is desirable to resect areas of the GI tract involved with the extensive lymphoma. At the resection, it is desirable to perform complete staging of the abdomen (Ondreyco et al. 1982).

A second benefit of surgery is splenectomy in some patients who exhibit hypersplenism. A splenectomy enables these patients to undergo more extensive chemotherapy (Schreiber et al. 1985).

RADIATION THERAPY

Before beginning radiation therapy, it is essential to carefully stage NHL patients. The goal of radiation therapy should be to control disease within the confines

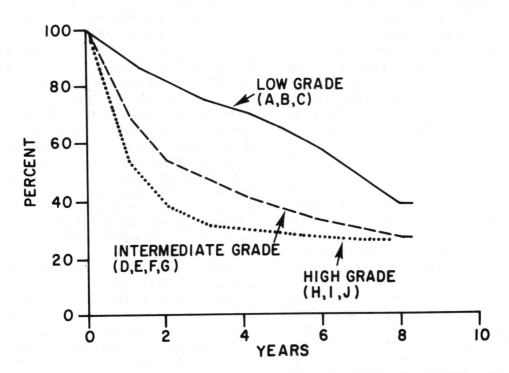

Fig. 28.7. Non-Hodgkin's lymphoma. Survival of patients classified by the working-formulation histologic subgroups.

of the clinically evident disease and not to irradiate adjacent areas. Fields utilized in the treatment of HD are often inappropriate for NHL. The Ann Arbor staging system is not satisfactory for definition of radiation therapy use. Stage II needs to be further refined into two subcategories: stage II_1 (localized), which can be managed by irradiation); and stage II_2 (bulky or disseminated, several sites on the same side of the diaphragm), which is similar to extensive stage III or stage IV disease when managed by radiation (Bush et al. 1977; Sweet and Golomb 1980).

The low-grade (favorable) lymphomas are generally highly responsive to irradiation. Local control rates exceeding 90% are achieved with 40 Gy administered to the involved field. Good control rates are usually achieved with doses in excess of 30 Gy. As indicated in table 28.9, it is uncommon for favorable-histology lymphomas to be localized at diagnosis; frequently the marrow or other sites are involved.

Two reports (Paryani et al. 1983; Gospodarowicz et al. 1981) of long-term follow-up after involved or extended field therapy for localized disease (stage I and stage II low-grade lymphomas) indicate a 10-year survival and freedom from relapse of greater than 50%, especially among younger patients. However, in these indolent diseases, late relapses can occur. Studies involving total lymphoid irradiation given alone or combined with chemotherapy, as well as whole-body irradiation, have been used to treat patients with stages III and IV disease. These therapeutic approaches produce a high remission rate, but there is no proof that they have curative potential in low-grade lymphomas (Glatstein et al. 1977; Hoppe et al. 1981).

In contrast to low-grade NHLs, intermediate- and high-grade lymphomas present approximately equally in localized stages I and II versus disseminated stages III and IV (see table 28.9). They also much more commonly arise in extranodal sites including the GI tract, bone marrow, CNS, and skin. Before the introduction of effective combination chemotherapy, radiation therapy was the standard means of treatment for patients with stages I and II large-cell lymphomas. The results of several controlled trials demonstrate long-term disease-free survival of over 50% for patients treated with radiation therapy alone (Hoppe 1985b; Bush and Gospodarowicz 1982). Patterns of relapse are less predictable than with Hodgkin's disease, and relapses are more common with systemic disease or other organ involvement. Also, local control rates with radiation therapy are not as predictable as with HD. These features have led to trials combining chemotherapy with radiation therapy for localized NHL.

Irradiation has to be highly tailored to the site of origin of the localized NHL. This includes careful treatment of Waldeyer's ring for patients with disease arising in the nasopharynx, tonsillar, or base of the tongue. For the gastrointestinal tract, the majority of patients are initially treated with surgical resection followed by low-dose whole-abdominal irradiation with

shielding of the kidneys, followed by a boost to the adjacent nodal sites. For primary bone lymphomas, radiation should involve the entire bone with adjacent local node treatment. The thyroid gland, a frequent site of localized E non-Hodgkin's lymphoma, is treated by irradiating the entire thyroid bed on both sides of the neck and the superior mediastinum. Radiation therapy is also a mainstay in the treatment of primary CNS non-Hodgkin's lymphoma. Long-term disease control appears to be less than with many other sites.

Radiation therapy is effective for the palliation of symptoms in patients with advanced NHLs of low-, intermediate-, and high-grade histologies. These situations include relieving superior vena cava obstruction, alleviating spinal cord compression, treating ureter occlusion, and to treat any painful tumor mass.

Electron beam radiation therapy has been extensively used in the management of patients with early stage mycosis fungoides. This is an effective palliative modality (Hoppe, Fuks, and Bagshaw 1979) because individual tumor nodules are highly responsive.

CHEMOTHERAPY

The non-Hodgkin's lymphomas frequently present as disseminated diseases and relapse with disseminated involvement following localized radiation therapy, so the prime means of treatment is chemotherapy. Useful chemotherapeutic agents useful are similar to those used in the treatment of HD (see table 28.4). The choice of the agent or combination is based on histology, stage, and general patient information such as age and performance status.

Low-grade non-Hodgkin's lymphoma typically is diagnosed as a systemic disease; approximately 90% of patients demonstrate stage III or stage IV disease. Newer staging techniques are showing more frequent bone marrow, spleen, or liver involvement, and that the peripheral blood is frequently involved with circulating monoclonal lymphoma cells. Although generally regarded as indolent diseases, they are ultimately fatal. Most of these patients retain their follicular histology, although some will advance to high-grade lymphoma histology when followed over time. The natural history of the low-grade lymphomas demonstrates that with minimal therapy, a median survival of 7.5 to 9 years can be expected. Thus, the decision to initiate therapy has to be weighed carefully. The quality of life is usually good, with long periods of symptom-free survival (Rosenberg 1979).

Treatment with a variety of programs, including single agents, COP, MOPP, CHOP, MACOP-B, m-BACOD, and ProMACE-CytaBOM, has been used (tables 28.4, 28.5, 28.6, 28.10, 28.11, 28.12, 28.13, 28.14). Unfortunately, although there is a high remission rate, the average remission is only approximately two to three years in duration. After succeeding relapses, the remissions induced with second courses of therapy are generally shorter. Data for all therapies indicate little evidence of

Table 28.10
COP REGIMEN

Agent	Dose/Administration Route	Day
Cyclophosphamide	400 mg/m² PO	1 to 5
	or 700 mg/m² IV	1
Vincristine	1.4 mg/m² IV	1
Prednisone	100 mg/m² PO	1 to 5

Repeat cycle every 21 days, usually for 6 or more cycles

Table 28.11
CHOP REGIMEN

Agent	Dose/Administration Route	Day
Cyclophosphamide	750 mg/m² IV	1
Doxorubicin	50 mg/m² IV	1
Vincristine	1.4 mg/m² IV	1
Prednisone	100 mg PO	1 to 5

Repeat cycles at 21 to 28 days, usually for 6 or more cycles

Table 28.12
MACOP-B REGIMEN

Agent	Dose/Administration Route	Week
Methotrexate	400 mg/m² IV (4 hrs)	2, 6, 10
Leucovorin	15 mg PO q 6 hr x 6	after Mtx
Doxorubicin	50 mg/m² IV	1, 3, 5, 7, 9, 11
Cyclophosphamide	350 mg/m² IV	1, 3, 5, 7, 9, 11
Vincristine	1.4 mg/m² IV	2, 4, 6, 8, 10, 12
Bleomycin	10 mg/m² IV	4, 8, 12
Prednisone	75 mg PO day	x 12 wks

Table 28.13
m-BACOD REGIMEN

Agent	Dose/Administration Route	Day
Cyclophosphamide	600 mg/m² IV	1
Doxorubicin	45 mg/m² IV	1
Vincristine	1.0 mg/m² IV	1
Bleomycin	4 mg/m² IV	1
Dexamethasone	6 mg/m² PO	1 to 5
Methotrexate	200 mg/m² IV	8 and 15
Leucovorin	10 mg/m² PO q 6 hr x 6	after Mtx

Repeat cycles every 21 days for 10 cycles

Table 28.14
ProMACE-CytaBOM REGIMEN

Agent	Dose/Administration Route	Day
Cyclophosphamide	650 mg/m² IV	1
Doxorubicin	25 mg/m² IV	1
Etoposide	120 mg/m² IV	1
Prednisone	60 mg/m² PO	1 to 14
Cytarabine	300 mg/m² IV	8
Bleomycin	5 mg/m² IV	8
Vincristine	1.4 mg/m² IV	8
Methotrexate	120 mg/m² IV	8
Leucovorin	25 mg/m² PO q 6 hr x 4	after Mtx

Repeat cycles every 21 days for 6 or more cycles

curability for stage III and stage IV disease (Portlock and Rosenberg 1979; McLaughlin et al. 1987; Ezdinli et al. 1985).

Current research questions for this patient population involve the application of progressive chemotherapy earlier in the course of the disease and/or biologic response modifiers used in combination with the chemotherapy or during maintenance (Young et al. 1988). It is too early to tell whether these treatment approaches will be successful.

Patients with unfavorable-histology (intermediate- and high-grade) NHLs have a much more aggressive disease that results in a rapid downhill course. For these groups, the median survival of several series with minimal treatments ranges from one to two years. However, this course has been dramatically changed by the introduction of aggressive combination chemotherapy that results in a high percentage of durable, long-term, disease-free survival—patients who are cured. For patients with bulky stage II, stage III, and stage IV unfavorable histology non-Hodgkin's lymphoma, initial aggressive systemic chemotherapy is the treatment of choice. Complete response rates with a variety of chemotherapy regimens vary from 40% to 80% (Coltman Jr. et al. 1977; Jones et al. 1979; Sweet et al. 1980; Jones et al. 1983; Cabanillas et al. 1983; Skarin et al. 1983; Fisher et al. 1983; Klimo and Connors 1985; Boyd et al. 1988; DeVita Jr. et al. 1988). A substantial portion of these patients who achieve a complete response rate, particularly among those with diffuse large-cell lymphoma, remain clinically disease-free for extended periods on a plateau phase of survival curves.

Chemotherapy regimens with the best potential to induce prolonged complete remissions are generally high-intensity regimens containing Adriamycin (Jones et al. 1979). The chemotherapy agents, frequency of administration, and doses vary considerably among regimens (see tables 28.10, 28.11, 28.12, 28.13, 28.14) and reports primarily on phase II trials give widely different complete response rates and claim superiority of one regimen over the other. A high-priority randomized prospective clinical trial of the National Cancer Institute is evaluating four combinations: CHOP, m-BACOD, ProMACE-CytaBOM, and MACOP-B (Fisher et al. 1987; Miller et al. 1987a). The results of representative cooperative group treatment using the four different regimens are given in table 28.15 (Miller et al. 1987b). Because of the intensity of treatment, the high incidence of life-threatening and potential toxicities associated with these complicated regimens clearly means they should be

Table 28.15
RESULTS OF REPRESENTATIVE COOPERATIVE GROUP TREATMENT USING 4 DIFFERENT REGIMENS

Regimen	No. Patients	No. Response Evaluable	CR %	Toxicity % LT	Fatal
CHOP	350	350	37 to 68	10	3
m-BACOD	84	84	65	31	6
ProMACE-CytaBOM	97	83	58	20	5
MACOP-B	72	68	56	28	2

LT = Life threatening

administered by qualified oncologists with extensive experience in treating these diseases.

Unfortunately, a significant number of patients with unfavorable non-Hodgkin's lymphomas either fail to respond or eventually have disease relapse. Prognosis then is uniformly poor and almost all can be expected to die of progressive lymphoma. Effective salvage chemotherapy with a variety of regimens can produce second remissions, but these are rarely of significant duration (Shipp, Takvorian, and Canellos 1984; Cabanillas, Hagemeister, and McLaughlin 1987). A number of investigational drugs are being evaluated for their ability to salvage these patients, but the most consistently reported effective salvage therapy for relapsing patients (excluding primary failures) seems to be bone marrow transplantation. Several centers have reported long-term disease-free survival either using cryopreserved autologous marrow or allogeneic marrow transplantation (Applebaum et al. 1987).

Some specific considerations are warranted in patients with non-Hodgkin's lymphomas. Increasing central nervous system involvement has been observed, especially with diffuse large-cell lymphomas and extensive marrow involvement. In these patients, the cerebrospinal fluid should be evaluated for lymphoma involvement; the patients should then either receive systemic agents at dose levels known to penetrate the CSF, or be given prophylactic intrathecal chemotherapy. Children have a higher incidence of aggressive histologic varieties with marrow and CNS involvement. Prophylactic treatment of the CNS appears warranted in most pediatric NHL patients. One particularly difficult problem has been the treatment of elderly patients with aggressive lymphomas. This category of NHL patients is growing larger as the incidence of lymphomas rises. Numerous studies have demonstrated that elderly patients have difficulty tolerating the aggressive chemotherapy regimens. However, because they can be cured with intensive therapy, new approaches are needed for this group.

COMBINED CHEMOTHERAPY AND RADIATION THERAPY

Localized stage I and minimal stage II large-cell lymphomas can be cured by local radiation therapy; survival rates range from 25% to 60%. The majority of patients who fail do so with foci of lymphoma outside of the treatment fields, although there are some failures within the treatment port. The best results of radiation therapy alone were achieved in surgically staged patients with 70% to 75% of stage I patients alive at five to 10 years, and about 50% of patients so staged with minimal stage II disease apparently cured.

The results of combination chemotherapy led to initial attempts to combine radiation therapy followed by chemotherapy. Although studies demonstrated a clearly superior outcome with this treatment approach (Nissen et al. 1983), several patients relapsed during the course of radiation therapy. Thus the next step was to reverse the treatment modalities. Initial chemotherapy followed by radiation therapy resulted in a better disease outcome in patients with stage I and stage II disease (Mauch et al 1985; Connors et al. 1987; Bonadonna 1985).

As the results of chemotherapy continue to improve, the most recent approach has been to investigate chemotherapy alone and reserve radiation therapy for patients who have incomplete responses (Miller and Jones 1984; Cabanillas 1985). Randomized prospective trials are currently evaluating chemotherapy alone versus chemotherapy followed by radiation therapy in the treatment of stage I and stage II large-cell lymphomas.

EXPERIMENTAL TREATMENTS

Approximately 30% to 40% of patients with aggressive non-Hodgkin's lymphomas do not respond to initial treatments with a complete remission, or they relapse early following initial chemotherapy and subsequently die from their disease. New therapies are needed in order to improve upon this outcome. Current research supports the concepts of dose intensity, with regimens employing

---

Table 28.16
GUIDELINES FOR TREATMENT OF THE NON-HODGKIN'S LYMPHOMAS

Grade	Recommended Therapy		Alternative Therapy
	Stage I, II₁*	Stages II₂,** III, IV	
Low	Localized irradiation	Observation until disease progression then palliative irradiation or single-agent or combination chemotherapy	Initial combination chemotherapy for stages III, IV
Intermediate	Combination chemotherapy with localized irradiation	Combination chemotherapy	Initial radiation followed by combination chemotherapy for stages I, II
High	Combination chemotherapy with localized irradiation	Combination chemotherapy	

*Stage II₁ — Nonbulky disease
**Stage II₂ — Bulky disease >10 cm or 1/3 diameter of chest

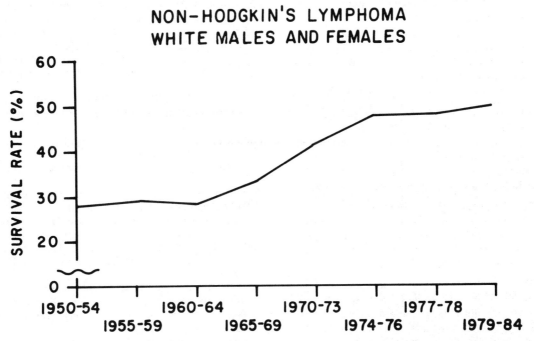

Fig. 28.8. Improvements in 5-year relative survival rates in the United States from 1950 to 1984: 28% to 49%.

higher doses and more drugs over a compressed time, resulting in better outcomes (DeVita Jr. et al. 1988). The role of biologicals such as lymphokines, tumor necrosis factor, and monoclonal antibodies is under intense investigation and these agents may be added to the current aggressive chemotherapy regimens. Better disease control may result.

This category of malignant disease has shown the way for advances in systemic chemotherapy and chemotherapy combined with radiation therapy (DeVita Jr. et al. 1987). Table 28.16 gives guidelines for treatment selection in patients with non-Hodgkin's lymphomas. Because of the marked differences in age, performance status, and ability to tolerate therapy, these suggestions must be individualized. The overall treatment results for non-Hodgkin's lymphomas have been steadily improving survival rates (fig. 28.8). Improved survival rates, however, are offset by the rising incidence rates, which has resulted in a slight rise in mortality rates (fig. 28.9)

Clearly the management of the malignant lymphomas has taught oncologists many lessons in the cure of malignant disease. Further advances and better control of these diseases will help the lessons be applied to other human malignancies.

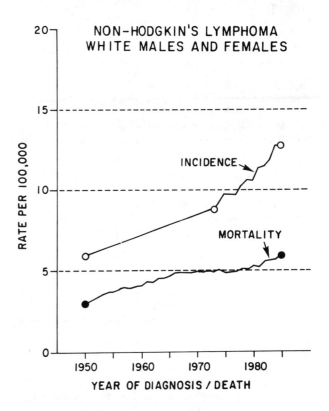

Fig. 28.9. Incidence rates (5.9-13.1 per 100,000) age adjusted to 1979 for non-Hodgkin's lymphoma have increased 123%. Mortality rates have doubled from 2.9 to 5.9 per 100,000.

REFERENCES

Aisenberg, A.C.; Krontiris, T.G.; and Mak, T.W. et al. 1985. Rearrangement of the gene for the beta chain of the T-cell receptor in T-cell chronic lymphocytic leukemia and related disorders. *N. Engl. J. Med.* 313:529.

Applebaum, F.R.; Sullivan, K.M.; and Buckner, C.D. et al. 1987. Treatment of malignant lymphoma in 100 patients with chemotherapy, total body irradiation and marrow transplantation. *J. Clin. Oncol.* 5:1340-47.

Behrendt, H.; Von Bunnigen, B.; and Van Leeuwen, E.F. 1987. Treatment of Hodgkin's disease in children with or without radiotherapy. *Cancer* 59:1870-73.

Bjorkholm, M.; Holm, G.; and Merk, K. 1982. Cyclic autoimmune hemolytic anemia as a presenting manifestation of splenic Hodgkin's disease. *Cancer* 49:1702-04.

Blayney, D.W.; Blattner, W.A.; Robert-Guroff, M. et al. 1983. The human T-cell leukemia/lymphoma virus (HTLV) in the Southeastern United States. *JAMA* 250:1048-52.

Bonadonna, G. 1985. Chemotherapy of malignant lymphomas. *Semin. Oncol.* 12:1.

Bonadonna, G.; Zucali, R.; and Monfardini, S. et al. 1975. Combination chemotherapy of Hodgkin's disease with Adriamycin, bleomycin, vinblastine, and imidazole carboximide vs. MOPP. *Cancer* 36:252-59.

Boyd, D.B.; Coleman, M.; and Papish, S.W. et al. 1988. COPBLAM III: infusion of combination chemotherapy for diffuse large-cell lymphoma. *J. Clin. Oncol.* 6:425-33.

Bush, R.S., and Gospodarowicz, M. 1982. The place of radiation therapy in the management of localized non-Hodgkin's lymphoma. In Rosenberg, S.A., and Kaplan, H.S. eds. *Malignant lymphomas: etiology, immunology, pathology, treatment.* pp. 485-502. Orlando: Academic Press.

Bush, R.S.; Gospodarowicz, M.; and Sturgeon, J. et al. 1977. Radiation therapy of localized non-Hodgkin's lymphoma. *Cancer Treat. Rep.* 61:1129-36.

Buzaid, A.C.; Lippman, S.M.; and Miller, T.P. 1987. Salvage therapy of advanced Hodgkin's disease. *Am. J. Med.* 83:523-32.

Cabanillas, F. 1985. Chemotherapy as definitive treatment of stages I-II large-cell and diffuse mixed lymphomas. *Hematol. Oncol.* 3:25.

Cabanillas, F.; Burgess, M.A.; and Bodey, G.P. et al. 1983. Sequential chemotherapy and late intensification for malignant lymphomas of aggressive histologic type. *Am. J. Med.* 74:382-88.

Cabanillas, F.; Hagemeister, F.B.; and McLaughlin, P. 1987. Results of MIME salvage regimen for recurrent or refractory lymphoma. *J. Clin. Oncol.* 5:407-12.

Canellos, G.P.; Nadler, L.; and Takvorian, T. 1988. Autologous bone marrow transplantation in the treatment of malignant lymphoma and Hodgkin's disease. *Semin. Hematol.* 25:58-65.

Carbone, P.P.; Kaplan, H.S.; and Mushoff, K. et al. 1971. Report of the Committee on Hodgkin's Disease Staging Classification. *Cancer Res.* 31:1860-61.

Case, D.C.; Hansen, J.A.; and Corrales, E. et al. 1976. Comparison of multiple *in vivo* and *in vitro* parameters in untreated patients with Hodgkin's disease. *Cancer* 38:1807-15.

Chabner, B.A.; Fisher, R.I.; and Young, R.C. et al. 1980. Staging of non-Hodgkin's lymphoma. *Semin. Oncol.* 7:285-91.

Chen, J.L.; Osborne, B.M.; and Butler, J.J. 1987. Residual fibrous masses in treated Hodgkin's disease. *Cancer* 60:407-13.

Clouse, M.E.; Harrison, D.A.; and Grassi, C.J. et al. 1985. Lymphangiography, ultrasonography, and computed tomography in Hodgkin's disease and non-Hodgkin's lymphomas. *J. Comput. Tomogr.* 9:1-8.

Coltman, C.A. Jr. 1980. Chemotherapy of advanced Hodgkin's disease. *Semin. Oncol.* 7:155-73.

Coltman, C.A. Jr., and Dixon, D.O. 1982. Second malignancies complicating Hodgkin's disease: a Southwest Oncology Group 10-year follow-up. *Cancer Treat. Rep.* 66:1023-33.

Coltman, C.A. Jr.; Luce, J.K.; and McKelvey, E.M. et al. 1977. Chemotherapy of non-Hodgkin's lymphoma: 10 year's experience in the Southwest Oncology Group. *Cancer Treat. Rep.* 61:1067-78.

Connors, J.M., and Klimo, P. 1984. Is it an E lesion or stage IV? an unsettled issue in Hodgkin's disease staging. *J. Clin. Oncol.* 2:1421-23.

Connors, J.M.; Klimo, P.; and Fairey, R.N. et al. 1987. Brief chemotherapy and involved field radiation therapy for limited stage, histologically aggressive lymphoma. *Ann. Intern. Med.* 107:25.

Cornbleet, M.A.; Vitolo, U.; and Ultmann, J.E. et al. 1985. Pathologic stages IA and IIA Hodgkin's disease: results of treatment with radiotherapy alone (1968-1980). *J. Clin. Oncol.* 3:758-68.

Cutler, S.J., and Young, J.C. eds. 1975. Third national cancer survey: incidence data. *Natl. Cancer Inst. Monogr.* 41:107-11.

Desser, R.K.; Golomb, H.M.; and Ultmann, J.E. et al. 1977. Prognostic classification of Hodgkin's disease in pathologic stage III, based on anatomic considerations. *Blood* 49:883-93.

Devesa, S.S.; Silverman, D.T.; and Young, J.L. et al. 1987. Incidence and mortality trends among whites in the United States, 1947-1984. *J. Natl. Cancer Inst.* 79:4.

DeVita, V.T. Jr.; Hubbard, S.M.; and Young, R.C. et al. 1988. The role of chemotherapy in diffuse aggressive lymphomas. *Semin. Hematol.* 25:2-10.

DeVita, V.T. Jr.; Jaffe, E.S.; and Hellman, S. 1985. Hodgkin's disease and the non-Hodgkin's lymphomas. In DeVita, V.T.; Hellman, S.; and Rosenberg, S.A. eds. *Cancer: principles and practice of oncology.* pp. 1623-1709. New York: J.B. Lippincott.

DeVita, V.T. Jr.; Longo, D.L,; and Hubbard, S.M. et al. 1987. The lymphomas: biologic implications of therapy and therapeutic implications of the new biology. In *Malignant lymphoma.* pp. 249-267. Baltimore: Williams & Wilkins.

DeVita, V.T. Jr.; Simon, R.M.; and Hubbard, S.M. et al. 1980. Curability of advanced Hodgkin's disease with chemotherapy: long-term follow-up of MOPP-treated patients at the National Cancer Institute (NCI). *Ann. Intern. Med.* 92:587-95.

Diehl, V.; Burrichter, H.; and Schaadt, M. et al. 1984. Hodgkin's disease: the remaining challenge. *Prog. Med. Virol.* 30:199-203.

Ezdinli, E.Z.; Anderson, J.R.; and Melvin, F. et al. 1985. Moderate vs. aggressive chemotherapy of nodular lymphocytic poorly differentiated lymphoma. *J. Clin. Oncol.* 3:769-75.

Farber, L.R.; Prosnitz, L.R.; and Cadman, E.C. et al. 1980. Curative potential of combined modality therapy for advanced Hodgkin's disease. *Cancer* 46:1509-17.

Fisher, R.I.; DeVita, V.T. Jr.; and Hubbard, S.M. et al. 1983. Diffuse aggressive lymphomas: increased survival after alternating flexible sequences of ProMACE and MOPP chemotherapy. *Ann. Intern. Med.* 98:304-309.

Fisher, R.I.; Miller, T.P.; and Dana, B.W. et al. 1987. Southwest Oncology Group clinical trials for intermediate and high-grade non-Hodgkin's lymphomas. *Semin. Hematol.* 24:21-25.

Foon, K.A.; Schroff, R.W.; and Gale, R.P. 1982. Surface markers on leukemia and lymphoma cells: recent advances. *Blood* 60:1-19.

Ford, R.J.; Mehta, S.; and Davis, F. et al. 1982. Growth factors in Hodgkin's disease. *Cancer Treat. Rep.* 66:633-38.

Glatstein, E.; Donaldson, S.S.; and Rosenberg, S.A. et al. 1977. Combined modality therapy in malignant lymphomas. *Cancer Treat. Rep.* 61:1199-1207.

Goffinet, D.R.; Warnke, R.; and Dunnick, N.R. et al. 1977. Clinical and surgical (laparotomy) evaluation of patients with non-Hodgkin's lymphomas. *Cancer Treat. Rep.* 61: 981-92.

Gospodarowicz, M.K.; Bush, R.S.; and Brown, T.C. et al. 1981. Prognostic factors in nodular lymphomas: a multivariate analysis based on the Princess Margaret Hospital experience. *Int. J. Radiat. Oncol. Biol. Phys.* 10:489-97.

Grufferman, S.; Cole, P.; and Levitan, T. 1979. Evidence against transmission of Hodgkin's disease in high schools. *N. Engl. J. Med.* 300:1006-11.

Grufferman, S.; Cole, P.; and Smith, P.G. et al. 1977. Hodgkin's disease in siblings. *N. Engl. J. Med.* 296:248-50.

Grufferman, S.; Duong, T.; and Cole, P. 1976. Occupation and Hodgkin's disease. *J. Natl. Cancer Inst.* 57:1193-95.

Henkelmann, G.C.; Hagemester, F.B.; and Fuller, L.M. 1988. Two cycles of MOPP and radiotherapy for stage III_1A and III_1B Hodgkin's disease. *J. Clin. Oncol.* 6:1293-1302.

Hesse, J.; Levine, P.H.; and Ebbesen, P. et al. 1977. A case-control study on immunity to two Epstein-Barr virus-associated antigens and to herpes simplex virus and adenovirus in a population-based group of patients with Hodgkin's disease in Denmark, 1971-1973. *Int. J. Cancer* 19:49-58.

Hoppe, R.T. 1980. Radiation therapy in the treatment of Hodgkin's disease. *Semin. Oncol.* 7:144-54.

Hoppe, R.T. 1985a. The management of stage II Hodgkin's disease with a large mediastinal mass: a prospective program emphasizing irradiation. *Int. J. Radiat. Oncol.* 11: 349-55.

Hoppe, R.T. 1985b. Role of radiation treatment in the management of NHL. *Cancer* 55:2176-83.

Hoppe, R.T.; Fuks, Z.; and Bagshaw, M.A. 1979. Radiation therapy in the management of cutaneous T-cell lymphomas. *Cancer Treat. Rep.* 63:625-32.

Hoppe, R.T.; Kushlan, P.; and Kaplan, H.S. et al. 1981. The treatment of advanced stage favorable histology non-Hodgkin's lymphoma: a preliminary report of a randomized trial comparing single agent chemotherapy, combination chemotherapy, and whole-body irradiation. *Blood* 58:592-98.

Jones, R.J.; Piantodosi, S.; and Mann, R.B. et al. 1990. High-dose cytotoxic therapy and base marrow transplantation for relapsed Hodgkin's disease. *J. Clin. Oncol.* 8:527-37.

Jones, S.E. 1980. Importance of staging in Hodgkin's disease. In Coltman, C.A. *Hodgkin's disease. Semin. Oncol.* 7:126-35.

Jones, S.E.; Grozea, P.N.; and Metz, E.N. et al. 1979. Superiority of Adriamycin-containing combination chemotherapy in the treatment of diffuse lymphoma. *Cancer* 43: 417-25.

Jones, S.E.; Grozea, P.N.; and Metz, E.N. et al. 1983. Improved complete remission rates and survival for patients with large-cell lymphoma treated with chemoimmunotherapy: a Southwest Oncology Group study. *Cancer* 51:1083-90.

Kadin, M.; Stites, D.P.; and Levy, R. et al. 1978. Exogenous origin of immunoglobulin in Reed-Sternberg cells of Hodgkin's disease. *N. Engl. J. Med.* 299:1208-14.

Kaplan, H.S. 1980a. *Hodgkin's disease.* 2nd ed. Cambridge: Harvard University Press.

Kaplan, H.S. 1980b. Hodgkin's disease: unfolding concepts concerning its nature, management, and prognosis. *Cancer* 45:2439-74.

Klimo, P., and Connors, J.M. 1985. MACOP-B chemotherapy for the treatment of diffuse large-cell lymphoma. *Ann. Intern. Med.* 102:596-602.

Leslie, N.T.; Mauch, P.M.; and Hellman, S. 1985. Stage IA to IIB supradiaphragmatic Hodgkin's disease: long-term survival and relapse frequency. *Cancer* 55:2072-78.

Lister, T.A.; Crowther, D.; and Sutcliffe, S.B. et al. 1989. Report of a committee convened to discuss the evaluation and staging of patients with Hodgkin's Disease: Cotswolds meeting. *J. Clin. Oncol.* 7:1630-36.

Longo, D.L.; Young, R.C.; and Wesley, M. et al. 1986. Twenty years of MOPP therapy for Hodgkin's disease. *J. Clin. Oncol.* 4:1295-1306.

Lukes, R.J.; Butler, B.B.; and Hicks, B.B. 1966. Natural history of Hodgkin's disease as related to its pathologic picture. *Cancer* 19:317-44.

Mauch, P.; Goodman, R.; and Hellman, S. 1978. The significance of mediastinal involvement in early stage Hodgkin's disease. *Cancer* 42:1039-45.

Mauch, P.; Leonard, R.; and Skarin, A. et al. 1985. Improved survival following combined radiation therapy and chemotherapy for unfavorable prognosis stages I-II non-Hodgkin's lymphomas. *J. Clin. Oncol.* 3:1301.

McLaughlin, P.; Fuller, C.; and Velasquez, W.S. et al. 1987. Stage III follicular lymphoma: durable remissions with a combined chemotherapy-radiotherapy regimen. *J. Clin. Oncol.* 5:867-74.

Miller, T.P.; Dahlberg, S.; and Jones, S.E. et al. 1987a. ProMACE-CytaBOM is active with acceptable toxicity in patients with unfavorable non-Hodgkin's lymphoma: a Southwest Oncology Group study. *ASCO* 6(abstr):197.

Miller, T.P.; Dana, B.W.; and Weick, J.K. et al. 1987b. Southwest Oncology Group clinical trials for intermediate- and high-grade non-Hodgkin's lymphomas. *Third Int. Conf. Malig. Lymph.* (abstr).

Miller, T.P., and Jones, S.E. 1984. Initial chemotherapy for clinically staged localized non-Hodgkin's lymphomas of unfavorable histology. In Ford, R.J.; Fuller, L.M.; and Hagemeister, F.B. eds. *Hodgkin's disease and non-Hodgkin's lymphoma: new perspectives in immunopathology, diagnosis, and treatment.* New York: Raven Press.

Moran, E.M., and Ultmann, J.E. 1974. Clinical features and course of Hodgkin's disease. *Clin. Haematol.* 3:91-129.

National Cancer Institute. 1988. *Annual cancer statistic review including cancer trends: 1950-1985.* Bethesda, Md.: National Cancer Institute.

Nissen, N.I.; Ersboll, J.; and Hansen, H.S. et al. 1983. A randomized study of radiotherapy vs. radiotherapy plus chemotherapy in stages I-II non-Hodgkin's lymphomas. *Cancer* 52:1.

Ondreyco, S.; Eyre, H.J.; and Kjeldsberg, C. et al. 1982. Abdominal lymphoma: lack of complete surgical staging. *Am. J. Surg.* 132:624-28.

Oppenheim, J.J.; Stadler, B.M.; and Siragnian, R. et al. 1982. Lymphokines—their role in lymphocyte responses: the role of interleukin-1. *Fed. Proc.* 41:257-62.

Paffenbarger, R. Jr.; Wing, A.L.; and Hyde, R.T. 1977. Characteristics in youth indicative of adult onset Hodgkin's disease. *J. Natl. Cancer Inst.* 58:1489-91.

Paryani, S.B.; Hoppe, R.T.; and Cox, R.S. et al. 1983. Analysis of non-Hodgkin's lymphomas with nodular and favorable histologies, stages I and II. *Cancer* 52:2300-2307.

Pinkus, G.S.; Thomas, P.; and Said, J.W. 1985. Leu-M1 a marker for Reed-Sternberg cells in Hodgkin's disease: an immunoperoxidase study of paraffin-embedded tissues. *Am. J. Pathol.* 119:244-52.

Portlock, C.S., and Rosenberg, S.A. 1979. No initial therapy for stages III and IV non-Hodgkin's lymphomas of favorable histologic types. *Ann. Intern. Med.* 90:10-13.

Proceedings of the symposium on Contemporary Issues in Hodgkin's Disease: biology, staging, and treatment. 1982. *Cancer Treat. Rep.* 66:601-1071.

Prosnitz, L.R.; Curtis, A.M.; and Knowlton, A.H. et al. 1980. Hodgkin's disease: significance of large mediastinal masses. *Int. J. Radiat. Oncol. Biol. Phys.* 6:809-14.

Prosnitz, L.R.; Montalva, R.L.; and Fisher, D.B. et al. 1978. Treatment of stage IIIA Hodgkin's disease: is radiotherapy alone adequate? *Int. J. Radiat. Oncol. Biol. Phys.* 4:781-87.

Redman, H.C.; Glatstein, E.; and Castellino, R.H. et al. 1977. Computed tomography as an adjunct in the staging of Hodgkin's disease and non-Hodgkin's lymphomas. *Radiology* 124:381-85.

Robertson, S.J.; Lowman, J.T.; and Grufferman, S. et al. 1987. Familial Hodgkin's disease: a clinical and laboratory investigation. *Cancer* 59:1314-19.

Rodriguez, M.A.; Pathak, S.; and Trujillo, J. et al. 1987. Structural abnormalities of chromosome 11q in patients with lymphoma. *Proc. Am. Assoc. Cancer Res.* 23:146 (abstr).

Rosenberg, S.A. 1979. Current concepts in cancer: non-Hodgkin's lymphoma—selection of treatment on the basis of histologic type. *N. Engl. J. Med.* 301:924-28.

Rosenberg, S.A.; Kaplan, H.S.; and Hoppe, R.T. et al. 1982a. The Stanford randomized trials of the treatment of Hodgkin's disease: 1967-1980. In Rosenberg, S.A., and Kaplan, H.S. eds. *Malignant lymphomas: etiology, immunology, pathology, treatment. Bristol-Myers cancer symposia.* vol. 3. New York: Academic Press.

Rosenberg, S.A.; Berard, C.W.; and Brown, B.W. et al. 1982b. National Cancer Institute sponsored study of classifications of non-Hodgkin's lymphomas: summary and description of a working formulation for clinical usage. *Cancer* 49:2112-35.

Rosenberg, S.A.; Diamond, H.D.; and Jaslowitz, B. et al. 1961. Lymphosarcoma: a review of 1,269 cases. *Medicine* 40: 31-84.

Rosenberg, S.A., and Kaplan, H.S. 1966. Evidence for an orderly progression in the spread of Hodgkin's disease. *Cancer Res.* 26:1225-30.

Rosenberg, S.A.; and Kaplan, H.S. eds. 1982. *Malignant lymphomas: etiology, immunology, pathology, treatment.* New York: Academic Press.

Rowley, J.D., and Ultmann, J.E. eds. 1983. *Chromosomes and cancer: from molecules to man.* Orlando: Academic Press.

Santoro, A.; Bonadonna, G.; and Valagussa, P. et al. 1987. Long-term results of combined chemotherapy-radiotherapy approach in Hodgkin's disease: superiority of ABVD plus radiotherapy vs. MOPP plus radiotherapy. *J. Clin. Oncol.* 5:27-37.

Santoro, A.; Bonfante, V.; and Bonadonna G. 1982. Salvage chemotherapy with ABVD in MOPP-resistant Hodgkin's disease. *Ann. Intern. Med.* 96:139-43.

Sarin, P.S., and Gallo, R.C. 1984. Retroviruses in human T-cell malignancies. *Cancer Invest.* 2:467.

Schreiber, D.P.; Jacobs, C.; and Rosenberg, S.A. et al. 1985. The potential benefits of therapeutic splenectomy for patients with Hodgkin's disease and non-Hodgkin's lymphomas. *Int. J. Radiat. Oncol. Biol. Phys.* 11:31-36.

Shipp, M.A.; Takvorian, R.C.; and Canellos, G.P. 1984. High-dose cytosine arabinoside: active agent in treatment of non-Hodgkin's lymphoma. *Am. J. Med.* 77:845-50.

Silverberg, E.; Boring, C.C.; and Squires, T. 1990. Cancer statistics, 1990. *CA* 40:7-24.

Skarin, A.T.; Canellos, G.P.; and Rosenthal, D.S. et al. 1983. Improved prognosis of diffuse histiocytic and undifferentiated lymphoma by use of high-dose methotrexate alternating with standard agents (m-BACOD). *J. Clin. Oncol.* 1:91-98.

Stein, R.S. 1981. Clinical features and clinical evaluation of Hodgkin's disease and the non-Hodgkin's lymphomas. In Bennett, J.M. ed. *Lymphomas I.* pp. 129-175. Boston: Marcus Nijhoff.

Strijk, S.P.; Wagener, D.J.; and Bogman, M.J. 1985. The spleen in Hodgkin's disease: diagnostic value of CT. *Radiology* 154:753-57.

Sweet, D.L., and Golomb, H.M. 1980. The treatment of histiocytic lymphoma. *Semin. Oncol.* 7:302-309.

Sweet, D.L.; Golomb, H.M.; and Ultmann, J.E. et al. 1980. Cyclophosphamide, vincristine, methotrexate with leucovorin rescue, and cytarabine (COMLA) combination sequential chemotherapy for advanced diffuse histiocytic lymphoma. *Ann. Intern. Med.* 92:785-90.

Symposium on contemporary issues in Hodgkin's disease: biology, staging and treatment. 1982. *Cancer Treat. Rep.* 66:601-1071.

Taylor, M.A.; Kaplan, H.S.; and Nelsen, T.S. 1985. Staging laparotomy with splenectomy for Hodgkin's disease: the Stanford experience. *World J. Surg.* 9:449.

Tucker, M.A.; Coleman, C.N.; and Cox, R.S. 1988. Risk of second cancers after treatment for Hodgkin's disease. *N. Engl. J. Med.* 318:76-81.

Ultmann, J.E., and Jacobs, R.H. 1985. The non-Hodgkin's lymphomas. *CA* 35:66-87.

Vianna, N.J., and Polan, A.K. 1978. Immunity in Hodgkin's disease: importance of age at exposure. *Ann. Intern. Med.* 89:550-56.

Vokes, E.E.; Ultmann, J.E.; and Golomb, H.M. et al. 1985. Long-term survival of patients with localized diffuse histiocytic lymphoma. *J. Clin. Oncol.* 3:1309.

Weingrad, D.N.; Decosse, J.J.; and Sherlock, P. et al. 1982. Primary gastrointestinal lymphoma: a 30-year review. *Cancer* 49:1258-1265.

Weiss, R.B.; Brunning, R.D.; and Kennedy, B.J. 1975. Hodgkin's disease in the bone marrow. *Cancer* 36:2077-83.

Young, R.C.; Corder, M.P.; and Hayes, H.A. et al. 1972. Delayed hypersensitivity in Hodgkin's disease. *Am. J. Med.* 52:63-72.

Young, R.C.; Longo, D.L.; and Glatstein, E. et al. 1988. The treatment of indolent lymphomas: watchful waiting vs. aggressive combined modality treatment. *Semin. Hematol.* 25:11-16

Zagars, G., and Rubin, P. 1985. Hodgkin's disease stages IA and IIA: a long-term follow-up study on the gains achieved by modern therapy. *Cancer* 56:1905-12.

Chapter 29

MULTIPLE MYELOMA

Glenn J. Bubley, M.D.
Lowell E. Schnipper, M.D.
Charles A. Dana Research Institute

Glenn J. Bubley, M.D.
Assistant Professor of Medicine
Harvard Medical School
Division of Hematology/Oncology, Beth Israel Hospital
Boston, Massachusetts

Lowell E. Schnipper, M.D.
Theodore W. and Evelyn G. Berenson Associate Professor of Medicine
Harvard Medical School
Chief, Oncology Division, Beth Israel Hospital
Boston, Massachusetts

Charles A. Dana Research Institute
Harvard-Thorndike Laboratory of Beth Israel Hospital
Hematology-Oncology Division/Harvard Medical School
Boston, Massachusetts

INTRODUCTION

Plasma cell dyscrasia (PCD) is a broad term for a family of clonal neoplastic disorders associated with the overproduction of a monoclonal antibody. The malignant cells in these disorders, plasma cells and plasmacytoid lymphocytes, are the most mature cells of B-lymphocyte origin. B-cell maturation is associated with a programmed rearrangement of DNA sequences in the process of encoding the structure of mature immunoglobulins. This development results in a myriad of plasma cell clones, each making an antibody specific for an almost infinite number of antigens. In PCD, one B-cell clone predominates and results in the production of large amounts of a single monoclonal immunoglobulin (Ig) (Waldenstrom 1970).

Multiple myeloma (MM) is the most common malignant PCD, in which monoclonal IgG, IgA, and/or light chains are overproduced. Waldenstrom's macroglobulinemia (WM), a malignant PCD with a different clinical spectrum than MM, is associated with overproduction of IgM. Often, otherwise healthy patients may produce an excess of a specific monoclonal antibody in the absence of a specific syndrome or symptom complex, and are thus characterized as having a monoclonal gammopathy of undetermined significance (MGUS). Patients in whom the amount of M-protein does not change over time and remain asymptomatic have a benign monoclonal gammopathy (BMG). Alternatively, MGUS may progress slowly (smoldering myeloma) to become a clinically evident disease associated with overproduction of a monoclonal protein or M-protein (e.g., MM, WM, amyloidosis, or non-Hodgkin's lymphoma). In almost all cases of PCDs, an M-protein can be detected in the serum or urine (Waldenstrom 1970).

ANTIBODY STRUCTURE

A general model of immunoglobulin structure is shown in fig. 29.1. This monomer is the basic structure of IgG, IgA, IgM, IgD, and IgE. It is made up of two identical dimeric units, each of which is composed of a heavy chain and a light chain held together by disulfide bonds (Rosen and Buxbaum 1986). Each polypeptide chain contains two general regions: an amino (NH_2) terminal variable (V) region, and a carboxy (CO_2H) terminal constant (C) region. The antigen recognition site is in the variable region and is composed of terminal heavy- and light-chain regions. It is called the fragment antigen binding (Fab) region (Natvig and Kunkel 1973) and also contains the amino acid sequence that defines the idiotype, that is, the unique antigenic structure of a specific immunoglobulin molecule. The other end of the molecule, the Fc region, is responsible for complement activation, cell binding, and placental transport (Natvig and Kunkel 1973).

Light chains have a single carboxy-terminal domain in contrast to heavy chains that have three or four constant (C_H) domains. Both heavy and light chains have one variable domain within which all hypervariable regions (areas of greater amino acid sequence diversity) lie (fig. 29.1);

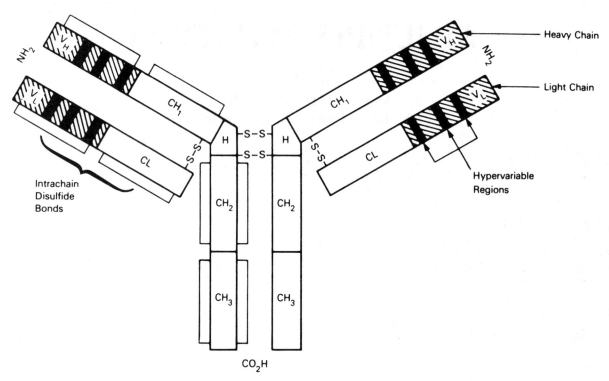

Fig. 29.1. Basic structure of immunoglobulin molecule. Each chain consists of variable regions, V_L or V_H, indicated by cross-hatched areas; hypervariable regions (solid black), characterized by minor variations in amino acid sequence; and constant regions (CL or CH). The amino-terminal variable or Fab region is responsible for antigen binding, and the constant carboxy-terminal region (Fc) has separate domains (CH_1, CH_2, or CH_3) responsible for cell or complement binding. H is the hinge region (Stamatoyannopoulos, Neinhuis, and Leder et al. [1987]).

each is made up of approximately 110 amino acids (Rosen and Buxbaum 1986; Natvig and Kunkel 1973).

The five major classes of human immunoglobulin — IgG, IgA, IgM, IgE, and IgD (Natvig and Kunkel 1973) — are each defined by a constant heavy chain (C_H) region that is specific for one of these classes. The light chain of the molecule is of two varieties, kappa or lambda. In normal development, B cells progress from producing an IgM molecule to an IgG or IgA by genetic recombination of a segment of DNA in the C_H region of chromosome 14. A similar process enables a single B-cell clone to produce antibodies of different IgG subclasses that have the same antigenic specificity. Genetic recombination, a process essential to the production of immunoglobulins, is one factor contributing to the amazing diversity of antibody molecules (Natvig and Kunkel 1973).

During B-cell maturation the first immunoglobulin produced is IgM; it is also the antibody produced during the primary immune response and is the antibody first produced by infants (Rosen and Buxboum 1973). The IgM structure is that of a pentameric ring formed by the attachment of a joining chain to the basic subunits at their Fc portion. Due to their large size these antibodies are called macroglobulins and are the M-protein overproduced in WM. These molecules efficiently bind complement and are restricted to the intravascular space.

IgG is the major immunoglobulin in the serum. It consists of four isotypic subclasses (IgG_{1-4}) that have

small differences in the heavy-chain regions that account for slightly different biologic properties. For example, IgG_1 and IgG_3 bind complement and mononuclear cells more effectively than IgG_2 and IgG_4. IgG_1 and IgG_3, when overproduced in MM, can be associated with hyperviscosity due to a propensity to form dimers. They have faster catabolic rates than the other IgG subclasses. IgG is normally produced during the secondary (anamnestic) immune response. It is the only immunoglobulin class that can be transported across the placenta and thereby provide passive immunity to the newborn (Rosen and Buxbaum 1986).

IgA is the chief antibody in saliva, tears, and the secretions of the GI and respiratory tract and serves as the first line of local defense against environmental agents. Its structure includes a secretory component that facilitates transport across the epithelial cell membrane (Rosen and Buxbaum 1986).

IgD and IgE are usually trace proteins in the plasma. IgD is thought to act as a cell-surface receptor that binds antigen and triggers B-cell proliferation and differentiation (Stamatoyannopoulos et al. 1987). IgE serum levels can be elevated during parasitic infection or in atopic individuals (Rosen and Buxbaum 1986). It binds with high affinity to receptors on basophils and mast cells, and may induce these cells to release vasoactive amines as part of an allergic response.

IgG makes up the largest proportion of immunoglobulins in adult plasma, followed by IgA and IgM (Natvig and Kunkel 1973). The distribution of these proteins in normal serum has a parallel in the observed distribution of M-protein types in PCDs (table 29.1). This holds true for the IgG subtypes as well. For example, IgG$_1$ makes up about 65% of the IgG concentration in normal serum and is the M-protein in a comparable percentage of IgG myelomas (Frei and Holland 1981). These observations suggest that any B-cell clone has an equal chance of evolving into a malignant clone.

B-LYMPHOCYTE DEVELOPMENT

The assembly of mature immunoglobulin molecules is the result of several genetic-recombination events that occur at identifiable stages of B-cell development and contribute to generating antibody diversity (Cooper 1975; Foon and Todd 1986). B-cell ontogeny begins when a lymphoid stem cell is committed to development as a progenitor B cell, and ends several developmental steps later at the stage of a plasma cell or (plasmacytoid) lymphocyte (fig. 29.2). A malignant B-cell clone producing monoclonal Ig in PCD has undergone a similar pattern of development, although heavy- and light-chain production may be unbalanced.

At least two different gene segments contribute to each constant and variable region of both the heavy and light chains (Cooper 1987). The DNA segments encoding the heavy-chain gene family are on chromosome 14, kappa light chains are encoded on chromosome 2, and lambda light chains on chromosome 22.

Table 29.1
FREQUENCY OF M-PROTEIN CLASSES PRODUCED BY PLASMA CELL NEOPLASMS

		%
A.	M-proteins containing both H and L chains	
	1. IgG	52
	2. IgA	21
	3. IgM	12
	4. IgD	2
	5. IgE	0.01
B.	M-proteins containing only L chains (κ or λ)	11
C.	M-proteins containing only H chains (γ, α, μ, δ, or ε)	1
D.	2 or more M-proteins	0.5
E.	No M-protein in serum or urine	1
		100

From data on 1,827 patients compiled by Pruzanski and Ogryzlo (Frei and Holland [1981]).

The first step in immunoglobulin production is the heavy-chain rearrangement on chromosome 14 that marks the cell's commitment to B-cell lineage. Initially, one of the 20 or more diverse (D) genes is transposed next to one of six joining (J) region genes on both chromosomes 14. If a DJ rearrangement is completed successfully, then one of at least 50 variable (V) region genes on only one of the chromosomes is translocated (fig. 29.3) to form a continuous VDJ$_H$ complex (Rosen and Buxbaum 1986; Cooper 1987). This genetic complex can encode the entire variable region of the heavy chain.

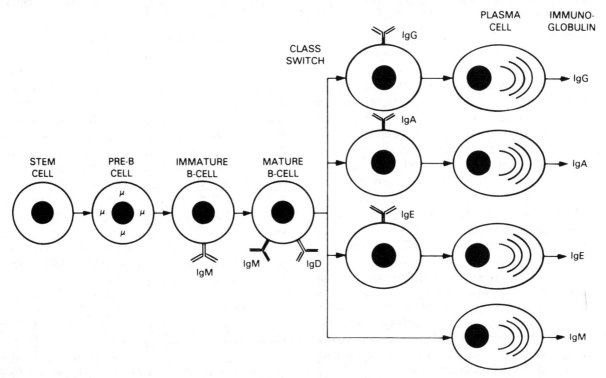

Fig. 29.2. Differentiation of B lymphocytes and plasma cells. A pleiotropic stem cell gives rise to the pre-B cell that has acquired the capacity to synthesize heavy chains (μ). The immature B cell can synthesize light chains so that a complete IgM molecule is formed and expressed on the cell surface. Mature B cells express both IgM and IgD on their surface. These cells can either mature into IgM-secreting plasmacytoid lymphocytes, or undergo a class switch to express IgG, IgA, or IgE on their cell surfaces. The latter cells can undergo terminal differentiation into IgG-, IgA-, or IgE-secreting plasma cells (Stamatoyannopoulos, Neinhuis, and Leder et al. [1987]).

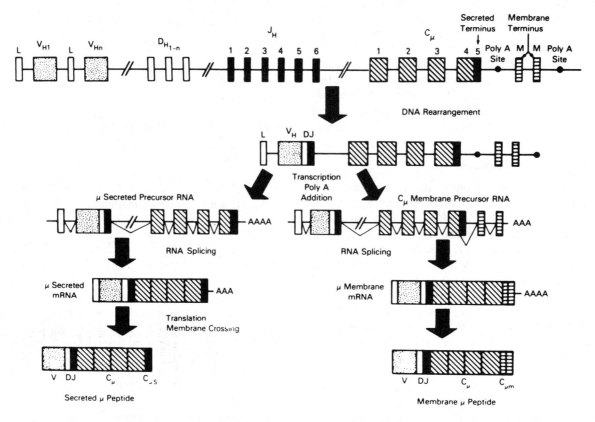

Fig. 29.3. Model of the DNA structure and rearrangement of the human heavy-chain gene. The region consists of multiple (300) V_H regions, families of diverse (D_H) segments, six joining (J_H) segments, and a single constant (C) gene made up of a number of domains. Single V_H-D_H- and J_H region gene subsegments are joined at the DNA level. Both secreted and membrane forms of IgM can be derived from a single constant region locus by addition of sites of poly-A residues (adenines added to the end of mRNA) and RNA splicing (Stamatoyannopoulos, Neinhuis, and Leder et al. [1987]).

Transcription into RNA is another mechanism for differential gene expression. When RNA is transcribed from DNA, both coding regions (exons) and noncoding intervening sequences (introns) are transcribed. Splicing is the process by which introns are removed prior to translation. Following removal of introns between the VDJ_H complex and the heavy-chain constant region ($C\mu$), the IgM heavy-chain region can be translated (Rosen and Buxbaum; Cooper 1981). Splicing, or removal, of different intervening DNA segments can also result in a B cell producing both cytoplasmic or surface IgM, or both (figs. 29.2 and 29.3).

Expression of the heavy or μ chain identifies the pre-B cell phase of development (Foon and Todd 1986). If a nonproductive rearrangement in the VDJ_H complex occurs on one of the pair of chromosomes 14, then rearrangement activity will shift to the other chromosome. This process, termed allelic exclusion, is repeated during light-chain development and ensures that a B lymphocyte can make only one type of antibody. Cells that do not undergo a functional heavy-chain rearrangement on either chromosome will not initiate light-chain production.

The next step in the gene rearrangement cascade occurs on chromosome 2, which encodes the variable region of the kappa gene. DNA fragments from two separate DNA segments, V and J, undergo a rearrangement to encode the kappa light-chain variable region. If a productive VJ rearrangement does not occur, then rearrangement will shift to the VJ region of the lambda light-chain region on chromosome 22. Successful production of a κ or λ light chain allows it to bind to the heavy chain to make a complete IgM monomer. This molecule is then transported to the cell surface where its expression marks the early stage of B-cell development (Rosen and Buxbaum 1986; Cooper 1986).

The result of multiple genetic rearrangements encoding slight alterations in DNA sequence, especially in the regions joining different segments, is production of millions of different B-cell clones (Cooper 1987). These enter the circulation from the bone marrow to migrate to the spleen and other lymphoid tissue, where further development depends on antigenic stimulation. If a specific B cell is exposed to an antigen that binds specifically to the variable region of the antibody expressed on its cell surface, the cell will internalize and digest the fragment. The antigen will then be expressed on the surface of the cell with MHC class II antigens. This complex can be recognized by helper T cells that produce factors promoting proliferation and differentiation, allowing the B cell to progress through further stages of B-cell development. When antigen-stimulated B cells lose surface IgD and IgM and begin to accumulate cytoplasmic IgG, they become intermediate and mature B cells, the final step prior to maturation into plasma cells (fig. 29.2). Plasma cells are terminally differentiated. The continued production of antibody depends on the continued presence of antigenic stimulation. Following removal of the antigen, antibody production depends on the life span of the plasma cell and the half-life of the immunoglobulin protein (Cooper 1987).

B lymphocytes in an individual clone can switch from IgM to IgG or IgA production with identical variable-region antigen-binding specificity. This process, termed a class switch, probably results from a deletion on chromosome 14 of DNA between the VDJ complex and the C_H region domain specific for another Ig class (Stamatoyannopoulos et al. 1987; Cooper 1987).

In general, the proliferation of B cells and production of immunoglobulin in PCD follows the pattern of normal development. In PCD, however, antibody production from one B-cell clone continues in the absence of an obvious antigenic stimulus. The production of other immunoglobulins may be reduced and the normal antibody responses to antigens may be blunted. Occasionally, the antibody produced in PCD is specific for a known antigen, such as a bacterial or viral surface protein (Seligmann and Brouet 1973).

ETIOLOGY

The etiology of PCD is not completely understood; however, there is now intriguing evidence about a specific factor that may induce growth of a B-cell clone (Kawano et al. 1985). There is also evidence that the abnormal proliferation of plasma cells may be programmed as early as the pre-B stage of development (Pilarski et al. 1985).

In an attempt to understand etiological factors for PCD, an animal model of this disease has been developed in specific strains of mice (Potter 1986). In this model, chronic intraperitoneal injection of an antigenic stimulus such as mineral oil leads to the formation of granulomas that progress to multiple plasmacytomas, with an associated diffuse hypergammaglobulinemia. This progresses to a monoclonal gammopathy, suggesting that a specific clone may outgrow and retard the growth of other B-cell clones. Consistent with this observation in humans is the demonstration that malignant plasma cells release a factor that binds to macrophages and induces these cells to release a soluble factor that suppresses helper B-cell function (Katzmann 1978; Krakauer 1977). The release of this factor may contribute to the suppression of normal gamma globulin production in MM, and suggests a possible mechanism of PCD-induced hypogammaglobulinemia.

Chromosomal translocations affecting genes encoding the immunoglobulin loci and the *myc* gene have been detected in DNA from mice having undergone experimentally induced PCD (Potter 1986). Translocations of these same genes in man are associated with another B-cell neoplasm, Burkitt's lymphoma (Foon and Todd 1986). Occasionally, Burkitt's and other non-Hodgkin's lymphomas have been associated with a monoclonal gammopathy (Frei and Holland 1981). No specific chromosomal abnormality involving the immunoglobulin loci or *myc* gene has been detected in MM in humans, although abnormalities have been frequently noted on chromosomes 1, 3, 6, 11, 16, and 17 (DeWald et al. 1985; Festi 1984).

In the mouse plasmacytoma model, host-genetic factors determine susceptibility to malignancy. For instance, only specific strains such as BALB/c and C3H mice develop plasmacytomas following mineral oil instillation (Potter 1986). A possible extension to humans is represented by the increased frequency of PCD that has been noted among close relatives of individuals with this disease (Maldonado and Kyle 1974).

Chronic antigenic stimulation has been implicated in the etiology of PCD. In the mouse model, the mineral oil injected into the peritoneum is not metabolized and serves as a nidus for chronic inflammation. Administration of anti-inflammatory agents such as indomethacin delays the progression of plasmacytomas. In man, a benign monoclonal gammopathy is sometimes preceded by polyclonal hyperglobulinemia in patients with recurrent or chronic inflammatory disorders such as osteomyelitis or pyelonephritis (Osserman and Takatsuki 1965). A self-limited or reversible form of PCD can also occur in patients with viral hepatitis or drug hypersensitivity. Monoclonal gammopathies can also be associated with nonlymphoid malignancies (Zawadski and Edwards 1972), in which case one may speculate that the tumor acts as a chronic antigenic stimulus for a B-cell clone.

A viral etiology has been suggested for PCD. In the mouse model, BALB/c mice infected with a specific RNA virus, MLV-A, have a shorter latent period prior to developing mineral-oil-induced plasmacytomas (Potter, Sklar, and Rowe 1973; Warner, Potter, and Metcalf 1974). It has been suggested that the virus may transform B lymphocytes and put them at greater risk for malignant transformation. Although viral particles have been visualized using electron microscopy in mouse plasmacytomas, the particles have not been seen in human myeloma.

Growth factors may play a role in the pathogenesis of PCD. The lymphokine B-cell stimulatory factor-2 (BSF-2), also called interleukin-6, was shown to be the active component facilitating growth of murine plasmacytomas (Hirano et al. 1987). Human myeloma cells in culture both produce and have a receptor for this hormone, which supports the hypothesis of an autocrine or self-stimulating loop in the pathogenesis of human myeloma (Kawano et al. 1988).

DIAGNOSTIC CONSIDERATIONS AND DETECTIONS OF PLASMA CELL DYSCRASIAS

The clinical presentation of multiple myeloma is suggested by the combination of bone pain (often in the

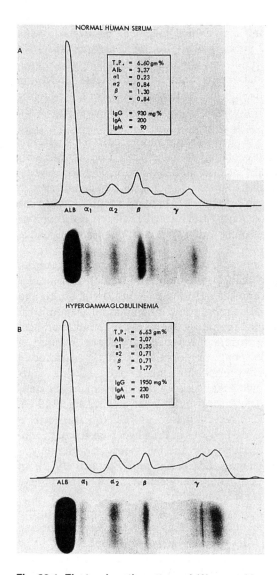

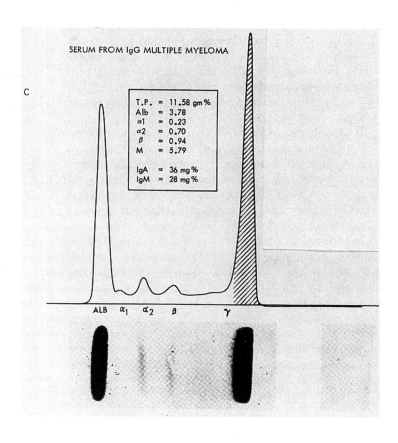

Fig. 29.4. Electrophoretic pattern of (A) normal human serum, (B) hypergammaglobulinemia, and (C) IgG multiple myeloma. (From: Wintrobe et al. eds. [1981].)

back) and anemia in a middle-aged or elderly patient. It is difficult to specify many clinical syndromes typical of MM or other PCDs since their presentation is highly variable, related to sites of infiltration by the neoplastic cells and the biochemical properties of the protein being overproduced. Frequently, patients are asymptomatic and the diagnosis is suggested by detection of an abnormal protein on the serum electrophoresis.

The most important means of detecting PCDs are electrophoretic measurements of immunoglobulin in both serum and urine. Examination of the urine for immunoglobulin is necessary because many patients with light-chain disease will not have a detectable M-spike in the serum (Kyle 1975). Reliable methods are available for detecting, quantitating, and determining the precise biochemical properties of an M-protein.

Serum protein electrophoresis (SPEP) is a useful screen for detecting M-proteins (Alper 1974). Proteins migrating on the basis of their mobility from left to right are: albumin, and alpha 1, alpha 2, beta, and gamma globulin (fig 29.4). Antibodies are found primarily in the beta and gamma globulin regions. An M-protein detected by SPEP usually appears as a sharp spike, and may represent a complete immunoglobulin or a subunit such as a light chain. In unusual cases two spikes may appear, possibly indicating a rare biclonal gammopathy. In a polyclonal elevation of Ig, a broad-based band will be demonstrated in the beta-to-gamma region.

Immunoelectrophoresis (IEP), a technique that differentiates proteins on the basis of electrophoretic and immunologic characteristics, is a sensitive method to type and confirm a monoclonal protein observed on SPEP (Kyle and Garton 1986). This technique is generally performed by allowing monoclonal antisera specific for any of the five immunoglobulin heavy chains and two light chains to diffuse into an electrophoretic gel following electrophoretic separation. At the point where the protein and antisera meet, a precipitin arc is formed that can be quantitated.

Other techniques such as immunofixation or radial immunodiffusion are available to quantitate plasma immunoglobulin levels. Immunofixation is a sensitive technique that is especially helpful in identifying an IgM spike in WM (Ritchie and Smith 1976), and for detecting and quantitating M-spikes in urine (Whicher, Hawkins, and Higginson 1980).

Dipstick tests of the urine are not reliable for detecting urinary light chains because they often identify only albumin. The use of sulfosalicylic acid or Exton's test is valuable for screening a spot urine sample for light chains (Kyle and Garton 1986). If light chains are present, an IEP is performed on a 24-hour collection of concentrated urine, and reacted with anti-kappa or anti-lambda antibody to determine if the light chain is a monoclonal spike (as in PCD) or a polyclonal broad-based band. As in the serum, the amount of M-protein in the urine correlates with plasma cell burden (Durie and Salmon 1975). In some cases immunofixation will detect a monoclonal urinary light-chain peak in the presence of a large amount of protein, including albumin. This finding raises the possibility of primary amyloidosis or amyloidosis secondary to multiple myeloma.

CLINICAL ASPECTS OF MULTIPLE MYELOMA

Multiple myeloma is a malignant neoplasm that results from monoclonal proliferation of plasma cells. Its clinical consequences result from an increasing tumor cell mass in bones, bone marrow, and extraosseous sites, and the production of vast excesses of monoclonal immuno-globulin. The pathophysiologic basis for the clinical sequelae of MM is best understood by thinking of them as resulting from an expanding plasma cell mass on the one hand, and from humoral factors — monoclonal immunoglobulin overproduction and osteoclast activating factor (OAF) — on the other (table 29.2).

The differential diagnosis of PCD includes an abundance of benign and several malignant disorders, as shown in table 29.3. Monoclonal gammopathies are frequent in the elderly, being observed in 5% of individuals over age 70, and are well-known in patients with autoimmune diseases (Papadopoulos et al. 1982). A monoclonal protein, most frequently an IgM, is detected in approximately 5% of patients with B-cell lymphomas.

The appearance of a monoclonal gammopathy may not represent the development of a malignant diathesis, although as many as 11% of patients with benign monoclonal gammopathy (BMG) will develop MM when followed for five years. Monoclonal gammopathies of undetermined significance (MGUS) have been classified into four categories by Kyle (1978) in accordance with the outcomes observed in a large group of patients followed because of the presence of an asymptomatic M-component (table 29.4). Over a 10-year period, the initial levels of monoclonal IgG and hemoglobin had no predictive value for identification of patients who would demonstrate rising M-components that evolve into MM. Most M-proteins were under 3 g/dL at diagnosis, only 28% had depression of normal Ig's, and urinary light-chain excretion was rare. In Group 1 there was no

Table 29.2
PATHOPHYSIOLOGY OF MULTIPLE MYELOMA

ORGAN SYSTEM	SECONDARY TO CELL PROLIFERATION	SERUM PROTEIN ABNORMALITIES
A. SKELETAL	1. Isolated plasmacytomas 2% to 10% of patients 2. Widespread lytic lesions or diffuse osteoporosis (more common) 3. Severe bone pain	1. Hypercalcemia—production of osteoclast activating factor (not an immunoglobulin)
B. HEMATOLOGIC	1. Bone marrow infiltration or replacement by plasma cells, resulting in: 2. Neutropenia and/or 3. Anemia and/or 4. Thrombocytopenia	1. Anemia—antibody mediated hemolysis (rare) 2. Bleeding—M-components may specifically interact with clotting factors, or coat platelets leading to defective aggregation, may interfere with fibrin polymerization 3. Hypogammaglobulinemia as a result of plasmacytoma-induced macrophage substance (PIMS) suppression of B-cell function
C. RENAL	1. Hyperuricemia due to plasma cell turnover—uric acid nephropathy 2. Hypercalcemic nephropathy 3. Renal infiltration by plasma cells	1. Myeloma kidney—light-chain nephropathy 2. Amyloidosis 3. Glomerulosclerosis
D. NERVOUS SYSTEM	1. Radiculopathy/cord compression due to skeletal destruction and nerve compression 2. Intracranial plasma cell masses	1. Amyloid infiltration of nerves—neuropathy
E. GENERAL		**Hyperviscosity Syndrome:** infrequent in MM, occurs with IgG$_1$, IgG$_3$, or IgA MM; sludging in capillaries due to aggregation of Ig's—purpura, retinal hemorrhage, papilledema, coronary ischemia, CNS symptoms (vertigo, seizures, confusion) **Cryoglobulinemia:** reversible precipitation of serum protein in the cold—Raynaud's phenomenon, thrombosis and gangrene in extremities

Table 29.3
DIFFERENTIAL DIAGNOSIS OF MONOCLONAL GAMMOPATHIES

1. Neoplasms of Immunoglobulin-Producing Cells
   A. Multiple myeloma (IgG, IgA, IgD, or IgE + free light chain; free light chain alone; rarely (1%) no detectable immunoglobulin abnormality; very rarely bi- or oligoclonal. Malignancy of plasma cells.

   B. Macroglobulinemia (IgM + free light chain). Malignancy of cells apparently transitional between lymphocytes and plasma cells.

   C. Heavy-chain diseases (and/or chain or fragment thereof). Malignancies of plasma cells or lymphoid precursors.

   D. Primary amyloidosis (IgG, IgA, IgM, or IgD — free light chain; free light chain alone, occasionally no detectable immunoglobulin abnormality). Question: special form of multiple myeloma?

2. Lymphoreticular Neoplasms
   Non-Hodgkin's lymphoma, chronic lymphocytic leukemia (often hypogammaglobulinemia; M-component when present often IgM, occasionally IgG). B lymphocytes in these disorders occasionally produce M-component.

3. Nonlymphoreticular Neoplasms
   Cancer of colon, prostate, breast, stomach and other sites (no consistent pattern of M-components). Occasional monoclonal immunoglobulin production is seen in this setting, presumably in reaction to the tumor.

4. Diseases With Autoimmune Features
   A. Mixed cryoglobulinemia (homogeneous IgM acting as anti-IgG)

   B. Hypergammaglobulinemic purpura (homogeneous IgG acting as anti-IgG)

   C. Cold agglutinin disease (IgM, predominantly)

   D. Sjogrens disease (IgM)

   E. Lupus and related disorders

5. Disorders of Varying and Unknown Etiology
   Chronic infections, parasitic diseases, cirrhosis of the liver, carcinoid, polycythemia vera, renal tubular acidosis (no consistent pattern of M-components); Gaucher's disease (IgG), pyoderma gangrenosum (IgA), lichen myxedematosus (IgG, predominantly). Usually polyclonal, rarely monoclonal reactions are part of underlying disorder.

6. No Associated Disease
   Monoclonal Gammopathy of Undetermined Significance (MGUS).

progression in the magnitude of the M-protein in the majority of patients over two decades; the gammopathy was truly benign. In a smaller proportion, the M-component slowly and progressively increased, indicating a gradual clonal expansion, but MM did not develop (Group 2). In Group 4 classical multiple myeloma developed, at a median follow-up of eight years, and the disease made up 70% of the tumors. The diagnostic criteria for MM is shown in table 29.5. The remainder of Group 4 individuals developed Waldenstrom's macroglobulinemia, or amyloidosis. As a rule, the most consistent sign that an MGUS is evolving into MM is a progressive rise in the level of the paraprotein, which is a rough correlation with plasma cell mass (Maldonado and Kyle 1974). Hence, serial measurement of the M-component on at least a yearly basis provides adequate follow-up.

INCIDENCE

MM is an infrequent disease that accounts for 1% of the hematologic malignancies in the United States. It is age-dependent, with less than 2% of cases occurring before age 40 (Hewell and Alexanian 1976), after which the incidence rises continuously through the eighth decade (Turesson et al. 1984). The disease is more common in blacks than whites by approximately 14 to 1. This may be due to the higher average immunoglobulin

levels in blacks, which represent a larger pool of B cells at risk for undergoing neoplastic transformation (Cutler and Young 1975).

OSSEOUS DISEASE

The vast majority of MM patients will develop skeletal manifestations that result from diffuse or focal areas of osteolysis in anatomic relation to an expanding mass of plasma cells. They present with localized areas of bone pain and/or swelling in conjunction with marked tenderness. Back pain is particularly common and is occasionally punctuated by episodes of severe, intractable discomfort that may represent a pathologic fracture. Compression fractures of the vertebrae are common and can cause the patient to lose several inches in height.

Table 29.4
MONOCLONAL GAMMOPATHIES OF UNDETERMINED SIGNIFICANCE (MGUS)

A. Monoclonal protein:	IgG <3.5 g/dL
	IgA ≤2.0 g/dL
	BJ ≤1.0 g/24 hr
B. <10% B.M. plasma cells	
C. No bone lesions	
D. No symptoms	

Table 29.5
MULTIPLE MYELOMA — CRITERIA

1.   Major Criteria
     A. Plasmacytoma on tissue biopsy

     B. B.M. plasmacytosis >30% plasma cells

     C. Monoclonal globulin spike on SPEP
          IgG >3.5 g/dL
          IgA >2.0 g/dL

     D. K or light chain >1.0 g/24 hr on urine electrophoresis

2.   Minor Criteria
     A. B.M. plasmacytosis 10% to 30%

     B. Monoclonal globulin spike, less than above levels

     C. Lytic bone lesions

     D. Hypogammaglobulinemia or suppression of antibody
        production other than monoclonal spike

On x-ray, the most frequent observation is the appearance of lucent lesions having clearly demarcated borders, the so-called punched out lesions. There is little osteoblastic activity or periosteal reaction, unlike the situation in most other neoplasms having metastases to bone. In some patients, bone x-rays demonstrate diffuse osteoporosis; however, if microradiography were performed, it would reveal extensive bone destruction. It is widely acknowledged that bone scintigraphy is considerably less sensitive than routine x-rays in demonstrating bone involvement by MM, presumably due to the minimal osteoblastic activity and hypovascularity associated with this disease (Frank et al. 1982). Where there is bone pain and normal routine radiography of the skeleton, high-resolution computed tomography (CT) often permits visualization of lesions that are present early in the course of the illness (Solomon et al. 1984).

A variant of the skeletal disease associated with MM is that of solitary osseous myeloma (SOM). These myelomas will present in 3% to 5% of cases of plasma cell neoplasia as pain and tenderness at the site of the bone lesion (Conklin and Alexanian 1975). Often there is radiologic evidence of bone destruction and accompanying neurologic signs such as nerve-root compression and radiculopathy or spinal-cord compression. Many of these patients (75%) do not have a demonstrable M-component; among those that do, it is usually less than 1.5 g/dL. The detectable paraprotein often disappears following radiation therapy. Unfortunately, 70% of patients develop typical MM within 10 years.

A frequent accompaniment of myelomatous bone involvement is hypercalcemia. Whereas the osseous lesions of MM are secondary to an expanding neoplastic cell mass, elevations in serum calcium have a humoral basis. Myeloma cells secrete osteoclast activating factor (OAF), a lymphokine that activates osteoclasts to produce organic acids that demineralize bone (Raisz 1975; Mundy et al. 1974). Serum calcium is elevated in 30% of presenting patients and rises above normal in another 30% throughout the course of the illness, roughly correlating with a large tumor burden (Bergsagel et al. 1967). Hypercalcemia is often precipitated by the enforced bed rest resulting from painful bone lesions, and can be exacerbated by dehydration. Consequently, both bed rest and dehydration are to be avoided if possible.

HEMATOLOGIC CONSEQUENCES OF MM

The most frequent finding is a normocytic, normochromic anemia, which is often present at the inception of the clinical illness, but which has developed insidiously. Rouleaux formation is discernible in the peripheral blood of patients with high levels of immunoglobulins, often in conjunction with a blue background on the smear due to the elevated concentrations of this protein. The reticulocyte count is typically low, and the erythrosuppression may worsen as a function of disease progression or chemotherapy. Leukopenia and thrombocytopenia are frequent, especially as the myeloma cell burden expands in the narrow space, or the patient is exposed to radiation or chemotherapy. Although serious bleeding can often be avoided by platelet transfusions, bleeding will occasionally occur because of nonspecific interactions between the M-component and clotting factors, or defective platelet function secondary to nonspecific coating of platelets by immunoglobulins (Perkins et al. 1970).

Severe neutropenia is an important contributor to the development of bacterial infection, a predisposition that is enhanced by the hypogammaglobulinemia that is so often present. The mechanisms underlying the impairment in humoral immunity are twofold: the increased rate of immunoglobulin catabolism, and the production by plasma cells of a factor (PC factor) that stimulates macrophages to produce PIMS (plasmacytoma-induced macrophage substance), which inhibits B-cell function (Ullrich and Zolla-Pazner 1982).

RENAL MANIFESTATIONS OF MM

MYELOMA CAST NEPHROPATHY

Dense tubular casts are a hallmark of MM and are observed in 75% of patients, all of whom are excreting free light chains, or Bence-Jones proteins (Hill et al. 1983). The large, hard casts cause compression atrophy of the tubular epithelium. The tubular basement membrane may then rupture and result in interstitial inflammation, subsequent fibrosis, and, ultimately, renal failure. The tubular casts stain positively for immunoglobulin light chains, but contain mucoproteins as well. Acute renal failure can be precipitated in MM patients by acute dehydration, which may occur during preparation for an x-ray study employing iodinated dyes; fever secondary to infection; or hypercalcemia (Cohen et al. 1984). Dehydration facilitates precipitation of light chains in tubules, which sometimes is compounded by coprecipitation with calcium. Although light-chain nephropathy is an ominous development, acute renal failure arising in this setting is often partially reversible by restoration of renal perfusion and cautious use of loop diuretics.

GLOMERULAR LESIONS

Twenty-five percent of patients develop cumulative deposition of the paraprotein in the mesangium that results in glomerulosclerosis. The morphology is characterized by coarse granular deposits, which stain with antibodies to kappa chains, and are located at the inner aspect of the glomerular basement membrane. The mechanism by which glomerular damage is produced is not understood.

Another glomerular lesion found in MM patients is renal amyloid deposits, present in 30% of patients. This material can be found in tubular basement membranes, renal vessels, the interstitium, and glomeruli. The latter can be associated with nephrosis in which mixed serum proteins including albumin are excreted in the urine, along with light chains.

Renal failure in MM often occurs when dehydration, hypercalcemia, and light-chain excretion are present. Management of acute renal failure that arises in the face of excessive light-chain production may be supplemented with plasmapheresis to rapidly lower the burden of light chains. The institution of hemodialysis in MM patients with irreversible, profound renal failure is entirely justified, if the prospects for systemic control of the disease are good. This important management approach has ameliorated the dire consequences otherwise imposed by this complication.

NEUROLOGIC COMPLICATIONS

Spinal-cord compression is almost always secondary to osseous involvement of ribs or vertebrae in association with an epidural mass. Back pain or radicular pain lasting for many months and increasing in severity is a frequent prelude to this dreaded complication. The importance of prompt diagnosis cannot be overstated, as the appearance of neurologic deficits often progresses to paraplegia within hours or days. Suspicion of cord compression based on new neurologic signs should stimulate the prompt initiation of CAT scans or myelography to delineate the upper and lower extent of the lesion or lesions. In particularly challenging clinical situations, nuclear magnetic resonance imaging (MRI) studies may provide definitive identification of an epidural lesion causing cord compression.

The usual emergency therapy for spinal-cord compression is high-dose decadron, followed by radiation therapy once the lesion's anatomic extent is known. Laminectomy is indicated in the circumstance of relapsing cord compression, when radiation is contraindicated, or in situations in which an isolated osseous lesion is associated with the neurologic deficit.

UNUSUAL NEUROLOGIC MANIFESTATIONS

Intracranial myeloma is a distinctly rare event that can occur due to extension of a lesion involving the cranium. When myelomatous masses invade the meninges, plasma cells are easily observed in the cerebrospinal fluid (CSF); immunoelectrophoresis of the CSF will demonstrate the paraprotein. Management consists of detailed analysis of the mass by CT or MRI exam, followed by surgical decompression or resection, if necessary, and radiotherapy.

Sensorimotor neuropathy occurs in about 1% of myeloma patients, and may precede the onset of the illness by years. When it occurs, it is more common in individuals with solitary osseous plasmacytomas, and resembles the syndrome occasionally seen in patients who ultimately develop lung or stomach cancer (Davis and Drachman 1972).

The hyperviscosity syndrome (HVS) is caused by elevated levels of serum proteins having a high intrinsic viscosity, and is usually manifest at serum viscosity levels greater than 4 centipoises (Cp). It is most common in the setting of Waldenstrom's macroglobulinemia, which is characterized by marked overproduction of monoclonal IgM protein. In MM it is associated with overproduction of IgG_1 and IgG_3 proteins, as the relevant heavy-chain classes within these categories have a propensity to aggregate (Hall and Abraham 1984). HVS is also observed in IgA myeloma, particularly when the M-component exceeds 5 gm%. The likelihood of these immunoglobulins aggregating is enhanced if the protein is temperature-sensitive, such that exposure to cold might precipitate HVS. The clinical picture is characterized by fatigue, headache, sluggish mentation, and visual disturbances. These symptoms can be compounded by vascular effects of sludging, such as myocardial ischemia, and by defects in platelet aggregation. It is important to be alert for the signs of HVS because plasmapheresis can be lifesaving, even in those cases of IgG MM in which the paraprotein is distributed throughout the intra- and extravascular space (unlike IgM which is entirely intravascular).

TUMOR KINETICS AND STAGING

The amount of monoclonal immunoglobulin produced in MM closely correlates with the tumor mass of plasma cells; therefore, serial measurement of the M-protein can be used to assess changes in tumor burden over time or following treatment. The ability to measure the M-protein reliably serves as a tumor marker that has been useful in providing a model for the growth kinetics of a human malignancy.

Durie and Salmon have developed a method to quantitate tumor burden in MM, defined as total-body myeloma-cell number (Durie, Salmon, and Moon 1980). Their investigation of a large series of MM patients at presentation has led to a staging system that correlates clinical characteristics with total mass of myeloma cells. The latter can be calculated by this formula:

$$\text{Total-body myeloma cell number} = \frac{\text{Total-body M-component synthetic rate}}{\text{M-component synthetic rate per myeloma cell}}$$

The total-body M-component synthetic rate can be calculated from the determination of the M-component serum concentration, the plasma volume, and the predicted catabolic rate for the Ig monoclonal protein in question. The M-component synthetic rate per cell is determined by growing myeloma cells obtained from bone marrow in short-term culture. From quantitation of the number of cells in culture and determination of their rate of immunoglobulin production, the synthetic rate per cell can be calculated.

Correlations of total-body myeloma-cell burden has been correlated with specific clinical characteristics, and has led to the identification of three stages of the disease (table 29.6): high cell mass ($>1.2 \times 10^{12}$ myeloma cells/m^2) stage III; intermediate cell mass (0.6-1.2 $\times$ $10^{12}/m^2$) stage II; and low cell mass (0.6 $\times 10^{12}/m^2$) stage I (Conklin and Alexanian 1975). Important prognostic implications (table 29.7) are based on these stages, and on the added subclassification for renal failure (Durie, Salmon, and Moon 1980). Furthermore, the staging system does not require extensive laboratory techniques.

Another important prognostic variable is based on the determination of the number of dividing cells in a population of myeloma cells. This technique, termed the labeling index (L.I.), also depends upon the ability to grow myeloma cells from a patient in short-term culture. It is performed by labeling cells with tritiated thymidine for one hour and counting the number of cells that have taken up the radioactive precursor (Mundy et al. 1974).

Most patients with MM have an L.I. between 1% and 5% at presentation. A L.I. greater than 3% correlates with a poor prognosis, especially if it is associated with a high tumor-cell burden. The group of patients with a L.I. of less than 1% have a relatively good prognosis. Patients with MGUS often have a L.I. of less than 0.5%.

Measurement of L.I. has permitted several observations about the kinetics of MM following treatment (Durie, Salmon, and Moon 1980). Patients who have a high L.I. respond more rapidly to chemotherapy, but their responses are often of short duration and their disease tends to grow back quickly. Conversely, patients with a low L.I. take longer to respond to therapy, but have a longer response-duration and survival.

Following effective therapy, the M-component falls until it reaches a plateau. The plateau phase lasts a fixed period of time, even if therapy is continued, until the M-component again starts to increase (Salmon 1973). In this relapse phase, about two-thirds of patients have a higher L.I. than they did at presentation, indicating an increasing growth fraction of probably drug-resistant cells (Drewinko et al. 1971). Other relapsing patients can have high tumor masses but low L.I.'s (Hobbs 1969). In these cases, the malignant mass of plasma cells increases in size and the tumor outgrows its blood supply. Growth then slows, resulting in a prolonged doubling time. This pattern of faster growth at smaller tumor volumes is called Gompertzian kinetics and may explain the presumed rapid subclinical growth of MM. Gompertzian kinetics obviously does not apply to all cases of PCD. In MGUS, the growth of plasma cells is halted or slowed at low-plasma cell masses (Kyle 1982). Progression of growth may be controlled by poorly understood host factors.

Another useful prognostic indicator in MM is the measurement of beta-2 microglobulin (β_2M) levels (Norfolk et al. 1979; Bataille et al. 1982). This protein has a structure similar to the constant region of the light chain. If renal function is normal, β_2M levels closely reflect tumor load in PCD. The measurement of β_2M is especially useful in patients with light-chain disease or rare nonsecretory myelomas for which the measurement of M-component levels over time may be problematic or impossible.

Table 29.6
MYELOMA STAGING SYSTEM

Stage	Criteria	Measured Myeloma Cell Mass, cells x $10^{12}/m^2$

I.	ALL of the following
	1. Hemoglobin value >10 g/100 mL
	2. Serum calcium value normal (<12 mg/100 mL)
	3. On x-ray, normal bone structure (scale 0) or solitary bone plasmacytoma only
	4. Low M-component production rates
	  a. IgG value <5 g/100 mL
	  b. IgA value <3 g/100 mL
	  c. Urine light chain M-component on electrophoresis <4 g/24 hr
		<0.6 (low)

II.	Fitting neither stage I nor stage III	>0.6-1.20 (intermediate)

III.	One or more of the following:
	1. Hemoglobin value 8.5 g/100 mL
	2. Serum calcium value >12 mg/100 mL
	3. Advanced lytic bone lesions (scale 3)
	4. High M-component production rates
	  a. IgG value >7 g/100 mL
	  b. IgA value >5 g/100 mL
	  c. Urine light chain M-component on electrophoresis >12 g/24 hr
		>1.20 (high)

Subclassification:
A = Relatively normal renal function (serum creatinine value 2.0 mg/100 mL)
B = Abnormal renal function (serum creatinine value 2.0 mg/100 mL)

Table 29.7
MYELOMA CELL MASS AND SURVIVAL IN 160 PATIENTS

Cell Mass Category (Cells/m²)	No. of Patients		Median Survival (Months)	p Values
	Alive	Dead		
High 1.2×10^{12}	38	57	32.6	0.05 0.002
Intermediate $0.6-1.2 \times 10^{12}$	20	20	54.5	0.05 0.10
Low 0.6×10^{12}	16	9	76.5	0.10 0.002

(From: Durie [1982].)

THERAPY FOR MULTIPLE MYELOMA

Conventional treatment for MM is palliative and fraught with long-term dangers. As a result, observation is appropriate for patients without anemia, bone pain, osteolysis, or renal failure. When therapy is indicated, the mainstay of chemotherapy has been melphalan (M), usually given on an intermittent schedule, e.g., 0.25 mg/kg/d for 4 days, in conjunction with prednisone (P), 2 mg/kg/d (Alexanian 1980). The addition of the steroid to melphalan increases the response rate substantially, but it does not have a large effect on survival. Melphalan is well-absorbed orally, and can be administered in standard doses to patients with renal failure. Melphalan therapy can be discontinued after the maximal response has been achieved.

Cyclophosphamide is an alkylating agent (AA) that is structurally different from melphalan, is not cross-resistant with it, and can be used when drug resistance to melphalan has developed (Bergsagel et al. 1972). It is equally effective in producing remissions in MM, is well-tolerated systemically, and can be administered in standard doses to patients with renal failure. Cyclophosphamide is less toxic to thrombopoiesis than are other alkylating agents and therefore can be used with greater safety in patients with thrombocytopenia.

The superiority of multiple-drug regimens has not been demonstrated when compared to MP. Combinations of melphalan, cyclophosphamide, BCNU, vincristine, prednisone, or alternating combinations of subsets of these agents, are effective at inducing remissions, perhaps at faster but not at substantially higher rates than MP. No reproducible survival advantage has been shown to be a result of these more intensive regimens, and their additional toxicity and cost raise serious questions about their utility.

Approximately 40% of patients are unresponsive to alkylating agents at the start of therapy, and virtually all who initially enjoy tumor regression will ultimately manifest AA resistance. A useful salvage regimen is composed of high-dose corticosteroids (prednisone or dexamethasone), and continuous infusions of vincristine and doxorubicin. Seventy percent of refractory MM will undergo an objective regression that may persist for approximately nine months (Hall et al. 1986). Numerous other regimens employing very intensive doses of non-AA chemotherapy have been attempted, with little success. Occasional objective responses with recombinant alpha interferon have been reported, but in the aggregate there is little to bolster enthusiasm for this biologic response modifier in MM (Ohno et al. 1985).

Bone marrow transplantation has been attempted in a few cases of MM without success, in part because of the inability to completely eradicate the malignant clone. The recent advent of treatment strategies employing extremely high doses of an AA such as melphalan (i.e., 180 mg/m² IV) has resulted in a substantial number of complete responses in untreated patients. Innovative approaches designed to extend this observation include conventional remission-induction therapy, followed by harvest of autologous bone marrow, high-dose melphalan therapy, and subsequent reinfusion of the bone marrow that has been purged with an antibody specific for plasma cells. It will require several years to determine whether this adventurous approach will alter the natural history of the disease.

A feared long-term consequence of standard therapy for MM is the development of acute leukemia. This secondary neoplasm results from prolonged exposure to AAs, and has been reported at a frequency of 20% after 50 months of follow-up (Bergsagel 1982). Secondary ANLL often begins as a myelodysplastic syndrome, demonstrating characteristic karyotypic abnormalities affecting chromosomes 5 and 7. Within several months of the onset, the disease progresses to frank acute leukemia, which generally responds poorly to established methods of therapy.

REFERENCES

Alexanian, R. 1980. Treatment of multiple myeloma. *Acta Haematol.* 63:237.

Alper, C. 1974. Plasma protein measurements as a diagnostic aid. *N. Engl. J. Med.* 29:287.

Bataille, R. et al. 1982. Serum beta-2microglobulin in multiple myeloma: relationship to presenting clinical features and clinical status. *Eur. J. Cancer Clinic. Oncol.* 18:59.

Bergsagel, D.E. et al. 1967. The treatment of plasma cell myeloma. *Adv. Cancer Res.* 10:311.

Bergsagel, D.E. et al. 1972. Plasma cell myeloma: response of melphalan-resistant patients to high dose intermittent cyclophosphamide. *Can. Med. Assoc. J.* 107:851.

Bergsagel, D.E. 1982. Plasma cell neoplasms and acute leukemia. *Clin. Haematol.* 11:221.

Cohen, D.J. et al. 1984. Acute renal failure in patients with multiple myeloma. *Am. J. Med.* 76:247.

Conklin, R., and Alexanian, R. 1975. Clinical classification of plasma cell myeloma. *Arch. Int. Med.* 135:139.

Cooper M. 1987. Current concepts—B lymphocytes: normal development and function. *N. Engl. J. Med.* 317:1452-55.

Cutter, S.J., and Young, J.L. 1975. *Third national cancer survey: incidence data.* Washington, D.C.: U.S. Government Printing Office.

Davis, L.E., and Drachman, D.B. 1972. Myeloma neuropathy: successful treatment of 2 patients and review of cases. *Arch. Neurol.* 25:507.

DeWald, G. et al. 1985. The clinical significance of cytogenetic studies in 100 patients with multiple myeloma, plasma cell leukemia or amyloidosis. *Blood* 66:380.

Drewinko, B.; Brown, B.; and Humphrey, R. et al. 1971. Effect of chemotherapy on the labeling index of myeloma cells. *Cancer* 34:526.

Durie, B., and Salmon, S. 1975. A clinical staging system for multiple myeloma: correlation of measured myeloma cell mass with presenting clinical features, response to treatment, and survival. *Cancer* 36: 842-54.

Durie, B.; Salmon, S.; and Moon, T. 1980. Pretreatment tumor mass, cell kinetics, and prognosis in multiple myeloma. *Blood* 55:364-72.

Festi, A. et al. 1984. Cytogenetic study in multiple myeloma. *Cancer Genet. Cytogenet.* 12:247.

Foon, K., and Todd, R. F. 1986. Immunologic classification of leukemia and lymphoma. *Blood* 68:1-31.

Frank, J.W. et al. 1982. The value of bone imaging in multiple myeloma. *Eur. J. Nucl. Med.* 7:502.

Frei, E., and Holland, J. eds. 1981. *Cancer medicine.* Philadelphia: Lea and Febiger.

Hall, C.G., and Abraham, G.N. 1984. Reversible self-association of a human myeloma protein: thermodynamics and relevance to viscosity effects and solubility. *Biochemistry* 23:5123.

Hall, A. et al. 1986. Melphalan resistance in myeloma. *Br. J. Haematol.* 63:1.

Hewell, G.M., and Alexanian, R. 1976. Multiple myeloma in young persons. *Ann. Int. Med.* 84:441.

Hill, G.S. et al. 1983. Renal lesions in multiple myeloma: their relationship to associated protein abnormalities. *Am. J. Kidney Dis.* 2:423.

Hirano, T. et al. 1987. Human B-cell differentiation factor defined by an anti-peptide antibody and its possible role in autoantibody production. *Proc. Natl. Acad. Sci. USA* 84: 228-31.

Hobbs, J. 1969. Growth rates and responses to treatment in human myelomatosis. *Br. J. Haematol.* 16:607.

Katzmann, J. 1978. Myeloma induced immunosuppression: a multistep mechanism. *J. Immunol.* 121:1405.

Kawano, M.; Hirano, T.; and Matusda, T. et al. 1988. Autocrine generation and requirement of BSF/IL-6 for human multiple myelomas. *Nature* 332:83-85.

Krakauer, R.S. et al. 1977. Hypogammaglobulinemia-experimental myeloma: the role of suppressor factors for mononuclear phagocytes. *J. Immunol.* 118:1385.

Kyle R. 1975. Multiple myeloma: review of 869 cases. *Mayo Clin. Proc.* 50:29.

Kyle, R., and Garton, J. 1986. Laboratory monitoring of myeloma proteins. *Semin. Oncol.* 13:310-17.

Kyle, R. 1982. Monoclonal gammopathy of undetermined significance (MGUS): a review. *Clin. Haematol.* 11:123.

Kyle, R. 1978. Monoclonal gammopathy of undetermined significance: natural history in 241 cases. *Am. J. Med.* 64:814.

Maldonado, J., and Kyle, R. 1974. Familial myeloma: report of eight families and a study of serum proteins in their relatives. *Am. J. Med.* 57:875.

Mundy, G.R. et al. 1974. Evidence for the secretion of an osteoclast stimulating factor in myeloma. *N. Engl. J. Med.* 291:1041.

Natvig, J.B., and Kunkel, H. 1973. Human immunoglobulins: classes, subclasses, genetic variants and idiotypes. *Adv. Immunol.* 16:1-59.

Norfolk, D. et al. 1979. Serum B$_2$-microglobulin in myelomatosis: potential valve in stratification and monitoring. *Br. J. Cancer* 39:510.

Ohno, R. et al. 1985. Treatment of multiple myeloma with recombinant human leukocyte A interferon. *Cancer Treat. Rep.* 69:1433.

Osserman, E., and Takatsuki, K. 1965. Considerations regarding the pathogenesis of the plasmacytic dyscrasias. *Ser. Haematol.* 4:28.

Papadopoulos, N.M. et al. 1982. Incidence of gamma globulin binding in a healthy population by high resolution electrophoresis. *Clin. Chem.* 28:707.

Perkins, H.A. et al. 1970. Hemostatic defects in dysproteinemias. *Blood* 35:695.

Pilarski, L.M. et al. 1985. Pre-B cells in peripheral blood of multiple myeloma patients. *Blood* 66:416.

Potter, M.; Sklar, M.; and Rowe, W. 1973. Rapid viral induction of plasmacytomas in pristine-primed BALB/c mice. *Science* 182:592.

Potter, M. 1986. Plasmacytomas in mice. *Semin. Oncol.* 13: 275-81.

Raisz, L.G. et al. 1975. Effect of osteoclast activating factor from human leukocytes on bone metabolism. *J. Clin. Invest.* 56:408.

Ritchie, R., and Smith, R. 1976. Immunofixation III: application to the study of monoclonal proteins. *Clin. Chem.* 22:1982.

Rosen, S.M.; Buxbaum, J.N.; and Frangione, B. 1986. Structures of immunoglobulins and their genes, DNA rearrangement and B-cell differentiation, molecular anomalies of some monoclonal immunoglobulins. *Semin. Oncol.* 13:260-74.

Salmon, S. 1973. Immunoglobulin synthesis and tumor kinetics of multiple myeloma. *Semin. Hematol.* 10:135.

Seligmann, M., and Brovet, J. 1973 Antibody activity of human myeloma globulins. *Semin. Hematol.* 10:163.

Solomon, A. et al. 1984. Multiple myeloma: early vertebral involvement assessed by computerized tomography. *Skeletal Radiol.* 11:258.

Stamatoyannopoulos, G.; Neinhuis, A.; and Leder, P. et al. eds. 1987. *The molecular basis of blood diseases.* Philadelphia: W.B. Saunders.

Turesson, I. et al. 1984. Comparison of trends in the incidence of multiple myeloma in Malmo, Sweden, and other countries, 1950-1979. *N. Engl. J. Med.* 310:421.

Ullrich, S.; and Zolla-Pazner, S. 1982. Immunoregulatory circuits in myeloma. *Clin. Haematol.* 11:87.

Waldenstrom, J. 1970. *Diagnosis and treatment of multiple myeloma.* New York: Grune and Stratton Inc.

Warner, N.; Potter, M.; and Metcalf, D. 1974. *Multiple myeloma and related immunoglobulin producing neoplasms.* UICC Technical Report Series vol. 13. Geneva: Internal Union Against Cancer.

Whicher, J.; Hawkins, L.; and Higginson, J. 1980. Clinical applications of immunofixation: a more sensitive technique for the detection of Bence-Jones protein. *J. Clin. Pathol.* 33:779-80.

Zawadski, Z., and Edwards, G. 1972. Nonmyelomatous monoclonal immunoglobulinemia. *Prog. Immunol.* 1:105.

Chapter 30

ADULT LEUKEMIAS

Anna J. Mitus, M.D.
David S. Rosenthal, M.D.

Anna J. Mitus, M.D.
Instructor in Medicine
Hematology Division
Brigham and Women's Hospital
Harvard Medical School
Boston, Massachusetts

David S. Rosenthal, M.D.
Hematologist
Brigham and Women's Hospital
Harvard Medical School
Harry K. Oliver Professor of Hygiene
Harvard University
Boston, Massachusetts

INTRODUCTION

The adult leukemias constitute about 10% of all cancers and are a heterogenous group of diseases broadly divided into acute and chronic disorders. In general, the acute leukemias are characterized by autonomous proliferation of undifferentiated cells, whereas the chronic leukemias are distinguished by uncontrolled expansion of mature cells. Acute nonlymphocytic leukemia (ANLL), often referred to as acute myelogenous leukemia (AML); acute lymphoblastic leukemia (ALL); chronic myelogenous leukemia (CML); and chronic lymphocytic leukemia (CLL) all involve the hematopoietic system and lead to disruption of normal hematopoiesis. Leukemia is a clonal disease affecting lymphoid progenitors in ALL and CLL and the pluripotent hematopoietic stem cell in ANLL and CML. Elimination of the neoplastic clone can be achieved in the acute forms of leukemia by intensive chemotherapy, while treatment of the chronic disorders is rarely curative.

Patients with leukemia develop infection, hemorrhage, and fatigue arising from neutropenia, thrombocytopenia, and anemia. Traditional morphologic and histochemical criteria have been supplemented by cytogenetic, immunologic, and molecular diagnostic methods, enabling more precise classification of the various disorders. Chemotherapy and supportive management have led to improved survival. Indwelling intravenous catheters, broad spectrum antibiotics, and intensive blood-product availability have all proved invaluable in this regard. Allogeneic bone marrow transplant (BMT) offers improved chance of cure for many of the leukemias and, as toxicities are reduced, will undoubtedly be used more frequently to treat these disorders.

ACUTE NONLYMPHOCYTIC LEUKEMIA

Acute nonlymphocytic leukemia makes up a group of heterogenous disorders characterized by uncontrolled proliferation of primitive hematopoietic cells. Massive accumulation of leukemic cells, or blasts, may occur, giving rise to the original description of this disease as *weisses blut* (white blood) by Virchow (1897). The ensuing disruption of normal hematopoiesis leads to severe pancytopenia and often life-threatening infections and bleeding. The French-American-British (FAB) classification, proposed in 1976 and subsequently modified, has divided ANLL into seven groups based on morphologic, cytochemical, and immunologic features. In each subtype, myeloid, monocyte, erythroid, or megakaryocyte cells predominate; however, the term acute myelogenous leukemia (AML) is often used nonspecifically to encompass this entire group. While ANLL remains highly lethal, significant improvement in survival has been achieved with intensive chemotherapy and bone marrow transplantation as well as by the increased availability of antibiotic and blood-product support. While three out of four patients will achieve remission, ultimately only one-fourth will be cured (Bloomfield 1987).

INCIDENCE AND EPIDEMIOLOGY

ANLL affects 2.3 individuals per 100,000 without predilection for sex or race. The incidence of ANLL increases with age, rising from less than 1 case per 100,000 in individuals under the age of 30, to greater than 14 per 100,000 for those older than 75 (Sandler 1987).

ETIOLOGY

Of all the leukemias, ANLL has perhaps the strongest etiologic link to toxin exposure and to a variety of underlying congenital and hematologic disorders (table 30.1).

Exposure to radiation, chemicals, or drugs can predispose to the development of ANLL. The leukemogenic potential of radiation was recognized decades ago with an early epidemiologic study showing a 9-fold increase in radiologists (March 1950; March 1961). The largest experience with radiation is in Japanese atomic bomb survivors. A 50-fold increase in the incidence of leukemia occurred in those individuals with the highest exposure, peaking at five to seven years, but continuing for up to 13 to 14 years (Moloney 1955; Heysell 1960; Hiroo 1982).

The best-documented chemical leukemogen is benzene, first shown to be associated with acute leukemia in 1928 (Borgomano 1928; Cronkite 1987). Most cases of benzene-induced leukemia are characterized by a prodromal phase of marrow aplasia. Chromosomal abnormalities have been documented, some resembling those found after radiation exposure.

Drugs have also been linked to the development of ANLL. Most notorious among this group are the alkylating agents whose leukemogenic potential was initially described in patients with multiple myeloma receiving prolonged courses of melphalan. Subsequently, many other alkylators have been shown to induce leukemia when used to treat neoplastic or benign conditions. Nonchemotherapy agents such as chloramphenicol and phenylbutazone are more tenuously linked with ANLL. Preceding marrow aplasia and cytogenetic abnormalities characterize these cases (Casciato 1979).

Several congenital and acquired disorders may terminate in ANLL (Bloomfield 1976). The best recognized of these, Down's syndrome, has a 20-fold increased incidence of leukemia (Miller 1968; Rowley 1981).

Malignancies such as multiple myeloma, ovarian cancer, and Hodgkin's disease may increase the risk of acute leukemia. It is difficult to separate this phenomenon from the potential leukemic effect of prescribed chemotherapy (Valagussa 1986; Coleman 1986). Nonneoplastic hematologic diseases are also linked to the development of ANLL. The myelodysplastic syndromes are notable among this group. These disorders, also referred to as preleukemia or refractory dysmyelopoietic anemias, have recently been classified morphologically. The incidence of ANLL approaches 30% for certain subgroups, and is particularly refractory to therapy (Rosenthal 1984).

Activation of oncogenes, and genetic control of hematopoietic growth factors and their receptors are major areas of ongoing interest and research (Vallenga 1987; Cheng 1988).

CLINICAL CHARACTERISTICS

Fatigue, weakness, shortness of breath, weight loss, fever, easy bruisability, and bleeding are prominent initial complaints of patients with ANLL. Certain presentations are distinctive, suggesting the leukemic subtype. Infiltration of skin, gums, and other soft tissues is particularly common in the monocytoid forms of leukemia, while hemorrhage due to disseminated intravascular coagulation (DIC) poses a serious complication of promyelocytic leukemia. Central nervous system (CNS) involvement by leukemia is detected in approximately 2% of cases at presentation and should be suspected when patients develop headache, nausea, vomiting, or cranial neuropathies. Symptoms of leukostasis including change in mentation and shortness of breath occur with high blast counts and constitute medical emergencies. Isolated collections of myeloblasts known as myeloblastomas, granulocytic sarcomas, or chloromas arise in various soft tissues, and in some cases precede bone marrow involvement. When present, these tumors should be treated with aggressive systemic as well as local antileukemic therapy (Eshghabadi 1986).

The physical findings in patients with acute leukemia often include fever, pallor, ecchymoses, purpura, and petechiae. Sinusitis, pneumonia, perirectal cellulitis, and skin abscesses are common localized infections. As previously noted, gingival hyperplasia, skin infiltrates, lymphadenopathy, and splenomegaly characterize monocytic variants.

CLASSIFICATION

Acute leukemia is defined by the presence of at least 30% immature cells in the bone marrow. The FAB classification categorizes ANLL into seven groups, M1 to M7 (Bennett 1976; 1985a). Distinct morphologic and histochemical features of the blasts form the basis of this classification, although cytogenetic and immunologic parameters have also been described for each subgroup (Bloomfield 1987; Griffin 1983). Table 30.2 summarizes the criteria for M1 to M7, including a partial listing of chromosomal and phenotypic data.

Table 30.1
PATHOGENESIS OF ACUTE LEUKEMIA

I. Toxins
  A. Radiation
  B. Chemicals: benzene
  C. Drugs:
    1. Alkylating agents: melphalan, cyclophosphamide, chlorambucil, busulfan, thiotepa, CCNU
    2. Chloramphenicol
    3. Phenylbutazone
II. Congenital Diseases
  A. Down's syndrome
  B. Fanconi's anemia
  C. Kleinfelter's syndrome
  D. Turner's syndrome
  E. Bloom's syndrome
  F. Wiskott-Aldrich syndrome
III. Acquired Disorders
  A. Malignancies
  B. Myeloproliferative:
    1. Polycythemia vera
    2. Primary thrombocytosis
    3. Agnogenic myeloid metaplasia
  C. Myelodysplastic syndromes
  D. Paroxysmal nocturnal hemoglobinuria (PNH)

Proliferation of undifferentiated myeloblasts defines M1 leukemia. Maturing granulocytes are rare and constitute less than 10% of nonerythroid cells. Granules in blasts are scant, and Auer rods are uncommon.

M2 leukemia, the most common form of ANLL, is characterized by myeloblasts that mature to the promyelocyte stage. Blasts show heavy granulation with frequent Auer rods (fig. 30.1A).

M3, or promyelocytic leukemia (APL), is distinguished by the predominance of heavily granulated promyelocytes, where clusters of Auer bodies or Auer rods may obscure the cytoplasm (fig. 30.1B). The t(15; 17) translocation is invariably associated with APL and is now felt to be a requisite for diagnosis (Rowley 1988). A microgranular variant of M3 has also been described with this translocation (Golomb 1980). Disseminated intravascular coagulation (DIC) complicates the course of APML in many cases, and is felt to arise from release of a procoagulant from these cells.

Monocytic forms of ANLL make up the M4 and M5 subtypes. M4, or myelomonocytic leukemia (AMML), is defined by the presence of both myeloblastic and monocytic components in the marrow. Monocytes at various stages of differentiation comprise greater than 20% of nonerythroid marrow cells and may constitute greater than 5,000/mm³ of circulating WBC count.

Myelomonocytic leukemia with eosinophilia (M4 with eo) has been classified as a distinct entity (LeBeau 1983). In this subgroup, abnormal eosinophils with unsegmented, monocytoid nuclei constitute 5% or more of the nonerythroid cells. In contrast to normal eosinophils, basophilic granules may be seen. Most important, abnormalities of chromosome 16, such as inversion or translocation, are found in virtually all cases of M4 with eosinophilia.

When greater than 80% of nonerythroid cells in the bone marrow are monocytes, the diagnosis of M5, or acute monocytic leukemia, is made (fig. 30.1C). Two subgroups of M5 have been described: a poorly differentiated form, M5a, where large, immature, nucleolated monoblasts are the predominant cell type, and a differentiated form, M5b, where there is an admixture of promonocytes and mature monocytes (monoblasts comprising less than 20% of cells).

It is often difficult to distinguish M4 and M5 leukemias from M2; use of histochemical stains is helpful (table 30.2). When gingival, skin, and lymph-node infiltration is found upon physical examination, and when elevated serum and urinary lysozyme concentrations are detected, monocytic leukemia is likely. Profound hypokalemia and renal dysfunction may ensue as a consequence of lysozymuria.

Table 30.2
CLASSIFICATION OF ANLL

FAB	MORPHOLOGY	HISTOCHEMISTRY	CYTOGENETICS	SURFACE MARKERS	OTHER
M1	Minimal maturation Scant granules and Auer rods	Peroxidase (+) 3-5% cells Sudan Black (+) 3-5% cells PAS, NSE* (−)	t(9;22) + 8 del(5), del(7)	Ia, CD13, CD33 (+) CD14, CD11b (+)	
M2	Greater maturation Granules and Auer rods	Peroxidase (+) Sudan Black (+) PAS, NSE (−)	t(8;21) + 8 del(5), del(7)	Ia, CD13, CD33 (+) CD14, CD11b (−)	
M3	Promyelocytes with prominent granules and Auer rods.	Peroxidase (+ +) Sudan Black (+ +) PAS, NSE (+/−)	t(15;17)	CD33, CD13 (+) Ia (−) CD11b (+/−)	DIC common
M4	Myelomonocytic blasts	Peroxidase (+) NSE (+), SE (+)*	t(4;11), t(9;11) + 8 del(5), del(7)	CD13, CD11b (+) Ia, CD14 (−)	Increased lysozyme
M4-eo	Myelomonocytic blasts >5% eosinophils	Esterase and PAS may be (+) in eosinophils	inv(16)		
M5 a	Undifferentiated monoblasts	Peroxidase (−) SE (−), NSE (+)	t(9;11) + 8 del(5), del(7)	CD13, CD11b (+) Ia, CD14 (−)	Increased lysozome
b	Differentiated monocytes	Peroxidase (−) SE (−), NSE (+)			
M6	Erythroblasts with dysplasia	PAS coarsely (+)	+ 8 del(5), del(7)	Glycophorin (+)	
M7	Pleomorphic megakaryoblasts	Platelet peroxidase (+) Peroxidase, Sudan Black (−) PAS, Esterase (+/−)		Factor VIII (+) Gp Ib, IIb/IIIa (+)**	Marrow fibrosis common

* NSE — Nonspecific esterase: α naphthyl acetate or α naphthyl butyrate esterase
SE — Specific esterase: naphthyl ASD chloracetate esterase
** Platelet glycoproteins

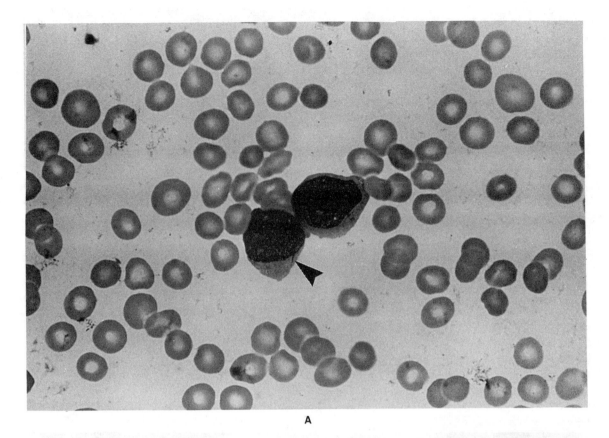

A

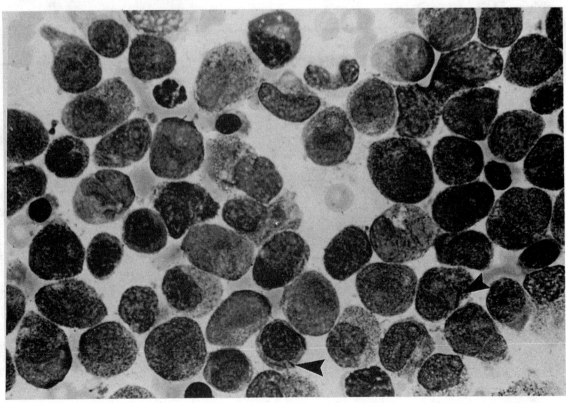

B

Fig. 30.1. A = M2 leukemia—myeloblasts with granules and Auer rods (1000x). B = M3 leukemia—promyelocytes with prominent granules and Auer rods (1000x).

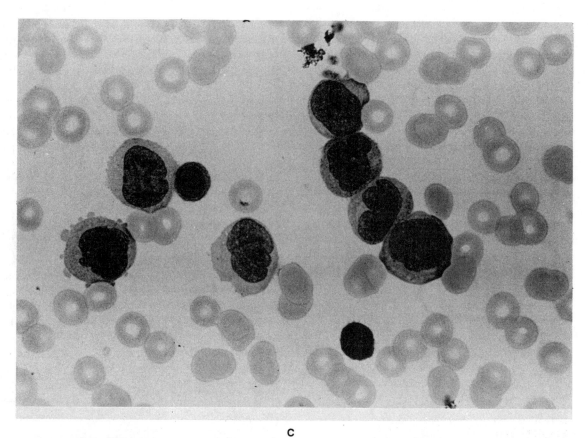

C

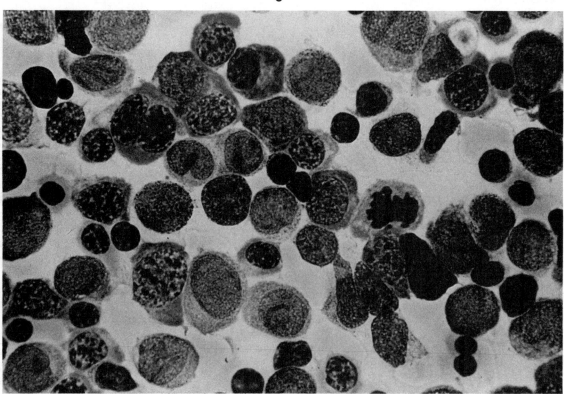

D

Fig. 30.1. C = M5 leukemia—monoblasts with folded nuclei (1000x). D = M6 leukemia—dysplastic erythroblasts with multiple nuclei (1000x).

M6 is also referred to as erythroleukemia or Di Guglielmo's disease syndrome. The presence of both erythroblasts (constituting 50% of nucleated cells) and myeloblasts (comprising greater than 30% of nonerythroid elements) is required to establish the diagnosis. Erythroid cells are dysplastic, and megalobloid often with multiple nuclei and distinctive gigantism, nuclear "pulverization," and fragmentation (fig. 30.1D).

The most recent addition to the FAB classification system is M7 or acute megakaryocytic leukemia (Bennett 1985b). Bone marrow fibrosis is characteristic of this disorder and the terms acute myelofibrosis or myelosclerosis are often used interchangeably with M7. Megakaryoblasts are undifferentiated and pleomorphic with one to three prominent nucleoli and occasional cytoplasmic blebbing. Megakaryocyte fragments and large, abnormal platelets can be found in the peripheral circulation. Because megakaryoblasts may be difficult to identify on a morphologic basis, electron microscopy (EM) and immunologic studies provide vital adjuncts to the diagnosis. The platelet peroxidase reaction (localized to the nuclear membrane and endoplasmic reticulum by EM) and monoclonal antibodies directed against the factor VIII antigen, and platelet glycoproteins Ib and IIb/IIIa, serve as helpful tools.

LABORATORY DATA

Some degree of anemia, thrombocytopenia, and neutropenia is uniform to all types of leukemia. Elevated WBC counts and circulating blasts are usually present, although with APL or early in the disease course of other leukemias, mild pancytopenia may be the only abnormality.

Multiple biochemical abnormalities occur in ANLL (O'Regan 1977). Both hyponatremia secondary to SIADH-like (Schwartz-Bartter) syndromes and hypernatremia due to diabetes insipidus have been reported. Hypercalcemia complicates up to 2.5% of all cases of leukemia, and is multifactorial in origin. Direct bony erosion by leukemic cells and PTH-like substances have been implicated, but, thus far, no osteoclast activating factor (OAF) has been identified in myeloblasts. Massive necrosis of malignant cells may develop during the initial phase of treatment for leukemia. This phenomenon, known as the tumor lysis syndrome, can lead to life-threatening metabolic derangements including hyperkalemia, hyperphosphatemia, hyperuricemia, hypomagnesemia, hypocalcemia, and acidosis. Prophylactic hydration with alkaline solutions is given to counteract these changes.

PROGNOSIS

ANLL is a highly lethal disease, with untreated median survival of only two months. Over the past two decades, advances in therapy and supportive care have improved the outlook. Remission induction rates now approach 75%, but 5-year disease-free survival remains disappointing, at 20% to 25%. Factors that carry a worse prognosis in ANLL include increased age, obesity, leukocytosis, leukostasis, renal insufficiency, or other complicating medical conditions. The pre-existence of a myelodysplastic syndrome portends a particularly poor outcome; only 20% to 40% of this group of patients achieve remission with standard induction therapy. Individuals with M3 leukemia and M4 with eosinophilia seem to enjoy more favorable long-term outcomes (Champlin 1987; Mertelsmann 1980). Generally, the prognosis for myelomonocytic, monocytic, erythroid, and megakaryocytic leukemias is worse than for M2 or M3 (Sultan 1981).

TREATMENT

Intensive chemotherapy is given in an attempt to eradicate the neoplastic clone. The two most effective agents used are cytosine arabinoside (Ara-C) and daunorubicin. The majority of studies show that once remission has been achieved (defined by <5% blasts in the bone marrow), additional consolidation or maintenance chemotherapy is required to further reduce leukemic cell burden and the incidence of relapse. Numerous trials have been conducted attempting to define an optimal regimen of treatment. Recent data favors the use of several short courses of intensive chemotherapy over prolonged administration of less myelosuppressive drugs (Sultan 1981).

Seventy-five percent of patients achieving remission will eventually relapse. Multiple agents have been used with varied success in attempt to reinduce remission, including repeated courses of daunorubicin, and Ara-C, mitoxantrone, amsacrine, 5-azacytidine, and etoposide. Overall, remission rates with any of these drugs is low (about 20%) and 5-year survival is less than 5% (Sultan 1981).

Allogeneic bone marrow transplantation (BMT) has been performed both in remission and during relapse of ANLL. The best results are obtained in young patients with HLA/MLC identical matches during first remission. Overall 2- to 5-year disease-free survival approaches 45% to 65%, a clear improvement over standard chemotherapy (fig. 30.2). For older patients, in whom toxicities are significant, and for individuals with relapsed disease, outcome with allogeneic bone marrow transplant is worse (Hurd 1987). Because the use of allogeneic BMT is limited by the patient's age and the availability of compatible donors, recent interest in autologous bone marrow transplantation has arisen. During this procedure, bone marrow is harvested when the disease is in remission, cryopreserved, then reinfused into the patient who has received ablative doses of chemotherapy or radiation therapy. As undetected leukemic cells may contaminate the marrow, a variety of chemotherapeutic and immunologic agents have been used to eradicate residual tumor cells. Bone marrow transplantation following marrow treatment with the drug 4-hydroperoxycyclophosphamide (4-HC) has yielded encouraging results. Patients with ANLL in second or third remission or those in first remission deemed to be at high risk achieved a 31% disease-free survival at a median of 21 months of follow-up (Santos 1989).

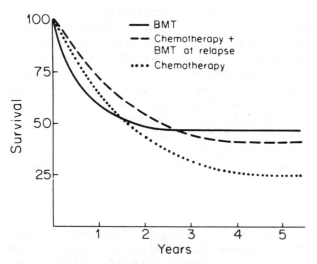

Fig. 30.2. Results of bone marrow transplantation and postremission chemotherapy for adult patients with AML. The dashed line indicates projected survival for patients initially receiving postremission chemotherapy with bone marrow transplantation as salvage therapy at the time of relapse. (Reprinted with permission from: Champlin [1987].)

Anticipated complications during treatment of ANLL are numerous. Infection is a major source of morbidity and mortality. Prolonged neutropenia, resulting from the leukemia itself or chemotherapy, renders patients susceptible to a variety of bacterial, viral, and/or fungal organisms. Most infections arise endogenously (from the patient's own bacterial flora), and frequent pathogens include gram-negative rods, particularly *Klebsiella, E. coli* and *Pseudomonas,* and the gram-positive organism *Staph epidermidis.* Immediate institution of antibiotic therapy in the setting of fever and neutropenia is mandatory, but the choice of agents, duration of treatment, and timing of empiric antifungal drugs remains controversial (Schiffer 1987). The use of granulocyte transfusions has been disappointing. Because of associated toxicity, this blood product is reserved for those patients with severe, culture-positive infection unresponsive to therapy, who are anticipated to recover from leukopenia (Strauss 1981). Prophylactic administration of oral antibiotics during neutropenic nadirs has been shown to reduce the incidence of severe infections, although not improve survival (Kapp 1987).

CNS involvement by leukemic cells, usually meningeal infiltration, occurs in 5% to 10% of patients with acute leukemia at some stage of the disease, most often at the time of bone marrow relapse. Cranial irradiation and intrathecal instillation of Ara-C and/or methotrexate are used to treat leukemic meningitis, although intravenous (as opposed to intrathecal) administration of high doses of Ara-C and methotrexate may be effective alternatives (Gale 1987). At this time, prophylactic treatment of the CNS in adults with ANLL is not recommended (Simone 1984).

Leukostasis occurs in ANLL or CML when blast counts exceed 100,000/mm^3. Alteration in mental status, respiratory distress, retinal hemorrhage, and priapism may occur and have been attributed to arteriolar plugging by large, nonpliable myeloblasts. Cranial irradiation, high doses of rapidly cytolytic drugs, and/or leukopheresis are instituted as emergent therapies.

Serious hemorrhagic and, less frequently, thrombotic, complications may arise from DIC in promyelocytic leukemia. Heparin is effective in controlling this bleeding diathesis; however, there is evidence that intensive blood product support with red cells, fresh frozen plasma, and platelets may suffice (Goldberg 1987).

CHRONIC MYELOGENOUS LEUKEMIA

The earliest description of chronic myelogenous leukemia (CML) has been credited to Virchow (1845), Craigie (1845), and Bennett (1845). Craigie's report perhaps best illustrates the cardinal features of this disease: "listlessness, . . . swelling and hardness in the left epigastric region . . . perspiration at night . . . blood vessels filled with grumus and clots containing lymph or purulent matter." Indeed, CML is characterized by profound myeloid hyperplasia, splenomegaly, and eventual evolution to acute leukemia (called blast crisis). It has gained additional attention as the first human disorder associated with a consistent cytogenetic abnormality, the Philadelphia (Ph) chromosome. Studies of isoenzymes in women with CML, heterozygous for glucose-6-phosphate dehydrogenase (G6PD), as well as cytogenetic analysis of leukemic cells, have afforded unequivocal evidence that CML is a clonal disorder, arising from neoplastic transformation of a single pluripotent hematopoietic stem cell. Landmark studies performed by Fialkow in the 1960s revealed that erythroid and granulocytic cells derived from CML patients heterozygous for G6PD, expressed only one isoenzyme (Fialkow 1967). Additionally, red cells, granulocytes, monocytes, megakaryocytes, macrophages, and some B-lymphocytes from leukemic patients are, characteristically, Ph chromosome-positive, underlining the fact that they share a common neoplastic progenitor. Whether T-lymphocytes may also be derived from the malignant clone remains uncertain, as the Ph chromosome and monoclonal expression of G6PD isoenzymes have not been consistently demonstrated in this cell type. The occasional finding of T-lymphocyte blast crisis, however, suggests their involvement in this disease (Draezen 1988). Fibroblasts and other stromal cells are not part of the leukemic, Ph chromosome-positive clone.

CML is a chronic myeloproliferative disorder characterized by excessive growth and expansion of differentiated cells. The granulocytes and erythrocytes in patients with CML require the addition of growth factors to proliferate *in vitro,* suggesting partial retention of normal regulatory mechanisms in this disease (Metcalf 1974). This phenomenon is in contrast to the generally uncontrolled, autonomous growth of undifferentiated cells seen in the acute leukemias.

INCIDENCE AND EPIDEMIOLOGY

CML comprises approximately 0.4% of all cases of cancer in the United States and about 20% of all cases of leukemia in Western countries with an incidence of 1 per 100,000 new cases per year (Koeffler 1981; Spiers 1984). Peak age of onset is 50 to 60 years, although cases of CML have been reported in childhood. There is no sex predominance.

ETIOLOGY

The etiology of CML remains unknown. Both benzene exposure and high doses of radiation have been linked to its development. CML comprised approximately 20% of leukemias occurring in spondylitic patients treated with low-dose radiation in Great Britain and one-third of cases occurring in Japanese atomic-bomb survivors (Court Brown 1955; Moloney 1987). No other environmental or genetic factors, however, have been clearly implicated as causal in this disease. The hallmark finding of the Philadelphia chromosome in 95% of CML cases has led to much speculation and interest as to its possible etiologic role in this disorder. Originally described by Nowell and Hungerford (1960) as a "minute chromosome" subsequent investigations have shown that this cytogenetic abnormality represents reciprocal translocation of genetic material (fig. 30.3) between chromosome 22 and chromosome 9 (t9;22) (q34.1;q11.21).

It has been discovered that two oncogenes are involved in the formation of the Ph¹ chromosome. The

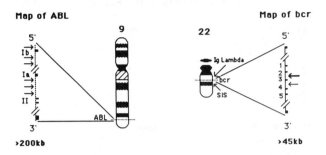

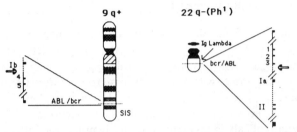

Fig. 30.4. Molecular analysis of the chromosome translocation in CML. A partial map of the *ABL* proto-oncogene on chromosome 9 (dashed line) and *bcr* on chromosome 22 (solid line). The exons are indicated by small black squares. The arrows in the upper portion of the figure indicate translocation breakpoints; those in *bcr* tend to cluster between exons 2 and 3 (heavy arrow), whereas those in *ABL* occur anywhere within the 200 kb intron that is 5' of exon II. The genetic consequences of one translocation are shown in the lower portion. *ABL* distal to exon Ib is translocated to the Ph¹ chromosome, whereas *bcr* distal to exon 3 is translocated to the 9q+ chromosome, resulting in fusion genes on both translocation partners. (Reprinted with permission from: Rowley [1988].)

oncogene c-*abl* is translocated from chromosome 9 to 22 while C-*sis*, found on chromosome 22, can be reciprocally translocated to chromosome 9 or to a variety of other chromosomes (Silver 1986). Breakpoints on chromosome 9 occur at a variable distance from the C-*abl* gene, whereas the breakpoint on chromosome 22 occurs within a narrow 5.8-kilobase-pair region (fig. 30.4) named the "breakpoint cluster region" (bcr). There is increasing evidence that even Ph chromosome-negative cases of CML will show evidence of *bcr-abl* gene fusion, when examined at a molecular level, making this rearrangement a possible *sine qua non* of the disorder (Weidemann 1988). A novel 8-kilobase mRNA has been identified and shown to represent the transcript of the chimeric gene created between *bcr* and C-*abl*. The role of the *bcr-abl* related protein, a 210 kd tyrosine kinase, and its possible relationship to the etiology of CML remains the focus of intense ongoing study (Weidemann 1988; Groffen 1984; Rowley 1988).

CLINICAL CHARACTERISTICS AND STAGING

CML is divided into three stages: chronic or stable phase, accelerated phase, and acute phase or blast crisis (table 30.3). Early in the course of the disease, clinical symptoms are mild and nonspecific. Complaints include

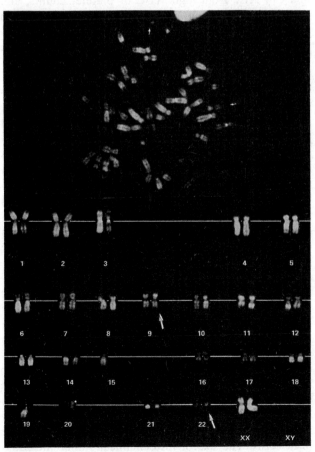

Fig. 30.3. Typical karyotype demonstrating t(9;22) found in CML.

Table 30.3
CLINICAL AND LABORATORY FEATURES OF CML DURING 3 PHASES OF THE DISEASE

PHASE	STABLE	ACCELERATED	BLAST CRISIS
Symptoms*	None/minimal	Moderate	Pronounced
Splenomegaly	Mild	May increase	May be marked
WBC	Elevated	Erratic	High or low
Hct	Normal	May decrease	Low
Platelets	High/normal	Erratic	Low
Differential	<1% to 2% blasts spectrum WBC	Increasing basophils and immaturity**	Circulating blasts Often >25%
LAP score	Low	May increase	Normal
Bone marrow	<10% immature	Increased immaturity	>30% blasts
Cytogenetics	Ph^1 (+)	Ph^1 (+), addt'l abn	Ph^1 (+), addt'l abn
Median survival	3 to 4 years	6 to 24 months	2 to 4 months

*Fever, bony pain, night sweats, fatigue, weight loss
**Promyelocytes and myeloblasts

malaise, fatigue, decreased exercise tolerance, weight loss, low-grade fever, night sweats, early satiety, left upper quadrant discomfort or fullness, and bony pain. Bleeding and easy bruising may arise from dysfunctional platelets, even if counts are normal or high. Splenomegaly is noted in 50% of patients at diagnosis, while hepatomegaly is less common and lymphadenopathy is rare. The simple finding of abnormal blood counts on routine testing frequently leads to the diagnosis of CML in chronic phase. Within an average of three to four years, most patients undergo transformation to blast crisis, often heralded by an accelerated phase. During the accelerated phase, fever, bony pain, and weight loss become more prominent. Erratic fluctuations in white blood cell (WBC) and platelet counts, increasing basophilia, rising leukocyte alkaline phosphatase (LAP) score, greater marrow immaturity, and additional cytogenetic abnormalities may also accompany acceleration of the disease.

Blast crisis represents evolution to acute leukemia. Two forms of blast crisis are generally seen: myeloid in two-thirds of cases and lymphoid in fewer than one-third. Rarely, acute erythrocytic or megakaryocytic leukemias occur (Rosenthal 1977b; Bain 1977). Constitutional symptoms are pronounced during this period, and splenomegaly may increase dramatically. Isolated foci of leukemic cells, known as myeloblastomas, granulocytic sarcomas, or chloromas, can involve skin, lymph nodes, bones, and/or the CNS. If very high blast counts are present (i.e., >100,000/mm³), symptoms of leukostasis including cerebral dysfunction and pulmonary compromise may occur. Papilledema, retinal hemorrhage, and priapism have also been reported. The prognosis for blast crisis is very poor, worse than for *de novo* forms of AML or ALL. A small percentage of patients with CML will convert to a myelofibrotic phase characterized by pancytopenia, massive splenomegaly, and extramedullary hematopoiesis (Moloney 1978).

LABORATORY FEATURES

The most characteristic laboratory finding at presentation is an elevated WBC count encompassing a full spectrum of circulating early myeloid precursors. A normal hematocrit or mild anemia is usual, and one-third of patients will develop thrombocytosis. A typical peripheral smear in stable phase CML will reveal orderly progression of WBC from myeloblasts (comprising less than 1% to 2% of cells), to mature neutrophils (fig. 30.5). Circulating nucleated red blood cells, large platelets, or megakaryocyte fragments may also be found. Basophilia and eosinophilia are common. WBC and platelet counts may fluctuate in 30- to 60-day cycles, a feature important to remember in assessing responsiveness to therapy (Chikkappa 1976; Vodopick 1972).

Abnormalities of serum chemistries include elevated uric acid and lactic dehydrogenase. Pseudohyperkalemia can arise from high WBC or platelet counts, and may be diagnosed by checking plasma (rather than serum) potassium values. As with other myeloproliferative disorders, vitamin B_{12} and B_{12} binding capacity are elevated, probably due to increased production of transcobalamin I by mature granulocytes.

The finding of a low leukocyte alkaline phosphatase (LAP) score is unique in CML, distinguishing this disease from other myeloproliferative disorders and leukemoid reactions. The LAP score is determined by rating peripheral blood neutrophils for intensity of staining after treatment with alkaline phosphatase. In CML, as well as in paroxysmal nocturnal hemoglobinuria and hypophosphatemia, this histochemical analysis will be abnormally low. As CML evolves into an accelerated phase, or blast crisis, or when associated with ongoing infection, the LAP score may become normal.

Morphological examination of the bone marrow usually adds little to the evaluation of CML, as the diagnosis is suggested by review of the peripheral blood smear in conjunction with physical findings and laboratory data. Typically, the bone marrow is hypercellular with marked increase in the myeloid-to-erythroid (M:E) ratio. In the chronic phase, myeloblasts and promyelocytes comprise less than 10% of the differential, but as the disease progresses, the proportion of immature cells increases. When blasts comprise greater than 30% of nucleated cells, acute leukemia has evolved. It may be difficult to distinguish myeloid from lymphoid blast crisis. The use of histochemical stains, including terminal deoxynucleotidyl transferase (TdT), and

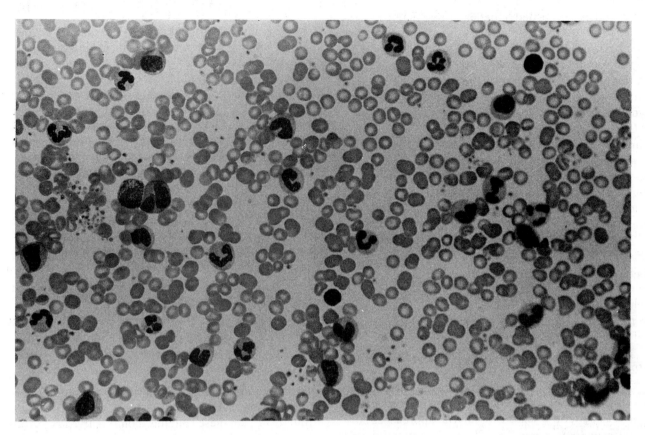

Fig. 30.5. Blood smear in CML with orderly progression of WBC maturation (40x).

immunologic markers such as the common acute lymphocytic leukemia antigen (CALLA), help define lymphoid leukemic conversion. An unusual feature of the bone marrow of some CML patients is the presence of pseudogaucher cells, which represent the collection of excess glucocerebroside within macrophages. They are morphologically indistinguishable from the cells found in the congenital disorder, Gaucher's disease. Additional bone marrow findings in CML include increased numbers of dysplastic and clustered megakaryocytes. Fibrosis may develop later in the course of the disease and is detected by distortion of bone marrow architecture and increased reticulin staining.

PROGNOSIS

The overall prognosis of CML is poor, although with bone marrow transplantation a percentage of patients are cured. The median survival is three to four years, with less than 30% of patients living five years after diagnosis. Overall, the risk of leukemic conversion approaches 10% per year, and thus, a small subset of patients may achieve prolonged survival. With the onset of accelerated phase, and blast crisis, life expectancy decreases to six to 24 months and two to four months, respectively (Champlin 1985). The lymphoid variant of blast crisis carries a somewhat better prognosis; 60% of patients attain transient remissions prolonging survival to six to eight months (Rosenthal 1977a).

TREATMENT

Therapy in chronic phase is generally palliative, directed simply at the control of WBC and platelet count. The most commonly used agents, hydroxyurea and busulfan, are both effective in this regard. However, they do not eliminate the neoplastic clone, as Ph chromosome-positive cells persist. There have been rare reports of the disappearance of the Ph chromosome after unintentional overdoses of busulfan, but this is not the rule with standard treatment. Hydroxyurea given at doses of 0.5 g to 2.0 g per day is usually preferable to busulfan because of the latter's toxicities, including pulmonary fibrosis, an Addisonian-like syndrome, xerostomia, and, rarely, bone marrow hypoplasia. Hydroxyurea, unlike busulfan, must be used in compliant patients who are able to take daily medication and have blood counts monitored frequently. Before the introduction of busulfan in the 1950s, splenic irradiation constituted first-line therapy in CML. Rarely, it is still used to control hypersplenism or painful splenomegaly. Splenectomy has not been shown to prolong survival or delay onset of blast crisis (Wolf 1978). High-dose intensive chemotherapy in the chronic phase offers, at best, transient disappearance of the Philadelphia clone and does not afford improved chance of cure (Clarkson 1985). Recently, alpha interferon has been evaluated in the treatment of CML. This biologic response modifier induces hematologic remissions in up to 80% of cases, and, in 56% of these, the number of Ph-chromosome metaphases is reduced (Talpaz 1988). Further long-term studies are needed to define its role in this disease.

Once blast crisis has evolved, cure or re-establishment of chronic phase is unlikely. Aggressive regimens including anthracyclines and Ara-C have been used during myelogenous blast crisis, with significant morbidity and remission rates of only 10% to 20%. The lymphoid variant is more responsive to therapy. As in ALL, treatment with vincristine and steroids alone or in conjunction with other chemotherapy, induces transient remissions in approximately 60% of cases. Intensive chemotherapy followed by autologous infusion of chronic phase cryopreserved peripheral blood or bone marrow has likewise proved disappointing in the treatment of acute phase CML (Goldman 1982).

An unexpected improvement in the peripheral counts of a patient with CML treated with mithramycin for hypercalcemia led to investigation of its use in blast crisis (Koller 1986). Patients with myeloid leukemia may achieve a return to chronic phase when treated with mithramycin and hydroxyurea, but this finding has not yet been widely reproduced (Koller 1986).

To date, allogeneic bone marrow transplantation offers the only potential cure for CML. Recent experience has shown that transplant is most successful and least toxic when undertaken in young patients in chronic phase. Long-term disease-free survival approaches 50% to 60% in these cases (fig. 30.6). Transplant-related complications, including graft vs. host disease, leukemic relapse, and interstitial pneumonitis, pose significant risks; the decision of who should undergo transplant and at what stage of their disease remains unsettled. Most authorities favor transplantation early in chronic phase for those patients under age 40 with a full HLA/MLC matched sibling donor, while some centers perform transplantation up to age 55 (Thomas 1986; O'Reilly 1983; Thomas 1989).

ACUTE LYMPHOBLASTIC LEUKEMIA

Acute lymphoblastic leukemia (ALL) comprises 90% of childhood leukemia but is uncommon in adults. It is a heterogenous disorder, whose classification rests on both morphologic and immunologic criteria (Champlin 1989). Remission rates of 60% to 80% and long-term survival of 40% have been achieved in adults, rendering ALL the most curable form of leukemia (Hoelzer 1987). Intensive chemotherapy and CNS prophylaxis are largely responsible for improved outcome, and bone marrow transplantation affords additional chance of cure for patients with relapsed disease. Prognostic factors that identify high-risk groups in ALL may allow further tailoring of therapy and increased survival (Clarkson 1985; Canellos 1984).

INCIDENCE AND EPIDEMIOLOGY

ALL comprises 20% of leukemia in adults. A slight male predominance has been identified, and, in the United States, whites are more frequently affected than blacks (Pendergrass 1985).

ETIOLOGY

Radiation exposure has been linked with the development of ALL, though the association has only been found in Japanese atomic bomb survivors. Ataxia telangiectasia has one of the best-documented propensities for leukemic evolution, but other congenital diseases such as Down's syndrome and Fanconi's anemia likewise predispose to this neoplasm (Toledano 1980). Concurrent development of leukemia in monozygotic twins approaches 20%, usually within months of one another (Miller 1968). The role of cytogenetic abnormalities and possible involvement of oncogenes in the pathophysiology of this disease are areas of ongoing investigation. The t(8;14) translocation, also seen in

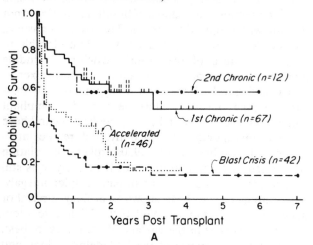

A

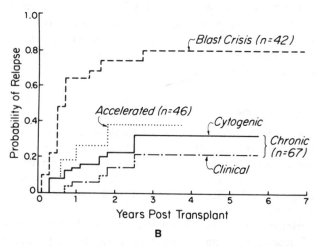

B

Fig. 30.6. A = Kaplan-Meier product limit estimates for survival after marrow transplantation for patients given allogeneic grafts in the first chronic phase (solid line), second chronic phase (broken line with dots), accelerated phase (dotted line), or blastic phase (broken line). The tick marks and solid circles indicate surviving patients. B = Kaplan-Meier product limit estimates for probability of relapse after allogeneic marrow grafting for patients transplanted in blastic phase (broken line) or accelerated phase (dotted line). The probability of relapse for patients transplanted in first chronic phase is shown as cytogenetic relapse (solid line), or clinical relapse (broken and dotted line). (Reprinted with permission from: Thomas [1986].)

Burkitt's lymphoma, is of particular interest. In these cases, the oncogene *c-myc* has been shown to be translocated from chromosome 8 to chromosome 14 where it is strategically positioned adjacent to the immunoglobulin heavy-chain locus. How this phenomenon relates to the development and progression of disease in Burkitt's lymphoma and ALL remains to be determined (Look 1985).

CLINICAL CHARACTERISTICS

Presentation is generally abrupt with symptoms of malaise, fatigue, bony pain (especially sternal), sweats, bleeding, and easy bruisability. Headache and/or cranial neuropathies imply CNS involvement, seen in a high proportion of patients with the T-cell subtype but also observed in the other common variants.

Physical findings include pallor, petechiae, and ecchymoses. Lymphadenopathy, splenomegaly, and hepatomegaly may be noted but are usually mild. The presence of a mediastinal mass typifies the T-cell subtype of ALL, while bulky abdominal adenopathy similarly characterizes the L3 or Burkitt's-like subgroup.

CLASSIFICATION

ALL is classified both on a morphologic and immunologic basis. The FAB system divides this disease into three groups: L1, L2, and L3 (Bennett 1976; 1981). L1, seen most frequently in childhood, is characterized by small, homogenous lymphoblasts with scant cytoplasm and regular nuclei. Nucleoli are not prominent; cytoplasmic vacuolization may be present (fig. 30.7A). In the most common form of adult ALL, L2, the lymphoblasts appear larger and more heterogenous. Nuclei are irregular; they contain one or more indistinct nucleoli; and the cytoplasm is more abundant (fig. 30.7B). Large lymphoblasts with deeply basophilic and vacuolated cytoplasm typify the L3 subgroup. Nucleoli are prominent (fig. 30.7C). This group is morphologically similar to the cells of Burkitt's lymphoma.

Myeloid and lymphoid leukemias may, on occasion, be difficult to differentiate; histochemistry has proven very useful in making the distinction. Myeloperoxidase and Sudan Black stains, positive in most myeloblasts, will not label lymphoblasts. Coarse PAS staining occurs in 75% of cases of ALL, while acid phosphatase reactivity localized to the Golgi distinguishes some of the T-cell variants. The most useful marker of lymphoblasts is terminal deoxynucleotidyl transferase (TdT), an intracytoplasmic protein normally found in early lymphocytes of the thymus and bone marrow. Over 80% of lymphoblasts will be TdT positive (Bollum 1979).

Immunologic techniques have been used to further classify cell lineage in ALL (Foon 1980; Foon 1986; Schroff 1982). Four major subtypes have been defined. Most easily identified are T-cell ALL (CD2+, CD5+, CD7+) and B-cell ALL (smIg+, CD20+) which make up 15% to 20% and 2% to 7% of cases, respectively. The remaining 75% to 80% of lymphoblasts whose surfaces mark neither as T nor B cells, were initially labelled *nonT-nonB* or *null* cells. With the advent of molecular genetic techniques, however, immunoglobulin gene rearrangements, characteristic of primitive B cells, have been identified in virtually all of these cases (Korsmeyer 1983). Cytoplasmic (as opposed to surface) immunoglobulin may also be detected or induced by maturation agents in some cells. Thus the terms null cell or nonT-nonB cell ALL have been largely replaced by *pre-* or *early pre-B cell* ALL. The glycoprotein common acute lymphoblastic antigen (CALLA) identifies an important subset of patients with ALL. This so-called common or CALLA (+) type constitutes about one-half of adult forms of leukemia and carries a somewhat better prognosis.

Correlation between morphologic and immunologic subtypes in ALL is not always possible (table 30.4). Furthermore, lineage infidelity, the expression by malignant cells of both myeloid and lymphoid surface markers, may occur in up to one-third of cases of adult ALL and gives rise to so-called biphenotypic or hybrid leukemias (Champlin 1989). A small number will remain unclassifiable by all diagnostic methods available, and may be referred to as undifferentiated leukemia.

LABORATORY DATA

As with other forms of leukemia, pancytopenia develops secondary to marrow replacement by tumor. Two-thirds of patients present with elevated WBC counts, at times greater than 100,000/mm³, and blasts are frequently found in the circulation. Elevated lactic dehydrogenase and uric acid correlate with large tumor burden. More than one-half of cases demonstrate cytogenetic abnormalities; t(9;22), t(4;11), t(8;14) carry an unfavorable prognosis (Bloomfield 1981; Bloomfield 1986). The Philadelphia (Ph) chromosome, t(9;22), is the most common abnormality in adult ALL, found in 17% to 25% of cases. Breakpoints on chromosome 22 may occur outside the usual *bcr* region and new distinct *bcr-abl* hybrid gene products have been reported (Klein 1986).

PROGNOSIS

Life expectancy has improved in ALL, with overall 5-year disease-free survival approaching 35% to 45%.

Multiple large series have identified factors which adversely affect outcome (table 30.5): male gender, older age, elevated WBC count at diagnosis (usually defined as >15-30,000/mm³), prolonged induction (>4 weeks), L3 cell type, B-cell and CALLA (−) phenotypes, and the t(9;22), t(8;14), and t(4;11) translocations (Hoelzer 1988; Baccarani 1982). Splenomegaly, high numbers of circulating blasts, thrombocytopenia, and CNS or mediastinal involvement are also reported to reduce rate or duration of remission (Jacobs 1984). While prolonged survival for standard risk groups reaches 60% to 70%, it drops to 20% to 25% for patients with unfavorable disease characteristics.

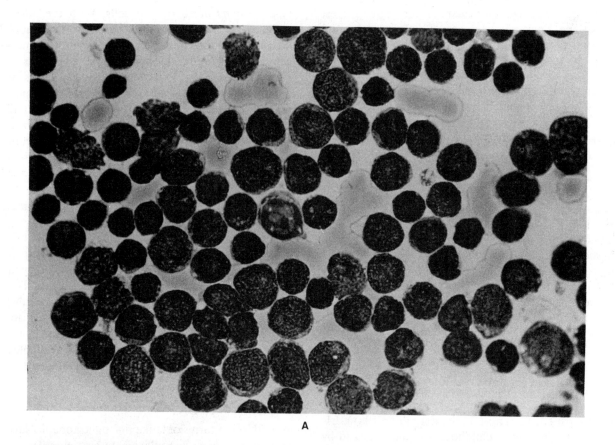

A

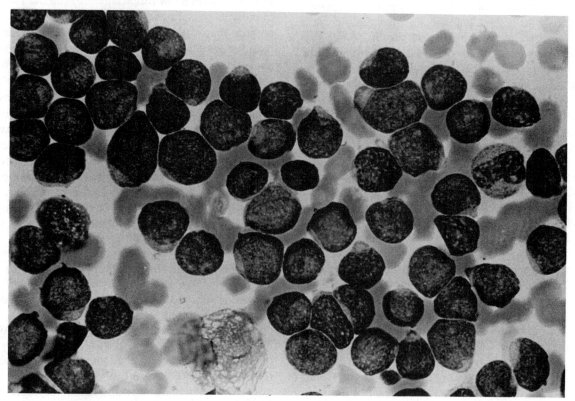

B

Fig. 30.7. A = L1 — small homogenous lymphoblasts with scant cytoplasm (1000x). B = L2 — larger lymphoblasts with irregular nuclei, and nucleoli (1000x).

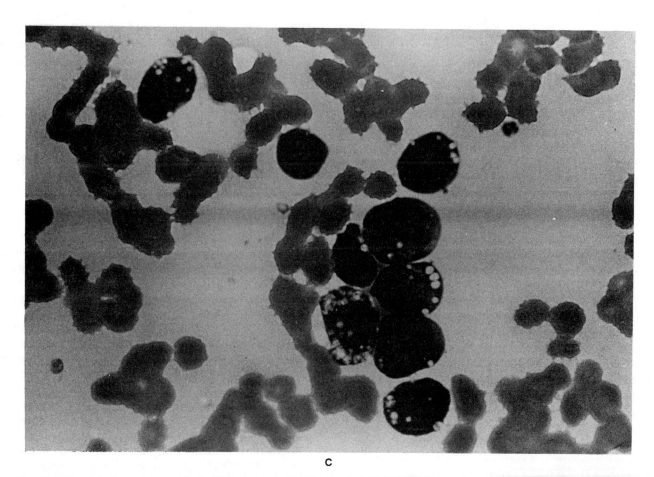

C

Fig. 30.7. C = L3—large lymphoblast with prominent vacuoles and nucleoli (1000x).

TREATMENT

Treatment programs for adult ALL are fashioned upon regimens used in childhood, which achieve remission rates of greater than 90%. Aggressive multidrug regimens, which include anthracyclines, vincristine, corticosteroids, cyclophosphamide, asparaginase, methotrexate, and 6-mercaptopurine, have been used in various combinations. Therapy consists of two stages: induction, designed to reduce leukemic burden to undetectable levels; and consolidation or maintenance, directed at the eradication of residual tumor and prevention of relapse. Remission rates of 60% to 90% and 5-year disease-free survival of 35% to 45% have been reported in large series (Schauer

1983; Barnett 1986; Linker 1987). In contrast to ANNL, where six months or less of postremission chemotherapy appears adequate, two to two- and-one-half years of treatment is the rule in ALL.

The incidence of CNS involvement in adults appears lower than in children. T-cell phenotype, L3 morphology, and high WBC count at presentation predispose to meningeal disease, which occurs in approximately 10% of patients at diagnosis. Prophylactic treatment with cranial irradiation and intrathecal chemotherapy (cytosine arabinoside, methotrexate, and/or dexamethasone) reduces the rate of CNS relapse but does not affect duration of remission or overall survival (Omura 1980).

Table 30.4
CLASSIFICATION OF ACUTE LYMPHOBLASTIC LEUKEMIA IN ADULTS

SUBTYPE	CLINICAL FEATURES	SURFACE MARKERS	MORPHOLOGY
T-cell (15% to 20%)	Mediastinal mass CNS involvement Poor prognosis	CD2 (Leu 5) (+) CD7 (Leu 9) (+) CD5 (Leu 1) (+)	L1, L2
Pre-B-cell (75% to 80%)		Ia (HLA-DR) (+) 100% CD19 (B4) (+) 95% CALLA (CD10) (+) 75% CD20 (B1) (+) 50% Cytoplasmic μ chain (+) 15%	L1, L2
B-cell (2% to 7%)	Abdominal masses CNS involvement Poor prognosis	Surface membrane Ig (smIg) CD20 (+) CD19 (+) Ia (+)	L3

Table 30.5
POOR PROGNOSIS IN ALL

Male sex
Age >9 years, or <2 years
WBC >15,000-30,000/mm³
Induction of remission >4 weeks from treatment
Phenotype: L3 morphology, B-cell, CALLA (−)
Chromosome: t(9;22), t(8;14), and/or t(4;11)

Fifty percent of adults with ALL will relapse and approximately one-half of these patients will attain a second remission, with standard agents. Allogeneic bone marrow transplantation was initially performed only in cases of resistant or multiple-relapsed leukemia, with long-term survival of 10% to 20%. Transplantation is now done earlier in the disease course and is generally felt to be the treatment of choice for patients in second remission where 2- to 4-year disease-free survival is 30% to 40% (Champlin 1989). Its role in first remission or for high-risk groups remains unresolved, awaiting large randomized trials (Nesbit 1985; Champlin 1987).

Autologous bone marrow transplant offers an alternative for older patients or for those without identical HLA matches. Leukemic relapse constitutes a major complication of this procedure and, consequently, various techniques designed to eliminate residual (subclinical) leukemic cells have been devised. Monoclonal antibodies directed at CALLA, as well as other B-cell antigens, have been used with limited success in adults (Ramsay 1985).

CHRONIC LYMPHOCYTIC LEUKEMIA

Chronic lymphocytic leukemia (CLL) is an indolent lymphoproliferative disorder characterized by lymphocytosis, lymphadenopathy, and splenomegaly. It has been described by Dameshek (1967) as an "accumulation of immunologically incompetent lymphocytes." In 95% of cases, CLL is a B-cell disorder; T-cell CLL represents a somewhat different disease with unique clinical and laboratory features. B-cell CLL has a variable course and prognosis, depending on the stage of the disease. Associated autoimmune phenomena (hemolytic anemia and thrombocytopenia), hypogammaglobulinemia, and other forms of B- and T-cell dysfunction highlight the underlying derangement of immune regulation in CLL.

INCIDENCE AND EPIDEMIOLOGY

CLL constitutes approximately 0.8% of all cancers and one-quarter of all leukemias, with an incidence of 2.7 per 100,000 in the United States. CLL occurs more frequently in men and in the elderly; 90% of cases affect persons older than 50 (Williams 1983).

ETIOLOGY

As with other forms of leukemia, the etiology of CLL remains unknown. It is the only form of leukemia not associated with radiation exposure, and neither drugs nor chemicals have been causally implicated. There appears to be a strong familial tendency, with some studies reporting up to a 16-fold increased incidence in relatives of CLL patients (Videback 1947). CLL is seen in the setting of various immunodeficiency states (e.g., Wiskott-Aldrich Syndrome, ataxia telangiectasia, and chronic immunosuppression following organ transplant), raising the possibility of immune dysregulation as etiologic in this disease. Numerous abnormalities in T-cell and B-cell function characterize CLL, but it is unclear whether they represent secondary phenomena or set the stage for evolution to leukemia (Kay 1986).

CLINICAL CHARACTERISTICS AND STAGING

Patients with CLL frequently present incidentally with the finding of an elevated, and otherwise unexplained, absolute lymphocyte count (>15,000/mm³). Fatigue, weight loss, shortness of breath, night sweats, and bleeding reflect more advanced disease. An exaggerated, but rarely fatal, response to insect bites (particularly that of mosquitoes) remains unexplained. Hypogammaglobulinemia is a major complication of CLL and leads to repeated infections. The incidence of herpes zoster approaches 20%, and diseases caused by bacteria (particularly pyogenic organisms) and fungi are also common.

A subset of 3% to 10% of patients with CLL develop a fulminant form of large cell lymphoma, a phenomenon first described by Richter in 1928. Fever, rapidly evolving lymphadenopathy, weight loss, and abdominal pain herald conversion to this high-grade lymphoma, and involvement of liver, bone, gastrointestinal tract, and other extranodal sites is not uncommon. Prognosis is poor; few patients respond to aggressive therapy (Trump 1980).

Lymphadenopathy and splenomegaly are present in approximately 75% of patients at diagnosis; hepatomegaly and skin infiltration are seen less frequently.

Used to establish prognosis and indications for therapy, staging in CLL combines physical findings with laboratory abnormalities. The Rai system (table 30.6), introduced in 1975, determines stage by the presence of adenopathy, splenomegaly, anemia, and thrombocytopenia (Rai 1975). Based on the finding that anemia and thrombocytopenia are the most important risk factors in CLL, Binet et al. (table 30.7) proposed a simplified schema. (Binet 1981a). This system was adopted by the international workshop on CLL and is now used in conjunction with the Rai classification: A (O, I or II), B (I or II), and C (III or IV) (Binet 1981b).

LABORATORY FEATURES

The hallmark finding in CLL is an unexplained absolute lymphocytosis (>15,000/mm³). When uncontrolled, lymphocyte counts as high as 1,000,000/mm³ have been recorded. Review of the peripheral smear shows mature and well-differentiated lymphocytes and characteristic smudge cells (fig. 30.8). Surface-marker phenotyping defines the lymphocytes as mature B-cells in 95% of cases. Low-intensity, monoclonal immunoglobulin is

Table 30.6
RAI STAGING OF CLL

STAGE	FINDINGS	SURVIVAL*
0	Lymphocytosis alone **	>150
I	Lymphocytosis and adenopathy	101
II	Lymphocytosis with splenomegaly and/or hepatomegaly	71
III	Lymphocytosis with anemia (Hb <11 g/dL)***	19
IV	Lymphocytosis with thrombocytopenia (plt <100,000/mm)***	19

*Median survival from diagnosis in months
**Peripheral blood >15,000/mm^3, bone marrow >40%
***May occur on a hypoproliferative or immune basis

found on the cell surface, with IgM alone being most frequent and IgM with IgD, IgG, or IgA seen less commonly. The presence of a single light chain, kappa or lambda, in the lymphocyte population confirms the monoclonal origin of CLL. Such studies can help establish the diagnosis of CLL even when there is only minimal lymphocytosis. The B-cell antigens CD20 (B1,Leu16) and CD21 (C3d receptor, B2) mark virtually all cells. The T-cell antigen CD5 (Leu1,T1) present on less than 5% of normal B-cells, is a unique finding on the CLL B-cell.

Anemia and thrombocytopenia are noted in 35% and 25% of cases at diagnosis, respectively, and may result from marrow replacement by lymphocytes or autoimmune destruction. Approximately 20% of patients with CLL develop a positive Coomb's (antiglobulin) test, but only one-half of these evolve a hemolytic process. (Rozman 1984). Immune thrombocytopenia is also seen although it occurs less frequently than autoimmune hemolytic anemia.

Elevated levels of serum uric acid and lactic dehydrogenase, characteristic of rapid tumor growth, are not typical of CLL. Hypogammaglobulinemia is notable in one-half of patients, while monoclonal gammopathies, IgG or IgM, occur in 10% of cases without relation to absolute globulin concentration.

The bone marrow is always involved in CLL. Four patterns of lymphocytic infiltration have been identified and touted to be of prognostic significance: diffuse replacement suggests worse outcome than nodular patterns. The role of bone marrow examination in addition to clinical staging remains unsettled (Montserrat 1987; Rozman 1984; Han 1984a). One-half of patients have chromosomal abnormalities; trisomy 12 is the most common and early finding. Additional cytogenetic derangements characterize more advanced disease and portend a worse prognosis (Han 1984b). When performed, lymph node biopsies demonstrate a morphologic pattern indistinguishable from well-differentiated lymphocytic lymphoma.

PROGNOSIS

The prognosis of CLL is variable. Early stage patients have a median survival of 10 to 12.5 years, whereas, for patients with advanced disease, survival may be as short as 19 to 24 months (Binet 1986). In an analysis of 41 clinical and laboratory features other than those involved in clinical staging, weight loss, performance status, degree of leukocytosis, elevated LDH, uric acid, and alkaline phosphatase were shown to be among important adverse predictors of outcome. This is perhaps because they reflect increased tumor burden. Hypogammaglobulinemia does not seem to affect overall prognosis (Lee 1987).

TREATMENT

There is still some controversy over optimal treatment for the various stages of CLL. It is generally agreed that patients with early disease do not benefit from therapy. As symptoms, anemia, or thrombocytopenia develop, treatment with single-agent alkylating drugs with or without corticosteroids is initiated. Chlorambucil has become the agent of choice, and, while prednisone seems to increase its efficacy, a paradoxical transient elevation of WBC counts can occur. Remissions are achieved in 70% of cases, enabling patients to remain off any medication for a period of time. Advanced stages of CLL often require more intensive chemotherapy. Cyclophosphamide, vincristine, and prednisone (CVP) constitute effective second-line management. A cooperative group study evaluated response of patients with CLL to a variety of therapeutic regimens. No significant differences in survival were found between chlorambucil and observation in stage A, or between chlorambucil and CVP in stage B. On the other hand, patients with stage C disease experienced an improved 2-year survival (44% vs. 77%) when Adriamycin was added to CVP (Binet 1986). Fludarabine may be a promising

Table 30.7
INTERNATIONAL STAGING OF CLL

STAGE	FINDINGS
A	Lymphocytosis alone with enlargement of less than 3 lymph node groups*
B	Lymphocytosis with enlargement of 3 or more lymph node groups
C	Lymphocytosis with presence of anemia (Hb <10 g/dL) or thrombocytopenia (plt <100,000/mm^3), regardless of number of enlarged lymph node groups

*Lymph node group is defined by axillary, cervical, or inguinal adenopathy, whether it occurs bilaterally or unilaterally. Enlargement of liver and spleen is also counted as a separate lymph node group.

agent for patients with advanced CLL, especially those who have failed prior therapy (Keating 1989).

Biologic response modifiers such as monoclonal antibodies and interferon have been tested but have not proved to be effective therapy (Foon 1986; O'Connell 1986). Ongoing studies may yet define a role for these agents in CLL.

Total body irradiation (TBI) has not shown an advantage over standard therapy (Jacobs 1987). Palliative radiation to spleen and/or bulky lymph nodes can be valuable when conventional treatment is unsuccessful. Extracorporeal radiation and leukopheresis offer short-lived improvement in leukocyte counts, but are not often used.

The secondary complications of hypogammaglobulinemia, autoimmune phenomena, and immunization problems pose particular challenges. The role of intravenous immunoglobulin replacement remains unsettled, but there is some evidence supporting reduction of infection with its use (Besa 1984; Bunch 1987; Bunch 1988). The treatment of autoimmune hemolytic anemia and immune thrombocytopenia may be problematic. High-dose corticosteroids, splenectomy, and/or gamma-globulin infusions are used in conjunction with treatment aimed at the underlying leukemia (alkylating drugs). Vaccinations against *pneumococcus, H. influenza,* and *meningococcus* ought to be given to patients with CLL; however, immunologic response may be suboptimal. Live viral vaccines should never be administered, because they may cause localized necrotizing vasculitis or fatal systemic disease (disseminated vaccinia).

CLL VARIANTS

PROLYMPHOCYTIC LEUKEMIA

Prolymphocytic leukemia (PLL) was described as a distinct clinical variant of CLL by Galton in 1974. While there are similarities between these two disorders, patients with PLL tend to be older and tend to develop more pronounced constitutional symptoms. Massive splenomegaly is often present, but lymphadenopathy is absent or minimal. Lymphocytosis is usually marked, at times greater than $1,000,000/mm^3$ (Bearman 1978). Prolymphocytes are larger than normal lymphocytes and have a prominent nucleolus and condensed nuclear chromatin (fig. 30.9). Immunophenotyping is similar to classic CLL but surface immunoglobulin staining is more intense (Melo 1987). A T-cell form of PLL has also been described (Matutes 1986). The course of PLL is more aggressive than CLL, and is less responsive to treatment (Hollister 1982).

HAIRY CELL LEUKEMIA

Hairy cell leukemia (HCL), previously known as leukemic reticuloendotheliosis, is a chronic B-cell disorder with a 4:1 male predominance (Catovsky 1974). Patients typically present with splenomegaly, scant lymphadenopathy, and

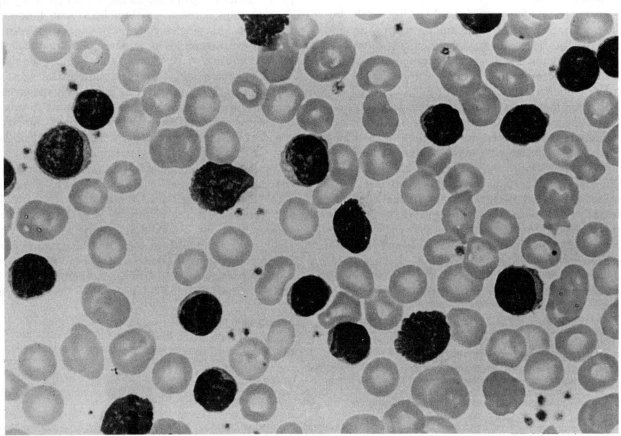

Fig. 30.8. Blood smear in CLL with mature lymphocytes and smudge cells (40x).

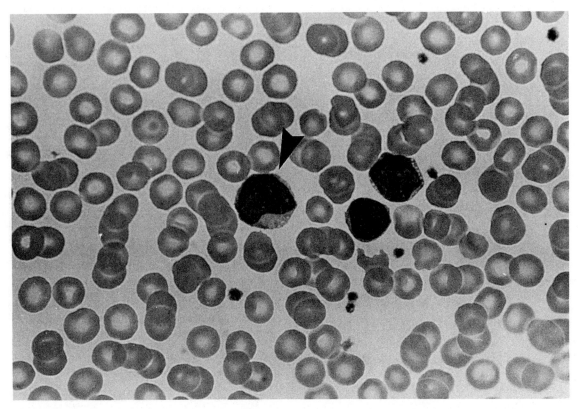

Fig. 30.9. Prolymphocyte: larger than CLL lymphocyte with prominent nucleolus (1000x).

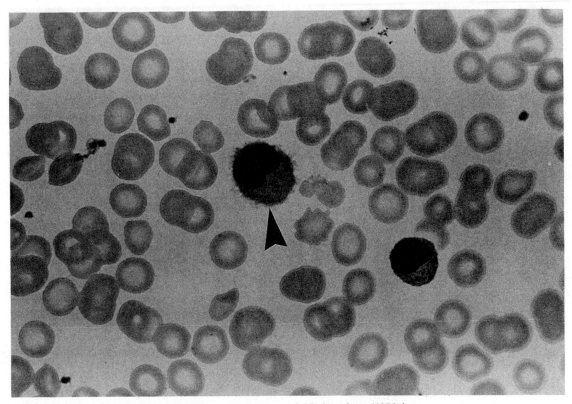

Fig. 30.10. Hairy cell: "hairy" cytoplasmic projections and folded nucleus (1000x).

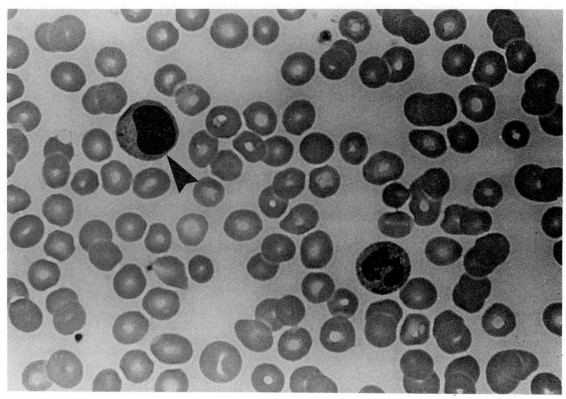

Fig. 30.11. Large granular lymphocyte: larger than CLL lymphocyte with cytoplasmic granules (1000x).

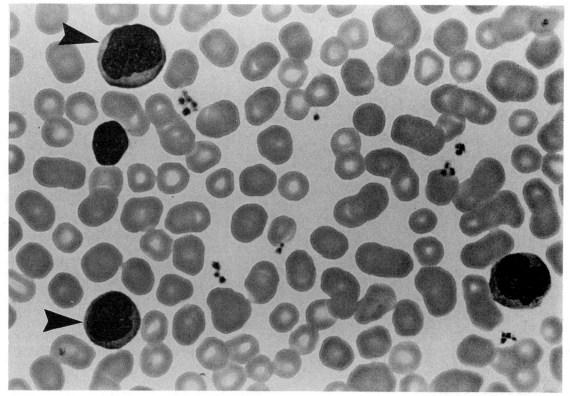

Fig. 30.12. Sezary cell with cerebriform nucleus (1000x).

pancytopenia. Distinctive circulating lymphocytes with "hairy" cytoplasmic projections and a folded nuclear structure (fig. 30.10) are found in the peripheral blood. The diagnosis is confirmed histochemically by the finding of tartrate-resistant acid phosphatase activity in lymphocytes, in conjunction with bone marrow infiltration by these unique-appearing cells. While bone marrow aspirates are usually "dry taps," the biopsy is pathognomonic for this disease.

HCL is an indolent disease; 20% of patients may have prolonged survival without therapeutic intervention (Golomb 1978). Pancytopenia often arises from hypersplenism; therefore splenectomy has been traditional first-line therapy. Improvement in blood counts results in up to 80% of cases, even when the spleen is only minimally enlarged; however one-half of patients relapse after surgery. The recent use of alpha-interferon and low-dose deoxycoformycin (pentostatin) has yielded encouraging results and, unlike splenectomy, has succeeded in eliminating hairy cells from the circulation and bone marrow (Golomb 1986; Spiers 1987). Future trials will determine whether these agents should replace surgery as initial management for HCL and will outline optimal duration of therapy.

T-CELL CLL

T-cell variants of CLL comprise a heterogenous group of diseases with a number of distinctive clinical and laboratory findings. The features of B-cell chronic leukemia, including male predominance, lymphocytosis, and bone marrow infiltration, are common. Splenomegaly is usually more prominent, while lymphadenopathy is less marked (Brouet 1975). Skin infiltration by lymphocytes may occur, although not as frequently as in the T-cell leukemia-lymphomas. Some circulating T-cell lymphocytes (fig. 30.11) are larger than usual, with prominent azurophil granules leading to their description as large granular lymphocytes (LGL) (Loughran 1985). Surface immunophenotyping in T-cell CLL reveals the presence of many subtypes including cells that mark as helper, suppressor, or natural killer cells. In some instances, two separate clones seem to be involved (Pandolfi 1982). It is unclear whether these subsets represent distinct disease entities or whether they form a spectrum of one disorder. Cytopenias are seen, but mechanisms may be different than in B-cell CLL. Direct bone marrow suppression of erythropoiesis and autoimmune-induced neutropenia are particularly characteristic of T gamma CLL (Reynolds 1984). Similar to the B-cell disorder, T-cell CLL is generally indolent, although more fulminant forms have been reported.

T-CELL LEUKEMIA-LYMPHOMA

Sèzary's syndrome and HTLV-I-associated adult T-cell leukemia-lymphoma (ATLL) both present with a leukemic component that is occasionally difficult to distinguish from CLL.

Sèzary's syndrome represents the leukemic phase of mycosis fungoides. Skin infiltration by malignant cells takes the form of a diffuse erythroderma or of isolated scaling plaques. Circulating Sèzary cells are morphologically distinguished by cerebriform nuclei (fig. 30.12) and mark as helper (CD4+) lymphocytes. Topical treatment may be effective in early stages, but advanced states may require lymphoma regimens (Knobler 1986). Extracorporeal photophoresis is an innovative modality for treating resistant forms of skin disease (Edelson 1987).

Adult T-cell leukemia-lymphoma is the first human malignancy causally linked with a viral infection, HTLV-I. It is characterized by an unusually aggressive course punctuated by nodular skin infiltrates, lymphadenopathy, hepatosplenomegaly, lytic bone lesions, and hypercalcemia. Its notable geographic distribution, with endemic areas of Japan, southeastern United States, Africa, and the Caribbean, has attracted particular attention. Circulating T-lymphocytes mark as helper cells, but can be distinguished from Sèzary cells by their more convoluted nuclei and the presence of the interleukin-2 receptor (TAC; CD25) on their surface. Despite treatment with aggressive chemotherapy, the disease course is fulminant, with average survival of 11 months after diagnosis (Koeffler 1986).

REFERENCES

Baccarani, M. 1982. Adolescent and adult acute lymphoblastic leukemia: prognostic features and outcome of therapy. A study of 293 patients. *Blood* 60:677-84.

Bain, B. 1977. Megakaryoblastic transformation of chronic granulocytic leukemia. *J. Clin. Path.* 30:235-42.

Barnett, M. 1986. Treatment of acute lymphoblastic leukemia in adults. *Br. J. Haematol.* 64:455-68.

Bearman, R. 1978. Prolymphocytic leukemia. *Cancer* 42:2360-72.

Bennett J. 1981. The morphologic classification of acute lymphoblastic leukemia: concordance among observers and clinical correlations. *Br. J. Haematol.* 47:553-61.

Bennett, J. 1976. Proposals for the classification of the acute leukemias. *Br. J. Haematol.* 33:451-58.

Bennett, J. 1985a. Proposed revised criteria for the classification of acute myeloid leukemia. *Ann. Intern. Med.* 103: 626-29.

Bennett, J. 1985b. Criteria for the diagnosis of acute leukemia of megakaryocyte lineage M7. *Ann. Intern. Med.* 103:460-62.

Bennett, J.H. 1845. Case of hypertrophy of the spleen and liver, in which death took place from suppuration of the blood. *Edinburgh Med. Surg. J.* 64:413-23.

Bennett, J.M. 1976. Proposals for the classification of the acute leukemias: French-American-British Cooperative Group. *Br. J. Haematol.* 33:451-58.

Besa, E. 1984. Use of intravenous immunoglobulin in chronic lymphocytic leukemia. *Am. J. Med.* 76(3A):209-18.

Binet, J. 1981a. A new prognostic classification of chronic lymphocytic leukemia derived from a multivariate survival analysis. *Cancer* 48:198-206.

Binet, J. 1981b. Chronic lymphocytic leukemia: proposals for a revised prognostic staging system. *Br. J. Haematol.* 48: 356-67.

Binet, J. 1986. Effectiveness of "CHOP" regimen in advanced untreated chronic lymphocytic leukemia. *Lancet* I:1346-49.

Bloomfield, C. 1976. Acute leukemia as a terminal event in nonleukemic hematopoietic disorders. *Semin. Oncol.* 3: 297-312.

Bloomfield, C. 1986. Chromosomal abnormalities identify high-risk and low-risk patients with acute lymphoblastic leukemia. *Blood* 67:415-20.

Bloomfield, C. 1981. Chromosomal abnormalities in acute lymphoblastic leukemia. *Cancer Res.* 41:4838-43.

Bloomfield, C. 1987. Introduction: acute myeloid leukemia. *Semin. Oncol.* 14:357-8.

Bloomfield, C. 1987. Chromosome abnormalities in acute nonlymphocytic leukemia: clinical and biologic significance. *Semin. Oncol.* 14:372-83.

Bollum, F. 1979. Terminal deoxynucleotidyl transferase as a hematopoietic cell marker. *Blood* 54:1203-15.

Borgomano, D. 1928. Leucemie aigue au cours de l'intoxication benzenique. *J. de Medecine de Lyon* 9:227-33.

Brouet, J. 1975. Chronic lymphocytic leukemia of T-cell origin. *Lancet* II:890-93.

Bunch, C. 1987. Intravenous immunoglobulin reduces bacterial infections in chronic lymphocytic leukemia: a controlled randomized trial. *Blood* 70:224a.

Bunch, C. 1988. Intravenous immunoglobulin for the prevention of infection in chronic lymphocytic leukemia. *N. Engl. J. Med.* 319:902-907.

Canellos, G. 1985. Chronic granulocytic leukemia: the heterogeneity of stem cell differentiation within a single disease entity. *Semin. Oncol.* 12:281-88.

Canellos, G. 1984. Acute lymphoblastic leukemia in adults. *Ann. Intern. Med.* 101:552-54.

Casciato, D. 1979. Acute leukemia following prolonged cytotoxic agent therapy. *Medicine* 58:32-46.

Catovsky, D. 1974. Leukemic reticuloendotheliosis ("hairy" cell leukemia): a distinct clinicopathological entity. *Br. J. Haematol.* 26:9-27.

Champlin, R. 1987. Bone marrow transplantation for acute leukemia: recent advances and comparison with alternative therapies. *Semin. Hematol.* 24:55.

Champlin, R. 1987. Bone marrow transplantation for acute leukemia: recent advances and comparison with alternative therapies. *Semin. Hematol.* 24:55-67.

Champlin, R. 1987. Acute myelogenous leukemia: recent advances in therapy. *Blood* 69:1551-55.

Champlin, R. 1989. Acute lymphoblastic leukemia: recent advances in biology and therapy. *Blood* 73:2051-66.

Champlin, R. 1985. Chronic myelogenous leukemia: recent advances. *Blood* 65:1039-47.

Cheng, G. 1988. Structure and expression of genes of GM-CSF and G-CSF in blast cells from patients with acute myeloblastic leukemia. *Blood* 71:204-208.

Chikkappa, G. 1976. Periodic oscillation of blood leukocytes, platelets, and reticulocytes in a patient with chronic myelocytic leukemia. *Blood* 47:1023-30.

Clarkson, B. 1985. Acute lymphoblastic leukemia in adults. *Semin. Oncol.* 12:160-79.

Clarkson, B. 1985. Chronic myelogenous leukemia: is aggressive treatment indicated? *J. Clin. Oncol.* 3:135-39.

Coleman, N. 1986. Secondary malignancy after treatment for Hodgkin's disease: an evolving picture. *J. Clin. Oncol.* 4:821-24.

Court-Brown, W.M. 1955. The incidence of leukemia in ankylosing spondylitis treated with X-rays. *Lancet* I:1283-85.

Craigie, D. 1845. Case of disease of the spleen in which death took place in consequence of the presence of purulent matter in the blood. *Edinburgh Med. Surg. J.* 64:400-13.

Cronkite, E. 1987. Chemical leukemogenesis: benzene as a model. *Semin. Hematol.* 24:2-11.

Dameshek, W. 1967. Chronic lymphocytic leukemia: an accumulative disease of immunologically incompetent lymphocytes. *Blood* 29:566-83.

Draezen, O. 1988. Molecular biology of chronic myelogenous leukemia. *Semin. Hematol.* 25:35-49.

Edelson, R. 1987. Treatment of cutaneous T-cell lymphoma by extracorporeal photochemotherapy. *N. Engl. J. Med.* 316: 297-303.

Eshghabadi, M. 1986. Isolated granulocytic sarcoma: report of a case and review of the literature. *J. Clin. Oncol.* 4:912-17.

Fialkow, P. 1967. Clonal origin of chronic myelocytic leukemia in man. *Proc. Natl. Acad. Sci. USA* 58:1468-71.

Foon, K. 1980. Immunologic classification of acute lymphoblastic leukemia: implication for normal lymphoid differentiation. *Blood* 56:1120-26.

Foon, K. 1986. Recent advances in the immunologic classification of leukemia. *Semin. Hematol.* 23:257-83.

Foon, K. 1986. Alpha interferon treatment of low-grade B-cell non-Hodgkin's lymphomas, cutaneous T-cell lymphomas and chronic lymphocytic leukemia. *Semin. Oncol.* 13:35-43.

Gale, P. 1987. Therapy of acute myelogenous leukemia. *Semin. Hematol.* 24:40-54.

Galton, D. 1974. Prolymphocytic leukemia. *Br. J. Haematol.* 27:7-20.

Goldberg, M. 1987. Is heparin administration necessary during induction chemotherapy for patients with acute promyelocytic leukemia? *Blood* 69:187-91.

Goldman, J. 1982. New approaches in chronic granulocytic leukemia. *Semin. Hematol.* 19:241-56.

Golomb, H. 1978. Hairy cell leukemia. *Ann. Intern. Med.* 89:677-83.

Golomb, H. 1986. Alpha-2 interferon therapy of hairy cell leukemia: a multicenter study of 64 patients. *J. Clin. Oncol.* 4:900-905.

Golomb, H. 1980. "Microgranular" acute promyelocytic leukemia: a distinct clinical, ultrastructural and cytogenetic entity. *Blood* 55:253-59.

Griffin, J. 1983. Surface marker analysis of acute myeloblastic leukemia: identification of differentiation-associated phenotypes. *Blood* 62:557-63.

Groffen, J. 1984. Philadelphia chromosomal breakpoints are clustered within a limited region, *bcr* on chromosome 22. *Cell* 36:93-99.

Han, T. 1984a. Bone marrow infiltration patterns and their prognostic significance in chronic lymphocytic leukemia. *J. Clin. Oncol.* 2:562-70.

Han, T. 1984b. Prognostic importance of cytogenetic abnormalities in patients with chronic lymphocytic leukemia. *N. Engl. J. Med.* 310:288-92.

Heyssel, R. 1960. Leukemia in Hiroshima atomic bomb survivors. *Blood* 15:313-31.

Hiroo, K. 1982. Studies of the mortality of A-bomb survivors. *Radiat. Res.* 90:395-432.

Hoelzer, D. 1987. Acute lymphoblastic leukemia in adults: recent progress, future directions. *Semin. Hematol.* 24: 27-39.

Hoelzer, D. 1988. Prognostic factors in a multicenter study for treatment of acute lymphoblastic leukemia in adults. *Blood* 71:123-31.

Hollister, D. 1982. Treatment of prolymphocytic leukemia. *Cancer* 50:1687-89.

Hurd, D. 1987. Allogeneic and autologous bone marrow transplantation for acute nonlymphocytic leukemia. *Semin. Oncol.* 14:407-15.

Jacobs, A. 1984. Recent advances in the biology and treatment of acute lymphoblastic leukemia in adults. *N. Engl. J. Med.* 311:1219-31.

Jacobs, P. 1987. A randomized prospective comparison of chemotherapy to total body irradiation as initial treatment for the indolent lymphoproliferative diseases. *Blood* 69: 1642-46.

Kapp, J. 1987. Oral norfloxacin for prevention of gram-negative bacterial infections in patients with acute leukemia and granulocytopenia. *Ann. Intern. Med.* 106:1-7.

Kay, N. 1986. Defective T-cell responsiveness in chronic lymphocytic leukemia: analysis of activational events. *Blood* 67:578-81.

Klein, A. 1986. *Bcr* rearrangement and translocation of the c-*abl* oncogene in Philadelphia positive acute lymphoblastic leukemia. *Blood* 68:1369-75.

Knobler, R. 1986. Cutaneous T cell lymphoma. *Med. Clin. North Am.* 70:109-38.

Koeffler, P. 1986. Adult T-cell leukemia-lymphoma. *Clin. Hematol.* 15:695-726.

Koeffler, P. 1981. Chronic myelogenous leukemia: new concepts. *N. Engl. J. Med.* 304:1201-1209.

Koller, C. 1986. Preliminary observation in the therapy of the myeloid blast phase of chronic granulocytic leukemia with plicamycin and hydroxyurea. *N. Engl. J. Med.* 315:1433-38.

Korsmeyer, S. 1983. Immunoglobulin gene rearrangement and cell surface antigen expression in acute lymphocytic leukemias of T-cell and B-cell precursor origins. *J. Clin. Invest.* 71:301-13.

LeBeau, M. 1983. Association of an inversion of chromosome 16 with abnormal marrow eosinophils in acute myelomonocytic leukemia. *N. Engl. J. Med.* 309:630-36.

Lee, J. 1987. Prognosis of chronic lymphocytic leukemia: a multivariate regression analysis of 325 untreated patients. *Blood* 69:929-36.

Linker, C. 1987. Improved results of treatment of adult acute lymphoblastic leukemia. *Blood* 69:1242-48.

Look, T. 1985. The emerging genetics of acute lymphoblastic leukemia: clinical and biologic implications. *Semin. Oncol.* 12:92-104.

Loughran, T. 1985. Leukemia of large granular lymphocytes: association with clonal chromosomal abnormalities and autoimmune neutropenia, thrombocytopenia, and hemolytic anemia. *Ann. Intern. Med.* 102:169-75.

March, C. 1950. Leukemia in radiologists in a 20 year period. *Am. J. Med. Sci.* 220:282-85.

March, C. 1961. Leukemia in radiologists, 10 years later. *Am. J. Med. Sci.* 242:137

Matutes, E. 1986. The morphologic spectrum of T-prolymphocytic leukemia. *Br. J. Haematol.* 64:1111.

Melo, J. 1987. Chronic lymphocytic leukemia and prolymphocytic leukemia: a clinicopathological reappraisal. *Blood Cells* 12:339-53.

Mertelsmann, R. 1980. Morphological classification, response to therapy, and survival in 263 adult patients with acute nonlymphoblastic leukemia. *Blood* 56:773-81.

Metcalf, D. 1974. Responsiveness of human granulocytic leukemia cell to colony-stimulating factor. *Blood* 43:847-59.

Miller, R. 1968. Deaths from childhood cancer in siblings. *N. Engl. J. Med.* 279:122.

Miller, W. 1968. Relation between cancer and congenital defects: an epidemiologic evaluation. *J. Natl. Cancer Inst.* 40:1079-84.

Moloney, W. 1978. Chronic myeloid leukemia. *Cancer* 42:865-73.

Moloney, W. 1955. Leukemia in survivors of atomic bombing. *N. Engl. J. Med.* 253:88-90.

Moloney, W. 1987. Radiogenic leukemia revisited. *Blood* 70:905-908.

Montserrat, E. 1987. Bone marrow biopsy in chronic lymphocytic leukemia: a review of its prognostic importance. *Blood Cells* 12:315-26.

Nesbit, M. 1985. Bone marrow transplantation for acute lymphocytic leukemia. *Semin. Oncol.* 12:149-59.

Nowell, P. 1960. Chromosome studies on normal and leukemic human leukocytes. *J. Natl. Cancer Inst.* 25:85-93.

O'Connell, M. 1986. Clinical trial of recombinant leukocyte alpha interferon as initial therapy for favorable histology non-Hodgkin's lymphomas and chronic lymphocytic leukemia. *J. Clin. Oncol.* 4:128-36.

O'Regan, S. 1977. Electrolyte and acid-base disturbances in the management of leukemia. *Blood* 33:345-53.

O'Reilly, R. 1983. Allogeneic bone marrow transplantation: current status and future directions. *Blood* 62:941-64.

O'Reilly, R. 1986. New promise for autologous marrow transplants in leukemia. *N. Engl. J. Med.* 315:186-88.

Omura, G. 1980. Combination chemotherapy of adult acute lymphoblastic leukemia with randomized central nervous system prophylaxis. *Blood* 55:199-204.

Pandolfi, F. 1982. Immunologic evaluation of T chronic lymphocyte leukemia cells: correlations among phenotype, functional activities, and morphology. *Blood* 59:688-93.

Pendergrass, T. 1985. Epidemiology of acute lymphoblastic leukemia. *Semin. Oncol.* 12:80-91.

Rai, K. 1975. Clinical staging of chronic lymphocytic leukemia. *Blood* 46:219-34.

Ramsay, N. 1985. Autologous bone marrow transplantation for patients with acute lymphoblastic leukemia in second or subsequent remission. *Blood* 66:508-13.

Reynolds, C. 1984. T-lymphoproliferative disease and related disorders in humans and experimental animals: a review of the clinical, cellular, and functional characteristics. *Blood* 64:1146-58.

Richter, M.N. 1928. Generalized reticular cell sarcoma of lymph nodes associated with lymphatic leukemia. *Am. J. Pathol.* 4:285.

Rosenthal, D. 1984. Refractory dysmelopoietic anemia and acute leukemia. *Blood* 63:314-18.

Rosenthal, S. 1977a. Blast crisis of chronic granulocytic leukemia, morphologic variants, and therapeutic implications. *Am. J. Med.* 63:542-7.

Rosenthal, S. 1977b. Erythroblastic transformation of chronic granulocytic leukemia. *Am. J. Med.* 63:116-24.

Rowley, J. 1988. Chromosomal abnormalities in leukemia. *J. Clin. Oncol.* 6:194-202.

Rowley, J. 1981. Down's syndrome and acute leukemia: increased risk may be due to trisomy 21. *Lancet* II:1020-22.

Rowley, J. 1988. Chromosome abnormalities in leukemia. *J. Clin. Oncol.* 6:194-202.

Rozman, C. 1984. Bone marrow histologic pattern—the best single prognostic parameter in chronic lymphocytic leukemia: a multivariate survival analysis of 329 cases. *Blood* 64:642-48.

Sandler, D. 1987. Epidemiology of acute myelogenous leukemia. *Semin. Oncol.* 14:359-64.

Santos, G.W.; 1989. Marrow transplantation in acute nonlymphocytic leukemia. *Blood* 74:901-908.

Schauer, P. 1983. Treatment of acute lymphoblastic leukemia in adults: results of the L-10 and L-10M protocols. *J. Clin. Oncol.* 1:462-70.

Schiffer, C. 1987. Supportive care: issues in the use of blood products and treatment of infection. *Semin. Oncol.* 14:454-67.

Schroff, R. 1982. Immunologic classification of lymphocytic leukemias based on monoclonal antibody-defined cell surface antigens. *Blood* 59:207-14.

Silver, R. 1986. Chronic myeloid leukemia. *Am. J. Med.* 80:1137-48.

Simone, J. 1984. Treatment of meningeal leukemia. *J. Clin. Oncol.* 2:357-58.

Spiers, A. 1984. Chronic granulocytic leukemia. *Med. Clin. North Am.* 68:713-27.

Spiers, A. 1987. Remissions in hairy cell leukemia with pentostatin (2'-deoxycoformycin). *N. Engl. J. Med.* 316:825-30.

Strauss, R. 1981. A controlled trial of prophylactic granulocyte transfusions during initial induction chemotherapy for acute myelogenous leukemia. *N. Engl. J. Med.* 305:597-602.

Sultan, C. 1981. Distribution of 250 cases of acute myeloid leukemia (AML) according to FAB classification and response to therapy. *Br. J. Haematol.* 47:545-51.

Talpaz, M. 1988. Therapy of chronic myelogenous leukemia: chemotherapy and interferons. *Semin. Hematol.* 25:62-73.

Thomas, E.D. 1989. Indications for marrow transplantation in chronic myelogenous leukemia. *Blood* 73:861-64.

Thomas, D. 1986. Marrow transplantation for the treatment of chronic myelogenous leukemia. *Ann. Intern. Med.* 104: 155-63.

Toledano, S. 1980. Ataxia-telangiectasia and acute lymphoblastic leukemia. *Cancer* 45:1675-78.

Travade, P. 1987. New trends in CLL treatment. *Blood Cells* 12:485-96.

Trump, D. 1980. Richter's syndrome: diffuse histiocytic lymphoma in patients with chronic lymphocytic leukemia. *Am. J. Med.* 68:539-48.

Valagussa, P. 1986. Second acute leukemia and other malignancies following treatment for Hodgkin's disease. *J. Clin. Oncol.* 4:830-37.

Vallenga, E. 1987. The biology of acute myeloblastic leukemia. *Semin. Oncol.* 14:356-71.

Videback, A. 1947. *Heredity in human leukemia and its relation to cancer.* London: H.R. Lewis.

Virchow, R. 1897. Weisses blut und milztumoran. *Med. Ztg.* 16:9-15.

Virchow, R. 1845. Weisses blut. *Frolep. Notizen* 36:151-56.

Vodopick, H. 1972. Spontaneous cyclic leukocytosis and thrombocytosis in chronic granulocytic leukemia. *N. Engl. J. Med.* 2286:284-90.

Weidemann, L. 1988. The correlation of breakpoint cluster region rearrangement and p210 *phl/abl* expression with morphologic analysis of Ph-negative chronic myeloid leukemia and other myeloproliferative diseases. *Blood* 71: 349-55.

Williams, W. 1983. *Hematology.* pp. 982. New York: McGraw-Hill.

Wolf, D. 1978. Splenectomy in chronic myeloid leukemia. *Ann. Intern. Med.* 89:684-89.

Yeager, A. 1986. Autologous bone marrow transplantation in patients with acute nonlymphocytic leukemia, using *ex vivo* marrow treatment with 4-hydroperoxycyclophosphamide. *N. Engl. J. Med.* 315:141-47.

Chapter 31

CHILDHOOD LEUKEMIAS

Ching-Hon Pui, M.D.
Gaston K. Rivera, M.D.

Ching-Hon Pui, M.D.
Member, Department of Hematology-Oncology
St. Jude Children's Research Hospital
Memphis, Tennessee
Professor of Pediatrics
University of Tennessee, Memphis, College of Medicine
Memphis, Tennessee

Gaston K. Rivera, M.D.
Member, Department of Hematology-Oncology
St. Jude Children's Research Hospital
Memphis, Tennessee
Professor of Pediatrics
University of Tennessee, Memphis, College of Medicine
Memphis, Tennessee

This work was supported in part by grants CA-20180 and CA-21765 from the National Cancer Institute and by the American Lebanese Syrian Associated Charities (ALSAC).

INTRODUCTION

Leukemia is the most common form of childhood cancer, affecting approximately 2,500 children each year in the United States. Acute lymphoblastic leukemia (ALL) accounts for about 80% of the leukemias in children and acute myeloid (nonlymphoblastic) leukemia (AML) for most of the remainder. The increased precision of diagnostic methods, more effective therapy administered in controlled clinical trials, and better supportive care have dramatically improved the outlook for children with leukemia. Today, 60% of children with ALL will be in continuous complete remission for five years or more after diagnosis, and most of them will be cured. Developing effective treatment for AML and relapsed ALL, however, remains a major challenge. Also, the late sequelae of treatment in long-term survivors pose new therapeutic problems that are expected to increase as this population grows.

The study of leukemia in children has yielded benefits that extend beyond improvements in cure rates. Leukemic cells are readily obtained from the blood and bone marrow, and their analysis over the past two decades has contributed many of the principles that underlie the understanding of tumor cell biology. Because of its relatively high incidence, childhood leukemia was one of the first malignant diseases for which large-scale therapeutic trials were conducted. The knowledge gained from these comparative studies has greatly influenced treatment strategies for cancers of all types.

MORPHOLOGICAL AND CYTOCHEMICAL CLASSIFICATION

Precise classification of the childhood leukemias is essential in order to understand their pathophysiology and to develop more specific methods of therapy. The childhood leukemias can be classified broadly as acute, chronic, or congenital. The terms *acute* and *chronic* originally referred to survival duration, but with the advent of effective chemotherapy they have taken on new meanings. Acute leukemia now refers to the malignant proliferation of immature (blastic) cells, and chronic leukemia to the proliferation of predominantly more mature (more differentiated) cell types. Unlike leukemia in adults, childhood leukemia is almost always acute. Congenital or neonatal leukemias are those diagnosed in the first four weeks of life. A related category, preleukemia, is a heterogenous condition, generally characterized by peripheral blood cytopenias and ineffective hematopoiesis with dysmorphic maturation of the hematopoietic elements, which may evolve into frank acute leukemia (Kobrinsky et al. 1982; Wegelius 1986).

The acute leukemias are classified as lymphoid or myeloid by their morphologic characteristics on Romanowsky-stained bone marrow smears and by their cytochemical staining properties. Most childhood leukemias are lymphoblastic (ALL). In general, lymphoblasts have a smooth, homogeneous nuclear chromatin pattern with indistinct nucleoli and scanty cytoplasm, without

Table 31.1
CLASSIFICATION OF CHILDHOOD LEUKEMIAS, FRENCH-AMERICAN-BRITISH (FAB) CRITERIA

FAB Designation	Percent (%)	Prominent Features
ALL		
L1	86	Small blasts with scanty cytoplasm and inconspicuous nucleoli
L2	13	Larger blasts with increased cytoplasm, irregular nuclear membranes, and prominent nucleoli
L3	1	Basophilic cytoplasm with vacuolization
AML		
M1	20	Poorly differentiated myeloblasts with occasional Auer rods
M2	29	Myeloblastic with differentiation and more prominent Auer rods
M3	7	Promyelocytic with heavy granulation and bundles of Auer rods
M4	22	Myeloblastic and monoblastic differentiation in various proportions
M5	19	Monoblastic
M6	1	Erythroleukemic with bizarre dyserythropoiesis and megaloblastic features
M7	2	Megakaryoblastic with bone marrow fibrosis

granules. Granular ALLs are unusual. In 60% to 90% of cases, lymphoblasts contain large aggregates of periodic acid-Schiff (PAS)-positive material. Lymphoblasts are myeloperoxidase-negative and are usually, but not always, nonreactive with Sudan black B (Stass, Pui, and Melvin et al. 1984). Myeloblasts are larger, with abundant granular cytoplasm and one or more distinct nucleoli. Auer rods, a coalescence of azurophilic granules, are pathognomonic for AML. The PAS stain may be weakly positive, with a diffuse pattern in one-third of AML cases. Myeloperoxidase is positive in approximately 80% of AMLs (Pui, Behm, and Kalwinsky et al. 1987) and Sudan black B positivity usually parallels that of myeloperoxidase.

In 1976, an international French-American-British (FAB) cooperative group devised a classification scheme based on the morphologic features and cytochemical staining properties of bone marrow blast cells (Bennett, Catovsky, and Daniel et al. 1976) (table 31.1). Lymphoblastic leukemias are classified as L1, L2, and L3; most childhood ALLs are L1. Although the biologic significance of L1 and L2 morphology is not clear, L3 is clearly distinct and associated with B-cell ALL and a poor prognosis. FAB classification includes seven major groups of AML: M1 through M7. The M1 variant is the least differentiated form of AML and can be morphologically indistinguishable from L2 ALL; the distinction requires myeloperoxidase staining. M2 blasts show differentiation beyond the promyelocyte stage (>30% blasts and promyelocytes). M3 has the largest amount of Auer rods seen in any FAB group. Clinically, M3 AML is associated with severe disseminated intravascular coagulation, older age, and bleeding (Cordonnier et al. 1985). In the M4 group, >20% of nonerythroid bone marrow cells are monoblastic, as shown by the presence of α-naphthyl butyrate esterase activity in the cytoplasm. In the M5 subtype, 80% or more of the nonerythroid cells in the bone marrow must be monoblasts, promonocytes, or monocytes. The M4 and M5 subtypes often occur in young children, particularly infants, and are characterized by hyperleukocytosis and a propensity for extramedullary involvement (Tobelem et al. 1980; Pui, Kalwinsky, and Sehell et al. 1988). The presence of spectrin or surface expression of

erythroid-associated antigens leads to the diagnosis of FAB M6 (erythroleukemia, or DiGuglielmo's syndrome). This form is extremely rare in children. In M7, known as acute megakaryoblastic leukemia, the blast cells are typically positive for α-naphthyl acetate esterase but are negative for α-naphthyl butyrate esterase. The presence of factor VIII-related antigens (by immunohistochemical techniques) or platelet peroxidase (by ultrastructural cytochemistry) is supportive of the diagnosis (Bennett, Catovsky, and Daniel 1985). Recently, monoclonal antiplatelet antibodies have helped in diagnosing acute megakaryoblastic leukemia. This subtype is often associated with pancytopenia and reticulin fibrosis of bone marrow (Pui, Rivera, and Mirro et al. 1985).

Morphology and cytochemistry cannot fully characterize a small population (<5%) of childhood leukemias and in these cases electron microscopy, with or without immunologic studies, establishes the diagnosis. The recognition of acute mixed lineage leukemia (AMLL) is a relatively recent development.

EPIDEMIOLOGY

In the United States, the annual incidence of leukemia in people under 15 years of age is about 4 per 100,000. The ratio of ALL to AML in children is 4:1 — almost the reverse of that in adults. In ALL, the peak age of occurrence is between 3 and 4 years; no age peak has been observed for AML (Fraumeni, Manning, and Mitus 1971). The incidence of ALL is higher among whites than among nonwhites (1.8:1). The distribution of leukemia subtypes varies geographically. In Turkey, acute myelomonocytic leukemia, often with ocular chloroma, accounts for approximately 35% of cases, in contrast to 5% in the United States. In Shanghai, China, nearly half of childhood leukemias are AMLs.

Caucasians have a risk of approximately 1 in 2,880 of developing leukemia in the first 15 years of life. Siblings of affected children have a fourfold increase in risk during the first decade of life (Miller 1967). When leukemia occurs in one monozygous twin, the chance that the disease will develop in the other twin during the first six years of life is 20% (usually within months of the first case); thereafter, the risk is the same as that for other siblings. Concordant leukemia in monozygotic infant twins may reflect a common prezygotic determinant, shared intrauterine event, or metastasis from one twin to the other.

An increased risk has been linked to a variety of disorders (table 31.2). Children with Down's syndrome have a 10- to 30-fold increased incidence; their leukemic cell types follow the usual distribution (Robinson et al. 1984). Compared to other children with ALL, those with Down's syndrome have a significantly lower remission rate and a higher mortality rate from complications during induction therapy. Autosomal recessive genetic diseases associated with chromosomal instability and predisposition to acute leukemia include Fanconi's anemia, Bloom's syndrome, and ataxia telangiectasia. In isolated instances, leukemia has developed in patients with Poland's syndrome, Klinefelter's syndrome, Rubinstein-Taybi syndrome, Blackfan-Diamond syndrome, incontinentia pigmenti, and various other congenital malformations. Children with a constitutional or acquired immune defect are also at increased risk.

Studies cite an association between leukemia and exposure to ionizing radiation (Kato and Schull 1982) and hydrocarbons such as benzene (Rinsky et al. 1987). Reports of AML as a second malignancy are increasing, especially in patients who have received combined therapy with radiation and alkylating agents (Kantarjian and Keating 1987). With wider use of intensive chemotherapy, lineage switch (lymphoid to myeloid or the reverse) has been noted in leukemia patients who relapse in marrow (Stass, Mirro, and Melvin et al. 1984; Pui, Raimondi, and Behm et al. 1986; Pui, Behm, and Raimondi et al. 1989). The exact mechanism underlying this finding is not known.

ETIOLOGY

Several predisposing or contributing factors have been identified, but the cause of human leukemia remains unknown. Leukemia has been induced in experimental animals with different strains of retroviruses. Occasional reports of leukemia clusters in well-defined geographic areas and the association of Epstein-Barr virus (EBV) with Burkitt's lymphoma suggest that infectious agents play a role in human leukemogenesis. Considerable effort has been devoted to establishing the relationship between viruses and leukemia. Human T-cell lymphotropic virus (HTLV)-I is associated with adult T-cell leukemia (Gallo 1984), and HTLV-II with an adult hairy cell leukemia (Kalyanaraman, Sarngadharan, and Robert-Guroff 1982). However, virus-induced leukemia has not been identified in children.

Recently, researchers have hypothesized that spontaneous mutation is the major cause of childhood ALL (Greaves 1988). The target cells for ALL, lymphoid precursor cells, have a high proliferative rate and increased propensity for gene rearrangement during early childhood and are more susceptible to mutation. One or, more likely, two sequential mutations arising spontaneously in key regulatory genes in a cell population under proliferative stress could occur at sufficient frequency to account for most cases of childhood ALL. Research on oncogenes and tumor-suppressing genes promises to increase understanding of the complex process of leukemogenesis and may lead to improved methods of cancer detection and treatment (Bishop 1988).

PATHOPHYSIOLOGY

The prevailing theory is that a single mutant progenitor cell, capable of indefinite self-renewal, gives rise to malignant, poorly differentiated hematopoietic precursors. Evidence from several lines of research support this concept. The finding of similar chromosomal abnormalities in multiple leukemic blast cells at diagnosis and at relapse supports the clonal origin of leukemia (Zuelzer et al. 1976). In G6PD studies, the existence of a single type of G6PD in the malignant cells of heterozygous patients who have a double-enzyme pattern in their normal tissues can demonstrate the unicellular origin of neoplasms (Fialkow, Jacobson, and Papayannopoulou 1977). Determination of the methylation patterns of X-linked restriction-fragment-length polymorphisms in heterozygous females is another sensitive method of analysis based on the same principle (Fearon et al. 1986; Pui, Raskind, and Kitchingman et al. 1989). Gene mapping

Table 31.2
RECOGNIZED CONGENITAL DISORDERS ASSOCIATED WITH AN INCREASED RISK OF LEUKEMIA

Congenital Disorders	Associated Leukemias
Down's syndrome	ALL, AML
Fanconi's anemia	AMMoL
Bloom's syndrome	AL
Ataxia telangiectasia	ALL
Neurofibromatosis	ALL, AML, CML
Kostman's infantile agranulocytosis	AMoL
Wiskott-Aldrich syndrome	AML
IgA deficiency	ALL
Variable immunodeficiency	ALL, AML
Schwachman's syndrome	ALL, AML
Congenital X-linked agammaglobulinemia	ALL

Abbreviations not defined in the text: AMMoL = acute myelomonocytic leukemia; AL = acute leukemia; AMoL = acute monoblastic leukemia.

with DNA probes specific for immunoglobulin heavy- or light-chain genes, or T-cell receptor genes, provides an alternative means of demonstrating the monoclonal origin of leukemia (Korsmeyer et al. 1981; Waldmann et al. 1985). Finally, demonstration of monoclonal immunoglobulin idiotypes and light-chain types is useful in B-cell malignancies (Sklar et al. 1984; Levy et al. 1977). In fact, in some patients differentiated cells originated from the same leukemic clone (Fearon et al. 1986).

The accumulation of blast cells in the marrow inhibits the normal production of granulocytes, erythrocytes, and platelets, resulting in infection, anemia, and hemorrhage. Moreover, leukemic cells can infiltrate virtually any organ and cause enlargement and dysfunction.

ACUTE LYMPHOBLASTIC LEUKEMIA (ALL)

CLINICAL AND LABORATORY FEATURES

The clinical presentation of ALL is quite variable. Symptoms may appear insidiously or acutely (table 31.3). Some patients have life-threatening infections or hemorrhage at diagnosis. In others the onset of leukemia is asymptomatic and detected during routine physical examination. Most patients, however, have some history of illness before diagnosis. The disease manifests in one or more of the following signs and symptoms: pallor, easy bruisability, lethargy, malaise, anorexia, intermittent fever, bone pain, arthralgia, abdominal pain, and bleeding (Pui and Rivera 1987). These symptoms may have been present for a few days to a few months.

Physical examination reveals fever, pallor, petechiae and ecchymoses on skin or mucous membrane, retinal hemorrhage, enlarged lymph nodes, hepatosplenomegaly, nephromegaly, and/or bone tenderness. Less common presenting features include subcutaneous nodules (leukemia cutis), enlarged salivary glands (Mikulicz's syndrome), painless enlargement of the testes, cranial nerve palsy with papilledema, painful swelling of the joints, and priapism due to marked leukocytosis. Rarely, epidural spinal cord compression may result in paraparesis or paraplegia, an oncologic emergency requiring immediate treatment (Pui, Dahl, and Hustu et al. 1985). In some patients, infiltration of the tonsils, adenoids, appendix, or mesenteric lymph nodes leads to surgical intervention before diagnosis of leukemia.

Initial blood cell counts show a wide spectrum of abnormalities. Anemia, abnormal leukocyte and differential counts, and thrombocytopenia are usually present at diagnosis. Very rarely, children have normal blood counts. Leukocyte counts range from 0.1 to 1000 x 10^9/L (median, 13 x 10^9/L), often with absolute granulocytopenia. Approximately two-thirds of the patients have leukocyte counts <25 x 10^9/L. (See table 31.3.)

The majority of cells in blood smears are lymphoblasts or lymphocytes. The white blood cell count at diagnosis is one of the most important prognostic features in childhood ALL; in general, counts >25 x 10^9/L indicate a worse prognosis. Because the morphology of the blast cells in peripheral blood smears may differ from that of those in bone marrow, the peripheral smears should not decide a definitive diagnosis. Hypereosinophilia may be present at diagnosis and is generally considered as reactive (Nelken and Stockman 1976). Hemoglobin levels range from 2 to 15 g/dL (median, 7.6 g/dL), and reticulocyte counts are normal or low. The platelet count varies from normal to extremely low with a median of 50 x 10^9/L. Disseminated intravascular coagulation, usually mild, can occur with T-cell ALL (Ribeiro and Pui 1986). Elevated serum uric acid level commonly indicates large leukemic cell mass. Patients with massive renal involvement may have increased serum urea and creatinine; hypercalcemia and hypercalciuria are rare. Urinalysis may reveal microscopic hematuria and the presence of uric acid crystals.

Definitive diagnosis rests on examination of bone marrow, which is usually completely replaced by leukemic lymphoblasts. Fibrosis or tightly packed marrow can lead to difficulties with bone marrow aspiration, necessitating biopsy (Hann et al. 1978). A touch preparation of the biopsied tissue can be stained for morphologic diagnosis. A small proportion of patients have bone marrow necrosis, usually in association with severe bone

Table 31.3
PRESENTING FEATURES IN 584 CHILDREN WITH ALL

Feature	Percent (%)
Age (yr)	
≤1	3
2-9	72
≥10	25
Male	59
Symptoms	
Fever	55
Malaise	50
Bleeding	42
Bone or joint pain	27
Anorexia	20
Abdominal pain	10
Lymphadenopathy	35
Liver edge below costal margin (cm)	
1-5	47
>5	19
Spleen edge below costal margin (cm)	
1-5	38
>5	19
Mediastinal mass	13
CNS leukemia	5
Leukocyte count (x 10^9/L)	
<25	64
25-49	12
50-100	10
>100	14
Hemoglobin (g/dL)	
<7	40
7-9	28
>10	32
Platelet count (x 10^9/L)	
<10	11
10-49	38
50-100	21
>100	30

(Source: Pui and Rivera [1987.] Used with permission.)

pain and tenderness, a very high serum lactic dehydrogenase level, and fever (Pui, Stass, and Green 1985). Bone marrow scans are sometimes necessary to guide attempts to obtain viable tissue; rarely, a lymph node biopsy may be required. For the most part, a marrow aspirate can promptly establish the diagnosis of childhood ALL. In children, the usual sites for marrow aspiration are the posterior or anterior iliac crest.

A chest roentgenogram should be performed to detect mediastinal nodal enlargement, thymic enlargement, or pleural effusion. Pulmonary infiltrates are occasionally detected and can indicate pneumonia, pulmonary edema, or, rarely, leukemic infiltration. Fifty percent of patients have a variety of skeletal lesions, including generalized rarefaction of bones, transverse radiolucent bands in metaphyses of long bones, periosteal new bone formation, cortical osteolytic lesions, osteosclerosis, and vertebral collapse (Ribeiro, Pui, and Schell 1988; Aur, Westbrook, and Riggs 1972). These changes have no independent prognostic significance; thus, skeletal survey is not necessary unless there are clinical indications (Aur, Westbrook, and Riggs 1972).

Cerebrospinal fluid should be examined because it contains leukemic blasts in 3% to 5% of patients, regardless of the presence or absence of neurologic manifestations. Concern that this practice may facilitate seeding of the CNS has not been substantiated.

IMMUNOLOGIC MARKERS

Differences in surface membrane or cytoplasmic components of T and B lymphocytes identify and classify lymphoproliferative diseases by cell origin and stage of differentiation (Crist, Grossi, and Pullen et al. 1985). These studies help in establishing the diagnosis and selecting an effective treatment plan. Childhood ALL can be classified as early pre-B (64%), pre-B (20%), B-cell (1%), or T-cell (15%). Blast cells from T-cell ALL express sheep erythrocyte receptor or T-cell surface antigens, or both. Male gender, older age, large leukemic cell mass reflected by high leukocyte count and elevated serum lactic dehydrogenase level, and a mediastinal mass often characterize this disease (Pullen et al. 1984; Pui, Behm, and Singh et al. 1990a) (table 31.4). B-cell ALL usually presents with a massive extramedullary tumor and with marrow replacement by blasts having L3 morphology and expressing surface immunoglobulin. B-cell ALL probably represents advanced Burkitt's lymphoma in a phase of leukemic

evolution (Magrath and Ziegler 1980). Most of the ALL cases have been classified as early pre-B, based on the leukemic cell surface expression of B-cell restricted-differentiation antigens or immunoglobulin gene rearrangements, or both (Crist, Grossi, and Pullen et al. 1985). Approximately 90% of children with early pre-B ALL have blasts that express the common ALL antigen (CALLA); generally this group is known as "common" ALL. Compared to patients with common ALL, those with CALLA-negative ALL have greater leukemic cell burden, are more likely to be infants, and have a high frequency of unfavorable blast cell chromosomal features (Pui, Williams, and Raimondi et al. 1986). In pre-B ALL, more than 10% of the blast cells contain cytoplasmic immunoglobulin μ heavy chains (Volger et al. 1978). Children with pre-B ALL have higher serum lactic dehydrogenase levels and are more likely to have unfavorable cytogenetic features than those with early pre-B ALL (Pui, Williams, and Kalwinsky et al. 1986).

GENETIC FEATURES

The fundamental changes associated with neoplastic transformation include chromosomal changes. Clonal cytogenetic abnormalities have been identified in more than 90% of patients with ALL (Pui, Williams, and Roberson et al. 1988), and a growing number of specific chromosomal changes is associated with certain subtypes of leukemia (Pui, Williams, and Roberson et al. 1988; Williams et al. 1984; Sandberg 1986) (table 31.5). Several chromosomal abnormalities, such as the t(9;22)(q34;q11) (Philadelphia [Ph] chromosome) and 9p− are not associated with specific immunophenotypes but are frequent findings, occurring in 5% and 10% of cases, respectively. These chromosomal markers have diagnostic, prognostic, therapeutic, and biologic importance. The recently established Morphology-Immunology-Cytogenetics (MIC) classification better reflects the intrinsic pathobiology of various ALL subtypes by combining information obtained from three fields of leukemia research (First MIC Cooperative Study Group 1986).

Specific chromosomal translocations, presumably involving reciprocal exchanges of DNA, appear to be the most biologically and clinically significant karyotypic change in human leukemia. The most consistently observed association between immunophenotype and chromosomal translocation occurs in B-cell leukemia.

Table 31.4
COMPARATIVE FEATURES OF THE IMMUNOLOGIC SUBCLASSES OF ALL

Feature	Phenotype			
	Early pre-B	Pre-B	B	T
Median age (yr)	4.4	4.4	8.7	7.5
Median WBC (x 10^9/L)	12.7	13.7	9.0	100
Median LDH (IU/L)	341.0	560.0	1600.0	1624.0
% Male	57	54	75	68
% Mediastinal mass	1	1	0	55
% CALLA positivity	90	91	47	30
% Hyperdiploidy >50	30	18	0	5
% Chromosomal translocation	35	59	100	40

Virtually all B-cell ALLs have one of three specific translocations: t(8;14), t(2;8), or t(8;22). These rearrangements consistently bring together the c-*myc* proto-oncogene on chromosome 8(q24) and a transcriptionally active gene for the immunoglobulin heavy chain on 14q32, the kappa light chain on 2p11-p12, or the lambda light chain on 22q11, leading to aberrant activation of c-*myc* (Croce 1986). Recent studies suggest that the genes encoding the T-cell receptor gene α-chain at 14q11-q13, β-chain at 7q32-q36, γ-chain at 7p15 and Δ-chain at 14q11) may also participate in proto-oncogene activation in T-cell ALL, in a manner similar to that observed in B-cell lymphoid malignancies (Isobe et al. 1988). These studies offer the exciting possibility of defining the molecular pathogenetic mechanisms leading to immortalization of malignant cells.

PROGNOSTIC FACTORS

The initial leukemic cell burden, as reflected by the leukocyte count and the degree of organomegaly, is closely linked with treatment outcome. There is a direct linear relationship between the presenting leukocyte count and likelihood of survival (Robison et al. 1980). The serum lactic dehydrogenase level may be an even more reliable estimate of the total body burden of leukemic cells than a leukocyte count alone and also appears to have a linear relationship to prognosis (Pui, Dodge, and Dahl et al. 1985).

Age at diagnosis is a consistently reliable predictor. Patients older than 10 years or younger than 12 to 18 months fare much worse than children in the intermediate age group (Reaman et al. 1985; Crist et al. 1986; Crist, Pullen, and Boyett et al. 1988). More extensive disease at diagnosis and unfavorable leukemic cell karyotype and immunophenotype, which usually lacks CALLA expression, partly explain the poor prognosis of infants (Reaman et al. 1985; Pui, Raimondi, and Murphy et al. 1987). Compared to patients between 1 and 10 years old, adolescents with ALL are more likely to have a higher leukocyte count, mediastinal mass, T-cell disease, and to be males; their leukemic cells are more likely to have L2 morphology, CALLA negativity, and unfavorable cytogenetic features (Crist, Pullen, and Boyett et al. 1988).

Although ALL occurs less often in black children, they fare worse than white children, despite modern chemotherapy (Falletta et al. 1984). Leukemia in blacks is usually associated with an increased leukocyte count, presence of a mediastinal mass, L2 morphology, CALLA negativity or pre-B phenotype, and pseudodiploidy.

Among the immunophenotypic subtypes of ALL, early pre-B cases have the most favorable treatment outcome; B-cell ALL cases, particularly those with CNS involvement, fare the worst (Crist, Grossi, and Pullen et al. 1985). Larger initial leukemic cell mass and unfavorable leukemic cell cytogenetic features partly explain the poorer prognosis of pre-B and T-cell cases, compared to early pre-B cases.

Chromosomal abnormalities have important prognostic value in ALL. Hyperdiploid stem lines, with >50 chromosomes per leukemic cell, comprise about 30% of children with ALL and have the most favorable prognosis (Pui, Williams, and Roberson et al. 1988; Williams, Tsiatis, and Brodeur et al. 1982). Analysis of cellular DNA content by flow cytometry, an alternative method of cytogenetic analysis for establishing leukemic cell ploidy, identifies this group of patients (Look et al. 1985). Pseudodiploidy (46 chromosomes with structural abnormalities) and hypodiploidy (<46 chromosomes) have been shown to correlate with a poorer outcome (Pui, Williams, and Raimondi et al. 1987). Finally, cases with a Ph chromosome have a particularly poor prognosis (Ribeiro, Abromourtch, and Raimondi et al. 1987).

Among FAB subtypes of ALL, L1 cases appear to have the best prognosis and L3 the worst (Miller et al. 1985). Other less-important presenting features that correlate with poor prognosis include male gender, low economic class, presence of mediastinal mass, low serum immunoglobulin levels, the presence of initial CNS leukemia, higher hemoglobin levels, lower platelet counts, larger renal size, lower levels of glucocorticoid receptors in leukemic blast cells, higher pretreatment blast cell proliferative activity, lower PAS positivity in blast cells, and the presence of hand mirror cells (Pui and Crist 1987).

Because the prognostic factors in ALL are highly interrelated, multivariate analyses are necessary to identify those with independent significance. Among the

Table 31.5
CONSISTENT PRIMARY STRUCTURAL CHROMOSOME ABNORMALITIES IN ALL

Abnormality	FAB Type	Immunophenotype
t(8;14)(q24;q32.3)	L3	B
t(8;22)(q24;q11)	L3	B
t(2;8)(p11-p12;q24)	L3	B
t(1;19)(q23;p13)	L1, L2	Pre-B, rarely early pre-B
t(8;14)(q24;q11)	L1, L2	T
t(10;14)(q24;q11)	L1, L2	T
t(11;14)(p13-p15;q11-q13)	L1, L2	T
t(7)(q32-q36)	L1, L2	T
del(6)(q21q25)	L1, L2	CALLA+ early pre-B
del/t(12p)	L1, L2	CALLA+ early pre-B
dic(9;12)(p11-p12;p12)	L1, L2	CALLA+ early pre-B, pre-B
t(11)(q23)*	L1, L2	CALLA− early pre-B

*Cases of t(4;11)(q21;q23) tend to coexpress lymphoid and myeloid markers (i.e., acute mixed lineage leukemia).

clinical features, leukocyte count, age, and race consistently emerge as independent indicators of treatment outcome. As improved chromosome banding and immunophenotyping techniques become more widely available, these features will probably become useful prognostic indicators. Improved therapy lessens the utility of many of the determinants for childhood ALL, so the prognostic factors should be evaluated in the context of the therapy (Miller et al. 1983; Pui, Ochs, and Kalwinsky et al. 1984).

High serum interleukin-2 receptor and CD8 antigen (marker for suppressor/cytotoxic T-cells) levels at diagnosis were recently associated with a poor treatment outcome in childhood ALL (Pui, Ip, and Iflah et al. 1988; Pui, Ip, and Dodge et al. 1988). Because interleukin-2 and suppressor/cytotoxic T-cells are important immune modulators, these findings suggest that host immunity may affect the progression of tumors.

DIFFERENTIAL DIAGNOSIS

The initial manifestations of ALL are similar to those of several other disorders. The acute onset of petechiae, ecchymoses, and bleeding may suggest idiopathic thrombocytopenia, which is often associated with a recent viral infection, large platelets in blood smears, and no evidence of anemia. Both ALL and aplastic anemia may present with pancytopenia and complications associated with bone marrow failure. In aplastic anemia, hepatosplenomegaly and lymphadenopathy are unusual, and the skeletal changes associated with leukemia do not occur. Bone marrow aspirations and biopsy usually establish the diagnosis. Distinguishing between the two diseases in a child whose ALL presents with a hypocellular marrow that lymphoblasts later replace may be difficult (Breatnach, Chessells, and Greaves 1981). Childhood infectious mononucleosis and other viral infections, especially those associated with thrombocytopenia or hemolytic anemia, may be confused with leukemia. Atypical lymphocytes and increased viral titers help to establish the correct diagnosis. Children with pertussis or parapertussis may have marked lymphocytosis; leukocyte counts have been as high as 50×10^9/L, but the affected cells are mature lymphocytes rather than leukemic lymphoblasts. Bone pain, arthralgia, and occasionally arthritis may mimic juvenile rheumatoid arthritis, rheumatic fever, other collagen vascular diseases, and osteomyelitis. Some patients with presumed systemic lupus erythematosus have ALL (Saulsbury et al. 1984). Therefore, bone marrow aspiration should be done to exclude leukemia before beginning steroid treatment for rheumatic diseases. If bone marrow is replaced by metastatic tumor (for example, neuroblastoma, rhabdomyosarcoma, or retinoblastoma), the malignant cells are usually in clumps, and a primary tumor can be found.

THERAPY

REMISSION INDUCTION AND CONSOLIDATION

Inadequate reduction of the initial leukemia cell burden allows regrowth of drug-resistant cells and results in treatment failure. Theoretically, anticancer drugs could cure if treatments were sufficiently intense to eradicate malignant cells before drug resistance developed (Lampkin and Wong 1986). Approaches to intensification of chemotherapy include multiple agents for early treatment, repeated administration of drug combinations within an otherwise standard regimen, administration of single agent at increased dosage, and rapid rotation of effective drug pairs (Rivera and Mauer 1987). Intensive early therapy has been the hallmark of several recent successful clinical trials (Steinherz et al. 1986; Clavell et al. 1986; Dahl et al. 1987; Riehm, Feikert, and Lampert 1986; Gaynon et al. 1988; Camitta et al. 1989). One study suggested that a late intensification phase cannot compensate for inadequate early therapy (Pui, Aur, and Bowman et al. 1984).

Most induction therapy regimens include prednisone, vincristine, daunorubicin, and asparaginase. With modern chemotherapy, 95% of children with ALL attain a complete remission; that is, the absence of clinical signs and symptoms of disease and the presence of normal blood counts and a normocellular bone marrow with less than 5% of blasts. Induction failure, seen in 2% to 5% of cases, is due to primary drug resistance or toxicity of therapy. For drug-resistant patients, teniposide and cytarabine produces a 65% complete remission rate (Rivera et al. 1980). The value of postremission consolidation therapy is controversial, especially for patients with favorable prognosis, but most clinical trials have included this phase of treatment.

SUBCLINICAL (PROPHYLACTIC) CNS TREATMENT

The importance of subclinical CNS therapy is universally accepted but concern about its adverse effects has prompted a reappraisal of therapeutic strategies (Rivera and Mauer 1987). Newer approaches being studied include lower doses of cranial irradiation (18 Gy) with intrathecal methotrexate; triple intrathecal therapy with methotrexate, cytarabine, and hydrocortisone; intermediate-dose methotrexate with concomitant intrathecal methotrexate; high-dose methotrexate alone; periodic intrathecal methotrexate with intensive systemic therapy; or pharmacokinetically derived drug dosage regimen. In general, CNS irradiation is now reserved for patients who have initial CNS leukemia or are at high risk of CNS relapse. It is also recognized that the efficacy of systemic chemotherapy affects subclinical CNS therapy.

CONTINUATION THERAPY

Regardless of whether an intensive consolidation regimen is used early in remission, continuation treatment is always given, but the optimal regimen and the duration of therapy have not been established. Until recently, oral daily mercaptopurine and weekly methotrexate, with or without prednisone and vincristine reinforcement, were the most common components of continuation treatment. For patients with poor-prognosis leukemia, most investigators now recommend more intensive continuation therapies (single agents at increased dosage or multiple drugs in an intermittent or rotating schedule).

All drugs induce undesirable toxic effects, so chemotherapy cannot be administered indefinitely. Prolonged exposure to the same agents may ultimately lead to emergence of drug-resistant leukemia, and the maximum antileukemic effect of any drug combination is probably reached in a finite period. Common practice has been to discontinue all therapy in patients who have been in continuous complete remission for 24 months or longer. Before cessation of therapy, patients should have bone marrow and cerebrospinal fluid examination. Elective testicular biopsy to detect occult leukemia, previously a common practice, is probably of little value with improved treatments (Pui, Dahl, and Bowman et al. 1985). After cessation of chemotherapy, children should be evaluated for their school, social, and vocational development as well as their remission status.

RELAPSED ALL

Relapse is the reappearance of leukemia at any site in the body. Although most relapses occur during treatment or within the first two years after therapy has stopped, initial relapses have been observed as long as 10 years after diagnosis. Anemia, leukocytosis, leukopenia, thrombocytopenia, enlargement of liver or spleen, bone pain, fever, or a sudden decrease in tolerance to chemotherapy may signal bone marrow relapse. The outlook for children who relapse in bone marrow during or shortly after treatment is extremely poor; most of these patients have short second remissions and eventually die (Rivera et al. 1978). When relapse occurs more than six months after elective cessation of therapy, the prospects for inducing and maintaining a new remission are clearly better (Rivera et al. 1976; Rivera et al. 1979; Pui, Bowman, and Ochs et al. 1988). Intensified chemotherapy regimens at the time of relapse have resulted in longer durations of second remission and even cures in some patients (Rivera et al. 1986). In some relapsed patients, especially those with a short initial marrow remission (<18 months), allogeneic bone marrow transplantation with hyperfractionated total-body irradiation and ablative chemotherapy is more effective than chemotherapy alone (Butturini et al. 1987; Brochstein et al. 1987; Coccia et al. 1988; Ramsay and Kersey 1990).

Central nervous system relapse may occur despite subclinical therapy. Some patients have repeated episodes of CNS leukemia while the bone marrow remains in initial remission. With the routine examination of cerebrospinal fluid throughout the treatment course and the availability of effective subclinical therapy, overt meningeal leukemia is uncommon today. It is usually diagnosed when leukemic cells are found on routine examination of the cerebrospinal fluid, before symptoms of increased intracranial pressure develop. Five or more mononuclear cells/μL with unquestionable leukemic blasts identified in cytospin examination of cerebrospinal fluid identify CNS relapse. Chemotherapy by lumbar puncture or via an Ommaya reservoir usually clears leukemic cells from cerebrospinal fluid within a few weeks (Bleyer and Poplack 1979). However, cranial or craniospinal irradiation is the only current way to eradicate overt CNS leukemia (Kun et al. 1984). Intensive systemic chemotherapy is also needed for these patients because they are at high risk of subsequent bone marrow relapse (Simone 1981). The outcome of a CNS relapse occurring as the first adverse event during initial remission depends upon the type of subclinical CNS therapy. Children who initially received suboptimal CNS prophylaxis are much more readily salvageable than those who were adequately treated (Nesbit, Sather, and Ortega 1981).

Leukemic infiltration of the testes presents as painless swelling of one or both gonads. Although testicular relapse may occur during therapy, particularly in patients with high leukocyte counts or T-cell leukemia at presentation, most relapses occur within the first year or so after elective cessation of therapy (Nesbit et al. 1980). The disease may be apparent in one testicle only, but the other testicle is frequently involved. As a result of overall improvement in therapy for childhood ALL (especially the use of intermediate-dose methotrexate), the frequency of testicular relapse has decreased substantially (Freeman et al. 1983). Children with overt testicular relapse during continuation therapy tend to have a poor prognosis with rapid involvement of bone marrow or other extramedullary sites, whereas treatment has been generally successful for those who have relapse after cessation of therapy (Bowman et al. 1984). Treatment should include local irradiation to both testes and systemic combination chemotherapy.

Leukemic relapse occasionally occurs at other extramedullary sites in patients in hematologic remission (Bunin et al. 1986). The sites vary widely and include the eye, ovary, bone, tonsil, kidney, mediastinum, and paranasal sinus. As with bone marrow relapse, recurrence during therapy confers a poor prognosis.

BONE MARROW TRANSPLANTATION

Intensive chemoradiotherapy followed by allogeneic or autologous marrow transplantation is an increasingly common treatment of ALL (Kersey et al. 1987; Ramsey and Kersey 1990). This approach mainly treats patients who have had a bone marrow relapse. With better definition of prognostic factors, bone marrow transplantation has also been employed to treat patients with newly diagnosed ALL whose presenting features (for example, specific chromosomal translocation) predict a poor response to chemotherapy (Herzig et al. 1987). The important issue of the relative efficacies and complications of transplantation and chemotherapy has been difficult to address because of the lack of large randomized studies comparing these two modalities.

COMPLICATIONS

The most frequent acute complications of leukemia therapy include nausea and vomiting, stomatitis, diarrhea, alopecia, and bone marrow suppression. Metabolic complications in children with ALL can result from spontaneous or drug-induced leukemic cell lysis and may be life-threatening for patients with a large burden of leukemic cells (Bunin and Pui 1985). The rapid release of blast cell components can cause hyperuricemia, hyperphosphatemia, and hyperkalemia. Some patients develop uric acid nephropathy or nephrocalcinosis. Rarely, urolithiasis with ureteral obstruction occurs after treatment for leukemia (Pui, Roy, and Noe 1986). Hydration, administration of allopurinol and aluminum hydroxide, and the judicious use of urinary alkalinization may prevent or correct these complications.

Diffuse leukemic infiltration of the kidneys can also lead to renal failure. Vincristine or cyclophosphamide therapy may increase the release of antidiuretic hormone. Hyperglycemia develops in 10% of patients after treatment with prednisone and asparaginase and may require short-term use of insulin (Pui, Burghen, and Bowman et al. 1981).

Because of the myelosuppressive and immunosuppressive effects of ALL and its chemotherapy, children with this disease are more susceptible to infections than normal, healthy children. The types of infections in immunosuppressed children with leukemia vary with the treatment and stage of the disease (Hughes et al. 1985). Most early infections are bacterial, manifested by sepsis, pneumonia, cellulitis, and otitis media. *Staphylococcus epidermidis, Escherichia coli, Staphylococcus aureus, Pseudomonas aeruginosa, Klebsiella pneumonia, Proteus mirabilis,* and *Hemophilus influenza* are the organisms usually responsible for sepsis. Any febrile patient with severe granulocytopenia should be considered septic and should be treated with broad-spectrum antibiotics. Granulocyte transfusions may be used for patients with absolute granulocytopenia and documented gram-negative septicemia.

With the use of intensive chemotherapy and prolonged exposure to antibiotics or hydrocortisone, disseminated fungal infections attributable to *Candida* or *Aspergillus* become more frequent, although the organisms can be difficult to culture from blood. Computed tomography (CT) scans are useful for documenting the involvement of the visceral organs. Abscesses of lung, liver, spleen, kidney, paranasal sinus, or skin suggest fungal infection; diagnosis can usually be established by demonstrating the organism in biopsy samples. Amphotericin B is the treatment of choice for suspected or biopsy-proven fungal infections; 5-Fluorocytosine and rifampin sometimes potentiate its effect.

Pneumocystis carinii pneumonia developing during remission of ALL was once a devastating complication, but it has become rare with routine use of trimethoprim-sulfamethoxazole as chemoprophylaxis (Hughes et al. 1987). Viral infections in leukemia patients — particularly those due to varicella virus, cytomegalovirus, herpes simplex virus, and measles virus — may overwhelm the patient's immune defenses. Zoster immune globulin given within 96 hours of exposure usually prevents or modifies the clinical manifestations of varicella (Balfour and Groth 1979). Although adenine arabinoside and acyclovir are both effective against varicella, the latter is less toxic in leukemia patients. Varicella vaccine has been safely administered to children receiving chemotherapy for ALL, with a 90% to 100% seroconversion rate (Gershon et al. 1984). Nevertheless, a large proportion of patients still receiving chemotherapy lack detectable antibody at 18 months after immunization. Other live virus vaccines (poliomyelitis, mumps, measles, and rubella) should not be administered to leukemia patients who receive immunosuppressive therapy. Siblings and other children who have frequent contact with patients should have inactivated rather than live oral poliomyelitis vaccine, and can be immunized against measles, mumps, and rubella (LaForce 1987).

ALL or its treatment can lead to thrombocytopenia. Hemorrhagic manifestations are common in children with this disease, but are usually limited to the skin and mucous membranes. Overt bleeding in the CNS, lungs, or gastrointestinal tract is rare but can be life-threatening. Patients with extremely high leukocyte counts at diagnosis are more likely to develop these complications (Ribeiro and Pui 1986; Bunin and Pui 1985). Coagulopathy attributable to disseminated intravascular coagulation, hepatic dysfunction, or chemotherapy in ALL is usually mild (Ribeiro and Pui 1986). Cerebral thromboses, peripheral vein thromboses, or both, occur in 1% or 2% of children after remission induction treatment with prednisone, vincristine, and asparaginase (Pui, Jackson, and Chesney et al. 1987). The pathogenesis of this complication has been attributed to a drug-induced hypercoagulable state. In general, drugs that can cause impaired platelet function, such as salicylates, should be avoided in patients with leukemia. Irradiation of blood products before transfusion prevents graft-vs.-host disease.

With the success of treatment for ALL, much attention has shifted to the late effects of therapy. Subclinical CNS therapy and intensified systemic treatment have been implicated as causative factors in leukoencephalopathy, mineralizing microangiopathy, seizures, and intellectual impairment in some children (Packer et al. 1987). Leukemia patients also have a significant risk of developing a second malignancy. Reports of brain tumors developing in these patients are of particular concern. Other late effects include impaired growth and dysfunction of gonads, thyroid, liver, and heart (Wheeler et al. 1988). Little information is available on the teratogenic and mutagenic effects of antileukemic therapy; however, no evidence exists of an increase in defects of either kind among children born to parents previously treated for leukemia (Aviles and Niz 1988).

ACUTE MYELOID (NONLYMPHOBLASTIC) LEUKEMIA (AML)

CLINICAL AND LABORATORY FEATURES

The presenting symptoms and signs of AML are similar to those of ALL: fever, pallor, bone or joint pain, fatigue, anorexia, and cutaneous or mucosal bleeding (table 31.6). Prodromal symptoms last for two days to twelve months (median, six weeks). Patients with transient symptoms usually have fever, bleeding, infection, or gastrointestinal symptoms; those with longer prodromes often present with fatigue and recurrent infection. Unexplained menorrhagia is a common presenting feature in teenage girls. Half of the patients have some degree of hepatosplenomegaly. Granulocytic sarcoma (chloroma), consisting of tumorous growth of granulocytic or monocytic precursor cells in the skin or other organs, is also common, especially in infants (Pui, Kalwinsky, and Schell et al. 1988). Occasionally, it precedes the development of leukemia by a few weeks or as long as three years (Meis et al. 1986). Some children have presented with ptosis from periorbital chloroma, cauda equina syndrome, or paraparesis from epidural tumor (Pui, Dahl, and Hustu et al. 1985).

Presenting leukocyte counts range from 0.8 to 750 x 10^9/L (median, 24 x 10^9/L), platelet counts from 1 to 520 x 10^9/L (median, 58 x 10^9/L), and hemoglobin levels from 2 to 15 g/dL (median, 7 g/dL). Disseminated intravascular coagulation or increased fibrinolytic activity associated with hemorrhagic complications may occur in any subtype of AML but is more common in the promyelocytic (M3), myelomonoblastic (M4), or monoblastic (M5) subtypes (Ribeiro and Pui 1986). Several mechanisms account for the coagulopathy observed in these patients; the release of thromboplastin from blast cells is probably the most important. Central nervous system leukemia at diagnosis, manifested by leukemia cells in cerebrospinal fluid, occurs in 5% to 20% of patients (Pui, Dahl, and Kalwinsky et al. 1985). Usually asymptomatic, it occasionally presents as cranial nerve palsy or intracerebral chloroma. An age of less than 2 years, initial leukocyte counts above 25 x 10^9/L, an M4 or M5 leukemia subtype, and an inversion or deletion of chromosome 16(q22) are associated with an increased frequency of CNS involvement (Pui, Dahl, and Kalwinsky et al. 1985; Holmes et al. 1985). A chest x-ray may demonstrate infiltrates caused by pulmonary edema, leukemic infiltration, or pneumonia (Bunin and Pui 1985). Patients with monoblastic or myelomonoblastic leukemia have elevated serum and urine levels of muramidase, a hydrolytic enzyme in the primary granules of myeloblasts or monoblasts causing renal tubular dysfunction with secondary hypokalemia (Osserman and Lawlor 1986). Although metabolic complications are relatively infrequent in AML, children with very high leukocyte counts (>200 x 10^9/L) may present with lactic acidosis and severe compromise of the CNS,

lungs, and kidney secondary to leukostasis (Bunin and Pui 1985). Such patients would benefit from leukaphoresis or exchange transfusion.

Although ALL and AML are not easily distinguishable on the basis of presenting clinical findings, certain subtypes of AML have distinctive manifestations. Acute promyelocytic leukemia is often associated with disseminated intravascular coagulation and serious hemorrhage (Cordonnier et al. 1985). High leukocyte count, gum hypertrophy, skin nodules, and frequent CNS involvement characterize acute monoblastic or myelomonoblastic leukemia (Tobelem et al. 1980).

The definitive diagnosis of AML requires that 30% of the cells seen on bone marrow examination be nonlymphoid blasts; the morphology of the blast cells and their cytochemical staining properties are usually adequate for classification (Bennett et al. 1976). In some difficult cases, electron microscopy may demonstrate myeloperoxidase activity in myeloblastic leukemia and platelet peroxidase in megakaryoblastic leukemia. Bone marrow biopsy is often needed to establish the diagnosis of megakaryoblastic leukemia because of the associated myelofibrosis (Pui, Rivera, and Mirro et al. 1985; Pui, Williams, and Scarborough et al. 1982).

IMMUNOLOGIC MARKERS

The monoclonal antibodies that have identified immunologic subtypes of ALL have in general not reacted

Table 31.6
PRESENTING FEATURES OF 184 CHILDREN WITH AML

Features	Percent (%)
Age (yr)	
<2	19
2-9	34
>10	47
Male	54
Symptoms	
Fever	30
Bleeding	33
Bone or joint pain	18
Lymphadenopathy	20
Liver edge below costal margin (cm)	
1-5	41
>5	12
Spleen edge below costal margin (cm)	
1-5	30
>5	19
Chloroma	16
Central nervous system leukemia	20
Leukocyte count (x 10^9/L)	
<25	53
25-49	17
50-100	13
>100	17
Hemoglobin (g/dL)	
<7	18
7-9	38
>10	44
Platelet count (x 10^9/L)	
<10	9
10-49	36
50-100	28
>100	27
Auer rods	46
Coagulopathy	18

(Source: Pui and Rivera [1987.] Used with permission.)

with the blast cells in AML. Although useful in classifying unusual cases of leukemia and in confirming the AML diagnosis, detection of cell surface markers is not by itself sufficient for the diagnosis of this disease. Moreover, attempts to correlate immunophenotyping results with FAB types have had only limited success (Drexler 1987).

Immunophenotyping studies have disclosed considerable diversity in the expression of surface antigens among AML cells (Griffin et al. 1986). The more undifferentiated cases tend to express early granulocytic antigens, such as CD33 (MY9) or CD13 (MY7). Several antigens, such as CD14 (MY4) and CD11b (Mol), have correlated with the M4 and M5 subtypes of AML. Leukemic myeloid cells tend to express surface antigens in patterns characteristic of immature normal myeloid cells in various stages of development. This suggests that AML originates in either a multipotent myeloid stem cell (CFU-GEMM) or a more mature committed precursor (Griffin et al. 1981). Although immunologic classification appears to have some correlation with clinical outcome in adult patients (Griffin et al. 1986), its prognostic significance in children remains unknown.

GENETIC FEATURES

Most cases of childhood AML have acquired chromosomal abnormalities (Raimondi et al. 1989). Table 31.7 provides a list of the currently recognized, consistent, primary abnormalities (Second MIC Cooperative Study Group 1988). The most frequent alteration, the t(8;21)(q22;q22), is more common in boys and is associated with a higher initial remission rate (Fourth International Workshop 1984). The t(15;17) occurs almost uniformly in cases of M3 AML and its variant form, but has not been reported in other cases. Abnormalities involving the 11q23 region, particularly the t(9;11)(p21-p22;q23), characterize a group of AML cases with predominantly monocytic components. An inversion or deletion of 16(q22) is associated with M4 leukemia, bizarre eosinophilia, and longer periods of relapse-free survival, despite higher frequency of CNS leukemia (Avilés and Niz 1988). The Ph chromosome, t(9;22)(q34;q11), is relatively rare in AML. In contrast to chronic myeloid leukemia, cases of AML with this chromosome have a substantial population of normal diploid cells at diagnosis, and all Ph chromosome-positive cells disappear once remission is induced. Monosomy 7 appears in 4% of children with AML, with or without a preleukemic phase (Weiss et al. 1987). Treatment outcome is extremely poor in this subgroup, for whom bone marrow transplantation should be a prime consideration.

Oncogenes have been implicated in the origin of many human cancers, but none linked to the genesis of AML. The CSF-1 growth factor receptor, encoded by the c-*fms* proto-oncogene, participates in a chemical signaling network that controls the proliferation of monocytes and their committed precursors (Roussel et al. 1987). CSF-1 receptors have been seen on either granulocytic or monocytic blast cells from about 40% of patients with AML (Ashmun et al. 1987). Apparently, the granulocytic cases aberrantly expressed CSF-1 receptors, as they lacked other cytochemical or morphologic features associated with monocytic differentiation. Further study is needed to determine the mechanism of aberrant c-*fms* gene expression in AML and its possible link to the abnormal cell growth. The effects of other hemopoietins, GM-CSF, G-CSF, and IL-3, are also mediated by high-affinity receptors expressed by normal and malignant myeloid cells (Metcalf 1985). Identification and cloning of the genes that encode these receptors will enable their contributions to leukemogenesis to be assessed.

PROGNOSTIC FACTORS

Prognostic factors in AML have not been as clearly defined as they have in ALL. Monocytic leukemia, a young age, a high leukocyte count, large spleen size, coagulopathy, and small megakaryocyte size are among the presenting clinical features that indicate poor treatment outcome (Ribeiro and Pui 1986; Jackson and Dahl 1983; Grier et al. 1987). The cytogenetic subtypes of inv/del(16)(q22) and t(8;21) indicate a somewhat more favorable prognosis (Holmes et al. 1985; Fourth International Workshop 1984). The drug sensitivity of clonogenic leukemic progenitors *in vitro* correlates with treatment outcome in some studies (Dow et al. 1986). Despite these associations, no factors have had sufficient predictive strength to warrant modifications in therapy.

DIFFERENTIAL DIAGNOSIS

The same considerations that apply to the differential diagnosis of ALL apply to AML. In addition, the megaloblastic changes in some patients with AML may mimic those related to folic acid or vitamin B_{12} deficiency (Kobrinsky et al. 1982). Occasionally, AML in children evolves from pre-existing myeloproliferative disorders, or preleukemic syndromes, characterized by a long period of progressive marrow failures (Kobrinsky et al. 1982; Wegelius 1986). Because of the typically small number of blast cells in marrow aspirates, the

Table 31.7
PRIMARY CHROMOSOMAL ABERRATIONS IN AML

Abnormality	Type of leukemia
t(8;21)(q22;q22)	M2
t(15;17)(q22;q12)	M3, M3v
t/del(11)(q23)	M5, M4
inv/del(16)(q22)	M4 with eosinophilia (M4Eo)
t(9;22)(q34;q11)	M1, M2
t(6;9)(p21-p23;q34)	M2 or M4 with basophilia
inv(3)(q21q26)	M1, M2, M4, M7 with thrombocytosis
t(8;16)(p11;p13)	M5 with phagocytosis
t/del(12)(p11-13)	M4 or M2 with eosinophilia
+4	M4, M2
-5/del(5q)	Secondary AML
-7/del (7q)	Secondary AML

diagnosis of malignancy may require demonstration of abnormal karyotypes in the bone marrow cells.

THERAPY

REMISSION INDUCTION

The effective antineoplastic agents for AML have a limited number and narrow therapeutic index. The most effective remission induction regimens include daunorubicin or doxorubicin and cytarabine, with or without 6-thioguanine (Champlin and Gale 1987). Daunorubicin is preferable to doxorubicin during remission induction because of its less severe gastrointestinal toxicity. Approximately 70% to 80% of children with AML attain complete remission; half of the failure cases acquire drug-resistant blasts, while the others succumb to the complications of the disease or its treatment (Weinstein et al. 1983; Lampkin et al. 1987; Creutzig et al. 1985). The intensification of remission induction therapy has led to improved measures of supportive care. Such advances are largely responsible for the higher induction rates achieved.

SUBCLINICAL CNS TREATMENT

Approximately 10% to 30% of children with AML develop CNS leukemia at diagnosis or at relapse (Pui, Dahl, and Kalwinsky et al. 1985; Weinstein et al. 1983; Lampkin et al. 1987). However, there is no definitive prospective clinical trial demonstrating the efficacy of preventive CNS treatment and its use in patients without identifiable leukemic cells in cerebrospinal fluid at diagnosis is still in question. When the duration of hematologic remission improves, the value of CNS prophylaxis may become apparent. Because monocytic or myelomonocytic leukemia and a young age are associated with an increased risk of CNS relapse, these patients should probably receive some form of preventive CNS treatment.

CONTINUATION THERAPY

In patients who achieve remission, further cytoreduction by consolidation therapy is probably required to prevent relapse (Champlin and Gale 1987). However, the value of continuation therapy in frequent courses of less myelosuppressive treatment over several months or years is unclear. The addition of nonspecific immunotherapy or early splenectomy has failed to improve treatment outcome. Only 35% to 40% of children in first complete remission remain disease-free with available chemotherapy (Weinstein et al. 1983; Lampkin et al. 1987; Creutzig et al. 1985; Dahl et al. 1982; Buckley et al. 1989; Amadori et al. 1987).

RELAPSED AML

Several chemotherapy regimens have led to second hematologic remission in about 50% of patients. Patients who relapse while off therapy generally have a longer second remission than do those who relapse while receiving therapy. With chemotherapy alone, very few patients survive long-term after a hematologic relapse. In contrast, CNS relapse in AML does not preclude long-term survival; about a third of these patients will attain a prolonged second remission and cure (Pui, Dahl, and Kalwinsky et al. 1985).

BONE MARROW TRANSPLANTATION

Allogeneic bone marrow transplantation from an HLA-identical donor, most often a sibling, is an alternative approach to therapy for AML and, for some patients, may be the preferred treatment (Champlin and Gale 1987). Several reports indicate that 50% to 60% of children with AML survive after bone marrow transplantation performed soon after they attained a complete remission (Sanders et al. 1985; Dinsmore et al. 1984). Graft-vs.-host disease and interstitial pneumonia account for most of the deaths in the transplantation group. For patients who have had a hematologic relapse, bone marrow transplantation is clearly the treatment of choice. Some investigators have reported long-term leukemia-free survival in as many as 30% of children transplanted early in second remission (Brochstein et al. 1987; Appelbaum et al. 1983). Recurrent leukemia is the major problem of bone marrow transplantation during second remission. Autologous marrow transplantation, with the patient's own bone marrow harvested during remission, is another promising approach (Hurd 1987; Yeager et al. 1986; Gorin et al. 1986; Ball et al. 1986). Since remission marrow is likely to contain leukemic cells, several agents including 5-hydroperoxycyclophosphamide, mafosfamid (ASTA-Z), and monoclonal antibodies have been used to eliminate residual malignant cells before reinfusion of the bone marrow (Yeager et al. 1986; Gorin et al. 1986; Ball et al. 1986). However, the need for this purging procedure is controversial. Preliminary results suggest that one-third of the patients receiving an autologous marrow transplant achieve long-term relapse-free survival. Recently, bone marrow transplantation with family donors mismatched for only a single HLA antigen or unrelated HLA-identical donors has been attempted with partial success (Beatty et al. 1985; Gingrich et al. 1985; Ash et al. 1990).

COMPLICATIONS

Metabolic complications seldom create problems in AML patients. Infection is the major cause of death during the first 10 weeks of intensive chemotherapy treatment. Susceptibility to bacterial, fungal, or viral infection arises from granulocytopenia and immunosuppression due to leukemia and chemotherapy and from the breakdown of anatomical barriers as a result of oral or gastrointestinal mucositis and venous access. Some patients develop typhlitis or necrotizing enterocolitis, a specific syndrome consisting of right-lower-quadrant abdominal pain with rebound tenderness and distension, vomiting, and sepsis (Lea et al. 1980). Typhlitis is most likely due to neutropenia and mucosal breakdown of the ileocecal area with secondary infection. Serious hemorrhagic complications also occur, particularly in cases of acute promyelocytic or monoblastic leukemia associated with disseminated intravascular coagulation (Ribeiro and Pui 1986). Leukostasis often occurs in AML patients with very high initial leukocyte counts, reflecting the failure of myeloblasts to circulate readily through small vessels (Bunin and Pui 1985). Intracerebral hemorrhage and respiratory distress resulting from leukostasis have been fatal in some patients with hyperleukocytosis. Leukaphoresis, exchange transfusion, and administration of hydroxyurea have all been used to reduce large masses of leukemic cells in order to decrease the morbidity and mortality associated with hyperleukocytosis.

ACUTE MIXED LINEAGE LEUKEMIA (AMLL)

The availability of extensive panels of cytochemical and immunologic tests has enabled identification of blast cells expressing both lymphoid- and myeloid-associated cell surface antigens in as many as 20% of children with acute leukemia (Pui, Dahl, and Melvin et al. 1984; Mirro et al. 1985; Pui, Mirro, and Woodruff et al. 1986; Pui, Behm, and Singh et al. 1990b). Dual-staining techniques disclose simultaneous expression of lymphoid and myeloid characteristics on individual blast cells. Acute mixed lineage leukemia (AMLL) is the term most often applied to these cases, although the terms biphenotypic leukemia, hybrid phenotype, lineage infidelity, and mixed lymphoid-myeloid phenotype are also used. The first designation appears to be more appropriate, because of findings that extend the dual-lineage classification to the genomic level (Mirro et al. 1985). Mixed lineage cases are more common in patients with 11q23 karyotypic abnormalities, such as the t(4;11) or t(9;11). Malignant transformation of a pluripotent stem cell capable of development along either a myeloid or a lymphoid pathway, or aberrant gene expression resulting from the leukemogenic event, or immortalization of rare progenitor cells coexpressing features of both lineages have explained such interlineage heterogeneity (Greaves 1986; McCulloch 1983).

The clinical significance of acute mixed lineage leukemia is only starting to emerge. In an earlier study by the Pediatric Oncology Group, myeloid-associated antigen expression in ALL was associated with a low remission induction rate (Weiner et al. 1985). However, a recent study suggested that, in the context of contemporary intensive multiagent treatment, expression of myeloid-associated antigens on lymphoblasts have no apparent prognostic significance in childhood ALL (Pui, Behm, and Singh et al. 1990b). Children with AML characterized by low levels of myeloperoxidase activity and expression of a T-cell-associated antigen (CD2) appear to respond poorly to induction therapy for AML (Pui, Behn, Kalwinsky et al. 1987) but may achieve remission with prednisone, vincristine, and asparaginase, drugs that are usually reserved for ALL.

CHRONIC MYELOGENOUS LEUKEMIA (CML)

Excessive growth of myeloid cells and their progenitors characterizes chronic myelogenous leukemia, a rare hematologic malignancy that accounts for about 2% to 4% of all childhood leukemias. Two types of CML, juvenile and adult, occur in children. Although both forms present with an increased number of differentiated myeloid cells in the blood, fetal hemoglobin level, leukocyte alkaline phosphatase activity, and other features distinguish them (table 31.8).

ADULT-TYPE CML

CLINICAL AND LABORATORY FEATURES
The presenting signs and symptoms of adult-type CML reflect the excessive accumulation of both mature and immature granulocytic cells. Malaise, abdominal discomfort, bleeding diathesis, and bone and joint pain are the most common presenting features. Occasionally, leukocytosis found on routine examination leads to the diagnosis of CML. Splenomegaly is present in most patients; hepatomegaly and lymphadenopathy are less common. Most patients present with a leukocyte count >100 x 10^9/L and thrombocytosis. Leukostasis syndrome manifested by papilledema, strokes, cerebellar signs, respiratory distress, or priapism is common (Castro-Malaspina et al. 1983; Rowe and Lichtman 1984). In addition to decreased alkaline phosphatase activity, neutrophils from these patients display many biochemical and functional abnormalities (Pederson 1982). Bone marrow examination discloses granulocytic hyperplasia, frequently associated with dysplastic eosinophils and basophils. Occasional findings are megakaryocytic hyperplasia or Gaucher-like cells.

Although CML usually remains stable for several months to years, it eventually transforms to a disorder called blast crisis, characterized by an increased number of immature cells. This phase occurs at a median of about three years from the date of diagnosis and may be heralded by a transitional phase of several months duration, with fever, weight loss, basophilia, thrombocytosis or thrombocytopenia, leukocytosis, anemia, splenomegaly, karyotypic evolution, and/or myelofibrosis (Marks et al. 1978; Clough et al. 1979). The predominant blast cell may be either myeloid (70%) or lymphoid (30%) (Rosenthal et al. 1977; Bakhshi et al. 1983). Myeloid blast crisis is heterogenous; myeloblastic, erythroid, and megakaryocytic variants have all been observed. In lymphoid crisis, the blasts have surface markers similar to those of *de novo* ALL (that is, common ALL or pre-B phenotype) and many have increased terminal deoxynucleotidyl transferase activity.

Table 31.8
PRESENTING FEATURES OF ADULT AND JUVENILE FORMS OF CHRONIC MYELOID LEUKEMIA

Feature	Adult	Juvenile
Median age (yr)	14	2
M:F ratio	6:1	2:1
Philadelphia chromosome	Present	Absent
Physical findings		
Skin rash	Unusual	Common
Bleeding	Unusual	Common
Bacterial infection	Unusual	Common
Lymphadenopathy	Unusual	Common with tendency to suppuration
Splenomegaly	Marked	Variable
Laboratory Findings		
Leukocyte count >100 x 10^9/L	Common	Unusual
Thrombocytopenia	Unusual	Common
Anemia	Variable	Common
Monocytosis	Unusual	Common
Eosinophilia and basophilia	Common	Unusual
Fetal hemoglobin level	Normal	15-70%
Erythrocyte I antigen	Normal	Decreased
Decreased leukocyte alkaline phosphatase	Common	Variable
Ineffective erythropoiesis	Absent	Common
Marrow M:E ratio	10:1 to 50:1	2:1 to 5:1
Nature of colony formation	Predominantly granulocytic	Nearly exclusively monocytic
Urine and serum muramidase	Slightly increased	Markedly increased
Immunologic abnormalities	None	Increased immunoglobulin levels, high frequency of antinuclear and anti-IgG antibodies
Clinical Course:		
Median survival (yr)	4-5	1-2
Blastic phase	Common	Unusual

(Source: Pui and Rivera [1987.] Used with permission.)

GENETIC FEATURES

More than 90% of patients have the Ph chromosome, a shortened chromosome 22 that forms by a reciprocal translocation of DNA material between chromosomes 9 and 22, t(9;22)(q34;q11). The cytogenetic abnormality is limited to hematopoietic cells; bone marrow fibroblasts and other mesenchymal tissues do not appear to be involved. The Ph chromosome usually persists during hematologic remission, although it may decrease in frequency. Variant translocations form in some patients, but it always involves chromosomes 9 and 22 (Hagemeijer et al. 1984). Several consistent secondary chromosome abnormalities, including +Ph, +8, i(17q), +19 and −Y, accompany the accelerated or blastic phase (Bernstein 1988).

The molecular consequence of Ph chromosome is the translocation of the c-abl oncogene on chromosome 9 to a 5.8-kb breakpoint cluster region (bcr) on chromosome 22 (Bartrum et al. 1983). This region of chromosome 22 is within a gene called bcr. This mechanism leads to the formation of a new chimeric transcriptional unit containing genetic information from both c-abl and bcr genes; the resulting transcript is a new fused mRNA of about 8.5 kb (Shtivelman et al. 1985). The translational product of this hybrid mRNA is a 210-kd phosphoprotein with tyrosine kinase activity, which apparently plays a role in the pathogenesis of CML (Konopka, Watanabe, and Witte 1984; Daley et al. 1990). Although Ph chromosomes in acute and chronic leukemia appear similar cytogenetically, they constitute a heterogenous group at the molecular level (Kurzrock et al. 1988; Lugo et al. 1990).

PATHOPHYSIOLOGY

G6PD isoenzyme analyses and cytogenetic studies have shown that CML is a clonal disorder of pluripotent hematopoietic stem cells. A monoclonal pattern of G6PD isoenzyme expression or the Ph chromosome has been identified in granulocytes, monocytes, macrophages, basophils, eosinophils, megakaryocytes, erythrocytes, and their committed progenitors (Fialkow, Jacobson, and Papayannopoulou 1977). B-lymphocytes also originate from the malignant clone; several reports of T-lymphoblast crisis suggest that the disease may involve a stem cell capable of differentiating to T-lymphocytes as well.

DIFFERENTIAL DIAGNOSIS

Occasionally, patients with severe infections, congenital heart disease, or metastatic cancer present with a leukemoid reaction. In these disorders, the leukocyte counts are lower than in CML, the differential counts rarely reveal blasts, and leukocyte alkaline phosphatase scores and karyotypes are normal. Some patients with adult-type CML may present in lymphoid blast crisis; in most instances, molecular studies can distinguish these cases from Ph-positive ALL (Clark et al. 1987; Kurzrock et al. 1988; Lugo et al. 1990).

TREATMENT

The lack of differential drug sensitivity of the malignant and normal hematopoietic cells in CML is the major obstacle to successful treatment. The median survival of patients with Ph-positive CML, about three years, has not been altered by chemotherapy. During the chronic phase, busulfan or hydroxyurea controls symptoms or signs by suppressing the growth of malignant cells. Hydroxyurea is sometimes preferred because it is less toxic. Recent clinical trials indicate that recombinant human alpha interferon is effective in inducing hematologic remission in most patients in chronic phase and in suppressing the Ph chromosome in some patients (Talpaz et al. 1986). Treatment for blast crisis has been disappointing. Although 60% of patients with lymphoid and 20% with myeloid blast crisis can achieve remission with chemotherapy, the remissions are generally brief. Bone marrow transplantation, currently the only treatment capable of eradicating the leukemic clone, has produced the most encouraging results (McGlave et al. 1987).

JUVENILE CML

Juvenile CML occurs during the first few years of life. Common presenting features are skin rashes, prominent lymphadenopathy, bleeding, persistent infections, pulmonary symptoms, fever, and failure to thrive (Castro-Malaspina et al. 1984). Patients have various degrees of leukocytosis (generally <100 x 10^9/L), thrombocytopenia, and anemia. Monocytosis in the peripheral blood, bone marrow, or both, is a striking finding. Bone marrow examination reveals myeloid hyperplasia and decreased megakaryocytes. Fetal erythropoiesis, which manifests as increased fetal hemoglobin and fetal-type antigens and enzymes, often characterizes this disease (Travis 1983). Leukocytes from the blood and the bone marrow in these patients form predominately monocytic colonies *in vitro* (Suda et al. 1982), in contrast to the myelocytic colony formation in patients with adult-type CML. Although different cytogenetic abnormalities appear, the Ph chromosome is not present in these cases (Castro-Malaspina et al. 1984; Brodeur, Dow, and Williams 1979). Congenital viral infections or persistent Epstein-Barr virus infection may induce a clinical picture mimicking juvenile CML and should be ruled out (Herrod, Dow, and Sullivan 1983). Children with juvenile CML have a more acute course of disease compared to patients with adult-type CML; their diseases do not respond to busulfan or hydroxyurea. Although cytarabine and mercaptopurine have produced responses in some patients, most of them survived only one to two years (Lilleyman, Harrison, and Black 1977). Intensive AML-type combination chemotherapy recently induced a remission in four patients, three of whom have relapsed (Chan et al. 1987). Bone marrow transplantation has produced long-term survival in some patients and is the treatment of choice for patients with a histocompatible donor (Sanders et al. 1988).

CONGENITAL LEUKEMIA

Congenital leukemia is rare; approximately 100 cases have been reported in the medical literature, the majority being AML (Weinstein 1978). Hyperleukocytosis, hepatosplenomegaly, nodular skin infiltrates, and respiratory distress secondary to pulmonary leukostasis generally mark this form of leukemia. Laboratory findings are similar to those of older children with leukemia. Most newborns with AML have the monocytic subtype (Odom and Gordon 1984), although occasional cases of pre-B ALL have been reported as congenital (Spier et al. 1984). Congenital leukemia has been associated with Down's syndrome, Turner's syndrome, trisomy 9, mosaic monosomy 7, Klippel-Feil syndrome, congenital heart disease, and a variant of Ellis-van Creveld syndrome. A variety of disorders in newborns may mimic leukemia. Leukoerythroblastic reaction from bacterial infection, hypoxia, or hemolytic disease should be considered. Other differential diagnoses include intrauterine infection by toxoplasmosis, syphilis, rubella virus, herpesvirus, or cytomegalovirus, and neuroblastoma. Treatment outcome in patients with congenital leukemia has been poor. Complete remissions are usually of short durations, and most patients die within a few months. Recently, several newborns with monocytic leukemia responded well to epipodophyllotoxin therapy (Odom and Gordon 1984).

The leukemoid reaction in neonates with Down's syndrome or trisomy 21 mosaicism poses a unique problem. This condition usually resolves spontaneously over a matter of weeks or months, but some patients with the presumed leukemoid reaction have developed leukemia (Wong et al. 1988). Leukemoid reactions and leukemia are common in children with Down's syndrome and the occurrence of both conditions in a patient may be coincidental. Because it cannot be distinguished with certainty the neonates with true congenital leukemia from those with leukemoid reaction, judicious supportive care and monitoring for a few weeks should be the preferred initial treatment.

REFERENCES

Amadori, S.; Ceci, A.; and Comelli, A. et al. 1987. Treatment of acute myelogenous leukemia in children: results of the Italian cooperative study AIEOP/LAM 8204. *J. Clin. Oncol.* 5:B56-63.

Appelbaum, F.R.; Clift, R.A.; and Buckner, C.D. et al. 1983. Allogeneic marrow transplantation for acute nonlymphoblastic leukemia after first relapse. *Blood* 61:949-53.

Ash, R.C.; Casper, J.T.; and Chitamber, C.R. et al. 1990. Successful allogeneic transplantation of T-cell-depleted bone marrow from closely HLA-matched unrelated donors. *N. Engl. J. Med.* 322:485-94.

Ashmun, R.A.; Look, A.T.; and Roberts, W.M. et al. 1989. Monoclonal antibodies to the human CSF-1 receptor (c-*fms* proto-oncogene product) detect epitopes on normal mononuclear phagocytes and on human myeloid leukemic blast cells. *Blood* 73:827-37.

Aur, R.J.A.; Westbrook, H.W.; and Riggs, W. Jr. 1972. Childhood acute lymphocytic leukemia: initial radiological bone involvement and prognosis. *Am. J. Dis. Child.* 124:653-54.

Avilés, A., and Niz, J. 1988. Long-term follow-up of children born to mothers with acute leukemia during pregnancy. *Med. Pediatr. Oncol.* 16:3-6.

Bakshi, A.; Minowada, J.; and Arnold, A. et al. 1983. Lymphoid blast crisis of chronic myelogenous leukemia represent stages in the development of B-cell precursors. *N. Engl. J. Med.* 309:826-31.

Balfour, H.H. Jr., and Groth, K.E. 1979. Zoster immune plasma prophylaxis of varicella: a follow-up report. *J. Pediatr.* 94:743-46.

Ball, E.D.; Mills, L.E.; and Coughlin, C.T. et al. 1986. Autologous bone marrow transplantation in acute myelogenous leukemia: *in vitro* treatment with myeloid cell-specific monoclonal antibodies. *Blood* 68:1311-15.

Bartram, C.R.; de Klein, A.; and Hagemeijer, A. et al. 1983. Translocation of c-*abl* oncogene correlates with the presence of a Philadelphia chromosome in chronic myelocytic leukaemia. *Nature* 306:277-80.

Beatty, P.G.; Clift, R.A.; and Mickelson, E.M. et al. 1985. Marrow transplantation from related donors other than HLA-identical siblings. *N. Engl. J. Med.* 313:765-71.

Bennett, J.M.; Catovsky, D.; and Daniel, M.T. et al. 1976. Proposals for the classification of the acute leukemias. *Br. J. Haematol.* 33:451-58.

Bennett, J.M.; Catovsky, D.; and Daniel, M.T. 1985. Criteria for the diagnosis of acute leukemia of megakaryocyte lineage (M7): a report of the French-American-British cooperative group. *Ann. Intern. Med.* 103:460-62.

Bernstein, R. 1988. Cytogenetics of chronic myelogenous leukemia. *Semin. Hematol.* 25:20-34.

Bishop, J.M. 1988. The molecular genetics of cancer: 1988. *Leukemia* 2:199-208.

Bleyer, W.A., and Poplack, D.G. 1979. Intraventricular vs. intralumbar methotrexate for central nervous system leukemia: prolonged remission with the Ommaya reservoir. *Med. Pediatr. Oncol.* 6:207-13.

Bowman, W.P.; Aur, R.J.A.; and Hustu, H.O. et al. 1984. Isolated testicular relapse in acute lymphocytic leukemia of childhood: categories and influence on survival. *J. Clin. Oncol.* 2:924-29.

Breatnach, F.; Chessells, J.M.; and Greaves, M.F. 1981. The aplastic presentation of childhood leukaemia: a feature of common ALL. *Br. J. Haematol.* 49:387-93.

Brochstein, J.A.; Kernan, N.A.; and Groshen, S. et al. 1987. Allogeneic bone marrow transplantation after hyperfractionated total-body irradiation and cyclophosphamide in children with acute leukemia. *N. Engl. J. Med.* 317:1618-24.

Brodeur, G.M.; Dow, L.W.; and Williams, D.L. 1979. Cytogenetic features of juvenile chronic myelogenous leukemia. *Blood* 53:812-19.

Buckley, J.D.; Chard, R.L.; and Baehner, R.L. et al. 1989. Improvement in outcome for children with acute nonlymphocytic leukemia: a report from the Children's Cancer Study Group. *Cancer* 63:1457-65.

Bunin, N.J., and Pui, C.-H. 1985. Differences in complications of hyperleukocytosis in childhood acute lymphoblastic vs. nonlymphoblastic leukemia. *J. Clin. Oncol.* 3:1590-95.

Bunin, N.J.; Pui, C.-H.; and Hustu, H.O. et al. 1986. Unusual extramedullary relapses in children with acute lymphoblastic leukemia. *J. Pediatr.* 109:665-68.

Butturini, A.; Bortin, M.M.; Rivera, G.K.; and Gale, R.P. 1987. Which treatment for childhood acute lymphoblastic leukemia in second remission? *Lancet* I:429-32.

Camitta, B.; Leventhal, B.; and Lauer, S.; et al. 1989. Intermediate-dose intravenous methomexate and mercaptopurine therapy for non-T, non-B acute lymphocytic leukemia of childhood: a Pediatric Oncology Group study. *J. Clin. Oncol.* 7:1539-44.

Castro-Malaspina, H.; Schaison, G.; and Briere, J. et al. 1983. Philadelphia chromosome-positive chronic myelocytic leukemia in children: survival and prognostic factors. *Cancer* 52:721-27.

Castro-Malaspina, H.; Schaison, G.; and Passe, S. et al. 1984. Subacute and chronic myelomonocytic leukemia in children

(juvenile CML): clinical and hematologic observations and identification of prognostic factors. *Cancer* 54:675-86.

Champlin, R., and Gale, R.P. 1987. Acute myelogenous leukemia: recent advances in therapy. *Blood* 69:1551-62.

Chan, H.S.L.; Estrov, Z.; and Weitzman, S.S. et al. 1987. The value of intensive combination chemotherapy for juvenile chronic myelogenous leukemia. *J. Clin. Oncol.* 5:1960-67.

Clark, S.S.; McLaughlin, J.; and Crist, W.M. et al. 1987. Unique forms of the *abl* tyrosine kinase distinguish Ph[1]-positive CML from Ph[1]-positive ALL. *Science* 235:85-88.

Clavell, L.A.; Gelber, R.D.; and Cohen, H.J. et al. 1986. Four-agent induction and intensive asparaginase therapy for treatment of childhood acute lymphoblastic leukemia. *N. Engl. J. Med.* 315:657-63.

Clough, V.; Geary, C.G.; and Hashmi, G.K. et al. 1979. Myelofibrosis in chronic granulocytic leukaemia. *Br. J. Haematol.* 42:515-26.

Coccia, P.F.; Strandjord, S.E.; and Warkentin, P.I. et al. 1988. High-dose cytosine arabinoside and fractionated total body irradiation: an improved preparative regimen for bone marrow transplantation of children with acute lymphoblastic leukemia in remission. *Blood* 71:888-93.

Cordonnier, C.; Vernant, J.P.; and Brun, B. et al. 1985. Acute promyelocytic leukemia in 57 previously untreated patients. *Cancer* 55:18-25.

Creutzig, U.; Ritter, I.; and Riehm, H. et al. 1985. Improved treatment results in childhood acute myelogenous leukemia: a report of the German Cooperative Study, AML-BFM-78. *Blood* 65:298-304.

Crist, W.M.; Grossi, C.E.; and Pullen, J. et al. 1985. Immunologic markers in childhood acute lymphocytic leukemia. *Semin. Oncol.* 12:105-21.

Crist, W.M.; Pullen, J.; and Boyett, J. et al. 1986. Clinical and biologic features predict a poor prognosis in acute lymphoid leukemias in infants: a Pediatric Oncology Group study. *Blood* 67:135-40.

Crist, W.M.; Pullen, J.; and Boyett, J. et al. 1988. Acute lymphoid leukemia in adolescents: clinical and biologic features predict a poor prognosis: a Pediatric Oncology Group study. *J. Clin. Oncol.* 6:34-43.

Croce, C.M. 1986. Chromosome translocations and human cancer. *Cancer Res.* 46:6019-23.

Dahl, G.V.; Kalwinsky, D.K.; and Murphy, S. et al. 1982. Cytokinetically based induction chemotherapy and splenectomy for childhood acute nonlymphocytic leukemia. *Blood* 60:856-63.

Dahl, G.V.; Rivera, G.K.; and Look, A.T. et al. 1987. Teniposide plus cytarabine improves outcome in childhood acute lymphoblastic leukemia presenting with a leukocyte count >100 x 10^9/L. *J. Clin. Oncol.* 5:1015-21.

Daley, G.Q.; van Etten, R.A.; and Baltimore. 1990. Induction of chronic myelogenous leukemia in mice by the P210[bcr/abl] gene of the Philadelphia chromosome. *Science* 247:824-30.

Dinsmore, R.; Kirkpatrick, D.; and Flomenberg, N. et al. 1984. Allogeneic bone marrow transplantation for patients with acute nonlymphocytic leukemia. *Blood* 63:649-56.

Dow, L.W.; Dahl, G.V.; and Kalwinsky, D.K. et al. 1986. Correlation of drug sensitivity *in vitro* with clinical responses in childhood acute myeloid leukemia. *Blood* 68:400-405.

Drexler, H.G. 1987. Classification of acute myeloid leukemias: a comparison of FAB and immunophenotyping. *Leukemia* 1:697-705.

Falletta, J.M.; Boyett, J.; and Pullen, D.J. et al. 1984. Clinical and phenotypic features of childhood acute lymphocytic leukemia in whites, blacks, and hispanics: a Pediatric Oncology Group study. In Magrath, I.T.; O'Connor, G.T.; and Ramot, B. eds. *Pathogenesis of leukemias and lymphomas: environmental influences.* pp. 191-95. New York: Raven Press.

Fearon, E.R.; Burke, P.J.; and Schiffer, C.A. et al. 1986. Differentiation of leukemia cells to polymorphonuclear leukocytes in patients with acute nonlymphocytic leukemia. *N. Engl. J. Med.* 315:15-24.

Fialkow, P.J.; Jacobson, R.J.; and Papayannopoulou, T. 1977. Chronic myelocytic leukemia: clonal origin in a stem cell common to the granulocyte, erythrocyte, platelet and monocyte macrophage. *Am. J. Med.* 63:125-30.

First MIC Cooperative Study Group. 1986. Morphologic, immunologic, and cytogenetic (MIC) working classification of acute lymphoblastic leukemias. *Cancer Genet. Cytogenet.* 23:189-97.

Fourth International Workshop on Chromosomes and Leukemia. 1984. *Cancer Genet. Cytogenet.* 11:249-360.

Fraumeni, J.F. Jr.; Manning, M.D.; and Mitus, W.J. 1971. Acute childhood leukemia: epidemiologic study by cell type of 1,263 cases at the Children's Cancer Research Foundation in Boston, 1947-65. *J. Natl. Cancer Inst.* 46:461-70.

Freeman, A.I.; Weinberg, V.; and Brecher, M.L. et al. 1983. Comparison of intermediate-dose methotrexate with cranial irradiation for the post-induction treatment of acute lymphocytic leukemia in children. *N. Engl. J. Med.* 308:477-84.

Gallo, R.C. 1984. Human T-lymphotropic retroviruses. In Gallo, R.C.; Essex, M.E.; and Gross, L. eds. *Human T-cell leukemia/lymphoma virus.* pp. 1-8. New York: Cold Spring Harbor Laboratory.

Gaynon, P.S.; Steinherz, P.G.; and Bleyer, W.A. et al. 1988. Intensive therapy for children with acute lymphoblastic leukaemia and unfavourable presenting features: early conclusions of study CCG-106 by the Children's Cancer Study Group. *Lancet* II:921-24.

Gershon, A.A.; Steinberg, S.P.; and Gelb, L. et al. 1984. Live attenuated varicella vaccine: efficacy for children with leukemia in remission. *JAMA* 252:355-62.

Gingrich, R.; Howe, C.; and Guekin, N. et al. 1985. Successful bone marrow transplantation with partially matched unrelated donors. *Transplant. Proc.* 17:450-52.

Gorin, N.C.; Douay, L.; and Laporte, J.P. et al. 1986. Autologous bone marrow transplantation using marrow incubated with ASTA-Z 7557 in adult acute leukemia. *Blood* 67:1367-76.

Greaves, M.F. 1986. Differentiation-linked leukemogenesis in lymphocytes. *Science* 234:697-704.

Greaves, M.F. 1988. Speculations on the cause of childhood acute lymphoblastic leukemia. *Leukemia* 2:120-25.

Grier, H.E.; Gelber, R.D.; and Camitta, B.M. et al. 1987. Prognostic factors in childhood acute myelogenous leukemia. *J. Clin. Oncol.* 5:1026-32.

Griffin, J.D.; Davis, R.; and Nelson, D.A. et al. 1986. Use of surface marker analysis to predict outcome of adult acute myeloblastic leukemia. *Blood* 68:1232-41.

Griffin, J.D.; Ritz, J.; and Nadler, L.M. et al. 1981. Expression of myeloid differentiation antigen on normal and malignant myeloid cells. *J. Clin. Invest.* 68:932-41.

Hagemeijer, A.; Bartram, C.R.; and Smit, E.M.E. et al. 1984. Is the chromosomal region 9q34 always involved in variants of the Ph[1] translocation? *Cancer Genet. Cytogenet.* 13:1-16.

Hann, I.M.; Evans, D.I.; and Marsden, H.B. et al. 1978. Bone marrow fibrosis in acute lymphoblastic leukaemia of childhood. *J. Clin. Pathol.* 31:313-15.

Herrod, H.G.; Dow, L.W.; and Sullivan, J.L. 1983. Persistent Epstein-Barr virus infection mimicking juvenile chronic myelogenous leukemia: immunologic and hematologic studies. *Blood* 61:1098-1104.

Herzig, R.H.; Bortin, M.M.; and Barrett, A.J. et al. 1987. Bone marrow transplantation in high-risk acute lymphoblastic leukaemia in first and second remission. *Lancet* I:786-89.

Holmes, R.; Keating, M.J.; and Cork, A. et al. 1985. A unique pattern of central nervous system leukemia in acute myelomonocytic leukemia associated with inversion (16)(p13;q22). *Blood* 65:1071-78.

Hughes, W.T.; Feldman, S.; and Gigliotti, F. et al. 1985. Prevention of infectious complications in acute lymphoblastic leukemia. *Semin. Oncol.* 12:180-91.

Hughes, W.T.; Rivera, G.K.; and Schell, M.J. et al. 1987. Successful intermittent chemoprophylaxis for *Pneumocystis carinii* pneumonitis. *N. Engl. J. Med.* 316:1627-32.

Hurd, D.D. 1987. Allogeneic and autologous bone marrow transplantation for acute nonlymphocytic leukemia. *Semin. Oncol.* 14:407-15.

Isobe, M.; Russo, G.; and Haluska, F.G. et al. 1988. Cloning of the gene encoding the δ-subunit of the human T-cell receptor reveals its physical organization within the α-subunit locus and its involvement in chromosome translocations in T-cell malignancy. *Proc. Natl. Acad. Sci. USA* 85:3933-37.

Jackson, C.W., and Dahl, G.V. 1983. Relationship of megakaryocyte size at diagnosis to chemotherapeutic response in children with acute nonlymphocytic leukemia. *Blood* 61:867-70.

Kalyanaraman, V.S.; Sarngadharan, M.G.; and Robert-Guroff, M. 1982. A new subtype of human T-cell leukemia virus (HTLV-II) associated with a T-cell variant of hairy cell leukemia. *Science* 218:571-73.

Kantarjian, H.M., and Keating, M.J. 1987. Therapy-related leukemia and myelodysplastic syndrome. *Semin. Oncol.* 14:435-43.

Kato, H., and Schull, W.J. 1982. Studies of the mortality of A-bomb survivors. 7: mortality, 1950-1978, part I: cancer mortality. *Radiat. Res.* 90:395-432.

Kersey, J.H.; Weisdorf, D.; and Nesbit, M.E. et al. 1987. Comparison of autologous and allogeneic bone marrow transplantation for treatment of high-risk refractory acute lymphoblastic leukemia. *N. Engl. J. Med.* 317:461-67.

Kobrinsky, N.L.; Nesbit, M.E. Jr.; and Ramsay, N.K.C. et al. 1982. Hematopoietic dysplasia and marrow hypocellularity in children: a preleukemic condition. *J. Pediatr.* 100:907-13.

Konopka, J.B.; Watanabe, S.M.; and Witte, O.N. 1984. An alternation of the human c-abl protein in K562 leukemia cells unmasks associated tyrosine kinase activity. *Cell* 37:1035-42.

Korsmeyer, S.J.; Hieter, P.A.; and Ravetch, J.V. et al. 1981. Developmental hierarchy of immunoglobulin gene rearrangements in human leukemic pre-B-cell. *Proc. Natl. Acad. Sci. USA* 78:7096-7100.

Kun, L.E.; Camitta, B.M.; and Mulhern, R.K. et al. 1984. Treatment of meningeal relapse in childhood acute lymphoblastic leukemia. I: results of craniospinal irradiation. *J. Clin. Oncol.* 2:359-64.

Kurzrock, R.; Gutterman, J.U.; and Talpaz, M. 1988. The molecular genetics of Philadelphia chromosome-positive leukemias. *N. Engl. J. Med.* 319:990-98.

LaForce, F.M. 1987. Immunizations, immunoprophylaxis, and chemoprophylaxis to prevent selected infections. *JAMA* 257:2464-70.

Lampkin, B.C., and Wong, K.Y. 1986. Indications for and benefits of intensive therapies in treatment of childhood cancers. *Cancer* 58:481-87.

Lampkin, B.C.; Masterson, M.; and Sambrano, J.E. et al. 1987. Current chemotherapeutic treatment strategies in childhood acute nonlymphocytic leukemia. *Semin. Oncol.* 14:397-406.

Lea, J.W. Jr.; Masys, D.R.; and Shackford, S.R. et al. 1980. Typhlitis: a treatable complication of acute leukemia therapy. *Cancer Clin. Trials* 2:355-62.

Levy, R.; Warnke, R.; and Dorfman, R.F. et al. 1977. The monoclonality of human B-cell lymphomas. *J. Exp. Med.* 145:1014-28.

Lilleyman, J.S.; Harrison, J.F.; and Black, J.A. 1977. Treatment of juvenile chronic myeloid leukemia with sequential subcutaneous cytarabine and oral mercaptopurine. *Blood* 49:559-62.

Look, A.T.; Roberson, P.K.; and Williams, D.L. et al. 1985. Prognostic importance of blast cell DNA content in childhood acute lymphoblastic leukemia. *Blood* 65:1079-86.

Lugo, T.G.; Pendergast, A.M.; and Muller, A.J. 1990. Tyrosine kinase activity and transformation potency of *bcr-abl* oncogene products. *Science* 247:1079-82.

McCulloch, E.A. 1983. Stem cells in normal and leukemic hemopoiesis (Henry Stratton Lecture 1982). *Blood* 62:1-13.

McGlave, P.; Arthur, D.; and Haake, R. et al. 1987. Therapy of chronic myelogenous leukemia with allogeneic bone marrow transplantation. *J. Clin. Oncol.* 5:1033-40.

Magrath, I.T., and Ziegler, J.L. 1980. Bone marrow involvement in Burkitt's lymphoma and its relationship to acute B-cell leukemia. *Leuk. Res.* 4:33-59.

Marks, S.M.; McCaffrey, R.; and Rosenthal, D.S. et al. 1978. Blastic transformation in chronic myelogenous leukemia: experience with 50 patients. *Med. Pediatr. Oncol.* 4:159-67.

Meis, J.M.; Butler, J.J.; and Osborne, B.M. et al. 1986. Granulocytic sarcoma in nonleukemic patients. *Cancer* 58:2697-2709.

Metcalf, D. 1985. The granulocyte-macrophage colony-stimulating factors. *Science* 229:16-22.

Miller, D.R.; Krailo, M.; and Bleyer, W.A. et al. 1985. Prognostic implications of blast cell morphology in childhood acute lymphoblastic leukemia: a report from the Children's Cancer Study Group. *Cancer Treat. Rep.* 69: 1211-21.

Miller, D.R.; Leikin, S.; and Albo, V. et al. 1983. Prognostic factors and therapy in acute lymphoblastic leukemia of childhood, CCG-141: a report from Children's Cancer Study Group. *Cancer* 51:1041-49.

Miller, R.W. 1967. Persons with exceptionally high risk of leukemia. *Cancer Res.* 27:2420-23.

Mirro, J.; Zipf, T.F.; and Pui, C.-H. et al. 1985. Acute mixed lineage leukemia: clinicopathologic correlations and prognostic significance. *Blood* 66:1115-23.

Nelken, R.P., and Stockman, J.A. III. 1976. The hypereosinophilic syndrome in association with acute lymphoblastic leukemia. *J. Pediatr.* 89:771-73.

Nesbit, M.E.; Robison, L.L.; and Ortega, J.A. et al. 1980. Testicular relapse in childhood acute lymphoblastic leukemia: association with pre-treatment, patient characteristics and treatment. *Cancer* 45:2009-16.

Nesbit, M.E.; Sather, H.N.; and Ortega, J. 1981. Effect of isolated central nervous system leukemia on bone marrow remission and survival in childhood acute lymphoblastic leukemia. *Lancet* I:1386-89.

Odom, L.F., and Gordon, E.M. 1984. Acute monoblastic leukemia in infancy and early childhood: successful treatment with an epipodophyllotoxin. *Blood* 64:875-82.

Osserman, E.T., and Lawlor, D.P. 1986. Serum and urinary lysozyme (muramidase) in monocytic and myelomonocytic leukaemia. *J. Exp. Med.* 124:921-51.

Packer, R.J.; Meadows, A.T.; and Rorke, L.B. et al. 1987. Long-term sequelae of cancer treatment on the central nervous system in childhood. *Med. Pediatr. Oncol.* 15: 241-53.

Pedersen, B. 1982. Functional and biochemical phenotype in relation to cellular age of differentiated neutrophils in chronic myeloid leukaemia. *Br. J. Haematol.* 51:339-44.

Pui, C.-H.; Aur, R.J.A.; and Bowman, W.P. et al. 1984. Failure of late intensification therapy to improve a poor result in childhood lymphoblastic leukemia. *Cancer Res.* 44:3593-98.

Pui, C.-H.; Behm, F.G.; and Kalwinsky, D.K. et al. 1987. Clinical significance of low levels of myeloperoxidase positivity in childhood acute nonlymphoblastic leukemia. *Blood* 70:51-54.

Pui, C.-H.; Behm, F.G.; and Raimondi, S.C. et al. 1989. Secondary acute myeloid leukemia in children treated for acute lymphoid leukemia. *N. Engl. J. Med.* 321:136-142.

Pui, C.-H.; Behm, F.G.; and Singh, B. et al. 1990a. Hetero-

geneity of presenting features and their relation to treatment outcome in 120 children with F cell acute lymphoblastic leukemia. *Blood* 75:174-79.

Pui, C.-H.; Behm, F.G.; and Singh, B. et al. 1990b. Myeloid-associated antigen expression lacks prognostic value in childhood acute lymphoblastic leukemia treated with intensive multiagent chemotherapy. *Blood* 75:198-202.

Pui, C.-H.; Bowman, W.P.; and Ochs, J. et al. 1988. Cyclic combination chemotherapy for acute lymphoblastic leukemia recurring after elective cessation of therapy. *Med. Pediatr. Oncol.* 16:21-26.

Pui, C.-H.; Burghen, G.A.; and Bowman, W.P. et al. 1981. Risk factors for hyperglycemia in children with leukemia receiving L-asparaginase and prednisone. *J. Pediatr.* 99: 46-50.

Pui, C.-H., and Crist, W.M. 1987. High risk lymphoblastic leukemia in children: prognostic factors and management. *Blood Rev.* 1:25-33.

Pui, C.-H.; Dahl, G.V.; and Bowman, W.P. et al. 1985. Elective testicular biopsy during chemotherapy for childhood leukemia is of no clinical value. *Lancet* II:410-12.

Pui, C.-H.; Dahl, G.V.; and Hustu, H.O. et al. 1985. Epidural spinal cord compression as a presenting feature of childhood acute leukemia and non-Hodgkin's lymphoma. *J. Pediatr.* 106:788-92.

Pui, C.-H.; Dahl, G.V.; and Kalwinsky, D.K. et al. 1985. Central nervous system leukemia in children with acute nonlymphoblastic leukemia. *Blood* 66:1062-67.

Pui, C.-H.; Dahl, G.V.; and Melvin, S. et al. 1984. Acute leukaemia with mixed lymphoid and myeloid phenotype. *Br. J. Haematol.* 56:121-30.

Pui, C.-H.; Dodge, R.K.; and Dahl, G.V. et al. 1985. Serum lactic dehydrogenase level has prognostic value in childhood acute lymphoblastic leukemia. *Blood* 66:778-82.

Pui, C.-H.; Ip, S.H.; and Dodge, R.K. et al. 1988. Serum levels of CD8 antigen in childhood lymphoid malignancies: a possible indicator of increased suppressor cell activity in poor-risk patients. *Blood* 72:1015-21.

Pui, C.-H.; Ip, S.H.; and Iflah, S. et al. 1988. Serum interleukin-2 receptor levels in childhood acute lymphoblastic leukemia. *Blood* 71:1135-37.

Pui, C.-H.; Jackson, C.W.; and Chesney, C.M. et al. 1987. Involvement of von Willebrand factor in thrombosis following asparaginase-prednisone-vincristine therapy for leukemia. *Am. J. Hematol.* 25:291-98.

Pui, C.-H.; Kalwinsky, D.K.; and Schell, M.J. et al. 1988. Acute nonlymphoblastic leukemia in infants: clinical presentation and outcome. *J. Clin. Oncol.* 6:1008-13.

Pui, C.-H.; Mirro, J.; and Woodruff, L. et al. 1986. Expression of phagocytic activity and myeloid-associated cell surface antigens by blast cells in acute lymphoblastic leukemia. *Med. Pediatr. Oncol.* 14:12-16.

Pui, C.-H.; Ochs, J.; and Kalwinsky, D.K. et al. 1984. Impact of treatment efficacy on the prognostic value of glucocorticoid receptor levels in childhood acute lymphoblastic leukemia. *Leuk. Res.* 8:345-50.

Pui, C.-H.; Raimondi, S.C.; and Behm, F.G. et al. 1986. Shifts in blast cell phenotype and karyotype at relapse of childhood lymphoblastic leukemia. *Blood* 68:1306-10.

Pui, C.-H.; Raimondi, S.C.; and Murphy, S.B. et al. 1987. An analysis of leukemic cell chromosomal features in infants. *Blood* 69:1289-93.

Pui, C.-H.; Raskind, W.H.; and Kitchingman, G.R. et al. 1989. Clonal analysis of childhood acute lymphoblastic leukemia with "cytogenetically independent" cell populations. *J. Clin. Invest.* 83:1971-77.

Pui, C.-H., and Rivera, G. 1987. Leukemia. In Rudolph, A.M., and Hoffman, J.I. eds. *Pediatrics.* 18th ed. pp. 1096-1104. East Norwalk, Conn.: Appleton and Lange.

Pui, C.-H.; Rivera, G.; and Mirro, J. et al. 1985. Acute megakaryoblastic leukemia: blast cell aggregates simulating metastatic tumor. *Arch. Pathol. Lab. Med.* 109:1033-35.

Pui, C.-H.; Roy, R. III; and Noe, H.N. 1986. Urolithiasis in childhood acute leukemia and non-Hodgkin's lymphoma. *J. Urol.* 136:1052-54.

Pui, C.-H.; Stass, S.; and Green, A. 1985. Bone marrow necrosis in children with malignant disease. *Cancer* 56: 1522-25.

Pui, C.-H.; Williams, D.L.; and Kalwinsky, D.K. et al. 1986. Cytogenetic features and serum lactic dehydrogenase level predict a poor treatment outcome for children with pre-B-cell leukemia. *Blood* 67:1688-92.

Pui, C.-H.; Williams, D.L.; and Raimondi, S.C. et al. 1986. Unfavorable presenting clinical and laboratory features are associated with CALLA-negative non-T, non-B lymphoblastic leukemia in children. *Leuk. Res.* 10:1287-92.

Pui, C.-H.; Williams, D.L.; and Raimondi, S.C. et al. 1987. Hypodiploidy is associated with a poor prognosis in childhood acute lymphoblastic leukemia. *Blood* 70:247-53.

Pui, C.-H.; Williams, D.L.; and Roberson, P.K. et al. 1988. Correlation of karyotype and immunophenotype in childhood acute lymphoblastic leukemia. *J. Clin. Oncol.* 6:56-61.

Pui, C.-H.; Williams, D.L.; and Scarborough, V. et al. 1982. Acute megakaryoblastic leukaemia associated with intrinsic platelet dysfunction and constitutional ring 21 chromosome in a young boy. *Br. J. Haematol.* 50:191-200.

Pullen, D.J.; Boyett, J.M.; and Crist, W.M. et al. 1984. Pediatric Oncology Group utilization of immunologic markers in the designation of acute lymphocytic leukemia subgroups: influence on treatment responses. *Ann. N.Y. Acad. Sci.* 428:26-48.

Raimondi, S.C.; Kalwinsky, D.K.; and Hayashi, Y.; et al. 1989. Cytogenetics of childhood acute nonlymphocytic leukemia. *Cancer Genet. Cytogenet.* 40:13-27.

Ramsay, N.K.C., and Kersey, J.H. 1990. Indications for marrow transplantation in acute lymphoblastic leukemia. *Blood* 75:815-18.

Reaman, G.; Zeltzer, P.; and Bleyer, W.A. et al. 1985. Acute lymphoblastic leukemia in infants less than one year of age: a cumulative experience of the Children's Cancer Study Group. *J. Clin. Oncol.* 3:1513-21.

Ribeiro, R.C.; Abromourtch, M.; and Raimondi, S.C. et al. 1987. Clinical and biologic hallmarks of the Philadelphia chromosome in childhood acute lymphoblastic leukemia. *Blood* 70:948-53.

Ribeiro, R.C., and Pui, C.-H. 1986. The clinical and biological correlates of coagulopathy in children with acute leukemia. *J. Clin. Oncol.* 4:1212-18.

Ribeiro, R.C.; Pui, C.-H.; and Schell, M.J. 1988. Vertebral compression fracture as a presenting feature of acute lymphoblastic leukemia in children. *Cancer* 61:589-92.

Riehm, H.; Feickert, H.-J.; and Lampert, F. 1986. Acute lymphoblastic leukemia. In Bloom, H.J. ed. *Cancer in children: clinical management.* 2nd ed. pp. 2-30. Heidelberg, Berlin, New York:Springer-Verlag.

Rinsky, R.A.; Smith, A.B.; and Hornung, R. et al. 1987. Benzene and leukemia: an epidemiologic risk assessment. *N. Engl. J. Med.* 316:1044-50.

Rivera, G.; Aur, R.J.A.; and Dahl, G.V. et al. 1979. Second cessation of therapy in childhood lymphocytic leukemia. *Blood* 53:1114-20.

Rivera, G.; Buchanan, G.; and Boyett, J.M. et al. 1986. Intensive retreatment of childhood acute lymphocytic leukemia in first bone marrow relapse: a Pediatric Oncology Group study. *N. Engl. J. Med.* 315:273-78.

Rivera, G.; Dahl, G.V.; and Bowman, P. et al. 1980. VM-26 and cytosine arabinoside combination chemotherapy for initial induction failures in childhood lymphocytic leukemia. *Cancer* 46:1727-30.

Rivera, G.K., and Mauer, A.M. 1987. Controversies in the management of childhood acute lymphoblastic leukemia: treatment intensification, CNS leukemia, and prognostic factors. *Semin. Oncol.* 24:12-26.

Rivera, G.; Murphy, S.B.; and Aur, R.J.A. et al. 1978. Recurrent childhood lymphocytic leukemia: clinical and cytokinetic studies of cytosine arabinoside and methotrexate for maintenance of second hematologic remission. *Cancer* 42:2521-28.

Rivera, G.; Pratt, C.B.; and Aur, R.J.A. et al. 1976. Recurrent childhood lymphocytic leukemia following cessation of therapy: treatment and response. *Cancer* 37:1679-86.

Robison, L.L.; Nesbit, M.E. Jr.; and Sather, H.N. et al. 1984. Down's syndrome and acute leukemia in children: a 10-year retrospective survey from Children's Cancer Study Group. *J. Pediatr.* 105:235-42.

Robison, L.; Sather, H.; and Coccia, P. et al. 1980. Assessment of the interrelationship of prognostic factors in childhood acute lymphoblastic leukemia. *Am. J. Ped. Hematol. Oncol.* 2:5-13.

Rosenthal, S.; Canellos, G.P.; and DeVita, V.T. Jr. et al. 1977. Characteristics of blast crisis in chronic granulocytic leukemia. *Blood* 49:705-14.

Roussel, M.F.; Dull, T.J.; and Rettenmeier, C.W. et al. 1987. Transforming potential of the *c-fms* proto-oncogene (CSF-1 receptor). *Nature* 325:549-52.

Rowe, J.M., and Lichtman, M.A. 1984. Hyperleukocytosis and leukostasis: common features of childhood chronic myelogenous leukemia. *Blood* 63:1230-34.

Sandberg, A.A. 1986. The chromosomes in human leukemia. *Semin. Oncol.* 23:201-17.

Sanders, J.E.; Buckner, C.D.; and Thomas, E.D. et al. 1988. Allogeneic marrow transplantation for children with juvenile chronic myelogenous leukemia. *Blood* 71:1144-46.

Sanders, J.E.; Thomas, E.D.; and Buckner, C.D. et al. 1985. Marrow transplantation for children in first remission of acute nonlymphoblastic leukemia: an update. *Blood* 66: 460-62.

Saulsbury, F.T.; Sabio, H.; and Conrad, D. et al. 1984. Acute leukemia with features of systemic lupus erythematosus. *J. Pediatr.* 105:57-59.

Second MIC Cooperative Study Group. 1988. Morphologic, immunologic and cytogenetic (MIC) working classification of the acute myeloid leukaemias. *Br. J. Haematol.* 68: 487-94.

Shtivelman, E.; Lifshitz, B.; and Gale, R.P. et al. 1985. Fused transcript of *abl* and *bcr* genes in chronic myelogenous leukaemia. *Nature* 315:550-54.

Simone, J.V. 1981. Leukaemia remission and survival. *Lancet* II:531.

Sklar, J.; Cleary, M.L.; and Thielemans, K. et al. 1984. Biclonal B-cell lymphoma. *N. Engl. J. Med.* 311:20-27.

Spier, C.M.; Kjeldsberg, C.R.; and O'Brien, R. et al. 1984. Pre-B cell acute lymphoblastic leukemia in the newborn. *Blood* 64:1064-66.

Stass, S.; Mirro, J.; Melvin, S. et al. 1984. Lineage switch in acute leukemia. *Blood* 64:701-706.

Stass, S.; Pui C.H.; and Melvin, S. et al. 1984. Sudan black B positive acute lymphoblastic leukaemia. *Br. J. Haematol.* 57:413-21.

Steinherz, P.G.; Gaynon, P.; and Miller, D.R. et al. 1986. Improved disease-free survival of children with acute lymphoblastic leukemia at high risk for early relapse with the New York regimen: a new intensive therapy protocol (report from the Children's Cancer Study Group). *J. Clin. Oncol.* 4:744-52.

Suda, T.; Miura, Y.; and Mizoguchi, H. et al. 1982. Characterization of hemopoietic precursor cells in juvenile-type chronic myelocytic leukemia. *Leuk. Res.* 6:43-53.

Talpaz, M.; Kantarjian, H.M.; and McCredie, K. et al. 1986. Hematologic remission and cytogenetic improvement induced by recombinant human interferon alpha$_A$ in chronic myelogenous leukemia. *N. Engl. J. Med.* 314:1065-69.

Tobelem, G.; Jacquillat, C.; and Chastany, C. et al. 1980. Acute monoblastic leukemia: a clinical and biologic study of 74 cases. *Blood* 55:71-76.

Travis, S.F. 1983. Fetal erythropoiesis in juvenile chronic myelocytic leukemia. *Blood* 62:602-605.

Vogler, L.B.; Crist, W.M.; and Bockman, D.E. et al. 1978. Pre-B-cell leukemia: a new phenotype of childhood lymphoblastic leukemia. *N. Engl. J. Med.* 298:872-78.

Waldmann, T.A.; Davis, M.M.; and Bonjiovanni, K.F. et al. 1985. Rearrangements of genes for the antigen receptor on T cells as markers of lineage and clonality in human lymphoid neoplasms. *N. Engl. J. Med.* 313:776-83.

Wegelius, R. 1986. Preleukaemic states in children. *Scand. J. Haematol.* 36:133-39.

Weiner, M.; Borowitz, M.; and Boyett, J.M. et al. 1985. Clinical pathologic aspects of myeloid antigen positivity in pediatric patients with acute lymphoblastic leukemia (ALL). *Proc. ASCO* 4:172.

Weinstein, H.J. 1978. Congenital leukaemia and the neonatal myeloproliferative disorders associated with Down syndrome. *Clin. J. Haematol.* 7:147-54.

Weinstein, H.J.; Mayer, R.J.; and Rosenthal, D.S. et al. 1983. Chemotherapy for acute myelogenous leukemia in children and adults: VAPA update. *Blood* 62:315-19.

Weiss, K.; Stass, S.; and Williams, D. et al. 1987. Childhood monosomy 7 syndrome: clinical and *in vitro* studies. *Leukemia* 1:97-104.

Wheeler, K.; Leiper, A.D.; and Jannoun, L. et al. 1988. Medical costs of curing childhood acute lymphoblastic leukaemia. *Br. Med. J.* 296:162-66.

Williams, D.L.; Harber, J.; and Murphy, S.B. et al. 1986. Chromosomal translocations play a unique role in influencing prognosis in childhood acute lymphoblastic leukemia. *Blood* 68:205-12.

Williams, D.L.; Look, A.T.; and Melvin, S.L. et al. 1984. New chromosomal translocations correlate with specific immunophenotypes of childhood acute lymphoblastic leukemia. *Cell* 36:101-9.

Williams, D.L.; Tsiatis, A.; and Brodeur, G.M.; et al. 1982. Prognostic importance of chromosome number in 136 untreated children with acute lymphoblastic leukemia. *Blood* 60:864-71.

Wong, K.Y.; Jones, M.M.; and Srivastava, A.K. et al. 1988. Transient myeloproliferative disorder and acute nonlymphoblastic leukemia in Down's syndrome. *J. Pediatr.* 112:18-22.

Yeager, A.M.; Kaizer, H.; and Santos, G.W. et al. 1986. Autologous bone marrow transplantation in patients with acute nonlymphocytic leukemia using *ex vivo* marrow treatment with 4-hydroperoxycyclophosphamide. *N. Engl. J. Med.* 315:141-47.

Zuelzer, W.W.; Inoue, S.; and Thomspon, R.I. et al. 1976. Long-term cytogenetic studies in acute leukemia of children: the nature of relapse. *Am. J. Hematol.* 1:143-90.

Chapter 32

PEDIATRIC SOLID TUMORS

Ching-Hon Pui, M.D.
William M. Crist, M.D.

Ching-Hon Pui, M.D.
Member, Departments of Hematology-Oncology, and Pathology and Laboratory Medicine
St. Jude Children's Research Hospital
Professor of Pediatrics
University of Tennessee, Memphis, College of Medicine
Memphis, Tennessee

William M. Crist, M.D.
Member and Chairman
Department of Hematology-Oncology
St. Jude Children's Research Hospital
Professor of Pediatrics and Chief of Division of Pediatric
Hematology-Oncology
University of Tennessee, Memphis, College of Medicine
Memphis, Tennessee

This work was supported in part by grants CA-23099 and CA-21765 from the National Cancer Institute and by the American Lebanese Syrian Associated Charities (ALSAC).

INTRODUCTION

Approximately 6,000 children in the United States are diagnosed as having cancer each year. Despite steady improvements in therapy, one-third of them will die. The spectrum of cancer in children differs markedly from that in adults. Malignant diseases in adults are generally epithelial in origin, and environmental carcinogens are often the cause. Lung, breast, prostate, skin, and many other cancers common in adults are almost never seen in children. Childhood cancers usually involve the hematopoietic system, nervous system, and connective tissue (Young et al. 1978; table 32.1). Neuroblastoma, Wilms' tumor, retinoblastoma, and hepatoma are rarely found in adults. Following is a discussion of the more common childhood cancers, except for brain tumors (see Chapter 24).

EPIDEMIOLOGY

In the United States, cancer is the second leading cause of death in persons under 15 years of age. The estimated annual incidence of childhood cancer is 124 per million whites and 98 per million blacks (Young and Miller 1975). With the exception of Wilms' tumor, the incidence of childhood cancer varies widely around the world (Editorial, *Lancet* 1973). Israel and Nigeria have the highest incidence, and Japan and India have the lowest (Doll, Meier, and Waterhouse 1970). Some childhood cancers have an unusually high incidence in certain areas, e.g., hepatoma in the Far East, retinoblastoma in India, neuroblastoma in Western Europe, Burkitt's lymphoma in Uganda, and orbital chloroma in Turkey and Uganda. The U.S. incidence of certain cancers also differs racially; for example, Ewing's sarcoma, testicular cancer, and melanoma are extremely rare in blacks.

Most cases of neuroblastoma, Wilms' tumor, retinoblastoma, rhabdomyosarcoma, primary liver cancers, and sacrococcygeal teratoma occur in children under 5 years of age. Many of the tumors in this age group are embryonal in nature, constituting about 40% of childhood cancers. Approximately 9% of cancers in patients under 15 years of age are diagnosed in the first year of life (Brader and Miller 1979). Some of these neoplasms

Table 32.1
FREQUENCY OF MAJOR CANCERS IN CHILDREN UNDER 15 YEARS OF AGE BY RACE IN UNITED STATES*

Category	Percentage of Total	
	White	Black
Leukemia	30.9	24.1
Central nervous system	18.3	21.6
Lymphoma	13.8	11.3
Sympathetic nervous system	7.8	7.2
Soft tissue	6.2	8.6
Kidney	5.8	9.0
Bone	4.7	3.6
Retinoblastoma	2.5	4.1
Gonadal and germ cell	2.0	3.6
Miscellaneous	8.0	6.9

*(Adopted from Young, Heise, and Silverberg et al. [1978].)

may have developed prenatally due to prezygotic or intrauterine events. The non-Hodgkin's lymphomas (NHLs) are more common than Hodgkin's disease (HD) in the first decade of life, but HD becomes more common than the NHLs in adolescents and young adults. The incidence of ovarian, testicular, bone, and thyroid tumors increases during the adolescent years. Several cancers, including Hodgkin's disease, osteosarcoma, testicular cancer, and certain brain tumors, have more than one prominent age peak in incidence; such bimodal or multimodal age peaks suggest heterogenous causes (Gutensohn 1982).

Cancer occurs more often in males than females (1.2:1) in both children and adults. Although gonad and skin cancers are more frequent in females, lymphomas and medulloblastomas occur more often in males. Lymphomas have the highest male-to-female ratio (2 to 3:1), a finding partly accounted for by the X-linked immunodeficiency disorders associated with a markedly increased incidence of malignant lymphomas (Young and Miller 1975).

ETIOLOGY

PRENATAL FACTORS

Maternal cancer is seldom transmitted across the placenta to the fetus, although rare cases of melanoma, lymphoma, and bronchogenic carcinoma have spread in this manner. One study found an almost 1.5-fold increase in childhood cancers to be associated with prenatal exposure to diagnostic irradiation, but other investigators have not been able to substantiate this finding. Moreover, no significant increase in mortality from cancer was noted in progeny of atomic bomb survivors who had prenatal exposure to irradiation (Jablon and Kato 1970).

Several drugs and chemicals have been implicated as carcinogens after *in utero* exposure. A relationship between *in utero* exposure to diethylstilbestrol (DES) or its structurally similar synthetic analogs during the first half of pregnancy and subsequent development of clear-cell adenocarcinoma of the vagina or cervix is well established (Herbst et al. 1977). Also, some males exposed to DES *in utero* have developed seminomas. Some children with fetal hydantoin syndrome have developed neuroblastomas; hepatoma, neuroblastoma, and adrenocortical carcinoma have been associated with fetal alcohol syndrome. Because of the apparent correlation between exposure to mutagenic and carcinogenic agents and increased incidence of cancers, laboratory screening tests for carcinogens in humans, such as the Ames test, are useful for evaluating new drugs (Ames et al. 1973). However, most childhood cancer cases have no history of prenatal exposure to known carcinogens.

HEREDITY

The great majority of children with cancer have no obvious underlying disorder. However, subgroups of children with certain heritable diseases, chromosomal disorders, or constitutional syndromes are at increased risk of developing a cancer (table 32.2). Most of these patients have distinctive clinical or laboratory features that permit diagnosis before the development of an associated cancer. Patients with genetic forms of cancer have several features in common: earlier disease onset, higher frequency of multifocal lesions within one organ, bilateral involvement in paired organs, or multiple primary cancers. These observations have led to the so-called two-hit hypothesis that malignant transformation occurs after at least two cellular mutational events (Knudson 1971). In hereditary cancers, the first (germinal) mutation presumably occurs prezygotically and, therefore, the first genetic change is present in all somatic cells. Cancer subsequently arises in one or several somatic cells that undergo a second mutation. In the nonhereditary cases, both hits presumably develop as chance events in the same somatic cell. The model fits the age pattern and laterality of retinoblastoma, Wilms' tumor, and neuroblastoma. It also predicts that about 40% of retinoblastomas and smaller percentages of Wilms' tumors and neuroblastomas are heritable. Penetrance is estimated as 95% for the retinoblastoma gene and considerably lower for Wilms' tumor and neuroblastoma genes.

Many forms of childhood cancer occasionally repeat within families. These clusters may result from polygenic inheritance, a single gene defect, exposure to common carcinogens, or a combination of these and other factors. When cancer has occurred in one child, the risk of cancer in siblings is approximately twice that of the general population (Draper, Heaf, and Kinnier-Wilson 1977). If two siblings develop childhood cancer, the risk to other siblings may be even higher. Although the cancers usually have the same form, dissimilar neoplasms have also been reported to aggregate in young siblings. Some families have more than 25% of members affected with cancer at sometime during their lives. The cancers may be of the same histology, developing at a single site or multiple sites in the same organ or paired organs, or of different histology within one organ system. Tumors occur in these family members years or decades earlier than in the general population, and vertical transmission in consecutive generations is consistent with autosomal dominant inheritance patterns. In some families, diverse patterns of cancer develop in both children and adults.

ENVIRONMENT

Cancer incidence is higher in survivors of nuclear bombing, workers exposed to radiation, and patients irradiated for diverse medical conditions (Kohn and Fry 1984). Quality of radiation, total dose, fraction size, dose rate, and other exposure variables affect cancer induction. Type of cancer and rate of occurrence are related to age at exposure. Carcinomas of skin, thyroid,

Table 32.2
CONDITIONS ASSOCIATED WITH AN INCREASED RISK
OF DEVELOPING CHILDHOOD CANCERS

Condition	Associated Tumor
Cutaneous Syndrome	
Nevoid basal cell carcinoma syndrome	Basal cell carcinoma, medulloblastoma
Familial trichoepithelioma syndrome	Basal cell carcinoma
Tylosis (palmar-plantar keratosis)	Esophageal squamous cell carcinoma
Xeroderma pigmentosum	Basal and squamous cell carcinoma, melanoma
Albinism	Squamous cell carcinoma
Werner's syndrome (adult progeria)	Soft-tissue sarcomas, carcinoma
Epidermodysplasia verruciformis	Basal and squamous cell carcinoma
Polydysplastic epidermolysis bullosa	Squamous cell carcinoma
Congenital dyskeratosis	Squamous cell carcinoma, mucous membrane carcinomas
Familial atypical mole-malignant melanoma syndrome	Melanoma, breast, colon, leukemia, lymphoma, sarcoma
Neurocutaneous Syndrome	
Neurofibromatosis	Brain, pheochromocytoma, neuroblastoma, medullary thyroid carcinoma, Wilms' tumor, leukemia, rhabdomyosarcoma, neurosarcoma
Tuberous sclerosis	Brain
von Hippel-Lindau	Brain, pheochromocytoma, hypernephroma
Chromosomal Syndrome	
Down's syndrome (trisomy 21)	Leukemia
Klinefelter's syndrome (47 XXY)	Breast, leukemia, lymphoma, teratoma
Female XY mosaicism (47 XO/46 XY)	Gonadoblastoma
13q-syndrome	Retinoblastoma
11p-, Aniridia-Wilms' tumor syndrome	Wilms' tumor
t(3;8)	Renal cell carcinoma
Bloom's syndrome	Leukemia, lymphoma, colon, squamous cell carcinoma
Fanconi's anemia	Leukemia, hepatoma, squamous cell carcinoma
Ataxia telangiectasia	Leukemia, lymphoma, Hodgkin's disease, brain, gastric, ovarian
Primary Immunodeficiency Syndrome	
X-linked agammaglobulinemia (Bruton's)	Lymphoma, leukemia, brain
X-linked lymphoproliferative disease (Duncan's)	Lymphoma
Severe combined immunodeficiency	Lymphoma, leukemia
Wiskott-Aldrich syndrome	Lymphoma, leukemia, brain
IgA deficiency	Lymphoma, leukemia, brain, gastrointestinal
DiGeorge syndrome	Brain, oral squamous cell carcinoma
Common variable immunodeficiency	Lymphoma, gastrointestinal, brain
IgM deficiency	Lymphoma
Gastrointestinal Syndrome	
Polyposis coli	Colon
Gardner's syndrome	Colon, soft tissue, bone, thyroid, adrenal
Turcot's syndrome	Colon, brain
Peutz-Jeghers syndrome	Gastrointestinal, ovarian, breast
Inflammatory bowel disease	Colorectal
Miscellaneous	
Hemihypertrophy	Wilms' tumor, hepatoma, adrenocortical carcinoma
Renal dysplasia	Wilms' tumor
Sporadic aniridia	Wilms' tumor
Beckwith-Wiedemann syndrome	Wilms' tumor, hepatoma, adrenocortical carcinoma
Gonadal dysgenesis	Gonadoblastoma
Cryptorchidism	Testicular
Multiple endocrine adenomatosis I (Werner's syndrome)	Schwannoma
Multiple endocrine adenomatosis II (Sipple's syndrome)	Thyroid carcinoma, pheochromocytoma
Enchondromatosis	Chondrosarcoma
Chediak-Higashi syndrome	Lymphoma
Schwachman's syndrome	Leukemia
21-hydroxylase deficiency congenital adrenal hyperplasia	Adrenocortical, testicular, mesodermal, neurogenic
Galactosemia	Liver
Hereditary tyrosinemia	Liver
Type I glycogen storage	Liver
Hypermethioninemia	Liver
Alpha-1-antitrypsin deficiency	Liver
Familial cholestatic cirrhosis of childhood	Liver

breast, and salivary glands; sarcomas of bones and soft tissues; and brain tumors and lymphomas may occur in irradiated sites. The latent period between radiation exposure and the development of a secondary solid tumor is several years to more than 20 years.

Certain individuals have increased risk to radiation-induced cancer because of genetic susceptibility. After unusually short latent periods, sarcomas may develop in patients treated for bilateral retinoblastoma, and skin cancers may develop in patients with nevoid basal cell carcinoma syndrome after radiation therapy for medulloblastoma. Patients with ataxia telangiectasia have a defect in DNA repair and are susceptible to lymphoid malignancy and acute radiation toxicity. Sunlight increases risk for skin cancer, but this does not usually occur in young individuals unless they have a genetic predisposition, such as xeroderma pigmentosum or another congenital defect in DNA repair mechanisms.

More than 50 chemical agents have been identified as probable human carcinogens (Report of an IARC Working Group 1980). Children may be exposed to these agents by transplacental passage; contamination of food, water, and air by-products such as aflatoxin B_1; and treatment for benign and malignant conditions. Table 32.3 summarizes a few of the medications and chemicals implicated as carcinogens in humans. The chemotherapeutic agents are usually alkylating agents such as cyclophosphamide, melphalan, busulfan, nitrosoureas, chlorambucil, nitrogen mustard, and procarbazine.

A few human cancers have been associated with specific infections (table 32.4). The association of Epstein-Barr virus (EBV) with lymphoproliferative disease, especially in patients with congenital or acquired immunosuppression, is the most compelling evidence for a viral cause of certain childhood cancers. Exposure to EBV may cause uncontrolled proliferation of polyclonal B cells, which increases the number of B cells at risk for mutational events and may lead to monoclonal B-cell lymphoma. Epidemiologic, serologic, and molecular evidence link this DNA virus to nasopharyngeal carcinoma (lymphoepithelioma) in children. Prolonged hepatitis B antigenemia has been associated with the development of hepatocellular carcinoma. Recently, NHL, Kaposi's sarcoma, and primary lymphoma of the brain have been associated with children who have acquired immunodeficiency syndrome (AIDS) (Kamani, Kennedy, and Brandsma 1988). Papovaviruses (types 6 and 11) are found in the lesions of laryngeal papillomatosis and condylomata acuminata. Types 16 and 18 papovaviruses

Table 32.3
DRUGS AND CHEMICALS WITH CARCINOGENIC POTENTIAL

Drugs or Chemicals	Associated Neoplasms
Chemotherapeutic Agents	
Cyclophosphamide	Leukemia, bladder cancer
Melphalan	Leukemia
Busulfan	Leukemia
Nitrosoureas	Leukemia
Chlorambucil	Leukemia
Nitrogen mustard	Leukemia
Procarbazine	Leukemia
Etoposide	Leukemia
Radioisotopes	
Radium	Osteogenic sarcoma
Thorium dioxide	Liver tumors
Radioactive iodine	Thyroid cancer
Hormones	
Prenatal diethylstilbestrol	Vaginal adenocarcinoma, seminoma
Androgenic steroids	Liver tumor
Estrogen compounds	Endometrial carcinoma
Others	
Immunosuppressive therapy	Lymphoma
Aromatic amines	Bladder cancer
Phenacetin	Bladder and renal pelvic cancer
Inorganic arsenicals	Skin cancer
Coal tar ointments	Skin cancer
Phenytoin	Lymphoma
Chloramphenicol	Leukemia
Phenylbutazone	Leukemia
Intramuscular iron	Sarcoma at injection site

Table 32.4
INFECTIOUS AGENTS ASSOCIATED WITH TUMOR

Agent	Associated Neoplasms
Epstein-Barr virus	African Burkitt's lymphoma, lymphoepithelioma
Hepatitis B virus	Hepatocellular carcinoma
Human T lymphotropic retrovirus (HTLV-I)	T-cell leukemia
Human immuno-deficiency virus (HIV)	Non-Hodgkin's lymphoma, Kaposi's sarcoma, brain lymphoma
Papovaviruses	Laryngeal papillomatosis, condylomata acuminata, cervical cancer
Chlonorchis sinensis	Biliary tract cancer
Schistosoma haematobium	Bladder cancer

may also be agents in carcinoma of the uterine cervix. Other suspected oncogenic viruses in humans include herpesvirus type 2 in cervical cancer, herpesvirus type 1 in certain head and neck cancers, and RNA virus type B in breast cancer.

Nonviral infectious agents with carcinogenic potential include *Clonorchis sinensis* for biliary tract cancer in China and *Schistosoma haematobium* for bladder cancer in North Africa.

GENETICS OF ONCOGENESIS

ONCOGENES AND TUMOR-SUPPRESSING GENES

Proto-oncogenes are heterogenous, normal cellular genes whose protein products are involved in normal cellular growth or differentiation (Friend, Dryja, and Weinberg 1988). Somatic mutations affect these genes or their regulatory elements in specific target tissues and convert them into oncogenic alleles. The classic examples of proto-oncogenes are N-*myc* in neuroblastoma and c-*myc* in Burkitt's lymphoma.

Retroviruses have clear causal roles in a small number of human cancers (Bishop 1985). The viral oncogenes transform target cells after incorporation into their genomes. Certain viruses acquire oncogenes from the genomes of host cells by transduction. Single oncogenes acquired by target cells through mutation or viral infection do not suffice to convert these cells into malignant cells. Instead, transformation of normal cells into primary tumors may require a multistep genetic process involving different classes of proto-oncogenes or other mutant genes. More than 20 distinct retroviral oncogenes and more than 30 cellular proto-oncogenes have been identified.

The term anti-oncogenes (tumor-suppressing genes) was introduced to describe DNA sequences that restrain or confine normal cellular proliferation and seem to behave as dominant repressors of cancer (Friend, Dryja, and Weinberg 1988; Knudson 1985). Both alleles must be lost or rendered inactive to permit tumor development. Experimental fusion of normal and cancer cells suppresses the neoplastic phenotype, suggesting that the cancer cells are missing cellular materials required for the regulation of the normal phenotype.

In childhood cancers, the presence of tumor-suppressing genes is best exemplified in retinoblastoma and Wilms' tumor. In retinoblastoma, ablational mutations affect the two homologous copies of a single gene, Rb, which is mapped to band q14 of human chromosome 13. The deletion of this chromosomal region is associated with predisposition to retinoblastoma. Similarly, deletion of 11p13 is associated with predisposition to Wilms' tumor. Recessive genetic lesions have also been described in some cases of osteosarcoma (13q14), neuroblastoma (1p32-pter), and embryonal tumors (11p15.5-pter) in patients with Beckwith-Wiedemann syndrome. The molecular mechanisms by which oncogenes or tumor-suppressing genes cause or control cancer are likely to lead to new approaches to diagnosis, prognosis, and therapy.

CANCER CYTOGENETICS

Specific chromosomal translocations, identified in particular types of cancers, may provide useful diagnostic and prognostic information. Childhood solid tumors are technically difficult to characterize cytogenetically, but a growing number of consistent abnormalities (table 32.5) have been revealed (Heim and Mitelman 1987). These consist of numerical changes (gain or loss of whole chromosomes) and structural changes (translocations, deletions, insertions, inversions, isochromosomes, duplications). From a genetic point of view, there are three main types of abnormalities. The first is translocation, in which a chromosomal segment has moved from one chromosome to another. This genetic change is often specific for tumor type. The second is a gain of specific genetic material, either by duplication of a chromosome(s) or a portion of a chromosome, or by gene amplification, which is manifested as extrachromosomal double-minute chromatin bodies or as chromosomally integrated, homogeneously staining regions. Gene amplification is a common mechanism for activating oncogenes and is generally associated with more aggressive disease. Neuroblastoma is the classic example of a human tumor that often shows gene amplification. The third type involves loss of genetic material from a specific chromosomal band or region. DNA ablation may involve the loss of tumor-suppressing genes. Deletion of chromosome 1, commonly found in

Table 32.5
CHARACTERISTIC KARYOTYPIC ABNORMALITIES IN SOLID TUMORS

Tumor Type	Karyotype
Rhabdomyosarcoma	t(2;13)(q35;q14)
Wilms' tumor	t/del(11)(p13)
Ewing's sarcoma	t(11;22)(q24;q12)
Malignant melanoma	t/del(1)(p12-p22)
	t(1;19)(q12;p13)
	t/del(6q)/i(6p)
	Trisomy 7
Neuroblastoma	del(1)(p31-p32)
Retinoblastoma	del(13)(q14)/-13
	i(6p)

solid tumors, may confer a growth advantage as part of the multistep process of tumorigenesis.

PRINCIPLES OF DIAGNOSIS

The early diagnosis of a childhood cancer is often overlooked because of atypical course or presentation of what appears to be a common childhood disease. Symptoms of prolonged fever, unexplained pain, or growing masses, especially in association with weight loss, should initiate appropriate tests to rule out cancer.

When a cancer is suspected, the immediate goal is to determine its nature and extent. It is always appropriate to search for metastatic disease before deciding to remove the tumor surgically. When metastatic disease is present, a diagnosis of cancer can often be reached with less invasive procedures such as bone marrow aspiration. Because management of each cancer is distinctive, adequate tissue must be obtained to establish the specific subtype. In rare exceptions a biopsy may be life-threatening, but the tumor location or a urine or serum marker is pathognomonic. The diagnosis should be established by an experienced pathologist who is adept in discerning histologic features. The small round-cell tumors of childhood (i.e., neuroblastoma, rhabdomyosarcoma, Ewing's sarcoma, primitive neuroectodermal tumor, lymphoma) are frequently difficult to distinguish pathologically.

It is important to assess the extent of the cancer to determine prognosis and treatment plan. Staging of solid tumors involves surgery, biochemical studies, and diagnostic imaging techniques. A coordinated approach involving the surgeon and the pathologist is crucial to determining the extent of tumor invasion.

In general, stage I indicates a completely resectable tumor; stage II, microscopically detectable residual disease; stage III, grossly unresectable tumor; and stage IV, widespread metastatic dissemination. A comprehensive approach to patients with solid tumors also includes extensive biologic studies of tumor tissue, including monoclonal antibody analysis and special stains to determine the phenotype, and cytogenetic and molecular analyses directed at determining mechanisms of malignant transformation.

Several presenting clinical features have prognostic value in a variety of childhood cancers. For example, age of less than 1 year is associated with a favorable prognosis in neuroblastoma.

PRINCIPLES OF THERAPY

Modern management of a child with cancer requires a well-coordinated multidisciplinary team approach that draws on the skills of physicians, nurses, psychiatrists, social workers, recreation therapists, dietitians, teachers, and chaplains. Today, most children with cancer in the United States are treated according to research protocols designed to provide the best treatment and to systematically collect information that will improve therapy. Treatment programs involve various combinations of chemotherapy, surgery, irradiation, and biologic therapy.

Surgery is the oldest form of therapy and may be curative alone for localized tumor. For example, surgery is often curative for completely resectable local neuroblastoma in infants, a small Wilms' tumor localized to the interior of one kidney, or a small hepatoma confined to one lobe of the liver. Radiation therapy is especially useful for localized but unresectable tumors such as Hodgkin's disease that tend to spread predictably to contiguous sites.

For most childhood cancers, including some apparently totally resected tumors, chemotherapy is an essential treatment component. Based on a mathematical (Goldie-Coldman) model, many front-line therapies include aggressive early therapy that rotates several noncross-resistant effective single agents or drug pairs in the highest doses possible to increase the fractional kill of malignant cells before drug resistance develops (Goldie, Coldman, and Gudauskas 1982). Therapies are improving because of research efforts. Prolonged intravenous infusion has improved the efficacy of methotrexate and cytarabine and lessened the toxicity of anthracyclines and cisplatin. Continuation therapy is now shortened for certain cancers such as B-cell lymphoma.

Chemotherapy is selected from several classes of agents, including alkylating agents, antimetabolites, antibiotics, plant alkaloids, and hormones. New agents with apparent antitumor activity can be identified after first establishing their effects against tumor cell lines and animals. The few agents of promise are then studied in patients with refractory cancer in a phase I study to assess the maximal tolerated dose (MTD) of the new compound and feasibility of administration by gradually escalating the dosages. After the MTD is determined, the drug is then studied (phase II) as a single agent (or drug pair) in patients with a wide variety of tumors to determine its range of effectiveness. Finally, phase III trials include the agent as part of the combination chemotherapy for use in newly diagnosed patients.

Although marrow transplantation is an important advance in the treatment of refractory cancers, it is still too early to assess its overall impact on survival in children with solid tumors. It is also associated with significant morbidity and mortality (O'Reilly 1983). Graft-vs.-host disease, interstitial pneumonitis, and infection remain serious post-transplantation problems. Current methods of allogeneic bone marrow transplantation require an HLA-matched donor, usually a sibling. Bone marrow transplantation using marrow from partially matched family donors or matched, unrelated donors is investigational. Another approach for patients who lack matched family donors has been autologous bone marrow transplantation (Kaizer and Chow 1984). After a patient's own marrow is harvested, supralethal irradiation or high-dose chemotherapy is administered

to ablate all tumor. The stored marrow is then reinfused to repopulate the bone marrow. Autologous transplantation has been studied in a number of childhood cancers with some early successes.

Researchers are investigating various biologic response modifiers, such as monoclonal antibodies, interferons, interleukins, and colony-stimulating factors. Interleukin-2 treatment, by enhancing host antitumor immune response, has produced tumor regression in some adults with refractory cancers (Rosenberg et al. 1985). Recombinant granulocyte-macrophage or granulocyte-colony stimulating factor can enhance bone marrow recovery and decrease marrow suppression by chemotherapy (Nienhuis 1988). These hormones may make patients better able to tolerate more chemotherapy, with the expectation of better treatment response. These approaches show great promise.

SUPPORTIVE CARE

The disease and its treatment cause complications. In lymphoid malignancies with large tumor burdens, expeditious management is required to correct severe metabolic derangements such as hyperuricemia, hypercalcemia, hyperphosphatemia, hyperkalemia, and lactic acidosis. Frequently, bone marrow is suppressed in children with cancer, and transfusions of blood products are needed. In immunosuppressed patients, irradiated blood products are indicated to prevent graft-vs.-host disease. Broadspectrum antibiotics in combination should be used in neutropenic patients with fever. Because of generalized immunosuppression, these patients are also predisposed to viral and fungal infections. Fungal infection is a particular concern in neutropenic children who have received prolonged antibiotic therapy.

Attention should also be paid to proper nutrition, adequate pain control, and management of chemotherapy-induced nausea and vomiting. The development of the indwelling vascular catheter and other venous access devices has dramatically improved therapy delivery (Hickman et al. 1979). Physicians should be sensitive to cancer's emotional impact on patients and their families. Care of adolescents with cancer is particularly difficult because of the anticipated physical changes and the limitations on daily activities after cancer treatment. Honesty, as well as a positive and hopeful attitude, are important in dealing with child and parents. Whenever possible, the child should remain in school and with classmates.

Physicians should also be familiar with drug-induced toxicities (table 32.6). Unfortunately, therapy may produce serious late sequelae, such as hormonal deficiency, neurologic dysfunction, liver cirrhosis, pulmonary fibrosis, cardiomyopathy, renal dysfunction, and hearing or visual impairment. Second cancers that may occur 10 to 15 years after treatment are a particular concern. Children who have been treated for cancer should be followed routinely.

Table 32.6
COMMON TOXICITIES ASSOCIATED WITH ANTICANCER AGENTS

Agent	Toxicities
Antimetabolites	
Methotrexate	Myelosuppression, mucositis, hepatitis
Cytarabine	Myelosuppression, mucositis, hepatitis, fever, vomiting
6-thioguanine	Myelosuppression
6-mercaptopurine	Myelosuppression, mucositis, vomiting, hepatitis
Alkylating Agents	
Cyclophosphamide	Myelosuppression, hemorrhagic cystitis, sterility, vomiting, carcinogenisis
Nitrogen mustard	Myelosuppression, phlebitis, vomiting, sterility, carcinogenesis
Chlorambucil/ melphalan/busulfan	Myelosuppression, immunosuppression, carcinogenesis
Procarbazine	Myelosuppression, mucositis, neuropathy
Antibiotics	
Doxorubicin/ daunorubicin	Myelosuppression, cardiomyopathy, vomiting, mucositis, alopecia, tissue necrosis from extravasation
Actinomycin D	Myelosuppression, vomiting, mucositis, alopecia, radiation sensitization
Bleomycin	Vomiting, pulmonary fibrosis, dermatitis, alopecia
Vinca Alkaloids	
Vincristine	Peripheral neuropathy, alopecia, constipation, tissue necrosis from extravasation, inappropriate ADH secretion
Vinblastine	Myelosuppression, vomiting, mucositis
Miscellaneous Agents	
Teniposide/etoposide	Myelosuppression, hypersensitivity, fever, hypotension, mucositis
L-asparaginase	Hypersensitivity, hyperglycemia, pancreatitis, coagulopathy, hepatic dysfunction
Cisplatin	Vomiting, nephrotoxicity, ototoxicity
Hydroxyurea	Myelosuppression
Steroids	Cushing's syndrome, diabetes mellitus, osteoporosis, hypertension, peptic ulcer, pancreatitis, personality changes

NON-HODGKIN'S LYMPHOMA

Non-Hodgkin's lymphoma (NHL) designates a heterogenous group of malignant lymphoproliferative disorders. They may resemble Hodgkin's disease (HD) in clinical presentation, but they differ histologically in clinical behavior and pattern of spread and require different therapies. The follicular types of NHL, frequently encountered in adults, are rarely seen in children, who instead have diffuse, high-grade neoplasms.

EPIDEMIOLOGY

NHL occurs one and one-half times more frequently in children than does HD, and its relative incidence increases throughout childhood. The disease occurs more often in males than in females (2 to 3:1). Constitutional and acquired aberrations in the immune system have been linked to increased risk of lymphomas (Fraumeni and Hoover 1977). Childhood NHL constitutes more than half the neoplasms associated with inborn immunodeficiency; B-cell lymphomas account for most of these tumors. The inherited immunodeficiencies associated with lymphoid malignancy include ataxia telangiectasia, Wiskott-Aldrich syndrome, common variable immunodeficiency, severe combined immunodeficiency, isolated deficiencies of IgA and IgM, X-linked lymphoproliferative syndrome, Bloom's syndrome, and other familial immunodeficiency states (Filipovich, Spector, and Kersey 1980). The incidence of lymphoma is also increased in immunosuppressed patients after renal transplantation. In patients with immunodeficiency, chronic immunostimulation by an infectious agent may cause uncontrolled proliferation of lymphoid cells and eventually lead to lymphomatous transformation. Chronic immunostimulation by malaria and intestinal parasite infestation in Africa and the Middle East, respectively, has been cited as a potential cofactor in triggering NHL.

EBV has been linked to African Burkitt's lymphoma. Tumor cells from these patients usually have integrated viral DNA and express EBV nuclear antigens, and patients have high antibody titers against the virus. Some cases of T-cell lymphoma and leukemia have been associated with human T-cell lymphotropic virus (HTLV-I) (Blayney et al. 1983). NHL has been found in patients with human immunodeficiency virus (HIV) infection (Ziegler et al. 1984). The exact mechanisms by which viral infections are linked to the development of NHL remains to be determined, but it is important to emphasize that most cases of childhood NHL have no known predisposing factor.

PATHOLOGY AND CLASSIFICATION

Childhood NHL is divided into three major subgroups: undifferentiated or small noncleaved-cell, lymphoblastic, and large cell (table 32.7). Undifferentiated lymphomas are composed of small, round, noncleaved

Table 32.7
CLASSIFICATION OF CHILDHOOD NHL

Histologic Type	Approximate Frequency (%)	Immunophenotype
Undifferentiated (small noncleaved cell) Burkitt's Non-Burkitt's	30-40	B
Lymphoblastic Convoluted Nonconvoluted	30-40	Usually T, rarely pre-B
Large cell Cleaved cell Noncleaved cell Immunoblastic	20-30	Usually B, few T, rarely of true histiocyte
Unclassifiable	5-10	

lymphoid cells, predominantly involving extranodal tissues, especially of the gastrointestinal tract, retroperitoneal and pelvic viscera, kidneys, gonads, jaws, thyroid gland, and central nervous system (CNS). The tumors are invariably of B-cell origin, and the cells typically display monoclonal surface immunoglobulin.

Lymphoblastic lymphomas are composed of small, round, immature cells with scant cytoplasm that lacks granules. Nuclei are round with varying degrees of convolution and slightly condensed chromatin. These cells are morphologically indistinguishable from the blast cells of acute lymphoblastic leukemia. The immunophenotype of most lymphoblastic lymphoma in children corresponds to that of cortical thymocytes, predominantly at the middle or late stage of thymic differentiation. Thymus, lymph nodes, liver, spleen, and bone marrow are common sites of involvement. A minority of lymphoblastic lymphomas in childhood are of pre-B-cell phenotype and have apparent skin primaries.

The large-cell lymphomas have been inappropriately called histiocytic. The tumor cells generally have characteristics of large transformed lymphocytes or immunoblasts and only rarely are derived from histiocytes. Most large cell lymphomas are B-cell derived, but a minority bear T-cell markers and some are devoid of identifiable surface characteristics. Common anatomic origins of large-cell lymphomas are lymph nodes, tonsils, adenoids, or Peyer's patches; a minority involve the skin, mediastinum, bone, and other sites. A minority of childhood NHLs are difficult to classify.

GENETICS

Recent advances in cytogenetics and molecular biology have furthered an understanding of the NHL biology. In Burkitt's lymphoma and related B-cell NHL, three reciprocal chromosomal translocations have been detected (table 32.8). In most cases, the distal end of the long arm of chromosome 8 translocates to the long arm of chromosome 14, with breakpoints at 8q24.1 and 14q32.3. In the remaining cases, the translocation involves the same region of chromosome 8 and the long arm of chromosome 22 or the short arm of chromosome 2. In the t(8;14), the c-*myc* oncogene moves from its native site on chromosome 8 to the site of the immunoglobulin heavy-chain gene. In the less frequent t(2;8) and t(8;22), kappa and lambda immunoglobulin light-chain genes translocate from their normal positions on chromosomes 2 and 22, respectively, to the region of the c-*myc* oncogene on chromosome 8. As a result, transcriptional deregulation of the c-*myc* oncogene occurs

Table 32.8
NONRANDOM CHROMOSOMAL
TRANSLOCATIONS IN B-CELL NEOPLASIA

Karyotype	Frequency (%)	Involved Immunoglobulin Gene
t(8;14)(q24.1;q32.3)	75	μ at 14q32
t(8;22)(q24.1;q11)	16	λ at 22q11
t(2;8)(p11-p12;q24.1)	9	κ at 2p11-13
c-*myc* mapped to 8q24.1		

Table 32.9
NONRANDOM CHROMOSOMAL
TRANSLOCATIONS IN T-CELL MALIGNANCY

Karyotype	Involved T-cell Receptor Gene
t(11;14)(p13;q13)	α/δ at 14q11-q13
t(10;14)(q24;q11)	α/δ at 14q11-q13
inv(14)(q11;q32.3)	α at 14q11-q13
t(8;14)(q24;q11)	α/δ at 14q11-q13
t(7;11)(q36;p13)	β at 7q34-q36
t(7;9)(q34-q36;q32-q34)	β at 7q34-q36
t(7;19)(q35;p13)	β at 7q34-q36

and leads to expression at increased levels, an apparently crucial step in the establishment and maintenance of the tumor (Croce and Nowell 1985).

Novel chromosomal aberrations in regions containing the loci for polypeptide chains of the T-cell receptor for antigen have been described (table 32.9) in T-cell NHL (Mecucci et al. 1988). The genes for the α, β, and γ chains of the receptor have been mapped to chromosomal regions 14q11-q13, 7q32-q36, and 7p15, respectively. The first two are the most frequently reported breakpoints associated with T-cell neoplasia. In some cases, molecular alterations have been demonstrated at either the α-chain or β-chain gene locus, suggesting that common mechanisms of chromosome rearrangement involving regions of the T-cell receptor genes result in deregulation of genes important in malignant cell transformation (Finger et al. 1986).

PRESENTATION AND DIAGNOSIS

In children, NHL can arise in any site of lymphoid tissue. Most NHLs grow rapidly; the duration of signs and symptoms before diagnosis is typically a few days to a few weeks. Painless, rapidly progressive lymphadenopathy in the head and neck region is one of the most common presenting signs. The axilla or groin may also be primary sites of tumor. The nodes are nontender and firm, discrete in the early phases of growth, but often confluent later. Patients with an anterior mediastinal mass may rapidly develop respiratory distress from compression of the airway or pleural effusion and signs of superior vena cava (SVC) obstruction, a medical emergency.

Gastrointestinal tumors, most commonly involving the distal ileum, appendix, or cecum, may produce symptoms of obstruction or mimic appendicitis. Intussusception may occur with the lymphoma as the lead point and NHL should be considered in children 5 years of age or older who develop intussusception. NHLs are among the most rapidly proliferating tumors with a high rate of spontaneous cell death and metastatic dissemination. As a result, patients frequently present with serious metabolic complications, including increased serum levels of uric acid, phosphate, and potassium.

Lymphoma of bone produces local or diffuse bone pain. Meningeal involvement may present signs of increased intracranial pressure. Cranial nerve palsies and paraplegia from epidural tumor compression may also be presenting signs. Occasionally, primary intracerebral lymphoma may develop, especially in patients with immunodeficiency.

The definitive diagnosis depends on biopsy, and, in general, the least invasive procedures should be used. Patients who present with massive mediastinal involvement may be very poor candidates for surgery because of airway compression and SVC syndrome. Because these patients often have cervical or supraclavicular adenopathy, a biopsy under local anesthesia should be obtained from these sites. Some patients may have involvement of the bone marrow despite normal blood counts. A bone marrow examination should be done before resorting to thoracotomy. For patients with pleural effusion, thoracocentesis demonstrating malignant cells is often diagnostic. Similarly, cytologic examination of ascitic fluid or bone marrow samples may obviate the need for surgical biopsy in patients with massive abdominal lymphoma. However, if a diagnostic laparotomy has been performed, an attempt should be made to excise all gross tumor.

Before starting therapy, the physician should complete a staging workup, including careful physical examination, a complete blood count, tests of renal and hepatic function, chest x-ray, an abdominal computerized tomograph (CT), examinations of bone marrow and spinal fluid, and a bone scan to determine the disease extent. Staging laparotomy and splenectomy are not indicated. The most common staging scheme is that of St. Jude Children's Research Hospital (Murphy 1980). Children with localized NHL in favorable sites have stage I disease. A single tumor with regional node involvement, a localized primary gastrointestinal tumor, or two tumors on the same side of the diaphragm represent stage II disease. Stage III includes disseminated disease on both sides of the diaphragm, extensive unresectable intra-abdominal disease, and all primary epidural or anterior mediastinal tumors without bone marrow or CNS involvement. Initial CNS or bone marrow involvement (<25% blast cells) in addition to other tumor sites indicate stage IV.

TREATMENT AND PROGNOSIS

The appropriate treatment program varies with the tumor histology and disease stage. Surgery can establish the diagnosis by biopsy and excise localized lymphoma of bowel. Recognition of the rapidly progressive and disseminated nature of childhood NHL led to the application of systemic multidrug therapy, which dramatically improved disease control (Murphy et al. 1989). All children, regardless of stage or tumor histology, should receive combination chemotherapy. For the one-third of patients with localized disease, a number of treatment regimens have produced excellent cure rates, with approximately 90% long-term disease-free survival (Meadows et al. 1989). Researchers are trying to reduce therapy for patients with limited disease in order to decrease acute and late effects. A recent trial showed that six weeks of intensive therapy with prednisone, vincristine, cyclophosphamide, and doxorubicin fol-

lowed by six months of maintenance therapy with 6-mercaptopurine and methotrexate, without radiation therapy, resulted in prolonged disease-free survival in over 85% of cases (Link et al. 1987). CNS prophylaxis was not required for patients who did not have head and neck lymphoma.

General therapy principles for advanced lymphoblastic lymphomas are similar to those that have been successful in high-risk forms of childhood lymphoblastic leukemia (Dahl et al. 1985). The current 2-year disease-free survival is in the range of 60% to 75%.

Management of advanced B-cell lymphomas is based on short-term (three to eight months) intensive combination chemotherapy, including high-dose cyclophosphamide, high-dose methotrexate, doxorubicin, cytarabine, vincristine, and intensive intrathecal chemoprophylaxis. Survival rates of more than 60% have been observed (Patte et al. 1986).

Appropriate treatment for advanced large-cell lymphomas is less clear. In general, multidrug regimens have yielded a survival rate of almost 70%, and the risk of primary CNS relapse appears to be lower. The indications for involved-field irradiation in children with advanced NHL are diminishing because of the effectiveness of chemotherapy regimens.

The outcome for patients who relapse while on treatment is extremely poor. However, current trials using allogeneic or autologous bone marrow transplantation suggest that this may be curative in a fraction of patients.

The most reliable prognostic factors in childhood NHL have been the stage of disease at diagnosis and serum lactic dehydrogenase level (LDH), a reliable indicator of the total burden of malignant cells. More recently, serum interleukin-2 receptor level was found to have independent prognostic value, even after adjustment for stage and LDH level (Pui et al. 1987). Serum interleukin-2 receptors may compete for ligands with the cellular receptors, suppressing the host antitumor response. Children with CNS involvement at diagnosis have a particularly unfavorable outcome.

HODGKIN'S DISEASE

Hodgkin's disease (HD) is a malignant lymphoma with distinctive clinical and pathologic characteristics, possessing features of a neoplasm, an infectious granulomatous disease, and an immunologic disorder. HD is considered a malignancy because the giant cells have aneuploid karyotypes and produce tumors when heterotransplanted into athymic mice (Kaplan 1981). The heterogenous cellular infiltration represents nonmalignant reactions to the tumor cells.

EPIDEMIOLOGY

In the United States, HD is rare in children younger than 5 years and gradually increases in frequency thereafter. The annual incidence in children under 15 years old is 6 cases per million. The disease has a bimodal age distribution, with peaks between 15 and 34 years of age and again over 50. From age 5 to 11, males outnumber females 3:1. The percentage of males declines until age 17, when the adult male-to-female ratio of 1.5:1 is reached. The change in the ratio is due to a sharp increase in incidence among females at the time of puberty.

Progressively better socioeconomic conditions are associated with decreased rates of HD in children, a corresponding rise among young adults, and a shift of histologic subtypes. In Third World countries and lower socioeconomic groups, the onset is earlier, the peak incidence is in the early teens, and the mixed cellularity subtype predominates. Compared with the general population, close relatives of patients with HD have a modestly increased risk of developing the disease, and many cases of "familial HD" have been described. Several surveys have found some degree of association of HD with specific HLA antigens. Neighbor-pairs and occasional clusters have also been reported. Although the cause is not yet established, genetic susceptibility and some environmental agents, including viruses, may influence the development of HD.

PATHOLOGY AND CLASSIFICATION

HD almost always arises in lymph nodes; extranodal primary sites occur in fewer than 1% of patients. The malignant cells normally compose less than 1% of the involved tissue, a feature that has made their isolation and study difficult. These cells are collectively called Hodgkin's cells and include the classical Reed-Sternberg (RS) cells and their mononuclear variants. Cells resembling RS cells have been reported in infectious mononucleosis, rubeola, and phenytoin-induced pseudolymphomatous adenopathy; thus, examination by an experienced hematopathologist is essential to establish the diagnosis.

The histologic features may include sparse to abundant concentrations of neoplastic, inflammatory, reactive, and stromal cells; and lymphocytes, collagen, and fibrous tissue. The Rye classification includes four major histologic categories: lymphocyte predominant, nodular sclerosis, mixed cellularity, and lymphocyte depletion (Lukes et al. 1966).

In the lymphocyte predominant variety, almost all of the cells appear to be mature lymphocytes or a mixture of lymphocytes and benign histiocytes, with only an occasional RS cell. This type affects 10% to 20% of patients and is associated with an early stage disease with the best prognosis.

In nodular sclerosis HD, affecting 50% of patients, islands of RS cells and associated lymphocytes, eosinophils, and histiocytes are surrounded by areas of fibrosis. Clear spaces surround so-called lacunar cells, which are variants of the Reed-Sternberg cell. Because of the amount of collagen, the radiographic appearance of these lesions, especially in the mediastinum, may be slow to return to normal, even when the patient is responding to therapy. Nodular sclerosing HD exhibits a typical regional disease, most frequently involving the anteriosuperior mediastinum and the scalene, supraclavicular, and lower cervical regions.

Mixed cellularity HD, affecting 30% of patients, is characterized by increased numbers of RS cells. Foci of necrosis may be present and extranodal involvement at the time of diagnosis is likely.

The lymphocyte depletion variety affects fewer than 10% of patients. Reed-Sternberg cells predominate the cellular infiltration of the lymph nodes. This type of HD is associated with advanced disease and a relatively poor prognosis.

The HD cell of origin remains controversial. Hodgkin's cells perhaps are the neoplastic counterparts of interdigitating reticulum cells or so-called dendritic cells, the antigen-trapping and presenting cells normally found in the paracortical T-dependent zones of the lymph nodes and the spleen. Studies of cell surface markers and cell cultures have implicated the mononuclear phagocyte system as the source of Hodgkin's cells. Reports based on results of immunoglobulin gene or T-cell receptor gene rearrangements have suggested a lymphoid origin (Sundeen et al. 1987; Brinker et al. 1987). All studies may be flawed because they were performed on cell lines or on mixed-cell populations in which it is not clear which cell type is responsible for the predominant picture. The Hodgkin's cell is possibly a unique cell type derived from a primitive stem cell.

IMMUNOLOGY

More than half of HD patients have defective cell-mediated immunity, as disclosed by impaired reactions to delayed hypersensitivity skin testing, impaired ability to reject skin homografts, and depressed lymphoproliferative responses to T-cell mitogens *in vitro* or in mixed lymphocyte culture (Romagnani, Ferrini, and Ricci 1985). Intrinsic lymphocyte abnormalities, immunosuppressive factors in serum or plasma, increased suppressor monocyte activity, and increased suppressor T-cell activity have all been implicated as causes of the depressed cellular immunity associated with HD (Romagnani, Ferrini, and Ricci 1985). Familial traits of decreased cellular immunity suggest that HD is more likely to develop in hosts with defective immunity. The severity of immunocompromise increases with more advanced disease, less-favorable histologic subtypes, and disease progression or recurrence. The immunosuppressive effects of radiation therapy and chemotherapy worsen the impairment, which is demonstrable even in successfully treated patients in long-lasting, unmaintained remission. The lymphocytes around the RS cells are mostly CD4-positive helper/inducer cells, and there is a corresponding decrease of these cells in the circulating blood. Whether these changes are primary or reactive is unclear. More recently, high serum levels of CD8 antigen, a surface membrane component of suppressor/cytotoxic T cells, were correlated with advanced disease (Pui et al. 1989).

PRESENTATION AND DIAGNOSIS

More than 90% of patients present with painless, unexplained lymphadenopathy involving cervical (60% to 80%), axillary (6% to 20%), and inguinal nodes (6% to 12%). Enlargement of single or multiple lymph nodes is firm, usually discrete, and often first noticed by the patient or parents. Characteristically, no regional inflammation can be found to explain the lymphadenopathy. The apparent growth rate of the lymph nodes is variable; the size of the nodes may wax and wane. Signs and symptoms may be present for a few weeks or many months before diagnosis. About 20% to 30% of children present with symptoms of fatigue, fever, weight loss, night sweats, and pruritus; the likelihood of systemic symptoms increases with clinical extent of disease. Fever may be cyclic, continuous, or intermittent. Rarely, classical Pel-Ebstein fever occurs. These cyclic bouts of high fever last one to two weeks and are separated by afebrile intervals of similar duration.

The tumor spreads initially to contiguous lymphoid areas and later involves extranodal tissues such as the liver, lung, bone marrow, and CNS. Mediastinal or hilar disease is found in approximately one-half of the patients and may cause dyspnea, cough, dysphagia, and SVC compression. Liver involvement is associated early with intrahepatic biliary obstruction and later with hepatocellular disease, but hepatosplenomegaly does not necessarily correlate with organ involvement by HD. Bone marrow involvement may result in pancytopenia. The tumor occasionally extends through neural foramina to compress the spinal cord, causing paraparesis or quadraparesis.

All patients should undergo careful clinical, laboratory, and diagnostic imaging evaluations to define the disease extent. Laboratory studies should include a complete blood count, erythrocyte sedimentation rate, and routine liver and renal function tests. In localized HD, blood counts are normal. With progression, neutrophilic leukocytosis, microcytic hypochromic anemia, thrombocytopenia, and lymphopenia may develop. Rarely, a Coombs'-positive hemolytic anemia, idiopathic thrombocytopenic purpura, or the nephrotic syndrome occurs. The sedimentation rate and serum copper or ferritin levels are useful indicators and should fall to normal levels with successful treatment. These tests could be repeated regularly to detect early recurrence. Bone marrow biopsy, rather than needle aspiration, is necessary to demonstrate HD.

The usefulness of chest x-rays is limited in HD; however, thoracic computerized tomography (CT) has become a critical part of staging. This is the only technique that can accurately assess pericardial, chest wall, and lung extension of disease associated with a mediastinal mass. Magnetic resonance imaging (MRI) may provide even more detail of a mediastinal mass. Abdominal-pelvic CT scan and pedal lymphangiography are complementary in evaluating disease below the diaphragm. CT scanning does not show abnormal lymph nodes in the retroperitoneal area clearly in young children because of the paucity of fat. Bipedal lymphangiography does not delineate the nodes of the celiac axis but allows visualization of the pelvic and lower abdominal, retroperitoneal nodes. There is a high risk of oil embolism following injection of the contrast medium in patients who have massive mediastinal lymphadenopathy or parenchymal pulmonary involvement.

In general, skeletal surveys, liver-spleen scans, bone scans, gallium scans, and intravenous pyelography have limited utility in staging. Although the role of surgical staging laparotomy with splenectomy is controversial, it is widely recommended because the findings of this procedure will alter the clinical stage in approximately one-third of children. Polyvalent pneumococcal vaccine is indicated for patients undergoing splenectomy.

The 1965 Rye symposium on HD offered guidelines for defining lymph node groups, and table 32.10 shows the current staging system for HD that was formulated during an international meeting at Ann Arbor, Michigan, in 1971 (Kaplan 1980; Carbone et al. 1971).

TREATMENT AND PROGNOSIS

Both radiation therapy and chemotherapy are highly effective in the treatment of HD. Radiation therapy has two major disadvantages. First, a staging laparotomy with splenectomy is often necessary to establish the disease's localized nature. Second, the high radiation dose required affects skeletal growth, and, in younger children, extended-field radiation therapy can be unacceptably disfiguring. However, radiation therapy avoids the systemic toxicity and late complications of chemotherapy.

Table 32.10
STAGING OF HODGKIN'S DISEASE*

Stage I	Involvement of a single lymph node region (I) or of a single extralymphatic organ or site (I$_E$).
Stage II	Involvement of two or more lymph node regions on the same side of the diaphragm (II), or localized involvement of extralymphatic organ or site, and of one or more lymph node regions on the same side of the diaphragm (II$_E$).
Stage III	Involvement of lymph node regions on both sides of the diaphragm (III), which may also be accompanied by a localized involvement of extralymphatic organ or site (III$_E$), or by involvement of the spleen (III$_S$) or both (III$_{SE}$).
Stage IV	Diffuse or disseminated involvement of one or more extralymphatic organs or tissues with or without associated lymph node enlargement.

* Each stage can be subdivided into A (no systemic symptoms) or B (presence of symptoms). Patients with B symptoms have one of the following: unexplained weight loss of more than 10% of body weight in the 6 months before admission; unexplained fever with temperatures above 38.5°C; and night sweats.

Stage III disease has been further subdivided into Stage III$_1$, in which disease is limited to the upper abdomen, i.e., spleen, splenic, celiac, or portal nodes; and Stage III$_2$, which includes all other intra-abdominal nodes, i.e., mesenteric, para-aortic, iliac nodes, with or without upper abdominal involvement.

The standard chemotherapy is the 6-cycle MOPP regimen (mechlorethamine, Oncovin [vincristine], procarbazine, and prednisone) developed at the National Cancer Institute (DeVita, Hubbard, and Moxley 1983). An alternative, noncross-resistant 4-drug combination, ABVD (Adriamycin [doxorubicin], bleomycin, vinblastine, and dacarbazine) is equivalent to MOPP in effectiveness for untreated patients with advanced HD, producing a 75% complete response in patients failing MOPP (Bonadonna 1982). The major advantages of systemic chemotherapy, especially in early stage disease, are circumventing a staging laparotomy and obviating the skeletal effects of radiation therapy. However, chemotherapy is associated with late relapses at the site of initial bulky disease, secondary leukemia and sterility after the MOPP regimen, and cardiopulmonary dysfunction for the ABVD regimen.

Radiation therapy has been used for patients with stages I or IIA disease; chemotherapy, with or without radiation therapy, has been used for those with stages IIB, III, or IV disease. In some studies, combined modalities are used for clinically early stage disease to obviate the need for a staging laparotomy. Because local recurrence is a problem with chemotherapy alone, some investigators give additional lower-dose irradiation to large tumors in patients with advanced disease. The goal is to design optimal treatment for patients in various prognostic groups using the minimum therapy needed for cure. Recently, ^{131}I antiferritin antibody and autologous bone marrow transplantation have been tested in adults with advanced disease.

Because of the immune defects, children with HD are susceptible to a variety of infectious complications, such as herpes zoster and *Pneumocystis carinii* pneumonia. It is important to constantly bear in mind that fever may be the only sign of overwhelming sepsis in children who have been splenectomized. Prompt cultures and antibiotic therapy are mandatory until the fever's origin is established. Physicians caring for these children should also recognize the other potential long-term sequelae from treatment, such as thyroid dysfunction, pericarditis, pulmonary fibrosis, ovarian and testicular failure, growth retardation, and a second cancer.

Progress in the treatment of HD has yielded an initial complete remission rate of over 90% and a cure rate approaching 80%. The stage of disease and type of treatment are currently the most important prognostic factors available. The serum interleukin-2 receptor and CD8 antigen levels have important prognostic value and appear to provide much-needed biologic markers of aggressive disease (Pui et al. 1989).

NEUROBLASTOMA

Neuroblastoma stands out among childhood cancer because of its relative frequency, intriguing age-related biologic behavior, and formidable therapeutic challenge. Neuroblastoma represents about 7% of all cases of childhood cancer, yet results in 15% of deaths related to pediatric cancer. This tumor, ordinarily highly malignant, often pursues a paradoxically benign course in infants. There is a high incidence of neuroblastoma *in situ* in infants under 3 months of age. Autopsies performed on infants who died of other causes showed that 0.5% of cases had clusters of primitive neuroblasts in the adrenal gland (Beckwith and Perrin 1963). Based on this figure, the actual incidence of clinically apparent neuroblastoma is approximately 40-fold less than anticipated. Moreover, autopsies of older children fail to demonstrate either neuroblastoma *in situ* or neuroblastoma comparable to the incidence in young infants. Thus, neuroblastoma *in situ* may represent normal embryological structures that usually disappear without progression. Another unusual characteristic of neuroblastoma is its ability to occasionally regress spontaneously.

EPIDEMIOLOGY

Neuroblastoma is the most common malignant tumor in infants, accounting for 50% of all neonatal malignancies and 30% of infant cancers. Congenital and even fetal neuroblastoma have been described. Approximately 50% are diagnosed during the first two years of life, and over two-thirds are diagnosed during the first five years of life. It is uncommon during the second decade of life or later. Neuroblastoma is slightly more common in white children than in black children and slightly more common in boys. Approximately 50 instances of familial neuroblastomas have been reported. There may be a link between neuroblastoma and neural-crest-derived disorders such as neurofibromatosis, pheochromocytoma, tuberous sclerosis, Hirschsprung's disease, and heterochromia of the iris. There are case reports of neuroblastoma in patients with the fetal hydantoin and fetal alcohol syndromes. The geographic distribution of neuroblastoma differs, most notably in a remarkably low incidence of this tumor in the Burkitt's lymphoma belt of Africa.

PATHOLOGY AND CLASSIFICATION

Neuroblastoma originates from neural crest cells that normally develop into the adrenal medulla and the sympathetic ganglia. These cells, sympathogonia, are pluripotent and may develop into ganglion cells, pheochromocytes, or neurofibrous tissue. Tumors derived from this tissue reflect their different stages in differentiation and include neuroblastoma, ganglioneuroblastoma, ganglioneuroma, pheochromocytoma, and neurofibroma. Neuroblastomas have been reported to evolve into ganglioneuroblastomas or ganglioneuromas spontaneously or following chemotherapy or radiation therapy.

Most neuroblastomas consist of small, round cells with little evidence of differentiation. The presence of rosette formation or neurofibrils is a useful diagnostic feature. In contrast to Ewing's sarcoma and rhabdomyosarcoma, neuroblastomas do not contain glycogen and are therefore negative for periodic acid-Schiff stain.

Electron microscopy reveals distinctive features: peripheral dendritic processes containing longitudinally oriented microtubules; and small, spherical, membrane-bound neurosecretory granules with electron-dense cores, representing cytoplasmic accumulation of catecholamines. Shimada and associates have described a histopathologic classification for neuroblastoma based on the degree of tumor cell differentiation and stromal tissue organization pattern (Shimada et al. 1984).

GENETICS

Some neuroblastomas are characterized cytogenetically by deletions of the short arm of chromosome 1 and by evidence of gene amplification in the form of double-minute (DM) chromosomes or chromosomal homogeneously staining regions (HSR) (Gilbert et al. 1982; Brodeur and Seeger 1986). Neuroblastomas are characterized by partial monosomy of the short arm of chromosome 1 in the region 1p32-1pter. One or more genes in this region may be important in the normal regulation of growth and differentiation in neuroblasts. Absence or inactivation of this putative neuroblastoma suppression gene on both chromosomes is associated with malignant transformation. However, deletion of 1p has yet to be identified as a constitutionally predisposing abnormality to neuroblastoma.

Extrachromosomal DMs are found in about 20% to 30% of primary, unrelated tumors and in almost 50% of neuroblastoma cell lines. HSRs are only rarely described in primary neuroblastoma tissue, but they are found in more than one-half of the established cell lines. HSRs may break down and give rise to DMs, which in turn reintegrate into chromosomes in an apparently nonspecific distribution to reform HSRs. Because of the homology to the c-myc oncogene, the amplified DNA segment in neuroblastoma cells is designated N-myc; the normal single copy is on chromosome 2. The mechanism of amplification is unknown, but correlation was excellent between the presence of DMs or HSRs cytogenetically and demonstration of N-myc amplification by DNA hybridization studies. The presence of N-myc amplification is associated with advanced stages of disease, rapid progression, and a poor prognosis (Seeger et al. 1985). Tumors that have a single copy of N-myc per cell at diagnosis rarely, if ever, develop amplification later in their disease course. Thus, tumors with N-myc amplification may represent a genetically distinct subset of neuroblastoma.

IMMUNOLOGY

Neuroblastoma may elicit both cell-mediated and humoral immune responses. Cytotoxic lymphocytes against neuroblastoma have been demonstrated in some patients. Research has found a correlation between a high circulating lymphocyte count, a high percentage of lymphoblasts in the bone marrow, or increased lymphoid infiltrates in the tumor itself, and a more favorable prognosis. Some patients produce antibodies directed against tumor-associated antigens in response to the presence of neuroblastoma. However, some immune responses may interfere with tumor control. Some patients with advanced neuroblastoma appear to have a "blocking factor" in their sera that inhibits the cytotoxic effect of host lymphocytes. Although no clinically useful immunotherapy has yet been demonstrated in neuroblastoma, these findings suggest that manipulation of the immune system may be an alternative treatment.

PRESENTATION AND DIAGNOSIS

Symptoms and signs of neuroblastoma are largely attributable to local problems from the primary tumor or metastases. Neuroblastoma can arise anywhere along the sympathetic nervous system. The most common site is in the retroperitoneal region in either the adrenal gland (40%) or in a paraspinal ganglion (25%). The thorax is the primary site in about 15% of patients, the pelvis in about 5%, and the neck in about 4%. The remaining tumors arise in unusual sites, including the nasopharynx (esthesioneuroblastoma), liver, and intracranial region. In a few children, the primary site is unidentifiable.

The most common presenting symptoms are pain, abdominal mass, lesions other than in the abdomen, and malaise. Abdominal distention may result either from an enlarging primary tumor or from hepatomegaly caused by tumor invasion. The abdominal enlargement may be asymptomatic, but more frequently is associated with anorexia, malaise, vague abdominal pain, and diarrhea. Presacral tumor may result in increased urinary frequency or bladder obstruction. Neuroblastoma that arises from a paravertebral ganglion tends to grow through the intervertebral foramen, resulting in epidural spinal cord compression. This is an oncologic emergency requiring immediate treatment. Neuroblastoma that arises in the posterior mediastinum can cause dyspnea or pneumonia due to airway obstruction. A thoracic primary lesion may be found on routine chest x-ray. Tumor arising from the cervical sympathetic ganglion can produce a Horner's syndrome (miosis, ptosis, enophthalmos, and anhidrosis). When the tumor arises in the ophthalmic sympathetic nerve, heterochromia irides may result. A primary tumor in the nasopharynx usually presents with unilateral epistaxis or occlusion of the nose.

In about two-thirds of patients, the initial findings are related to metastatic disease; these include lymph node enlargement, bone pain, subcutaneous nodules, periorbital ecchymosis with proptosis, pancytopenia, fever, fatigue, and anorexia. Disseminated disease is found in 70% of children older than 1 year of age and in 50% younger than 1 year. Some patients have intractable diarrhea due to tumor secretion of an enterohormone, a vasoactive intestinal polypeptide. Rarely, patients present with an encephalopathy involving the cerebellum (opsomyoclonus syndrome) characterized by progressive ataxia and titubation of the head, myoclonic jerks, chaotic conjugate jerking movements of the eyes, and progressive dementia. Episodes of unexplained flushing and sweating are common, but hypertension is relatively rare. The systemic syndromes occur in patients with all stages of disease and do not necessarily reflect disseminated disease or poor prognosis (Rosen et al. 1984).

Each patient should have a complete blood count, skeletal survey, chest x-rays, bone scan, bone marrow examination, coagulation screen, liver and kidney function tests, and urinary catecholamine determination performed. For abdominal tumors, CT scan has replaced intravenous pyelograms, arteriograms, and inferior venocavograms. Helpful findings include stippled calcifications within the tumor (80% of cases), displacement of the kidney with little or no distortion of the pyelocalyceal system, and occasionally, hydronephrosis resulting from compression of the ureter. On CT scan, neuroblastomas generally have mixed solid and cystic components from hemorrhage or necrosis. CT scan of the head and orbit, chest, or abdomen helps to determine disease extent. MRI may be more useful than CT in evaluating epidural spinal cord compression and may be obtained in conjunction with a metrizamide myelogram. Newer diagnostic scanning with ^{131}I-meta-iodo-benzyl-guanidine (MIBG) may supersede other methods. MIBG is taken up by adrenergic secretory vesicles and is handled by the cells in the same manner as norepinephrine. In most patients, ^{131}I-MIBG is taken up both in the primary tumor and by metastases.

Excessive production and excretion of catecholamines and their metabolites — vanillylmandelic acid (VMA), metanephrine, and homovanillic acid (HVA) — characterizes many neuroblastomas. Analysis of urinary excretion of the molecules is a useful diagnostic procedure, because almost 90% of the cases will have elevated levels at presentation. A high VMA/HVA ratio (>1:5) is believed to correlate with a better prognosis, and a low level of urinary excretion of the amino acid cystathionine has also been correlated with a more favorable outcome. Other useful serum markers include lactic dehydrogenase, ferritin, and neuron-specific enolase.

Increased levels of these markers are generally associated with more advanced disease and poor outcome.

Table 32.11 outlines the most common staging systems. The Evans staging system is based on the tumor size and extent; it does not include lymph node status, operability criteria, or completeness of removal as a determining factor (Evans, D'Angio, and Randolph 1971). The Pediatric Oncology Group staging system is based partially on clinical and radiologic findings; for localized disease, it is based entirely on surgical and pathological findings. Recently, an international group of conferees has proposed a new staging system taking into account the most important elements of current but inconsistent systems and standardized criteria for response to treatment (Brodeur et al. 1988). Of interest are those infants with apparently widely disseminated disease (Evans stage IV-S) whose tumors may completely regress even in the absence of systemic therapy. Stage IV-S disease is associated with low serum ferritin level and generally lacks N-*myc* oncogene amplification. Although some investigators suggest that IV-S neuroblastoma represents a benign polyclonal proliferative disorder, a recent study demonstrated it to be clonal and hyperdiploid, both accepted criteria of malignancy (Look et al. 1984).

TREATMENT AND PROGNOSIS

For clinically localized tumors, excision of the primary tumor mass will cure over 90% of patients (Matthay et al. 1989; Nitschke et al. 1988). The presence of microscopic residual tumor does not affect outcome and the addition of adjuvant chemotherapy or radiation therapy does not improve this excellent cure rate. For unresectable regional disease, the degree and nature of the local extension should be established by regional lymph node and liver biopsies. The value of surgical resection of the primary tumor in patients with demonstrable metastases has not been established. Extensive and potentially morbid procedures are not warranted because a majority of tumors are initially responsive to chemotherapy. A

Table 32.11
STAGING SYSTEMS FOR NEUROBLASTOMA

Stage	Criteria
Evans Staging	
I	Tumors confined to the organ or structure of origin.
II	Tumors extending in continuity beyond the organ or structure of origin but not crossing the midline; regional lymph nodes on the ipsilateral side may be involved.
III	Tumors extending in continuity beyond the midline; regional lymph nodes may be involved bilaterally.
IV	Remote disease involving the skeleton, parenchymatous organs, soft tissue, distant lymph node groups.
IV-S	Patients who would otherwise be stage I or II but who have remote disease confined to liver, spleen, or bone marrow and who have no radiologic evidence of bone metastases on complete skeletal survey.
Pediatric Oncology Group Staging	
A	Complete gross excision of primary tumor, margins histologically negative or positive. Intracavitary lymph nodes not intimately adhered to and removed with resected tumor must be histologically free of tumor. If primary tumor is in abdomen (includes pelvis), liver must be histologically free of tumor.
B	Incomplete gross resection of primary tumor. Lymph nodes and liver must be histologically free of tumor as in stage A.
C	Complete or incomplete gross resection of primary tumor. Intracavitary nodes* histologically positive for tumor. Liver histologically free of tumor.
D	Disseminated disease beyond intracavitary nodes.

*Intracavitary nodes = nodes in same cavity as primary.

"second look" procedure after reduction of tumor mass may be the treatment of choice.

Chemotherapeutic agents that cause tumor regression, in order of decreasing effectiveness, are cyclophosphamide, cisplatin, doxorubicin, teniposide and etoposide, vincristine, and dacarbazine. Although irradiation may provide local symptomatic relief of disseminated tumor, total-body irradiation or extensive irradiation to treat systemic disease has been disappointing. Experimental treatments include targeted radiation therapy using MIBG or monoclonal antibodies as carriers, bone marrow transplantation, and biologic response modifiers.

The prognosis depends largely on the age at diagnosis and the stage of disease (Green and Hayes 1987). Infants younger than 1 year have a better prognosis than older patients. For patients older than 1 year, the prognosis depends primarily on disease stage. Eighty percent of patients with disseminated disease will die of the disease despite aggressive therapy. As the cure rate improves, other factors may become significant. Regional lymph node involvement and increased serum level of ferritin or neuron-specific enolase at diagnosis correlate with a poor prognosis. The DNA content of tumor cells is important, and hyperdiploidy is associated with a better outcome in infants (Look et al. 1984). Also, amplification of the N-*myc* proto-oncogene in tumor cells is associated with advanced stage and poor outcome (Seeger et al. 1985). There may be two biologically different populations of patients with neuroblastoma; the most favorable prognosis is for infants with hyperdiploid tumors that lack N-*myc* gene amplification.

WILMS' TUMOR

Wilms' tumor, or nephroblastoma, is a malignant embryonal neoplasm of the kidney that usually occurs in young children. It was the first childhood cancer in which combining surgery, radiation therapy, and chemotherapy attained significant cure rates. Through design of a surgicopathologic staging system and recognition of the prognostic significance of certain histologic subtypes, treatment programs were developed to maximize the cure rate and minimize toxicity for most patients. The overall cure rate is now over 80% (Wilimas et al. 1988).

EPIDEMIOLOGY

The incidence of Wilms' tumor is remarkably constant throughout the world and has been used as a marker against which to measure the incidence of other tumors. The annual incidence is 5.0 to 7.8 per million children under 15 years of age. It affects males and females equally. Most children are 1 to 5 years of age (median, 3.1 years) at diagnosis. The tumor is rare before the age of 8 months; most primary renal tumors in these infants represent mesoblastic nephroma, a benign, spindle cell tumor. Bilateral Wilms' tumor occurs in 5% to 10% of patients; these patients are significantly younger than children with unilateral renal involvement (Pastore et

al. 1988; Coppes et al. 1989). Some patients present at a very young age with a single tumor and subsequently develop a contralateral tumor. Thus, young children presenting with unilateral Wilms' tumor should have a careful follow-up of the contralateral kidney for at least three to four years, as most contralateral tumors will develop during this period (Coppes et al. 1989).

Wilms' tumor occurs in both heritable and sporadic forms. In children with the heritable form, the neoplasm develops earlier and is more likely to be bilateral and multicentric. All bilateral cases and approximately 20% of unilateral cases represent a heritable form of the disease. Familial cases are inherited in an autosomal dominant fashion, with incomplete (approximately 40%) penetrance. In the two-hit model of carcinogenesis of the heritable form, the first hit is inherited and the second hit is acquired. In the sporadic form, both hits are acquired. An estimated 8% of the offspring of patients with unilateral, unifocal disease and 20% to 30% of the offspring of those with bilateral or known familial disease will develop Wilms' tumor.

About 15% of patients with Wilms' tumor have congenital anomalies, including genitourinary anomalies (5%), hemihypertrophy (2%), and aniridia (1%). Patients with bilateral disease are more likely to have congenital anomalies. Genitourinary anomalies associated with Wilms' tumor include ectopic and solitary kidney, horseshoe kidneys, ureteral duplication, hypospadias, and cryptorchidism. Hemihypertrophy is usually idiopathic, may occur ipsilateral or contralateral to the tumor site, and may be present at diagnosis or emerge later. Wilms' tumor has developed in children or siblings of patients with hemihypertrophy.

Patients with another syndrome of tissue growth, the Beckwith-Wiedemann syndrome (omphalocele, macroglossia, and visceromegaly), have a 10% risk of neoplasm; in one report, 14 neoplasms occurred in these patients and Wilms' tumor accounted for six cases. Sporadic bilateral aniridia occurs in 1% of patients with Wilms' tumor, compared with 0.01% frequency in the general population. Children with sporadic aniridia have a one in three chance of developing a Wilms' tumor and should be evaluated frequently using abdominal ultrasonography. Familial aniridia is more common than sporadic aniridia, but it is rarely associated with Wilms' tumor. Several cases of neurofibromatosis with Wilms' tumor have also been described.

PATHOLOGY AND CLASSIFICATION

Most of the tumors have standard histology consisting of a mixed blastoma (undifferentiated spindle cells), epithelial differentiation (tubules), and stromal elements. Abortive glomeruli, smooth and striated muscle, myxomatous tissue, fat, bone, or cartilage may also appear. Foci of persistent blastemal cells, which appear as subscapular nodules or as sheets of primitive metanephric epithelium, have been found in kidneys containing a Wilms' tumor and in uninvolved contralateral kidneys. When the nodules are small and localized, the condition is called nodular renal blastema; the diffuse form is called nephroblastomatosis. They may be precursor lesions of Wilms' tumor and represent the first mutation in the sequence that leads to cancer; some patients with these lesions have subsequently developed Wilms' tumor. About 12% of cases have a more aggressive and prognostically unfavorable histology: clear-cell sarcoma (6%), anaplastic (4%), or rhabdoid sarcoma (2%) (Beckwith 1986). Clear-cell sarcomas have relatively inconspicuous cytoplasm, which may be optically clear. The disease occurs more often in boys and has a propensity for bony metastasis. Although this histologic subtype carried a poor prognosis, intensification of chemotherapy by adding doxorubicin has improved the outcome substantially (Beckwith 1986).

Cellular pleomorphism, nuclear enlargement, hyperchromatism, and the presence of bizarre mitotic figures indicate anaplastic tumor. Children with anaplastic Wilms' tumor are generally one to two years older at diagnosis, are more likely to be black, and have a higher frequency of local recurrence and pulmonary metastases. Hyperdiploidy and complex chromosomal rearrangements are characteristic features of anaplastic tumors (Douglass et al. 1986).

Rhabdoid tumor has cells with fibrillar eosinophilic inclusions and was originally considered a sarcomatous variant of Wilms' tumor. However, it has appeared in extrarenal sites, including the posterior fossa of the brain and the mediastinum. This tumor type is found most often in very young patients (median age, 18 months). It carries an extremely poor prognosis because of early metastases to liver, lungs, and many other sites.

GENETICS

Several chromosomal anomalies including 11p-, trisomy 8, trisomy 18, and XX/XY mosaicism have been associated with Wilms' tumor. Interstitial deletion of chromosome 11 at band p13 (11p13), aniridia, ambiguous genitalia, and mental retardation defines Aniridia-Wilms' tumor association (AWTA), described in patients with Wilms' tumor. Analysis of cytogenetic abnormalities in Wilms' tumor indicates that deletion or rearrangements involving the short arm of chromosome 11, including 11p13, may occur in 30% to 40% of cases (Slater et al. 1985). These relationships suggest the existence of a putative Wilms' tumor suppressive gene that resides in the 11p13 band. Recombinant DNA analysis based on restriction-fragment-length polymorphisms demonstrated loss of genetic material and resultant homozygosity for the 11p region in Wilms' tumor cells derived from patients with normal constitutional phenotype and genotype (Koufos et al. 1984). The chromosomal events leading to homozygosity for 11p may constitute the second hit in the Knudson model of tumorigenesis.

PRESENTATION AND DIAGNOSIS

Most patients (85%) present with an abdominal or flank mass first noticed by a parent. Abdominal pain occurs in 40% of patients and is severe enough in about 10% to suggest a possible acute surgical abdomen. Hypertension, usually mild, is found in 60% to 90% of patients and is often associated with elevated plasma renin levels. About one-fourth of patients have fever, sometimes in association with a urinary tract infection. Gross hematuria is rare, but about one-third of children have microscopic hematuria. Other rarer symptoms include weight loss, nausea, vomiting, anorexia, bone pain, dysuria, and polyuria. The usual site of metastasis is in the lung; dyspnea and tachypnea may occur in children with advanced disease.

The laboratory evaluation should include a complete blood count, liver and kidney function tests, chest x-rays, and CT scans of the chest and abdomen. On CT scan without enhancement, the Wilms' tumors appear as an unhomogenous mass with areas of low density indicating necrosis. Areas of hemorrhage and small focal calcifications are less common and less prominent than in neuroblastoma. Contrast medium shows a slight enhancement of tumors, with a sharp demarcation from normal renal parenchyma. CT scan can establish the intrarenal origin of the tumor, determine the extent of tumor, detect multiple masses, and evaluate the opposite kidney. Abdominal ultrasonography can evaluate patency of the inferior vena cava. With the advent of the CT scan and ultrasonography, an intravenous pyelogram is no longer considered essential. However, if performed, the characteristic findings include intrarenal distortion of calices and displacement of the urinary collection system; nonvisualization of the kidney may be present. CT of the lungs is more sensitive than a plain chest x-ray in detecting metastasis, but about half of the lesions found are benign.

Radionuclide bone scan and skeletal survey should be performed for patients with documented pulmonary metastasis or with clear-cell sarcoma. Similarly, bone marrow examination should be reserved for patients with tumor of unfavorable histology.

An abnormal protein-polysaccharide complex has been detected in the serum, urine, and cell-free tumor extracts. Although serum lactic dehydrogenase and renin may be elevated, neither of these markers is sensitive nor specific for Wilms' tumor. Certain rare paraneoplastic syndromes may be associated with Wilms' tumor. The neoplasm may produce erythropoiesis leading to polycythemia, and secondary hypercalcemia has been reported.

Surgery is the primary modality for diagnosis and staging of Wilms' tumor, and it often provides adequate local therapy. The procedure should include a thorough examination of the abdominal cavity and a biopsy of adjacent lymph nodes and any suspicious areas in the liver and opposite kidney. The surgical findings and the pathologist's report determine the surgicopathologic stage. Table 32.12 shows the staging system that the National Wilms' Tumor Study Group used. Preoperative chemotherapy or radiation therapy has been advocated as a means of shrinking very large tumors and

Table 32.12
CLINICAL STAGING CLASSIFICATION FOR WILMS' TUMOR*

Stage	Criteria
I	Tumor limited to kidney and completely excised.
II	Microscopic residual tumor. Tumor is completely excised but penetrates through the capsule or into perirenal soft tissues. Local spillage of tumor is confined to the flank.
III	Gross residual tumor confined to the abdomen (lymph node involvement, diffuse peritoneal contamination, peritoneal implants, tumor extends beyond the surgical margins, tumor incompletely excised).
IV	Hematogenous metastases to lung, noncontiguous liver, bone, or brain.
V	Bilateral involvement at diagnosis.

*The patient should be characterized by both stage of the disease and histology of the tumor, e.g., stage II, unfavorable histology or stage III, favorable histology. Unfavorable histologic subtypes are focal or diffuse anaplasia and sarcomatous histology.

facilitating surgical removal. However, it is associated with a 6% false diagnosis rate, changes of histologic pattern, and alteration of eventual stage from resolution of intra-abdominal metastases.

TREATMENT AND PROGNOSIS

Treatment should begin with transabdominal radical nephrectomy and abdominal exploration with staging. The transabdominal approach has the advantage of providing adequate exposure, permitting a thorough exploration of the abdominal contents and opposite kidney, and a sweeping dissection of the attached renal fossa for removal of the involved kidney and associated lymph nodes. Careful attention to the inferior vena cava and renal vein is needed to avoid dislodging any tumor that may be propagating intraluminally.

Surgery may also be useful in second-look procedures after chemotherapy or radiation therapy in patients who have massive unresectable tumor at diagnosis or who have bilateral tumors. A second-look surgical procedure can either document a complete response or convert a partial response to a complete response by removing residual tumor.

Only three chemotherapeutic agents are clearly effective for Wilms' tumor: vincristine, dactinomycin, and doxorubicin. For patients with stage I disease (28%), a combination of vincristine and dactinomycin without irradiation results in more than 90% 2-year disease-free survival and presumed cure. Optimal length of therapy has yet to be defined. For patients with stage II disease (28%), intensive administration of vincristine and dactinomycin without irradiation for at least six months can yield an approximately 90% 2-year disease-free survival. Preliminary results show an approximately 76% 2-year disease-free survival in the 29% of patients with stage III disease after treatment with vincristine, dactinomycin, and doxorubicin, together with 10 Gy irradiation to the tumor bed (D'Angio et al. 1984). For the 15% of patients with stage IV disease, the same triple chemotherapy combined with 12 Gy bilateral lung irradiation for lung metastasis and higher-dose irradiation to the tumor bed attain an approximate 70% 2-year disease-free survival. For patients with clear-cell histology, triple chemotherapy and 10 Gy irradiation to the tumor bed are recommended for all stages. Optimal therapy for patients with

an anaplastic cancer remains unclear, although the addition of cyclophosphamide may be beneficial.

The treatment of patients with bilateral cancer is complicated because functional kidney tissue must be preserved. A variety of approaches has been used: nephrectomy of the more involved kidney plus heminephrectomy or biopsy of the other; bilateral heminephrectomy; and bilateral biopsy followed by chemotherapy with second-look surgery. Recent treatment has resulted in 75% long-term disease-free survival (Coppes et al. 1989). Time and site of relapse, tumor histology, and treatment history should determine therapy for patients with recurrent disease. These patients should undergo a complete re-evaluation. Surgery should be strongly considered to confirm the diagnosis and to remove all gross recurrent disease, especially in children with apparent isolated pulmonary recurrence. Radiation should be considered for all previously unirradiated sites of recurrence. Doxorubicin and/or cyclophosphamide may be given to patients who have not received these agents. Ifosfamide, etoposide, and cisplatin are also useful for patients with recurrent Wilms' tumor. With intensive salvage therapy, approximately 30% of children will have 3-year postrelapse survival (Grundy et al. 1989).

In general, the prognosis is better for patients diagnosed before the age of 2 years and for those with tumors weighing less than 250 g. The most important adverse prognostic factors are sarcomatous or anaplastic histology and advanced disease stage. Hyperdiploidy, multiple complex translocations, and multiple stem lines of tumor cells confer a poor prognosis in patients with Wilms' tumor and may reflect genetic instability of tumor cells, which increases the likelihood of developing drug resistance (Douglass et al. 1986).

RHABDOMYOSARCOMA

Rhabdomyosarcoma is the most common soft-tissue cancer in childhood. Although frequently described as a tumor of striated muscle origin, it most likely arises from primitive or undifferentiated mesenchyme and has the capacity to differentiate into muscle. These tumors can originate virtually anywhere in the body, and they tend to disseminate early.

EPIDEMIOLOGY

The annual incidence of rhabdomyosarcoma among children under 15 years of age in the United States is an estimated 4.4 per million white children and 1.3 per million black children. It peaks in children 2 to 6 years old and again in adolescents 15 to 19 years old. The early peak is due primarily to the occurrence of tumors in the head and neck region and genitourinary tract (prostate, bladder, and vagina); the latter peak is in tumors of the male genitourinary tract, particularly of testes or paratesticular tissue. The male-to-female ratio is 1.4:1.

Rhabdomyosarcoma has been associated with neurofibromatosis, fetal alcohol syndrome, and Gorlin's basal cell nevus syndrome. There appears to be a familial aggregation of rhabdomyosarcoma with other sarcomas. Relatives of children with rhabdomyosarcoma have a high frequency of carcinoma of the breast and other sites. Patients with rhabdomyosarcoma are often found in cancer families, in which there is a high incidence of brain tumor and breast cancer at an early age, particularly when such tumors occur in parents.

PATHOLOGY AND CLASSIFICATION

Rhabdomyosarcoma is usually associated with extensive necrosis and hemorrhage and often has ill-defined margins. The characteristic cellular element is the rhabdomyoblast, a primitive skeletal muscle cell with eosinophilic cytoplasm and cross-striations or longitudinal myofibrils. Glycogen granules may be present in the cytoplasm. Rhabdomyoblasts can vary in morphology within individual tumors and have been described as round cells, tadpole cells, spindle cells, spider-web cells, and multinucleated giant cells. Definitive pathologic diagnosis may require additional studies. Electron microscopy reveals cells with eccentric nuclei, abundant mitochondria, and large numbers of thick and thin cytoplasmic filaments that tend to form so-called Z-bands. Desmin, an intermediate protein, is a useful marker for distinguishing rhabdomyosarcoma from other round-cell tumors of childhood (Altmannsberger et al. 1985).

Traditionally, the tumors are classified into four histologic groups based on tissue patterns: embryonal, alveolar, pleomorphic, and undifferentiated. The embryonal subtype accounts for 50% to 60% of cases. A variable number of large acidophilic myoblasts and many primitive round and spindle-shaped cells with little myoblastic differentiation characterize it; cross-striations within the cytoplasm may be found. This subtype is found most commonly in the head, neck, and genitourinary tract. Sarcoma botryoides is a polypoid variant of embryonal rhabdomyosarcoma and usually has a grapelike appearance. The botryoid variant accounts for 5% of rhabdomyosarcomas and is commonly seen in younger children. It affects the vagina, uterus, bladder, nasopharynx, and middle ear.

The alveolar subtype accounts for about 20% of cases and is characterized by a pseudoalveolar growth pattern reminiscent of the alveoli of fetal lung. It is more common in older children in the extremities and perineal sites. It tends to metastasize to lymph nodes, and has a poor prognosis.

Pleomorphic rhabdomyosarcoma is rare in children (1% of cases) and almost always arises in the extremities. About 10% to 20% of patients are considered to have undifferentiated tumor. The first International Rhabdomyosarcoma Study (IRS-I) included three additional tumor types: sarcoma of undetermined histogenesis, and special undifferentiated types I and II (extraskeletal Ewing's sarcoma) (Maurer et al. 1977). A more recent classification, based on cytologic features, has defined three variants: anaplastic, monomorphous round cell, and mixed (Palmer and Foulkes 1983). The first two variants make up 20% of all cases and represent unfavorable histology.

GENETICS

Abnormalities of the short arm of chromosome 3 are found in some rhabdomyosarcomas. Recent studies revealed the t(2;13) as specific for this tumor. Although this translocation did not correlate with specific histology, it appeared to be associated with more advanced disease (Douglass et al. 1987). The loss of heterozygosity for chromosome 11 in two cases of rhabdomyosarcoma suggested that a tumor-suppressing gene is involved in some cases (Koufos et al. 1985).

PRESENTATION AND DIAGNOSIS

Clinical presentations depend on the site of tumor origin, rapidity of tumor growth, and presence of metastases. The most common presenting feature is a mass, which may be painful. The main sites of origin are the head and neck including the orbit (37%), genitourinary tract (21%), extremities (20%), retroperitoneum (8%), trunk (7%), gastrointestinal tract (2%), perineum-anus (2%), and intrathoracic area (2%) (Maurer et al. 1988). One percent of patients are diagnosed as having disseminated disease involving the bones and bone marrow, without an identifiable primary tumor site.

Young children with orbital tumor present with proptosis, periorbital edema, and ptosis. Tumors of the middle ear are associated with ear pain, chronic otitis media, or hemorrhagic discharge from the ear canal. Tumors of the nasopharynx can present with airway obstruction, local pain, sinusitis, epistaxis, or dysphagia. Parameningeal lesions, such as those in the nasal cavity, paranasal sinuses, nasopharynx, and middle ear, may extend into the middle cranial fossa in 35% of cases and result in cranial nerve paralysis, meningeal symptoms, and signs of brain-stem compression (Gasparini et al. 1983).

Rhabdomyosarcoma of the trunk or extremities appears as enlarging soft-tissue masses, frequently first noticed after trauma and possibly mistaken for a hematoma. Genitourinary tract involvement may produce hematuria, recurrent urinary tract infection, incontinence, or obstruction of the lower urinary tract.

Paratesticular tumor presents as a rapidly growing mass in the scrotum. Vaginal or uteral rhabdomyosarcoma may present as a grapelike mass bulging through the vaginal orifice.

Rhabdomyosarcoma may spread by local extension or through the venous or lymphatic systems. The most frequent sites of metastases are the regional lymph nodes, lung, liver, bone marrow, bones, and brain. The paratesticular tumors are most commonly associated with regional lymph node involvement (40%), probably because of the rich lymphatic supply of the testes. By contrast, orbital tumors rarely have regional lymphatic involvement because of the paucity of lymphatic vessels. Bone invasion is frequent and extensive involvement may produce symptomatic hypercalcemia.

Initial studies should include a complete blood count, liver and kidney function tests, a skeletal survey, bone scan, chest x-ray, bone marrow examination, and other appropriate radiographic studies, depending on the region of origin. For patients with parameningeal tumors, CT and MRI are the primary imaging modalities for evaluating intracranial extension and bony involvement at the base of the skull. The cerebrospinal fluid should be examined to rule out meningeal seeding. For abdominal tumors, CT scan with contrast medium and ultrasonogram can help delineate tumors. CT scan and ultrasonography are useful for genitourinary tract tumors, with the addition of cystourethrogram in those with bladder tumors. MRI is useful for imaging extremity tumors. Finally, a gallium scan may help detect nodal metastases.

The most common staging system (table 32.13) in the United States was developed by the Intergroup Rhabdomyosarcoma Study Group (Maurer et al. 1988). This system is based upon local disease status, the involvement of regional lymph nodes, the extent of residual tumor after primary surgery, and distant metastases. Approximately 15% of patients have resected, localized disease (Group I); 25% have residual microscopic disease with or without lymph node involvement (Group II); 41% have gross residual local-regional disease (Group III); and 19% have metastases at diagnosis.

TREATMENT AND PROGNOSIS

Total excision of the primary lesion is a desirable goal if it will not result in unacceptable deformity. Radiation therapy to areas of known residual tumor and systemic multiagent chemotherapy are also indicated. In general, in Group I, complete local excision is followed by chemotherapy. For Groups II and III, surgery should be followed by local irradiation and systemic chemotherapy. The treatment of patients with Group IV tumors relies principally on systemic chemotherapy. Intrathecal therapy may be indicated in patients with parameningeal tumor if there is extension into the adjacent CNS. Radiation therapy is given in large volumes and relatively high doses (40 Gy to 50 Gy) over six weeks. The most effective drugs are cyclophosphamide, vincristine, dactinomycin, and doxorubicin. Etoposide, cisplatin, and dacarbazine also have some activity against this tumor. The most commonly used chemotherapeutic regimens involve combinations of vincristine, dactinomycin, and cyclophosphamide.

The use of the combined modality treatment has substantially improved the proportion of long-term, disease-free survivors. However, patients with advanced disease at diagnosis remain a therapeutic challenge (table 32.13). Once a patient relapses, survival is extremely poor regardless of local, regional, or distant recurrence; 32% of such patients survived one year and 17% survived two years, despite retreatment with aggressive surgery, radiation therapy, and adjuvant chemotherapy.

The most important prognostic factor (table 32.13) is the extent of disease at diagnosis (Maurer et al. 1988). Primary site is also important, because tumors arising in locations that produce early symptoms are associated with a better prognosis than are those arising in deep, poorly confined areas. The prognosis is good for patients whose primary tumor is orbit, bladder, or prostate, but patients with intrathoracic or retroperitoneal primaries have a poor outcome (Crist et al. 1982; Crist et al. 1985). Children with the sarcoma botryoides variant of embryonal rhabdomyosarcoma have the best survival rates; those with alveolar histology have the

Table 32.13
STAGING AND OUTCOME OF RHABDOMYOSARCOMA*

Stage	Criteria	Proportion of patients (%)	8-year disease-free survival (%)
I	Localized disease, completely resected (regional nodes not involved); confined to muscle or organ of origin; contiguous involvement with infiltration outside the muscle or organ of origin, as through fascial planes.	15	74
II	Grossly resected tumor with microscopic residual disease; no evidence of gross residual tumor; no evidence of regional node involvement. Regional disease, completely resected (regional nodes involved or extension of tumor into an adjacent organ); all tumor completely resected with no microscopic residual tumor. Regional disease with involved nodes; grossly resected, but with evidence of microscopic residual disease.	25	65
III	Incomplete resection or biopsy with gross residual disease.	41	40
IV	Distant metastatic disease present at diagnosis (lung, liver, bones, bone marrow, brain, and distant muscle and nodes).	19	15

*(Based on data from the Intergroup Rhabdomyosarcoma Study I. Maurer et al. [1988].)

worst outcome. Mixed histology is more favorable than the anaplastic and monomorphous round-cell variants (Palmer and Foulkes 1983). Older children have worse prognoses than younger ones, probably because they have a greater frequency of extremity primaries and of alveolar histology.

OSTEOSARCOMA

Osteosarcoma, also known as osteogenic sarcoma, is a malignant tumor of mesenchymal origin that forms neoplastic osteoid. It is the most common bone tumor in children and adolescents. The disease is more common in teenagers than in young children, and it primarily involves the distal portion (metaphysis) of long bones. Osteosarcoma usually occurs during the second decade of life, a time when body image is of utmost importance. Because therapy usually involves mutilating surgery, psychological support is especially essential for these patients.

EPIDEMIOLOGY

The occurrence of osteosarcoma appears to correlate with linear bone growth. Incidence is rare in prepubertal children, but rises after puberty and peaks between 15 and 19 years of age. During the first 13 years of life, boys and girls have the same incidence of osteosarcoma. After this age, the incidence continues to increase for males, but girls reach a plateau. The result is a male-to-female ratio of 1.5:1. The relationship between the adolescent growth spurt and the tumor development suggests that high growth rate increases the risk of somatic mutation, leading to neoplastic tumor formation. Indeed, osteosarcoma occurs most commonly in long bones at the metaphyseal ends, regions of bone with the most active growth and reconstruction.

Children with the hereditary form of retinoblastoma have a 500-fold increase in risk of developing osteosarcoma. Although these osteosarcomas most often develop in the field of irradiation, disease has occurred in bones outside of the radiation field and in multiple sites. With use of DNA markers for chromosome 13, molecular analysis reveals deletion of genetic material at band 13q14 in hereditary retinoblastoma, osteosarcoma associated with retinoblastoma, and sporadic osteosarcoma (Hansen, Koufos, and Gallie 1985). A recessive tumor-suppressing gene on chromosome 13 may be involved in tumor development. Other conditions associated with osteosarcoma include multiple hereditary exostoses, multiple osteochondromatosis (Ollier's disease), polyostotic fibrous dysplasia, osteogenesis imperfecta, Paget's disease of bone, and exposure to ionizing irradiation. Familial cases of osteosarcoma have been reported occasionally.

PATHOLOGY AND CLASSIFICATION

Osteosarcoma generally arises within the medullary canal and breaks through the cortex and periosteum to form a soft-tissue mass that may reach a considerable size. The tumor may also extend along the medullary cavity. In about 20% of cases, tumor deposits develop quite far from the primary tumor.

Histologically, the tumor contains primitive spindle cells that form osteoids. Approximately 75% of the cases are considered classic osteosarcoma which, depending on the predominant matrix, can be subdivided into osteoblastic, fibroblastic, and chondroblastic types. The remaining 25% form a heterogenous group of variants, each with unique features and some of which have different prognoses. Telangiectatic osteosarcoma is an unusual variant that characteristically appears as a lytic lesion on radiographs with little calcification or bone formation. Pathologic fractures are common in this variant, and it seems to have a particularly poor prognosis. Periosteal osteosarcoma arises from the bone periosteum and grows away from it without cortical invasion. It usually occurs in the proximal metaphysis of the tibia, is most common in adolescents, is less aggressive, and may require only wide resection (Hall et al. 1985). Periosteal osteosarcoma is most common in older patients (median age, 30 years) and occurs in the metaphyseal region of the femur. It often surrounds the bone shaft without involvement of the cortical structure. The tumor's growth is relatively slow, but local recurrence and metastasis can occur. Low-grade intraosseous osteosarcoma is a rare variant confined to the marrow cavity, and it has a very low potential to metastasize. Small-cell osteosarcoma resembles Ewing's sarcoma histologically but produces osteoid. Multifocal sclerosing osteosarcoma may appear simultaneously in many sites with a predominantly osteoblastic pattern.

PRESENTATION AND DIAGNOSIS

The usual presenting symptom is localized pain with or without a mass overlying the involved bone. Pain often increases with activity. Occasionally, trauma precedes the pain. In some patients, diagnosis is delayed because pain is attributed to the injury. An x-ray should be done on any patient with prolonged, unexplained bone pain. Depending on the tumor site, the mass may or may not be palpable. Tenderness, local erythema, or limitation of movement is encountered occasionally. Pathological fractures are uncommon, but they may occur in almost 30% of patients with telangiectatic osteosarcoma. Metastasis of osteosarcoma is usually to the lungs, without respiratory symptoms unless extensive pulmonary involvement occurs as well. Occasionally, bone or brain metastases occur. Lymphatic spread is present in only 3% of patients.

Approximately 60% to 80% of osteosarcomas occur around the knee (distal femur or proximal tibia or fibula) and 10% to 15% in the proximal humerus. Central axis involvement accounts for less than 10% of cases.

The initial workup should include plain x-rays of the involved bone, which are often diagnostic. X-rays demonstrate destruction of the normal bony trabecular pattern, with indistinct margins. A soft-tissue mass is common, and there is usually intense periosteal new-bone formation. The eroded cortex may be transversed by horizontal bone spicules that extend into the surrounding soft tissue, resulting in the sunburst sign in 60% of cases. At the tumor margins, a triangular region of periosteal new bone (Codman's triangle) is often present. CT scan and MRI can delineate the extent of the cortical bone involvement and the presence of intramedullary spread, as well as the presence of skip lesions and soft-tissue extensions. These determinations are important for planning surgical treatments. Arteriographs are needed to evaluate the relationship between the tumor and major vessels in patients who are candidates for limb salvage procedures.

At diagnosis, 10% to 20% of patients have metastasis, which can usually be detected by routine chest x-rays or CT scans. CT is more sensitive but occasionally yields false-positive results. The role of MRI in detection of metastasis is under study. Bone scan and skeletal survey are indicated to rule out bone metastases. At diagnosis, about 60% of patients have increased serum alkaline phosphatase levels that are associated with an increased likelihood of subsequent pulmonary metastasis.

TREATMENT AND PROGNOSIS

Surgical removal of the affected bone and surrounding soft tissue, whether by amputation or limb salvage procedure, is crucial for local tumor control. The choice between the two surgical procedures depends on the patient's age; anatomical location, extent and size of tumor; soft-tissue and neurovascular involvement; surgical expertise; expected function; and the patient's attitude and preference.

Historically, transosseous amputation was performed for distal femoral tumors, above-knee amputations for proximal tibia or fibula tumors, and below-knee amputations for distal tibia lesions. Shoulder disarticulation or fore-quarter amputations are performed for proximal humerus lesions, and hemipelvectomy for tumors of the proximal femoral neck or ilium. The usual practice is to have a tumor-free margin of 7 cm to 10 cm. After amputation, early rehabilitation of the patient with immediate fitting of prosthesis is extremely important.

Limb salvage is increasingly favored as an alternative to amputation (Marcove and Rosen 1980). Patients are often given chemotherapy intravenously or intra-arterially before the operation. In these procedures, the tumor-bearing bone is resected *en bloc* and replaced with a cadaver allograft or a custom-made prosthesis. Complications include infections, breaking of the inserted rod from metal fatigue, decreased functional activity, and local tumor recurrence. Many patients undergoing this procedure eventually require conventional amputation because of complications. For patients with bone metastases, surgery has little role except to relieve pain or resect grossly disfiguring metastatic lesions.

The beneficial effects of chemotherapy in osteosarcoma have been controversial. A recent controlled clinical trial clearly demonstrated that adjuvant chemotherapy improves the chances of relapse-free survival from approximately 20% to 60% (Link et al. 1986; Eilber et al. 1987). Effective chemotherapeutic agents for osteosarcoma include methotrexate, melphalan, cisplatin, doxorubicin, 5-fluorouracil, cyclophosphamide, and mitomycin-C.

Osteosarcoma is a radioresistant tumor. Several biological response modifiers, including transfer factor and interferons, have been tested, but none was proven to be beneficial.

Aggressive surgical treatment for patients who develop pulmonary metastases is warranted. Some patients require repeated resection of metastases. Aggressive use of multiple or bilateral thoracotomies has resulted in prolonged survival and potential cure in 25% of these patients (Meyer et al. 1987).

Locations of the primary lesion and metastatic or multifocal disease are important prognostic variables for osteosarcoma. In general, the further the primary is away from the axial skeleton, the better the prognosis. Tumor size also appears to be important, with a larger tumor (>15 cm in diameter) conferring a poorer prognosis. Histologically, a relatively good outcome is reported for periosteal, parosteal, and low-grade intraosseous osteosarcoma; the telangiectatic variant is associated with poor prognosis. Pre-existing Paget's disease, irradiation-induced malignancy, age less than 10 years, male sex, short duration of symptoms, and high levels of alkaline phosphatase are also adverse indicators. Osteosarcomas with near-diploid stem lines respond significantly better to adjuvant chemotherapy than do tumors with only hyperdiploid lines (Look, Douglass, and Meyer 1988).

EWING'S SARCOMA

Since the first description of this tumor in 1921, the cell of origin has not been clearly delineated. It is thought to arise from the primitive mesenchyme of the medullary cavity. Extraosseous Ewing's sarcoma is a tumor of similar morphology that arises from soft tissue near bone. Ewing's sarcoma involves flat bones in 40% of the reported cases (Nesbit, Robinson, and Dehner 1984).

EPIDEMIOLOGY

Ewing's sarcoma is most common in early adolescence, often between 11 and 15 years (median age, 13 years). It represents approximately 1% of childhood cancers and 30% of all bone tumors in this age group. It occurs more often in males than in females (1.6:1) and is exceedingly rare in blacks (Fraumeni and Glass 1970). Familial cases have been described.

PATHOLOGY

The tumors, often soft and friable, consist of undifferentiated, small round cells with scanty cytoplasm and little or no surrounding stroma. Coagulative necrosis may be prominent and calcification is rare. The periodic acid-Schiff reaction can demonstrate glycogen in 80% of the samples. Although electron microscopy discerns no diagnostic feature for Ewing's sarcoma, it is useful for ruling out other childhood tumors.

GENETICS

Cytogenetic analysis of cell lines or fresh tumors have demonstrated a subtle but characteristic chromosomal abnormality, t(11;22)(q24;q12) (Whang-Peng et al. 1986). An apparently identical reciprocal translocation has also been described in neuroepitheliomas and Askin's tumor, both of which may be closely related to Ewing's sarcoma. Although the c-*sis* oncogene at 22q13 is involved in this translocation, it is not rearranged or activated at the molecular level. Whether the c-*ets*-1 oncogene, normally located in 11q23-25, is translocated or in any other way functionally rearranged in Ewing's sarcoma is unknown.

PRESENTATION AND DIAGNOSIS

Initial findings are localized pain in the affected bone with subsequent swelling, tenderness, and heat later in the course. At times it is difficult to differentiate from osteomyelitis. Various laboratory abnormalities, such as leukocytosis, anemia, and an elevated sedimentation rate also suggest infection. When the diagnosis of osteomyelitis is questionable and the cultures are negative, a diagnosis of Ewing's sarcoma should always be considered.

The tumor can occur in any bone and is found most frequently in the midshaft (diaphysis) of long bones. The femur is the bone most frequently involved, followed in decreasing order by the ilium-pubis, tibia, humerus, fibula, ribs, scapula, hand and foot bones, vertebra, sacrum, clavicle, skull and facial bones, radius, and ulna.

Up to one-third of patients will have evidence of metastatic disease in the lungs or other bones at presentation. Patients with a primary tumor in the proximal extremity or central axis have a higher incidence of metastasis than those with tumor in the distal extremity (50% and 10%, respectively). Primary tumors of the rib may be quite massive and result in respiratory distress. In rare instances (<2% of cases), soft-tissue extension of vertebral disease can cause epidural spinal cord compression.

Anemia, leukocytosis with a shift to the left, elevated erythrocyte sedimentation rate, and increased serum lactic dehydrogenase levels may occur in some patients, but they are nonspecific findings. The radiographic appearances of Ewing's sarcoma vary, but a diffuse lytic lesion with periosteal reaction and a soft-tissue mass is the most common finding. Sclerotic lesions may occur, and the so-called onion-skin appearance thought to be characteristic of Ewing's sarcoma is seen in only a minority of cases. CT of the primary lesion, especially in

the pelvic region, is important because the tumor is often grossly underestimated by usual radiographic methods. Bone scans show increased uptake, and gallium scans are positive in approximately 80% of cases. CT, plain x-rays of the chest, skeletal survey, bone scan, and bone marrow aspiration can exclude metastatic disease.

TREATMENT AND PROGNOSIS

Amputation is not indicated in patients with Ewing's sarcoma because the tumor is sensitive to chemotherapy and radiation therapy (Hayes et al. 1983; Hayes et al. 1989). Treatment regimens usually begin with chemotherapy (cyclophosphamide, doxorubicin, vincristine, and dactinomycin) to reduce tumor bulk and to eradicate micrometastases. Radiation therapy can then be delivered through a smaller port, sparing normal tissue, and using a lower dose in some cases. For expendable bones, complete surgical excision is preferred. With current therapy, 70% of patients with localized tumor and 30% to 50% of those with metastatic disease at diagnosis can enjoy long-term survival. Late relapses can occur. For some patients with advanced tumor, autologous bone marrow transplantation and sequential half-body irradiation with adjuvant chemotherapy have been successful (Berry et al. 1986).

The presence of metastatic disease indicates a poor prognosis, and primary tumors in the flat bones or proximal extremity have a poorer prognosis than those occurring in distal long bones. A large tumor (>8 cm or 100 cc), regardless of site, carries a bad prognosis.

RETINOBLASTOMA

Retinoblastoma is a malignant tumor arising from primitive neuroectodermal tissue within the nuclear layer of the retina (Kyritsis et al. 1984). Histologically, it is similar to neuroblastoma, medulloblastoma, and pineoblastoma, three other malignant neoplasms of neural origin. A so-called trilateral retinoblastoma syndrome has been reported in patients with bilateral ocular retinoblastoma and a pineal tumor. Interesting features of retinoblastoma include instances of spontaneous regression, multicentric origin in some cases, a high frequency of secondary malignancy, and a pattern of inheritance.

EPIDEMIOLOGY

Retinoblastoma is relatively rare and has an annual incidence of 3.4 per million. About 200 children in the United States develop retinoblastoma each year. It usually occurs in children younger than 2 years of age. The mean age at diagnosis is 8 months for bilateral cases and 26 months for unilateral cases.

PATHOLOGY

Retinoblastoma is an undifferentiated small-cell tumor with deeply staining nuclei and scant cytoplasm, or of larger cells that form rosettes around a central cavity. The blood supply is invariably inadequate, and patchy necrosis and degeneration with calcium deposition are characteristic. It may grow into the vitreous cavity (endophytic) or into the subretinal space (exophytic). Tumor fragments may break off from the endophytic tumor and float free in the vitreous to seed unaffected parts of the retina. Retinoblastoma can grow into the choroid, sclera, optic nerve, or subarachnoid space and seed along the base of the brain and spinal cord. Involvement of the periglobal tissue can result in hematogenous spread of tumor to the bone marrow, bones, lymph nodes, and liver.

GENETICS

Retinoblastoma occurs in two forms, one sporadic (60% of patients) and the other inherited. About 30% of patients have bilateral involvement and an inherited predisposition to retinoblastoma. Usually, the tumor is first diagnosed in one eye only; the tumor in the other eye appears several months to years later. About 15% of patients with unilateral retinoblastoma also have a genetic predisposition. The attack rate of the hereditary form is 40%, consistent with an autosomal dominant pattern with 80% penetrance (Nussbaum and Puck 1976). Studies by cytogenetic and DNA restriction-fragment-length polymorphism analyses indicate that the malignant tumors are generated by recessive mutations (Friend et al. 1986). In the heritable form, one of the genetic loci, Rb, at 13q14, has been mutated or otherwise rendered nonfunctional in the germ line. A single event inactivating the homologous locus in the unaffected chromosome is sufficient to generate the tumor in a predisposed individual. In sporadic cases, two separate somatic events have to inactivate both alleles.

Most patients with retinoblastoma have a normal constitutional karyotype. A small number of cases have the 13q-syndrome characterized by mental retardation, growth failure, characteristic facies, microcephaly, skeletal deformities, congenital heart disease, and eye defects. The deletion of the long arm of chromosome 13 is present in all body cells. Fifty percent of patients with the 13q-syndrome develop retinoblastoma. The retinoblastoma gene also carries an increased risk of other tumors; about 15% of survivors of the hereditary form of retinoblastoma develop a second cancer, with a median latent period of 11 years. Most are osteosarcomas that develop at both irradiated sites and nonirradiated sites, often multifocally.

PRESENTATION AND DIAGNOSIS

Sporadic retinoblastomas are rarely diagnosed early because signs and symptoms are not obvious in the young patient. Only 3% of cases have been identified on routine ocular examination. Nonetheless, early diagnosis is important to improve treatment outcome and to decrease morbidity. The parents are usually the first to notice an eye abnormality in the child. Cat's eye reflex, a whitish appearance of the pupil, is the most common presenting sign. Strabismus is the next most common sign and can occur early if the tumor develops in the macula. A red and painful eye, with or without glaucoma, indicates extensive disease. Limited vision or loss of vision, proptosis, buphthalmos, and increased intracranial pressure are late signs.

All patients should receive meticulous ophthalmoscopic examinations under general anesthesia. A number of eye conditions must be differentiated from retinoblastoma. These include persistent hyperplastic primary vitreous, cysticercus, visceral larva migrans, retrolental fibroplasia, Coat's disease, and bacterial panendophthalmitis. Staging procedures also include CT of the head. If advanced disease is suspected, cerebrospinal fluid examination, chest x-ray, skeletal survey, and bone marrow examination may be indicated as well (Pratt et al. 1989). The finding of calcium on high-resolution thin-section CT scan of the orbit is characteristic in over 80% of cases. An anterior chamber paracentesis may identify tumor cells in some cases. CT scan of the head should be part of the workup because of the possibility of trilateral retinoblastoma syndrome. Table 32.14 shows the staging system common for retinoblastoma (Bedford, Bedotto, and Macfaul 1971).

TREATMENT AND PROGNOSIS

Every effort should be made to preserve sight by irradiation, photocoagulation, or cryotherapy. Eyes with extensive tumor destruction of the retina or neovascular glaucoma are enucleated with an attempt made to resect as much of the optic nerve as possible (>10 mm). Radiation therapy should be given to the orbit if there is regional extraocular tumor extension. If tumor is advanced or extrabulbar extension has occurred, chemotherapy (cyclophosphamide, doxorubicin, vincristine) should be considered along with radiation therapy.

The prognosis depends on tumor size and location and the presence and degree of ocular and extraocular involvement. The cure rates for patients with Group I to IV retinoblastoma are over 90%. Group V patients have

Table 32.14
STAGING FOR RETINOBLASTOMA

Stage	Criteria
Group I	Solitary or multiple tumors, <4 disc diameters in size, at or behind the equator.
Group II	Solitary or multiple tumors, 4-10 disc diameters in size, at or behind the equator.
Group III	Any lesion anterior to the equator. Solitary tumors >10 disc diameters, behind the equator.
Group IV	Multiple tumors; some >10 disc diameters, any lesion extending anterior to the ora serrata.
Group V	Massive tumors involving over one-half of the retina. Vitreous seeding.
Group VI	Residual orbital disease; optic nerve involvement and extrasclera extension (metastatic disease).

a 5-year survival rate of 85%. Once the tumor has extended into the optic nerve, the cure rate decreases to about 50%. Survival rates decrease to 25% with extraocular extension. Cure for widespread metastatic disease is rare. Spontaneous regression occurs in 1.8% of patients. Bilateral retinoblastoma carries a significantly higher mortality rate, mostly due to second cancers (Abramson et al. 1985).

GERM CELL TUMOR

Germ cell tumors are benign or malignant neoplasms originating from the primordial germ cell, which may undergo germinomatous or embryonic differentiation. The totipotentiality of germ cells results in a wide array of neoplastic histologic patterns. The migration pattern of the primordial germ cells during embryonic development explains the usual occurrence of germ cell tumors in midline sites (e.g., sacrococcyx, neck, mediastinum, retroperitoneum, pineal gland).

EPIDEMIOLOGY

Germ cell tumors account for about 2% to 3% of childhood cancers. Sacrococcygeal teratoma is the most common solid tumor in newborns and has a higher incidence in females. Tumors in the sacrococcygeal and head and neck regions often have an early peak incidence, between birth and 3 years of age. During puberty there is an increase in the incidence of ovarian and testicular tumors. Boys with cryptorchid testes have a 50-fold greater risk of developing malignant testicular tumors, which may occur even in the surgically descended testis. Gonadal dysgenesis is the underlying defect for patients who develop gonadoblastoma.

PATHOLOGY AND CLASSIFICATION

These tumors are generally classified by the most malignant component when they contain a mixture of cell types. Pure germ cell tumors are called germinomas (seminoma and dysgerminoma). The embryonic differentiation may result in embryonal carcinoma or teratoma and extraembryonic differentiation in endodermal sinus tumor (yolk sac tumor) or choriocarcinoma. Mixed germ cell tumors with various histologic types are also seen. Germinoma occurs most commonly in the ovary of an early pubertal or adolescent girl or in the pineal region of an adolescent boy. It is less common in the anterior mediastinum or testis. Embryonal carcinoma, a highly anaplastic tumor that retains the potential to develop along either embryonal or extraembryonal lines, is rare in children. Teratomas contain derivatives of at least two of three germ layers: ectoderm, endoderm, and mesoderm. Although benign, they may undergo malignant change, most frequently to endodermal sinus tumor. Endodermal sinus tumor with histologic features resembling the yolk sac is most commonly found in the ovary, testes, and sacroccygeal areas. Choriocarcinoma resembling the chorion layer of the placenta usually occurs as a nongestational tumor of the pineal region, the anterior mediastinum, or the ovary in early childhood. Gestational choriocarcinoma occurs most commonly in girls between 15 and 19 years of age.

PRESENTATION AND DIAGNOSIS

Sacrococcygeal teratoma is usually detected during infancy and frequently at birth. Signs are an external midline sacrococcygeal mass, a pelvic mass, or unilateral gluteal enlargement. Depending on the involvement, patients may have paralysis, constipation, diarrhea, bladder distension, or recurrent urinary tract infections. Associated clinical features include congenital anomalies involving the lower vertebrae, genitourinary system, or anorectum. The testicular tumors are most common in boys younger than 5 years of age and present as painless, unilateral masses. They are rarely inflamed and a hydrocele is frequently present. Ovarian tumors are usually large and can cause pain, nausea, and vomiting. Patients who have ovarian torsion may have acute abdominal pain.

The physical examination can delineate the anatomic extent of the primary tumor, especially sacrococcygeal tumors. CT scans have replaced most conventional x-ray studies. X-rays of the tumor may show calcification and, in the case of a teratoma, even bone or teeth. All patients should have x-ray studies, CT scans of the chest, and bone scans to detect metastatic disease. The most helpful clinical laboratory studies for diagnosis and follow-up are the serum biomarkers, alpha-fetoprotein (AFP), and the beta subunit of human chorionic gonadotropin (HCG). The former is increased in embryonal carcinoma and endodermal sinus tumor; the latter in embryonal carcinoma and choriocarcinoma (Kurman et al. 1977).

TREATMENT AND PROGNOSIS

Tumors should be completely excised if possible and the surgical specimen carefully studied for the presence of malignant components that may occupy only a small portion of the tumor. It is imperative to remove the sacrococcygeal tumor as soon as possible because the incidence of cancer increases with age. For tumors with malignant components, chemotherapy (vincristine, cyclophosphamide, dactinomycin, vinblastine, bleomycin, and cisplatin) and/or radiation therapy should be given after surgery (Green 1983; Richie and Garnick 1984). Patients with pure germinomas are frequently treated only with radiation therapy.

The disease extent is the most important prognostic factor. Histologically, choriocarcinoma is associated with the poorest treatment outcome and germinoma with the best. Infants have a high cure rate probably because of the high age-related incidence of presacral teratomas and localized yolk sac tumors.

LANGERHANS CELL HISTIOCYTOSIS

Recognition of the histologic and clinical interrelationships between eosinophilic granuloma, Hand-Schüller-Christian syndrome, and Letterer-Siwe syndrome led to grouping all three syndromes under the term "Histiocytosis X" (Lichtenstein 1953). The involved Langerhans cells are dendritic cells derived from bone marrow, and the disease is now correctly called Langerhans cell histiocytosis (The Writing Group of the Histiocyte Society 1987). Some evidence suggests that the disorder is a manifestation of an immunologic aberration. Although traditionally treated by oncologists, it is probably not a cancer; it is neither monoclonal in origin, nor does it show cellular atypia.

EPIDEMIOLOGY

This disease is rare, at least 20 times less common than acute leukemia in children, and the exact incidence is unknown. The peak in mortality in infants and reported occurrence of disease in siblings or twins suggest the importance of hereditary, constitutional, or genetic factors in this disorder.

PATHOLOGY

The typical lesion is granulomatous and is composed of Langerhans cells and variable numbers of granulocytes and lymphocytes. The Langerhans cells are large and have lobulated, folded, and grooved nuclei. They are characterized by the presence of Birbeck granules (intracytoplasmic, rodlike, lamellar organelles) detected by electron microscopy and by the presence of antigenic surface markers that react with the monoclonal antibody OKT6/Leu-6.

PRESENTATION AND DIAGNOSIS

The clinical manifestations vary according to the tissue and organ infiltration. Solitary- or multiple-bone involvement (eosinophilic granuloma) occurs in older children, especially in the skull and long bones. Exophthalmos, diabetes insipidus, and membranous bone defects (Hand-Schüller-Christian syndrome) are rarely seen together. These patients may have chronically draining ears, with destruction of the mastoid area or cholesteatomas. The skin may have seborrheic-like lesions. Diabetes insipidus may be present at the time of diagnosis or may occur later in the course of the disease.

Some patients have aggressive disease (Letterer-Siwe disease) that often is fatal, particularly in children younger than 2 years of age and those with dysfunctional livers, lungs, or hematopoietic systems. Liver enlargement does not indicate a poor prognosis unless it is accompanied by hypoalbuminemia, hyperbilirubinemia, or edema. The presence of dyspnea, tachypnea, cyanosis, pneumothorax, or pleural effusion, not x-ray findings, demonstrate pulmonary dysfunction. Hematopoietic dysfunction is defined as hemoglobin <10 g/dL (not due to iron deficiency or infection), leukopenia $<4 \times 10^9/L$, or thrombocytopenia $<100 \times 10^9/L$. Prominent cervical lymphadenopathy, a rash resistant to conventional therapy, persistent hepatosplenomegaly, prolonged fever, weight loss, lethargy, diarrhea, and therapy-resistant gingival lesions resembling thrush are seen in some patients.

The diagnosis is based on histologic examination of a biopsy often taken from skin, gingiva, lymph nodes, or skeleton. A biopsy of liver or lung is rarely indicated. A complete excisional biopsy and curettage is both diagnostic and therapeutic for a solitary bone lesion. To assess the extent of disease, complete blood counts, a skeletal survey, chest x-rays, and liver function tests should be performed. If indicated, bone marrow biopsy or pulmonary function tests should also be done.

TREATMENT AND PROGNOSIS

The optimal treatment for children with multifocal involvement is unknown, but it usually includes systemic chemotherapy (e.g., vinblastine, prednisone, methotrexate). Low-dose radiation may be given to selected cases, such as single bone lesions, by preference or when the response to chemotherapy is less than adequate. Good supportive care is essential for these children because secondary bacterial infection, especially otitis media, is frequent. Prophylactic trimethoprim-sulfamethoxazole is recommended to prevent *Pneumocystis carinii* pneumonia in children with extensive disease. Children with diabetes insipidus require replacement therapy with vasopressin.

Impaired hematopoietic, hepatic, or pulmonary function is the most important prognostic factor (Berry et al. 1986). Younger patients have a poor outcome because they tend to have more widespread disease.

REFERENCES

Abramson, D.H.; Ellsworth, R.M.; and Grumbach, N. et al. 1985. Retinoblastoma: survival, age at detection and comparison 1914-1958, 1958-1983. *J. Pediatr. Ophthalmol. Strabismus* 22:246-50.

Altmannsberger, M.; Weber, K.; and Droste, R. et al. 1985. Desmin is a specific marker for rhabdomyosarcomas of human and rat origin. *Am. J. Pathol.* 118:85-95.

Ames, B.N.; Durston, W.E.; and Yamasaki, E. et al. 1973. Carcinogens are mutagens: a simple test system combining liver homogenates for activation and bacteria for detection. *Proc. Natl. Acad. Sci.* 70:2281-85.

Beckwith, J.B. 1986. The John Lattimer Lecture: Wilms' tumor and other renal tumors of childhood, an update. *J. Urol.* 136:320-24.

Beckwith, J.B., and Perrin, E.V. 1963. *In situ* neuroblastoma: a contribution to the natural history of neural crest tumors. *Am. J. Pathol.* 43:1089-1104.

Bedford, M.A.; Bedotto, C.; and Macfaul, P.A. 1971. Retinoblastoma: a study of 139 cases. *Br. J. Ophthalmol.* 55:19-27.

Berry, D.H.; Gresik, M.V.; and Humphrey, G.B. et al. 1986. Natural history of histiocytosis X: a Pediatric Oncology Group Study. *Med. Pediatr. Oncol.* 14:1-5.

Berry, M.P.; Jenkin, R.D.; and Harwood, A.R. et al. 1986. Ewing's sarcoma: a trial of adjuvant chemotherapy and sequential half-body irradiation. *Int. J. Radiat. Oncol. Biol. Phys.* 12:19-24.

Bishop, J.M. 1985. Viral oncogenes. *Cell* 42:23-38.

Blayney, D.W.; Jaffe, E.S.; and Blattner, W.A. et al. 1983. The human T-cell leukemia/lymphoma virus associated with American adult T-cell leukemia/lymphoma. *Blood* 62:401-405.

Bonadonna, G. 1982. Chemotherapy strategies to improve the control of Hodgkin's disease: The Richard and Hinda Rosenthal Foundation Award Lecture. *Cancer Res.* 42: 4309-20.

Brader, J.L., and Miller, R.W. 1979. U.S. cancer incidence and mortality in the first year of life. *Am. J. Dis. Child.* 133: 157-59.

Brinker, M.G.L.; Poppema, S.; and Buys, C.H.C.M. et al. 1987. Clonal immunoglobulin gene rearrangements in tissues involved by Hodgkin's disease. *Blood* 70:186-91.

Brodeur, G.M., and Seeger, R.C. 1986. Gene amplification in human neuroblastomas: basic mechanisms and clinical implications. *Cancer Genet. Cytogenet.* 19:101-11.

Brodeur, G.M.; Seeger, R.C.; and Barrett, A. et al. 1988. International criteria for diagnosis, staging, and response to treatment in patients with neuroblastoma. *J. Clin. Oncol.* 6:1874-81.

Carbone, P.P.; Kaplan, H.S.; and Musshoff, K. et al. 1971. Report of the Committee on Hodgkin's Disease Staging Classification. *Cancer Res.* 31:1860-61.

Coppes, M.J.; de Kraker, J.; and van Dijken, P.J. et al. 1989. Bilateral Wilms' tumor: long-term survival and some epidemiologic features. *J. Clin. Oncol.* 7:310-15.

Crist, W.M.; Raney, R.B., Jr; and Newton, W. et al. 1982. Intrathoracic soft tissue sarcomas in children. *Cancer* 50: 598-604.

Crist, W.M.; Raney, R.B., Jr; and Tefft, M. et al. 1985. Soft tissue sarcomas arising in the retroperitoneal space in children: a report from the Intergroup Rhabdomyosarcoma Study (IRS) Committee. *Cancer* 56:2125-32.

Croce, C.M., and Nowell, P.C. 1985. Molecular basis of human B cell neoplasia. *Blood* 65:1-7.

D'Angio, G.J.; Evans, A.E.; and Breslow, N. et al. 1984. Results of the Third National Wilms' Tumor Study (NWTS-3): a preliminary report. *Proc. Ann. Meet. Am. Assoc. Cancer Res.* 25:183.

Dahl, G.V.; Rivera, G.; and Pui, C.-H. et al. 1985. A novel treatment of childhood lymphoblastic non-Hodgkin's lymphoma: early and intermittent use of teniposide plus cytarabine. *Blood* 66:1110-14.

Dahlin, D.C., and Coventry M.B. 1967. Osteosarcoma: a study of six hundred cases. *J. Bone Joint Surg.* 49A:101-10.

DeVita, V.T., Jr.; Hubbard, S.M.; and Moxley, J.H., III. 1983. The cure of Hodgkin's disease with drugs. *Adv. Intern. Med.* 28:277-302.

Doll, R.; Meier, C.; and Waterhouse, J. 1970. *Cancer incidence in five continents.* vol. II. New York: Springer-Verlag.

Douglass, E.C.; Look, A.T.; and Webber, B. et al. 1986. Hyperdiploidy and chromosomal rearrangements define the anaplastic variant of Wilms' tumor. *J. Clin. Oncol.* 4:975-81.

Douglass, E.C.; Valentine, M.; and Etcubanas, E. et al. 1987. A specific chromosomal abnormality in rhabdomyosarcoma. *Cytogenet. Cell. Genet.* 45:148-55.

Draper, G.J.; Heaf, M.M.; and Kinnier-Wilson, L.M. 1977. Occurrence of childhood cancers among sibs and estimation of familial risks. *J. Med. Genet.* 14:81-90.

Editorial. 1973. Nephroblastoma: an index reference cancer. *Lancet* II:651.

Eilber, F.; Giuliano, A.; and Eckardt, J. et al. 1987. Adjuvant chemotherapy for osteosarcoma: a randomized prospective trial. *J. Clin. Oncol.* 5:21-26.

Evans, A.E.; D'Angio, G.J.; and Randolph, J. 1971. A proposed staging for children with neuroblastoma: Children's Cancer Study Group A. *Cancer* 27:374-78.

Filipovich, A.H.; Spector, B.D.; and Kersey, J. 1980. Immunodeficiency in humans as a risk factor in the development of malignancy. *Prev. Med.* 9:252-59.

Finger, L.R.; Harvey, R.C.; and Moore, R.C.A. et al. 1986. A common mechanism of chromosomal translocation in T- and B-cell neoplasia. *Science* 234:982-85.

Fraumeni, J.F. Jr., and Glass, A.G. 1970. Rarity of Ewing's sarcoma among U.S. Negro children. *Lancet* 1:366-67.

Fraumeni, J.F. Jr., and Hoover, R. 1977. Immunosurveillance and cancer: epidemiologic observations. *Natl. Cancer Inst. Monogr.* 47:121-26.

Friend, S.H.; Bernards, R.; and Rogelj, S. et al. 1986. A human DNA segment with properties of the gene that predisposes to retinoblastoma and osteosarcoma. *Nature* 323:643-46.

Friend, S.H.; Dryja, T.P.; and Weinberg, R.A. 1988. Oncogenes and tumor-suppressing genes. *N. Engl. J. Med.* 318: 618-22.

Gasparini, M.; Lombardi, F.; and Gianni, C. et al. 1983. Childhood rhabdomyosarcoma with meningeal extension: results of combined therapy including central nervous system prophylaxis. *Am. J. Clin. Oncol.* 6:393-98.

Gilbert, F.; Balaban, G.; and Moorhead, P. et al. 1982. Abnormalities of chromosome 1p in human neuroblastoma tumors and cell lines. *Cancer Genet. Cytogenet.* 7:33-42.

Green, A.A., and Hayes, F.A. 1987. Neuroblastoma. In Rudolph, A.M., and Hoffman, J.I. eds. *Pediatrics.* 18th ed. pp. 1113-16. East Norwalk, Conn.: Appleton and Lange.

Green, D.M. 1983. The diagnosis and treatment of yolk sac tumors in infants and children. *Cancer Treat. Rev.* 10: 265-88.

Goldie, J.H.; Coldman, A.J.; and Gudauskas, G.A. 1982. Rationale for the use of alternating noncross-resistant chemotherapy. *Cancer Treat. Rep.* 66:439-49.

Grundy, P.; Breslow, N.; and Green, D.M. et al. 1989. Prognostic factors for children with recurrent Wilms' tumor: results from the Second and Third National Wilms' Tumor Study. *J. Clin. Oncol.* 7:638-47.

Gutensohn, N.M. 1982. Social class and age at diagnosis of Hodgkin's disease: new epidemiologic evidence for the "two-disease hypothesis." *Cancer Treat. Rep.* 66:689-95.

Hall, R.B.; Robinson, L.H.; and Malawar, M.M. et al. 1985. Periosteal osteosarcoma. *Cancer* 55:165-71.

Hansen, M.F.; Koufos, A.; and Gallie, B.L. 1985. Osteosarcoma and retinoblastoma: a shared chromosomal mechanism revealing recessive predisposition. *Proc. Natl. Acad. Sci. USA* 82:6216-20.

Hayes, F.A.; Thompson, E.I.; and Hustu, H.O. et al. 1983. The response of Ewing's sarcoma to sequential cyclophosphamide and Adriamycin induction therapy. *J. Clin. Oncol.* 1:45-51.

Hayes, F.A.; Thompson, E.I.; and Meyer, W.H. et al. 1989. Therapy for localized Ewing's sarcoma of bone. *J. Clin. Oncol.* 7:208-13.

Heim, S., and Mitelman, F. 1987. *Cancer cytogenetics.* New York: Alan R. Liss.

Herbst, A.L.; Cole, P.; and Colton, T. et al. 1977. Age-incidence and risk of diethylstilbestrol-related clear-cell adenocarcinoma of the vagina and cervix. *Am. J. Obstet. Gynecol.* 128:43-50.

Hickman, R.O.; Buckner, C.D.; and Clift, R.A. et al. 1979. A modified right atrial catheter for access to the venous system in marrow transplant recipients. *Surg. Gynecol. Obstet.* 148:871-75.

Jablon, S., and Kato, H. 1970. Childhood cancer in relation to prenatal exposure to atomic-bomb radiation. *Lancet* II: 1000-1003.

Kaizer, H., and Chow, H.S. 1984. Autologous bone marrow transplantation (ABMT) in the treatment of cancer. *Cancer Invest.* 2:203-13.

Kamani, N.; Kennedy, J.; and Brandsma, J. 1988. Burkitt lymphoma in a child with human immunodeficiency virus infection. *J. Pediatr.* 112:241-44.

Kaplan, H.S. 1980. *Hodgkin's disease.* 2nd ed. p. 429. Cambridge, Mass.: Harvard University Press.

Kaplan, H.S. 1981. Hodgkin's disease: biology, treatment, prognosis. *Blood* 57:813-22.

Knudson, A.G., Jr. 1971. Mutation and cancer: statistical study of retinoblastoma. *Proc. Natl. Acad. Sci.* 68:820-23.

Knudson, A.G., Jr. 1985. Hereditary cancer, oncogenes, and antioncogenes. *Cancer Res.* 45:1437-43.

Kohn, H.I., and Fry, R.J. 1984. Radiation carcinogenesis. *N. Engl. J. Med.* 310:504-11.

Koufos, A.; Hansen, M.F.; and Copeland, N.G. et al. 1985. Loss of heterozygosity in three embryonal tumours suggests a common pathogenetic mechanism. *Nature* 316:330-34.

Koufos, A.; Hansen, M.F.; and Lampkin, B.C. et al. 1984 Loss of alleles at loci on human chromosome 11 during genesis of Wilms' tumour. *Nature* 309:170-72.

Kurman, R.J.; Scardino, P.T.; and McIntire, K.R. et al. 1977. Cellular localization of alpha-fetoprotein and human chorionic gonadotropin in germ cell tumors of the testis using an indirect immunoperoxidase technique: a new approach to classification utilizing tumor markers. *Cancer* 40:2136-51.

Kyritsis, A.P.; Tsokos, M.; and Triche, T.J. et al. 1984. Retinoblastoma: origin from a primitive neuroectodermal cell? *Nature* 307:471-73.

Lichtenstein, L. 1953. Histiocytosis X: integration of eosinophilic granuloma of bone, "Letterer-Siwe disease," and "Schüller-Christian disease" as related manifestations of a single nosologic entity. *Arch. Pathol.* 56:84-102.

Link, M.P.; Donaldson, S.S.; and Berard, C.W. et al. 1987. High cure rate with reduced therapy in localized non-Hodgkin's lymphoma (NHL) of childhood. *Proc. Ann. Meet. Am. Soc. Clin. Oncol.* 6:190.

Link, M.P.; Goorin, A.M.; and Miser, A.W. et al. 1986. The effect of adjuvant chemotherapy on relapse-free survival in patients with osteosarcoma of the extremity. *N. Engl. J. Med.* 314:1600-1606.

Look, A.T.; Douglass, E.C.; and Meyer, W.H. 1988. Clinical importance of near-diploid tumor stem lines in patients with osteosarcoma of an extremity. *N. Engl. J. Med.* 318:1567-72.

Look, A.T.; Hayes, F.A.; and Nitschke, R. et al. 1984. Cellular DNA content as a predictor of response to chemotherapy in infants with unresectable neuroblastoma. *N. Engl. J. Med.* 311:231-35.

Lukes, R.J.; Craver, L.F.; and Hall, T.C. et al. 1966 Report of the nomenclature committee. *Cancer Res.* 26:1311.

Marcove, R.C., and Rosen, G. 1980. *En bloc* resections for osteogenic sarcoma. *Cancer* 45:3040-3044.

Matthay, K.K.; Sather, H.N.; and Seeger, R.C. et al. 1989. Excellent outcome of stage II neuroblastoma is independent of residual disease and radiation therapy. *J. Clin. Oncol.* 7:236-44.

Maurer, H.M.; Moon, T.; and Donaldson, M. et al. 1977. The Intergroup Rhabdomyosarcoma Study: a preliminary report. *Cancer* 40:2015-26.

Maurer, H.M.; Beltangady, M.; and Gehan, E.A. et al. 1988. The Intergroup Rhabdomyosarcoma Study I: a final report. *Cancer* 61:209-20.

Meadows, A.T.; Sposto, R.; and Jenkin, R.D.T. et al. 1989. Similar efficacy of 6 and 18 months of therapy with four drugs (COMP) for localized non-Hodgkin's lymphoma of children: a report from the Children's Cancer Study Group. *J. Clin. Oncol.* 7:92-99.

Mecucci, C.,; Louwagie, A.; and Thomas, J. et al. 1988. Cytogenetic studies in T-cell malignancies. *Cancer Genet. Cytogenet.* 30:63-71.

Meyer, W.H.; Schell, M.J.; and Kumar, A.P.M. et al. 1987. Thoracotomy for pulmonary metastatic osteosarcoma: an analysis of prognostic indicators of survival. *Cancer* 59:374-79.

Murphy, S.B. 1980. Classification, staging and end results of treatment of childhood non-Hodgkin's lymphomas: dissimilarities from lymphomas in adults. *Semin. Oncol.* 7:332-39.

Murphy, S.B., Fairclough, D.L.; and Hutchison et al. 1989. Non-Hodgkin's lymphomas of childhood: an analysis of the histology, staging, and response to treatment of 338 cases at a single institution. *J. Clin. Oncol.* 7:186-93.

Nesbit, M.E. Jr.; Robison, L.L.; and Dehner, L.P. 1984. Round cell sarcomas of bone. In Sutow, W.W.; Fernbach, D.J.; and Vietti, T.J. eds. *Clinical pediatric oncology.* pp. 710-33. St. Louis: C.V. Mosby.

Nienhuis, A,W. 1988. Hematopoietic growth factors: biologic complexity and clinical promise (Editorial). *N. Engl. J. Med.* 318:916-18.

Nitschke, R.; Smith, E.I.; and Schochat et al. 1988. Localized neuroblastoma treated by surgery: a Pediatric Oncology Group study. *J. Clin. Oncol.* 6:1271-79.

Nussbaum, R., and Puck, J. 1976. Recurrence risks for retinoblastoma: a model for autosomal dominant disorders with complex inheritance. *J. Pediatr. Ophthalmol.* 13:89-98.

O'Reilly, R.J. 1983. Allogeneic bone marrow transplantation: current status and future directions. *Blood* 62:941-46.

Palmer, N.F., and Foulkes, M. 1983. Histopathology and prognosis in the Second Intergroup Rhabdomyosarcoma Study (IRS-II). *Proc. Ann. Meet. Am. Soc. Clin. Oncol.* 2:229.

Pastore, G.; Carli, M.; and Lemerle, J. et al. 1988. Epidemiological features of Wilms' tumor: results of studies by the International Society of Paediatric Oncology (SIOP). *Med. Pediatr. Oncol.* 16:7-11.

Patte, C.; Philip, T.; and Rodary, C. et al. 1986. Improved survival rate in children with stage III and IV B-cell non-Hodgkin's lymphoma and leukemia using multiagent chemotherapy: results of a study of 114 children from the French Pediatric Oncology Society. *J. Clin. Oncol.* 4:1219-26.

Pratt, C.B.; Meyer, D.; and Chenaille, P. et al. 1989. The use of bone marrow aspirations and lumbar puncture at the time of diagnosis of retinoblastoma. *J. Clin. Oncol.* 7:140-43.

Pui, C.-H.; Ip, S.H.; and Thompson, E. et al. 1989. High serum interleukin-2 receptor levels correlate with poor prognosis in children with Hodgkin's disease. *Leukemia* 3:481-84.

Pui, C.-H.; Ip, S.H.; and Thompson, E. et al. 1989. Increased serum CD8 antigen level in childhood Hodgkin's disease relates to advanced stage and poor treatment outcome. *Blood* 73:209-13.

Pui, C.-H.; Ip, S.H.; and Kung, P. et al. 1987. High serum interleukin-2 receptor levels are related to advanced disease and a poor outcome in childhood non-Hodgkin's lymphoma. *Blood* 70:624-28.

Report of an IARC Working Group. 1980. An evaluation of chemicals and industrial processes associated with cancer in humans based on human and animal data. IARC Monographs. vols. 1-20. *Cancer Res.* 40:1-12.

Richie, J.P., and Garnick, M.B. 1984 Changing concepts in the treatment of nonseminomatous germ cell tumors of the testis. *J. Urol.* 131:1089-92.

Romagnani, S.; Ferrini, P.L.; and Ricci, M. 1985. The immune derangement in Hodgkin's disease. *Semin. Hematol.* 22:41-55.

Rosen, E.M.; Cassady, J.R.; and Frantz, C.N. et al. 1984. Neuroblastoma: the Joint Center for Radiation Therapy/Dana Farber Center Institute/Children's Hospital Experience. *J. Clin. Oncol.* 2:719-32.

480   *Textbook of Clinical Oncology*

Rosenberg, S.A.; Lotze, M.T.; and Muul, L.M. et al. 1985. Observations on the systemic administration of autologous lymphokine-activated killer cells and recombinant interleukin-2 to patients with metastatic cancer. *N. Engl. J. Med.* 313:1485-92.

Seeger, R.C.; Brodeur, G.M.; and Sather, H. et al. 1985. Association of multiple copies of the N-*myc* oncogene with rapid progression of neuroblastomas. *N. Engl. J. Med.* 313:1111-16.

Shimada, H.; Chatten, J.; and Newton, W.A. et al. 1984. Histopathologic prognostic factors in neuroblastic tumors: definition of subtypes of ganglioneuroblastoma and an age-linked classification of neuroblastomas. *J. Natl. Cancer Inst.* 73:405-16.

Slater, R.M.; de Kraker, J.; and Voute, P.A. et al. 1985. A cytogenetic study of Wilms' tumor. *Cancer Genet. Cytogenet.* 14:95-109.

Sundeen, J.; Lipford, E.; and Uppenkamp, M. et al. 1987. Rearranged antigen receptor genes in Hodgkin's disease. *Blood* 70:96-103.

The Writing Group of the Histiocyte Society. 1987. Histiocytosis syndromes in children. *Lancet* I:208-209.

Whang-Peng, J.; Triche, T.J.; and Knutsen, T. et al. 1986. Cytogenetic characterization of selected small round cell tumors of childhood. *Cancer Genet. Cytogenet.* 21:185-208.

Wilimas, J.A.; Douglass, E.C.; and Lewis, S. et al. 1988. Reduced therapy for Wilms' tumor: analysis of treatment results from a single institution. *J. Clin. Oncol.* 6:1630-35.

Young, J.L. Jr.; Heise, H.W.; and Silverberg, E. et al. 1978. *Cancer incidence, survival and mortality for children under 15 years of age.* New York: American Cancer Society Professional Education Publications.

Young, J.L. Jr., and Miller, R.W. 1975. Incidence of malignant tumors in U.S. children. *J. Pediatr.* 86:254-58.

Ziegler, J.L.; Beckstead, J.A.; and Volberding, P.A. et al. 1984. Non-Hodgkin's lymphoma in 90 homosexual men: relation to generalized lymphadenopathy and the acquired immunodeficiency syndrome. *N. Engl. J. Med.* 311:565-70.

Chapter 33

GYNECOLOGIC CANCERS

S. B. Gusberg, M.D.
Carolyn D. Runowicz, M.D.

S.B. Gusberg, M.D.
Distinguished Service Professor and Chairman Emeritus
Department of Obstetrics-Gynecology and Reproductive Science
Mount Sinai School of Medicine
New York, New York

Carolyn D. Runowicz, M.D.
Director of Gynecologic Oncology and Associate Professor
Albert Einstein School of Medicine
New York, New York

Acknowledgments
Parts of this chapter are based on earlier published chapters in the text Female Genital Cancer, *Gusberg, S.B.; Shingleton, H.M.; and Deppe, G. eds. 1988, published by Churchill Livingstone. We wish to express our gratitude to the authors and publisher of that work for their permission to excerpt from it.*

INTRODUCTION

The genital organs are among the most common sites of cancer in women. Gynecologic cancers account for more than 73,000 new cases and approximately 23,000 deaths in the United States each year. These figures do not include the 45,000 new cases of carcinoma *in situ* of the uterine cervix that occur annually.

Gynecologic cancer is one area in which screening of asymptomatic women is particularly rewarding in terms of effecting a cure. Virtually all cervical and other gynecologic cancers (with the exception of ovarian cancer) are curable if treated in an *in situ* or precancerous stage. A 90% cure rate can be achieved if the cancers are diagnosed and treated when they are less than 1 cm in diameter, and even more-advanced cancers can be cured 80% of the time provided they are confined to the primary site of origin. This compares with estimates that 50% of all cancers could be cured if treated early.

The concept of screening healthy, asymptomatic women for early gynecologic cancer is now well-accepted, thanks largely to the development of the Papanicolaou (Pap) smear. The steady decline in mortality from cervical cancer is attributed to widespread Pap smear screening.

Educational campaigns that focus on early detection and prevention are also a powerful means of reducing the incidence of most gynecologic cancers. As long as elimination of all carcinogens from our environment remains a remote ideal, measures that lead to early detection represent the best hope for effective cancer control.

Post-treatment management of gynecologic cancer has some specific challenges, as in the area of the patient's sexuality. Because treatment often affects both physical and psychological aspects of sexual function and may lead to reduced libido, chronic anxiety, and other disorders, sexual counseling should be routinely offered to gynecologic cancer patients as an integral part of rehabilitation.

CERVICAL CANCERS

Due to widespread screening programs, more than two-thirds of cervical cancers in the United States are now detected in the *in situ* stage. Consequently, mortality from this type of malignancy has dropped sharply. It remains a leading cause of death in relatively young women in developing countries, where screening is less prevalent. The American Cancer Society estimated there would be 13,500 new cases of invasive cervical cancer for 1990, and an estimated 6,000 deaths.

In its early stages, cancer of the cervix is a highly curable disease, with a favorable outlook similar to that of skin cancer. With the present level of knowledge and technology, cervical cancer could be controlled worldwide if adequate funds and political support were channeled towards this task. Early detection is the key to reducing mortality rates, but extensive epidemiologic data pointing to a viral etiology suggest that antiviral strategies, such as vaccination, are not to be excluded.

Most cervical cancers are squamous cell carcinomas, although some are adenocarcinomas. The principles of diagnosis and treatment apply to both types.

EPIDEMIOLOGY

Cervical cancer is now considered to be generally a sexually transmittable disease (STD). Probable agents are human papillomaviruses, mostly types 16 and 18. There is also indirect evidence, based primarily on serologic and immunologic data, showing that herpes simplex virus type 2 may be a cofactor.

Sexual history and socioeconomic status are the major criteria that define groups at high risk for developing cancer of the cervix. However, because there are no data to make this definition specific enough, all adult women and sexually active adolescents must be included in efforts aimed at prevention and early detection.

Onset of sexual activity before age 20 and multiple sexual partners increase risk. Many reports have shown prostitutes to have at least a 4-fold relative risk, whereas no cases of cervical cancer were found in a study of 13,000 nuns (Gagnon 1952).

Incidence appears to be higher among women of low socioeconomic status. Diet may be a factor, but there is no clear evidence to support this. Recent studies have suggested that women who develop cervical cancer are deficient in vitamin A (specifically beta carotene), vitamin C, folic acid, or all three, but further investigations are needed. Cigarette smoking is also regarded as a cofactor.

Family history and menstrual pattern have no bearing on the prevalence, nor is there any evidence of endocrine dysfunction with cancer of the cervix. There appears to be no hormonal correlation, and women treated for cervical cancer can receive estrogen replacement therapy if needed.

The incidence of invasive cervical cancer appears to rise sharply until age 45 and peaks between 45 and 55 years, with an average age of 48 (Gusberg and McKay 1971). For carcinoma *in situ,* the peak occurs approximately 10 years earlier; for endometrial cancer, 10 years later. In the past two decades, more and more younger women have presented with dysplasia, carcinoma *in situ,* and invasive cervical cancer.

DIAGNOSIS

At the onset of the disease, abnormal cellular growth is slow. Preclinical, preinvasive phases, referred to as cervical intraepithelial neoplasia (CIN), last as long as eight to 10 years. During this stage, malignant cells lack the ability to penetrate the underlying tissues or to metastasize. Once microinvasion and invasive cancer develop, the tumor grows rapidly and can cause death within two to three years.

Screening should start at age 18, or earlier if a woman is sexually active. Subsequent frequency of Pap-smear monitoring has been a controversial issue in the gynecologic community. Concerns have been expressed that in high-risk women the transit time from dysplasia to invasive cancer is shorter, but as yet there are no firm data to support such claims. On the other hand, quality of testing in some commercial laboratories remains a problem, and even an experienced clinician may miss the affected area or apply the spray fixative imperfectly. An additional factor is the occasional mislabeled specimen (Shingleton and Gore 1988). In view of these potential drawbacks, it seems appropriate that women be advised to have three or four annual Pap smears initially, and then every two or three years.

Varying degrees of atypia and dysplasia can be detected in a Pap smear specimen (Shingleton and Orr 1987). A colposcopic examination is recommended when the smear is atypical. A cervix that appears grossly normal usually indicates that it only harbors a preinvasive or microinvasive cancer, unless the lesion is entirely endocervical. The cervix may contain an erosion or ectropion, which is an inverted transformation zone. Colposcopically directed biopsy is crucial for definite diagnosis. To enhance its accuracy, this procedure should include endocervical curettage (Shingleton and Gore 1988).

An invasive tumor usually presents in a so-called cauliflower shape, with a generally friable texture and a hard nodular edge. Ulcers occur on the surface and are surrounded by necrosis when the stroma is destroyed by an invasive tumor. The tumor's extension is determined by palpating the mass vaginally, and by conducting a rectovaginal palpation. A complete investigation must include intravenous pyelogram (IVP), cystoscopy, and sigmoidoscopy. All test findings must be correlated when the final diagnosis is made.

There is no characteristic symptom for cervical cancer. Bleeding, the only significant symptom, is caused by ulceration — a breakthrough on the epithelial surface — but unfortunately some tumors spread without ulcerating the surface altogether. Although it is not always a reliable indicator, abnormal bleeding signals the need for an immediate examination because it can lead to early diagnosis.

Persistent aching pain may occur in the low quadrants or low back when a tumor has reached the pelvic side wall and presses against nerve trunks and the sacral plexus. Extensive tumors infiltrate the parametrium and may obstruct the ureters, causing hydronephrosis with renal pain or uremia.

STAGING

Staging provides important information that can affect the choice of treatment protocol and assist the oncologist in making a correct prognosis. It is also helpful in comparing and assessing the results of different therapies.

For many years, staging of cervical cancer was based on clinical examination because patients were mostly treated by radiotherapy without operation. In the past three decades, there has been an increased interest in surgical staging. An analysis of six reports between 1971 and 1981 involving 971 patients (Shingleton and Orr 1987) demonstrated that surgical staging was more accurate than clinical staging in up to 42.9% of cases. However, a risk-benefit analysis of pretreatment surgical

Table 33.1
INTERNATIONAL STAGING OF CANCER OF THE CERVIX

Stage	Description/Features
0	Carcinoma *in situ,* intraepithelial carcinoma (cases of stage 0 should not be included in any therapeutic statistics for invasive carcinoma)
I	Carcinoma strictly confined to the cervix; extension to the corpus should be disregarded
	a. Preclinical carcinomas of the cervix; that is, those diagnosed only by microscopy
	Ia1. Minimal microscopically evident stromal invasion
	Ia2. Lesions detected microscopically that can be measured; the upper limit of the measurement should not show a depth of invasion of more than 5 mm taken from the base of the epithelium, either surface or glandular, from which it originates, and a second dimension, the horizontal spread must not exceed 7 mm; larger lesions should be staged as Ib
	Ib. Lesions of greater dimension than stage Ia2, whether seen clinically or not; space involvement should not alter the staging, but should be specifically recorded so as to determine whether it should affect treatment decisions in the future
II	Carcinoma extending beyond the cervix, but not onto the pelvic wall; involves the vagina, but not the lower one-third
	a. No obvious parametrial involvement
	b. Obvious parametrial involvement
III	Carcinoma extending onto the pelvic wall; (on rectal examination, there is no cancer-free space between the tumor and the pelvic wall; the tumor involves the lower one-third of the vagina; all cases with a hydronephrosis or nonfunctioning kidney)
	a. No extension onto the pelvic wall
	b. Extension onto the pelvic wall; urinary obstruction of one or both ureters on intravenous pyelogram (IVP) without the other criteria for stage III disease
IV	Carcinoma extending beyond the true pelvis or clinically involving the mucosa of bladder or rectum (a bullous edema, as such, does not permit a case to be allotted to stage IV)
	a. Spread to adjacent organs
	b. Spread to distant organs

staging by exploratory laparotomy should be carried out before the procedure enters common practice.

The first international classification of cervical cancer was adopted by the International Federation of Gynecology and Obstetrics (FIGO) in 1961. With this type of malignancy, stage refers to clinical extent, class to the cytologic interpretation, and grade to the histologic differentiation of the tumor. Table 33.1 shows the most current FIGO staging; it may be used alone or in combination with the TNM (tumor, node, metastasis) system.

Preclinical stage I lesions, invading to 3 mm, are usually diagnosed by conization and are rarely associated with lymph node metastases. All other stage I cases are designated as stage IB. Although some hospitals also distinguish a IC stage for tumors over 2.5 cm in diameter, FIGO has not accepted such a refinement in the classification.

Surgical experience has given physicians extensive knowledge of the distribution and incidence of nodal metastases in relationship to disease stage. Stage I disease demonstrates microscopically positive lymph nodes in approximately 15%; stage II in about 25%; stage III in 36% to 50%; and stage IVA in over 50% of cases (Shingleton and Orr 1987). An increase in stage leads to a greater involvement of secondary nodes (table

33.2) along the common iliac vessels and the aorta (Kavanagh, Ruffolo, and Marsden 1985).

APPROACHES TO TREATMENT

The extent of disease is a critical factor for prognosis. The cure rate is about 100% in stages 0 and IA; 90% in stage IB (small); 70% in stage IC (large); 50% to 60% in stage II; 30% to 40% in stage III; and possibly 5% in stage IV (Gusberg and Shingleton 1988).

Staging also determines the choice of treatment, which lies between radical surgery and irradiation; adjuvant chemotherapy is only used experimentally. Surgery is generally done through stage IIA, while patients with stage IIB and stage III (AB) are usually managed in the United States with radiation therapy. Virulence factors, including depth of stromal invasion, grade, involvement of vascular spaces, and local migration of lymphocytes to form a round collar around the tumor, are less important than disease stage, but they can also be factored into the treatment protocol (tables 33.3 and 33.4).

Other relevant factors include the tumor's sensitivity to radiation, the technical expertise of the personnel, and the patient's general health. Thus, highly individualized and complex judgments are involved in the treatment of each patient.

Table 33.2
INCIDENCE OF PARA-AORTIC NODE INVOLVEMENT IN THE VARIOUS STAGES OF CERVICAL CARCINOMA

INVESTIGATORS	CLINICAL STAGE OF TUMOR				
	I	II	III	IV	OVERALL
Averette et al. (1972)	3/40	4/18	2/20	1/2	10/80 (12%)
Buchsbaum (1972)	0/23	1/12	7/20	1/2	9/57 (16%)
Nelson et al. (1977)	—	9/63	15/39	0/2	24/104 (23%)
Sudasanam et al. (1978)	11/53	7/43	5/19	0/3	23/218 (11%)
Lagasse et al. (1980)	8/143	23/80	19/64	1/4	51/291 (18%)
Total	22/259	44/216	48/162	3/13	117/750 (16%)
	(8%)	(20%)	(30%)	(23%)	

(From: Cavanaugh, D.; Ruffolo, E.H.; and Marsden, D.E. eds. 1985. *Gynecologic cancer: a clinicopathologic approach.* Norwalk, Conn.: Appleton-Century-Crofts.)

Table 33.3
VIRULENCE FACTOR, LYMPHATIC INVASION, AND
CURE RATE WITH GOOD RST

Lymphatics	STAGE I		STAGE II		TOTAL	
	N	%	N	%	N	%
Negative	28	87.5	53	85.1	81	86.0[a]
Positive	14	53.9	20	30.0	34	39.4[a]

[a]Significant at 0.01 level
RST = radiosensitivity test
(Source: Gusberg, Shingleton, and Deppe [1988]. p. 287.)

Precursor lesions can be treated by conservative therapy on an outpatient basis if they are well-demarcated and do not involve more than two quadrants of the portio. Excision of CIN may be accomplished by cryosurgery, electrocautery, or laser vaporization. Some physicians favor cryosurgery over electrocautery because of greater patient acceptance (Shingleton and Kim 1988), but electrocautery is no less effective in eradicating the lesions (Chanene and Rome 1983; Schuurmans, Ohlke, and Carmichael 1984). Laser vaporization is more costly, but it allows for greater precision in the destruction of the lesion than does cryosurgery (Shingleton et al. 1983a).

Other techniques for treating precursor lesions include excisional biopsy, conization, and hysterectomy. In patients with CIN, the estimated 3.5% recurrence rate after conization is not all that different from the 0.5% to 2% recurrence rates following hysterectomy (Shingleton et al. 1983b). However, hysterectomy should be considered if the woman is unlikely to return for adequate follow-up visits or has completed childbearing and desires sterilization.

Stromal invasion to less than 1 mm is treated by therapeutic conization or total hysterectomy (abdominal or vaginal). Invasion to less than 3 mm below the basement membrane is treated by conventional hysterectomy. When stromal invasion exceeds 3 mm, radical hysterectomy is accompanied by pelvic node dissection and aortic node assessment (Shingleton and Kim 1988).

In stage I disease, radiation therapy or radical surgery achieve similar cure rates. However, radiation is associated with a number of delayed complications and post-treatment sexual dysfunction (Abitol and Davenport 1974). Radical surgical excision of stage IB disease is preferred, especially in premenopausal women.

For patients with invasive cancer, a treatment protocol must be determined on the basis of a comprehensive evaluation that includes a careful physical examination to evaluate pelvic extent of disease, and abdominal palpation. Chest radiography, IVP, and barium enema may be required for women over 50 or those with a history of gastrointestinal disease. Endoscopic tests (cystoscopy, sigmoidoscopy) must also be conducted, and hematologic and blood chemistry findings must be taken into account. Evaluation may include several optional tests, such as computed tomography (CT), retrograde pyelography, and coagulation studies.

Two types of radiation therapy are used to treat cervical cancer: brachytherapy (intracavity and interstitial) and external pelvic radiation therapy. Brachytherapy is directed towards the primary tumor site and immediate paracervical and vaginal extensions of the lesion. In the intracavity method, an applicator which has colpostats that are approximated to the vaginal fornices is inserted into the uterine cavity. With this technique, high tumoricidal doses of radiation are delivered directly to the cervix with minimal complications to the adjacent organs.

The distortion of vaginal anatomy associated with advanced cancer of the cervix may preclude the placement of intracavity applicators. To circumvent this problem, a group of 18-gauge hollow steel needles may be inserted into the parametrium, theoretically representing modified interstitial colpostats. The interstitial method may increase morbidity, and long-term studies are needed to determine whether it leads to improved survival rates.

Extension of the tumor into the extrauterine pelvic soft tissue and lymph nodes is treated by external radiation therapy. The beam is aimed at the region that reaches the upper end of the fifth lumbar vertebra (L5) and includes all vaginal extension of tumor and the entire obturator fossa.

Both modes of radiation therapy are used in combination. For example, an invasive tumor may be externally radiated until it shrinks and creates conditions for placement of intracavity equipment. Schedule and dose of radiation should be adjusted to each patient depending on her age, stage of disease, nutritional status, anatomical factors, and concomitant systemic disease.

Radiation therapy, particularly when delivered in high doses, inevitably affects organs adjacent to the cervix. For example, 83 complications (8%) were reported among 1,030 patients with stage I and II cervical cancer treated at M.D. Anderson Hospital (Strockbine, Hancock, and Fletcher 1970); however, only 22 patients (2%) had serious complications, such as bladder or rectal fistula, vaginal vault necrosis, or obstruction.

Acute complications, such as serious skin reaction, acute radiation cystitis, proctosigmoiditis, and enteritis, are common during the course of radiation treatment, but are usually transient. Delayed side effects, which appear six to 24 months after completion of therapy, include varying degrees of vaginal and cervical fibrosis which can cause sexual dysfunction, vaginal stenosis, dyspareunia, and proctitis. Such complications as

Table 33.4
BIOPSY LYMPHATICS AND LYMPH NODES IN
CANCER OF THE CERVIX

CERVICAL LYMPHATICS	POSITIVE LYMPH NODES	
	N	%
Positive (N = 36)	16	44
Negative (N = 67)	3	4

(Source: Gusberg, Shingleton, and Deppe [1988]. p. 287.)

rectovaginal fistula, bladder fistula, and small bowel injury may require surgical intervention.

New methods for administering radiation therapy under investigation include interstitial implants, high linear energy transfer (LET) radiation, and hypoxic cell sensitizers.

Because advanced cervical cancer is highly metastatic, hope lies in a therapy that would combine surgery, radiation therapy, and adjuvant chemotherapy. Studies of hydroxyurea used in combination with radiation therapy have had some promising results (Piver et al. 1983). Preliminary results with cisplatin administered simultaneously with pelvic irradiation in locally advanced cervical cancer have also been excellent (Runowicz et el. 1989).

The disease-free interval after treatment depends on the stage of the tumor when first detected, the adequacy of the initial treatment, and other factors. In patients whose cervical cancer ultimately recurs, tumors tend to appear at distant sites, in the retroperitoneal spaces, or in the central pelvis (Shingleton et al 1983b). Prognosis is poor for most patients with recurrence, and the great majority of deaths occur within the first three years (Shingleton and Kim 1988).

ENDOMETRIAL CANCERS

Endometrial tumor is the most common type of female genital cancer in the United States and is one of the six leading causes of cancer death. While in the first half of the twentieth century cancer of the cervix was three to six times more prevalent than cancer of the endometrium, this trend has reversed. According to the American Cancer Society, 33,000 new endometrial cancers were expected to occur in 1990, as opposed to only 13,500 new cases of cervical cancer.

The sharp rise in the relative prevalence of endometrial tumors probably has been due to the aging population, high-calorie and high-fat diets, and the popularity of estrogen therapy without progestational modification in the 1960s and early 1970s. However, the cure rate for endometrial cancer is very high because these tumors tend to be well-differentiated and localized (Gusberg 1988a). In 1990, endometrial tumor was expected to result in only 4,000 deaths in the United States, as compared with approximately 6,000 deaths from the less-common cervical cancer, 44,000 breast cancer deaths, and 50,000 female lung cancer deaths.

Adenocarcinoma of the endometrium is the predominant malignant neoplasm of the uterus that originates in the endometrial epithelium. However, a variety of other tumors of mixed origin can arise in the body of the uterus, the most common of which are: sarcoma of the endometrium, mixed mesodermal tumors, rhabdomyosarcoma, leiomyosarcoma, hemangioendothelioma, adenosquamous carci noma, clear cell carcinoma, and papillary serous carcinoma.

EPIDEMIOLOGY AND RISK FACTORS

Endometrial cancer mostly affects postmenopausal women: 75% of cases occur after age 50, and only 4% before age 40. The incidence peaks at 58 to 60 years of age, approximately 10 years later than invasive cervical cancer or adenomatous hyperplasia, the precursor of endometrial cancer.

Although no genetic marker is known, in 12% to 28% of cases the tumor has occurred in families. In this respect it is similar to breast cancer. The disease has also occurred in identical twins at about the same age.

Women with endometrial cancer tend to be of a higher socioeconomic status, although in the United States this tendency has been disappearing as the so-called class differences are being evened out. Geographically, frequency is higher in industrialized countries and lower in developing countries, while the distribution of cervical cancer follows an inverse pattern and is lower in developed countries and higher in developing nations, Japan being the only exception. Both the socioeconomic and geographical patterns are now attributed to differences in diet, as a high incidence of endometrial cancer is related to high intake of dietary fat.

Women at a high risk of developing endometrial cancer tend to be obese and have a large body frame, a finding that has been confirmed by epidemiologic studies (Wynder, Escher, and Mantel 1966). Women who are 50 lb (22.5 kg) overweight have a 9-fold risk of developing the disease. Other risk factors include diabetes and hypertension, although the relationship with these disorders appears to be casual and not causal. However, a young, slender, nondiabetic, normotensive woman can have endometrial cancer. Constant estrogenic stimulation and a deficit in progestational modification necessary to protect the endometrium (Gusberg 1947) are other risk factors. Yet, although the hormone dependency of endometrial cancer has been a long-established fact, almost 40% of endometrial tumors appear to be autonomous and unrelated to endocrine dysfunction, and their etiology remains unknown.

Infertility due to failure of ovulation is one of the hormone-related disorders characteristic of the high-risk group. Absence of ovulation creates a deficit in progestin, resulting in an endocrinologic imbalance. Menstrual aberration, common in the history of women with endometrial cancer, is another symptom also frequently related to anovulation. Another significant characteristic is dysfunctional bleeding during the menopause, which indicates overstimulation of the endometrium by irregular estrogen secretion without modification by progesterone.

Finally, prolonged exogenous estrogen administration has been shown to increase the risk of endometrial cancer. Studies have demonstrated that women taking estrogen for more than two years had a 4- to 14-fold risk of developing the tumor compared with age-matched controls.

DIAGNOSIS

Because of its clearly defined risk factors, the initiation of a screening activity for endometrial cancer would seem appropriate, although few such attempts have been made. While screening for cervical cancer is directed towards younger women especially, detection programs for endometrial tumors should be aimed primarily at the perimenopausal and postmenopausal age groups. Due to the long preclinical stage, suggested by its development late in life, and the recognition of its precursor lesions, the development of this tumor is highly preventable. In addition to screening all women at menopause, preventive measures must include restriction of promiscuous use of estrogen and appropriate treatment of precursor lesions.

Various techniques are available for detection and diagnosis of endometrial tumors and precursor lesions. Aspiration curettage, which can be performed with minimum discomfort on an outpatient basis, is widely performed in the United States. Fractional curettage under anesthesia is a highly accurate technique that offers a complete biopsy for analysis. The Pap smear, which is very accurate for cervical cancer, has only a 50% accuracy in the detection of endometrial tumors. Cytologic samples taken through a cannula from the endometrial cavity have a considerable degree of accuracy, but usually not for precursor lesions. Cytologic samples obtained by abrasion also frequently supply histologic fragments that are diagnostically useful.

The only significant clinical sign is bleeding, which signals ulceration. In postmenopausal women, bleeding indicates a malignancy in one-third of cases and a benign condition in about another one-third; it has an unknown etiology in the remaining one-third. In pre- and perimenopausal women bleeding is associated with endometrial cancer in a small minority of cases.

Pain usually appears only in widespread disease, and is not helpful for early detection. Pelvic examination is of little use because the uterus frequently retains its normal size and shape.

STAGING

Adenomatous hyperplasia has been recognized as an endometrial cancer precursor since the 1940s (Gusberg 1947). If left untreated, it can progress to invasive cancer in 20% to 25% of cases. Depending on the extent of histopathologic changes, grades I, II, and III of adenomatous hyperplasia are distinguished. Grade III may be called stage 0 carcinoma of the endometrium.

Staging of endometrial cancer previously was based on the extent of the tumor. However, studies conducted in the 1960s have shown the importance of incorporating major virulence factors—size of uterine cavity, involvement of cervix, and histologic differentiation—into the classification scale. The staging proposed by the FIGO committee in 1971, which includes these factors and is now widely accepted, is shown in table 33.5. A new surgical staging is now proposed.

Table 33.5
FIGO CLASSIFICATION OF VIRULENCE FACTORS IN ENDOMETRIAL CANCER

STAGES	DESCRIPTION/FEATURES
IA GI, II, III	Tumor limited to endometrium
IB GI, II, III	Invasion to < ½ myometrium
IC GI, II, III	Invasion > ½ myometrium
IIA GI, II, III	Endocervical glandular involvement only
IIB GI, II, III	Cervical stromal invasion
IIIA GI, II, III	Tumor invades serosa and/or adnexae and/or positive peritoneal cytology
IIIB GI, II, III	Vaginal metastases
IIIC GI, II, III	Metastases to pelvic and/or para-aortic lymph nodes
IVA GI, II, III	Tumor invasion of bladder and/or bowel mucosa
IVB	Distant metastases including intra-abdominal or inguinal lymph node

Histopathology—Degree of Differentiation
Cases of carcinoma of the corpus should be grouped with regard to the degree of differentiation of the adenocarcinoma as follows:
G1 = 5% or less of a nonsquamous or nonmorular solid growth pattern
G2 = 6%-50% of a nonsquamous or nonmorular solid growth pattern
G3 = more than 50% of a nonsquamous or nonmorular solid growth pattern

Notes on Pathological Grading
(1) Notable nuclear atypia, inappropriate for the architectural grade, raises the grade of a grade I or grade II tumor by 1
(2) In serous adenocarcinomas, clear cell adenocarcinomas, and squamous cell carcinomas, nuclear grading takes precedence
(3) Adenocarcinomas with squamous differentiation are graded according to the nuclear grade of the glandular component

Rules Related to Staging
(1) Since corpus cancer is now surgically staged, procedures previously used for determination of stages are no longer applicable, such as the finding of fractional D&C to differentiate between stage I and stage II
(2) It is appreciated that there may be a small number of patients with corpus cancer who will be treated primarily with radiation therapy; if that is the case, the clinical staging adopted by FIGO in 1971 would still apply but designation of that staging system would be noted
(3) Ideally, width of the myometrium should be measured along with the width of tumor invasion

The rate of metastasis varies greatly, but no more than 15% of tumors develop quickly and lethally. The adenocarcinoma tends to spread along the surface of the uterine cavity before progressing to deeper invasion. It can then spread in several ways: directly into the myometrium; to the ovary or peritoneal cavity via cells escaping from the fallopian tubes; to lung, bone, or other sites through the blood vessels; and through the lymphatic system.

APPROACHES TO TREATMENT

A woman's age and reproductive needs determine the choice of treatment for adenomatous hyperplasia (Gusberg 1988b). Lesions caused by hormonal imbalances are often reversible. In young women it is frequently due to failure of ovulation, and may disappear when a progestin is administered or ovulation is restored. In perimenopausal women grades I and II may be treated effectively by a progestin; however, hysterectomy is recommended in more intense cases of grade II and especially grade III forms. In the postmenopausal woman adenomatous hyperplasia is often the result of estrogen therapy. In this case, estrogen must be discontinued and, if this is not enough, a progestin should be administered before going on to surgery.

Treatment protocol for endometrial cancer is highly individualized, a trend that was launched by our reports in the early 1960s and reinforced by Wade, Kohorn, and Morris (1967), Nelson and Koller (1969), Stallworthy (1971), and Rutledge (1974), among others. Virulence factors and parameters of tumor aggression are taken into consideration, as are volume of tumor growth, involvement of the cervix or isthmus, myometrial invasion, and node penetration. More aggressive tumors and extensive involvement require more aggressive treatment.

SURGERY

The mainstay of treatment for endometrial cancer in the United States and in most other parts of the world is hysterectomy, with or without irradiation, although the question of optimum therapy remains open. In most cases, the operation should be conducted through a vertical suprapubic or paramedian incision, and not through the cosmetic Pfannenstiel incision. Vaginal hysterectomy is inadequate because it provides limited exposure, which rules out an assessment of the pelvis and upper abdomen. Radical hysterectomy with lymphadenectomy is performed only under special circumstances because it is associated with greater operative morbidity and has not been shown to increase the cure rate as compared with more conventional treatment. Conservative hysterectomy, with pelvic and aortic node dissection reserved for the most virulent tumors, is the preferred treatment.

RADIATION

Radiation therapy is used as adjuvant treatment in combination with surgery, and in the infrequent inoperable patient. Earlier reports (Arneson 1953; Gusberg

1966) appeared to show a clear advantage of therapy including preoperative radiation over surgical treatment alone, but more studies are needed to reach a well-based conclusion. Nor is there sufficient evidence concerning the advantages and disadvantages of preoperative vs. postoperative radiation, as cure rates with both approaches appear to be the same (Graham 1963). Increasingly, postoperative irradiation is reserved for patients with tumors of high virulence. These patients are also subjected to pelvic and aortic lymphadenectomy.

Irradiation can be performed internally or externally. An internal method employs the traditional technique known as Stockholm Packing, in which tubes containing radium or a radium equivalent are inserted into the endometrial cavity. Postoperative radium irradiation of the vaginal vault is another example of the internal technique. External radiotherapy, which is becoming more common as both preoperative and postoperative treatment, covers the entire pelvic area at risk.

In contrast with treatment for cancer of the cervix, the presently used doses present little risk of significant radiation injury if radiation is carefully directed and adjusted to avoid exposure of vital organs. In current practice, surgery followed by irradiation only for patients at high risk of recurrence (approximately 30%) is the preferred treatment.

HORMONAL THERAPY AND CHEMOTHERAPY

Hormonal treatment with a progestin has induced regression of metastases, particularly those to the lung, in about one-third of patients. Differentiated lesions are more responsive, and best results are achieved with recurrent disease; primary metastases are more resistant.

Hormonal treatment of primary endometrial tumors has been advocated for young women with the aim of preserving their fertility, but it is still considered as investigational. There have been favorable reports about hormonal treatment used as adjuvant therapy in primary disease after surgery, but these results are still tentative, especially those with positive steroid receptors.

Chemotherapy appears to be most effective in poorly differentiated tumors that are not hormone-dependent. It may also be of help in patients with positive para-aortic lymph nodes. Adriamycin and 5-fluorouracil, used as single agents or in combinations, have been the most frequently studied drugs in the management of advanced or recurrent endometrial carcinoma.

Survival figures are difficult to analyze because not all studies use a virulence type of clinical classification, but the best broad-based view is offered by the Stockholm annual report (table 33.6).

OVARIAN CANCERS

Among gynecologic tumors, ovarian cancer is the most difficult to prevent or cure because it is notoriously silent at the outset and usually presents in stage III, when it is very difficult to control. It is the sixth most

Table 33.6
CARCINOMA OF THE ENDOMETRIUM

INSTITUTION (CITY)	NO. TREATED	% SURVIVED AFTER 5 YRS
Melbourne	279	64.1
Vienna	312	52.5
Saskatchewan	262	84.8
Toronto	560	78.6
Vancouver	445	83.7
Winnipeg	370	81.7
Brno, Czech.	235	78.6
Helsinki	253	74.7
Leipzig	204	63.5
Kiel	229	72.6
Munich, 1st Clinic	226	57.1
Munich, Grosshadern	264	66.0
Debrecen, Hungary	215	70.3
Oslo	678	84.1
Lodz	200	83.2
Gothenburg	508	77.8
Stockholm	541	80.2
New Haven	211	76.5
Leningrad	201	88.6
Ljubljana	310	73.7
Zagreb	236	80.5

(Source: FIGO Annual Report [1985].)

common cancer in women, and one of the most deadly: 12,400 women were expected to die of this tumor in 1990, more than the deaths due to endometrial and cervical cancers combined.

Two-thirds of all ovarian neoplasms and more than three-fourths of all malignant ovarian tumors derive from different types of epithelial cells (Deppe and Lawrence 1988a). Germ-cell tumors account for fewer than 5% of all ovarian cancers (Weiss, Homonchuk, and Young 1977), but in females younger than 20 they represent approximately two-thirds of malignant ovarian tumors (Deppe and Lawrence 1988a).

EPIDEMIOLOGY AND RISK FACTORS

Epithelial ovarian cancer is far more common in Western industrialized nations than anywhere else in the world. In the United States, it is primarily encountered among older Caucasian women of Northern European descent (Deppe and Lawrence 1988a). Such a distribution is probably due to dietary and environmental factors, since studies show that the incidence of ovarian cancers increases when emigrants move from developing to better-developed countries (Smith and Ol 1984; Greene, Clark, and Blayney 1984). Studies also suggest that a diet rich in vitamin A and fiber reduces the risk of ovarian tumor (Byers et al. 1983).

Nongerm-cell ovarian cancer is a disease of older women because its risk increases with the number of ovulations. Pregnancy before age 25, early menopause, and the use of oral contraceptives, which reduces the frequency of ovulation, appear to be protective against ovarian cancer (Dicker et al. 1983). Conversely, women with more than 40 ovulation years belong to the high-risk group; women with a late menopause, or those over 45 with nulliparity or first pregnancy after 30, are at a significant risk (Smith and Ol 1984).

Ovarian cancer is known to run in families. In women who have a mother or sister with this disease, the risk is increased 20-fold (Franceschi, LaVecchia, and Mangioni 1982). It has been suggested that women with a family history of the tumor should undergo prophylactic oophorectomy when they plan to have no more children, but some studies have suggested that this procedure does not prevent the development of carcinoma (Tobacman et al. 1982).

The common occurrence of ovarian tumor at the same time or shortly before the development of breast, colon, or endometrial cancer suggests that these malignancies may have a common etiology (Reimer et al. 1978; Eifel et al. 1982).

DIAGNOSIS

To detect ovarian cancer early when it is still curable, skilled physicians would have to conduct regular and thorough abdominal-pelvic examinations of women at high risk. Pelvic ultrasonography—especially by vaginal probe—may be useful as well, particularly in obese women. Elevated serum markers CEA and CA 125 may also signal a developing ovarian cancer (Shingleton and Gore 1988).

In the absence of these measures early detection is highly unlikely, since a routine gynecologic examination can reveal ovarian lesions but clinical symptoms develop only when the disease is well-advanced. In approximately two-thirds of cases, at the time of diagnosis ovarian carcinoma has spread to involve pelvic and abdominal organs (Deppe and Lawrence 1988a).

Symptoms of early ovarian cancer, which are not always present and which can be very mild, include vague abdominal discomfort, dyspepsia, flatulence, bloating, and digestive disturbances (Barber 1984). Symptoms of advanced disease include abdominal distention and pain, and abdominal and pelvic masses or ascites which are often discovered by patients themselves. Barber (1984) notes that a physician must always pay attention to persistent, unexplained gastrointestinal symptoms, particularly if the woman is 35 or older and has a long history of ovarian imbalance and malfunction.

Germ-cell ovarian malignancies are characterized by rapid growth, frequent production of tumor markers, lymphatic and hematogenous spread, frequent mixture of germ cell types, and predominantly unilateral development (Deppe and Lawrence 1988a). Dysgerminomas are bilateral in 10% to 15% of patients. Some germ-cell tumors, such as nongestational ovarian choriocarcinoma, initially produce symptoms that may be confused with signs of intra- or extrauterine pregnancy, so pregnancy should first be ruled out by ultrasound.

The diagnostic procedure must start with a complete history and physical examination, including a Pap smear and rectovaginal examination. Laboratory evaluation should include a complete blood cell (CBC) count, and hepatic and renal function tests. If a germ-cell tumor is suspected, serum markers such as alpha-fetoprotein

(AFP) and human chorionic gonadotropin (hCG), should be ordered. CA 125 is a useful tumor marker in patients with ovarian cancer. It is an antigenic determinant which is elevated (>35 units/mL) in approximately 80% of patients with epithelial ovarian tumors.

Laparoscopy permits direct vision of the abdominal and pelvic viscera, but its use is limited because a laparotomy is usually required.

STAGING

Definitive staging usually includes surgery accompanied by histologic and cytologic tests if effusions are present. FIGO also recommends that biopsies be taken from suspicious areas outside the pelvis. However, surgical staging can be preceded by an array of preoperative tests. These include a chest radiograph, which must always be performed prior to an operation, an IVP, a barium enema, an upper GI series, and an endoscopic bowel examination. The procedures must be chosen on the basis of good clinical judgment, so that exploratory laparotomy is not delayed.

Tumor masses can also be defined by ultrasound, CT, and lymphangiogram, but these techniques only detect masses larger than 1 cm in diameter and do not replace surgical staging. Table 33.7 shows the staging system approved by FIGO in 1985.

Ovarian tumor cells spread most commonly by intraperitoneal implantation and usually grow on the surfaces of the involved organs (Deppe and Lawrence 1988a). They can also spread through the lymphatic and hematogenous systems, although the latter dissemination appears to occur late in the disease process (Larson et al. 1986).

During the surgical procedure, any ascites must be aspirated and sent for cytologic evaluation. If no free fluid is present, washings for cytologic examination must be obtained from the cul-de-sac, both lateral and para-colic gutters, and the subdiaphragmatic areas. If it is not clear whether the tumor is malignant, it is resected and sent for frozen-section examination. If the tumor is unequivocally malignant, biopsies must be obtained from all visible lesions, and scrapings for cytology must be made from all visceral and parietal surfaces.

APPROACHES TO TREATMENT

In each case, the physician must determine the potential usefulness and extent of surgical debulking. For example, some cancers spread so aggressively that significant debulking is impossible. If surgery is undertaken, its goal is to remove as much of the tumor as possible, leaving masses no larger than 2 cm in diameter, or none at all. While improved survival rates may be explained by successes in cytoreductive surgery (Griffiths, Parker, and Fuller 1975; Wharton and Herson 1981; Hacker et al. 1983; Stehman et al. 1983), more studies are needed to make a definitive assessment of surgical debulking.

All patients with known or suspected ovarian tumor must undergo a mechanical and antibiotic bowel prep, as adequate debulking may involve bowel resection. Para-aortic and pelvic lymphadenectomy is important when the disease is grossly confined to the ovaries, so that its proper stage can be determined (Deppe and Lawrence 1988a).

Postoperative treatment of ovarian cancer includes chemotherapy and/or radiation (table 33.8). Similar survival rates have been observed with single-agent and combination chemotherapy, although the response rate was greater with combination regimens (Young, Chabner, and Hubbard 1978; Delgado et al. 1979; Trope 1981; Omura et al. 1983). A trial conducted by the Gynecologic Oncology Group has recently demonstrated that the most effective combination regimens contain cisplatin (Omura et al. 1986). In patients who had failed chemotherapy once, second-line single agents

Table 33.7
FIGO STAGING SYSTEM FOR PRIMARY CARCINOMA OF THE OVARY

STAGE	DESCRIPTION/FEATURES
I	Growth limited to the ovaries
IA	Growth limited to one ovary; no ascites; no tumor on the external surface; capsule intact
1B	Growth limited to both ovaries; no ascites; no tumor on the external surfaces; capsules intact
IC[a]	Tumor either stage IA or IB but with tumor on the surface of one or both ovaries; or with capsule ruptured; or with ascites present containing malignant cells; or with positive peritoneal washings
II	Growth involving one or both ovaries with pelvic extension
IIA	Extension and/or metastases to the uterus and/or tubes
IIB	Extension to other pelvic tissues
IIC[a]	Tumor either stage IIA or IIB, but with tumor on surface of one or both ovaries; or with capsule(s) ruptured; or with ascites present containing malignant cells; or with positive peritoneal washings
III	Tumor involving one or both ovaries with peritoneal implants outside the pelvis and/or positive retroperitoneal or inguinal nodes; superficial liver metastasis equals stage III; tumor limited to the true pelvis but with histologically proven malignant extension to small bowel or omentum
IIIA	Tumor grossly limited to the true pelvis with negative nodes but with histologically confirmed microscopic seeding of abdominal peritoneal surfaces
IIIB	Tumor of one or both ovaries with histologically confirmed implants of abdominal peritoneal surfaces, none exceeding 2 cm in diameter; nodes negative
IIIC	Abdominal implants greater than 2 cm in diameter and/or positive retroperitoneal or inguinal nodes
IV	Growth involving one or both ovaries with distant metastases; if pleural effusion present, there must be positive cytology to allot a case to stage IV; parenchymal liver metastasis equals stage IV

[a] To evaluate the impact on prognosis of the different criteria for alotting cases to stage IC or IIC, it would be of value to know whether (1) rupture of the capsule was spontaneous or caused by the surgeon, or (2) the sources of malignant cells detected was peritoneal washings or ascites.

Table 33.8
POSTOPERATIVE TREATMENT IN PATIENTS WITH EPITHELIAL OVARIAN CANCER

Stage	Grade	
IA	1	No therapy
IA IB,C	2 1,2 (and residual disease < 2 cm)	Cisplatin Cyclophosphamide
IIA,B,C		±Doxorubicin or Abdominopelvic radiation or Intraperitoneal ^{32}P
IA,B,C	3 (and residual disease < 2 cm)	Cisplatin
IIA,B,C IIIA,B		Cyclophosphamide ±doxorubicin or Abdominopelvic radiation
IA,B,C	3 (and/or residual disease > 2 cm)	Cisplatin
IIA,B,C IIIC IV		Cyclophosphamide ±doxorubicin

or combination regimens appear to have no effect on long-term survival. Second-look operative exploration in patients who appear clinically well after chemotherapy has been used to determine the need for future therapy.

A promising avenue of research is the intraperitoneal administration of chemotherapeutic agents. It may help patients with microscopic or minimal residual disease (<2 cm). The technique decreases general toxicity because the drug is applied directly to the tumor.

The major alternative to chemotherapy in the treatment of ovarian cancer is external radiotherapy, which has been explored in several studies (Smith, Rutledge, and Delclos 1975; Dembo et al. 1979; Dembo 1984; Peters et al. 1986). Ovarian cancer spreads to all peritoneal surfaces, so the whole abdomen is usually irradiated, using one of two methods. In the moving strip technique, the radiation field is moving and affects only one segment of the abdominal cavity at a time. In the open-field technique, the treatment covers the entire abdomen simultaneously.

The choice of postoperative therapy is dictated by the properties of the tumor and the age and reproduction status of the patient; her general well-being must always be considered. Epithelial and germ-cell tumors vary and may require individualization of treatment.

More than half of common epithelial tumors have estrogen and/or progesterone receptors, therefore attempts have been made to treat ovarian cancer with megestrol acetate (Sikic et al. 1986; Geisler 1985; Geisler 1983), medroxyprogesterone acetate (Slayton, Pagano, and Creech 1981), and antiestrogen tamoxifen (Meyers, Moore, and Major 1981; Schwartz et al. 1982). Some of these studies have demonstrated a palliative or stabilizing effect of hormonal therapy, but the number

of patients has thus far been too limited to draw any conclusions.

A high risk of relapse in an ovarian cancer patient is associated with a poorly differentiated tumor, a large tumor mass prior to start of chemotherapy, and advanced-stage disease. The overall 5-year survival rate in this disease is approximately 30%. Survival depends on stage of the disease, grade of the lesion, and amount of residual disease following surgery. In patients with stage I disease, the 5-year survival is approximately 70%, while for stage IV disease it stands at approximately 4%.

VULVAR CANCERS

A variety of neoplasms, benign tumors, and malignant growths can appear on the vulva. They include dystrophies, intraepithelial neoplasia, bowenoid papulosis, vulvar condyloma, and squamous cell carcinoma.

Vulvar dystrophies—often subdivided into hyperplastic dystrophy with and without atypia, lichen sclerosis, and mixed dystrophy—are lesions that appear as leukoplakia, or thick white plaques. They are treated by topical application of fluorinated hydrocortisone cream, 2% testosterone cream, or combination of the two.

Vulvar intraepithelial neoplasia is a preinvasive disease that was previously known as Bowen's disease and is also referred to as vulvar carcinoma *in situ.* Two-thirds of patients develop pruritus, the lesion's most common symptom, but one-third may be symptom-free. Lesions can be white, red, or darkly pigmented. The incidence has apparently been increasing, and nearly 50% of newly diagnosed patients are 20 to 40 years old. However, older women have a higher risk of developing invasive cancer (Deppe and Lawrence 1988b). Treatment must be individualized, and can consist of topical application of chemotherapeutic cream, local excision, cryosurgery, laser evaporation, or vulvectomy.

Bowenoid papulosis is believed to be a self-limited benign disease (Berger and Hori 1978), characterized by pigmentation and usually treated by surgical excision or local destructive methods (Patterson et al. 1986). The etiology of this condition, which was originally described in the skin of the penis (Wade, Kopf, and Ackerman 1978), is unclear.

Vulvar condyloma, or condyloma acuminata, is also known as genital warts and is probably the most common benign vulvar lesion (Deppe and Lawrence 1988b). It is transmitted by human papillomavirus, and is believed to be in a causal relationship with vulvar squamous cell carcinoma (Daling et al. 1984).

Squamous cell carcinoma accounts for 90% to 95% of primary vulvar tumors. It is more common in older women, although some observations suggest that the average age of affected women is getting lower, while the incidence of the disease is on the rise (Hacker et al. 1983a; Wilkinson 1985). Lesions usually occur on the labia majora, clitoris, and periurethral areas, and begin to ulcerate as they grow larger. In advanced stages, they manifest as exophytic fungating masses that have spread to the labia, urethra, vagina, and rectum. Vulvar biopsy, performed with a Keyes cutaneous punch, is the best diagnostic technique.

The cancer spreads primarily by lymphatic dissemination. The current staging approved by FIGO is shown in table 33.9. Cystoscopy, sigmoidoscopy, chest radiography, and, in advanced disease, liver and bone scan, skeletal radiography, and CT scan, are recommended prior to treatment.

Surgical treatment must be individualized depending on tumor size, location, and lymph node involvement. Investigators differ on the extent of surgery as optimal therapy, but most agree that pelvic irradiation should be considered as adjuvant therapy if groin lymph nodes are positive. Exenterative vulvectomy is recommended only if no distant metastases have been located. The trend appears to be towards multimodality therapy, so that

extremely radical treatment can be eliminated. Table 33.10 shows treatment recommendations for different stages of the disease. Most-frequent early complications of radical vulvectomy and groin dissection include wound separation, infection, and necrosis. Delayed complications include leg edema and lymphangitis (Podratz 1983). None of these complications, however, cancels the value of radical vulvectomy.

Due to the success of surgery, radiation therapy is seldom used alone as primary treatment of vulvar squamous cell carcinoma in the United States, although it has been shown to achieve good results (Frischbier 1986). In some cases, irradiation is given preoperatively or postoperatively, and more studies are needed to determine its role in the treatment of vulvar cancer. There have been very few studies on the use of chemotherapy in treating this type of malignancy.

Table 33.9
CLINICAL STAGES OF INVASIVE CARCINOMA OF THE VULVA[a]

Stage	Tumor Classification			Description
		Invasive Carcinoma of the Vulva (FIGO Classification)		
0				Carcinoma *in situ*
I	T1	N0	M0	All lesions confined to the vulva with a maximum diameter of
	T1	N1	M0	2 cm or less and no suspicious groin lymph nodes
II	T2	N0	M0	All lesions confined to the vulva with a diameter greater than
	T2	N1	M0	2 cm and no suspicious groin lymph nodes
III	T3	N0	M0	Lesions extending to the urethra, vagina, anus, or perineum,
	T3	N1	M0	but without grossly positive groin lymph nodes
	T3	N2	M0	
	T1	N2	M0	Lesions of any size confined to the vulva and having suspi-
	T2	N2	M0	cious lymph nodes
IV	T1	N3	M0	Lesions with grossly positive groin lymph nodes regardless of
	T2	N3	M0	extent of primary
	T3	N3	M0	
	T4	N3	M0	
	T4	N0	M0	Lesions involving mucosa of the rectum, bladder, urethra, or
	T4	N1	M0	involving bone
	T4	N2	M0	
	M1A			All cases with pelvic or distant metastases
	M1B			

Invasive Carcinoma of the Vulva (TNM Classification)

N	Regional lymph nodes	T	Primary tumor
N0	No palpable lymph nodes	T1	Tumor confined to the vulva, 2 cm or less in diameter
N1	Palpable lymph nodes in either groin, not enlarged, mobile (not clinically suspicious for neoplasm)	T2	Tumor confined to the vulva, more than 2 cm in diameter
N2	Palpable lymph nodes in either one or both groins, enlarged, firm and mobile (clinically suspicious for neoplasm)	T3	Tumor of any size with adjacent tumor spread to the urethra and/or vagina, and/or anus
N3	Fixed or ulcerated lymph nodes	T4	Tumor of any size infiltrating the bladder mucosa and/or the rectal mucosa or both, including the upper part of the urethral mucosa and/or fixed to the bone
M	Distant metastases		
M0	No clinical metastases		
M1A	Palpable deep pelvic lymph nodes		
M1B	Other distant metastases		

[a]If cytology or histology of lymph nodes reveals malignant cells, the symbol + (plus) should be added to N; if such examinations do not reveal malignant cells, the symbol − (minus) should be added to N.

Table 33.10
TREATMENT OPTIONS FOR INVASIVE CARCINOMA OF THE VULVA

Stage	Description
I	Radical vulvectomy and groin lymph node dissection Radical local excision for lesions less than 1 mm in depth
II	Radical vulvectomy and groin lymph node dissection
III	Radical vulvectomy and groin lymph node dissection Deep pelvic lymph node dissection or groin and pelvic lymph node irradiation if inguinal lymph nodes are positive
IV	Radical vulvectomy and pelvic exenteration Surgery followed by radiation therapy Radiation of large primary lesion to improve resectability followed by radical surgery

(Source: Gusberg, Shingleton, and Deppe [1988]. p. 240.)

Lymph node involvement is the major prognostic factor. Metastases usually develop within the first two years after treatment (Deppe and Lawrence 1988b). The overall 5-year survival rate of patients with squamous cell carcinoma of the vulva is 46.3% (Annual Report on the Results of Treatment in Gynecological Cancer 1985). Improvement in this survival rate would necessitate clarifying the etiology of the disease, educating the public about early symptoms, performing immediate biopsy of vulvar lesions, and providing timely and adequate therapy.

VAGINAL CANCERS

Vaginal dysplasia-carcinoma *in situ* (vaginal intraepithelial neoplasia, or VIN) occurs much less frequently than neoplasia of the cervix. It usually produces no symptoms, although some patients suffer from dyspareunia, vaginal spotting, or leukorrhea. Diagnosis is based on an abnormal Pap smear and a colposcopically directed biopsy (Benedet and Sanders 1984).

Local surgical excision and partial or complete vaginectomy, which used to be the mainstay of treatment, have given way to a more individualized approach that takes into consideration the patient's age and the extent of abnormalities in the vagina. Current treatment modalities include laser vaporization, cryosurgery, electrocautery, and intravaginal chemotherapeutic cream. Local excision is performed in the case of unifocal lesions; radiotherapy and extensive surgery are recommended for patients with recurrent multifocal lesions unresponsive to other treatments (Deppe and Lawrence 1988c). Vaginal intraepithelial neoplasia can progress to invasive squamous cancer of the vagina.

Primary tumors of the vagina are very rare, accounting for approximately 2% of all gynecologic cancers. Most often, tumors spread from the cervix and endometrium, and in rare cases ovarian cancer first manifests itself in the vagina.

Squamous cell carcinoma represents close to 95% of these malignancies (Plentl and Friedman 1971). Other types include adenocarcinoma, verrucous carcinoma, small-cell carcinoma, diethylstilbestrol (DES)-associated clear cell adenocarcinoma, sarcoma, melanoma, and the rare childhood neoplasms rhabdomyosarcoma and endodermal sinus tumor.

The etiology of vaginal squamous cell carcinoma is unknown, but it has been suggested that genital viruses (Weed, Lozier, and Daniel 1983) or chronic irritation (Rutledge 1967; Herbst, Green, and Ulfelder 1970) may trigger the disease. In two-thirds of cases it affects women over age 50, and is most common during the sixth and seventh decades of life. Women who have had hysterectomies are believed to be at a higher risk (Deppe and Lawrence 1988c).

Women usually present with vaginal bleeding, and may also complain of vaginal discharge and pelvic pain (Monaghan 1985; Underwood and Smith 1971). However, some have no symptoms. The most common site is the upper third of the vagina's posterior wall. An abnormal vaginal Pap smear must be investigated by colposcopy and iodine staining of the vagina, while a definitive diagnosis is established by biopsy. Any suspicious visible or palpable lesion must be biopsied. In making the diagnosis, it is important to exclude metastases from other genital or extragenital sites.

Table 33.11 shows the FIGO staging of vaginal carcinoma. Therapy depends on the tumor's stage and location, the patient's age, and the desire to preserve a functional vagina. In most cases the major treatment modality is radiation (Rubin, Young, and Mikuta 1985; Perez and Camel 1982; Pride et al. 1979; Johnston, Klotz, and Boutselis 1983; Kucera et al. 1985). Intracavitary or interstitial radiation is used in small superficial stage I disease; external beam radiation in extensive stage I and in stage II disease; and a combination of internal and external radiation in stages III and IV.

Radical hysterectomy, vaginectomy, and pelvic lymphadenectomy are sometimes performed in stage I disease. Exenterative surgery is recommended in the case of recurrent radiation-resistant tumor. Chemotherapy has proven ineffective in the treatment of disseminated squamous cell carcinoma of the vagina.

Survival rates with this type of malignancy are at 64% to 90% for stage I; 29% to 66% for stage II; and 0% to 40% for stages III and IV disease (Monaghan 1985). Fortunately, vaginal carcinoma occurs infrequently.

Table 33.11
STAGING SYSTEM FOR PRIMARY VAGINAL CANCER

FIGO[a] Stage	Degree of Involvement
0	Carcinoma *in situ*, intraepithelial carcinoma
I	Carcinoma limited to the vaginal wall
II	Carcinoma involving the subvaginal tissue but not extending onto the pelvic wall
III	Carcinoma extending onto the pelvic wall
IV	Carcinoma extending beyond the true pelvis or involving the mucosa of the bladder or rectum (bullous edema, as such, does not permit a case to be allotted to stage IV)
IVA	Spread of the growth to adjacent organs and/or direct extension beyond the true pelvis
IVB	Spread to distant organs

[a]FIGO = International Federation of Gynecology and Obstetrics

CANCER OF THE FALLOPIAN TUBES

Primary carcinoma of the fallopian tube is very rare (Deppe, Malone, and Lawrence 1988), accounting for only 0.31% (Hu, Taymor, and Hertig 1950) to 1.8% (Hurlbutt and Nelson 1963) of all gynecologic cancers. The incidence peaks in the fifth decade, with a mean age of 52 years, but the tumor has been reported in women of all ages.

The main diagnostic challenge is distinguishing tubal carcinoma from cancer of the ovary and uterus. Difficulty is compounded by anatomic proximity and histologic similarities; as a result, diagnosis is usually established only at the time of exploratory laparotomy performed for an adnexal or pelvic mass. Finn and Javert (1949) have suggested the following criteria for differentiating tubal as opposed to ovarian origin of the tumor:

1. The tubal carcinoma should originate in the endosalpinx;

2. The histologic pattern should resemble the epithelium of the tubal mucosa;

3. Transition from benign to malignant epithelium should be present; and

4. The endometrium and ovaries should be normal or should contain a malignant neoplasm that by its histological appearance, small size, and distribution appears to be metastatic from a tubal primary.

The most frequent type of malignancy in the fallopian tube is papillary adenocarcinoma. Less common types include squamous cell carcinoma, sarcoma, and choriocarcinoma.

There is no official staging system, but because its spread and anatomic location appear to be similar to ovarian cancer, some experts have proposed a system based on the FIGO staging for ovarian carcinomas. One such suggestion, put forward by Dodson, Ford, and Averette (1970), is shown in table 33.12.

Treatment of choice for tubal carcinoma consists of cytoreductive surgery, including an abdominal hysterectomy and bilateral salpingo-oophorectomy. Cytologic samples of the pelvis and peritoneal organs and biopsies of selective lymph nodes are necessary to rule out the spread of the disease. Radiotherapy is frequently used in the management of tubal malignancy, but results are difficult to evaluate because of discrepancies in dosages and techniques employed in different studies. In the past, chemotherapy was mostly used in patients who had failed prior irradiation and surgery (Boronow 1973). Cisplatin combination therapy may have a potential benefit.

Because fallopian tube carcinoma is rare, sufficient data are lacking to establish a pattern of its recurrence. Five-year survival figures range from 40% to 69% in stage I; 27% to 60% in stage II; and 15% to 29% in stage III (Deppe, Malone, and Lawrence 1988).

GESTATIONAL TROPHOBLASTIC DISEASE AND GESTATIONAL CHORIOCARCINOMA

Gestational trophoblastic disease (GTD) refers to all neoplastic disorders arising from the human placenta, including partial and complete hydatidiform mole, placental site tumor, invasive mole (chorioadenoma destruens), and gestational choriocarcinoma. These neoplasms

Table 33.12
STAGING OF FALLOPIAN TUBE CARCINOMA

Stage	Description
I	Growth limited to the tubes
IA	Growth limited to one tube; no ascites
	No tumor on the external surface; capsule intact
IB	Growth limited to both tubes; no ascites
	No tumor on the external surface; capsule intact
IC[a]	Tumor either stage IA or IB but with tumor on surface of one or both tubes; or with capsule ruptured; or with ascites present containing malignant cells; or with positive peritoneal washings
II	Growth involving one or both tubes with extension into adjacent pelvic structures
IIA	Extension and/or metastases to the uterus and/or ovaries
IIB	Extension to other pelvic tissues
IIC	Tumor either stage IIA or IIB, but with tumor on surface of one or both tubes; or with capsule(s) ruptured; or with ascites present containing malignant cells; or with positive peritoneal washings
III	Tumor involving one or both tubes with peritoneal implants outside the pelvis and/or positive retroperitoneal or inguinal nodes
	Superficial liver metastasis equals stage III
	Tumor limited to the true pelvis but with histologically proven malignant extension to small bowel or omentum
IIIA	Tumor grossly limited to the true pelvis with negative nodes, but with histologically confirmed microscopic seeding of abdominal peritoneal surfaces
IIIB	Tumor of one or both tubes with histologically confirmed implants of abdominal peritoneal surfaces, none exceeding 2 cm in diameter; nodes negative
IIIC	Abdominal implants greater than 2 cm in diameter and/or positive retroperitoneal or inguinal nodes
IV	Growth involving one or both tubes with distant metastases
	If pleural effusion present, there must be positive cytology to allot a case to stage IV
	Parenchymal liver metastases indicate stage IV

[a]To evaluate the impact on prognosis of the different criteria for allotting cases to stage IC or IIC, it would be of value to know whether (1) rupture of the capsule was spontaneous or caused by the surgeon, and (2) the source of malignant cells detected was peritoneal washings or ascites.

are unique because they mainly contain paternal chromosomal markers.

Partial and complete hydatidiform moles are benign forms of GTD. They occur much more frequently in developing than in industrialized developed nations, which may be due to racial differences and nutritional factors. Ultrasound produces a characteristic image of the mole and is currently the preferred diagnostic method, in combination with measurement of the beta subunit chorionic gonadotropin (B-hCG) levels, which are elevated in patients with the disease. Suction curettage, or dilation and curettage, are techniques recommended for termination of molar pregnancy (Stone and Bagshawe 1979).

As complete hydatidiform moles lead to malignant GTD in 10% to 30% of cases (Soper and Hammond 1988), all patients should be monitored following molar evacuation. Monitoring can be conducted by means of physical examinations, chest radiography, and measuring of human chorionic gonadotropin (hCG), which is secreted by malignant gestational trophoblastic neoplasms.

Malignant GTD occurs after molar pregnancy in 50% of cases, after abortion or ectopic pregnancy in approximately 25% of cases, and after gestation in the remaining 25% (Soper and Hammond 1988). Initial clinical symptoms may include gastrointestinal or urologic bleeding, hemoptysis, or cerebral hemorrhage. Diagnosis is supported by serum hCG testing.

GTD often spreads to the lung, brain, or liver. Therefore, it should be considered in any woman of reproductive age who has metastases at these sites from an unknown primary site of cancer. The following is the anatomic staging system of the disease proposed by FIGO (Goldstein and Berkowitz 1984): stage I, confined to the uterine corpus; stage II, vaginal or pelvic metastases; stage III, pulmonary metastases; stage IV, other extrapelvic metastases. GTD can also be classified as metastatic or nonmetastatic disease, or as having good or poor prognosis.

Before effective chemotherapeutic agents were developed, GTD was treated with either surgery or irradiation, and overall survival was poor (Brewer et al. 1971). Current treatment is primarily by chemotherapy, and the disease is responsive to a variety of chemotherapeutic regimens. Surgery is now used as primary therapy only in selected patients, and is usually reserved for isolated metastases or resection of drug-resistant foci of disease.

Methotrexate and actinomycin D have been the main single agents used since the late 1950s in low-risk (nonmetastatic and metastatic with good prognosis) gestational trophoblastic disease. Oral etoposide has been recently administered to GTD patients with good results. Treatment of nonmetastatic disease usually produces a 100% cure rate. The cure rate for good-prognosis metastatic GTD also approaches 100%, although approximately 40% will require treatment with another regimen to achieve a cure.

Patients who have a risk score greater than 7, which is calculated on the basis of duration of the disease, pretherapy titer, metastatic sites, and other factors are considered as having poor-prognosis metastatic disease. They have a better survival rate when treated initially with multiagent chemotherapeutic regimens (Hammond et al. 1973; Lurain et al. 1982).

GTD, and especially poor-prognosis disease, can recur, so maintenance chemotherapy is recommended as a preventive measure. Pregnancy following GTD therapy should be deferred for at least one full year of hCG-titer surveillance (Soper and Hammond 1988).

CANCER IN PREGNANCY

Cancer is estimated to occur in 1 of every 1,000 pregnancies (Potter and Schoeneman 1970), although the precise rate of occurrence is unknown. Invasive cancer is rare in pregnant women (Schwartz 1988). It is a highly traumatic event as it concerns two patients, the mother and fetus, and the mother is usually young and unprepared for the situation.

One population-based epidemiologic study has shown that pregnant women had a lower incidence of cancer as compared with nonpregnant ones (Haas 1984). These data suggest that occult cancer may hamper conception, but there is also a possibility that incomplete reporting by physicians may have skewed the study's results.

Cancer of the cervix is the most common type of malignancy encountered in pregnant women, followed by cancers of the breast, vulva, ovary, and vagina. Only rarely do tumors spread from mother to fetus, and those that do are usually melanomas.

Treatment is complicated by the need not only to cure the mother but to avoid abortion and minimize damage to the fetus. In some cases, earlier delivery is recommended to reduce fetal exposure to effects of therapy. Survival, and the baby's quality of life, should be a guiding principle in the choice of treatment protocol.

In the case of all three standard therapies—surgery, radiation, and chemotherapy—the fetus is most vulnerable during the first trimester, and utmost caution must be used during this period. Surgery, particularly intra-abdominal surgery, may lead to spontaneous abortion if performed early, and when possible should be delayed to the second trimester. To avoid anesthetic complications, anesthesiologists must always consider pregnant patients as having a full stomach no matter how long they fasted, and choose their approach accordingly (Roberts and Shirley 1979).

Radiation therapy is also most damaging to the fetus between the first and tenth weeks of gestation, when it can lead to growth retardation, malformations, and death. Dekaban (1968) reported that the incidence of congenital anomalies was highest during this time, but declined significantly between the eleventh and twentieth weeks. After the twentieth week, the effects observed were far less serious.

The dose, rate, and site of radiation must also be taken into account. Pelvic radiation usually induces spontaneous abortion. Supradiaphragmatic irradiation is relatively safe in early pregnancy due primarily to internal radiation scatter, but it may cause unacceptable fetal injury in later pregnancy.

Cytotoxic chemotherapy must be avoided during the first trimester because it can lead to spontaneous abortion or cause teratogenic damage to the fetus (Nicholson 1968; Sweet and Kinzie 1976). During the second and third trimesters, both single-agent and combination chemotherapy may be successfully used for the treatment of some malignancies, although their long-term effects remain unknown. Chemotherapy must be timed so that the patient is not excessively weakened during delivery.

REFERENCES

Abitol, M.M., and Davenport, J.H. 1974. Sexual dysfunction after therapy for cervical carcinoma. *Am. J. Obstet. Gynecol.* 119:181.

Annual report on the results of treatment in gynecological cancer. 1985. vol. 19. Radiumhemmet, Stockholm, Sweden: FIGO.

Arneson, A.N. 1953. An evaluation of the use of radiation in the treatment of endometrial cancer. *Bull. N.Y. Acad. Med.* 29:395.

Barber, H.R.K. 1984. Ovarian cancer: diagnosis and management. *Am. J. Obstet. Gynecol.* 150:910.

Benedet, J.L., and Sanders, J.H. 1984. Carcinoma *in situ* of the vagina. *Am. J. Obstet. Gynecol.* 148:695.

Berger, B.W., and Hori, Y. 1978. Multicentric Bowen's disease of the genitalia: spontaneous regression of lesions. *Arch. Dermatol.* 114:1698.

Boronow, R.C. 1973. Chemotherapy of disseminated tubal cancer. *Obstet. Gynecol.* 42:62.

Brewer, J.I.; Echman, T.R.; and Dolkart, R.E. et al. 1971. Gestational trophoblastic disease. *Am. J. Obstet. Gynecol.* 109:335.

Byers, T.; Marshall, J.; and Graham, S. et al. 1983. A case control study of dietary and non-dietary factors in ovarian cancer. *J. Natl. Cancer Inst.* 71:681.

Chanen, W., and Rome, R.M. 1983. Electrocoagulation diathermy for cervical dysplasia and carcinoma *in situ:* a 15-year survey. *Obstet. Gynecol.* 61:673.

Daling, J.R.; Chu, J.; and Weiss, N.S. et al. 1984. The association of condylomata acuminata and squamous carcinoma of the vulva. *Br. J. Cancer* 50:533.

Dekaban, A. 1968. Abnormalities in children exposed to x-irradiation during various stages of gestation: tentative timetable of radiation injury to the human fetus, part I. *J. Nucl. Med.* 9:471.

Delgado, G.; Schien, P.; and MacDonald, J. et al. 1979. L-PAM vs. cyclophosphamide, hexamethylmelamine, and 5-fluorouracil (CHF) for advanced ovarian cancer. *Proc. Am. Assoc. Cancer Res.* 20:434.

Dembo, A.J.; Bush, R.S.; and Beale, F.A. et al. 1979. Ovarian carcinoma: improved survival following abdominopelvic irradiation in patients with a completed pelvic operation. *Am. J. Obstet. Gynecol.* 134:793.

Dembo, A.J. 1984. Radiotherapeutic management of ovarian cancer. *Semin. Oncol.* 11:238.

Deppe G,; Malone, J.M. Jr.; and Lawrence, W.D. 1988. Cancer of the fallopian tube. In Gusberg, S.B.; Shingleton, H.M.; and Deppe, G. eds. *Female genital cancer.* pp. 427-34. New York: Churchill Livingstone.

Deppe, G., and Lawrence, W.D. 1988a. Cancer of the ovary. In Gusberg, S.B.; Shingleton, H.M.; and Deppe G. eds. *Female genital cancer.* pp. 379-425. New York: Churchill Livingstone.

Deppe, G., and Lawrence, W.D. 1988b. Vulvar dystrophy and neoplasia. In Gusberg, S.B.; Shingleton, H.M.; and Deppe, G. eds. *Female genital cancer.* pp. 223-51. New York: Churchill Livingstone.

Deppe, G., and Lawrence, W.D. 1988c. Cancer of the vagina including DES-related lesions. In Gusberg, S.B.; Shingleton, H.M.; and Deppe, G. eds. *Female genital cancer.* pp. 253-74. New York: Churchill Livingstone.

Dicker, R.C.; Webster, L.A.; and Layde, P.M. et al. 1983. Oral contraceptive use and the risk of ovarian cancer. *JAMA* 249:1596.

Dodson, M.G.; Ford, J.H. Jr.; and Averette, H.E. 1970. Clinical aspects of fallopian tube carcinoma. *Obstet. Gynecol.* 36:935.

Eifel, P.; Henriksson, M.; and Ross, J. et al. 1982. Simultaneous presentation of carcinoma involving the ovary and uterine corpus. *Cancer* 50:163.

Finn, W.F., and Javert, C.T. 1949. Primary and metastatic cancer of the fallopian tube. *Cancer* 2:803.

Franceschi, S.; LaVecchia, C.; and Mangioni, C. 1982. Familial ovarian cancer: eight more families. *Gynecol. Oncol.* 13:31.

Frischbier, H.J. 1986. Radiation therapy of vulvar carcinoma (Hamburg Method). In Zander, J., and Baltzer, J. eds. *Erkrankungen der Vulva.* Baltimore: Urban & Schwarzenberg.

Gagnon, F. 1952. The lack of occurrence of cervical cancer in nuns. *Proc. Natl. Cancer Conf.* 1:625.

Geisler, E.H. 1983. Megestrol acetate for palliation of advanced ovarian carcinoma. *Obstet. Gynecol.* 61:95.

Geisler, E.H. 1985. The use of high-dose megestrol acetate in the treatment of ovarian adenocarcinoma. *Semin. Oncol.* 12(Suppl 1):20.

Goldstein, D.P., and Berkowitz, R.S. 1984. Staging system for gestational trophoblastic tumors. *J. Reprod. Med.* 29:792.

Graham, J.B. 1963. Discussed in Boutelis et al. *Am. J. Obstet. Gynecol.* 85:994.

Greene, M.H.; Clark, J.W.; and Blayney, D.W. 1984. The epidemiology of ovarian cancer. *Semin. Oncol.* 11:209.

Griffiths, C.T.; Parker, L.M.; and Fuller, A.F. 1975. Surgical resection of tumor bulk in the primary treatment of ovarian carcinoma. *Natl. Cancer Inst. Monogr.* 42:101.

Gusberg, S.B., and Shingleton, H.M. 1988. Diagnosis and principles of treatment of cancer of the cervix. In Gusberg, S.B.; Shingleton, H.M.; and Deppe, G. eds. *Female genital cancer.* pp. 275-96. New York: Churchill Livingstone.

Gusberg, S.B. 1988a. Diagnosis and principles of treatment of cancer of the cervix. In Gusberg, S.B.; Shingleton, H.M.; and Deppe, G. eds. *Female genital cancer.* pp. 337-61. New York: Churchill Livingstone.

Gusberg, S.B. 1988b. Treatment of cancer of the endometrium. In Gusberg, S.B.; Shingleton, H.M.; and Deppe, G. eds. *Female genital cancer.* pp. 361-77. New York: Churchill Livingstone.

Gusberg, S.B., and McKay, D.G. 1971. Malignant lesions of the cervix and corpus uteri. In Danforth, D.N. ed. *Textbook of obstetrics and gynecology.* 2nd ed. New York: Harper & Row.

Gusberg, S.B. 1966. The problem of staging endometrial cancer. *Obstet. Gynecol.* 28:305.

Gusberg, S.B. 1947. Precursors of corpus carcinoma: estrogens and adenomatous hyperplasia. *Am. J. Obstet. Gynecol.* 54:905.

Haas, J.F. 1984. Pregnancy in association with a newly diagnosed cancer: a population-based epidemiologic assessment. *Int. J. Cancer* 34:229.

Hacker, N.F.; Berek, J.S.; and Lagasse, L.D. et al. 1983. Primary cytoreductive surgery for epithelial ovarian cancer. *Obstet. Gynecol.* 61:413.

Hacker, N.F.; Nieberg, R.K.; and Berek, J.S. et al. 1983. Superficially invasive vulvar cancer with nodal metastases. *Gynecol. Oncol.* 15:65.

Hammond, C.B.; Borchert, L.G.; and Tyrey, L. et al. 1973. Treatment of metastatic trophoblastic disease: good and poor prognosis. *Am. J. Obstet. Gynecol.* 115:4.

Herbst, A.L.; Green, T.H.; and Ulfelder, H. 1970. Primary carcinoma of the vagina: an analysis of 68 cases. *Am. J. Obstet. Gynecol.* 106:210.

Hu, C.Y.; Taymor, M.L.; and Hertig, A.T. 1950. Primary carcinoma of the fallopian tube. *Am. J. Obstet. Gynecol.* 59:58.

Hurlbutt, F.R., and Nelson, H.B. 1963. Primary carcinoma of the uterine tube: report on 12 new cases. *Obstet. Gynecol.* 21:730.

Johnston, G.A.; Klotz, J.; and Boutselis, J.G. 1983. Primary invasive carcinoma of the vagina. *Surg. Gynecol. Obstet.* 156:34.

Kavanagh, D.; Ruffoll, E.H.; and Marsden, D.E. eds. 1985. *Gynecologic cancer: a clinicopathologic approach.* East Norwalk, Conn: Appleton-Century-Crofts.

Kucera, H.; Langer, M.; and Smekal, G. et al. 1985. Radiotherapy of primary carcinoma of the vagina: management and results of different therapy schemes. *Gynecol. Oncol.* 21:87.

Larson, D.M.; Copeland, L.J.; and Moser, R.P. et al. 1986. Central nervous system metastases in epithelial ovarian carcinoma. *Obstet. Gynecol.* 68:746.

Lurain, J.R.; Brewer, J.I.; and Torok, E.E. et al. 1982. Gestational trophoblastic disease: treatment results at the Brewer Trophoblastic Disease Center. *Obstet. Gynecol.* 60:354.

Meyers, A.M.; Moore, G.E.; and Major, F. 1981. Advanced ovarian carcinoma: response to antiestrogen therapy. *Cancer* 48:2368.

Monaghan, J.M. 1985. The management of carcinoma of the vagina. In Shepherd, J.H., and Monaghan, J.M. eds. *Clinical gynaecological oncology.* Oxford: Blackwell Scientific Publications.

Nicholson, H.D. 1968. Cytotoxic drugs in pregnancy. *J. Obstet. Gynaecol. Br. Commonw.* 75:307.

Omura, G.A.; Morrow, C.P.; and Blessing, J.A. et al. 1983. A randomized comparison of melphalan vs. melphalan plus hexamethylmelamine vs. Adriamycin plus cyclophosphamide in ovarian carcinoma. *Cancer* 51:783.

Omura, G.A.; Blessing, J.A.; and Ehrlich, C.E. et al. 1986. A randomized trial of cyclophosphamide and doxorubicin with or without cisplatin in advanced ovarian carcinoma: a Gynecologic Oncology Group study. *Cancer* 57:1725.

Patterson, J.W.; Kao, G.F.; and Graham, J.H. et al. 1986. Bowenoid papulosis: a clinicopathologic study with ultrastructural observations. *Cancer* 57:823.

Perez, C.A., and Camel, H.M. 1982. Long term follow-up in radiation therapy of carcinoma of the vagina. *Cancer* 49:1308.

Peters, W.A. III; Blasko, J.C.; and Bagley, C.M. Jr. et al. 1986. Salvage therapy with whole-abdominal irradiation in patients with advanced carcinoma of the ovary previously treated by combination chemotherapy. *Cancer* 58:880.

Piver, M.S.; Barlow, J.J.; and Vongtama, V. et al. 1983. Hydroxyurea: a radiation potentiator in carcinoma of the uterine cervix. *Am. J. Obstet. Gynecol.* 147:803.

Plentl, A.A., and Friedman, E.A. 1971. *Lymphatic system of the female genitalia: the morphologic basis of oncologic diagnosis and therapy.* Philadelphia: W.B. Saunders.

Podratz, K.C.; Symmonds, R.E.; and Taylor, W.F. et al. 1983. Carcinoma of the vulva: analysis of treatment and survival. *Obstet. Gynecol.* 61:63.

Potter, J.F., and Schoeneman, M. 1970. Metastasis of maternal cancer to the placenta and fetus. *Cancer* 25:380.

Pride, G.L.; Schultz, G.E.; and Chuprevich, T.W. et al. 1979. Primary invasive squamous carcinoma of the vagina. *Obstet. Gynecol.* 53:218.

Reimer, R.R.; Hoover, R.; and Fraumeni, J.F. Jr. et al. 1978. Second primary neoplasms following ovarian cancer. *J. Natl. Cancer Inst.* 61:1195.

Roberts, R.B., and Shirley, M.A. 1979. Reducing the risk of acid aspiration during cesarean section. *Anesth. Analg.* 53:859.

Rubin, S.C.; Young, J.; and Mikuta, J.J. 1985. Squamous carcinoma of the vagina: treatment, complications, and long-term follow-up. *Gynecol. Oncol.* 20:346.

Rutledge, F. 1967. Cancer of the vagina. *Am. J. Obstet. Gynecol.* 97:635.

Rutledge, F. 1974. Role of radical hysterectomy in adenocarcinoma of the endometrium. *Gynecol. Oncol.* 2:331.

Schuurmans, S.N.; Ohlke, I.D.; and Carmichael, J.A. 1984. Treatment of cervical intraepithelial neoplasia with electrocautery: reports of 426 cases. *Am. J. Obstet. Gynecol.* 148:544.

Schwartz, P.E. 1988. Cancer in pregnancy. In Gusberg, S.B.; Shingleton, H.M.; and Deppe, G. eds. *Female genital cancer.* pp. 725-54. New York: Churchill Livingstone.

Schwartz, P.E.; Keating, G.; and MacLusky, N. et al. 1982. Tamoxifen therapy for advanced ovarian cancer. *Obstet. Gynecol.* 66:575.

Shingleton, H.M., and Gore, H. 1988. Principles of diagnosis. In Gusberg, S.B.; Shingleton, H.M.; Deppe, G. eds. *Female genital cancer.* pp. 197-221. New York: Churchill Livingstone.

Shingleton, H.M.; Hatch, K.D.; and Orr, J.W. Jr. et al. 1983a. Diagnosis and treatment of preinvasive and microscopically invasive squamous cell carcinoma of the cervix: including comments on surveillance of DES-exposed patients with cytologic atypias. *Cancer Bull.* 35:172.

Shingleton, H.M.; Gore, H.; and Soong, S-G. et al. 1983b. Tumor recurrence and survival in stage IB cancer of the cervix. *Am. J. Clin. Oncol.* 6:265.

Shingleton, H.M., and Kim, R.Y. 1988. Treatment of cancer of the cervix. In Gusberg, S.B.; Shingleton, H.M.; and Deppe, G. eds. *Female genital cancer.* pp. 297-335. New York: Churchill Livingstone.

Shingleton, H.M., and Orr, J.W. Jr. 1987. *Cancer of the cervix: diagnosis and treatment.* Edinburgh: Churchill Livingstone.

Sikic, B.I.; Scudder, S.A.; and Ballon, S.C. et al. 1986. High-dose megestrol acetate therapy of ovarian carcinoma: a phase II study by the Northern California Oncology Group. *Semin. Oncol.* 13:26.

Slayton, R.E.; Pagano, M.; and Creech, R.H. 1981. Progestin therapy for advanced ovarian cancer: a phase II Eastern Cooperative Oncology Group trial. *Cancer Treat. Rep.* 65:895.

Smith, L.H., and Ol, R.H. 1984. Detection of malignant ovarian neoplasms: a review of the literature. 1: detection of the patient at risk: clinical, radiological and cytological detection. *Obstet. Gynecol. Surv.* 39:313.

Smith, J.P.; Rutledge, F.N.; and Deldos, L. 1975. Postoperative treatment of early cancer of the ovary: a random trial between postoperative irradiation and chemotherapy. *Natl. Cancer Inst. Monogr.* 42:149.

Soper, J.T., and Hammond, C.B. 1988. Gestational trophoblastic disease and gestational choriocarcinoma. In Gusberg, S.B.; Shingleton, H.M.; and Deppe, G. eds. *Female genital cancer.* pp. 435-58. New York: Churchill Livingstone.

Stallworthy, J.A. 1971. Surgery of endometrial cancer in the Bonney tradition. *Ann. R. Coll. Surg. Engl.* 48:293.

Stehman, F.B.; Ehrlich, L.H.; and Einhorn, L.H. et al. 1983. Long-term follow-up and survival in stage III-IV epithelial ovarian cancer treated with cis-dichlorodiammineplatinum, Adriamycin, and cyclophosphamide (PAC). *Proc. Am. Soc. Clin. Oncol.* C-593.

Stone, M., and Bagshawe, K.D. 1979. An analysis of the influence of maternal age, gestational age, contraceptive method, and the primary mode of treatment of patients with hydatidiform mole and the incidence of subsequent chemotherapy. *Br. J. Obstet. Gynaecol.* 46:782.

Strockbine, M.F.; Hancock, J.G.; and Fletcher, G.H. 1970. Complications in 831 patients with squamous cell carcinoma of the intact cervix treated with 3,000 rads or more whole pelvic irradiation. *AJR* 108:293.

Sweet, D.L., and Kinzie, J. 1976. Consequences of radiotherapy and antineoplastic therapy for the fetus. *J. Reprod. Med.* 17:241.

Tobacman, J.K.; Tucker, M.A.; and Kase, R. et al. 1982. Intra-abdominal carcinomatosis after prophylactic oophorectomy in ovarian cancer prone families. *Lancet* II:795.

Trope, C. 1981. A prospective and randomized trial comparison of melphalan vs. Adriamycin-melphalan in advanced ovarian carcinoma. *Proc. Am. Soc. Clin. Oncol.* 22:469.

Underwood, P.B., and Smith, R.T. 1971. Carcinoma of the vagina. *JAMA* 217:41.

Wade, J.E.; Kohorn, E.I.; and Morris, J.Mc.L. 1967. Adenocarcinoma of endometrium. *Am. J. Obstet. Gynecol.* 99:869.

Wade, T.R.; Kopf, A.W.; and Ackerman, A.B. 1978. Bowenoid papulosis of the penis. *Cancer* 42:1890.

Weed, J.C.; Lozier, C.; and Daniel, S.J. 1983. Human papilloma virus in multifocal, invasive female genital tract malignancy. *Obstet. Gynecol.* 62:832.

Weiss, N.S.; Homonchuk; and Young, J.L. 1977. Incidence of the histologic type of ovarian cancer: the U.S. Third National Cancer Survey, 1969-1971. *Gynecol. Oncol.* 5:161.

Wharton, J.T., and Herson, J. 1981. Surgery for common epithelial tumors of the ovary. *Cancer* 48:582.

Wilkinson, E.J. 1985. Superficial invasive carcinoma of the vulva. *Clin. Obstet. Gynecol.* 28:188.

Wynder, E.L.; Escher, G.; and Mantel, N. 1966. An epidemiological investigation of cancer of the endometrium. *Cancer* 19:489.

Young, R.C.; Chabner, B.A.; and Hubbard, S.P. 1978. Prospective trial of melphalan (L-PAM) vs. combination chemotherapy (hexa-CAF) in ovarian adenocarcinoma. *N. Engl. J. Med.* 299:1261.

Chapter 34

NUTRITION AND
THE CANCER PATIENT

John M. Daly, M.D.
Michael Shinkwin, M.D.

John M. Daly, M.D.
Jonathan E. Rhoads Professor of Surgical Sciences
Chief, Division of Surgical Oncology
University of Pennsylvania School of Medicine
Philadelphia, Pennsylvania

Michael Shinkwin, M.D.
Fellow in Surgical Oncology
University of Pennsylvania School of Medicine
Philadelphia, Pennsylvania

INTRODUCTION

Progressive weight loss and nutritional depletion are common among cancer patients (Nixon, Heymsfield, and Cohen 1980; Theologides 1972; DeWys et al. 1980). The importance of malnutrition as a major source of morbidity and mortality is widely appreciated (Copeland, Daly, and Dudrick 1977; Smale et al. 1981). Furthermore, antineoplastic therapy modalities can exert a varying impact on the host's nutritional status, adding to the cachectic state caused by the tumor and leading to a more profound nutritional depletion (McAnena and Daly 1986) and increased morbidity. Malnourished cancer patients should be so recognized prior to initiation of antineoplastic treatment and efforts should be made to improve their nutritional status. This chapter outlines the causes of cancer cachexia, the impact of antitumor therapy on nutrition, the nutritional assessment of the cancer patient, and the provision of optimal nutritional support for each patient.

CANCER CACHEXIA

The term "cancer cachexia" describes a group of symptoms and signs that encompass inanition, anorexia, weakness, tissue wasting, and organ dysfunction. Cachexia, common in patients with advanced metastatic disease, also occurs in patients with localized disease. DeWys et al. (1980) noted substantial weight loss in 40% of patients with breast cancer and in 80% of patients with gastric or pancreatic carcinoma. The relationship of cachexia to tumor burden, disease stage, and cell type is inconsistent and no single theory satisfactorily explains the cachectic state. A variety of etiological factors can occur simultaneously or sequentially to produce cachexia.

DIMINISHED NUTRIENT INTAKE

Anorexia accompanies most neoplasms to some extent and is a major contributing factor in the development of the cachectic state. Often, loss of appetite is an important symptom of an underlying neoplasm. Several physiologic derangements have been cited as possible reasons for anorexia. Abnormalities in taste perception such as reduced threshold for sweet, sour, and salty flavors have been demonstrated. DeWys and Walters (1975) have shown that a reduced taste sensitivity for sucrose and urea is associated with reduced caloric intake; the reduced oral threshold for urea correlates with an aversion for red meat. In contrast, others have noted increased taste sensitivity in cancer patients. Deficiencies in zinc and other trace elements may contribute to altered taste sensation. Patients with hepatic metastases accompanied by some degree of hepatic insufficiency may develop anorexia and nausea as a result of difficulty in clearing lactate produced by anaerobic tumor metabolism of glucose. Substances released by the tumor or by the host's monocytes (cachectin) may act on the feeding center in the hypothalamus and cause anorexia. Recent studies have demonstrated the presence of cachectin in the plasma of tumor-bearing rodents that correlated with the onset of anorexia.

Many studies have been conducted to elucidate the specific metabolic processes that affect nutrient intake in cancer patients. Results of parabiosis studies performed by Lucke, Bornick, and Zeckwer (1952) indicate the presence of a humoral factor that produces in the nontumor-bearing rat characteristics of the tumor-bearing state. Theologides (1972) proposed that tumor peptides acting through neuroendocrine cells and neuroreceptors alter metabolic pathways. Nakahara (1960) described a "toxohormone" capable of mimicking the cancerous state when injected into normal animals. Toxohormone is a 75,000 d protein identified in several tumors such as melanoma and carcinoma; it leads to increased lipolysis and immunosuppression. Experiments in which rats were given cachectin intraperitoneally for five days show that cachectin causes decreased dietary intake with a corresponding decline in host weight. Rats given cachectin for 10 days developed tolerance to cachectin after five days (Stovroff and Norton 1987). When subsequently inoculated with tumor, these rats survived for a significantly longer period than control animals not pretreated with cachectin. This result strengthens the evidence that endogenously produced cachectin may mediate the development of cachexia in the tumor-bearing host. Krause and coworkers (1981) postulated that abnormalities in the central nervous system's metabolism of serotonin may be responsible for the cancer-associated anorexia.

The local effect of the tumor may lead to reduced food intake, especially when the tumor arises from or impinges on the alimentary tract. Patients with cancer of the oral cavity, the pharynx, or the esophagus may have reduced intake because of the odynophagia or dysphagia due to partial or complete obstruction. Patients with gastric cancer often have reduced gastric capacity or partial gastric outlet obstruction leading to nausea, vomiting, and an early feeling of fullness. Intestinal tumors can cause partial obstruction or blind-loop syndrome and interfere with nutrient absorption. Pancreatic carcinomas frequently lead to exocrine enzyme deficiencies, bile salt unavailability, and malabsorption syndromes.

Psychological factors such as depression, grief, or anxiety resulting from the disease or its treatment may lead to poor appetite, abnormal eating behavior, and learned food aversions, and thus to a diminished or unbalanced dietary intake.

ABNORMALITIES OF SUBSTRATE METABOLISM

Extensive changes in energy, carbohydrate, lipid, and protein metabolism have been demonstrated in patients with malignant disease (Brennan 1977; Brennan 1981). Increased energy expenditure and inefficient energy utilization are frequently cited causes of malnutrition in tumor-bearing hosts (Holroyde and Reichard 1981; Young 1977). The normal response to diminished food intake is a reduction in basal metabolic rate (BMR); the BMR or resting energy expenditure is basically the sum of all the energy-requiring processes of vegetative function and accounts for 75% of total energy expenditure in normal individuals.

There have been many studies of the energy requirements of cancer patients. Young (1977) reviewed a number of them and could not conclude that resting metabolism is consistently elevated in cancer patients, although the data did show increased resting energy expenditure in leukemia and lymphoma patients. One study demonstrated that increases in resting metabolic rate paralleled advancing disease and reduced nutrient intake (Warnold, Lundholm, and Schersten 1978).

Shike and colleagues (1984) demonstrated in a group of patients with small-cell lung carcinoma that basal energy expenditure was elevated. Responders to chemotherapy had a significant decrease in basal energy expenditure while nonresponders exhibited no change. In 1983, Knox and colleagues measured energy expenditure in 200 malnourished cancer patients by indirect calorimetry. Patients considered normal were also studied and exhibited resting energy expenditure levels within 10% of the value predicted by the Harris-Benedict equation. Only 41% of cancer patients had a normal resting energy expenditure (REE), while decreased and increased REE was observed in 33% and 26% of patients respectively (see fig. 34.1). Similarly, Heber and colleagues (1982) found no clear evidence of hypermetabolism in noncachectic lung cancer patients. They argued that since malnourished patients normally decrease BMR as an adaptation to starvation, even normal predicted metabolic rates are inappropriately elevated in malnourished cancer patients. Shaw, Humberstone, and Wolfe (1988) argued that the alteration in metabolic rate depends on the type of tumor. They demonstrate an elevated rate of energy expenditure in sarcoma-bearing patients associated with increased Cori cycle activity, glucose turnover, reduced glucose oxidation, and increased protein catabolism. Others have shown an elevation in resting energy expenditure with lymphomas, lung cancer, and head and neck cancers. Buzby and coworkers (1980) have shown a reduction in metabolic rate associated with pancreatic cancer. Patients with lower GI neoplasms tend to be metabolically similar to normal volunteers, whereas upper GI tumors result in an elevated metabolic rate.

Inefficient energy utilization by the tumor-bearing host was studied by Holroyde and Reichard (1981), who reported increased Cori cycle activity in patients with malignancy. This futile cycle, in which glucose is converted to lactic acid and subsequently reconverted to glucose by hepatocytes, is an energy-wasting process. The highest level of Cori cycle activity was observed in patients with the greatest energy expenditure and weight loss. Young (1977) has suggested that increased rates of protein turnover also result in significant energy losses due to the failure of normal adaptation to starvation. During the first two days of fasting, endogenous glycogen stores of muscle and the liver are depleted. Glucose utilization by the brain and erythrocytes continues, resulting in the breakdown of protein for gluconeogenesis. In noncancer patients, muscle protein breakdown is gradually replaced by fat fuel metabolism in which fatty acids are converted to ketone bodies. These are used for energy by peripheral tissues and eventually up to 95% of energy utilization by the brain; this results in decreased glucose utilization with secondary sparing of muscle protein. In cancer patients, these adaptive mechanisms do not occur, resulting in increased glucose production and protein catabolism.

Although cancer patients have normal levels of circulating insulin and glucose, they have impaired insulin

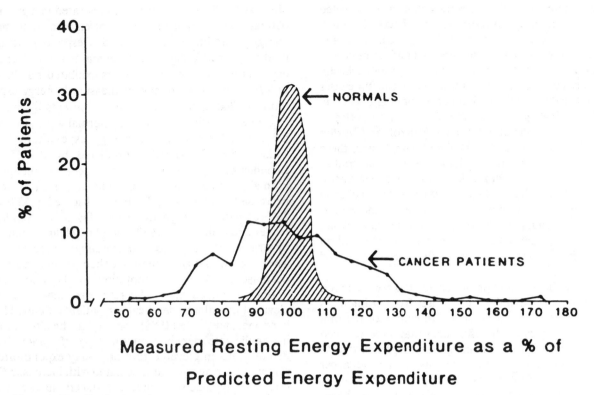

Fig. 34.1. The distribution of measured resting energy expenditure in "normals" and in 200 cancer patients. (Reproduced with permission from: Knox, Crosby, and Feurer et al. [1983].)

sensitivity. Glucose intolerance is documented by hyperglycemia and delayed clearance of blood glucose in cancer patients after oral or intravenous glucose administration (Holroyde and Reichard 1981; Heber et al. 1982; Schein et al. 1979). Glucose intolerance is due in part to decreased tissue sensitivity to insulin, but may also involve an attenuated secretory response to glucose (Schein et al. 1979; Marks and Bishop 1957). Cancer patients also exhibit increased gluconeogenesis from alanine and lactate. Using carbon-14 labeled alanine, Waterhouse and colleagues (1979) found that the apparent increase in gluconeogenesis from alanine reflected a very rapid glucose turnover. Feedback control of glucose production may be impaired because gluconeogenesis and Cori cycle activity are not inhibited by glucose administration in the cancer patient.

Alterations in lipid metabolism in cancer patients include changes in body composition and increased lipid mobilization (Lundholm et al. 1981; Brennan 1986). Decreases in total body fat are common among these patients and are most likely related to insulin deficiency. Increased oxidation of fatty acids also occurs. Glycerol and fatty acids, the byproducts of lipolysis, serve as substrates for gluconeogenesis and energy production, respectively, during periods of nutrient deprivation. Waterhouse (1963) found that fatty acids are the major substrates in patients with progressive malignant disease. Increased plasma clearance of endogenous fat stores and exogenously administered fat emulsions in cancer patients has been demonstrated (Waterhouse and Kemperman 1971; Edmonson 1966) in both fasting

and fed states. Patients with malignancy fail to suppress lipolysis after glucose administration and continue to oxidize fatty acids.

Several abnormalities of protein metabolism occur in cancer patients, including host nitrogen depletion, decreased muscle protein synthesis, and the occurrence of abnormal plasma aminograms (Brennan and Burt 1981; Blackburn et al. 1976). Nitrogen balance is negative in 30% to 100% of patients with progressive malignancy (Brennan and Burt 1981). Amino acid trapping by tumor cells has been demonstrated clinically and experimentally. In a study of sarcoma-bearing limbs, Norton and colleagues found that affected limbs released less than 50% of the amount of amino acids released from tumor-free limbs. Evidence obtained with whole body protein studies using nitrogen-15 (N-15) labeled glycine indicates that cancer patients have increased protein turnover, a circumstance that contributes to increased energy expenditure (Norton, Stein, and Brennan 1981).

Also associated with cachexia are changes in body composition such as increased extracellular fluid and total body sodium and decreased intracellular fluid and total body potassium. Cohn and others, using prompt gamma-neutron activation to evaluate total body nitrogen and a whole body counter to measure potassium-40, found that total body potassium was diminished out of proportion to total body nitrogen. On the basis of this finding, they concluded that endogenous nutrient losses in cancer patients were predominantly in the skeletal muscle compartment since muscle comprises 45% of total body nitrogen and 85% of total body potassium

(Cohn et al. 1980). A recent study, using potassium-40 and a whole body counter, measured body cell mass (BCM) in relation to body weight in normal volunteers, anorexia nervosa patients, and cancer patients. In the normal volunteers, body cell mass tended to decrease with increasing age as an absolute value and as a percentage of total body weight. In anorexia nervosa patients, there was a significant depletion of BCM but with relative sparing of the BCM when expressed as a percentage of body weight. This reflects the normal adaptation to starvation where fat utilization predominates and endogenous protein is spared. In cancer patients, there was a significant degree of weight loss accompanied by a proportional decline in BCM, indicating that protein is depleted to the same extent as fat stores (Moley et al. 1987).

THE IMPACT OF ANTITUMOR THERAPY ON NUTRITION

Antineoplastic therapy invariably affects the host, either by mechanical and physiologic alterations due to surgery, or at the cellular level with chemotherapy or radiation therapy (McAnena and Daly 1986). The effects of therapy may add to the cachexia of malignancy and leave the patient with a more severe nutritional deficiency.

Operative therapy is the primary treatment modality of many cancers, particularly those of the GI tract. The immediate metabolic response to surgery in patients with cancer is similar to that of patients who have surgery for benign disease: increased nitrogen losses and energy requirements (Stein and Buzby 1981; Brennan 1979). However, because cancer patients tend to have significant weight loss prior to surgery, their ability to cope with stress is impaired (Buzby et al. 1980),

resulting in increased morbidity and mortality. The physical insult, the associated pain, and the emotional response to surgery set off an integrated endocrine and metabolic reaction designed to maintain body functions. There is an increased output of catecholamines, glucagon, and cortisol that results in hypermetabolism, weight loss, negative nitrogen balance, and retention of sodium and water. As well as the general response to injury, operations on the oropharynx and GI tract have specific nutritional sequelae depending on the site of surgery (table 34.1).

Cancer chemotherapy may profoundly alter the host's nutritional state. The effects may be direct (by interfering with host cell metabolism or DNA synthesis and cellular replication), or indirect (by producing nausea, vomiting, changes in taste sensation, and learned food aversions). Most agents have the ability to stimulate the chemoreceptor trigger zone, resulting in nausea and vomiting. The rapid cell turnover in the alimentary tract mucosa makes it especially vulnerable to chemotherapy, resulting in stomatitis, ulceration, and decreased absorptive capacity. These effects result, in turn, in decreased intake and absorption of nutrients and further predispose the cancer patient to malnutrition. The bone marrow is another organ with a high cell turnover; toxicity is manifested by anemia, leukopenia, and thrombocytopenia. Neutropenia is, in turn, associated with an increased risk of sepsis.

Radiation therapy may affect the host's nutritional state by its effects on the gastrointestinal tract. The severity of the injury is related to the dose of radiation and the volume of tissue treated. The effects of radiation therapy are classified as early or late. Early effects are transient and are manifested by diarrhea, bleeding, nausea, vomiting, weight loss, mucositis, xerostomia, alterations in taste, and food aversions. Late effects include intestinal strictures, fistulae, and malabsorption.

Table 34.1
NUTRITIONAL CONSEQUENCES OF RADICAL OPERATIVE RESECTION

Organs Resected	Nutritional Sequelae
Oral cavity and pharynx Thoracic esophagus	Dependency on tube feedings Gastric stasis (secondary to vagotomy) Fat malabsorption Gastrostomy feedings in patients without reconstruction
Stomach	Dumping syndrome Fat malabsorption Anemia

Small intestine
  Duodenum
  Jejunum
  Ileum
  Massive (greater than 75%)
	Pancreatobiliary deficiency with fat malabsorption
	Decrease in efficiency of absorption (general)
	Vitamin B_{12} and bile salt absorption
	Fat malabsorption and diarrhea
	Vitamin B_{12} malabsorption
	Gastric hypersecretion

Colon (total or subtotal)	Water and electrolyte loss

(With permission from: Lawrence [1977].)

CONSEQUENCES OF MALNUTRITION IN THE CANCER PATIENT

The clinical relevance of severe malnutrition has been demonstrated by increased morbidity and mortality and poor treatment tolerance in malnourished tumor-bearing individuals (Copeland, Daly, and Dudrick 1977; Smale et al. 1981; Nixon, Heymsfield, and Cohen 1980). In 1932, after reviewing 500 autopsy reports on cancer patients, Warren found that malnutrition was a major factor contributing to their deaths. The protein-calorie malnutrition produced by the cancer-bearing state leads not only to obvious weight loss, but also to visceral and somatic protein depletion that compromises enzymatic, structural, and mechanical functions. Impairment of immunocompetence (Bistrian et al. 1975; Daly, Dudrick, and Copeland 1978) and increased susceptibility to infection frequently result. The effect on immune function may be further exacerbated by chemotherapy (Cosimi et al. 1972). Moreover, poor wound healing, increased wound infections, prolonged postoperative ileus, and longer hospital stays have all been linked to poor nutritional status in cancer patients. Meguid and coworkers (1986) demonstrated that in patients undergoing colorectal cancer operations, the return to adequate oral food intake was significantly delayed in those patients classified as malnourished based on preoperative assessment. In this study, the morbidity and mortality in malnourished patients was 52% and 12% respectively, compared with 31% and 6% in well-nourished patients.

In animal studies, severe protein restriction depresses both humoral and cellular immune responses. In 1976, Daly, Copeland, and Dudrick demonstrated that only 30% of tumor-bearing rats had a delayed hypersensitivity response to intradermal purified protein derivative after two weeks on an oral protein-free diet. Protein repletion with seven days of total parenteral nutrition (TPN) or oral *ad libitum* feeding restored the response in 91% and 78% of rats, respectively. Only 17% of animals who remained on protein-free diets for the further seven days showed a delayed hypersensitivity response. Law, Dudrick, and Abdou (1974) found reduced titers of antibodies, IgM-producing cells, reduced lymphocyte response to mitogens, and decreased delayed hypersensitivity in rats after six weeks on protein-free nutrition.

In human studies, there is evidence for increased morbidity and mortality with depressed immunocompetence. In addition, it has been documented that nutritional therapy reverses anergy. Harvey, Bath, and Blackburn (1979) reported on a group of 161 cancer patients undergoing nutritional support. Of these, 32 were anergic prior to therapy. In 27 of these patients anergy was reversed and three of this group died. Of the five patients who remained anergic, all died. Daly, Dudrick, and Copeland (1980) documented that 51% of anergic patients undergoing cancer treatment had restoration of skin test reactivity in response to intravenous (IV) hyperalimentation.

Surgery, chemotherapy, and radiation therapy all add further nutritional stress to patients with cancer cachexia.

Numerous retrospective studies have correlated severe malnutrition with adverse clinical outcome after major surgery (Mullen 1981). In a study by Mullen and coworkers (1982), TPN was shown to reduce weight loss, major complications, and mortality rates after cancer surgery. Patients were prospectively randomized to preoperative parenteral nutrition or to regular hospital diet for 10 days. The two groups were similar in terms of cancer site, stage of tumor, and type of operation. While the rates of postoperative wound infection, pneumonia, major complications, and mortality were lower in the parenteral nutrition group, the differences were significant only for major complications and mortality. These clinical differences were paralleled by improvement in serum proteins and immunocompetence. A retrospective review of operative therapy in 244 esophageal cancer patients also showed benefit in terms of reduced morbidity and longer survival postoperatively (fig. 34.2) in parenterally fed patients compared to patients not receiving parenteral nutrition (Daly et al. 1982).

A narrow margin of therapeutic safety exists for chemotherapeutic drugs and adequate levels of radiation therapy; cachexia may reduce the therapeutic index of those modalities. Animal studies indicate that protein depletion increases the toxicity and lethality of chemotherapy (Flanigen-Roat, Milholland, and Ip 1985). Furthermore, TPN (Souchon et al. 1975) or increased dietary protein (Flanigen-Roat, Milholland, and Ip 1985) reduces toxicity in animals, compared to regular or protein-depleted diets. In the 1970s, clinical reviews correlated malnutrition with a poor prognosis in patients with metastatic disease receiving chemotherapy. This suggested that nutritional support should increase therapeutic benefit and many trials using TPN as adjunctive therapy were initiated. In 1986, Chlebowski reviewed recent randomized trials and found no clear evidence that TPN alleviates chemotherapy-related toxicity, or enhances the response in man (table 34.2). Although randomized trials have failed to demonstrate an adjunctive role for TPN or a reduction in side effects, nutritional therapy is an important supportive measure. It may permit some patients, who are otherwise not candidates for treatment due to inanition, to undergo continuing chemotherapy and, potentially, achieve disease remission.

Some researchers have demonstrated reduced mortality and increased response rates in patients receiving extensive radiation therapy with adjunctive TPN, compared to patients not receiving nutritional support (Boethe et al. 1979; Valerio et al. 1978). However, these studies were carried out in small groups of patients. Donaldson reviewed these and other prospective trials in 1984 and failed to show that adequate nutritional support reduced the complication rates or improved local cancer control and survival. This suggests that TPN or enteral feeding is an important support measure in patients undergoing a planned course of radiation therapy, but does not sensitize the tumor to irradiation or prevent gastrointestinal side effects.

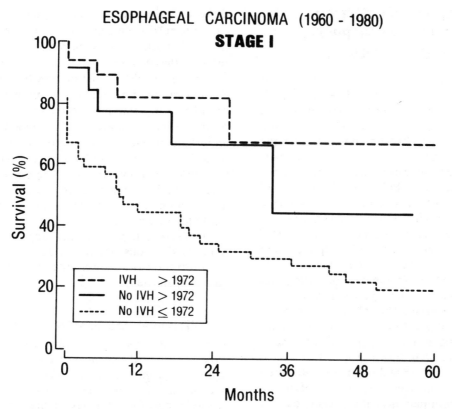

Fig. 34.2. Five-year survival curves for patients with stage I esophageal cancer show a significant improvement in survival with TPN over concurrent non-TPN patients treated from 1960 to 1972. (Adapted with permission from: Daly, Massar, and Giacco et al. [1982].)

Table 34.2
RANDOMIZED TRIALS OF TPN ADDITION TO CHEMOTHERAPY IN PATIENTS WITH CANCER

Tumor Type	Patients Entered	Summary Results	Reference
Lung cancer			
Small-cell	119	More febrile episodes (p 0.001) on TPN	Clamon et al. 1985
	49	No difference in outcome	Valdievieso et al. 1981
	19	No difference in outcome	Serrou et al. 1982
Non-small cell	26	Less myelosuppression on TPN	Issel et al. 1978
	65	*Decreased survival on TPN	Jordan et al. 1981
	31	No difference in outcome	Moghissi et al. 1977
	27	No difference in outcome	Lanzotti et al. 1980
Colon	45	*Decreased survival (p 0.03) on TPN	Nixon et al. 1981
Lymphoma	42	No difference in outcome	Popp et al. 1983
Testicular	30	Trend to more infections (p 0.07) on TPN	Samuels et al. 1981
Sarcoma	27	*Increased relapse (p 0.01) in patients on TPN made NED	Shamberger et al. 1984
Acute leukemia	24	No difference in outcome	Coquin et al. 1981
	21	More rapid bone marrow recovery on TPN	Hays et al. 1983
Pediatric malignancies	19	No difference in outcome	Van Eys et al. 1980

*Trials suggesting adverse effect of TPN addition to chemotherapy. NED = no evidence of disease. (With permission from: Chlebowski [1986].)

EFFECT OF MALNUTRITION AND NUTRITIONAL SUPPORT ON TUMOR GROWTH

Severe protein-calorie malnutrition inhibits tumor development and retards tumor growth in the experimental animal (Tannenbaum and Silverstone 1953; White 1961), but these apparent benefits are countered by loss of host body weight and impaired immune function (Daly, Dudrick, and Copeland 1978). Malnourished animals that undergo nutritional repletion orally (Steiger et al. 1975) or with TPN (Daly, Copeland, and Dudrick 1978) may have a significant increase in tumor growth. Stimulation of tumor growth does not appear to be selective, as evidenced by constant tumor weight-to-host weight ratios in nutritionally depleted and repleted animals (Daly, Copeland, and Dudrick 1978). Thus, it is of great concern in the clinical setting that nutritional support may promote tumor growth.

One of the most extensive clinical studies on nutritional support is that of Copeland and colleagues (1979). After following over 1,500 patients with cancer, they observed no increase in tumor growth attributable to nutritional support. Nixon and others in 1981 noted no direct clinical or biochemical evidence of tumor stimulation with TPN in patients with metastatic colon cancer, although they did note that survival duration was less in the patients given TPN. Tumor protein synthesis, as determined by N-15 glycine metabolism, shows no differences in patients on TPN and those fed orally, despite a substantial increase in protein and calorie intake in the TPN group (Mullen et al. 1980). To date, numerous retrospective and prospective studies in man have shown no enhanced tumor growth in response to increased nutritional intake. The issue is complicated by the fact that most patients studied were having antitumor treatment during their nutritional support. Also, the changes may be difficult to assess precisely by clinical or radiological methods. Malnutrition may affect tumor growth by impairing the host's antitumor immune response. In animal studies, the effects of nutritional repletion appear to vary specifically with tumor immunogenicity and the host's immune response. In animals that do not develop an immune response to the tumor, nutritional repletion results in enhanced tumor growth (Karpeh et al. 1987). Conversely, nutritional repletion in animals with an immunogenic tumor results in diminished tumor growth. Although increased nutritional intake may stimulate tumor growth in animal studies, it may decrease toxicity of chemotherapy without decreasing the response and lead to prolonged survival after treatment (Flanigen-Roat, Milholland, and Ip 1985).

NUTRITIONAL MANAGEMENT OF THE CANCER PATIENT

Nutritional support for cancer patients is time-consuming and costly, and has its own inherent complications. There is no doubt that in malnourished patients, nutritional support can restore body composition and substrate metabolism towards normal. It also reduces the morbidity and mortality associated with major surgery. Nutritional therapy has also allowed the administration of more intensive antineoplastic therapy or radical surgery to patients who might otherwise have been considered unacceptable candidates. Thus, it is important to assess cancer patients accurately prior to treatment, in order to identify those who may benefit from nutritional intervention. The object of nutritional assessment is to characterize the type and degree of malnutrition and relate these factors to the risk of morbidity and mortality.

The decision to nutritionally support a cancer patient requires decisions about the route and duration of administration and the formulation of the quantity and quality of nutrients.

NUTRITIONAL ASSESSMENT

The patient's history and physical examination may indicate the need for nutritional support. Once malnutrition is diagnosed, more precise measurements of nutritional status may be carried out. The patient's history allows for estimates of the rate and extent of weight loss and the quantity and quality of nutritional intake. Recent weight loss of more than 10% of body weight (over a period of 3 months) signifies substantial protein-calorie malnutrition. In Western society, where obesity is more the norm than the exception, the percent loss of body weight may be more relevant than comparison with ideal body weight standards. In 1936, Studley showed a strong correlation between preoperative weight loss and postoperative complications in 50 patients undergoing gastric surgery. The patient's history may also provide information regarding special diets; problems with taste, chewing, or swallowing; food allergies; medicine and alcohol intake; and learned food aversions. Physical examination may reveal dry, scaly, atrophic skin; muscle wasting; pitting edema; and loss of muscle strength. A thorough history and physical examination by an experienced clinician is the simplest, and perhaps the best, method of nutritional assessment.

As an initial test, serum albumin can give important information. Values less than 3.4 g/dL are associated with increased morbidity and mortality following therapy. Less than 3 g/dL indicates significant visceral protein depletion. Albumin with a half-life of 20 days changes slowly in response to additional stress, such as therapy, or in response to nutritional support. Serum prealbumin, retinal binding globulin, and transferrin, with half-lives of one-half, two, and eight days, respectively, may be more useful under these circumstances. Alterations in the serum levels of these proteins may occur with varying levels of hydration and it is not uncommon for serum albumin to fall initially on TPN. This decrease reflects increased hydration rather than a worsening malnourished state.

The degree of visceral protein depletion is also reflected by impaired cell-mediated immunity evaluated by determining recall antigen skin testing and by total lymphocyte count. Loss of immunocompetence is not a sensitive indicator because weight loss usually exceeds 10% before anergy develops. Therefore, anergy with malnutrition indicates a significant visceral protein depletion leading to higher morbidity and mortality in hospitalized patients. Anergy has been associated with decreased serum albumin and transferrin levels (Harvey et al. 1981). Delayed hypersensitivity (Christou, Meakins, and McLean 1981) is tested by the administration of subdermal injections of five antigens (purified protein derivative, candida, trichophytin, mumps skin test antigen, and streptokinose-streptodornase). A positive reaction with each antigen is defined as induration greater than 5 mm diameter at 24 hours after injection. A normal delayed hypersensitivity response is defined as two or more positive reactions. Anergy is defined as no reaction, and one reaction is relative anergy.

Anthropometric measurements are noninvasive methods of determining body compartments and relate to measurements of age- and sex-matched normal populations. Skinfold thicknesses measured over the triceps, scapular area, iliac crest, and thigh provide an estimate of subcutaneous and total body fat, since 50% of total body fat is in the subcutaneous layer. Midarm muscle circumference, calculated as arm circumference, is measured at a point midway between the tip of the shoulder and the olecranon, minus .314 triceps skinfold thickness. This is measured on the nondominant arm and reflects lean body mass, which makes up most of the body's protein. Creatinine height index, defined as the 24-hour creatinine urinary excretion divided by the expected 24-hour excretion of creatinine by a normal adult of the same height, provides another measurement of muscle protein mass in patients with normal renal function. Substantial protein-calorie malnutrition would be defined as a level less than 75% of standard. Skeletal muscle mass may also be determined using a whole body counter to detect potassium–40, which is present in small amounts, primarily intracellularly in skeletal muscle. From this value total body potassium, a reasonable estimate of lean body mass, can be calculated.

Nutritional measurements have proved accurate in population surveys but have varying sensitivity and lack specificity. For example, anergy can occur due to exogenous steroid administration, inhalation anesthetics, trauma, radiation therapy, or sepsis; anthropometric measurements may increase with edema; and changes in serum albumin may result from alterations in hydration. Thus, the value of nutritional measurements lies in supporting the clinical diagnosis of malnutrition. With each individual patient, these measurements can help define the nutritional status and allow objective assessment of the efficacy of nutritional therapy (table 34.3).

While the initial clinical assessment and blood tests select nutritionally depleted patients, complete nutritional assessment provides an estimate of body composition and quantifies the magnitude of malnutrition. This may be helpful in determining which patients may benefit from maintenance or anabolic nutritional therapy. These measurements have also been used individually or in various combinations as predictors of surgical risk, in order to select specifically those patients who would benefit from nutritional support. Examples are serum albumin (Forse and Shizal 1980), serum transferrin (Mullen et al. 1979), delayed hypersensitivity skin tests (Forse and Shizal 1980), and total lymphocyte count (Grant, Custer, and Thurlow 1981). Clinical judgment also plays a role in such assessments (Baker et al. 1982).

The key issue is whether there is a correlation between the risk of complications and the degree of malnutrition. Mullen and his coworkers developed an index of risk based on some nutritional parameters for patients undergoing surgery (Mullen et al. 1979; Buzby et al. 1980). The resulting formula was termed the prognostic nutritional index (PNI):

$$PNI = 158\% - 16.6(ALB) - 0.78(TSF) - 0.2(TFN) - 5.8(DH)$$

[ALB = albumin (g/dL); TSF = triceps skinfold thickness (mm); TFN = transferrin (mg/dL); DH = delayed hypersensitivity to any of 3 recall antigens graded from 0 to 2 where 0 is no reaction, 1 is a reaction less than 5 mm in diameter, and 2 is a reaction greater than 5 mm in diameter at 24 hours after injection.]

A PNI less than 30% (low risk) was associated with an 11.7% complication rate and a mortality of 2%. A PNI greater than 60% (high risk) was associated with an 81% complication rate and a mortality of 59%. In general, a PNI greater than 40% is regarded as an indication for nutritional support. Cancer patients with a PNI greater than 40% have been shown to have a significant decrease in postoperative mortality and morbidity if given total parenteral nutrition.

A simple, practical definition of significant malnutrition that can be applied clinically includes recent unexplained (i.e., not due to dieting) weight loss of 10% or more of body weight, a serum albumin less than 3.4

Table 34.3
SUMMARY OF NUTRITIONAL ASSESSMENT

Measurement	Body Compartment
Recent weight loss	Total body mass
Skinfold thickness over triceps, scapula, iliac crest	Total body fat
Midarm muscle circumference	Lean body mass
Creatinine height index	
Serum albumin, transferrin, retinal binding globulin, and prealbumin	Visceral protein
Total lymphocyte count	Immune competence
Delayed hypersensitivity to common skin antigens	

g/dL, and a serum transferrin less than 190 mg/dL (normal range 210-375 mg/dL). Any combination of two of these criteria is an indication for nutritional support. The efficiency of PNI for patient selection was assessed for cancer surgery in 1981 (Smale et al.). Based on the PNI, patients were allocated to high risk (PNI >40%) or low risk (PNI <40%) groups. Within each group patients were assigned to TPN or no nutritional support. In the low-risk group there was no operative mortality and similar complication rates in TPN and no-TPN groups. In the high-risk category patients without nutritional support had a complication rate of 66% and a mortality rate of 40% while in the TPN group the results were 31% and 15%, respectively. This study indicated that an adequate period of TPN is effective in reducing mortality and morbidity in cancer patients undergoing major surgery. The PNI, which is a nutritional composite representing fat stores, visceral protein, and immunocompetence, provides the clinician with an accurate and objective measure of risk for each individual.

DESIGNING NUTRITIONAL SUPPORT

ROUTE OF ADMINISTRATION

In the presence of a normal gastrointestinal tract, enteral feeding is preferred because it is more physiological, less expensive, and has fewer complications associated with it than does parenteral feeding. Animal experiments indicate that adequate caloric and protein intake lead to the same benefits in terms of weight gain and serum albumin levels, irrespective of whether the route of administration is enteral or intravenous (Daly et al. 1974; Kudsk et al. 1981). A recent study of surgical patients compared those on enteral feeding to patients not receiving nutritional support (Shukla et al. 1984). Sixty-seven patients were given a protein hydrolysate solution containing 3,500 to 4,000 calories/day by nasogastric feeding tube; 43 patients received no treatment. Results showed highly significant advantages with enteral nutritional support in terms of body weight, serum albumin, nitrogen balance, immunocompetence, morbidity, and mortality. An earlier study of 24 esophageal cancer patients compared preoperative enteral feeding per gastrostomy with TPN. Weight gain was greater in the TPN group; the percentage gain in serum albumin was similar in both groups (Lim et al. 1981). In a study of nonsurgical cancer patients randomized to TPN, jejunostomy feeding, or normal oral diet, the TPN and enterally fed groups appeared to stabilize nutritionally; no significant differences could be found between the enteral and parenteral groups of patients (Burt, Stein, and Brennan 1983). Overall, these studies indicate that enteral and parenteral methods are equally efficacious in supplying nutritional requirements, although if rapid repletion is required, intravenous methods are preferable.

In some patients, adequate intake may be achieved orally with aggressive dietary counseling; the normal diet can be supplemented with preparations containing high calorie content, amino acids, vitamins, and minerals. However, the presence of anorexia or upper GI cancers such as oropharyngeal or esophageal neoplasms may necessitate enteral tube feeding to achieve adequate nutritional intake.

For enteral feeding, nasogastric or nasoduodenal tubes, feeding gastrostomy, or jejunostomy routes provide access to the GI tract. Nasogastric tube feeding is the method most commonly used. Recent refinements in design have resulted in smaller-bore (6F-8F) and more pliable tubes made from silicone or polyurethane. These are available weighted or with a stylet to facilitate passage of the tip. They can be left in place for four to six weeks with fewer complications (such as mucosal irritation, erosions, and sinusitis) than with the large-bore, less-pliable nasogastric tubes. A large number of commercially prepared formulas are available that are homogenous and sterile, flow easily through small-bore tubes, and require little preparation.

If it is anticipated that the duration of enteral feeding will be longer than six weeks, gastrostomy or jejunostomy feeding should be considered. Large-bore gastrostomy tubes allow easy administration of bolus feeding but require operative insertion using local or general anesthesia. Endoscopic techniques permit insertion of smaller percutaneous gastrostomy tubes using a local anesthetic and sedation (Ponsky, Gauderer, and Stellato 1983). A jejunostomy tube is recommended when there is a proximal gastrointestinal obstruction or fistula. It is associated with less stomal leakage, skin erosion, nausea, vomiting, and bloating compared with gastrostomy feeding (Torosian and Rambeau 1980). The conventional feeding tubes are made of rubber or latex; needle insertion of small-bore polyurethane catheters has become popular. Small-bore jejunostomy feeding requires a continuous flow pump to avoid clogging of the tube. The main disadvantage with jejunostomy feeding is diarrhea. Administration of hyperosmolar solutions within the small intestine results in diffusion of water into the lumen. To reduce the incidence of diarrhea, jejunal feeding should commence with small volumes (25-30 mL/hr) of full-strength formula with a gradual increase in volume over three to five days depending on the patient's tolerance. If diarrhea persists, antiperistaltic agents may be administered in the feeding formula. Gastric feeding allows the stomach to dilute hyperosmolar solutions and reduces the incidence of diarrhea, but it carries the risk of regurgitation and pulmonary aspiration and is contraindicated in the presence of gastric outlet obstruction, obtundation, or laryngeal incompetence.

The candidate for TPN is a malnourished patient who cannot be renourished enterally and who is potentially responsive to antineoplastic therapy. TPN should also be given to patients with severe protein-calorie malnutrition (PNI >40%), who would be considered for treatment if their nutritional status improved. In these patients, severe visceral protein depletion may decrease the absorptive capacity of the intestine and delay the administration of treatment if enteral feeding methods are used. TPN is also indicated in patients who, as a result of their treatment, are unable to maintain their nutritional status by oral or enteral feeding. To administer sufficient calories and amino acids intravenously it is necessary to use hypertonic solutions, administered through a high-flow vein to prevent chemical endothelial phlebitis and thrombosis. The standard approach is central venous access using percutaneous, infraclavicular subclavian vein catheterization. In patients with emphysema, the risk of pneumothorax is high and access through the internal jugular vein is preferred, though it may be less comfortable.

NUTRITIONAL REQUIREMENTS

In normal individuals, calorie and nitrogen requirements can be calculated based on age, gender, height, and weight. Ideally, caloric requirement should be calculated for each patient by adjusting the calculated or measured resting energy expenditure (REE) for the level of physical activity and the degree of stress (table 34.4). Indirect calorimetry is a more precise measurement of REE in each patient. Calorie requirements can be conveniently calculated using the Harris-Benedict equation:

For women:

$$REE(kcal/day) = 655 + 9.6W + 1.7H - 4.7A$$

For men:

$$REE(kcal/day) = 66 + 13.7W + 5.0H - 6.8A$$
[W = weight (kg); H = height (cm); A = age (years).]

Nonprotein caloric intake in excess of 130% of the REE is necessary for positive energy balance and repletion of fat stores. Dempsey, Hurwitz, and Mullen (1985) found that increasing energy intake beyond 115% of REE did not improve nitrogen balance. Several studies have shown that provision of excessive caloric intake, especially in the form of hypertonic dextrose, leads to lipogenesis when the glycogen stores are repleted and results in impaired hepatic function (Sheldon, Peterson, and Sanders 1978; Greenlaw 1980). The concept has evolved of using both fat and carbohydrate for nonprotein calories to minimize the complications of administration of excessive glucose calories alone. Most organs use fat and carbohydrate for energy; the central nervous system, red blood cells, and the renal medulla preferentially metabolize glucose. To provide all the required calories as glucose results in simpler preparation and efficient utilization by all tissues; it spares the use of amino acids for gluconeogenesis. Hypertonic glucose solutions may result in high blood glucose levels leading to loss of glucose in the urine, resulting in an osmotic diuresis with electrolyte loss and tissue dehydration. Coadministration of insulin improves glucose uptake and utilization. High serum insulin levels, whether the result of exogenous administration or stimulated by high glucose levels, inhibit lipolysis and promote fat deposi-

tion, decreasing the availability of fat as an energy source. Glucose provides 4 kcal/g and utilization is optimal when it is given at rates of 4 mg/kg/min to 5 mg/kg/min. Administration at rates in excess of 7 mg/kg/min does not further increase glucose oxidation rates. Glycogenolysis is stimulated and excess glucose is converted to glycerol and fatty acids, leading to fat deposition in the liver. Insulin has an anabolic effect on skeletal muscle, increasing uptake and decreasing release of amino acids, that may bias protein repletion in favor of muscle protein at the expense of visceral protein. The provision of a lipid source of calories helps to overcome these problems. When plasma levels of fatty acids are elevated, they become the main source of energy for peripheral tissues, sparing glucose for tissues that preferentially metabolize it. In addition, using glucose alone as a caloric source results in an increase in carbon dioxide (CO_2) production (Askanazi et al. 1980), since glucose is oxidized with a respiratory quotient (RQ) of 1.0. Fat, on the other hand, has an RQ of 0.7 and fat oxidation produces less CO_2. Conversion of glucose to lipid is associated with an RQ of 8.0 and a substantial rise in CO_2 production. This requires the patient to increase minute ventilation to cope with rising CO_2 production and may cause respiratory distress with acidosis in patients with chronic obstructive airways disease. This is evidenced clinically by the fact that patients are more easily weaned off mechanical ventilators if they are receiving lipid in their diet or TPN solution.

Fat is usually given as lipid emulsions mainly made up of long-chain fatty acids with a caloric value of 9 kcal/g. Large quantities of long-chain fatty acids may impair neutrophil and reticuloendothelial macrophage function and reduce bacterial clearance (Hamany et al. 1985). Thus, long-chain fatty acids should be limited to a maximum of 1.5 g/kg/day. Medium-chain triglycerides are available and do not impair macrophage function. They do not contain essential fatty acids and thus a mixture of long- and medium-chain triglycerides is commonly used.

Administration of amino acids and calories adds to the circulating pool of amino acids supplying the liver

Table 34.4
DETERMINATION OF ENERGY REQUIREMENTS

1.	Resting energy expenditure; Harris-Benedict equation/indirect calorimetry	
2.	Stress factors:	
	Starvation	0.85
	Elective surgery	1.0–1.2
	Major sepsis	1.4–1.8
	Fever	1.0 + 0.13 per degree C
	Peritonitis	1.2–1.5
	Cancer	1.1–1.45
3.	Activity factor:	
	Confined to bed	1.2
	Mobile	1.3
4.	Total energy expenditure = REE x stress x activity	

(Adapted with permission from: Shanbhogue, Chwals, and Weintraub [1987].)

with substrates for protein synthesis and reduces protein catabolism for energy production. In the malnourished patient, pyruvate is converted to alanine in skeletal muscle, receiving an amino group from one of the branched-chain amino acids (BCAA), leucine, isoleucine, and valine. In the liver, alanine is deaminated to pyruvate and converted to glucose. The administration of BCAA has been advocated to improve nitrogen balance in hypercatabolic patients. However, because of high costs, the use of these solutions is not warranted.

In addition to protein and calorie requirements, minerals, trace elements, and vitamins must be supplied. The clinical course of the patient should be monitored closely. Each day the patient's temperature, weight, glucose excretion, fluid and electrolyte balance and physical findings should be reviewed. Serum urea, calcium, and phosphorus; and electrolyte concentrations, liver function, and blood glucose should be measured two or three times weekly to assess the effects of nutritional therapy on the patient. As part of the initial assessment, serum trace elements can be measured so that specific deficits can be corrected.

Numerous standard commercial solutions are available for TPN, some of which may be combined to provide the total daily nutrient requirements for each patient. The solutions can be combined into large bags containing up to three liters that can be changed once each day. This reduces the risk of contaminating the central venous line and is more convenient for the nursing staff. Mixing is carried out in the pharmacy under sterile conditions within a laminar flow hood. Standard amino acid TPN solutions are comprised of 500 cc 8.5% amino acids of which 30% to 50% are essential amino acids. Table 34.5 shows the composition of three typical standard amino acid solutions. For protein-depleted patients such as cancer cachexia patients, these solutions are available at 10% concentrations. Solutions varying from 3% to 14% amino acids are available, depending on the patients' needs. For renal failure patients, a 3% to 5% solution mainly made up of essential amino acids is usually used. Some of the amino acids, such as glutamine, degenerate in solution and are not included. In the future, glutamine should be added because it is an important amino acid for the maintenance of gastrointestinal mucosal integrity.

Nonprotein calories can be given as glucose or lipid. A combination of fat and carbohydrate minimizes the complications of excessive administration of glucose calories (Meguid et al. 1982). Fat emulsions also provide essential fatty acids. Intravenous fat emulsions are usually prepared from soybean or sunflower oils and are rich in polyunsaturated fatty acids. They are usually prepared as a 10% or 20% emulsion using egg phospholipid as the emulsifier and providing 1.1 kcal/mL or 2.2 kcal/mL, respectively. The commercially available emulsions are similar in composition and are therapeutically equivalent.

Glucose is usually administered as dextrose, a polymer of glucose which yields 3.4 kcal/g. Solutions are

Table 34.5
COMPOSITION OF 8.5% AMINO ACID SOLUTIONS

Amino Acids (g/L)	Freamine III	Aminosyn	Travasol
Essential			
Leucine	7.7	8.1	5.3
Isoleucine	5.9	6.2	4.1
Valine	5.6	6.8	3.9
Phenylalanine	4.8	3.8	5.3
Methionine	4.5	3.4	4.9
Lysine	6.2	6.2	4.9
Histidine	2.4	2.6	3.7
Threonine	3.4	4.6	3.6
Tryptophan	1.3	1.5	1.5
Non-Essential			
Alanine	6.0	11.0	17.6
Glycine	11.9	11.0	17.6
Arginine	8.1	8.5	8.8
Proline	11.2	7.5	3.6
Tyrosine	0	0.4	0.3
Serine	5.0	3.7	0
Cysteine	0.2	0	0
Glutamic Acid	0	0	0
Aspartic Acid	0	0	0

available from 5% to 70% concentrations (we usually use a 50% solution).

Nutritional and metabolic support includes electrolytes, vitamins, and trace elements. Daily intravenous requirements of minerals are as follows:

Sodium 60–140 mEq
Potassium 60–100 mEq
Chloride 60–120 mEq
Magnesium 8–10 mEq
Calcium 200–400 mg
Iron 1–2 mg

These must be provided daily, but the amounts administered must constantly be re-evaluated in light of existing deficits or abnormal losses.

Parenteral vitamin requirements for maintenance and repletion are poorly defined. The standard approach is to give the recommended daily allowance (RDA) of each vitamin as set down by the Food and Drug Administration (table 34.6). Dempsey and colleagues (1987) determined the prevalence of abnormal vitamin levels in adult hospitalized patients prior to receiving TPN and found abnormally low levels in 42% of the patients. Standard parenteral vitamin therapy resulted in marginal improvement. A higher repletion dose resulted in significant improvement

Table 34.6
FOOD AND DRUG ADMINISTRATION RECOMMENDED DAILY ALLOWANCE OF VITAMINS

Vitamin	RDA
A (IU)	4000-5000
D (IU)	400
E (IU)	12-15
C (mg)	45
B_1 (mg)	1.0-1.5
B_2 (mg)	1.1-1.8
B_6 (mg)	1.6-2.0
B_{12} (μg)	3
Folate (μg)	400
Niacin (mg)	12-30
Pantothenic acid (mg)	5-10
Biotin (μg)	150-300

in vitamins A and C, and pyridoxine. Commercially available multivitamin products contain more than the RDA, and the addition of one vial to the TPN solution each day is recommended. Vitamin K is not available in multivitamin preparations because vitamin K therapy is not required by all patients, such as those on anticoagulants. It is available as a separate parenteral injection as phytonadione. The recommended dosage is 10 mg once a week. Trace elements are also available commercially for TPN regimens and the daily requirements of zinc, copper, manganese, selenium, and chromium can be added to the TPN solution. These elements and others are also available individually and can be added for specific deficiencies. All the above can be added together in a 3-liter bag. Heparin (8,000-10,000 units) is added to reduce the incidence of subclavian vein thrombosis. More water may be added to make up the daily fluid requirements. Initially, the solution is given at 40 mL/hr to 50 mL/hr; the rate is gradually increased over two or three days until the full daily requirements are tolerated. Insulin can be added to the solution as required and six hourly blood sugars checked until they are stable. Suggested daily TPN regimen for an adult cancer patient is given in table 34.7.

SPECIFIC NUTRITIONAL MANIPULATION OF HOST AND TUMOR

Visceral protein and lean body mass depletion result in a worse prognosis than does fat depletion (Nixon, Heymsfield, and Cohen 1980). This is to be expected as proteins are the constituents of enzymes, hormones, immunoglobulins, and the contractile elements of muscle tissue. Using standard nutritional support, weight can be maintained or gained during repletion. This may not, however, represent true anabolism in most patients. Animal evidence suggests that increases in body weight in response to TPN are due to excess water and increased lipid stores (Popp, Morrison, and Brennan 1981). Most prospective studies using TPN have failed to detect a therapeutic benefit to the host in terms of prolonged survival or in tumor response to chemotherapy or radiation therapy. For nutritional therapy to be maximally effective, the aim should be to increase host protein while inhibiting, or at least not stimulating, tumor growth, as animal studies suggest.

In simple chronic starvation, the body adapts by relying on fat as its main energy source. Free fatty acids are used in muscle and liver metabolism for energy, and excess free fatty acids are converted to ketones by the liver to be used as an energy source in other tissues. In these tissues, the ketones are reconverted to acetyl coenzyme A and enter the Krebs cycle. This spares glucose utilization, the need for gluconeogenesis, and reduces nitrogen output. In the cancer cachectic state, these adaptive mechanisms are not effective and this results in continuous protein catabolism. Exogenously administered ketones have been given to normal humans as an external energy source; they produce a fall in urinary nitrogen excretion, reflecting protein conservation (Sherwin, Hendler, and Felig 1975). A number of tumors specifically metabolize glucose, and the administration of a lipid source of energy may reduce the substrate available to the tumor. Another approach is to use the nutrient-induced phase of tumor stimulation to enhance the effect of therapy. Torosian and coworkers (1984) have shown in animals that the percentage of cells in the S-phase increases significantly two hours after the commencement of TPN. This may enhance tumor response to cycle-specific chemotherapy.

Table 34.7
SUGGESTED DAILY TPN REGIMEN FOR AN ADULT CANCER PATIENT

A.	Protein-calorie		kcal
	700 mL 50% dextrose		1,190
	400 mL 20% lipid emulsion		880
	1000 mL 10% amino acid solution		400
	Total calories		2,470
	Total calorie:protein nitrogen ratio		154:1
	Total volume		2,100 mL
B.	Additives		
	Electrolytes	sodium chloride	60-140 mEq/day
		potassium chloride	60-100 mEq/day
		magnesium sulfate	8-10 mEq/day
		calcium gluconate	9 mEq/day
		potassium phosphate	30-45 mEq/day
	Trace minerals	copper	
		zinc	
		manganese	one vial/day
		chromium	
		selenium	
	Iron		1 mg/day
	Multivitamin preparation		one vial/day
	Vitamin K$_1$		10 mg/once weekly
	Heparin		8000 u/day
	Glutamic acid		4 g/day

An alternative approach to shifting nutritional balance in favor of the host is to reduce tumor metabolism by blocking the utilization of a substrate necessary for tumor growth. It has been noted that some animal and human tumors metabolize large amounts of glutamine. Increased activity of enzymes that utilize glutamine for the production of purines and pyrimidines in a variety of rodent tumors has also been shown. Acivicin is a potent inhibitor of this enzyme system and recent work has shown that acivicin reduces tumor growth in rats fed regular rat chow or on TPN (Chance et al. 1987). In addition, the TPN resulted in a significant gain in body weight in these animals. Thus, the specific nutritional requirements of tumors may be used as a weapon against tumor growth while the host benefits from TPN.

Tumor growth may be altered by dietary immunomodulation. Dietary supplementation with arginine demonstrated an inhibition of tumor growth in mice bearing C1300 neuroblastoma. This was associated with augmented specific antitumor immune response (Reynolds et al. 1988).

CONCLUSION

Frequently, cancer patients are malnourished at the time of diagnosis. These patients develop anorexia and reduced nutritional intake. Specific abnormalities in substrate metabolism and energy expenditure have been detected in patients and in tumor-bearing animals. Protein catabolism, increased lipolysis, and glucose availability help to create a milieu favorable to tumor growth at the host's expense. There is evidence that the tumor can control these changes through neurohumoral mechanisms. There is little doubt that malnutrition associated with cancer has a negative prognostic effect and can contribute directly to the patient's death. It can also increase postoperative morbidity and decrease tumor response and patient tolerance to all modalities of treatment.

Nutritional therapy is an important supportive measure for the patient undergoing antineoplastic treatment. It increases the patient's well-being and may permit the administration of more intensive therapies. There is no conclusive evidence that adequate nutritional support preferentially feeds the tumor and results in increased tumor growth in man. There is good evidence that effective nutritional repletion can reduce the postoperative complication and mortality rates after surgery. Weight gain is possible and immune status may be improved, but definite improvement in tumor response rates and patient survival following chemotherapy or radiotherapy remains unproven. In the future, more specific manipulation of substrates and hormones administered to the host may improve the results.

REFERENCES

Askanazi, J.; Rosenbaum, S.H.; and Hyman, A.I. et al. 1980. Respiratory changes induced by large glucose loads of total parenteral nutrition. *JAMA* 243:1444-47.

Baker, J.P.; Detsky, A.S.; and Wesson, D.E. et al. 1982. Nutritional assessment: a comparison of clinical judgment and objective measurements. *N. Engl. J. Med.* 306:969-72.

Bistrian, B.R.; Blackburn, D.L.; and Scrimshaw, N.S. et al. 1975. Cellular immunity in semi-starved states in hospitalized adults. *Am. J. Clin. Nutr.* 28:1148-55.

Blackburn, G.L.; Maini, B.S.; and Bistrian, B.R. et al. 1976. The effect of cancer on nitrogen, electrolyte, and mineral metabolism. *Cancer Res.* 36:3936-40.

Boethe, A. Jr.; Valerio, D.; and Bistrian, B.R. et al. 1979. Randomized control trial of hospital nutritional support during abdominal radiotherapy. *J. Parenteral Enteral Nutr.* 3:292.

Brennan, M.F., and Burt, M.E. 1981. Nitrogen metabolism in cancer patients. *Cancer Treat. Rep.* 65(Suppl):67-78.

Brennan, M.F. 1977. Uncomplicated starvation versus cancer cachexia. *Cancer Res.* 37:2359-64.

Brennan, M.F. 1979. Metabolic response to surgery in the cancer patient. *Cancer* 43:2053-64.

Brennan, M.F. 1981. Total parenteral nutrition in the cancer patient. *N. Engl. J. Med.* 305:375-81.

Brennan, M.F. 1986. Cancer cachexia and rate of whole body lipolysis. *Metabolism* 35:304-10.

Bucklin, D.L., and Gilsdorf, R.B. 1985. Percutaneous needle pharyngostomy. *J. Parenteral Enteral Nutr.* 9:68-70.

Burt, M.E.; Stein, T.P.; and Brennan, M.F. 1983. A controlled randomized trial evaluating the effects of enteral and parenteral nutrition on protein metabolism in cancer-bearing man. *J. Surg. Res.* 34:303-14.

Buzby, G.P.; Muller, J.L.; and Matthews, D.C. et al. 1980. Prognostic nutritional index in gastrointestinal surgery. *Am. J. Surg.* 139:160-67.

Chance, W.T.; Cao, L.; and Nelson, J.L. et al. 1987. Acivicin reduces tumor growth during TPN. *Surgery* 102:386-94.

Chlebowski, R.T. 1986. Effect of nutritional support on the outcome of antineoplastic therapy. *Clin. Oncol.* 5:365-79.

Christou, N.V.; Meakins, J.L.; and McLean, L.D. 1981. The predictive role of delayed hypersensitivity in preoperative patients. *Surg. Gynecol. Obstet.* 152:297-301.

Clamon, G.H.; Feld, R.; and Evans, W.K. et al. 1985. Effect of adjuvant central IV hyperalimentation on the survival and the response to treatment of patients with small-cell lung cancer: a randomized trial. *Cancer Treat. Rep.* 69:167-77.

Cohn, S.H.; Gartenhaus, W.; and Sawitsky, A. et al. 1980. Compartmental body composition of cancer patients by measurement of total body nitrogen, potassium, and water. *Metabolism* 30:222-29.

Copeland, E.M.; Daly, J.M.; and Dudrick, S.J. 1977. Nutrition as an adjunct to cancer treatment in the adult. *Cancer Res.* 37: 2451-56.

Copeland, E.M.; Daly, J.M.; and Ota, D.M. et al. 1979. Nutrition, cancer, and intravenous hyperalimentation. *Cancer* 43:2108-16.

Coquin, J.Y.; Maranichi, D.; and Gastant, J.A. et al. 1981. Influence of parenteral nutrition on chemotherapy and survival of acute leukemias: preliminary results of a randomized trial. *J. Parenteral Enteral Nutr.* 5(Abstr):357.

Cosimi, A.B.; Brunstetter, F.H.; and Kemmere, W.T. et al. 1972. Cellular immune competence of breast cancer patients receiving chemotherapy. *Arch. Surg.* 107:531-35.

Daly, J.M.; Copeland, E.M.; and Dudrick, S.J. 1978. Effect of intravenous nutrition on tumor growth and host immuno-competence in malnourished animals. *Surgery* 84:655-58.

Daly, J.M.; Dudrick, S.J.; and Copeland, E.M. 1980. Intravenous hyperalimentation: effect on delayed cutaneous hypersensitivity in cancer patients. *Ann. Surg.* 192:587-92.

Daly, J.M.; Massar, E.; and Giacco, G. et al. 1982. Parenteral nutrition in esophageal cancer patients. *Ann. Surg.* 196: 203-208.

Daly, J.M.; Steiger, E.; and Vars, H.M. et al. 1974. Postoperative oral and intravenous nutrition. *Ann. Surg.* 180:709-15.

Dempsey, D.T.; Hurwitz, S.; and Mullen, J.L. 1985. Selective repletion of fat and/or protein stores. *J. Parenteral Enteral Nutr.* 9:117.

Dempsey, D.T.; Mullen, J.L.; and Rombeau, J.L. et al. 1987. Treatment effects of parenteral vitamins in total parenteral nutrition patients. *J. Parenteral Enteral Nutr.* 11:229-37.

DeWys, W.D., and Walters, K. 1975. Abnormalities of taste sensation in cancer patients. *Cancer* 36:1888-96.

DeWys, W.D.; Begg, C.; and Lavin, P.T. et al. 1980. Prognostic effect of weight loss prior to chemotherapy in cancer patients. *Am. J. Med.* 69:491-97.

Donaldson, S.S. 1984. Nutritional support as an adjunct to radiation therapy. *J. Parenteral Enteral Nutr.* 8:302-309.

Edmonson, J.H. 1966. Fatty acid mobilization and glucose metabolism in patients with cancer. *Cancer* 19:277-80.

Flanigen-Roat, D.T.; Milholland, R.J.; and Ip, M.M. 1985. Effect of a high-protein, low-carbohydrate diet on toxicity and antitumor activity of 5-fluorouracil in mice. *J. Natl. Cancer Inst.* 74:705-10.

Forse, R.A., and Shizgal, H.M. 1980. The assessment of malnutrition. *Surgery* 88:17-24.

Grant, J.P.; Custer, P.B.; and Thurlow, J. 1981. Current techniques of nutritional assessment. *Surg. Clin. North Am.* 61:437-63.

Greenlaw, C.W. 1980. Liver enzyme elevation associated with total parenteral nutrition. *Drug Intell. Clin. Pharm.* 14:702-706.

Hamawy, K.J.; Moldawer, L.L.; and Georgieff, M. et al. 1985. Effect of lipid emulsions on the reticuloendothelial system function in the injured animal. *J. Parenteral Enteral Nutr.* 9:559-65.

Harvey, K.B.; Bath, A. Jr.; and Blackburn, G.L. 1979. Nutritional assessment and patient outcome during oncological therapy. *Cancer* 43(Suppl):2065-69.

Harvey, K.B.; Moldawer, L.L.; and Bistrian, B.R. et al. 1981. Biological measures for the formulation of a hospital prognostic index. *J. Clin. Nutr.* 34:1739-46.

Hays, D.M.; Merritt, R.J.; and White, L. et al. 1983. Effect of total parenteral nutrition on marrow recovery during induction therapy for acute nonlymphocytic leukemia in childhood. *Med. Pediatr. Oncol.* 17:134-40.

Heber, D.; Byerley, L.O.; and Chi, J. et al. 1986. Pathophysiology of malnutrition in the adult cancer patient. *Cancer* 58(Suppl):1867-73.

Heber, D.; Chlebowski, R.T.; and Ishibashi, D.E. et al. 1982. Abnormalities in glucose and protein metabolism in non-cachectic lung cancer patients. *Cancer Res.* 42:4815-19.

Holroyde, C.P., and Reichard, A. 1981. Carbohydrate metabolism in cancer cachexia. *Cancer Treat. Rep.* 65(Suppl):55-59.

Issel, B.F.; Valdievieso, M.; and Zaren, H.A. et al. 1978. Protection against chemotherapy toxicity by IV hyperalimentation. *Cancer Treat. Rep.* 62:1139-43.

Johnson, W.C.; Ulrich, F.; and Meguid, M.M. et al. 1979. Role of delayed hypersensitivity in predicting postoperative morbidity and mortality. *Am. J. Surg.* 137:536-42.

Jordan, W.M.; Valdievieso, M.; and Frankmann, C. et al. 1981. Treatment of advanced adenocarcinoma of the lung with ftorafur, doxorubicin, cyclophosphamide, and cisplatin (FACP), and intensive IV hyperalimentation. *Cancer Treat. Rep.* 63:197-205.

Karpeh, M.S.; Kehne, J.A.; and Choi, S.H. et al. 1987. Tumor immunogenicity, nutritional repletion, and cancer. *Surgery* 102:283-90.

Knox, L.S.; Crosby, L.O.; and Feurer, I.D. et al. 1983. Energy expenditure in malnourished cancer patients. *Ann. Surg.* 197:152-62.

Krause, R.; Humphreys, C.; and von Meyenfeldt, M. et al. 1981. A central mechanism for anorexia in cancer: a hypothesis. *Cancer Treat. Rep.* 65(Suppl 5):15-21.

Kudsk, K.A.; Stone, J.M.; and Carpenter, G. et al. 1981. Effects of enteral vs. parenteral feeding of malnourished rats on body composition. *Current Surg.* 38:322-23.

Lanzotti, V.; Copeland, E.M.; and Bhuchar, V. et al. 1980. A randomized trial of total parenteral nutrition with chemotherapy for non-oat cell lung cancer. *Proc. Am. Assoc. Cancer Res.* 21(Abstr):377.

Law, D.K.; Dudrick, S.J.; and Abdou, N.I. 1974. The effects of protein-calorie malnutrition on immunocompetence of the surgical patient. *Surg. Gynecol. Obstet.* 139:257-66.

Lawrence. W. Jr. 1977. Nutritional consequences of surgical resection of the gastrointestinal tract for cancer. *Cancer Res.* 37:2379-86.

Lim, S.T.; Choa, R.G.; and Lam, K.H. et al. 1981. Total parenteral nutrition vs. gastrostomy in the preoperative preparation of patients with carcinoma of the esophagus. *Br. J. Surg.* 68:69-72.

Lucke, B.; Borwick, M.; and Zeckwer, I. 1952. Liver catalase activity in parabiotic rats with one partner tumor bearing. *J. Natl. Cancer Inst.* 13:681-86.

Lundholm, K.; Edstron, S.; and Ekman, L. et al. 1981. Metabolism in peripheral tissues in cancer patients. *Cancer Treat. Rep.* 65(Suppl):79-83.

Marks, P.A., and Bishop, J.S. 1957. The glucose metabolism of patients with malignant disease and of normal subjects as studied by means of an intravenous glucose tolerance test. *J. Clin. Invest.* 36:254-64.

McAnena, O.J., and Daly, J.M. 1986. Impact of antitumor therapy on nutrition. *Surg. Clin. North Am.* 66(6):1213-28.

Meguid, M.M.; Mughal, M.M.; and Debonis, D. et al. 1986. Influence of nutritional status on the resumption of adequate food intake in patients recovering from colorectal cancer operation. *Surg. Clin. North Am.* 66(6):1167-76.

Meguid, M.M.; Schimmel, E.; and Johnson, W.C. et al. 1982. Reduced metabolic complications in total parenteral nutrition: pilot study using fat to replace one-third of glucose calories. *J. Parenteral Enteral Nutr.* 6:304-307.

Moghissi, K.; Hornshaw, J.; and Teasdale, P.R. et al. 1977. Parenteral nutrition in carcinoma of the esophagus treated by surgery: nitrogen balance and clinical studies. *Br. J. Surg.* 64:125-28.

Moley, J.F.; Aamodt, R.; and Rumble, W. et al. 1987. Body cell mass in cancer bearing and anorexic patients. *J. Parenteral Enteral Nutr.* 11:219-22.

Mullen, J.L. 1981. Consequences of malnutrition in the surgical patient. *Surg. Clin. North Am.* 61:465-73.

Mullen, J.L.; Buzby, G.P.; and Waldman, T.G. et al. 1979. Prediction of operative morbidity and mortality by preoperative nutritional assessment. *Surg. Forum* 30:80-82.

Mullen, J.L.; Buzby, G.P.; and Gertner, M.H. et al. 1980. Protein synthesis dynamics in human gastrointestinal malignancies. *Surgery* 87:331-38.

Muller, J.M.; Dienst, C.; and Brenner, U. et al. 1982. Preoperative parenteral feeding in patients with gastrointestinal carcinoma. *Lancet* I:68-71.

Nakahara W. 1960. A chemical basis for tumor host relations. *J. Natl. Cancer Inst.* 24:77-86.

Nixon, D.W.; Heymsfield, S.B.; and Cohen, A.E. 1980. Protein-calorie malnutrition in hospitalized cancer patients. *Am. J. Med.* 68:683-90.

Nixon, D.W.; Moffitt, S.; and Lawson, D.H. et al. 1981. Total parenteral nutrition as an adjunct to chemotherapy of metastatic colorectal cancer. *Cancer Treat. Rep.* 65(Suppl):121-28.

Norton, J.A.; Stein, T.P.; and Brennan, M.F. 1981. Whole body protein synthesis and turnover in normal and malnourished patients with and without known cancer. *Ann. Surg.* 194:123-28.

Ponsky, J.L.; Gauderer, M.W.; and Stellato, T.A. 1983. Percutaneous endoscopic gastrostomy. *Arch. Surg.* 118:913-14.

Popp, M.B.; Morrison, S.D.; and Brennan M.F. 1981. Total parenteral nutrition in a methylcholanthrene-induced rat sarcoma model. *Cancer Treat. Rep.* 65:137-43.

Popp, M.B.; Wagner, S.C.; and Brito, O.J. 1983. Host and tumor responses to increasing levels of intravenous nutritional support. *Surgery* 92:300-307.

Reynolds, J.V.; Zhang, S.; and Thom, A.K. et al. 1988. Arginine, protein malnutrition and cancer. *J. Surg. Res.* 45:513-22.

Samuels, M.L.; Selig, D.E.; and Ogden, S. et al. 1981. IV hyperalimentation and chemotherapy for stage II testicular cancer: a randomized study. *Cancer Treat. Rep.* 68:615-27.

Schein, P.S.; Kesner, D.; and Haller, D. et al. 1979. Cachexia of malignancy: potential role of insulin in nutritional management. *Cancer* 43:2070-76.

Serrou, B.; Cupissol, D.; and Plagne, R. et al. 1982. Follow-up of a randomized trial for oat-cell carcinoma, evaluating the efficacy of peripheral intravenous nutrition (PIVN) as adjunct treatment. *Recent Results Cancer Res.* 80:246-53.

Shamberger, R.C.; Brennan, M.F.; and Goodgame, J.T. Jr. et al. 1984. A prospective, randomized study of adjuvant parenteral nutrition in the treatment of sarcomas: results of metabolic and survival studies. *Surgery* 96:1-13.

Shanbhogue, L.K.; Chwals, W.J.; and Weintraub, M. et al. 1987. Parenteral nutrition in the surgical cancer patient. *Br. J. Surg.* 74:172-80.

Shaw, J.M.; Humberstone, D.M.; and Wolfe, R.R. 1988. Energy and protein metabolism in sarcoma patients. *Ann. Surg.* 207:283-89.

Sheldon, G.F.; Peterson, S.R.; and Sanders, R. 1978. Hepatic dysfunction during hyperalimentation. *Arch. Surg.* 113:504-508.

Sherwin, R.S.; Hendler, R.G.; and Felig, P. 1975. Effect of ketone infusions on amino acid and nitrogen metabolism in man. *J. Clin. Invest.* 55:1382-90.

Shike, M.; Russel, D.; and Detsky, A. et al. 1984. Changes in body composition in patients with small-cell lung cancer: the effect of TPN as an adjunct to chemotherapy. *Ann. Intern. Med.* 101:303-309.

Shukla, H.S.; Raja-Rao, R.; and Banu, N. et al. 1984. Enteral hyperalimentation in malnourished surgical patients. *Indian J. Med. Res.* 80:339-46.

Smale, B.F.; Mullen, J.L.; and Buzby, G.P. et al. 1981. The efficacy of nutritional assessment and support in cancer surgery. *Cancer* 47:2375-81.

Souchon, E.A.; Copeland, E.M.; and Watson P. et al. 1975. Intravenous hyperalimentation as an adjunct to cancer chemotherapy with 5-fluorouracil. *J. Surg. Res.* 18:451-54.

Steiger, E.; Oram-Smith, J.; and Miller, E. et al. 1975. Effects of nutrition on tumor growth and tolerance to chemotherapy. *J. Surg. Res.* 18:455-61.

Stein, J.P., and Buzby, G.P. 1981. Protein metabolism in surgical patients. *Surg. Clin. North Am.* 61:519-27.

Stovroff, M.C., and Norton, J.A. 1987. Cachectin: a mediator of cancer cachexia. *Surg. Forum* 413-15.

Studley, H.O. 1936. Percentage of weight loss: a basic indicator of surgical risk in patients with chronic peptic ulcer. *JAMA* 106:458-60.

Tannenbaum, A., and Silverstone, H. 1953. Nutrition in relation to cancer. *Adv. Cancer Res.* 1:451.

Theologides, A. 1972. Pathogenesis of cachexia in cancer. *Cancer* 29:484-88.

Torosian, M.H., and Rombeau, J.L. 1980. Feeding by tube enterostomy. *Surg. Gynecol. Obstet.* 150:918-27.

Torosian, M.H.; Tsou, K.C.; and Daly, J.M. et al. 1984. Alteration of tumor cell kinetics by pulse total parenteral nutrition. *Cancer* 53:1409-15.

Valdievieso, M.; Bodey, G.P.; and Benjamin, R.S. et al. 1981. Role of intravenous hyperalimentation as an adjunct to intensive chemotherapy for small-cell bronchogenic carcinoma. *Cancer Treat. Rep.* 5(Suppl):145-50.

Valerio D; Overett L; and Malcolm et al. 1978. Nutritional support of cancer patients receiving abdominal and pelvic radiotherapy. *Surg. Forum* 29:145-48.

Van Eys, J.; Copeland, E.M.; and Cangir, A. et al. 1980. A randomized controlled clinical trial of hyperalimentation in children with metastatic malignancies. *Med. Pediatr. Oncol.* 8:63-73.

Warnold, I.; Lundholm, K.; and Schersten, T. 1978. Energy balance and body composition in cancer. *Cancer Res.* 38:1801-1807.

Warren, S. 1932. The immediate cause of death in cancer. *Am. J. Med. Sci.* 184:610-15.

Waterhouse, C. 1963. Nutritional disorders in neoplastic diseases. *J. Chron. Dis.* 16:637-44.

Waterhouse, C.; Jeanpretre, N.; and Keilson, J. 1979. Gluconeogenesis from alanine in patients with progressive malignant disease. *Cancer Res.* 39:1968-72.

Waterhouse, C., and Kemperman, J.H. 1971. Carbohydrate metabolism in subjects with cancer. *Cancer Res.* 31:1273-78.

White, F.R. 1961. The relationship between underfeeding and tumor formation, transplantation, and growth in rats and mice. *Cancer Res.* 21:281-90.

Young, V.R. 1977. Energy metabolism and requirements in the cancer patient. *Cancer Res.* 37:2336-47.

Chapter 35

ONCOLOGIC EMERGENCIES

Donna Glover, M.D.
John H. Glick, M.D.

Donna Glover, M.D.
Chief of Hematology and Oncology
Department of Medicine
Presbyterian Medical Center
Philadelphia, Pennsylvania

John H. Glick, M.D.
Director, Cancer Center
University of Pennsylvania
Philadelphia, Pennsylvania

INTRODUCTION

Advances in radiotherapy, chemotherapy, and supportive care have increased the incidence of oncologic emergencies as survival of cancer patients improves. Before initiating treatment, several important management factors must be considered in evaluating and treating an oncologic emergency (see table 35.1).

Aggressive treatment is indicated when a histologic diagnosis of malignancy has not been established or if the patient has a good prognosis with either surgery, radiotherapy, or chemotherapy. A chance for cure or prolonged palliation may indicate radical treatment plans. In advanced malignancies the primary goal is often palliation and relief of symptoms, even if the patient has a limited life expectancy. Restoring functional status frequently leads to improved quality of life. If the oncologic emergency is directly due to the malignant process, the general approach is to treat the underlying malignancy if there is effective therapy and to initiate treatment promptly to prevent complications and permanent disability. However, for terminal cancer patients, withholding treatment and controlling pain may be the most appropriate decision.

Following is a review of the pathophysiology, clinical presentation, diagnostic evaluation, and therapy of common oncologic emergencies.

PERICARDIAL EFFUSIONS AND NEOPLASTIC CARDIAC TAMPONADE

At autopsy, up to 20% of cancer patients have cardiac or pericardial metastases (Theologides 1978; Goodie 1955; Thurber, Edwards, and Achoe 1962; Martini, Bains, and Beattie 1975). Cancers of the lung or esophagus grow by direct extension into the pericardium, while distant primary malignancies metastasize to the pericardium hematogenously. Lung and breast carcinomas, lymphoma, leukemia, melanoma, gastrointestinal primaries, and sarcomas are the most common primary cancers associated with malignant pericardial effusions (Thurber, Edwards, and Achoe 1962; Martini, Bains, and Beattie 1975).

PATHOPHYSIOLOGY

Tamponade usually occurs because of cardiac compression from large malignant pericardial effusions, although encasement of the heart by tumor or postirradiation pericarditis can mimic tamponade (Spodick 1967; Applefield et al. 1981). With cardiac tamponade, signs of circulatory collapse appear suddenly, even though the effusion or constriction may have developed gradually (Spodick 1967). The severity of tamponade depends on the rate of pericardial fluid formation and

Table 35.1
MANAGEMENT FACTORS IN THE EVALUATION AND TREATMENT OF AN ONCOLOGIC EMERGENCY

SYMPTOMS AND SIGNS
1. Are the symptoms and signs due to the tumor or to complications of treatment?
2. How quickly are the symptoms of the oncologic emergency progressing?

NATURAL HISTORY OF THE PRIMARY TUMOR
1. Is there a previous diagnosis of malignancy?
2. What is the disease-free interval between the diagnosis of the primary and the onset of the emergency?
3. Has the emergency developed in the setting of terminal disease?

EFFICACY OF AVAILABLE TREATMENT
1. No prior therapy vs. extensive pretreatment
2. Should treatment be directed at the underlying malignancy and/or the urgent complication?
3. Will the patient's general medical condition influence the ability to administer effective treatment?

TREATMENT AND GOALS
1. Potential for cure
2. Is prompt palliation required to prevent further debilitation?
3. What is the risk vs. benefit ratio of treatment?
4. Should treatment be withheld if the patient is terminal with minimal chance of response to available antitumor therapies?

the volume of fluid accumulated. Slow pericardial fluid accumulation may stretch the pericardium and cardiac contractility may not be impaired. However, if the pericardium is surrounded by tumor or radiation fibrosis, a small effusion may produce significant cardiac compression (Applefeld et al. 1981; Pories and Gaudiani 1975). Elevated pericardial pressures reduce ventricular expansion and diastolic filling. As stroke volume falls, hypotension, compensatory tachycardia, and equalization and elevation of the mean left atrial, pulmonary arterial and venous, right atrial, and vena caval pressures occur. Tachycardia and peripheral vasoconstriction develop in an attempt to maintain arterial pressure, increase blood volume, and improve venous return (Spodick 1967; Pories and Gaudiani 1975).

CLINICAL PRESENTATION

In a large autopsy series, fewer than 30% of patients with malignant pericardial effusions had symptoms of pericarditis. In most patients, the diagnosis of pericardial tumor is not made prior to death (Theologides 1978; Thurber, Edwards, and Achoe 1962). With tamponade or pericardial constriction, patients may complain of dyspnea, cough, and retrosternal chest pain relieved by leaning forward. When cardiac output falls, decreased cerebral blood, peripheral cyanosis, decreased systolic and pulse pressures, and pulsus paradoxsus occur (Theologides 1978). Occasionally patients with large effusions develop hoarseness, hiccups, nausea, vomiting, and epigastric pain. Physical examination may reveal engorged neck veins, distant heart sounds, edema, ascites, hepatosplenomegaly, and hepatojugular reflex (Theologides 1978).

DIAGNOSTIC EVALUATION

More than half the patients with pericardial effusions have cardiac enlargement, mediastinal widening, or hilar adenopathy that can be seen on chest x-ray. As the fluid increases, the mediastinum shortens and widens, the normal arcuate borders are lost, and the cardiac silhouette becomes globular (Spodick 1967; Hancock 1975; Martin et al. 1975). Electrocardiographic abnormalities are often nonspecific. With pericarditis, the electrocardiogram may have low QRS voltage in the limb leads, sinus tachycardia, ST elevations, and T wave changes (Spodick 1967; Niarchos 1975). Electrical alternans may occur with tamponade, but this is not a reliable diagnostic parameter (Lawrence and Cronin 1963). Echocardiography is the most specific and sensitive noninvasive test and an echocardiogram should be performed immediately if the diagnosis is suspected (Pories and Gaudiani 1975; Millman et al. 1977; Morris 1976). With posterior effusions, two distinct echoes are seen: one from the effusion and the other from the posterior heart border. The space between these echoes indicates the size of the effusion or thickness of the pericardium (Hancock 1975; Millman et al. 1977). Inconclusive physical examination and noninvasive

studies require that a right heart catheterization be performed to diagnose pericardial tamponade or constriction (Morris 1976; Hudson 1978).

Pericardiocentesis should be performed for both diagnostic and therapeutic purposes. The fluid is analyzed for cell count, cytology, and appropriate cultures. The cytology is usually positive in patients with metastatic carcinoma, but is frequently inconclusive with lymphoma and mesothelioma (Theologides 1978; Martini, Bains, and Beattie 1975; Krikorian and Hancock 1978; Zipf and Johnston 1972). If a histologic diagnosis is important and pericardial fluid cytologies are negative, a pericardial biopsy should be performed either under local anesthesia with a subxiphoid approach or under general anesthesia with an anterior thoracotomy. The latter procedure is more sensitive because more tissue can be obtained, but has higher morbidity and mortality (Hankins et al. 1980; Hill and Cohen 1970).

THERAPY

A significant decrease in cardiac output indicates emergency pericardiocentesis before initiating definite local therapy in order to prevent recurrent tamponade. Emergency pericardiocentesis must be performed when the patient develops: (1) cyanosis, dyspnea, shock, or impaired consciousness; (2) a pulsus paradoxus greater than 50% of the pulse pressure; (3) decrease of over 20 mm Hg in pulse pressure; or (4) peripheral venous pressures above 13 mm Hg (Spodick 1967; Hill and Cohen 1970). Oxygen should be administered but positive pressure breathing is contraindicated because of impaired venous return from increased intrapericardial and intrapleural pressures (Spodick 1967). If pericardiocentesis cannot be performed immediately, cardiac contractility and filling can be improved with isoproterenol and volume expansion (Theologides 1978).

Tamponade will reoccur generally within 24 to 48 hours unless promptly treated to prevent pericardial fluid reaccumulation. Therapeutic options depend on the primary tumor's sensitivity to systemic chemotherapy, hormonal therapy, or local radiotherapy; prior treatment; and life expectancy. Pericardial windows, sclerosing agents, radiotherapy, effective systemic antineoplastic drugs, and pericardiectomy have all produced excellent, long-term palliation in selected series. These treatments are difficult to compare because responses are not based on objective criteria. The durations of response and survival are influenced by the extent of metastatic disease, and the chance of response to concurrent systemic hormonal therapy or chemotherapy (Theologides 1978; Martini, Bains, and Beattie 1975; Hankins et al. 1980; Hill and Cohen 1970; Lajos et al. 1975; Davis et al. 1978; Rubinstein and Bolooki 1972).

Tamponade can be controlled by pericardial catheter drainage and sclerosis. An indwelling pericardial catheter is left in place until pericardial drainage stops. Tetracycline (500-1000 mg) is then instilled through the pericardial cannula and flushed with normal saline. The procedure is repeated every two to three days until there is no fluid drainage in the preceding 24 hours (Davis et al. 1978; Rubinstein and Bolooki 1972). The inflammatory response and fibrosis from intrapericardial tetracycline obliterates the space between the parietal and visceral pericardium and prevents fluid formation.

Recent reports have shown effective pericardial sclerosis with one installation of bleomycin (30 mg or 60 mg) through the catheter. Bleomycin is instilled after all the pericardial fluid has been evacuated for 24 hours, then the tube is clamped for 10 minutes and then withdrawn. In a recent study echocardiograms were performed one day, one week, and one month after the procedure and at various times during the patients' subsequent course. No major side effects were noted, except for one transient elevation in temperature which resolved in less than 12 hours. Bleomycin may have certain advantages over tetracycline, including fewer side effects (especially less pain). Severe fibrosis was not reported after local installation, nor was fibrous thickening of the pericardium found at autopsy. None of the patients in the study died from pericardial tamponade (Van Belle et al. 1987).

Palliation may also be obtained with pleural-pericardial windows. Under local anesthesia, inferior pericardiotomy provides immediate relief of cardiac compression and tissue for histologic diagnosis with complication rates under 2% (Hankins et al. 1980). Tamponade symptoms reoccur in less than 5% of patients. A thoracotomy may be required if the heart is encased with tumor, or if additional tissue is required for a diagnostic purpose (Hill and Cohen 1970).

Although radiotherapy has been reported to control over 50% of malignant pericardial effusions, the tumor's radiosensitivity will determine the response and duration of palliation. Radiation doses are given in 1.5 Gy to 2.0 Gy fractions to a total dose of 25 Gy to 30 Gy. Patients with lymphoma or leukemia may respond to lower doses (e.g., 15 Gy to 20 Gy over two weeks).

Pericardiectomy is necessary if radiation-induced pericardial disease is not controlled with conservative medical management, but it should not be performed when there is extensive pericardial tumor. With extensive pericardial metastases, life expectancy is short and surgical morbidity and mortality rates with pericardiectomy are high (Theologides 1978).

After the patient is clinically stable, systemic therapy should be administered if effective treatment is available. If a rapid chemotherapeutic response can be obtained (e.g., lymphoma, small-cell lung cancer), the patient may be treated with pericardial drainage and systemic chemotherapy (Theologides 1978).

Recent data suggests that cytotoxic therapy may be effective in chemotherapy-sensitive tumors such as lymphoma, leukemia, and breast cancer. Patients with lymphoma who have not received first-line therapy have an excellent response rate to combination chemotherapy for their pericardial effusions. In one series of three patients with malignant pericardial effusions due to breast cancer, control of effusion was achieved with single pericardiocentesis followed by systemic chemotherapy. No other local therapy was necessary. Similar results have also been observed in patients with effusions due to acute leukemia (Buzaid, Garewal, and Greenberg 1989).

SUPERIOR VENA CAVAL SYNDROME

ETIOLOGY AND PATHOPHYSIOLOGY

The superior vena cava (SVC) is easily compressed by adjacent, expanding masses (Theologides 1978). When obstructed, venous blockage produces pleural effusions and facial, arm, and tracheal edema. With severe SVC obstruction, brain edema and impaired cardiac filling may produce altered consciousness and focal neurologic signs. Symptoms depend on the extent and rapidity of SVC compression; table 35.2 lists the signs and symptoms of SVC syndrome. If the SVC is gradually compressed and collateral circulation develops, symptoms may be indolent and subtle (Perez, Presant, and Van Amburg 1978).

Most cases of SVC syndrome are caused by malignant, mediastinal tumors (Shimm, Logue, and Rigsby 1981; Ahmann 1984; Sculier and Feld 1985). More than 75% of malignant SVC obstructions are secondary to small-cell or squamous-cell lung cancers (Shimm, Logue, and Rigsby 1981; Ahmann 1984; Sculier and Feld 1985; Davenport et al. 1978). Ten percent to 15% of neoplastic SVC syndromes are secondary to mediastinal lymphomas, most often diffuse large-cell subtypes (Kane et al. 1976). Less than 15% are secondary to benign etiologies such as tuberculosis, aneurysms, and thrombus (Perez, Presant, and Van Amburg 1978; Sculier and Feld 1985; Schraufragel et al. 1981; Van Houtte and Fruhling 1981). The most common nonmalignant cause of SVC obstruction is thrombus in central venous catheters (Sculier and Feld 1985).

DIAGNOSTIC EVALUATION

Diagnosis of SVC obstruction is easy if facial edema, venous engorgement, and impaired consciousness are present. However, if SVC obstruction develops slowly, venography or radionuclide scans may be necessary to confirm the diagnosis. Angiographic or radionuclide studies also help to localize the site of obstruction and plan radiation portals (Van Houtte and Fruhling 1981;

Table 35.2
SUPERIOR VENA CAVAL SYNDROME SYMPTOMS AND SIGNS

FINDING	NUMBER	%
Thoracic vein distention	56	67
Neck vein distention	49	59
Edema of face	47	56
Tachypnea	34	40
Plethora of face	16	19
Cyanosis	13	15
Edema of upper extremities	8	9.5
Paralyzed true vocal cord	3	3.5
Horner's syndrome	2	2.3
Total No. of Patients	84	

(Reprinted with permission from: Perez et al. [1978].)

Gollub, Hirose, and Klauher 1980). Chest computerized tomography (CT) scans with intravenous contrast or magnetic resonance imaging (MRI) scans will provide excellent anatomic detail and help to define radiation portals (Sculier and Feld 1985).

Most patients with SVC syndrome do not present with a histologic diagnosis of malignancy (Perez, Presant, and Van Amburg 1978; Shimm, Logue, and Rigsby 1981). In such situations, the least invasive technique should be used to establish the diagnosis by biopsy or cytology. Sputum cytology, bronchoscopy with brushings and washings, and biopsy of palpable adenopathy provide the correct diagnosis in 70% of cases (Perez, Presant, and Van Amburg 1978). If small-cell lung cancer or lymphoma is suspected, bone marrow aspirates or biopsies may confirm the diagnosis. Fine needle biopsy of mediastinal masses under CT guidance may provide sufficient tissue for a cytologic diagnosis (Barek et al. 1982). If necessary, invasive diagnostic procedures (e.g., thoracotomy or mediastinoscopy) can be performed safely if the trachea is not obstructed (Ahmann 1984; Sculier and Feld 1985). In the past, invasive procedures were postponed a few days until radiotherapy was begun to prevent complications from bleeding or airway compromise. However, delaying diagnostic procedures several days after radiotherapy may yield only necrotic tissue (Shimm, Logue, and Rigsby 1981; Ahmann 1984).

Radiation therapy is very effective for most cases of superior vena caval syndrome due to malignancy. However, when the signs and symptoms of SVC are not relieved following radiation therapy, the persistent tumor outside the treatment portals must be suspected. In this setting, the use of invasive diagnostic procedures such as contrast venography should be used to establish the cause of treatment failure. Treatment could therefore be modified and thus achieve a higher chance of complete response. A superior vena cavagram, radionuclide vena cavagrams, or angiography may reveal almost complete obstruction of the superior or inferior vena cava, if this diagnosis is suspected because of pedal edema (Kumar and Good 1989).

THERAPY

Only a small percentage of patients with rapid onset of SVC obstruction are at risk for life-threatening complications (Ahmann 1984; Sculier and Feld 1985). Emergency treatment is indicated when there is brain edema, decreased cardiac output, or upper-airway edema. Most patients with malignant SVC obstruction are treated with radiotherapy, initially given in high daily fractions (4.0 Gy for three days), followed by 1.5 Gy to 2.0 Gy per day to a total dose of 30 Gy to 50 Gy. The radiation dose depends on the tumor size, radioresponsiveness, and probability of achieving a response with systemic therapy (Perez, Presant, and Van Amburg 1978; Ahmann 1984; Davenport et al. 1978). The radiation portal should include a 2 cm margin around the tumor. Patients with locally advanced nonsmall-cell lung cancer without distant metastases should have the medi-

astinal, hilar, and supraclavicular lymph nodes and any adjacent parenchymal lesions irradiated. Mantle irradiation may be preferable to mediastinal irradiation in selected cases of Hodgkin's disease or malignant lymphoma (Perez, Presant, and Van Amburg 1978; Davenport et al. 1978). During radiation, patients improve clinically before objective signs of tumor shrinkage are evident on chest x-rays (Davenport et al. 1978). Radiation palliates SVC obstruction in 70% of patients with lung carcinoma and over 95% with lymphoma (Davenport et al. 1978).

In a recent review of 125 patients with SVC syndrome due to malignancies, high initial dose radiation treatment (3 Gy to 4 Gy daily for 3 fractions) provided symptomatic relief in less than two weeks in 70% of patients. When conventional dose radiation treatment (2 Gy daily, 5 weekly fractions) was used, the same response was seen in 56% of patients. Combined radiation and chemotherapy did not improve response rate overall. However, this would be difficult to assess depending upon the types of tumors treated. In 13% of patients, SVC syndrome recurred. Treatment side effects were minimal, occurring in 26% of patients (Armstrong et al. 1987).

Chemotherapy may be preferable to radiation for patients with disseminated disease if a prompt response is anticipated. For example, small-cell anaplastic carcinoma and lymphoma respond to radiation (Perez, Presant, and Van Amburg 1978); however, these malignancies may respond rapidly to systemic chemotherapy (Kane et al. 1976; Perez-Soler et al. 1984; Miller et al. 1981). Sclerosing agents given to patients with SVC syndrome should not be injected into dilated arm veins. Anticoagulation may help relieve venous obstruction by preventing thrombus formation. Although anticoagulated patients improve more rapidly and have shorter hospitalizations, there is no difference in overall survival (Salsali and Cliffton 1965; Ghosh and Cliffton 1973). Generally, the risks of hemorrhage associated with antithrombotic therapy outweigh the temporary benefit if the venous obstruction is due to tumor rather than clot. Corticosteroids decrease edema associated with inflammatory reactions following tumor necrosis from irradiation. If clinical signs of venous obstruction progress shortly after radiotherapy is initiated, steroids are administered for three to seven days. When SVC obstruction is due to thrombus around a central venous catheter, patients may be treated with antifibrinolytics or anticoagulants. The catheter may need to be removed surgically (Sculier and Feld 1985).

SPINAL CORD COMPRESSION

ETIOLOGY AND PATHOPHYSIOLOGY

Spinal cord compression is always an emergency, especially when neurologic deterioration is rapid. Once the patient becomes paraplegic, there is little chance of regaining function. The most common tumors associated with spinal cord compression are carcinomas of the breast, lung, and prostate; multiple myeloma; and lymphoma (Rodriguez and Dinapoli 1980; Gilbert et al. 1977; Posner 1977). At autopsy, over 5% of patients with metastatic disease have epidural tumors (Posner 1977), which generally arise within the vertebral body and grow along the epidural space anterior to the spinal cord (Bruckman and Bloomer 1978). Patients with paraspinal tumors (e.g., lymphoma) may develop epidural metastases when the neoplasm grows through the intervertebral foramina from adjacent nodes. Spinal cord and nerve root compression can occur secondary to epidural tumor or vertebral collapse from destructive osseous metastases. Permanent neurologic dysfunction also may occur if vascular compromise produces prolonged ischemia or hemorrhage (Rodriguez and Dinapoli 1980; Bruckman and Bloomer 1978).

Symptoms and signs indicating spinal cord compression may be due to a number of noncompressive causes including paraneoplastic syndromes, carcinomatous myopathy or neuropathy, radiation myelopathy, herpes zoster, subacute myelopathy, pain from pelvic or long-bone metastases, anterior spinal artery occlusion, retroperitoneal tumor, or toxicity of cytotoxic drugs. Nonmalignant diseases such as herniated disks, osteoporotic vertebral fractures, and intraspinal abscess can also cause cord compression in the cancer patient. The cause of neurological symptoms are generally evaluated by plain film myelography, MRI, and CT scans.

CLINICAL PRESENTATION

Over 95% of patients with spinal cord compression complain of progressive central or radicular back pain. The pain is often aggravated by recumbency, weight bearing, coughing, sneezing, or the valsalva maneuver, and is relieved by sitting (Gilbert et al. 1977). The earliest neurologic symptoms are sensory changes, including numbness, paresthesias, and coldness. The incidence of motor dysfunction is less frequent due to earlier diagnosis and treatment. Although bladder and bowel dysfunction are rarely the first objective signs of cord compression, metastases to the cauda equina typically produce impaired urethral, vaginal, and rectal sensation, bladder dysfunction, saddle anesthesia, and decreased sensation in the lumbosacral dermatomes (Rodriguez and Dinapoli 1980; Gilbert et al. 1977; Bruckman and Bloomer 1978). The level of cord compression can be determined by pain elicited by straight leg raising, neck flexion, or vertebral percussion. The upper limit of the sensory level is often one or two vertebral bodies below the site of compression. Decreased rectal tone and perineal sensation are often observed when there is automatic dysfunction. Deep tendon reflexes may be brisk with cord compression and diminished with nerve root compression (Rodriguez and Dinapoli 1980; Posner 1977).

DIAGNOSTIC EVALUATION

Rodichuk et al. (1981) initiated a prospective clinical trial designed to diagnose spinal cord compression before irreversible neurologic damage occurred. In his series, over 90% of patients with epidural tumors had radiographic evidence of vertebral metastases (e.g., vertebral collapse, osteolytic lesions, pedicle erosion, or a paraspinal mass). However, in another series of cancer patients with vertebral compression, 15% had only benign disease on CT scan of the spine. There was a high correlation between posterior cortical bone discontinuity and the presence of epidural tumor (Redmond et al. 1988). Myelograms revealed epidural metastases in 81% of patients with x-ray abnormalities. However, only 14% of patients with negative bone films had positive myelograms regardless of neurologic deficits. Although bone scans were more sensitive in detecting early osseous metastases, up to 30% of abnormalities on bone scan may be due to benign disease; they are less accurate in predicting spinal cord compression (Rodichuk et al. 1981).

The majority of patients with solid tumors presenting with spinal cord compression have x-ray abnormalities on plain films, but myelography is essential in radiotherapeutic management. In a series reported by Calkins et al., plain films tended to result in an underestimation of the extent of disease in the spinal canal. Among 22 patients who had clinical examination and x-rays suggestive of a specific level of compression, the myelograms or metrizamide CT scans changed the treatment plans for radiation therapy in 69% of cases. Two patients had two areas of block that were unsuspected prior to myelography. Solid tumors have a much higher incidence of bony involvement than do hemotologic malignancies. Because abnormal bone radiographs were seen in only about one-third of patients with non-Hodgkin's lymphoma, Hodgkin's disease, or myeloma, there is a stronger role for metrizamide CT or myelography in patients with these malignancies (Calkins, Olson, and Ellis 1980).

The accuracy of MRI to detect metastatic compression of the spinal cord or cauda equina has been compared to findings at myelography, surgery, clinical follow-up, and autopsy results. Magnetic resonance imaging has been shown to have sensitivity of 93%, a specificity of 97%, and an overall accuracy of 95%. It also has a distinct advantage over myelography because no contrast injections are required. Patients with a complete or partial block of the spinal canal from an epidural metastasis may also have additional epidural deposits at other levels and MRI may show these multiple sites, which may not be obvious on the initial myelogram unless special attention is given to these areas. The detection of cord displacement, however, becomes less certain and more subjective when the spine is scoliotic. The use of a surface coil may improve image detail.

The disadvantage of MRI is the necessity for the patient to lie still in one position, which many patients with severe central back pain cannot maintain for long periods of time (Li and Poon 1988).

Today, MRI scans are the diagnostic procedure of choice to confirm the presence of cord compression.

THERAPY

All patients with suspected cord compression should have emergency myelography or a magnetic resonance imaging (MRI) scan of the spine. These radiographic studies are necessary to determine the proximal and distal extent of the epidural defect and to determine if there is more than one area of cord or nerve root compression. If a complete block is found on myelogram, a cisternal or lateral cervical puncture is required if the block's upper limit cannot be defined by air injection following lumbar pantopaque myelography (Katz et al. 1981). If there is not a complete block, cerebral spinal fluid (CSF) can be obtained safely. The CSF is sent for glucose, protein, cell count, cytology, and appropriate stains and cultures, if infection is suspected (Rodriguez and Dinapoli 1980). If there is a complete block, no more than 1 cc of CSF should be removed. If a myelogram is not performed, either an MRI scan or a metrizamide CT scan may delineate the subarachnoid space and define the area of block. MRI scans of the spine, spinal canal, vertebral foramina, and paravertebral soft tissues may also identify abnormalities that are not seen on plain films or myelography.

Suspected spinal cord compression requires immediate consultation of the radiation oncologist and the neurosurgeon. Treatment decisions must be based on the tumor's radiosensitivity, clinical expertise with surgical decompression, the level of cord compression, rate of neurologic deterioration, and prior radiotherapy. Radiotherapy is the primary treatment for most patients with epidural metastases and once the diagnosis of cord compression is confirmed, emergency radiotherapy should be given. Radiation portals include the entire area of block and two vertebral bodies above and below it. Radiation doses range from 30 Gy to 40 Gy given over two to three weeks. Radioresponsive tumors (e.g., lymphoma and multiple myeloma) have higher response rates to radiotherapy than do radioresistant tumors (e.g., melanoma) (Rodriguez and Dinapoli 1980; Gilbert et al. 1977; Posner 1977; Rubin, Mayer, and Poulter 1969). More than half of the patients with rapid neurologic deterioration improve with radiotherapy (Gilbert et al. 1977); however, the prognosis for patients with autonomic dysfunction or paraplegia is poor despite surgery or radiotherapy (Posner 1977; Wild and Parker 1963; White, Patterson, and Bergland 1971).

Laminectomy provides prompt decompression of the spinal cord and nerve roots. However, with a posterior laminectomy it is extremely difficult to remove the tumor, since most epidural metastases arise in the vertebral bodies anterior to the spinal cord. Because the tumor cannot be removed surgically, postoperative radiotherapy is given to decrease residual tumor, relieve pain, and improve functional status. Most ambulatory patients have improved neurologic function following surgical decompression, but those with severe preoperative neurologic deficits rarely benefit from surgery (Gilbert et al. 1977; Posner 1977; White, Patterson, and

Bergland 1971). Surgery is generally contraindicated when there are multiple areas of cord compression.

A recent review suggests that patients with vertebral collapse rarely benefit from surgical laminectomy due to a higher incidence of neurological complications. The data suggests that laminectomy in the presence of vertebral body collapse has a higher risk of major neurological deterioration by at least one grade (50% compared to 24% in patients without vertebral collapse). This is probably caused by the presence of a destructive lesion in the anterior spinal column, which results in further instability with posterior laminectomy. In most cases, laminectomy is contraindicated in the presence of a collapsed vertebral body, and alternate methods of treatment should be applied. Although radiation therapy should not affect spinal stability, there is no evidence that radiation therapy improves neurological results. The most logical approach may be to use an anterior surgical approach to the spine (i.e., transthoracic) and early mobilization (Findlay 1987).

In cases where there is no prior histologic diagnosis of malignancy or if infection or epidural hematoma must be ruled out, a laminectomy is required for both diagnosis and treatment. High cervical cord lesions can cause death from respiratory paralysis unless surgical decompression is accomplished. If surgery is not possible, the patient's neck should be stabilized in a halo. When neurological signs progress over 48 to 72 hours despite high-dose steroids and radiotherapy, emergency decompression should be attempted although operative results are generally poor when there is rapid neurologic progression. If there is a long interval following radiotherapy for spinal cord compression, surgery may be beneficial when the epidural tumor recurs.

Corticosteroids may promptly reduce peritumoral edema and improve neurologic function (Gilbert et al. 1977). Prior to emergency diagnostic procedures, patients with neurologic symptoms from possible cord compression should receive dexamethasone (10 mg). Generally, dexamethasone (4 mg to 10 mg every 6 hours) is continued during radiation therapy, then tapered. Steroids initially improve neurologic function, but it is not clear whether they affect the ultimate outcome following definitive therapy. The side effects of high-dose glucocorticoids (table 35.3) must be considered when drug doses are prescribed.

Chemotherapy rarely has a major therapeutic role in spinal cord compression but if the malignancy is sensitive to chemotherapy, the drug regimen can be administered concurrently with or soon after radiotherapy or surgery is complete.

Although the management of spinal cord compression due to multiple myeloma usually involves radiation, with or without decompressive surgery, chemotherapy may play a role in patients who have had prior radiation if they have a chance of response to chemotherapy. Six myeloma patients became ambulatory with melphalan and prednisone alone. Three of the patients had total paraplegia, two had moderate paresis, and one patient was ambulatory. Four patients had loss of bladder control. The duration of symptoms in these patients ranged from two weeks to two months. The time to begin full ambulation ranged between two weeks to eight months (Sinoff and Blumshohn 1989).

Although hormonal therapy or chemotherapy should not be the mainstay of treatment for oncology patients who have not had prior radiation therapy or surgery, systemic therapy may play a role in certain tumor types. Spinal cord compression due to lymphoma, malignant thymoma, and seminoma have been reported to respond to glucocorticoids alone but whether this is due to a nonspecific role by reducing edema or a direct antitumor effect is unclear (Greenberg, Kim, and Posner 1980). Neurologic recovery in patients with lymphoma and cord compression has been observed with single-agent chemotherapy. Paraplegia due to prostate cancer has been found to respond to hormonal manipulation without radiation treatment.

OBSTRUCTIVE UROPATHY

ETIOLOGY

Obstructive uropathy is frequently associated with intra-abdominal, retroperitoneal, and pelvic malignancies. The diagnostic procedures and therapeutic approach depend on whether the site of obstruction is in the bladder neck or ureter. Bladder outlet obstruction is often secondary to cancer of the prostate, cervix, or bladder, or to benign prostatic hypertrophy. Ureteral blockage is due to para-aortic malignancies such as lymphomas, sarcomas, and nodal metastases from carcinomas of the cervix, bladder, prostate, rectum, or ovary (Michigan and Catalano 1977; Garnick and Mayer 1978; Williams and Peet 1976).

Most cancer patients have obstructive nephropathy due to tumor, but benign conditions must be considered in the differential diagnosis. Chronic hypercalcemia, hyperuricemia, or urinary tract infection predisposes patients to renal calculi. Ureteral strictures are delayed complications of both surgery and radiotherapy. Following retroperitoneal surgery, abscesses or hematomas cause ureteral obstruction. Although the primary cause

Table 35.3
SIDE EFFECTS OF CORTICOSTEROIDS

LIFE-THREATENING SIDE EFFECTS
1. Diabetes
2. Proximal muscle weakness
3. Increased risk of infection
4. Edema
5. Peptic ulcer disease
6. Psychosis
7. Adrenal suppression
BOTHERSOME COSMETIC SIDE EFFECTS
1. Weight gain
2. Striae
3. Moon facies
4. Acne
RARE SIDE EFFECTS
1. Hiccups
2. Insomnia
3. Pseudorheumatoid arthritis

of acute hyperuricemic nephropathy is uric acid deposition in the renal tubules, ureteral obstruction from uric acid calculi has been reported in association with myeloproliferative disorders (Garnick and Mayer 1978; Kjellstrand et al. 1974). Bladder outlet obstruction may be secondary to clots, urethral strictures from radiation fibrosis, or cyclophosphamide cystitis. Patients with locally advanced bladder cancer or with metastases in the brain, spinal cord, or sacral roots may have impaired bladder emptying. Voiding problems may be secondary to medications that alter the central or autonomic nervous system (Herwig 1980; Gutman and Boxer 1982). Regardless of the etiology of obstruction, pathologic changes in the dilated structures proximal to the site ultimately culminate in renal failure and death (Gutman and Boxer 1982). The initial staging evaluation for patients with locally advanced pelvic or retroperitoneal malignancies should include studies to assure patency of the urinary tract.

CLINICAL PRESENTATION

Obstruction should be suspected when patients complain of urinary retention, flank pain, hematuria, or persistent urinary tract infections. Unfortunately, ureteral obstruction often is not diagnosed until renal failure results in obtundation, seizures, volume overload, and anuria (Garnick and Mayer 1978; Herwig 1980; Pillay and Dunea 1971). Ureteral obstruction and neurogenic bladders are recognized earlier than ureteral blockage. Impaired bladder emptying causes symptoms of hesitancy, urgency, nocturia, frequency, and decreased force of the urinary stream (Garnick and Mayer 1978; Herwig 1980; Gutman and Boxer 1982; Pillay and Dunea 1971). Partial kidney obstruction should be suspected when polyuria alternates with oliguria. Physical examination may reveal enlargement of the prostate or bladder, or a pelvic, flank, or renal mass. Decreased anal sphincter tone or diminished bulbocavernosus reflexes should suggest a neurogenic bladder (Herwig 1980).

DIAGNOSTIC EVALUATION

The diagnosis of obstructive uropathy can be made readily with intravenous pyelography (IVP), renal ultrasound (US), renal radionuclear scans, or computerized tomography (CT). The bladder must be catheterized to exclude urethral obstruction. Routine serum chemistries, including creatinine, electrolytes, blood urea nitrogen (BUN), calcium, phosphorous, uric acid, and hematologic profiles should be monitored frequently. Pyuria and bacteriuria suggest infection behind an obstruction that requires immediate drainage and parenteral antibiotics.

The obstruction site must be determined prior to planning appropriate therapy. Usually hydronephrosis is confirmed by renal ultrasonography, since the risks of contrast-induced nephrotoxicity are high. Renal US can demonstrate pelvic or retroperitoneal masses, ureteral dilatation, calculi, and the residual normal renal cortex (Russell and Resnick 1979). Unless the patient is allergic to contrast dye or has severe renal dysfunction, intravenous urograms will define the site of blockage in 80% of cases of acute urinary obstruction. However, a dilated collecting system does not always imply obstruction. These selected cases may require a repeat injection of contrast or a radionuclide scan after hydration and intravenous diuretics. Renal nuclear or US scans are preferable to IVP studies since nephrotoxic contrast is avoided. Computerized tomography is more expensive and less specific, but it can help differentiate hydronephrosis from renal cysts and identify obstructing masses (McClennan and Fair 1979).

Percutaneous antegrade pyelography has the advantage of both diagnosing and relieving obstruction without the risks of anesthesia. Under US guidance, a catheter is inserted in the dilated renal pelvis. Urine is aspirated and sent for analysis and culture. To localize the site of the obstruction, contrast is injected through the catheter. Once the site is determined, an attempt is made to advance the catheter through the obstruction to restore internal ureteral drainage. If internal drainage is ineffective, external drainage can be done through the percutaneous catheter until indwelling ureteral stents are placed with cystoscopy and retrograde pyelography (Hepperlen, Mardis, and Kammandel 1978).

Urodynamic and urethrocystography are helpful in differentiating bladder dysfunction secondary to neuromuscular or mechanical causes. Generally, transurethral or suprapubic cystoscopy is required to determine the cause of bladder outlet obstruction. The ureteral orifices must be visualized and urinary flow confirmed from each orifice. Appropriate biopsies and cytologies should be obtained (Herwig 1980).

THERAPY

Lower urinary tract obstruction can be temporarily relieved by an indwelling urethral catheter, suprapubic cystostomy, or cutaneous vesicotomy. If bladder outlet obstruction cannot be promptly corrected, suprapubic cystostomy is preferable to an indwelling urethral catheter. Suprapubic cystostomies are more comfortable, carry a lower risk of infections, and avoid prostatic swelling. For partially denervated bladders, parasympathomimetic drugs (e.g., bethanechol) can improve bladder contraction and prevent overflow incontinence. Low pressure incontinence can be treated with adrenergic agonists (e.g., ephedrine). Anticholinergics (e.g., Probanthine) are prescribed for patients with uninhibited or reflex neurogenic bladders (Herwig 1980). Generally, prostatic obstruction is corrected by transurethral resection. Obstructive symptoms from advanced prostate cancer can be relieved also by orchiectomy, hormonal therapy, or radiation. However, if transurethral resection is not performed, temporary urinary diversion is required because maximal benefit from hormonal manipulation or radiation is often delayed for a few weeks (Michigan and

Catalano 1977; Kraus et al. 1972; Megalli et al. 1974; Green et al. 1974).

Radiation therapy or chemotherapy may effectively relieve obstruction if the tumor has a good chance of response to these treatment modalities (Kopelson et al. 1981; Sise and Crichlow 1978; Grillo 1973). Appropriate dose adjustments must be made for renal insufficiency and nephrotoxic drugs (e.g., cisplatin and methotrexate) should be avoided. Cyclophosphamide and ifosphamide should not be given because severe damage to the uroepithelium occurs after prolonged exposure to the active urinary metabolites of these drugs. After the obstruction is relieved, appropriate intravenous or oral fluids are needed for a few days to compensate for the postobstructive diuresis.

Infection, hyperkalemia, and acidosis must be treated promptly. Unless obstruction is relieved promptly, permanent renal damage will result. The decision to relieve an obstructing lesion must be carefully considered in terminally ill patients, as patient survival, but not comfort, may be prolonged.

AIRWAY OBSTRUCTION

Tracheal or endobronchial tumors that cause significant airway obstruction must be treated promptly to prevent postobstructive pneumonia, respiratory distress, and irreversible lung collapse. Bronchial obstruction is usually caused by endobronchial malignancies (Sise and Crichlow 1978). However, tracheal obstruction is often secondary to benign etiologies such as tracheal stenosis, tracheomalacia, or edema from infection or recent irradiation (Grillo 1973). Usually, patients with head and neck cancers have elective tracheostomies performed prior to developing upper airway obstruction (Sise and Crichlow 1978).

Lung cancer is the primary cause of bronchial obstruction. At diagnosis, partial or complete bronchial obstruction is present on chest x-rays in 53% of patients with squamous cell carcinoma; 25% with adenocarcinoma; 33% with large-cell anaplastic carcinomas; and 38% with small-cell carcinoma (Miller 1977). Endobronchial tumor is seen in 70% of lung cancer patients at thoracotomy. Endobronchial lesions are found in the main stem and lobular bronchi in 20% and 50% of cases, respectively (Brewer 1977).

In contrast to primary bronchogenic carcinomas, significant endobronchial metastatic lesions are rare. Only 2% of cancer patients have significant endobronchial metastases. However, if patients with microscopic endobronchial disease are included, the incidence of endobronchial metastases ranges from 25% to 50% (Brewer 1977; Rosenblatt, Lisa, and Trinidad 1966; Braman and Whitcomb 1975; Baumgartner and Mark 1980). The most common malignancies that metastasize to the bronchial tree are carcinomas of the breast, colon, and kidney; sarcomas; melanomas; and ovarian cancer (Baumgartner and Mark 1980; Fitzgerald 1977).

CLINICAL PRESENTATION

Bronchial and tracheal obstruction are often difficult to differentiate on physical examination. Presenting symptoms include dyspnea, orthopnea, cough, wheezing, stridor, hoarseness, and hemoptysis. Symptoms of bacterial, post-obstructive pneumonia may be found with complete obstruction. High-pitched breathing or stridor are usually associated with laryngeal or tracheal obstruction. Wheezing and rhonchi may be audible or palpable over a partially obstructed airway. If the bronchus is significantly obstructed, the trachea will deviate toward the obstructed side. However, most patients are asymptomatic until at least 75% of the lumen is occluded (Sise and Crichlow 1978; Fitzgerald 1977).

DIAGNOSTIC EVALUATION

Lateral neck radiographs with soft tissue technique provide the best view of the upper third of the trachea, but tracheal narrowing may be seen on routine chest x-rays or bilateral oblique views. Before initiating treatment, overpenetrated tracheal films, tomography, and barium swallow should be obtained to evaluate tracheal narrowing (Weber and Grillo 1978b). If radiologic studies are not definitive, upper-airway obstruction can be confirmed with flow-volume loops using an 80% helium and 20% oxygen mixture. Tracheostomy and directed biopsies are usually needed to obtain a definitive histologic diagnosis.

With bronchial obstruction, chest x-rays may reveal atelectasis or segmental consolidation. Cultures should be obtained if fever or other signs of postobstructive pneumonitis are present. A definitive diagnosis is made with fiberoptic bronchoscopy, biopsy, and brushing (Baumgartner and Mark 1980; Weber and Grillo 1978).

THERAPY

Significant upper-airway obstruction requires immediate treatment to prevent respiratory failure and death. A low tracheostomy should be performed if the obstruction is in the hypopharynx, larynx, or upper one-third of the trachea. A long tracheostomy tube can be inserted after tracheal dilatation if there is lower tracheal obstruction (Sise and Crichlow 1978). Once the airway is secured, most patients are treated with emergency radiotherapy. Often high dose corticosteroids (dexamethasone 10 mg to 16 mg·a day) are administered to decrease edema during the initial days of radiation. Patients with neoplasms that are very sensitive to chemotherapy, such as small-cell anaplastic lung cancer or lymphoma, may have a prompter response with combination chemotherapy (Glover and Glick 1987).

Patients with tracheal tumors should be considered for surgical resection and reconstruction if there is no evidence of extratracheal metastases (Sise and Crichlow 1978; Grillo 1973; Glover and Glick 1987). When nonsmall-cell lung cancer obstructs a major bronchus, patients are rarely curable with surgical resection (Brewer 1977). When curative radiotherapy is used for obstructing nonsmall-cell lung cancer, initially it is difficult to plan radiation portals because of obstructing pneumonitis. As atelectasis resolves, the portal should be reduced. Patients with endobronchial obstruction from small-cell lung cancer may respond promptly to either combination chemotherapy or radiotherapy. If an endobronchial lesion regrows in the irradiated field, the patient may be palliated with laser therapy, iridium seed implantation, or cryosurgery (Glover and Glick 1987).

BRAIN METASTASES

Emergency measures are indicated when patients present with signs of increased intracranial pressure, herniation, or hemorrhage due to brain metastases. Even when patients have more gradual neurologic deterioration, prompt treatment is recommended to prevent permanent neurologic damage. The incidence of brain metastases has increased among patients with cancers of the breast, bladder, and lung because of prolonged survival with combination chemotherapy. Most chemotherapeutic drugs penetrate the blood-brain barrier poorly and brain metastases may develop without disease progression outside the central nervous system (Glover and Glick 1987; Shapiro, Chernik, and Posner 1973). Lung and breast cancers and melanoma are the most common malignancies that metastasize to the brain. Ten percent of patients with small-cell lung cancer have brain metastases at presentation; 80% of small-cell lung cancer patients who survive two years develop brain metastases unless prophylactic cranial irradiation is given (Bunn et al. 1976; Nugent et al. 1979). Up to one-third of patients with metastatic breast cancer have CNS involvement at autopsy (Yap et al. 1978).

Most neurologic deficits in cancer patients are secondary to CNS metastases, but benign etiologies must be excluded. Elderly patients may develop neurologic signs due to metabolic disturbances, cerebrovascular thrombosis, or hemorrhage. Meningitis and brain abscesses occur with increased frequency in immunosuppressed patients. When neurologic deficits recur long after high-dose whole-brain radiotherapy, it may be difficult to differentiate brain necrosis from recurrent metastatic disease (Glover and Glick 1987).

PATHOPHYSIOLOGY AND CLINICAL PRESENTATION

More than 60% of patients with a brain metastasis will have multiple lesions at autopsy (Weissman 1988); over 90% of brain metastases are in the cerebrum. Signs and symptoms depend on the lesion's location, the extent of brain edema, and the intracranial pressure. Extensive edema surrounding the brain metastasis or ventricular obstruction by tumor increases intracranial pressure with its characteristic symptoms of decreased mental status, vomiting, nausea, and headache. The headache is usually present before arising from bed and improves within one hour after arising. Engorged retinal veins lead to papilledema, which results in blurred vision (Glover and Glick 1987; Posner, Howeison, and Cvitkovic 1977). Seizures occur more frequently among patients with increased intracranial pressure, melanoma, or carcinomatous meningitis (Glover and Glick 1987; Posner, Howeison, and Cvitkovic 1977).

DIAGNOSTIC EVALUATION

Magnetic resonance imaging (MRI) scans or computerized tomography (CT) scans are the safest and most accurate tests. When CT scans are performed with and without contrast, most lesions over 1 cm in size are detected. MRI scans are more sensitive and do not require contrast, but they are usually more expensive than brain CT scans. Both scans will determine the lesion size, number, and location and whether there is significant edema, hemorrhage, shift of midline structures, or ventricular dilatation (Glover and Glick 1987; Posner, Howeison, and Cvitkovic 1977). Nuclear brain scans are much less sensitive (Kramer, Hendrickson, and Zelen 1977). Skull films may be helpful in the rare patient with increased intracranial pressure due to a skull metastasis that either occludes the sagittal sinus or produces focal neurologic signs because of extrinsic compression of the underlying brain. Angiograms may be necessary to determine the tumor's blood supply if surgery is planned (Glover and Glick 1987; Posner, Howeison, and Cvitkovic 1977).

Intraoperative fine needle aspiration biopsy (FNAB) of the brain performed through either a burr hole or a craniotomy is extremely useful in determining the type of central nervous system neoplasm. Immediate evaluation of stained smears can be performed to assess the adequacy of the specimen and in most cases may provide a rapid preliminary diagnosis, similar to a frozen section report. The cytologic preparation demonstrates superior cellular detail, without the architectural distortion seen on frozen section preparations. Fine needle aspiration biopsy allows a small amount of tissue to be used so that residual tissue can be used for permanent section. Special studies including electron microscopy and immunohistochemistry may be particularly valuable in patients who have lesions deep in the cerebrum where biopsy needles can now obtain tissue (Silverman 1986).

A panel of monoclonal antibodies may be useful to evaluate cytologic specimens from the CNS. These monoclonal antibodies have been used based on their specificities; U.J. 13:A stains most neoplastic and non-neoplastic cell types of neuroectodermal origin; 3 antiglial fibrillary acidic protein antibodies stain neoplastic glial cells; B 72.3 reacts with most carcinomas; 2D1 is a panleukocyte marker. These monoclonal antibodies were systematically applied using immunohistochemical techniques to a series of 53 specimens of cerebrospinal fluid in patients with CNS disease.

The monclonal antibody U.J. 13:A consistently recognizes benign brain tissue in CNS-derived tumors. There was strong staining with U.J. 13:A in primary brain tumors, especially those that were malignant. There was no staining in lymphoma or metastatic disease.

Monoclonal antibody B 72.3 stained tumor cells in six cases of adenocarcinoma and one large-cell cancer. This antibody was useful in distinguishing metastatic non-small-cell carcinoma from primary brain tumors, lymphoma, and leukemia. Metastatic melanoma did not stain with the panel of antibodies; however, the S100 protein is specific for melanoma. Lymphoma and leukemia cells and inflammatory cells stain with 2D1 antibody (Vic et al. 1987).

THERAPY

When patients have signs of increased intracranial pressure or rapid neurologic deterioration, high-dose corticosteroids (dexamethasone 10 mg four times a day) and emergency radiotherapy are indicated. If intracranial pressure does not decrease promptly, mannitol is given as a 50 g intravenous bolus or as a 20% infusion. If steroids, mannitol, and radiation fail to decrease the intracranial pressure, an emergency neurosurgical procedure should be performed. A ventricular needle or Scott cannula may be inserted through a burr hole. Ventriculoperitoneal shunts are indicated if there is significant ventricular obstruction (Glover and Glick 1987).

Although steroids initially may benefit 60% to 75% of patients, without radiotherapy or surgical resection patients will rarely survive more than a few weeks. Table 35.4 lists the possible mechanisms by which steroids may reduce brain edema. Symptoms may improve within four hours following steroids or may gradually improve over several days. Dexamethasone is recommended because of its minimal salt-retaining properties (Weissman 1988). If there are no signs of increased intracranial pressure, the initial daily dexamethasone dose is 16 mg in divided doses. If there is no clinical improvement, higher dexamethasone doses (up to 100 mg daily) may be required for several days (Glover and Glick 1987; Weissman 1988; Posner, Howeison, and Cvitkovic 1977). Common practice has been to continue steroids throughout radiation because of the fear of radiation-induced edema that exacerbates symptoms and/or herniation (Weissman 1988). After several days of radiation the steroid dose is gradually tapered but if neurologic deficits recur, the steroid dose may have to be increased temporarily. Although steroids improve neurologic deficits more quickly, they do not improve

Table 35.4
POSSIBLE MECHANISMS BY WHICH CORTICOSTEROIDS REDUCE BRAIN EDEMA

A. DECREASED EDEMA PRODUCTION
1. Decreased tumor capillary permeability
2. Anti-inflammatory effects by reducing oxygen free-radical damage
3. Alteration of sodium and water transport across endothelial cells
4. Antitumor effects
B. INCREASED EDEMA REABSORPTION
1. Decreased CSF production in the choroid plexus
2. Improved pressure gradient for edema fluid to pass from the extravascular space into the CSF

Table 35.5
POSSIBLE INDICATIONS FOR NEUROSURGICAL INTERVENTION OR CONSULTATION FOR BRAIN METASTASES

1. Diagnosis of brain metastases is uncertain
2. Solitary metastasis with small chance of postoperative neurologic deficit
3. Increased intracranial pressure from cerebellar or temporal lobe lesion
4. Ventricular obstruction
5. Radioresistant tumors
6. Long time interval between diagnosis of primary tumor and brain metastasis
7. Rapid neurologic deterioration despite osmotic therapy and radiation

the response rate to radiation or patient survival, unless there is significant increased intracranial pressure (Glover and Glick 1987; Posner, Howeison, and Cvitkovic 1977; Kramer, Hendrickson, and Zelen 1977). Anticonvulsants are not prescribed unless there is a history of seizures. When dilantin and corticosteroids are used concurrently, the doses may have to be increased because of increased drug metabolism (Posner, Howeison, and Cvitkovic 1977).

Radiation therapy provides prompt palliation for most patients with brain metastases. The indications for surgical consultation are listed in table 35.5. Surgical resection may be indicated if the diagnosis of brain metastases is uncertain, particularly in patients without a history of malignant disease. Patients with a solitary brain metastasis without other systemic metastases may be surgical candidates if resection would not produce neurologic defects. Emergency neurosurgical consultation is indicated for patients with increased intracranial pressure from cerebellar or temporal lobe lesions or ventricular obstruction. There is debate whether surgery or radiation is preferred for patients with (1) a solitary brain metastasis with a long time interval between the initial primary malignancy and the brain metastasis; (2) slow-growing radioresistant tumors; or (3) rapid neurologic deterioration despite mannitol and steroids (Posner, Howeison, and Cvitkovic 1977; Winston, Walsh, and Fisher 1980). Mortality rates with surgical resection range from 10% to 30%. Patients with poor performance status, cardiopulmonary insufficiency, or increased intracranial pressure are in the highest surgical risk group. Good prognostic factors that predict for a long survival following surgery for solitary brain metastasis include (1) minor neurologic deficits preoperatively; (2) a long interval between the diagnosis of the primary neoplasm and the brain metastasis; (3) total resection of the brain metastasis; and (4) postoperative radiotherapy (Winston, Walsh, and Fisher 1980).

Patients with brain metastases from metastatic melanoma appear to have improved survival with surgery. The median survival in 12 patients with a solitary brain metastasis treated with radiation therapy alone was 16 weeks. The median survival of 66 patients with brain metastasis after initiation of radiation therapy was 14 weeks. Survival was improved (median survival of 36 weeks) only in 10 patients who underwent subtotal or total resection of a solitary brain metastasis prior to radiation therapy (Rate, Solin, and Turisi 1988).

Almost all patients with brain metastases receive cranial irradiation, and because most patients have multiple metastases at autopsy, the whole brain is irradiated (Glover and Glick 1987; Posner, Howeison, and Cvitkovic 1977; Shehata, Hendrickson, and Hindo 1974). Most patients receive 30 Gy over two weeks or 40 Gy over three weeks (Kramer, Hendrickson, and Zelen 1977; Glover and Glick 1987). More than 69% of patients show improvement in neurologic deficits. Thirty-two percent to 66% of patients have resolution of all neurologic signs following radiotherapy. However, 30% to 50% die from recurrent brain metastases. Although patients may benefit from additional brain radiation, they must be warned of the risk of brain necrosis (Glover and Glick 1987; Weissman 1988; Winston, Walsh, and Fisher 1980).

CARCINOMATOUS MENINGITIS

ETIOLOGY AND CLINICAL PRESENTATION

Carcinomatous meningitis is increasing in frequency because of improved survival with systemic antineoplastic therapies and increased awareness of this problem among oncologists. At autopsy, 4% of patients have leptomeningeal spread, most commonly associated with lymphoma, leukemia, cancers of the breast and lung, and melanoma (Yap et al. 1978; Posner, Howeison, and Cvitkovic 1977; Wasserstrom, Glass, and Posner 1982; Bunn et al. 1981). Because most chemotherapy drugs fail to penetrate the blood-brain barrier, carcinomatous meningitis develops frequently in patients without signs of progressive systemic disease outside the CNS (Shapiro et al. 1977).

At autopsy, the brain and spinal cord may be covered by a sheet of malignant cells or the spinal and cranial nerve roots may have multifocal metastases. The malignant cells tend to settle in the basal cisterns where they interfere with cerebrospinal fluid flow and absorption, which may lead to obstructive hydrocephalus (Wasserstrom, Glass, and Posner 1982).

Carcinomatous meningitis should be suspected when neurologic signs indicate that more than one structural area of the nervous system is affected. Clinical symptoms depend on the extent of tumor involving the brain, cranial nerves, or spinal cord. Occasionally, neurologic symptoms may be subtle and exist for several weeks prior to diagnosis. Headache may be associated with nausea and vomiting, and mental status changes, lethargy, and decreased memory are frequent. The most common cranial nerve deficits cause diplopia, visual blurring, hearing loss, and facial numbness. Over 70% of patients have neurologic signs due to spinal cord or nerve root involvement and may have symptoms of spinal cord compression (Yap et al. 1978; Posner, Howeison, and Cvitkovic 1977; Wasserstrom, Glass, and Posner 1982).

DIAGNOSTIC EVALUATION

The diagnosis of carcinomatous meningitis is established by cytologic examination. At least 5 mL of cerebrospinal fluid (CSF) should be sent for cytology, although the initial fluid analysis may not be diagnostic. Repeated lumbar punctures are required to confirm the diagnosis. In retrospective series of carcinomatous meningitis, malignant cells were seen in the first, second, and third CSF samples in 42% to 66%, 60% to 87%, and 68% to 96% of cases, respectively. With obstruction of normal CSF pathways, patients may have repeatedly negative lumbar CSF cytologies, while cytologic examination of cisternal or ventricular fluid are positive (Wasserstrom, Glass, and Posner 1982; Kirkwood and Bankole 1981; Olsen, Chernik, and Posner 1974). More than half of the patients with carcinomatous meningitis have one or more of the following CSF abnormalities: opening pressure above 160 mm of water, increased white cell count, a reactive lymphocytosis, elevated CSF protein, and decreased glucose (Wasserstrom, Glass, and Posner 1982; Olsen, Chernik, and Posner 1974).

Computerized tomography (CT) scans may reveal contrast enhancement in the meninges and periventricular area, hydrocephalus, or brain metastases; concurrent brain metastases are present in 20% of patients (Wasserstrom, Glass, and Posner 1982). Emergency myelograms or MRI scans of the spine should be performed in patients with symptoms or signs due to metastases to the spinal cord or cauda equina.

THERAPY

Treatment for carcinomatous meningitis consists of intrathecal chemotherapy and radiation therapy to the areas of the neuroaxis responsible for the neurologic deficits. Without treatment, patients will die within four to six weeks. Therapeutic drug levels are not generally achieved in the CSF with parenteral chemotherapy. Intraventricular chemotherapy via an Ommaya reservoir generally is preferable to lumbar injections. With lumbar puncture, the drug may reach only the epidural or subdural spaces. Even when the chemotherapeutic drug reaches the subarachnoid space, therapeutic drug levels are rarely reached in the ventricles. Intraventricular injections via the Ommaya are also less painful than lumbar punctures and allow drug concentrations to follow the normal pathways for CSF flow (Bunn et al. 1981; Olsen, Chernik, and Posner 1974). Compared to retrospective series in which drugs were given by lumbar puncture, it appears that response rates are higher and longer in duration with intraventricular therapy and radiation therapy. In Wasserstrom's series, more than 60% of patients with leptomeningeal metastases from breast cancer, 100% with lymphoma, 50% with lung cancer, and 40% with melanoma improved or stabilized with therapy. In this series, the median survival was 5.8 months with a range from one to 29 months (Wasserstrom, Glass, and Posner 1982).

Ommaya reservoirs can be placed with less than 2%

Table 35.6 CHEMOTHERAPEUTIC DOSAGES FOR CARCINOMATOUS MENINGITIS

DRUG	LUMBAR PUNCTURE INJECTION	INTRAVENTRICULAR OMMAYA INJECTION
Methotrexate	12-15mg	10-12mg
Cytosine arabinoside	45mg	30-45mg
Thiotepa	15mg	10mg

morbidity and no mortality. If intracranial pressure is increased, an Ommaya reservoir can be placed and connected to a ventricular peritoneal shunt. The shunt has an on-off valve that allows it to be closed off for about four hours after intraventricular drug administration (Wasserstrom, Glass, and Posner 1982).

The most frequently used intrathecal drugs are methotrexate, thiotepa, and cytosine arabinoside. The chemotherapy drug doses are listed in table 35.6. Leucovorin (10 mg every 6 hours for 6 doses) will decrease methotrexate's systemic side effects. Methotrexate doesn't cross the blood-brain barrier so its antitumor efficacy in the CSF will not be effected.

Methotrexate and thiotepa are usually administered for solid tumors associated with carcinomatous meningitis. Cytosine arabinoside alone or with methotrexate is used in leukemic and lymphomatous meningitis. Intrathecal therapy is given twice a week until symptoms improve or stabilize and the cytology becomes negative. Intrathecal therapy may then be given weekly, and gradually spaced out to monthly injections if the cytologies are persistently negative (Yap et al. 1978; Wasserstrom, Glass, and Posner 1982).

Whole-brain and brain-stem irradiation are employed when there are cerebral or cranial nerve abnormalities. When spinal cord or nerve root signs are present, myelograms or MRI scans of the spine are required to plan radiation portals. Doses are usually 30 Gy over two weeks.

Lymphomatous and leukemic meningitis are more responsive to intrathecal therapy and may also respond to high-dose systemic methotrexate with leucovorin rescue. Because of the high incidence of leptomeningeal involvement, patients with acute lymphocytic leukemia, acute lymphoblastic lymphoma, and Burkitt's lymphoma receive prophylactic intrathecal chemotherapy via lumbar puncture and whole-brain irradiation after a complete remission is obtained.

METABOLIC EMERGENCIES

HYPERCALCEMIA

The most frequent metabolic emergency in oncology is hypercalcemia, which develops when the rate of calcium mobilization from bone exceeds the renal threshold for calcium excretion. Neoplastic disease is the leading cause of hypercalcemia among inpatients (Besarb and Caro 1978; Glover and Glick 1985; Massaferri, O'Dorisio, and LaBuglio 1978). The most common malignancies associated with hypercalcemia are carcinomas of the breast and lung, hypernephroma, multiple myeloma, squamous cell carcinoma of the head and neck and esophagus, and thyroid cancer (Glover and Glick 1985). Parathyroid carcinoma is a rare malignancy associated with intractable hypercalcemia due to elevated parathyroid hormone (PTH) levels.

Although more than 80% of patients with hypercalcemia have osseous metastases, the extent of bony disease does not correlate with the level of hypercalcemia (Glover and Glick 1985). During the course of their disease, about 40% to 50% of patients with breast carcinoma metastatic to the bones will develop hypercalcemia. In most settings hypercalcemia suggests disease progression, but patients with metastatic breast cancer involving bone may develop hypercalcemia when they are placed on hormonal therapy. Estrogen and antiestrogens stimulate breast cancer cells to produce osteolytic prostaglandins and to increase bone resorption (Mundy 1985). Within several days of initiating hormonal therapy for metastatic breast cancer, the calcium level may rise and the bone pain increase. This tumor flare, in response to hormonal therapy, usually implies that the patient will subsequently have an excellent antitumor response to hormonal treatment. However, the hormonal therapy must be temporarily held and the hypercalcemia corrected before the drug is reinstituted.

In the majority of patients with bone metastases, direct neoplastic bone resorption is felt to be the cause of hypercalcemia. However, 20% of solid tumors associated with hypercalcemia have no evidence of osseous spread. In these situations, investigators have demonstrated humoral substances, such as parathyroid-hormonelike substances or osteolytic prostaglandins, which are secreted by tumor cells. In multiple myeloma, hypercalcemia occurs because of production of osteoclast activating factor (OAF) by the abnormal plasma cells, rather than from a direct neoplastic bone effect (Glover and Glick 1985).

Bone metastases or the indirect effects of ectopic humoral substances directly stimulate osteoclast activity and proliferation. Although osseous metastases are frequently surrounded by a zone of osteoclasts, it is not clear whether hypercalcemia results from direct neoplastic bony destruction or from release of osteolytic substances from the malignant cells. *In vitro* studies have shown selective cancer cell lines that are capable of reabsorbing bone without increasing osteoclast activity (Glover and Glick 1985; Mundy 1985).

Patients with squamous cell carcinomas of the head and neck, lung, and esophagus may develop a clinical syndrome suggestive of hyperparathyroidism owing to ectopic secretion of parathyroid hormone or parathyrotropic substances. In association with hypercalcemia, patients develop hypophosphatemia, increased urinary cyclic AMP, and elevations in bone alkaline phosphatase (Glover and Glick 1985). It is clear that parathyroid carcinoma cells produce excessive parathyroid hormone, but in other tumor types recent data suggest that ectopic PTH production may be a less important cause of hypercalcemia than previously reported. Except in parathyroid carcinoma, extractable parathyroid hormone is rarely present in neoplastic tissues. Most cases of hypercalcemia, which were presumed to be secondary to ectopic PTH production, are now felt to be due to ectopic secretion of PTH-like substances that bind to PTH receptors. In contrast to hypercalcemia due to hyperparathyroidism, these patients have impaired production of 1,25-dihydroxy vitamin D and no evidence of renal bicarbonate wasting (Mundy 1985).

Osteolytic prostaglandins have been detected in hypercalcemic patients with carcinomas of the lung, kidney, and ovary (Brereton et al. 1974; Josse et al. 1981; Shane and Bilezikian 1982; Tashjian 1975). Animal studies have shown that inhibitors of prostaglandin synthesis (such as aspirin, indomethacin, and other nonsteroidal anti-inflammatory drugs, as well as corticosteroids) are successful therapies, but these agents are less effective in clinical practice (Mundy 1985; Shane and Bilezikian 1982; Tashjian 1975).

Osteoclast activating factor (OAF), a potent osteolytic peptide, causes bone reabsorption and secondary hypercalcemia in multiple myeloma and lymphoma (Besarb and Caro 1978; Bockman 1980; Mundy et al. 1974). However, despite the potent osteolytic activity of OAF *in vitro*, patients with elevated OAF levels do not always develop hypercalcemia unless there is renal dysfunction (Mundy 1985). Patients with lymphoma due to the human T-cell lymphotrophic virus (HTLV) present with severe hypercalcemia due to ectopic production of several osteotrophic factors (OAF, colony-stimulating factor, gamma interferon, and an active vitamin D metabolite) (Mundy 1985).

CLINICAL PRESENTATION AND DIAGNOSTIC EVALUATION

Hypercalcemia is rarely a presenting sign of malignancy, except in patients with parathyroid carcinoma, HTLV-I T-cell lymphoma, or multiple myeloma. Most hypercalcemic patients present with nonspecific symptoms of fatigue, anorexia, nausea, polyuria, polydipsia, and constipation. Neurologic symptoms from hypercalcemia begin with vague muscle weakness, lethargy, apathy, and hyporeflexia. Without treatment, symptoms progress to profound alterations in mental status, psychotic behavior, seizures, coma, and ultimately death. Patients with prolonged hypercalcemia eventually develop permanent renal tubular abnormalities with renal tubular acidosis, glucosuria, aminoaciduria, and hyperphosphaturia (Massaferri, O'Dorisio, and LaBuglio 1978). Sudden death from cardiac arrhythmias may occur when the serum calcium rises acutely (Besarb and Caro 1978; Glover and Glick 1985). Except for those with parathyroid cancer, hypercalcemic cancer patients rarely live long enough to develop signs of chronic hypercalcemia.

All hypercalcemic patients should have serial serum calcium phosphate, alkaline phosphatase, electrolytes, BUN, and creatinine level measurements. Elevated immunoreactive PTH levels in association with hypo-phosphatemia may suggest ectopic hormone production. In malnourished patients with low albumin levels, the ionized calcium value may be helpful in deciding on therapy, since hypercalcemic symptoms correlate with elevation in ionized rather than protein-bound calcium. Patients with multiple myeloma may have elevated serum calciums secondary to abnormal calcium binding to paraproteins without an elevation in ionized calcium, while malnourished patients with hypoalbuminemia may have symptoms of hypercalcemia with normal serum calcium levels. The electrocardiogram often reveals shortening of the QT interval, widening of the T wave, bradycardia, and PR prolongation (Glover and Glick 1985).

THERAPY

The cause of hypercalcemia, severity of associated clinical signs, and chance of response to effective antitumor therapy must be considered in choosing the most appropriate therapy. Mild hypercalcemia is frequently corrected with intravenous hydration alone. If effective antitumor therapy is available, the serum calcium will gradually decline as the tumor regresses. However, most hypercalcemic cancer patients require additional hypocalcemic therapy until an antitumor response is obtained. Calcium balance can be corrected by directly decreasing bone reabsorption, promoting urinary calcium excretion, and decreasing oral calcium intake. Patients should be mobilized to avoid osteolysis. Constipation should be corrected, and medications (such as thiazide diuretics and vitamins A and D) that may elevate calcium levels should never be used (Glover and Glick 1985).

All hypercalcemic patients are dehydrated because of polyuria from renal tubular dysfunction. Intravenous hydration with normal saline will increase urinary calcium excretion, since the urinary clearance rates for calcium parallel sodium excretion (Glover and Glick 1985). When hypercalcemia is life-threatening, aggressive hydration (e.g., 250-300 mL/hr) and intravenous furosemide should be administered to decrease reabsorption calcium (Glover and Glick 1985; Bockman 1980).

Corticosteroids, which block bone reabsorption due to OAF, have been effective in multiple myeloma, lymphoma, breast cancer, and leukemia. Corticosteroids block bone reabsorption due to OAF. High-dose steroids may also have hypocalcemic effects by increasing urinary calcium excretion, inhibiting vitamin D metabolism, decreasing calcium absorption, and after long-term use by producing negative calcium balance in bone (Glover and Glick 1985; Mundy 1985). High doses of corticosteroids are generally required for several days before an effective hypocalcemic response is seen; most patients require 40 mg to 100 mg of prednisone daily (Glover and Glick 1985; Bockman 1980).

The majority of hypercalcemic patients are treated with Mithracin (plicamycin), a chemotherapeutic agent that decreases bone reabsorption by reducing osteoclast number and activity. Mithracin is effective in patients with hypercalcemia from either bone metastases or from bone reabsorption from ectopic humoral substances (Elias and Evans 1972). The drug is a sclerosing agent and must be given as a bolus through a freshly started intravenous line. If extravasation occurs, patients will develop ulceration and ultimately fibrosis of the underlying tissues. Hypercalcemic patients will often require one or two injections of Mithracin (15-20 mcg/kg) per week, unless effective antitumor therapy is initiated. The serum calcium level will begin to fall within six to 48 hours. If no response occurs within the first two days, a second dose should be administered (Glover and Glick 1985; Massaferri, O'Dorisio, and LaBuglio 1978; Elias and Evans 1972; Perlia et al. 1970). Only low doses of Mithracin are necessary to control hypercalcemia and the majority of patients do not develop side effects (e.g., thrombocytopenia, coagulopathy, hypertension, liver function abnormalities, or nephrotoxicity) generally seen with high doses (Elias and Evans 1972; Perlia et al. 1970).

When hypercalcemia occurs following hormonal therapy for metastatic breast cancer, patients should be treated with hydration, steroids, and Mithracin if necessary. When severe hypercalcemia occurs after hormonal therapy for breast cancer, the hormone should be discontinued immediately. Once the calcium level normalizes, the hormone can be restarted in lower doses and gradually increased. When mild hypercalcemia is precipitated by hormonal therapy, the hormone frequently can be continued without undue risk while the patient is managed with hydration alone (Glover and Glick 1985).

Calcitonin promptly inhibits bone reabsorption causing a fall in serum calcium within hours of administration (Glover and Glick 1985; Binstock and Mundy 1980). Although a prompt hypocalcemic response is obtained, tachyphylaxis develops unless glucocorticoid therapy is given with calcitonin. For unclear reasons, if the serum calcium begins to rise with calcitonin, the drug may be temporarily held and then reinstituted; occasionally a secondary response will occur within 48 hours. Calcitonin is given in daily doses (3-6 Medical Research Council [MRC] units/kg) intravenously or twice daily in intermuscular or subcutaneous injection (100-400 MRC units/kg) (Glover and Glick 1985; Body 1984).

Although initial clinical trials suggested that inhibitors of prostaglandin synthesis (e.g., indomethacin or aspirin) were hypocalcemic agents, subsequent trials have failed to confirm the initial reports (Besarb and Caro 1978; Glover and Glick 1985; Bockman 1980). Clinical trials using diphosphonates have shown encouraging results in patients with breast cancer and multiple myeloma. Intravenous phosphate may rapidly decrease serum calcium, but is rarely employed because of the high incidence of severe complications (hypotension, hypocalcemia, renal failure, and death); maximal effect will occur five days later. With hypercalcemia associated with cardiac arrhythmias and coma, a 50 mmol infusion of mono- or dibasic anhydrous potassium phosphate may be administered over six to eight hours. Oral phosphates (1 g to 3 g of sodium acid phosphate/day) are effective and relatively safe in controlling mild hypercalcemia (Glover and Glick 1985).

Most patients are effectively managed with hydration, mobilization, effective antitumor therapy, and gradually tapering doses of either Mithracin, calcitonin, or corticosteroids. If effective antitumor therapy is not available, patients must be maintained on hypocalcemic therapy indefinitely and serum calcium levels should be monitored at least twice a week. If corticossteroids are used, the dose can be gradually tapered to the lowest effective therapeutic dose. When Mithracin is used chronically, the interval between injections generally can be lengthened. Similarly, if hypercalcemia is controlled with calcitonin, the injection interval can be gradually increased from 12 to 24 hours (Glover and Glick 1985).

URIC ACID NEPHROPATHY

Uric acid nephropathy is usually associated with malignancies that have an increased rate of cell turnover. Although it can occur spontaneously, the condition most frequently is reported as a complication following cytotoxic therapy that produces a rapid antitumor response. Rapid cell death increases uric acid production and results in hyperuricemia and uric acid crystal deposition in the urinary tract (Garnick and Mayer 1978; Kjellstrand et al. 1974; Klinenberg, Kippen, and Bluestone 1975). Hyperuricemia and associated renal uric acid deposition occur most commonly with the tumor lysis syndrome, which is often associated with Burkitt's lymphoma. Most episodes of uric acid nephropathy are associated with effective cytotoxic chemotherapy or radiation therapy, but spontaneous hyperuricemic nephropathy in hematologic malignancies has been occasionally reported in lymphoma and leukemia patients (Kjellstrand et al. 1974). Untreated leukemics have increased uric acid excretion. The degree and incidence of hyperuricemia correlates with the cytologic type of leukemia, rather than the degree of white count elevation. For example, uric acid excretion is typically higher in acute myelocytic leukemia than in chronic lymphocytic leukemia (Glover and Glick 1985; Garnick and Mayer 1978).

Uric acid stones are seen in fewer than 10% of patients in recent series and occur most often in patients with chronic hyperuricemia such as that associated with chronic myeloproliferative syndromes (Glover and Glick 1985; Kjellstrand et al. 1974).

The incidence and severity of hyperuricemic nephropathy have decreased with prophylactic treatment with allopurinol, vigorous hydration, and alkalinization of the urine. In previous studies, mortality rates from hyperuricemic nephropathy ranged from 47% to 100%. However, with current aggressive medical therapy, the majority of patients regain normal renal function within a few days of treatment, after the serum uric acid level falls below 10 mg/dL (Kjellstrand et al. 1974).

The most common tumors associated with hyperuricemia are leukemia and lymphoma, but case reports of uric acid nephropathy have been reported among patients with chronic myeloproliferative syndromes, multiple myeloma, and squamous-cell carcinomas of the head and neck (Glover and Glick 1985; Kjellstrand et al. 1974).

CLINICAL PRESENTATION AND DIAGNOSTIC EVALUATION

Patients rarely develop ureteral obstruction, so flank pain and gross hematuria are uncommon (Kjellstrand et al. 1974). The most common presentation is signs of uremia, including nausea, vomiting, lethargy, and oliguria. Early treatment provides an excellent chance of rapidly reversing renal dysfunction (Glover and Glick 1985; Kjellstrand et al. 1974; Klinenberg, Kippen, and Bluestone 1975). Often it is difficult to differentiate acute uric acid nephropathy from other causes of renal failure with secondary hyperuricemia. In acute uric acid nephropathy, the mean serum uric acid level at presentation was 20.1 mg/dL (ranging from 9.2 mg/dL to 92 mg/dL) (Glover and Glick 1985; Kjellstrand et al. 1974).

If flank pain or gross hematuria occurs, a renal ultrasound should be performed to exclude ureteral obstruction. Hyperuricemia increases the incidence of dye-induced renal dysfunction, so intravenous contrast should be avoided. In the tumor lysis syndrome, hyperphosphatemia and hypocalcemia often occur out of proportion to the degree of renal insufficiency (Kjellstrand et al. 1974). Serial blood studies for electrolytes, BUN, creatinine, calcium, phosphorus, and uric acid must be obtained. The urinalysis will be helpful if uric acid crystals are seen, but their absence does not exclude the diagnosis since crystalluria and hematuria occur only in the acute phase (Kjellstrand et al. 1974; Klinenberg, Kippen, and Bluestone 1975). Kelton has demonstrated that a urinary uric acid-to-creatinine ratio of >1 is relatively specific for hyperuricemia nephropathy (Glover and Glick 1985).

THERAPY

The primary goal of therapy should be the prevention of hyperuricemia. Patients at high risk should be treated with allopurinol, vigorous hydration, and urinary alkalinization for at least 48 hours prior to cytotoxic therapy. Drugs that block tubular reabsorption of uric acid (such as aspirin, radiographic contrast, probenecid, and thiazide diuretics) should be avoided. Prior to chemotherapy, the serum uric acid level should be normal, the urine pH above 7, and intravenous hydration given to ensure a urine volume of more than 3 liters per day (Glover and Glick 1985; Garnick and Mayer 1978; Kjellstrand et al. 1974; Klinenberg, Kippen, and Bluestone 1975). To alkalinize the urine, intravenous sodium bicarbonate, 100 mEq/m², should be given daily. When the urinary pH is above 7.5, uric acid solubility is maximal and it is not necessary to produce significant metabolic alkalosis, which may complicate the clinical situation (Kjellstrand et al. 1974; Klinenberg, Kippen, and Bluestone 1975; Seyberth et al. 1975). Serum potassium and magnesium levels should be followed closely and allopurinol administered in doses ranging from 300 mg/day to 800 mg/day to decrease uric production by competitively inhibiting xanthine oxidase (Garnick and Mayer 1978; Kjellstrand et al. 1974; Seyberth et al. 1975). Although high xanthine levels might precipitate xanthine stones, this has not been reported in patients treated for hyperuricemic nephropathy (Glover and Glick 1985; Klinenberg, Kippen, and Bluestone 1975). Prophylactic colchicine is not required when allopurinol is administered because patients rarely develop acute gouty arthritis.

If oliguria or anuria develops, ureteral obstruction must be excluded by renal US or antegrade or retrograde pyelography; nephrotoxic contrast must be avoided. Once ureteral obstruction is excluded, mannitol or high-dose furosemide should be given in an attempt to restore urine flow. A Foley catheter should be inserted to accurately measure urine output. If a prompt diuresis does not occur within a few hours, emergency hemodialysis will be necessary to reverse uric acid obstruction of the renal tubules (Kjellstrand et al. 1974).

A hollow-fiber kidney apparatus will decrease serum uric acid levels more rapidly than either peritoneal or coil hemodialysis (Glover and Glick 1985; Garnick and Mayer 1978). With hemodialysis, all patients in Kjellstrand's series had rapid normalization of renal function and a prompt diuresis when the serum uric acid level decreased below 10-20 mg/dL. Within six hours of hemodialysis, uric acid levels generally fall by 50%. Most patients will require six days of dialysis before hyperuricemia resolves and renal function returns to baseline normal values (Kjellstrand et al. 1974).

In patients undergoing dialysis, a low calcium dialysate should be used to prevent calcium phosphate precipitation, which theoretically would increase nephrotoxicity. Aluminum hydroxide antacids may help to decrease gastrointestinal phosphate absorption (Kjellstrand et al. 1974). If hemodialysis cannot be done, uric acid clearance can be improved by adding albumin to the peritoneal dialysis. Albumin will increase uric acid protein binding and removal. Alkalinizing the dialysate to a neutral pH with sodium bicarbonate will also enhance uric acid clearance (Knochel and Mason 1966). Fortunately, with aggressive measures for prevention and treatment, acute uric acid nephropathy now has an extremely low morbidity and mortality rate (Glover and Glick 1985; Kjellstrand et al. 1974).

HYPONATREMIA

Only 1% to 2% of patients with malignancy develop the syndrome of inappropriate antidiuretic hormone secretion (SIADH). Despite a low plasma osmolality, the urine is inappropriately concentrated with a high sodium level. This situation can also occur in renal disease, hypothyroidism, and adrenal insufficiency and these diseases must be excluded to confirm the diagnosis of SIADH (DeFronzo

and Thier 1980; Goldberg 1981; Trump 1981). The majority of patients are asymptomatic unless the serum sodium concentration falls abruptly (Glover and Glick 1985).

Ectopic antidiuretic hormone secretion has been confirmed in patients with bronchogenic carcinoma. Small-cell anaplastic carcinoma of the lung is the most common malignancy associated with SIADH (Glover and Glick 1985). At presentation, more than 50% of patients with small-cell lung cancer may develop hyponatremia following a water load, but fewer than 15% of patients will develop clinically significant hyponatremia (Glover and Glick 1985; Lockton and Thatcher 1986). Case reports of SIADH have also been published on patients with cancers of the prostate, adrenal cortex, esophagus, pancreas, colon, and head and neck; carcinoid; thymoma; lymphoma; and mesothelioma (Glover and Glick 1985; Trump 1981).

Because ectopic antidiuretic hormone production is rarely seen except in patients with small-cell carcinoma, SIADH is more frequently associated with pulmonary or CNS metastases. Inappropriate antidiuretic hormone secretion can also occur with medications including morphine, vincristine, and cyclophosphamide (DeFronzo and Thier 1980; Goldberg 1981). With advanced malignancy, patients may also develop hyponatremia due to a "reset osmostat" in which the serum sodium is usually mildly depressed and may be corrected to normal levels with effective antitumor therapy. Kerne and associates (1986) reported that SIADH secretion can occur with pituitary prolactinomas. These tumors may produce SIADH without detectable arginine vasopressin levels. In this setting, bromocriptine induces both tumor regression and correction of hyponatremia.

Adrenal insufficiency resulting from withdrawal of corticosteroids or metastases to the adrenal or pituitary glands may cause mild hyponatremia. In the setting of severe liver disease, heart failure, or acute renal insufficiency, patients may develop dilutional hyponatremia (DeFronzo and Thier 1980; Goldberg 1981). Vomiting, diarrhea, ascites, or diuretics may precipitate hyponatremia (Hudson 1978). Patients with plasma cell dyscrasias may have artifactual hyponatremia. Electrolytes should be followed when patients are treated with high-dose cisplatin with mannitol diuresis (Glover and Glick 1985; Brereton et al. 1974).

PATHOPHYSIOLOGY

With increased ADH secretion, excessive water is reabsorbed in the collecting ducts. This leads to increased distal sodium delivery by producing a mild increase in intravascular volume. Volume expansion also increases renal perfusion, decreases proximal tubular reabsorption of sodium, and decreases aldosterone effect (Brereton et al. 1974). Ectopic ADH secretion has been measured in patients with small-cell lung carcinoma (Spencer, Yarger, and Robinson 1976). In other conditions associated with increased ADH secretion, there is excessive production of ADH by the posterior pituitary (Glover and Glick 1985).

Dilutional hyponatremia occurs in volume overloaded states secondary to cardiac, hepatic, or renal dysfunction. Although the total body sodium and water content are increased, the circulating plasma volume is reduced. With impaired renal perfusion, there is greater reabsorption of water in the collecting duct and increased ADH secretion, resulting in a dilutional hyponatremic state (DeFronzo and Thier 1980). With dehydration, total body salt and water content are generally decreased which results in decreased renal perfusion and increased ADH secretion. Diuretics, interstitial renal disease, and mineralocorticoid deficiency are also associated with excessive renal sodium losses. Pseudohyponatremia is associated with elevated parathyroid levels in patients with plasma cell dyscrasias. Since the plasma sodium concentration is measured as the sodium concentration per unit of plasma, with elevated paraprotein levels, the percentage of water in plasma is decreased (DeFronzo and Thier 1980). With mannitol infusion or hyperglycemia, an osmotic gradient producing increases water movement into the extravascular spaces resulting in hyponatremia (Glover and Glick 1985).

CLINICAL PRESENTATION

With mild hyponatremia, patients may complain of anorexia, nausea, myalgias, and subtle neurological symptoms. When hyponatremia develops rapidly or the sodium falls below 115 mg/dL, patients frequently have alterations in mental status ranging from lethargy to confusion and coma. Seizures and psychotic behavior have also been reported. With profound hyponatremia, alterations in mental status, pathologic reflexes, papilledema, and rarely, focal neurological signs may be found on physical examination (Goldberg 1981; Trump 1981). The cause of hyponatremia must be determined before appropriate therapy can be initiated. If pseudohyponatremia due to hyperproteinemia, hyperlipidemia, or hyperglycemia is suspected, serum protein electrophoresis, lipids, and glucose levels should be checked. Medication records should be reviewed since chemotherapeutic agents (e.g., vincristine or cyclophosphamide), mannitol, morphine, diuretics, and abrupt steroid withdrawal may contribute to hyponatremia (Glover and Glick 1985).

A careful history, physical examination, and review of the patient's intake and output will help to determine whether the patient is volume expanded, dehydrated, or euvolemic. Serum and urine electrolytes, osmolality, and creatinine should be measured. With SIADH, there is inappropriate sodium concentration in the urine for the level of hyponatremia. The urine osmolality is greater than plasma osmolality, but is never maximally dilute. With SIADH, the BUN is usually low from volume expansion. Hypouricemia and hypophosphatemia may result from decreased proximal tubular reabsorption of these ions (Glover and Glick 1985; DeFronzo and Thier 1980; Goldberg 1981). Thyroid and adrenal dysfunction should be ruled out if laboratory studies suggest SIADH. Chest x-ray and CT scans of the brain may reveal pulmonary or neurologic disorders that may cause excessive ADH production.

THERAPY

Ideally, treatment should be given to correct the cause of the hyponatremia; SIADH will resolve when the underlying cause of excessive antidiuretic hormone production is removed. Following effective combination chemotherapy for small-cell lung cancer, the sodium will rise to normal levels. Corticosteroids and radiotherapy may alleviate SIADH due to brain metastasis. If drug-induced SIADH occurs, the serum sodium will correct once the offending agent is discontinued (Glover and Glick 1985). If the etiology of excessive ADH secretion cannot be corrected, the initial therapy is water restriction. If free water intake is restricted to 500 cc to 1,000 cc per day, the negative free water balance will correct the hyponatremia within seven to 10 days (Glover and Glick 1985; DeFronzo and Thier 1980; Goldberg 1981; Trump 1981). If the serum sodium does not correct with water restriction, demeclocycline may correct the hyponatremia by decreasing ADH's stimulus for free water reabsorption in the collecting ducts (DeFronzo and Thier 1980; Goldberg 1981; Lockton and Thatcher 1986; Skrabanek and Powell 1978). Demeclocycline produces a dose-dependent, reversible nephrogenic diabetes insipidus (DeFronzo and Thier 1980; Geheb and Cox 1980; Forrest et al. 1978).

With demeclocycline, despite liberal fluid intake, the average pretreatment serum sodium (121 mEq/L) rose above 130 mEq/L within three to four days of initiating treatment (Trump 1981). The only side effect of demeclocycline is reversible nephrotoxicity (Glover and Glick 1985; Trump 1981). Renal dysfunction develops in fewer than half of the patients and is generally mild. The majority of patients who experienced nephrotoxicity were either receiving other nephrotoxic drugs or higher doses of demeclocycline. Demeclocycline is excreted in the urine and bile; patients with renal or hepatic dysfunction should either avoid this drug or have reduced doses administered (Glover and Glick 1985; Trump 1981; Skrabanek and Powell 1978). The initial daily demeclocycline dose is 600 mg, unless the patient has liver or kidney dysfunction or is receiving other nephrotoxic drugs (Koff, Thrall, and Keyes 1979). Doses may be increased up to 1,200 mg daily if hyponatremia persists. The total drug dose is divided and given two or three times a day (Glover and Glick 1985).

Patients with coma or seizures from SIADH should receive 3% hypertonic saline or isotonic saline with intravenous furosemide 1 mg/kg (Glover and Glick 1985). In volume-expanded patients, hyponatremia will resolve if the associated cardiac, renal, or liver dysfunction can be corrected. Dehydrated hyponatremic patients are managed with intravenous isotonic saline solutions (DeFronzo and Thier 1980; Goldberg 1981).

HYPOGLYCEMIA

Fasting hypoglycemia occurs with insulinomas and rarely, with other islet cell tumors of the pancreas. Other tumors associated with hypoglycemia usually are large, bulky, slow-growing mesenchymal malignancies, including fibrosarcomas, mesotheliomas, and spindle-cell sarcomas (Glover and Glick 1985; Anderson and Lokich 1979; Kahn 1980; Smitz et al. 1985).

Normally, glucose homeostasis is maintained by appropriate hormonal regulation of gluconeogenesis and glycogenolysis in patients with adequate caloric intake (Glover and Glick 1985). Tumor-induced hypoglycemia may be caused by secretion of insulin or an insulinlike substance, increased glucose utilization by the tumor, or alterations in the regulatory mechanisms for glucose homeostasis. Although insulin levels are elevated in hypoglycemia from islet cell cancers, increased insulin secretion has not been observed with other neoplasms (Glover and Glick 1985; Kahn 1980). Using bioassays, increased levels of substances with insulinlike activity have been measured in serum samples from patients with hypoglycemia and nonislet-cell malignancies. These substances are now referred to as nonsuppressible insulinlike activity (NSILA). Only 5% to 10% of their insulinlike activity can be neutralized with anti-insulin antibodies. NSILA appears to be a combination of somatomedins A and C, high-molecular-weight glycoproteins, and low-molecular-weight growth factors. These substances have both the growth-promoting and metabolic effects of insulin. However, the growth-promoting effects of the low-molecular-weight substances are 54% greater than insulin's effects, while their metabolic effects are only 1% to 2% as potent. The high-molecular-weight substances have minimal growth-promoting capabilities but maintain their metabolic effects (Glover and Glick 1985).

Elevated levels of low-molecular-weight NSILA have been demonstrated in patients with nonislet-cell tumors causing hypoglycemia by both radioreceptor and bioassay techniques. Elevated levels of these substances have been observed in patients with hemangiopericytomas, hepatomas, pheochromocytomas, adrenocortical carcinomas, and large mesenchymal tumors. Low to normal levels of NSILA have been measured in patients with hypoglycemia in association with leukemia, lymphoma, or gastrointestinal primaries (Glover and Glick 1985; Kahn 1980). Most hypoglycemic patients with fibrosarcomas will have elevated high-molecular-weight NSILA levels (Glover and Glick 1985). When there is a rapid reduction in glucose levels in the normal patient, counterregulatory mechanisms should increase secretion of ACTH, glucocorticoids, growth hormone, and glucagon. However, in patients with tumor-induced hypoglycemia, the fall in glucose is usually not rapid enough to increase these hormone levels (Kahn 1980).

Cancer patients have reduced rates of hepatic gluconeogenesis-reduced glycogen breakdown following epinephrine or glucagon, and decreased hepatic glycogen stores (Glover and Glick 1985). These data suggest that impaired glucose homeostasis may contribute to tumor-induced hypoglycemia. In the past, increased glucose utilization by the tumor was thought to be one of the causes of hypoglycemia. However, increased glycogen breakdown and gluconeogenesis should compensate for increased glycolysis. Before assuming that the metabolic abnormality is caused by the malignancy, the more common causes of hypoglycemia (i.e., exogenous insulin use, oral diabetic agents, adrenal failure, pituitary insufficiency, alcohol abuse, or malnutrition) should be excluded (Glover and Glick 1985).

Most patients will complain of excessive fatigue, weakness, dizziness, and confusion. Patients will rarely have symptoms to suggest reactive hypoglycemia. Symptoms tend to occur after fasting in the early morning or late afternoon. If the blood sugar remains depressed below 40 mg/dL, seizures may result.

Fasting and late-afternoon glucose levels are most helpful in making the diagnosis. Patients with insulinomas will have increased insulin levels with fasting glucose levels below 50 mg/dL, while patients with nonislet-cell tumors will have normal to low insulin levels during the periods of hypoglycemia (Glover and Glick 1985; Kahn 1980). Leukemic patients with high leukocyte counts may have artifactual hypoglycemia when blood remains in collection tubes for prolonged periods (Glover and Glick 1985).

Insulinomas produce large amounts of proinsulin and have elevated proinsulin-to-insulin ratios. Higher proinsulin levels are seen with malignant insulinomas. If technically feasible, insulinlike plasma factors should be measured by bioassay or radioreceptor technique (Glover and Glick 1985).

Hypoglycemia is corrected rapidly with intravenous injections of 50% dextrose, which should be followed by a continuous infusion of 10% dextrose. Insulinomas are frequently cured by surgery, while the rare patient with an inoperable insulinoma can be managed with chemotherapy or diazoxide (Glover and Glick 1985).

If effective antitumor therapy is available for nonislet-cell tumors associated with hypoglycemia, the metabolic abnormalities should resolve with tumor regression. Following surgical resection of fibrosarcomas, hypoglycemia will resolve. Effective chemotherapy regimens for mesotheliomas have also corrected hypoglycemia (Kahn 1980). To prevent nocturnal hypoglycemia, patients should be awakened from sleep for meals and have frequent between-meal and bedtime snacks. Occasionally, corticosteroids may provide temporary relief. Patients have also benefitted from intermittent subcutaneous or long-acting intermuscular glucagon injections (Glover and Glick 1985).

SUMMARY

As antitumor therapy becomes more effective and less toxic, it is imperative to recognize potentially life threatening or permanently disabling complications that may be prevented or reversed by prompt action. Accurate diagnosis and treatment of oncologic emergencies can improve quality of life and prolong survival, allowing more patients to receive an adequate trial of definitive therapy designed to eradicate or effectively palliate their malignant disease.

REFERENCES

Ahmann, F.R. 1984. A reassessment of the clinical implications of the superior vena caval syndrome. *J. Clin. Oncol.* 2:961-69.

Anderson, N., and Lokich, J.J. 1979. Mesenchymal tumors associated with hypoglycemia: case report and review of the literature. *Cancer* 44:785-90.

Applefeld, M.M.; Slawson, R.G.; and Hall-Craigs, M. et al. 1981. Delayed pericardial disease after radiotherapy. *Am. J. Cardiology* 47:210-13.

Armstrong, B.A.; Perez, C.A.; and Simpson, J.R. et al. 1987. Role of irradiation in the management of superior vena caval syndrome. *Int. J. Radiat. Oncol. Biol. Phys.* 13:531-39.

Barbaric, Z.L. 1979. Interventional uroradiography. *Radiol. Clin. North Am.* 17:413-33.

Barek, L.; Lautin, R.; and Ledor, S. et al. 1982. Role of CT in the assessment of superior vena cava obstruction. *J. Comput. Tomogr.* 6:121-26.

Baumgartner, W.A., and Mark, J.B.D. 1980. Metastatic malignancies from distant sites to the tracheobronchial tree. *J. Thorac. Cardiovasc. Surg.* 79:499-503.

Besarb, A. and Caro, J.F. 1978. Mechanisms of hypercalcemia in malignancy. *Cancer* 41:2276-85.

Binstock, M.L., and Mundy, G.R. 1980. Effect of calcitonin and glucocorticoids in combination on the hypercalcemia of malignancy. *Ann. Intern. Med.* 93:269-72.

Bleyer, W.A., and Poplack, D.G. 1979. Intraventricular versus intralumbar methotrexate for central nervous system leukemia: prolonged remission with the Ommaya reservoir. *Med. Pediatr. Oncol.* 6:207-13.

Bockman, R.S. 1980. Hypercalcemia in malignancy. *Clin. Endocrinol. Metab.* 9:157-333.

Body, J.J. 1984. Cancer hypercalcemia: recent advances in understanding and treatment. *Eur. J. Cancer Clin. Oncol.* 20:865-69.

Borgelt, B.; Gelber, R.; and Kramer, S. et al. 1980. The palliation of brain metastases: final results of the first two studies by the Radiation Therapy Oncology Group. *Int. J. Radiat. Oncol. Biol. Phys.* 6:1-9.

Braman, S.S., and Whitcomb, M.E. 1975. Endobronchial metastases. *Arch. Intern. Med.* 135:543-47.

Brereton, H.D.; Halushka, P.V.; and Alexander, R.W. et al. 1974. Indomethacin-responsive hypercalcemia in a patient with renal cell adenocarcinoma. *N. Engl. J. Med.* 291:83-85.

Brewer, L.A. 1977. Patterns of survival in lung cancer. *Chest* 71:644-50.

Bruckman, J.E., and Bloomer, W.D. 1978. Management of spinal cord compression. *Semin. Oncol.* 5:135-40.

Bunn, P.; Rosen, S.; and Aisner, J. et al. 1981. Carcinomatous leptomeningitis in patients with small-cell lung cancer: a frequent, treatable complication. *Proc. Am. Assoc. Cancer Res., and ASCO* 231:641 (Abstr. C-39).

Bunn, P.A. Jr.; Schein, P.S.; and Banks, P.M. et al. 1976. Central nervous system complications in patients with diffuse histiocytic and undifferentiated lymphoma and leukemia revisited. *Blood* 41:3-10.

Buzaid, A.C.; Garewal, H.S.; and Greenberg, B.R. 1989. Managing malignant pericardial effusions. *West. J. Med.* 150:174-79.

Calkins, A.R.; Olson, M.A.; and Ellis, J.H. 1980. Impact of myelography on the radiotherapeutic management of malignant spinal cord compression. *Neurosurgery* 19:614-16.

Davenport, D.; Ferree, C.; and Blake, D. et al. 1978. Radiation therapy in treatment of superior vena caval obstruction. *Cancer* 42:2600-2603.

Davis, S.; Sharma, S.M.; and Blumberg, E.D. et al. 1978. Intrapericardial tetracycline for the management of cardiac tamponade secondary to malignant pericardial effusion. *N. Engl. J. Med.* 299:1113-14.

DeFronzo, R.A., and Thier, S.O. 1980. Pathophysiologic approach to hyponatremia. *Arch. Intern. Med.*; 140:897-902.

Dombernowsky, P., and Hanson, H. 1978. Combination chemotherapy in the management of superior vena caval obstruction in small cell anaplastic carcinoma of the lung. *Acta Med. Scand.* 204:513-16.

Elias, E.G., and Evans, J.T. 1972. Hypercalcemic crisis in neoplastic diseases: management of Mithracin. *Surgery* 71:615-35.

Findlay, G.F.G. 1987. The role of vertebral body collapse in the management of malignant spinal cord compression. *J. Neurol. Neurosurg. Psych.* 50:151-54.

Fitzgerald, R.H. 1977. Endobronchial metastases. *South Med. J.* 70:440-41.

Forrest, J.N. Jr.; Cox, M.; and Hong, C. et al. 1978. Superiority of demeclocycline over lithium in the treatment of chronic syndrome of inappropriate secretion of antidiuretic hormone. *N. Engl. J. Med.* 298:173-77.

Fowler, N.O. 1978. Diseases of the pericardium. *Curr. Prob. Cardiol.* 2:6-38.

Garnick, M.B., and Mayer, R.J. 1978. Acute renal failure associated with neoplastic disease and its treatment. *Semin. Oncol.* 5:156-65.

Geheb, M., and Cox, M. 1980. Renal effects of demeclocycline. *JAMA* 243:2519-20.

Gerber, W.L.; Brown, R.C.; and Culp, D.A. 1981. Percutaneous nephrostomy with immediate dilation. *J. Urol.* 125:169-71.

Ghosh, B.C., and Cliffton, E.E. 1973. Malignant tumors with superior vena cava obstruction. *N.Y. State J. Med.* 73:283-89.

Gilbert, H.A.; Kagan, A.R.; and Nussbaum, H. et al. 1977. Evaluation of radiation therapy for bone metastases: pain relief and quality of life. *Am. J. Roentgenol.* 129:1095-96.

Glover, D.J., and Glick, J.H. 1985. Oncologic emergencies and special complications. In Calabresi, P.; Schein, P.J.; and Rosenberg, S.A. eds. *Medical oncology: basic principles and clinical management of cancer.* pp. 1261-26. New York: MacMillian.

Glover, D.J., and Glick, J.H. 1987. Oncologic emergencies. *CA* 37:302.

Goldberg, M. 1981. Hyponatremia. *Med. Clin. N. Am.* 65:251-69.

Gollub, S.; Hirose, T.; and Klauher, J. 1980. Scintigraphic sequelae of superior vena caval obstruction. *Clin. Nucl. Med.* 5:89-93.

Goodie, R.B. 1955. Secondary tumors of the heart and pericardium. *Br. Heart J.* 17:183-88.

Green, N.; Melbye, R.W.; and George, F.W. III et al. 1974. Radiation therapy of inoperable localized prostatic carcinoma: an assessment of tumor response and complications. *J. Urol.* 3:662-64.

Greenberg, H.S.; Kim, J.H.; and Posner, J.B. 1980. Epidural spinal cord compression from metastatic tumor: results from a new treatment protocol. *Ann. Neurol.* 8:361-66.

Grillo, H.C. 1973. Obstructing lesions of the trachea. *Ann. Otol. Rhinol. Laryngol.* 82:770-77.

Gutman, F.D., and Boxer, R.J. 1982. Neoplasms involving the kidney or producing renal failure via urinary obstruction. In Rieselbach R.E., and Garnick, M.B. eds. *Cancer and the kidney.* pp. 594-624. Philadelphia: Lea and Febinger.

Hancock, E.W. 1975. Constrictive pericarditis: clinical clues to diagnosis. *JAMA* 232:176-77.

Hankins, J.R.; Scatterfield, J.R.; and Aisner, J. et al. 1980. Pericardial window for malignant pericardial effusion. *Ann. Thorac. Surg.* 30:465-71.

Hepperlen, T.W.; Mardis, H.R.; and Kammandel, H. 1978. Self-retained internal ureteral stents: a new approach. *J. Urol.* 119:731.

Herwig, K.R. 1980. Management of urinary incontinence and retention in the patient with advanced cancer. *JAMA* 244:2203-2204.

Hill, G.J. II, and Cohen, B.I. 1970. Pleural pericardial window for palliation of cardiac tamponade due to cancer. *Cancer* 26:81-93.

Hudson, R.E.B. 1978. Diseases of the pericardium. In Hurst, J.W.; Logue, R.B.; and Schlant, R.C. et al. eds. *The heart.* 4th ed. New York: McGraw-Hill.

Josse, R.G.; Wilson, D.R.; and Heersche, J.N.M. et al. 1981. Hypercalcemia with ovarian carcinoma: evidence of a pathogenetic role for prostaglandins. *Cancer* 48:1233-41.

Kahn, C.R. 1980. The riddle of tumor hypoglycemia revisited. *Clin. Endocrinol. Metab.* 9:335-60.

Kane, R.C.; Cohen, M.H.; and Broder, L.E. et al. 1976. Superior vena cava obstruction due to small cell anaplastic lung carcinoma *JAMA* 235:1717-19.

Katz, P.B.; Lee, Y.; and Wallace, S. et al. 1981. Myelography of spinal block from epidural tumor: a new approach. *Am. J. Radiol.* 136:945-47.

Kerne, P.A.; Robbins, R.J.; and Bichet, D. et al. 1986. Syndrome of inappropriate antidiuretics in the absence of arginine vasopressin. *J. Clin. Endocrinol. Metab.* 62:148-52.

Kirkwood, J.M., and Bankole, D.O. 1981. Carcinomatous meningitis at Yale 1970-1980. *Proc. Am. Assoc. Cancer Res. and ASCO* 22:633.

Kjellstrand, C.M.; Campbell, D.C. II; and Von Hartitzsch, B. et al. 1974. Hyperuricemic acute renal failure. *Arch. Int. Med.* 133:349-59.

Klinenberg, J.R.; Kippen, I.; and Bluestone, R. 1975. Hyperuricemic nephropathy: pathologic features and factors influencing urate deposition. *Nephron.* 14:99-115.

Knochel, J.P., and Mason, A.D. 1966. Effect of alkalinization on peritoneal diffusion of uric acid. *Am. J. Physiol.* 210:1160.

Koff, S.A.; Thrall, J.H.; and Keyes, J.W. 1979. Diuretic radionuclide urography: a non-invasive method for evaluation of nephroureteral dilatation. *J. Urol.* 122:451-54.

Kopelson, G.; Munsenrider, J.E.; Kelley, R.M.; and Shipley, W.V. 1981. Radiation therapy for ureteral metastases from breast carcinoma. *Cancer* 47:1976-79.

Kramer, S.; Hendrickson, F.; and Zelen, M. 1977. Therapeutic trials in the management of metastatic brain tumors by different time/dose fractionation schemes of radiation therapy. *Natl. Cancer Inst. Monogr.* 46:213-21.

Kraus, P.A.; Lytton, B.; and Weiss, R.M. et al. 1972. Radiation therapy for local palliative treatment of prostatic cancer. *J. Urol.* 108:612-14.

Krikorian, J.G., and Hancock, E.W. 1978. Pericardiocentesis. *Am. J. Med.* 65:808-14.

Kumar, P.P., and Good, R.R. 1989. Need for invasive diagnostic procedures in the management of superior vena cava syndrome. *JAMA* 81:41-47.

Lajos, T.Z.; Black, H.E.; and Cooper, R.G. et al. 1975. Pericardial decompression. *Ann. Thorac. Surg.* 19:47-53.

Lawrence, L.T., and Cronin, J.F. 1963. Electrical alternans and pericardial tamponade. *Arch. Intern. Med.* 112:415-18.

Levine, H.L., and Olmstead, E.J. 1979. Myelographic evaluation of non-traumatic spinal cord obstruction: a new approach. *Am. J. Radiol.* 133:715-18.

Li, K.C., and Poon, P.Y. 1988. Sensitivity and specificity of MRI in detecting malignant spinal cord compression and in distinguishing malignant from benign compression fractures of vertebrae. *MRI* 6:547-56.

Lockton, J.A., and Thatcher, N. 1986. A retrospective study of 32 patients with small cell bronchogenic carcinoma and inappropriate secretion of antidiuretic hormone. *Clin. Radiol.* 37:47-50.

Martin, R.G.; Ruckdeschel, J.C.; and Chang, P. et al. 1975. Radiation-related pericarditis. *Am. J. Cardiol.* 35:216-20.

Martini, N.; Bains, M.S.; and Beattie, E.J. Jr. 1975. Indications for pleurectomy in malignant effusion. *Cancer* 35:734-38.

Massaferri, E.L.; O'Dorisio, T.M.; and LaBuglio, A.F. 1978. Treatment of hypercalcemia associated with malignancy. *Semin. Oncol.* 5:141-53.

McClennan, B.L., and Fair, W.F. 1979. CT scanning in urology. *Urol. Clin. North Am.* 6:343-74.

Megalli, M.R.; Gursel, E.O.; and Demirag, H. et al. 1974. External radiography in ureteral obstruction secondary to locally invasive prostatic cancer. *Urology* 3:562-64.

Michigan, S., and Catalano, W.J. 1977. Ureteral obstruction from prostatic carcinoma: response to endocrine and radiation therapy. *J. Urol.* 118:733-38.

Miller, J.B.; Variakojis, D.; and Bitran, J.D. et al. 1981. Diffuse histiocytic lymphoma with sclerosis: a clinicopathologic entity frequently causing superior vena caval obstruction. *Cancer* 74:748-56.

Miller, W.E. 1977. Roentgenographic manifestations of lung cancer. In Straus, M.J. ed. *Lung cancer: clinical diagnosis and treatment.* New York: Grune & Stratton.

Millman, A.; Meller, J.; and Motro, M. et al. 1977. Pericardial tumor or fibrosis mimicking pericardial effusion by echocardiography. *Ann. Intern. Med.* 86:434-36.

Morris, A.L. 1976. Echo evaluation of tamponade. *Circulation* 53:746-47.

Mundy, G.R. 1985. Pathogenesis of hypercalcemia of malignancy. *Clin. Endocrin.* 23:705-14.

Mundy, G.R.; Raisz, L.G.; and Cooper, R.A. et al. 1974. Evidence for the secretion of an osteoclast stimulating factor in myeloma. *N. Engl. J. Med.* 291:1041-46.

Niarchos, A.P. 1975. Electrical alternans in cardiac tamponade. *Thorax* 30:228-33.

Nugent, J.L.; Bunn, P.A. Jr.; and Matthews, M.J. et al. 1979. CNS metastases in small-cell bronchogenic carcinoma: increasing frequency and changing pattern with lengthening survival. *Cancer* 44:1885-93.

Olsen, M.E.; Chernik, N.L.; and Posner, J.B. 1974. Infiltration of the leptomeninges by systemic cancer. *Arch. Neurol.* 30:122-37.

Perez, C.A.; Presant, C.A.; and Van Amburg, A.L. III. 1978. Management of superior vena caval syndrome. *Semin. Oncol.* 5:123-34.

Perez-Soler, R.; McLaughlin, P.; and Velasquez, W.S. et al. 1984. Clinical features and results of management of superior vena caval syndrome secondary to lymphoma. *J. Clin. Oncol.* 2:260-66.

Perlia, C.P.; Gubisch, N.J.; and Wolter, J. et al. 1970. Mithramycin treatment of hypercalcemia. *Cancer* 25:389-94.

Pillay, V.K.G., and Dunea, G. 1971. Clinical aspects of obstructive uropathy. *Med. Clin. North Am.* 55:1417-27.

Pories, W.J., and Gaudiani, V.A. 1975. Cardiac tamponade. *Surg. Clin. North Am.* 55:573-89.

Posner, J.B. 1977. Management of central venous system metastases. *Semin. Oncol.* 4:81-91.

Posner, J.B.; Howeison, J.; and Cvitkovic, E. 1977. Disappearing spinal cord compression: oncologic effect of corticosteroids (and other chemotherapeutic agents) on epidural metastases. *Ann. Neurol.* 2:409-13.

Rate, W.R.; Solin, L.J.; and Turrisi, A.T. 1988. Palliative radiation therapy for metastatic melanoma: brain metastasis, bone metastasis, and spinal cord compresison. *Int. J. Radiat. Oncol. Biol. Phys.* 15:859-64.

Redmond, J. III; Friedl, K.E.; and Cornett, P. et al. 1988. Clinical usefulness of an algorithm for the early diagnosis of spinal metastatic disease. *J. Clin. Oncol.* 6:154-57.

Rodichuk, L.D.; Harper, G.R.; and Ruckdeschel, J.C. et al. 1981. Early diagnosis of spinal epidural metastases. *Am. J. Med.* 70:1181-88.

Rodriguez, M., and Dinapoli, R.P. 1980. Spinal cord compression with special reference to metastatic epidural tumors. *Mayo Clin. Proc.* 55:442-48.

Rosenblatt, M.B.; Lisa, J.R.; and Trinidad, S. 1966. Pitfalls in the clinical and histologic diagnosis of bronchogenic carcinoma. *Dis. Chest* 40:297-404.

Rubin, P.; Mayer, E.; and Poulter, C. 1969. Extradural spinal cord decompression by tumor. I: high daily dose experience without laminectomy. *Radiology* 93:1248-60.

Rubinstein, R.M., and Bolooki, H. 1972. Intrapleural tetracycline for control of malignant pleural effusion: a preliminary report. *South Med. J.* 65:847-49.

Russell, J.M., and Resnick, M.I. 1979. Ultrasound in urology. *Urol. Clin. N. Am.* 6:445-68.

Salsali, M., and Cliffton, E.E. 1965. Superior vena caval obstruction with carcinoma of the lung. *Surg. Gynecol. Obstet.* 121:783-88.

Schraufragel, D.F.; Hill, B.; and Leech, J.A. et al. 1981. Superior vena caval obstruction: is it a medical emergency? *Am. J. Med.* 70:1169-74.

Sculier, J.P., and Feld, R. 1985. Superior vena cava obstruction syndrome: recommendations for management. *Cancer Treat. Rev.* 12:209-18.

Seyberth, H.W.; Sewgre, G.V.; and Morgan, J.L. et al. 1975. Prostaglandins as mediators of hypercalcemia associated with certain types of cancer. *N. Engl. J. Med.* 293:1278-83.

Shane, E., and Bilezikian, J.P. 1982. Parathyroid cancer: a review of 62 patients. *Endocrine Rev.* 3:218-26.

Shapiro, W.R.; Chernik, N.L.; and Posner, J.B. 1973. Necrotizing encephalopathy following intraventricular instillation of methotrexate. *Arch. Neurol.* 28:96-102.

Shapiro, W.R.; Posner, J.B.; and Ushio, Y. et al. 1977. Treatment of meningeal neoplasms. *Cancer Treat. Rep.* 61:733-43.

Shehata, W.M.; Hendrickson, F.R.; and Hindo, W.A. 1974. Rapid fractionation technique and retreatment of cerebral metastases by irradiation. *Cancer* 34:257-61.

Shimm, D.S.; Logue, G.L.; and Rigsby, L.C. 1981. Evaluating the superior vena cava syndrome. *JAMA* 245:951-53.

Silverman, J.F. 1986. Cytopathology of fine needle aspiration biopsy of the brain and spinal cord. *Diag. Cytopathol.* 2:312-18.

Sinoff, C.L., and Blumshon, A. 1989. Spinal cord compression in myelomatosis: response to chemotherapy alone. *Euvr. J. Cancer Clin. Oncol.* 25:197-200.

Sise, J.B., and Crichlow, R.W. 1978. Obstruction due to malignant tumors. *Semin. Oncol.* 5:213-24.

Skrabanek, P., and Powell, D. 1978. Ectopic insulin and Occam's razor: reappraisal of the riddle of tumor hypoglycemia. *Clin. Endocrinol.* 9:141-54.

Smitz, S.; Legros, J.; and Franchimont, P. et al. 1985. High molecular weight vasopressin: detection of a large amount in the plasma of a patient. *Clin. Endocrinol.* 23:379-84.

Spencer, H.W.; Yarger, W.E.; and Robinson, R.E. 1976. Alterations of renal function during dietary-induced hyperuricemia in the rat. *Kidney Int.* 9:489-500.

Spodick, D.H. 1967. Acute cardiac tamponade: pathologic physiologic, diagnosis, and management. *Prog. Cardiovasc. Dis.* 10:64-96.

Tashjian, A.H. 1975. Prostaglandins, hypercalcemia, and cancer. *N. Engl. J. Med.* 293:1317-18.

Theologides, A. 1978. Neoplastic cardiac tamponade. *Semin. Oncol.* 5:181-92.

Thurber, D.L.; Edwards, J.E.; and Achoe, R.W.P. 1962. Secondary malignant tumors of the pericardium. *Circulation* 26:228-41.

Trump, D.L. 1981. Serious hyponatremia in patients with cancer. *Cancer* 47:2908-12.

Van Belle, S.J.P.; Bolckaert, A.; and Taeymans, Y. et al. 1987. Treatment of malignant pericardial tamponade with sclerosis induced by instillation of bleomycin. *Int. J. Cardiol.* 16:155-60.

Van Houtte, P., and Fruhling, J. 1981. Radionuclide venography in the evaluation of superior vena caval syndrome. *Clin. Nucl. Med.* 6:177-83.

Vic, W.W.; Wikstrand, C.J.; and Bullard, D.E. et al. 1987. The use of a panel of monoclonal antibodies in the evaluation of cytologic specimens from the central nervous system. *Acta Cytologica* 31:815-29.

Wasserstrom, W.R.; Glass, J.P.; and Posner, J.B. 1982. Diagnosis and treatment of leptomeningeal metastases from solid tumors: experience with 90 patients. *Cancer* 49:722-59.

Weber, A.L., and Grillo, H.C. 1978. Tracheal tumors: a radiological, clinical and pathological evaluation of 84 cases. *Radiol. Clin. North Am.* 16:227-46.

Weissman, D.E. 1988.: Glucocorticoid treatment for brain metastases and epidural spinal cord compression: a review. *J. Clin. Oncol.* 6:543-51.

White, W.A.; Patterson, R.H.; and Bergland, R.M. 1971. Role of surgery in the treatment of spinal cord compression by metastatic neoplasm. *Cancer* 27:558-61.

Wild, W.O., and Parker, R.W. 1963. Metastatic epidural tumor of the spine: a study of 45 cases. *Arch. Surg.* 87:137-42.

Williams, G., and Peet, T.N.D. 1976. Bilateral ureteral obstruction due to malignant lymphoma. *Urology* 7:649-51.

Winston, K.R.; Walsh, J.W.; and Fisher, E.G. 1980. Results of operative treatment of intracranial metastatic tumors. *Cancer* 45:2639-45.

Yap, J.Y.; Yap, B.S.; and Tashima, C.K. et al. 1978. Meningeal carcinomatosis in breast cancer. *Cancer* 42:283-86.

Zipf, R.E. Jr., and Johnston, W.W. 1972. The role of cytology in the evaluation of pericardial effusions. *Chest* 62:593-96.

Chapter 36

AIDS-RELATED CANCER

Tony W. Cheung, M.D., F.A.C.P.
Frederick P. Siegal, M.D., F.A.C.P.

Tony W. Cheung, M.D., F.A.C.P.
Assistant Professor
Department of Medicine and Neoplastic Diseases
Mount Sinai Medical Center
New York, New York

Frederick P. Siegal, M.D., F.A.C.P.
Head, Section of Hematology Research
Division of Hematology-Oncology
Long Island Jewish Medical Center
New Hyde Park, New York

KAPOSI'S SARCOMA

INTRODUCTION

In early 1981, a new epidemic of Kaposi's sarcoma (KS) and *Pneumocystis carinii* pneumonia (PCP) was first reported in young men of homosexual or bisexual orientation (Siegal et al. 1981; Gottlieb et al. 1981; Hymes et al. 1981). The etiologic agent of this disease is a retrovirus of the lentivirus group known as human immunodeficiency virus type I, or HIV-I, subsequently referred to as HIV (Siegal 1987; Barre-Sinoussi et al. 1983; Gallo et al. 1983). This syndrome, now known as acquired immunodeficiency syndrome (AIDS), results from a virally induced, progressive depletion of cell-mediated immunity. The resulting immunologic deficiency predisposes the host to a variety of opportunistic infections and unusual neoplasms, especially Kaposi's sarcoma and aggressive lymphomas.

In addition, in transforming T-cell tropic retroviruses distantly related to HIV, the human T-cell leukemia viruses type I (HTLV-I) and type II (HTLV-II) have now been shown to be causally linked to adult T-cell leukemia-lymphoma (ATLL) (Poiesz et al. 1980) and, possibly, to some cases of hairy-cell leukemia (Kalyanaraman et al. 1982). These retroviruses can also predispose to immune deficiency, but they are principally recognized to immortalize and transform some of the cells they infect, leading after a long incubation to characteristic lymphoid tumors.

The appearance of certain neoplasms among patients with AIDS resembles closely the previously observed association of neoplastic processes with other states of immunodeficiency (see table 36.1). The pattern of neoplasms is sufficiently stereotyped to provide information about the role of the immune system in the containment of neoplasms in general. These patients do not seem to develop the common tumors of the breast, lung, and colon in increased frequency; instead, they are plagued with a limited group of neoplastic diseases: a variety of monoclonal non-Hodgkin's lymphomas, polyclonal lymphoid tumors (including some limited to the central nervous system), Hodgkin's disease, Kaposi's sarcoma, and squamous carcinomas of the skin. This peculiar disease spectrum appears to be associated with a viral role in tumor induction. In particular, human herpesviruses (including Epstein-Barr virus, herpes simplex, possibly human herpes virus type 6) and human papillomaviruses have been implicated. In the special case of common, variable immunodeficiency (acquired hypogammaglobulinemia), there is an additional unexplained increased incidence of colon and stomach cancers.

BACKGROUND

In 1872, Moritz Kohn Kaposi, a Hungarian dermatologist, first described Kaposi's sarcoma as an "idiopathic multiple pigmented sarcoma of the skin" (Kaposi 1872). From that time until the recent epidemic, classic KS remained a rare and unusual tumor (table 36.2). Most cases were seen in elderly men of Italian or Eastern European Jewish ancestry.

Table 36.1
EXAMPLES OF IMMUNE DEFICIENCY DISORDERS WITH INCREASED RISK FOR NEOPLASIA

Primary Immunodeficiency States
  Congenital or Genetically Determined
    Severe, combined immune deficiency
    X-linked agammaglobulinemia
  Acquired
    Common, variable immunodeficiency
    Syndrome of thymoma with immune deficiency
  Iatrogenic Immunosuppression
    Organ transplant recipients
Secondary Immunodeficiency States
    Chronic lymphocytic leukemia

Table 36.2
CLINICAL CLASSIFICATION OF KAPOSI'S SARCOMA

	AGE	RISK GROUPS	CLINICAL CHARACTERISTICS	COURSE
CLASSIC	50-80	Older men of Jewish and Italian origin M:F = 12:1	Skin lesions confined to lower extremities; later can spread cutaneously and to visceral organs	Indolent; survival 10-15 years
AFRICAN Nodular	25-40	Young black men in Central Africa M:F = 13:1	Localized nodular lesions, rarely involving bone and lymph nodes	Indolent
Florid	25-40		Fungating exophytic skin lesions, often involving bone (38%), but rarely lymph nodes	Locally aggressive
Infiltrative	25-40		Diffuse skin infiltration, always involving bone, but rarely lymph nodes	Locally aggressive
Lymphadenopathic	2-13	Children	Generalized lymphadenopathy (5%), rarely involving the skin	Rapidly progressive; survival 3 years
IMMUNOSUPPRESSIVE THERAPY-RELATED	Renal transplant patient or patients with autoimmune disease on immunosuppressive therapy M:F = 3:1		May be localized to skin or widespread with systemic involvement	Can be indolent or rapidly progressive; tumor may regress when immuno-suppressive therapy is discontinued
AIDS-EPIDEMIC	19-64	HIV infected patients; primarily homosexual men; few Haitians; IV drug users	Commonly presents with generalized mucocutaneous lesions often involving lymph nodes and visceral organs	Variable; without OI, 80% survival at 2 years; however, <20% survival if associated with OI

M = male; F = female; OI = opportunistic infection

Kaposi's sarcoma has been widespread among both children and older people in sub-Saharan Africa; in children, the disease tended to involve lymph nodes and appeared at a sex ratio of around 1:1; among African adults, the male-to-female ratio was around 11:1. In 1950, 43 cases of KS were reported from South Africa (Ackerman and Murray 1963). Since then, increasing numbers of KS were reported in Central Africa (Taylor et al. 1971).

Two distinct clinical forms were identified. An indolent variety is characterized by cutaneous plaque and nodular lesions. This benign type is similar in behavior to the classic (Western European) type in its clinical pattern, and is associated with a long survival. A more aggressive form of KS was observed in young, black Africans. If not treated appropriately, this type of tumor can kill the patient within a year. The aggressive form is subdivided morphologically into florid, infiltrative, and generalized lymphadenopathic types. The most aggressive "florid" lesions grow into fungating and exophytic masses and often invade the subcutaneous and surrounding tissues, including the underlying bone. Both the localized (indolent) and aggressive forms occur mostly in young male adults between the ages of 25 and 40.

KS has also been a known complication of iatrogenically induced or late-onset idiopathic (primary) immunodeficiencies associated with spindle-cell thymoma (Siegal 1988); interestingly, it occurred in the same ethnic groups as did classical KS, but at an earlier age, and tended to regress if the immune suppression could be eliminated. KS, in association with renal transplantation, was first described in 1969. Some renal allograft recipients receiving prednisone and azathioprine develop KS shortly after the onset of immunosuppressive therapy (Harwood et al. 1971). The tumors in these iatrogenically immunosuppressed patients often remain localized to the skin, although widespread dissemination with mucocutaneous or visceral organ involvement was sometimes observed. The extent of KS is related to the degree of depression of cellular immunity. Occasionally, the KS tumors have regressed as a result of reduction or cessation in immunosuppressive treatment (Harwood et al. 1971; Myers et al. 1974). KS has also been reported to develop after the use of immunosuppressive agents in the treatment of various autoimmune disease, such as rheumatoid arthritis (Yarboro 1987).

HISTOPATHOLOGY AND HISTOGENESIS

Kaposi's sarcoma is a vascular tumor arising from the middermis. It consists of interweaving bands of spindle cells and irregular slit-like vascular channels embedded in reticular and collagen fibers, infiltrations with mononuclear cells, and plasma cells. There are extravasated erythrocytes along with erythrophagocytosis and hemosiderin deposition.

However, there are many controversies regarding the cellular origin of KS. The following phenotypic markers strongly suggest that KS arises from lymphatic endothelial cells (Beckstead, Wood, and Fletcher 1985): positive for histochemical marker, HLA-DR (Ia), 5'-nucleotidase, and lectin binding protein Ulex europaeus I; weakly positive for factor VIII related antigen and monoclonal antibody EN-4 (Salahuddin et al. 1988). A relationship of KS to lymphatics would be consistent with the common appearance of extensive lymphedema, sometimes even in areas with little or no apparent skin involvement by tumor.

CLINICAL EXPRESSION

Kaposi's sarcoma usually presents on the skin as one or more asymptomatic red, purplish, or brown patches, plaques, or nodules (see table 36.2). Except for the African form, the KS lesions are localized mainly to one or both lower extremities. The disease commonly runs a relatively benign and indolent course for 10 or more years with slow enlargement of the original lesion, and gradual development of additional tumors and progressive edema, most likely related to obstruction of the normal lymphatic channels by tumor. Patients usually die from causes unrelated to KS. In contrast, the clinical manifestations and extent of dissemination seen in patients with underlying immune deficiency tends to relate to the degree of immune compromise, the genetics of the host, and factors that are largely unknown.

KAPOSI'S SARCOMA ASSOCIATED WITH AIDS

EPIDEMIOLOGY AND IMMUNOGENETIC DATA

The form of KS associated with the AIDS outbreak is sometimes referred to as epidemic KS or AIDS/KS. Approximately 96% of all cases of epidemic KS in the United States have been diagnosed in homosexual or bisexual men. The patients range in age from 19 to 64 years, with a mean age of 37.7 (CDC 1986). Very rarely, KS occurs in people with AIDS who are not homosexual or bisexual males. Only about 3% of all reportedly heterosexual intravenous drug users with AIDS and about 9% of Haitian AIDS patients develop this form of KS (CDC 1986; Pitchenik et al. 1983). The reason for this striking difference is still unclear. The observation of KS developing in some homosexual men who apparently are not HIV-infected could suggest that another transmissible agent, most common among homosexual males or selectively transmitted via anal intercourse, is involved in the induction of KS.

Early expression of AIDS/KS has been linked to the major histocompatibility cell-surface antigen, HLA-Dr5, among patients seen in New York City (Rubenstein et al. 1983). A significantly higher percentage of companions of homosexual men studied early in the epidemic expressed this antigen than did a normal control population; Dr5 was about three-fold more frequent among the companions. Dr5 was found with progressively less frequency in successive companions of affected men as the epidemic progressed, until in the most recently studied, the presence of the antigen was found to be less common than in the general population. This observation suggests that genetic factors play an important role in clinical expression of KS. A number of other studies failed to find as significant an association to Dr5, but they may have begun later than did the New York investigations.

CLINICAL FEATURES

The earliest presentation of AIDS/KS is often characterized by multifocal, widespread lesions. Sometimes, multiple lesions appear suddenly over the body surface. The skin, oral mucosa, lymph nodes, and visceral organs such as the submucosa of the gastrointestinal tract, lung, liver, and spleen may be involved. Because of its simultaneous development at multiple sites, the disease is generally not considered to be metastatic from a primary focus, but arising independently as a polyclonal disorder. No evidence for a clonal population of neoplastic cells has been reported in KS.

Systemic manifestations may be present simultaneously, or even precede the appearance of the tumor lesions by several months. These manifestations include persistent or intermittent fever, weight loss, diarrhea, malaise, and fatigue (Friedman-Kien 1981) and usually develop in the context of severe cellular immune deficiency, probably reflecting the presence of unrecognized opportunistic infections.

The sites of disease at presentation are much more varied in AIDS/KS. Widespread involvement is most common; the skin of the face, extremities, and torso are commonly affected, as are the mucous membranes of the oral cavity, especially the palate. Sixty-one percent of the patients have generalized lymphadenopathy at the time of the first examination; in at least some of these, the adenopathy will reflect the reactive lymphadenopathy of early HIV infection (progressive, generalized lymphadenopathy, or PGL), rather than nodal KS. In 45% of the patients in one study, KS lesions were found in one or more sites along the GI tract.

Untreated, almost all patients with KS develop progressive disease. A few localized or isolated mucocutaneous lesions can progress to more numerous and generalized skin, lymph node, and GI tract involvement. The development of pleuropulmonary KS is an ominous sign, usually leading to death within a median of two months (Meduri et al. 1986). The majority of AIDS/KS patients are male. However, rare cases of females with AIDS/KS have been reported. Preliminary data showed that these patients may have a higher incidence of visceral involvement and more aggressive disease (Cheung and Siegal 1989; Desmond-Hellmann et al. 1990).

The natural history of KS is highly variable, and is closely linked to the degree of coexisting cellular immune deficiency. In one study, patients with epidemic

KS who never developed an opportunistic infection had an actuarial survival of 80% at 28 months from diagnosis, as compared to less than 20% survival in those who had an opportunistic infection at some time during the course of their illness (Morris et al. 1982). The occurrence of opportunistic infection indicates a coexistent severe immune deficit.

Laboratory abnormalities are those found commonly in HIV infection, and usually reflect the stage of the viral infection at which KS develops: leukopenia (including lymphopenia) and mild anemia. Thrombocytopenia, as an expression of immune thrombocytopenic purpura (ITP), occurs sometimes as a further complication of the syndrome, but there is no evidence for a selective association of this complication of HIV infection and KS (Morris et al. 1982).

Kaposi's sarcoma can develop, in persons at risk, at almost any stage of HIV infection. Even though KS in an HIV-seropositive person is definitive for AIDS by the surveillance definition of the Centers for Disease Control (CDC), certain individuals fitting this definition through biopsy of skin lesions can remain well, apparently for many years, evidently because the factors that open the door to KS expression do not invariably include clinically significant immune deficiency. There is, however, in AIDS/KS a significant relationship between the absolute numbers of circulating T-helper (CD4, T4) cells and outcome, both with respect to the development of advancing KS and towards susceptibility to opportunistic infections. There is also a statistical correlation between the number of T-helper lymphocytes and the number of granulocytes and erythrocytes (Taylor et al. 1986; Mitsuyasu 1986). Hematocrit and the number of T-helper lymphocytes are useful independent prognostic factors (table 36.3) in this disease (Stahl 1982).

THERAPY FOR AIDS/KS

GENERAL
Therapeutic interventions in most neoplasms are based upon the extent of disease (table 36.4). In AIDS/KS, this approach is often not practical or straightforward, as the more extensive disease is frequently associated with severe immunodeficiency or myelosuppression, both of which limit tolerance for therapy. Patients with only a few cutaneous KS lesions may simply be observed or treated on protocol with experimental agents, exploring the role of antiretroviral drugs or biologic response

Table 36.3
POOR PROGNOSTIC INDICATORS OF AIDS-RELATED KAPOSI'S SARCOMA

1. Visceral involvement
2. Prior or coexistent opportunistic infection
3. Systemic symptoms (fever, night sweats, weight loss greater than or equal to 10% normal body weight, and unexplained diarrhea)
4. Low number of circulating T-helper (CD4) lymphocytes (<250/mm^3)
5. Low T-helper to T-suppressor (CD4:CD8) ratio (<0.2)
6. Low hematocrit (Volberding et al. [1984])
7. Presence of acid labile alpha-interferon (Vadhan-Raj et al. [1986])

modifiers. Multicenter studies, currently in progress under the AIDS Clinical Trials Group (ACTG), are investigating the use of zidovudine (AZT) alone, or in combination with interferon or interleukin-2 (IL2). Preliminary clinical experience seems to indicate that improvement in KS may follow the use of zidovudine alone. This may reflect a drug-mediated improvement in the underlying immune deficiency, and resemble the regression of KS in the context of organ transplantation when immunosuppressive drugs are withdrawn.

RADIATION THERAPY
KS tumors are generally very radiosensitive. Excellent palliation can be obtained with doses not much higher than 20 Gy. Good cosmetic results can be obtained, especially in patients with lymphedema. However, an increased risk of toxicity, especially severe mucositis, has been noted (Chak et al. 1988). The use of forms of radiation with limited potential for tissue penetration, i.e., electron beam, which affects tissues no deeper than 1.5 cm below the surface, appears to be a satisfactory and relatively nontoxic approach to dermal KS (Nobler, Leddy, and Huh 1987).

BIOLOGIC RESPONSE MODIFIERS
Among the biologic response modifiers, recombinant alpha-interferon has been studied most extensively. Alpha-interferon has been evaluated either at low dose (1 million–3 million units/m^2) or higher doses (20 million–36 million units/m^2), given intramuscularly three times weekly (Groopman et al. 1984; Rius et al. 1985; Krown et al. 1986; Kern et al. 1987; Abrams and Volberding 1987; Volberding et al. 1985). The response rates vary from 13% to 42%, with major responses occurring most frequently in patients receiving higher doses, and in those who have had better residual cellular immunity, limited disease and/or absence of other AIDS-related infectious complications (Groopman et al. 1984). Alpha-interferon was approved by the FDA for use in AIDS/KS in November 1988.

CHEMOTHERAPY
In the classic and African forms of KS, vinblastine has been the most commonly used chemotherapeutic agent. A response rate as high as 95% has been reported (Klein et al. 1980). In AIDS/KS, chemotherapy has presented major problems because of the patients' often severe neutropenia and advanced immune deficits; thus, regimens should be tailored to this special problem, using agents that are relatively marrow-sparing. Vinblastine used alone, or alternating with vincristine, produces objective responses in over one-quarter of patients (Laubenstein et al. 1984; Kaplan, Volberding, and Abrams 1986; Mintzer et al. 1985). Other active single agents include etoposide (VP-16), bleomycin, and methotrexate (Laubenstein et al. 1984; Wernz et al. 1986; Minor and Brayer 1986). Adriamycin appears to be one of the most effective agents; it can be used in combination with less myelosuppressive agents such as bleomycin, vincristine, or vinblastine.

Tumor response rates over 80% were initially reported with multidrug regimens; for example, a combination of doxorubicin, bleomycin, vinblastine, and dacarbazine (ABVD) was used early in the outbreak (Hymes et al. 1981). Preliminary results showed that a protocol including vincristine, bleomycin, and doxorubicin achieved superior response rates and duration of response than doxorubicin alone (Gill et al. 1986; Gill et al. 1988). Unfortunately, the majority of responses to chemotherapy (whether with a single agent or in a combination regimen yielding a high initial response rate) have been relatively short-lived, and long-term disease-free survival is rare (Gelmann et al. 1987).

Regimens with significant myelosuppression should be used with greater caution, because the already increased risk of opportunistic infections in this patient population may be compounded by leukopenia. In clinical practice, chemotherapy should probably be reserved for patients with extensive, visceral, or rapidly progressive disease (see table 36.4). Under other conditions, the role of chemotherapy is undefined and patients should be encouraged to participate in ongoing clinical trials, or be observed expectantly. For many, the chief objective is cosmetic improvement, and this can be accomplished by local irradiation.

MALIGNANT LYMPHOMA ASSOCIATED WITH AIDS

EPIDEMIOLOGY

In June 1985, case-definition criteria of AIDS were expanded to include individuals who have high-grade B-cell lymphomas with positive serologic or virologic evidence of infection with HIV (CDC 1985). Prior to that time, epidemiologic data had suggested that there was a statistical increase in the incidence of non-Hodgkin's lymphoma among intravenous drug users (Cheung and Silber 1982; Lowenthal et al. 1988) and among "never-married

men" (Ross et al. 1985). Although the overall incidence of lymphoma was inordinately high in this population group, the most significant increase was in the category of high-grade B-cell disease (Burkitt's lymphoma and immunoblastic sarcoma).

AIDS-related lymphomas have now been reported in intravenous drug abusers and hemophiliacs; however, most cases reported to date have occurred in homosexual men (Levine, Gill, and Rasheed 1986).

CLINICAL EXPRESSION

Although high-grade lymphoma may be the first manifestation of AIDS, a sizable number of these patients have already had another AIDS-defining illness (47%), opportunistic infections (25%), or Kaposi's sarcoma (11%) by the time of the expression of lymphoma (Ziegler et al. 1984). Many patients have developed an AIDS-related lymphoma in the setting of previously recognized AIDS related complex (ARC), or out of a background of persistent, generalized lymphadenopathy (PGL).

HISTOLOGY AND CYTOGENETICS

Approximately 60% to 80% of patients with AIDS-related lymphoma have had B-cell tumors of high-grade pathologic types (Ziegler et al. 1984; Levine et al. 1985). Histologically, these would include small, noncleaved lymphoma, either Burkitt's lymphoma or Burkitt-like, and immunoblastic lymphoma (immunoblastic sarcoma) (National Cancer Institute 1982). Intermediate-grade lymphomas were also reported in a smaller percentage of patients (Ziegler et al. 1984; Kalter et al. 1985; Knowles et al. 1988). In addition, cases of more clinically indolent low-grade lymphoma have been noted in HIV-positive patients (Chak et al. 1988), as have other lymphoproliferative malignancies including multiple myeloma, plasmacytoma, and B-cell acute lymphocytic leukemia (Burkitt's lymphoma, L-3).

Table 36.4
THERAPY GUIDELINES FOR EPIDEMIC KS

DISEASE CHARACTERISTICS	FIRST OPTION	SECOND OPTION
MINIMAL TUMOR EXTENT*, SLOW RATE OF PROGRESSION		
Favorable prognostic factors	Observation	Experimental immunomodulators and/or antiviral drugs; vinblastine/ vincristine
Unfavorable factors [+]	Vinblastine/vincristine or experimental immunomodulators and/or antiviral drugs; investigational agents	Observation
EXTENSIVE DISEASE, RAPID GROWTH		
Favorable prognostic factors	VP-16, Adriamycin, vinca alkaloids	Immunomodulators
Unfavorable factors	VP-16, Adriamycin	Vinca alkaloids or experimental chemotherapy
LOCALLY SYMPTOMATIC LESIONS		
Lymphedema or painful necrotic lesions	Radiation therapy	

* 25 cutaneous lesions, no known visceral involvement
[+] See table 36.3
(Adapted from Volberding [1987]).

Cytogenetic studies of AIDS-related Burkitt's lymphoma have shown a high frequency of t(8;14) and t(8;22) translocations. These associated chromosomal abnormalities occurred as frequently as in ordinary Burkitt's lymphoma. However, an unusual trisomy was observed in three of 13 AIDS-related Burkitt's lymphoma cases (Kalter et al. 1985; Bernheim and Berger 1988).

AIDS-RELATED CNS LYMPHOMA

Lymphoma of the central nervous system (CNS) has been considered an illness definitive for AIDS since the beginning of the epidemic. CNS lymphoma, previously well-described in other states of acquired or congenital immune deficiency, is recognized often to be an opportunistic complication in the immunocompromised host (Frizzera et al. 1980).

AIDS-related CNS lymphoma usually occurs relatively late in the course of HIV infection, and less commonly in patients with marked reduction of CD4+ T cells. The most common presenting features include headache, cranial nerve palsies, other focal neurologic deficits, or a seizure disorder. Altered mental status or a personality change may coexist with neurologic deficits, or be the only initial manifestation of disease (Gill et al. 1985; So, Beckstead, and Davis 1986; Poon, Matoso, and Datta 1988).

Clinically, lymphoma most often has to be differentiated from CNS toxoplasmosis or brain abscess. On radiographic evaluation by CT scanning, most patients have definite space-occupying lesions, which are isodense or hyperdense prior to the administration of contrast media, with varying degrees of edema and mass effect. With double contrast studies, most lesions appear as homogenous or heterogenous contrast enhancing masses. The ring-enhancing mass lesions are very similar to those seen in CNS toxoplasmosis. However, patients with toxoplasmosis are more likely to have multiple, smaller CNS lesions on CT scans (mean 1.5 cm, range 1-4 cm); they also generally have serologic evidence for prior infection with the organism. Those with primary CNS lymphoma tend to present with fewer, larger (mean 4.5 cm, range 3-5 cm) lesions (Gill, Graham, and Boswell et al. 1986). Nevertheless, a definitive diagnosis of lymphoma can only be made by brain biopsy. Lacking this, a trial of empirical therapy for toxoplasmosis, especially in the presence of a positive serologic test for *T. gondii,* may be justified.

Whole brain radiotherapy, with corticosteroids, is the standard treatment for CNS lymphoma, and is effective in some cases. Approximately 50% of patients do not respond to such treatment; their median survival has been less than six months. For the responders, the duration of remission is usually brief (So, Beckstead, and Davis 1986). The role of chemotherapy has yet to be defined, but in people with CNS lymphoma but without HIV infection, the use of drugs capable of crossing the blood-brain barrier (e.g., methotrexate, Ara-C) appears to provide some survival advantage. In rare cases of polyclonal B-cell lymphoproliferative brain disease, treatment with acyclovir has been reported

to be helpful. The causes of death may be lymphoma or multiple opportunistic infections occurring in the brain, as well as systemic sites.

SYSTEMIC AIDS-RELATED LYMPHOMA

The pattern of lymphoma expression often differs from that of the nodes usually involved in PGL. In the latter condition, axillary and inguinal/femoral nodes are preferentially involved, while epitrochlear, retroperitoneal, and intrathoracic nodes are usually not involved. Biopsies in PGL usually reveal polyclonal hyperplasia with germinal center activities (Burns, Wood, and Dorfman 1985). Lymphomatous nodes can also appear at these sites, but clinical clues to a malignant transformation include the development of rapidly enlarging, tender nodes; nodes at sites other than those common to PGL; or an extranodal mass with local symptoms, including intestinal obstruction. In addition to benign reactive adenopathy and lymphoma, such nodes can also harbor mycobacteria and other opportunistic pathogens.

Sixty percent to 70% of patients with AIDS-related lymphoma first present with systemic B symptoms, including fever, night sweats, and/or weight loss. Occasionally, some patients can present with a peripheral neurologic syndrome (Gold, Jimenez, and Zalusky 1988). In the experience of the group at the University of Southern California (USC) with 82 cases, 54 (66%) presented with stage IV disease, while 17 (21%) had stage IE, involving a single extranodal site; a total of 87% presented with extranodal disease (Levine 1988). The sites of extranodal disease are variable. Central nervous system involvement is seen in approximately 30% of those with systemic disease; bone marrow (25%), liver (12%), and gastrointestinal tract (26%) are also commonly involved (Constatine et al. 1982). Unusual sites of disease (e.g., heart, adrenals, rectum, small intestine) have been reported (Burkes et al. 1986; Ioachim et al. 1987; Estrin et al. 1987; Levine, Gill, and Muggia 1987).

THERAPY

Presently, the therapy of choice in AIDS-related non-Hodgkin's lymphomas is undefined; the therapy needs to be tailored to the specific situation. Treatment planning should consider the following problems: (1) these patients usually have high-grade, advanced disease requiring intensive multiagent chemotherapy; (2) because of underlying HIV-induced immunosuppression, the use of multiagent chemotherapy may lead to even greater risk of immune compromise and opportunistic infection (Gill et al. 1987); (3) it is also apparent that CNS prophylaxis must be administered, since about 40% of these patients have had documented CNS lymphoma at some time during the course of illness. Furthermore, in an autopsy series from the USC eight of 12 (66%) patients with systemic lymphoma were found to have involvement of the brain, which had been suspected clinically in only three.

Various chemotherapeutic regimens have been tried without significant success. At USC, a prospective study using a modified combination chemotherapeutic regimen, m-BACOD (methotrexate, bleomycin, Adriamycin [doxorubicin], cyclophosphamide, vincristine, and dexamethasone) was superior to a novel, intensive regimen that included high-dose cytosine arabinoside and high-dose methotrexate (Gill et al. 1987). However, Kalter has also shown that less intensive regimens may be effective (Kalter et al. 1985).

Recently, a group of 26 patients was treated with a variety of standard chemotherapeutic regimens and another group of 38 was treated with a novel regimen consisting of cyclophosphamide, vincristine, methotrexate, etoposide, and cytosine arabinoside (COMET-A) (Kaplan 1989). Although patients treated with COMET-A had a slightly higher complete response rate (58% vs. 46%), they had a significantly shorter median survival (5.2 months) than those treated with standard chemotherapy (11.3 months). In addition, patients receiving the higher doses of cyclophosphamide had significantly shorter survival. These data support the earlier suggestion (Gill et al. 1987) that more aggressive chemotherapy regimens may result in shorter survival.

Further studies are needed to define better tolerated and more efficacious protocols and to evaluate the optimal duration of therapy, the use of cytokines (e.g. granulocyte-macrophage colony-stimulating factor [GM-CSF]) in prevention of myelotoxicity), and the role of CNS prophylaxis.

HODGKIN'S DISEASE

Presently, there is no definitive epidemiologic proof that Hodgkin's disease (HD) is part of the spectrum of opportunistic diseases comprising AIDS. However, it is apparent that patients who are HIV-positive may present with HD, perhaps because the age-related frequency of these two diseases of the lymphoid system tend to overlap. HD is, additionally, a disorder considered in the past to appear in increased frequency among the immunocompromised. Patients with HD and concurrent HIV infection often present with systemic B symptoms and extensive stage III or stage IV disease. Further, unusual disease sites including skin and marrow may be seen (Scheib and Siegal 1985; Schoeppel et al. 1985; Robert and Schneiderman 1984). Such individuals also tolerate chemotherapy poorly; significant neutropenia and opportunistic infections can develop during their treatment (Baer, Anderson, and Wilkinson 1986). While complete remission rates may be similar to those for other patient groups, the median survival of HIV-positive patients has been shorter than usually expected.

OTHER MALIGNANCIES IN HIV-INFECTED INDIVIDUALS

Patients who have undergone organ transplantation, with subsequent use of long-term immunosuppressive agents to prevent graft rejection, are at increased risk for development of lymphomas; KS; squamous cell carcinomas of the cervix, vulva, anus, and skin; basal cell carcinoma of the skin; and lip cancers (Penn 1986). This may be due to the breakdown of normal immune surveillance and additional factors, such as the presence of various oncogenic viruses.

Although KS and high-grade lymphoma have already been linked epidemiologically with AIDS, the other cancers that have been noted in organ transplant recipients have not yet increased statistically in association with the HIV epidemic (Li, Osborn, and Cronin 1982; Daling et al. 1982; Croxson et al. 1984). Anecdotally, squamous cell carcinoma of the anus and cervix (Maiman et al. 1988), head and neck carcinoma, and basal cell carcinoma (Sitz, Kepper, and Johnson 1987) have been reported to occur in HIV-infected individuals. It is possible that such associations will be documented in future years.

In addition, single-case reports of adenosquamous carcinoma of the lung (Irwin, Begardy, and Moore 1984), adenocarcinoma of the colon and pancreas (Kaplan et al. 1987), and cloacagenic carcinoma (Cooper, Patchefsky, and Marks 1979) have been described in HIV-infected individuals. An increased incidence of testicular carcinoma has also been described in young homosexual men (Logothetis, Newell, and Samuels 1985; Kaplan et al. 1987). The significance of these reports is unclear.

OTHER RETROVIRUSES

In addition to HIV, there is very strong evidence that other related retroviruses can play an important role in the induction of neoplastic diseases. Human T-cell, leukemia virus type I (HTLV-I) is the primary etiologic agent of adult T-cell leukemia-lymphoma (Logothetis, Newell, and Samuels 1985). This retrovirus selectively infects and sometimes transforms and immortalizes the CD4 + T cell, leading to expression of receptors for IL2 and substantial IL2 production by the transformed cells. It is thought that an autocrine interaction of IL2 and IL2 receptors on the transformed cells provides them with a survival advantage, leading to lymphoproliferation that becomes monoclonal.

Human T-cell leukemia virus type II (HTLV-II) has been recovered from a number of cases of a helper T-cell variant of hairy-cell leukemia and appears to be important in the pathogenesis of this disorder (Kalyanaraman et al. 1982).

Adult T-cell leukemia-lymphoma (ATLL) was first described in 1977 (Uchiyama et al. 1977), and has been studied in detail in endemic areas in Southern Japan. The HTLV-I and its resulting disease were also found to be endemic in the West Indies and in Africa; it is also seen sporadically worldwide, including cases in Israel, the Pacific basin, and the Southeastern United States, where people of African descent are most often affected.

Patients characteristically present with leukemia, lymphadenopathy, and hepatosplenomegaly. They also have skin lesions showing leukemic infiltration with the morphologically typical leukemia cell of ATLL. This cell is a mature T-lymphocyte with a lobulated nucleus, and is usually of the CD4+ (helper) T-cell phenotype. Some of the earlier cases of ATLL were considered variants of Sezary syndrome. Hypercalcemia and eosinophilia are often seen. The disease is usually aggressive and leads to death in several months.

Recently, cases of HTLV-I infection, plus ATLL, and of coinfection with HIV and HTLV-I, have been described among intravenous drug abusers in New York City (Dosik et al. 1988; Robert-Guroff 1986). In addition, one case of CD8+ (suppressor phenotype) monoclonal lymphoproliferative disease has been described in a patient with coinfection by HIV and HTLV-I. In this so-far unique situation, the lymphoproliferative disorder apparently involved the CD8 cell as the target for transformation and immortalization by HTLV-I, in a setting in which CD4+ cells had been depleted, and may have represented an unusual opportunistic neoplasm of AIDS (Sohn et al. 1986).

Chemotherapy for ATLL has been generally disappointing, although combinations including pentostatin (deoxycoformycin) have shown encouraging results (Daenen et al. 1984).

The role of HTLV-II in human leukemogenesis has not been clear because only a few cases have been reported. HTLV-II was first isolated from a cell line derived from the spleen of a patient with hairy-cell leukemia (Kalyanaraman et al. 1982). Recently, HTLV-II was also isolated in a patient with T-cell prolymphocytic leukemia (Cervantes et al. 1986).

OVERVIEW

The management of AIDS-associated neoplasms is difficult. Care of the underlying disease with antivirals, appropriate prophylactic antimicrobials, patient education, and prompt recognition and intervention at the time of intercurrent opportunistic complications is essential, although this obvious principle is sometimes forgotten in the face of the administration of already complex chemotherapeutic protocols. Physicians managing persons infected with HIV can, to an extent, practice preventive medicine via surveillance for these neoplasms: compulsive history-taking; careful and repeated examination of lymphoid tissue, the entire skin surface, and the oral cavity; and the performance of frequent Pap smears.

REFERENCES

Abrams, D.I., and Volberding, P.A. 1987. Alpha-interferon therapy of AIDS-associated Kaposi's sarcoma. *Semin. Oncol.* 14 (Suppl 2): 43-47.

Ackerman, L.V., and Murray, J.F. 1963. Symposium on Kaposi's sarcoma. Basel: S. Karger.

Afrasiabi, R.; Mitsuyasu, R.T.; and Nishanian, P. et al. 1986. Characterization of a distinct subgroup of high-risk persons with Kaposi's sarcoma and good prognosis who present with normal T4 cell number and T4:T8 ratio and negative HTLV-III/LAW serologic test results. *Am. J. Med.* 81:696-973.

Ahmed, T.; Wormser, G.P.; and Stahl, R.E. et al. 1987. Malignant lymphomas in a population at risk for acquired immune deficiency syndrome. *Cancer* 60:719-23.

Baer, D.M.; Anderson, E.T.; and Wilkinson, L.S. 1986. Acquired immune deficiency syndrome in homosexual men with Hodgkin's disease. *Am. J. Med.* 80:738-40.

Barre-Sinoussi, F.; Chermann, J.C.; and Rey, F. et al. 1983. Isolation of T-lymphotropic retrovirus from a patient at risk for acquired immunodeficiency syndrome (AIDS). *Science* 220:868-71.

Beckstead, J.H.; Wood, G.S.; and Fletcher, V. 1985. Evidence for the origin of Kaposi's sarcoma from lymphatic endothelium. *Am. J. Pathol.* 119: 294-300.

Bernheim, A., and Berger, R. 1988. Cytogenetic studies of Burkitt's lymphoma-leukemia in patients with acquired immunodeficiency syndrome. *Cancer Genet. Cytogenet.* 32:67-74.

Burkes, R.L.; Meyer, P.R.; and Gill, P.S. et al. 1986. Rectal lymphoma in homosexual men. *Arch. Intern. Med.* 146: 913-15.

Burns, B.F.; Wood, G.S.; and Dorfman, R.F. 1985. The varied histopathology of lymphadenopathy in the homosexual male. *Am. J. Surg. Pathol.* 9:287-97.

Centers for Disease Control Update. 1986. Acquired immunodeficiency syndrome—United States. *M.M.W.R.* 35:757-65.

Centers for Disease Control. 1985. Revision of the case definition of acquired immunodeficiency syndrome for national reporting—United States. *Ann. Intern. Med.* 103: 402-403.

Cervantes, J.; Hussain, S.; and Jensen, F. et al. 1986. T-prolymphocytic leukemia associated with human T-cell lymphotropic virus II. *Clin. Res.* 34:454A.

Chak, L.Y.; Gill, P.S.; and Levine, A. et al. 1988. Radiation therapy for acquired immunodeficiency syndrome-related Kaposi's sarcoma. *J. Clin. Oncol.* 6:863-67.

Cheung, T.W., and Silber, R. 1982. Malignant lymphoma among drug addicts (Abstr). *Proc. Am. Soc. Clin. Oncol.* 1:4.

Cheung, T.W., and Siegal, F. 1989. Kaposi's sarcoma in women with AIDS (Abstr). *The Fifth International Conference on AIDS.* M.B.P. 297.

Constantino, A.; West, T.E.; and Gupta, M. et al. 1987. Primary cardiac lymphoma in a patient with acquired immune deficiency syndrome. *Cancer* 60:2801-2805.

Cooper, H.S.; Patchefsky, A.S.; and Marks, G. 1979. Cloacagenic carcinoma of the anorectum in homosexual men: an observation of four cases. *Dis. Colon Rectum* 22:557-58.

Croxson, T.; Chabon, A.B.; and Rorat, E. et al. 1984. Intraepithelial carcinoma of the anus in homosexual men. *Dis. Colon Rectum* 27:325-30.

Daenen, S.; Rojer, R.A.; and Smit, J.W. et al. 1984. Successful chemotherapy with deoxycoformycin in adult T-cell lymphoma-leukemia. *Br. J. Haematol.* 58:723-27.

Daling, J.R.; Weiss, N.S.; and Klopfenstein, L.L. et al. 1982. Correlation of homosexual behavior and the incidence of anal cancer. *JAMA* 247:1988-90.

DeAngelis, L.M.; Yahalom, J.; and Rosenblum, et al. 1987. Primary CNS lymphoma: managing patients with spontaneous and AIDS-related disease. *Oncology* 1:52-59.

Desmond-Hellmann S.D.; Mbidde, E.K.; and Kizito, A. et al. 1990. The epidemiology and clinical features of Kaposi's sarcoma in African women with HIV infection (Abstr). *The Sixth International Conference on AIDS.* S.B. 508.

Dosik, H.; Denic, S.; and Patel, N. et al. 1988. Adult T-cell leukemia- lymphoma in Brooklyn. *JAMA* 259:2255-57.

Estrin, H.M.; Farhi, D.C.; and Ament, A.A. et al. 1987. Ileoscopic diagnosis of malignant lymphoma of the small bowel in acquired immunodeficiency syndrome. *Gastroint. Endo.* 33: 390-91.

Friedman-Kien, A.E. et al. 1981. Disseminated Kaposi-like sarcoma syndrome in young homosexual men. *J. Am. Acad. Dermatol.* 5:468-71.

Frizzera, G.; Rosai, J.; and Dehner, L.P. et al. 1980. Lymphoreticular disorders in primary immunodeficiency: new findings based on an up-to-date histologic classification of 35 cases. *Cancer* 46:692-99.

Gallo, R.C.; Sarin, P.S.; and Gelmann, E.P. et al. 1983. Isolation of human T-cell leukemia virus in acquired immune deficiency syndrome (AIDS). *Science* 220:865-67.

Gelmann, E.P.; Longo, D.; and Lane, H.C. et al. 1987. Combination chemotherapy of disseminated Kaposi's sarcoma in patients with the acquired immune deficiency syndrome. *Am. J. Med.* 82: 456-62.

Gill, P.S., and Levine, A.M. 1988. HIV-related malignant lymphoma: clinical aspects, treatment, and pathogenesis. *Cancer Invest.* 6:413-16.

Gill, P.S.; Graham, R.A.; and Boswell, W. et al. 1986. A comparison of imaging, clinical, and pathologic aspects of space occupying lesions within the brain in patients with acquired immune deficiency syndrome. *Am. J. Physiol. Imaging* 1:134-41.

Gill, P.S.; Levine, A.M.; and Krailo, M. et al. 1987. AIDS-related malignant lymphoma: results of prospective treatment trials. *J. Clin. Oncol.* 5:1322-28.

Gill, P.S.; Deyton, L.R.; and Rarick, M. et al. 1986. Treatment of epidemic Kaposi's sarcoma (EKS) with vincristine, bleomycin, and low dose Adriamycin (Abstr). *Blood* 68(Suppl 1):126a.

Gill, P.S.; Levine, A.M.; and Meyer, P.R. et al. 1985. Primary central nervous system lymphoma in homosexual men: clinical, immunologic and pathologic features. *Am. J. Med.* 78:742-48.

Gill, P.S.; Krailo, M.; and Slater, L. et al. 1988. Randomized trial of ABV (Adriamycin, bleomycin, vincristine) vs. A in advanced Kaposi's sarcoma (KS): preliminary results (Abstr). *Proc. Am. Soc. Clin. Oncol.* 7:3.

Gold, J.E.; Jimenez, E.; and Zalusky, R. 1988. Human immunodeficiency virus-related lymphoreticular malignancies and peripheral neurologic disease. *Cancer* 61:2318-24.

Gottlieb, M.S.; Schroff, R.; and Schanker, H.M. et al. 1981. *Pneumocystitis carinii* pneumonia and mucosal candidiasis in previously healthy homosexual men: evidence of a new acquired cellular immunodeficiency. *N. Engl. J. Med.* 305:1425-31.

Groopman, J.E.; Gottlieb, M.S.; and Goodman, J. et al. 1984. Recombinant alpha-2 interferon therapy for Kaposi's sarcoma in the acquired immunodeficiency syndrome. *Ann. Intern. Med.* 100:671-76.

Harper, M.E.; Kaplan, M.H.; and Marselle, L.M. et al. 1986. Concomitant infection with HTLV-I and HTLV-III in a patient with T8 lymphoproliferative disease. *N. Engl. J. Med.* 315:1073-78.

Harwood, A.R.; Osoba, D.; and Hofstader, S.L. et al. 1971. Kaposi's sarcoma in recipients of renal transplants. *Am. J. Med.* 67:759-65.

Hymes, K.; Cheung, T.; and Greene, J.B. et al. 1981. Kaposi's sarcoma in homosexual men. *Lancet* II:598-600.

Ioachim, H.L.; Weinstein, M.A.; and Robbins, R.D. et al. 1987. Primary anorectal lymphoma: a new manifestation of acquired immune deficiency syndrome (AIDS). *Cancer* 60:1449-53.

Irwin, L.E.; Begandy, M.K.; and Moore, T.M. 1984. Adenosquamous carcinoma of the acquired immunodeficiency syndrome. *Ann. Intern. Med.* 100:158.

Kalter, S.P.; Riggs, S.A.; and Cabanillas, F. et al. 1985. Aggressive non-Hodgkin's lymphomas in immunocompromised homosexual males. *Blood* 66:655-59.

Kalyanaraman, V.S.; Sarngadharan, M.G.; and Robert-Guroff, M. et al. 1982. A new subtype of human T-cell leukemia virus (HTLV-II) associated with a T-cell variant of hairy cell leukemia. *Science* 218:571-73.

Kaplan, L.D.; Abrams, D.I.; and Feigal, E. et al. 1989. AIDS-associated non-Hodgkin's lymphoma in San Francisco. *JAMA* 261:719-24.

Kaplan, M.H.; Susin, M.; and Pahwa, S.G. et al. 1987. Neoplastic complications of HTLV-III infection: lymphomas and solid tumors. *Am. J. Med.* 82:389-96.

Kaplan, M.H.; Volberding, P.; and Abrams, D. 1986. Treatment of Kaposi's sarcoma in acquired immunodeficiency syndrome with an alternating vincristine-vinblastine regimen. *Cancer Treat. Rep.* 70: 1121-22.

Kaposi, M. 1872. Idiopathiches multiple pigment sarcom der Hant. *Arch. Dermatol. Syphil.* ([Berlin]) 4: 265-73.

Kern, P.; Meigel, W.; and Racz, P. et al. 1987. Interferon-alpha in the treatment of AIDS-associated Kaposi's sarcoma. *Onkologie* 10:50-52.

Klein, E.; Schwartz, R.A.; and Loar, Y. et al. 1980. Treatment of Kaposi's sarcoma with vinblastine. *Cancer* 45:427-31.

Klepp, O.; Dahl, O; and Stenwig, J.T. 1978. Association of Kaposi's sarcoma and prior immunosuppressive therapy. *Cancer* 42:2626-30.

Knowles, D.M.; Chamulak, G.A.; and Subar, M. et al. 1988. Lymphoid neoplasia associated with acquired immunodeficiency syndrome (AIDS). *Ann. Intern. Med. Quar.* 1:65-68.

Krown, S.E.; Real, F.X.; and Vadhan-Raj, S. et al. 1986. Kaposi's sarcoma and the acquired immune deficiency syndrome. *Cancer* 57:1662-65.

Laubenstein, L.J.; Krigel, R.L.; and Odajank, C.M. et al. 1984. Treatment of epidemic Kaposi's sarcoma (EKS) with etoposide or a combination of doxorubicin, bleomycin, and vinblastine. *J. Clin. Oncol.* 2:1115-20.

Levine, A.M.; Gill, P.S.; and Rasheed, S. 1986. AIDS-related B-cell lymphoma. In Broder, S. ed. *AIDS* p. 233. New York: Marcel Dekker.

Levine, A.M.; Gill, P.S.; and Meyer, P.R. et al. 1985. Retrovirus and malignant lymphoma in homosexual men. *JAMA* 254:1921-25.

Levine, A.M.; Gill, P.S.; and Muggia, F. 1987. Malignancies in the acquired immunodeficiency syndrome. *Curr. Prob. Cancer* 11(4):209-55.

Levine, A.M. 1988. Reactive and neoplastic lymphoproliferative disorders and other miscellaneous cancers associated with HIV infection. In DeVita, V.T.; Hellman, S.; and Rosenberg, S.A. *AIDS.* p. 263-76. Philadelphia: J.B. Lippincott.

Li, F.P.; Osborn, D.; and Cronin, C.M. 1982. Anorectal squamous carcinoma in two homosexual men. *Lancet* II:391.

Logothetis, C.J.; Newell, G.Y.; and Samuels, M.L. 1985. Testicular cancer in homosexual men with cellular immune deficiency: report of two cases. *J. Urol.* 133:484-86.

Lowenthal, D.A.; Straus, D.J.; and Campell, S.W. et al. 1988. AIDS-related lymphoid neoplasia: the Memorial Hospital experience. *Cancer* 61:2325-37.

Lozada, F.; Silverman, S. Jr.; and Conant, M. 1982. New outbreak of oral tumors, malignancies, and infectious disease strikes young male homosexuals. *Calif. Dent. Assoc. J.* 10:39-42.

Maiman, M.; Fruchter, R.G.; and Serur, E. et al. 1988. Prevalence of human immune deficiency virus in a colposcopy clinic. *JAMA* 260:2214.

Meduri, G.U.; Stover, D.E.; and Lee, M. et al. 1986. Pulmonary Kaposi's sarcoma in the acquired immune deficiency syndrome. *Am. J. Med.* 81:11-18.

Minor, D.R., and Brayer, T. 1986. Velban and methotrexate combination chemotherapy for epidemic Kaposi's sarcoma (Abstr). *Proc. Am. Soc. Clin. Oncol.* 5:1.

Mintzer, D.M.; Real, F.X.; and Jovino, L. et al. 1985. Treatment of Kaposi's sarcoma and thrombocytopenia with vincristine in patients with acquired immunodeficiency syndrome. *Ann. Intern. Med.* 102:200-202.

Mitsuyasu, R.T.; Glaspy, I.; and Taylor, J.M. et al. 1986. Heterogeneity of epidemic Kaposi's sarcoma: implications for therapy. *Cancer* 57 (Suppl 8):1657-61.

Morris, L.; Distenfeld, A.; and Amorosi, E. et al. 1982. Autoimmune thrombocytopenic purpura in homosexual men. *Ann. Intern. Med.* 96: 714-17.

Myers, B.D.; Kessler, E.; and Levi, D. et al. 1974. Kaposi's sarcoma in kidney transplant recipients. *Arch. Intern. Med.* 133: 307-11.

Nobler, M.P.; Leddy, M.E.; and Huh, S.H. 1987. The impact of palliative irradiation on the management of patients with acquired immune deficiency syndrome. *J. Clin. Oncol.* 5:107-12.

Non-Hodgkin's Lymphoma Pathologic Classification Project. 1982. National Cancer Institute sponsored study of classifications of non-Hodgkin's lymphomas: summary and description of a working formulation for clinical usage. *Cancer* 49:2112-35.

Penn, I. 1978. Immunosuppression and malignant diseases. In Towmey, J.J., and Good, R.A. eds. *Immunopathogenesis of lymphatic neoplasm. Comprehensive immunology.* vol. 4. pp. 223-37. New York: Plenum Press.

Penn, I. 1986. Cancers of the anogenital region in renal transplant recipients. *Cancer* 58:611-16.

Pitchenik, A.E.; Fischl, M.A.; and Dickinson, G.M. et al. 1983. Opportunistic infectious and Kaposi's sarcoma among Haitians: evidence of a new acquired immunodeficiency state. *Ann. Intern. Med.* 98:277-84.

Poiesz, B.J.; Ruscetti, F.W.; and Gazdar, A.F. et al. 1980. Detection and isolation of type C retrovirus particles from fresh and cultured lymphocytes of a patient with cutaneous T-cell lymphoma. *Proc. Natl. Acad. Sci. (USA)* 77:7415-19.

Pollack, M.S.; Safai, B.; and Dupont, B. 1983. HLA-Dr5 and Dr-2 are susceptibility factors for acquired immunodeficiency syndrome with Kaposi's sarcoma in different ethnic subpopulations. *Dis. Markers* 1:135-9.

Poon, T.P.; Matoso, I.M.; and Datta, B. 1988. Ultrastructural study of a primary cerebral lymphoma in acquired immunodeficiency syndrome. *N.Y. Med. Quar.* 1:65-68.

Rios, A.; Mansell, P.W.A.; and Newell, G.R. et al. 1985. Treatment of acquired immunodeficiency syndrome-related Kaposi's sarcoma with lymphoblastoid interferon. *J. Clin. Oncol.* 3:506-511.

Robert, N.J., and Schneiderman, H. 1984. Hodgkin's disease and the acquired immunodeficiency syndrome (letter). *Ann. Intern. Med.* 101:142-43.

Robert-Guroff, M.; Weiss, S.H.; and Giron, J.A. et al. 1986. Prevalence of antibodies to HTLV-I, II, and III in intravenous drug abusers from an AIDS endemic region. *JAMA* 255:3133-37.

Rosenblatt, J.D.; Golde, D.W.; and Wachsman et al. 1986. A second case of HTLV-II associated with atypical hairy-cell leukemia. *N. Engl. J. Med.* 315:372-77.

Ross, R.K.; Dworsky, R.L.; and Paganini-Hill, A. et al. 1985. Non-Hodgkin's lymphomas in never-married men in Los Angeles. *Br. J. Cancer* 52:785-87.

Rubenstein, P.; de Cordoba, S.; and Oestricher, R. et al. 1984. Immunogenetics and predisposition to Kaposi's sarcoma. In Groopman, J. ed. *Acquired immune deficiency syndrome.* pp. 309-18. New York: Alan R. Liss.

Rubinstein, O.; Walker, N.; and Moller, N. et al. 1983. Immunogenetic aspects of epidemic Kaposi's sarcoma in homosexual men. In Friedman-Kien, A., and Laubenstein, L. eds. *AIDS: the epidemic of Kaposi's sarcoma and opportunistic infections.* pp. 139-46. New York: Masson.

Salahuddin, S.Z.; Nakamura, S.; and Biberfeld et al. 1988. Angiographic properties of Kaposi's sarcoma derived cells after long-term culture *in vitro. Science* 242:430-33.

Scheib, R.G., and Siegal, R.S. 1985. Atypical Hodgkin's disease and the acquired immunodeficiency syndrome (letter). *Ann. Intern. Med.* 102:68-70.

Schoeppel, S.L.; Hoppe, R.T.; and Dorfman, F.T. et al. 1985. Hodgkin's disease in homosexual men with generalized lymphadenopathy. *Ann. Intern. Med.* 102:68-70.

Siegal F.P.; Lopez, C.; and Hammer G.S. et al. 1981. Severe acquired immunodeficiency in male homosexuals, manifested by chronic perianal ulcerative herpes simplex lesions. *N. Engl. J. Med.* 305:1439-44.

Siegal, F.P. 1988. Immunodeficiency diseases and thymoma. In Givel, J-Cl. ed. *Surgery of the thymus.* ch. 15. Heidelberg: Springer-Verlag.

Siegal, F.P. 1987. Immune deficiency of AIDS. In Wormser, G.P.; Stahl, R.E.; and Bottone, E.J. eds. *Acquired immune deficiency syndrome.* pp. 304-30. New Jersey: Noyes.

Sillman, F.H., and Sedlis, A. 1987. Anogenital papillomavirus infection and neoplasia in immunodeficient women. *Obstet. Gynecol. Clin. North Am.* 14:537.

Sitz, K.V.; Keppen, M.; and Johnson, D.F. 1987. Metastatic basal cell carcinoma in acquired immunodeficiency syndrome-related complex. *JAMA* 257:340-43.

So, Y.T.; Beckstead, J.H.; and Davis, R.L. 1986. Primary central nervous system lymphoma in acquired immune deficiency syndrome: a clinical and pathological study. *Ann. Neurol.* 20:566-72.

Sohn, C.C.; Blayne, D.W.; and Misset, J.L. et al. 1986. Leukopenic chronic T-cell leukemia mimicking hairy-cell leukemia: association with human retroviruses. *Blood* 67:949-56.

Specter, B.D.; Perry, G.S. III; and Good, R.A. et al. 1978. Immunodeficiency diseases and malignancies. In Towmey, J.J., and Good, R.A. eds. *Immunopathogenesis of lymphatic neoplasm. Comprehensive immunology* vol. 4. pp. 203-22. New York: Plenum Press.

Stahl, R.E.; Friedman-Kien, A.; and Dubin, R. et al. 1982. Immunologic abnormalities in homosexual men: relationship to Kaposi's sarcoma. *Am. J. Med.* 73:171-78.

Subar, M.; Chamulak, G.; and Dalla-Favera, R. et al. 1986. Clinical and pathologic characteristics of AIDS-associated Hodgkin's disease (Abstr). *Blood* 68:135a.

Tayler, J.; Afrasiabi, R.; and Fahey, J.L. et al. 1986. Prognostic significant classification of immune changes in AIDS with Kaposi's sarcoma. *Blood* 67:666-71.

Taylor, J.F.; Templeton, A.C.; and Vogel, C.L. et al. 1971. Kaposi's sarcoma in Uganda: a clinicopathologic study. *Int. J. Cancer* 8:122-35.

Uchiyama, T.; Yodoi, J.; and Sagawa, K. et al. 1977. Adult T-cell leukemia: clinical and hematologic features of 16 cases. *Blood* 50:481-92.

Vadhan-Raj, S.; Wong, G.; and Gnecco, C. et al. 1986. Immunological variables as predictors of prognosis in patients with Kaposi's sarcoma and the acquired immunodeficiency syndrome. *Cancer Res.* 46:417-25.

Volberding, P.A. 1987. The role of chemotherapy for epidemic Kaposi's sarcoma. *Semin. Oncol.* 14 (Suppl 3):23-26.

Volberding, P.A.; Kaslow, K.; and Bille, M. et al. 1984. Prognostic factors in staging Kaposi's sarcoma in the acquired immune deficiency syndrome (Abstr). *Proc. Am. Soc. Clin. Oncol.* 3:51.

Volberding, P.A.; Abrams, D.I.; and Conant, M. et al. 1985. Vinblastine therapy for Kaposi's sarcoma in the acquired immunodeficiency syndrome. *Ann. Intern. Med.* 103:335-38.

Wernz, J.; Laubenstein, L.; and Hymes, K. et al. 1986. Chemotherapy and assessment of response in epidemic Kaposi's sarcoma with bleomycin/Velban (Abstr). *Proc. Am. Soc. Clin. Oncol.* 5:5.

Yarboro, J.W. ed. 1987. Neoplasms in AIDS: the multidisciplinary approach to treatment. *Semin. Oncol.* 14 (Suppl 3):2.

Ziegler, J.L.; Beckstead, J.A.; and Volberding, P.A. et al. 1984. Non-Hodgkin's lymphoma in 90 homosexual men: relationship to generalized lymphadenopathy and acquired immunodeficiency syndrome (AIDS). *N. Engl. J. Med.* 311:565-70.

Chapter 37

SUPPORTIVE CARE
AND REHABILITATION OF
THE CANCER PATIENT

Robert J. McKenna, Sr., M.D.

Robert J. McKenna, Sr., M.D.
Clinical Professor of Surgery
Los Angeles County Medical Center
University of Southern California Medical School
Los Angeles, California

INTRODUCTION

In 1884, Ulysses S. Grant was diagnosed with throat cancer. He died nine months later without any attempt having been made at cure. Newspaper coverage of his long illness was uniformly gloomy, reinforcing the public perception of cancer as a fatal disease. The attitude toward Grant's illness is in sharp contrast with that of another U.S. president, 100 years later. Ronald Reagan's colon cancer was treated surgically with minimal inconvenience, a limited time away from work, and no residual disability. A team of specialists provided modern surgical therapy and excellent supportive care, enabling the patient to continue his presidential duties without restrictions. The public attitude was generally optimistic, despite some efforts by the press to play up fear of the illness.

In the United States today, modern medical care has made it possible to cure cancers in the majority (51%) of those with the disease. There is hope that, by the year 2000, the cure rate will reach 75%. More than 5 million Americans are alive today with a history of cancer, 3 million of them five years or more after their diagnosis. This statistic highlights a major contrast to the grim outlook at the turn of the century, when the disease was almost invariably fatal. However, large segments of the population today are skeptical about the efficacy of cancer treatment, in part because they have not kept abreast of medical advances, and in part because they have known people whose cancers have not been cured. Less-educated and less-affluent people may not obtain competent medical care for their cancer—or may not seek it. Others consult quacks or faith healers who promise a cure without complications.

QUALITY OF LIFE

Today's advanced therapies must be accompanied by supportive care in order to maintain quality of life. Physicians may concentrate all their expertise on the scientific application of modern oncological knowledge, and forget that emotional and psychosocial support are also essential. Such treatment may result in failure to obtain maximum rehabilitation for each and every patient. Oncologists must always be aware that their patients are human beings with individual goals, dreams, hopes, and concerns. The oncologist's role is not only to deliver the best quality cancer treatment, but also to consider the disease's impact on each patient's lifestyle, and to assist in returning the patient to his or her pretreatment state, or to a state as close as possible to it.

Simply asking a question such as "How does the patient feel?" is not a valid means of assessing a cancer patient's quality of life. The assessment must take into account issues such as symptoms, the side effects of treatment, physical functioning, psychological distress, social interaction, sexuality, self-image, and satisfaction with care. Moreover, these issues are not static, but change with the stage of the cancer, the passage of time, and the complications in morbidity associated with the disease process. Thus, no simple or single instrument can measure quality of life. The matrix shown in fig. 37.1 is a good expression of this aspect of care. Four dimensions are listed: physical side effects, which may be both general and a result of treatment; functional status, both personal and social; psychological morbidity, expressed in both distress and depression; and coping and/or satisfaction in work or social relationships.

Yancik and Yates (1986) emphasize that the care of cancer patients must encompass not only the patients' serious illness but also their social and psychological needs. They suggest that the use of toxic drugs, high dosages, and even some surgery and hospitalizations might be prevented if physicians treating cancer were better able to predict and monitor the course of the disease as it affects the patients' quality of life.

QUALITY OF LIFE DIMENSIONS

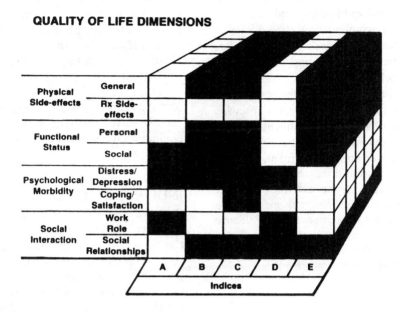

Fig. 37.1. Quality-of-life matrix includes dimensions of physical side effects, functional status, psychological morbidity, and social interaction. (Adapted from: Yancik and Yates [1986].)

CANCER REHABILITATION

GOALS

Almost all patients who have been treated for cancer need some measure of rehabilitation. A reason for this is the increase in survival. Nearly half of all cancer patients can now expect to live at least five more years, and many live out a normal lifespan. Even for those who are not so fortunate, rehabilitation is an integral part of good, comprehensive care.

In 1972, the National Cancer Institute identified four objectives for cancer rehabilitation: psychological support upon diagnosis; optimal physical functioning after treatment; vocational counseling, when indicated; and, the ultimate goal of cancer treatment and control, optimal social functioning. In its broadest sense, the goal of cancer rehabilitation is to enable patients to achieve as normal and full a life as possible in light of the effects of the disease and its treatment. Rehabilitation should begin upon diagnosis, continue throughout treatment, and be an integral part of follow-up. Attention must always be given to the physical, psychological, social, and vocational needs of the patient—to the quality of survival rather than to survival alone.

THE REHABILITATION TEAM

Rehabilitation is a team effort focusing on the whole person rather than on a cancer at a specific site, although the site is an important factor and will necessarily direct the emphasis of the rehabilitation plan. The physician directing the treatment team should be the one closest to the patient, either the primary physician, the oncologist, or another responsible physician. The support team may include oncology nurses, a psychologist or other mental health professional, a physiatrist, a physical therapist, a speech therapist, an occupational therapist, a social worker, home care nurses, clergy, and lay volunteers. The rehabilitation effort may also include ongoing counseling, hospice services, and other long- or short-term programs of supportive care. Not every patient needs the team's services, because patients' requirements, desires, and personal resources vary. However, the physician should be alert to any need for services, particularly when the cancer has not been cured.

Although effective rehabilitation recently has become more feasible, many patients still encounter difficulties in securing it. Physicians may be more familiar with diagnosis and treatment than with rehabilitation; community hospitals may lack the full complement of personnel for a team approach; social workers may be unaware of specific appropriate resources; and, in general, the readaptation needs of the cancer patient may be understood poorly. Effective coordination of services is essential for maximum rehabilitation and, in this respect, state and federal agencies are of little help. They traditionally assign a low priority to cancer patients, because of the stigma once attached to the disease, and because of a failure to recognize that most cancer patients now have a greatly improved outlook.

INTERVENTIONS

The rehabilitation goals must be realistic and individualized for each patient. They depend on the patient's functional abilities and the stage of the disease. Interventions may be preventive, restorative, supportive, or palliative.

Preventive interventions lessen the impact of an anticipated disability through patient training and education; for example, teaching a woman about to undergo a mastectomy the exercises she will need to perform after the operation to prevent swelling and loss of arm function. *Restorative* procedures aim to restore, as closely as possible, the patient's state before the treatment; for example, breast reconstruction following mastectomy. *Supportive* rehabilitation interventions may be provided for the patient who has a disabling condition as a result of the cancer and its treatment, who can learn to cope with that condition, and who retains control over many or most of the activities of daily living; for example, teaching esophageal speech to a patient who has had a total laryngectomy. *Palliative* interventions provide comfort, assistance in everyday functioning, and emotional support in those cases where cancer is advanced and recovery is not expected.

PATIENTS

The most fortunate patients are those with an early stage of cancer, who can be treated successfully, who have minimal disability, and who live out a normal lifespan free of recurrence. All of these people live in some fear of the unknown and with the major apprehension that the cancer may recur. They are, indeed, at risk for a second cancer and need continued checkups. Most patients fall into this category.

A second group is made up of people who have curable cancer from an anatomic standpoint, who have a total response to treatment, and who have an interval of time free from cancer before experiencing a recurrence, either locally or at a distant site. Some individuals in this group can be cured by further treatment and live out a normal lifespan. Others fail to respond and develop progressive disease and eventually die. Crises occur at all stages in the course of their treatment. These patients need major psychological support that emphasizes the hope that the treatment side effects will be short-lived.

Patients in a third group are those treated for cancer and cured, only to develop a second (or a third or fourth) cancer. Some of these later cancers are related to the lifestyle that caused the first; for example, tobacco-induced cancers in the oral cavity, larynx and lung, or alcohol-induced cancers in the oral cavity. Other second cancers are bilateral disease in the breast, which occurs in up to 20% of women over a 30-year follow-up, and multicentric disease in the colon, which develops frequently during the follow-up after the first cancer. Patients in this group are strong candidates for curative treatment and often tolerate their later cancer well. They are seasoned fighters in the battle against their malignancy and are some of the best participants in volunteer programs to help others with newly diagnosed cancer. This group will probably increase in size as more people are cured of their first cancer and as they live longer.

Patients in the last group present incurable disease at the onset and require palliative and supportive therapy to correct the complications caused by their cancer. It is often difficult for these individuals to accept their diagnosis. Such patients should always be offered worthwhile treatment modalities when a good probability of response exists. The aim should be an extension of useful quality of life at reasonable cost. Discomfort can usually be reduced and suffering minimized. Multidisciplinary care is especially appropriate for patients in this group.

INDIVIDUALIZED CASES

Each of the different sites at which cancer occurs presents specific problems because of the function of the body part involved and because of what it takes to cope with physiological and cosmetic changes. The problems of a woman who loses a breast will differ from those of a man who loses his rectum. Skin cancer is rarely a significant problem unless it is very advanced; it is easily treated with minimal cost and often without hospitalization. In contrast, cancer of the pancreas is almost never curable, has a fairly rapid progression, and is often associated with severe nutritional problems and pain. The experiences of the vast majority of people with cancer fall somewhere between these extremes. The need for individualization, both in treatment and in support systems, cannot be overemphasized. Some concepts that should be stressed are:

1. Individuals should be treated individually, with the right to accept or refuse offered treatment. (If the patient is a child, the parents should have this right.)

2. They may choose to discuss their cancer with others, or may refuse to do so if they prefer.

3. They should remain free of the stigma of cancer as a "dread disease."

4. They should be accepted for what they are and what they were before the diagnosis, not as patients who have or who have had cancer.

THE MEANING OF CANCER

Patients with cancer feel the disease's impact in many different ways and at many different times. Nevertheless, as a group they share some common, important concerns: the threatened loss of life; the threat posed by the disease to relationships with others; fears about loss of independence, job, and career; and concern about the integrity of the body and its functions. These fears, centering first on the threat to life itself and then on the quality of life, constitute the basic meaning of cancer for the patient. A patient's age and the extent to which the disease threatens life goals and activities modify that meaning. To an older person, cancer may predominantly mean becoming a burden to others in the course of a serious illness; for a younger patient, the disease threatens career, sexuality, and family life. Older individuals may display greater depression, while younger ones may show more anger and be less cooperative as an expression of their anger. At any age, disruption of function, even when temporary, becomes disturbing if it involves valued life activities or forces a change in goals.

Each individual's reactions to his or her cancer and treatment should be viewed as a sequence of related events. The sequence begins with the first appearance of symptoms. It continues through the realization that the diagnosis is cancer, to treatment, convalescence, and cure—or recurrence and death. Predicting a patient's reactions is very difficult and requires considerable knowledge of the individual's basic behavior patterns and of his or her ability to develop compensatory patterns.

Patients' behavior and emotions are usually appropriate to their view of what is happening and are designed to minimize or repair the damage of events. For example, delay in seeking help may be the patient's way of averting injury. Many who suspect cancer procrastinate in seeking care, maintaining that their symptoms are not real. They deny their symptoms to avoid the anxiety that acknowledging them would produce. People most likely to delay in seeking help are those whose attitudes toward cancer are characterized by shame, guilt, or extreme fear; the elderly; those with a family history of cancer; those who are uneducated or have a language barrier; and those who have no personal physician.

Some patients take their cancer as a sign of personal weakness or failure. Others believe that their stressful lives caused their disease, or that it is a punishment for some past wrongdoing. Such feelings may be compounded by friends' and families' uneasiness in dealing with cancer, leading to increased isolation of the patient.

THE PSYCHOSOCIAL IMPACT OF CANCER AND CANCER TREATMENT

STRESS

In a paper written in 1951 that has become a classic in the oncological literature, Arthur Sutherland emphasized that a cancer patient is a person under a special and severe form of stress: the threat of a disabling disease, mutilation or loss by surgery of an important body part, or death (Sutherland 1951). Stress due to cancer can disrupt important patterns of adaptation, defined by Sutherland as the beliefs and behavior designed to bring the individual's physical and emotional needs into harmony with the demands of the environment. When such patterns are threatened, much anxiety is generated and patients may believe that they are unable to meet environmental demands or fulfill their emotional needs. A loss of self-esteem commonly results.

In a study conducted by the California Division of the American Cancer Society (American Cancer Society 1979), the time period immediately following diagnosis was reported as the highest period of stress for 30.5% of patients. The period of hospitalization and initial treatment was the most upsetting for 16.7%; 11.1% reported release from the hospital as the most stressful. Some who had coped well with stress during the diagnosis and treatment phases experienced a delayed reaction six months or more after the end of treatment. They expressed this reaction by depression or heavy drinking.

A lot of stress is also due to the uncertain outcome after cancer. The person who has had cancer is a life-long patient, subject to the continuing threat of recurrence, to complications of the treatment, and to sequelae from altered anatomy and physiology. Some individuals are unable to overcome concern about their illness and remain physically and psychologically uncomfortable whenever the disease is discussed, even when treatment has been successful. Others are afraid to return to their normal activities and withdraw to their home environments.

TREATMENT CONCERNS

The average patient knows little about radiation therapy before the treatment is recommended, but almost all have strong preconceived notions about it. Some of these are erroneous. For example, many patients believe that they will lose hair all over the body, although only one area is being treated. They are understandably apprehensive about nausea, skin effects, loss of energy and appetite, and, depending on the site treated, may be concerned about dysphagia, cough, diarrhea, urinary frequency, or other problems. In addition to these fears, the coldness of the radiation room often conveys feelings of isolation, even of danger, and the sight of others who are much sicker than they leads to an expectation that the treatment will be very hard to bear.

Most patients are extremely fearful of chemotherapy. They associate the drugs with major side effects such as nausea, vomiting, diarrhea, and harm to the hemopoietic and immune systems. Many assume that it is never helpful or curative because they have known patients whose chemotherapy has not cured their cancer. Simply approaching the facility where the medications will be administered induces anticipatory nausea in many patients. Anxiety due to the disease process combined with anxiety about the treatment often causes patients to fail to complete treatment as planned. The lay public frequently advises the cancer patient that chemotherapy is dangerous and that alternative treatments that have less toxicity and a guaranteed cure are available for the asking.

Although surgery cures more cancer than any other modality of treatment, patients often look for an alternative in order to avoid disfigurement. Many associate cancer surgery with the word "radical," despite the fact that most procedures are far less radical than in the past. Those patients who believe that surgeons are all-powerful and that all cancers can be totally removed with an operation are equally misguided.

RELATIONSHIPS

Serious illness in one family member is reflected in stress in all. Children are particularly vulnerable and their anxieties may be expressed in ways that do not seem to be related to the illness in the family.

A patient who is without spouse or family usually has greater needs for supportive care than one with family support. Family members can be of great help to the patient in adjusting psychologically to diagnosis, treatment, and disability, and in ensuring compliance with treatment. A supportive family can also do much to prevent the seeking of multiple second opinions and unproven treatments. However, the presence of family members does not in itself mean that the patient is not isolated; some patients choose not to "burden" others with their fears and concerns, some find it very difficult to talk to anyone about their illness.

When the relationship between spouses has been strong, patients can expect continuing sympathy and support. A weak marriage may be disrupted by anxiety that seems intolerable, but some marriages become stronger under the stress of a spouse's cancer. When a child has cancer, stress on the parents results in a greater than 50% probability that the marriage will dissolve.

In the American Cancer Society study (1979), 23.2% (N = 810) of patients and 35.2% of families reported that patients' roles in the household changed as a result of their cancer. The changes reported most frequently were: a diminished role as a homemaker (119); loss of the role of breadwinner, either partially or entirely (94); inability to fill the role of companion, usually to a spouse (76); and a diminution of the parenting role (35). Adverse effects on household roles were more common in the lower than in the higher income groups.

A significant number of cancer patients (47 out of 567 in this study) reported sexual problems with their partners. Fear and misunderstanding often lead to impotence, frigidity, or loss of libido. When a partner has gynecological cancer, fear of contagion can make sexual relations very difficult. Abdominal perineal resection with a colostomy is associated with a high incidence of impotence. In other cases, there may be an actual sexual deficit caused by either the tumor or its treatment. Many patients are reluctant to discuss sexual problems with their physicians, but the sooner such problems are identified and addressed, the better the chance for resolution.

Other marital problems that commonly result from cancer include anger engendered by the diagnosis, financial burdens, neglect by the spouse, drinking or gambling or frequent absences on the part of the spouse, and the fear of contagion.

Friends can provide a cancer patient with much needed emotional support. Unfortunately, they sometimes abandon the patient, perhaps because they fear contagion, or because they assume that a bad lifestyle led to the illness, or because their own sense of security is threatened by the disease.

FINANCIAL PROBLEMS

Despite attempts to plan early discharge from the hospital and do many procedures on an outpatient basis, cancer care continues to be ever more costly. Patients often experience major economic stress due to the cost of the illness, loss of earning power, and physical or emotional disability.

More than 16% of patients sampled in the California study felt less secure financially in terms of the future as a result of their illness. There was no inverse correlation between the proportion adversely affected and income. When family income is less than $15,000 a year, it is often difficult to meet the needs of the household. Pre-illness lifestyles could not be maintained and dependents were affected in 13% of the patients sampled. This was more common in lower income and younger age groups.

Health insurance is a significant factor in reducing cancer's financial impact. Of those in this study, 40% reported that all hospital and medical costs were covered by insurance.

Among those who were employed at the time of this study, almost 20% were apprehensive that their cancer would adversely affect fringe benefits. Others reported that their disease effectively locked them into their current jobs.

EMPLOYMENT

Patients with cancer should have the right to employment befitting their skills, training, and experience. They should not have to accept jobs that they would not have considered before their illness. Hiring, promotion, and treatment in the workplace should depend on ability and qualifications.

Those cancer patients who return to work usually have adapted to treatment and disability. They often have stronger support systems than those who cannot continue working.

Some problems with employment are protected by Sections 503 and 504 of the Federal Rehabilitation Act of 1974, but many workers are not covered because of the specifics of their employment. Forty-seven states have statutes related to the employment of people with various illnesses; some of these statutes are cancer-specific. It is unfortunate that a cancer patient's ability to continue employment or to gain new employment without discrimination must so often depend on legislation (McKenna and Toghia 1989).

COMMUNICATION AND SUPPORT

Cancer forces major changes in functioning as a whole person and brings with it a wide variety of psychological problems and problems in living. Mobility and physical functioning are reduced; work and family roles are altered; needs for emotional and social support increase. Patients experience fear, uncertainty about the future, loss of self-esteem, high stress levels, disability, and pain. Good communication between patient and physician will bring such problems to light. In such cases, the communication helps to reduce fears and anxiety, assist the patient in completing treatment, counter feelings of isolation, and correct misconceptions. Poor communication, on the other hand, results in a high anxiety level and poor compliance — often in incomplete or inadequate treatment. The physician who is in too much of a hurry to stop and listen will not notice the patient's anxiety. Fear and tension will mount and may lead the patient, in desperation, to an unproven treatment. In dealing with the manifold problems of this serious illness, the physician will need assistance and should call upon the other medical and paramedical personnel who make up the treatment team.

Most patients will benefit psychologically by having an accurate conceptual framework with which to understand their cancer and assist them in making decisions about their treatment. Patient education is basically the responsibility of the physician, whether specialist or primary care physician. The primary care physician often has the advantage of a relationship with the patient and family that spans a number of years and a knowledge of their emotional strengths and weaknesses, as well as their other medical problems.

Patients should be told the truth about their condition, realistically but optimistically. Few patients are better off not knowing the facts or being deceived or knowing less than the full truth. Lies are invariably exposed and the patient who has been lied to will be unable to give the physician the trust that is essential for maximum cooperation. Frank, open discussion is mandatory. Such discussions should be conducted with patience and understanding; explanations should be clear and patients should be given as much, or as little, honest medical information as they desire. An essential part of good management rests with the physician's availability to answer questions at any time during the course of the illness.

There should be no discrepancy between the facts presented to the patient and those given to the family. The best way to accomplish this is to provide information to the family and patient together. Families sometimes claim that patients should be protected from the truth because they "won't be able to handle it." However, in such situations it is usually the family members who cannot deal with the facts.

It is characteristic of supportive families to encourage and maintain close communication with both the patient and the doctor about the disease and therapy. Many physicians support this process by including a family member — or other person significant to the patient — in all their discussions with the patient about his or her illness. This approach encourages further discussion in the physician's absence, eliminates suspicion of secrets, and makes misunderstandings less likely.

Presenting the diagnosis requires sensitivity and some knowledge of the patient's ability to handle stress. It may be useful to use the word "tumor" initially, saving "cancer" for later in the discussion or for a later meeting. Often only a portion of the information given at the first meeting is absorbed because of the emotional upheaval created by the diagnosis and the feared outcome. Patients need help in understanding the implications of the diagnosis and in dealing with fear.

A period of emotional turmoil generally follows patients' acceptance of their diagnosis. Anxiety, depression, insomnia, lack of appetite, and poor concentration should be expected; patients may also be unable to carry out the activities of daily living. Many patients express anger at what has happened to them and ask "Why me?" In most cases these problems gradually ease as treatment plans are developed and the patient gains confidence that there may be a solution to the threat of an aggressor disease.

Counseling focusing on issues of self-respect and self-image may be indicated when patients believe that their illnesses are caused by a weakness in their own characters. Depression should be treated in order to minimize sequelae such as drinking or feelings of general tiredness. Serious emotional deterioration is unusual, but an earlier psychiatric disturbance may be reactivated.

The laws governing informed consent apply to all modalities of cancer treatment. In presenting the choices of treatment and their possible side effects and complications, the physician must be honest but not overly alarming. Patients frequently have misconceptions about the risks and side effects of treatment; the encouragement and understanding of the physician and the entire staff is necessary for acceptance of, and compliance with, the best course of treatment.

For most patients, cancer treatment is a new experience. Unless plans and procedures are explained, as often as necessary, fear and anxiety will increase for both the patient and the family. Nurses and technicians should reinforce educational efforts daily. Support mechanisms are essential throughout the course of treatment to control side effects, maintain nutritional status, and preserve hope. Under no circumstances should technicians or laboratory personnel make remarks that could be interpreted to mean that the patient's situation is hopeless.

The majority of people cope with cancer fairly well, but at least 20% of hospitalized patients have significant emotional distress. A battery of psychological tests is not necessary to determine which patients might be expected to have difficulty handling illness-associated crises. Careful attention to what the patient says and a review of his or her past medical experiences will often give clues to anticipated problems. Psychological disturbances in patients undergoing cancer treatment include depression, anxiety, and central nervous system dysfunction. Some disturbances are due to analgesic agents, steroids, or chemotherapy agents that cause electrolyte imbalance, hypercalcemia, or altered brain function.

Some patients require mild antianxiety medications to help them through crises. The severely depressed or extremely anxious patient may need psychiatric care, especially from a professional skilled in the problems of cancer patients. Oncology nurses today are also often skilled in giving psychological and emotional support to the patient, and are in an excellent position to alleviate families' anxieties. Counseling by a volunteer from a support group is especially useful to those patients who must make major physical and emotional adjustments to their illness. A patient with a stoma, for example, often finds that talking with an ostomate allays many apprehensions.

Good doctor-patient communication is as essential in the follow-up period as in the initial treatment phase. Continued follow-up and monitoring for recurrence should be mandatory because those patients with a history of the disease are the people most commonly affected by it, in the form of a second or third cancer. Moreover, delayed effects of radiation therapy and chemotherapy often become apparent in the follow-up period and dysfunction may occur after surgical treatment and require revision.

All patients are anxious when coming for checkups and many experience significant anxiety about recurrence for years after they have been cured, despite freedom from any sign of the disease. Living with uncertainty is one of the most troublesome psychological problems associated with cancer; adaptation requires flexible adjustment to day-to-day changes and emotional fluctuations. Patients need the physician's constant reassurance that the disease is controlled or cured, and that the future is bright.

Communication with patient and family must be maintained through the final stages of the illness. Some patients wish to be told when death is near, some do not, and some know without being told. Physicians and members of the support team can greatly aid a patient's psychological adaptation to approaching death. Some physicians find it very difficult to continue to treat a terminally ill patient; abandonment is not uncommon. This may be because physicians' training prepares them poorly for the supportive role that they must provide cancer patients.

When a patient has advanced progressive cancer and has failed to respond to definitive local and systemic treatment, it is unlikely that further traditional therapy will be of benefit. The physician must then tell the patient and the family that attempts at heroic treatment are unwise and that the goal should now be relief of distressing symptoms. In such circumstances, also, the designation of a no-code or no-code blue is entirely ethical and proper (it is when there is uncertainty about treatment efficacy that this is much more problematic). The question of CPR should be discussed with the patient and family ahead of any imminent need. A decision not to resuscitate must be based on the patient's beliefs and value systems. A living will may provide pertinent evidence of the wishes of a patient who is no longer competent; if such a document does not exist, the decision must be discussed with the patient's family or surrogate. However, resuscitation should never be withheld simply because a patient has a form of cancer.

SUPPORTIVE SERVICES

Supportive services are those that assist patients and their families in dealing with the many emotional, physical, and practical problems that follow the diagnosis and treatment of cancer. Supportive and referral services are usually offered initially as the patient is being admitted to the hospital for the first course of treatment. At this time it is possible to start defining concerns and setting a course of action to meet some of the perceived needs.

In the California study, supportive and referral services were rated somewhat inadequate to grossly inadequate. Of those surveyed, 27% received literature about cancer and its treatment; 22% met with other cancer patients; 20% received visits from volunteers who themselves had cancer; 14% had visits from social workers; 12% had the services of a psychologist or psychiatrist. Only 9% of family members received psychological help. One-fourth of the patients used no support service, due to lack of knowledge of the service or rejection of the service offered. An overwhelming majority of patients stated that services, if available, could have been used at the time of diagnosis and treatment. Patients and families agreed that support to family members from medical personnel in times of crisis would be desirable.

The service most often reported as necessary (22% of the patients) was daily home help. This need was seen as a continuing one, although with time it became less severe. Whether this type of assistance was available was not related to ability to pay. Other service needs were marital or family counseling (1% to 3%); psychological counseling (5% to 10%); nursing care (4% to 7%); child care (2.5%); a live-in homemaker (1% to 5%); financial aid (4% to 6%); transportation (1.6%); financial planning (2.3%); and yard work or repairs (1% to 2%). Ranges are included in the above figures because the need is generally perceived to be acute at the time of diagnosis and early treatment, decreasing thereafter. The need for financial assistance, however, does not decrease with time.

Hotlines for information and services are provided by the American Cancer Society, by the cancer information services of the comprehensive cancer centers, and by community agencies. The questions received by the University of California at Los Angeles cancer hotline indicate the type and relative frequency of the psychosocial concerns of cancer patients and their families (see table 37.1).

HOME CARE

Cost-containment issues have limited hospitalization time and have made it essential that home care assumes a greater role in the management of the cancer patient. Creative coordination of home care and outpatient care can result in a significant decrease in the amount of time a patient is disabled, in an earlier return to work, and a better quality of life. The first three months following

Table 37.1
RELATIVE FREQUENCY OF PSYCHOSOCIAL
CONCERNS (N = 1071)

Rank	Concerns	Frequency	Percentages
1	Referral to support group	210	19.6
2	Anxiety/fear associated with illness	190	17.7
3	Family problems associated with illness	133	12.4
4	Patient-physician relationships	110	10.3
5	Sadness/depression associated with illness	105	9.8
6	Financial demands of illness	91	8.5
7	Death-related feelings, thoughts	82	7.6
8	Unproven methods/compliance	63	5.9
9	Coping with treatment and side effects	63	5.9
10	Referral to professional psychotherapy	56	5.2

(Reference: Personal communication, Helene Brown, UCLA Cancer Center.)

hospital discharge are a critical period during which problems tend to be most severe, but in many cases good home care can prevent rehospitalization.

In a randomized trial to evaluate home nursing care for patients with progressive lung cancer (McCorkle 1987), patients cared for by oncology nurses, rather than those who had regular home care nurses or office nurses, showed better control of symptoms and reduced rehospitalization. Reasons for rehospitalization included bleeding and infection, further treatment, palliation, and diagnostic workups. A major finding in this study was that a large number of complications and rehospitalizations occur over a 6-month period.

Parenteral nutrition, pain control, performance of activities of daily living, and physical therapy can be provided for many by home health care services, without jeopardizing rehabilitation. Unfortunately, in many communities such facilities are grossly lacking.

Successful management of cancer requires significant cooperation between health providers and patients' families. Most families can participate in home health care when provided with basic knowledge and some monitoring of their services. Difficulties arise, however, when a patient's spouse is elderly and other family members are not readily available.

Provision for transportation to treatment facilities goes hand-in-hand with home health care. Frequently a patient is rehospitalized when medical care is not available at home and the family is unable to provide transportation to the treatment facility or outpatient service.

HOSPICE

Hospice is an integral part of the broad spectrum of cancer care. It is defined as an integrated program of appropriate hospital and home care for the patient with a limited life expectancy (usually the eligibility guideline is six months or less). The usual goal is to help the patient live as fully as possible for whatever time remains, but not to perform heroic, uncomfortable, or meaningless treatments or procedures. A high degree of skilled professional services is required to provide symptom control. The program provides a physician-directed, nurse-coordinated, interdisciplinary approach to patient care, 24 hours a day, seven days a week. Medicare will reimburse for hospice care for people over 65 years of age.

Hospice is not necessary for every dying person, but it is an option. Whether it is appropriate and acceptable will depend largely on the patient's lifestyle, beliefs, and value systems (Jacob 1984). However, acceptance of hospice services is generally high among seriously ill patients. One of the accomplishments of hospice should be to increase the number of patients who die at home rather than in the hospital, which is at present the situation for 70% of all Americans.

Approximately 1,000 programs in the United States are designated as hospices. Some are free-standing units; others are hospice units within general hospitals; others are consultation teams within medical centers; still others are community-based home care programs. The concept is care, not location.

Much research remains to be done to determine the true role and effectiveness of hospice facilities. One study conducted at the hospice connected with the UCLA Medical Center was reported by Rainey and colleagues (1984). In this study, 115 patients were being treated for cancer and 74% of them were outpatients at the time. The study showed that there was considerable interest in hospice services among these patients although almost all expressed a desire to continue their involvement with their personal physicians during the period of hospice care. Their priorities for services are listed in table 37.2. It is interesting to note that bereavement care, which is an integral part of most hospice programs, was ranked last in importance by the patients.

PASTORAL CARE

Robert Hudnut (1971) once described organized religion in America as a "sleeping giant—a collection of individuals who might do a great deal of good in the world if only they would wake up." The involvement of organized religion in cancer care began about 15 years ago when the American Cancer Society started professional education programs for the clergy and produced its first training film on pastoral care. However, the

Table 37.2
PATIENT PRIORITIES FOR HOSPICE SERVICES

Rank	Service
1	Medical control of symptoms
2	Home nursing care
3	Psychological counseling
4	Nutrition evaluation
5	Respite care
6	Spiritual guidance
7	Home support services
8	Legal and financial advice
9	Occupational, physical, and speech therapy
10	Bereavement care

clergy, as a group, need greater basic knowledge about cancer, if they are to have a truly effective role in supportive care.

According to the Rev. Mark Peterson (1987), who works with patients in the Bayfront Medical Center, St. Petersburg, Florida, there are four reasons why cancer facilities and organized religion should work together. First, when people are sick, the goals of medicine and religion are much the same: cure, comfort, and care. Second, although many patients do not practice their religion before or after their hospitalization, once admitted to the hospital they generally become more concerned with spiritual matters. Third, all health care has a moral and ethical dimension. Finally, organized religion could serve as a valuable resource for practical aid in every community in America.

VOLUNTEER SUPPORT GROUPS

Volunteer support groups aiding in cancer patient rehabilitation fall into two general categories. One has as its primary focus helping cancer patients with the difficult periods of adjustment during and after treatment. The oldest group in this category is the International Association of Laryngectomies, founded in 1952. Its activities include the development of educational materials, assisting patients with speech therapy, and pre- and postoperative counseling. Another group with a similar focus is the Reach to Recovery program of the American Cancer Society. Volunteers in the program are women who have had a mastectomy and have been trained to help others receiving such treatment. Other support groups of this kind are ostomy clubs and the Leukemia Society of America (patients and family members). Volunteers can offer a patient the kind of support that comes only from personal experience with cancer at a specific site.

A second category focuses on broad issues of coping with cancer. Support groups include the American Cancer Society programs I Can Cope and CanSurMount; Make Today Count, another nationwide program for those who have experienced cancer, either themselves or in their families; and Candlelighters, a support organization of parents whose children have had cancer. Additional organizations that offer support programs for cancer patients include the American Red Cross, the Salvation Army, and the YMCA/YWCA.

SOME PROBLEMS IN REHABILITATION

NUTRITION

Cancer cachexia is characterized by anorexia, weight loss, early satiety, and asthenia. The common association of weight loss and cancer is the effect of a number of factors including anorexia, primary involvement of the gastrointestinal tract, infection, and tumor growth. A significant loss of taste and an aversion to meat are seen in many patients. Cachexia results in a decrease in caloric intake; depletion of essential nutrients; aberra-

tions in protein, fat, carbohydrate, mineral, and vitamin metabolism; and possibly a tumor-host competition for nutrients (Ota, Kleman, and Diamond 1986).

It should not be assumed that all cancer patients have good nutritional status prior to their diagnosis. For example, patients with oral or esophageal cancer are frequently heavy drinkers; excessive alcohol consumption, if associated with an inadequate food intake, predisposes to significant nutritional deficiencies. Therapy may have to be delayed in patients with a compromised nutritional status.

It is generally agreed that nutrition through the alimentary canal is preferable to intravenous feeding. Numerous commercially available enteral products can supplement or replace a patient's oral diet.

Dietitians can be extremely helpful in evaluating patients' food likes and dislikes and their ethnic preferences, as well as in recognizing the special problems that individuals have with cancer at certain sites. The use of a blender to liquefy an ordinary select diet is valuable for the person with dysphagia. The patient with a bowel obstruction is not a suitable candidate for an oral diet and will need intravenous alimentation.

Total parenteral nutrition (TPN), using central venous access, can create an anabolic state in patients who are incapable of adequate oral food intake, or who have significantly deficient absorption ability from the GI tract. Although expensive, TPN is indispensable in a number of situations, including extreme cachexia and prolonged nausea and vomiting, or where there are alimentary tract fistulas or significant complications from radiation therapy or chemotherapy.

The potential risks of IV hyperalimentation are subclavian vein thrombosis, thrombophlebitis, and sepsis. The risk of these complications may be decreased to about 2% when hyperalimentation is undertaken by a skilled cancer care team.

PAIN

For the patient with cancer, pain is the most feared complication of the disease process. However, when current knowledge is applied, pain can be controlled or even eliminated. Fear contributes greatly to the perception of pain; hypnosis, behavioral training, biofeedback, and relaxation training may be useful in such cases.

The goal of pain therapy for patients receiving active treatment is to provide relief sufficient for the tolerance of the necessary diagnostic and therapeutic approaches. In cases of advanced cancer, pain control should be sufficient to allow patients to function at a level of their choosing, or to die relatively free of pain. The oncologist must understand the physiology, pharmacology, and psychology of pain perception; must constantly monitor the effectiveness of treatment; and must change the pain medication as necessary.

The type of pain encountered in the cancer patient varies. Acute cancer pain may be related to the presence of the disease and the therapy which is given. Chronic pain may be associated with progression of the disease, or with treatment. Some patients have pre-existent chronic pain on which the cancer-related pain is superimposed. Many of those dying of cancer have pain which is controllable, but physicians and nurses may be reluctant to provide drugs in the dosages sufficient to give relief. In cancer patients with a past history of drug addiction, the problem of pain relief is a double one.

Non-narcotic analgesics are the first-line agents for the management of mild to moderate cancer pain. Where there is severe pain, these drugs serve to potentiate the effects of narcotic analgesics. Adjuvant analgesic drugs constitute a third group of medications and include several different categories: anticonvulsant drugs, phenothiazines, butyrophenones, tricyclic antidepressants, antihistamines, amphetamines, and steroids.

Some useful guidelines for the use of narcotic analgesics in cancer pain management are (Foley 1986):

1. Start with a specific drug and know its pharmacology;

2. Adjust the route of administration to the patient's needs;

3. Administer the analgesic on a regular basis after initial titration of the dose;

4. Use drug combinations to provide additive analgesic effect;

5. Avoid drug combinations that increase sedation without enhancing analgesia;

6. Anticipate and treat side effects such as sedation, respiratory depression, nausea, vomiting, and constipation;

7. Watch for the development of tolerance; if it develops, switch to an alternative narcotic analgesic;

8. Prevent acute withdrawal; and

9. Anticipate and manage complications such as overdose or seizures.

The use of intravenous morphine delivered either as a continual drip or by a patient-administered bolus has increased in the past 15 years. A major barrier to the use of continual infusions in the past was fear that drug addiction would result. However, this is not a serious problem for those who have honest, severe cancer pain.

Regional blocks were utilized extensively in the past but have gone into disfavor because fewer physicians feel comfortable with, or have had sufficient training in, nerve block administration. There is still a place for this approach. Neurosurgical approaches are also used, but infrequently.

VENOUS ACCESS

Cancer patients require frequent monitoring of hematologic toxicity, transfusions, and IV alimentation. Venous access is a problem when there is repeated venisection and the placement of a central line is becoming routine for all people with cancer who need continued therapy. Two choices exist: the standard percutaneous transneedle catheter bedside insertion, or the surgical placement of a tunnelled catheter such as a Broviac, Hickman, or Groshong. These latter catheters seem to be less irritating and appear to have fewer complications. They are mandatory if the venous access is expected to be needed for more than a month's time. Nursing care for these catheters has become routine and patients can easily be taught to manage them.

INFECTION

Infection is a major cause of morbidity and mortality among oncological patients and complicates all forms of treatment. The presence of infection may delay definitive tumor management.

Infection may be associated with diagnostic procedures and antitumor therapy, as well as with the tumor itself. Many cancer patients are immunocompromised, either because of their disease or because of its treatment. The multimodal treatment of cancer may render such patients vulnerable to opportunistic organisms. Nutritional deficits, although not a cause of infection, are often associated with it and influence its outcome. Infections can offset the significant gains that are being made in patient survival.

Gram-negative bacteria are the most significant and common cause of infection in cancer patients. Organisms such as *Pseudomonas, Bacteroides, E. Coli, Klebsiella,* and *Proteus* are frequently found to be responsible for infections in the lung, alimentary tract, and skin. Fungal infections are commonly caused by *Candida albicans, Aspergillus,* and *Cryptococci.* Herpesviruses cause a large number of infections and *Pneumocystis carinii,* a common protozoal parasite, is increasingly responsible for pulmonary infections in leukemia patients and those with AIDS.

Cultures with sensitivity should be done to determine which antibiotic to use to treat infection. While waiting for the cultures to be reported, a combination of carbenicillin and gentamicin should be given. This is considered to be the most effective treatment available at present. Amphotericin B is the most commonly used drug in the treatment of fungal infections. Isolation techniques are indicated when the patient is immunosuppressed.

In about one-fourth of the febrile episodes that occur in people with leukopenia, a septicemia is diagnosed on blood culture. Usually the organisms responsible are gram-negative bacilli or other major pathogens, but in some institutions gram-positive bacteria surpass gram-negative bacteria as the most frequent aerobic isolate. Mortality from septicemia generally runs from 20% to 40% but can be much higher when multiple microbial sepsis is present.

Although many patients with venous-access catheters have fever, only rarely does such a catheter need to be removed providing the appropriate treatment is instituted after blood cultures have established the offending organism.

Unexplained fever is present in about 50% of granulocytopenic patients. Empirical antibiotic therapy is mandatory in the absence of positive blood cultures.

Infection occurs most commonly when the host is compromised due to the cancer treatment. More than

80% of the organisms arise from the patient's endogenous microbial flora and nearly half of these organisms are acquired during hospitalization. Because many of the organisms for infection require a human vector, hand washing remains the most important preventive procedure. Isolation techniques offer very little protection against newly acquired infection. Total protective environments may be useful in special situations such as bone marrow transplantation.

Much remains to be learned about prevention as well as treatment for some of the more exotic infections that develop in the immunocompromised patient. Members of the oncology team need to consult with an infectious disease specialist about the management of these complex issues.

BLOOD PRODUCTS

Blood replacement is more often used in cancer therapy than in the treatment of any other medical condition. Patients with cancer may have anemia because of a depressed marrow production, nutritional deficiencies, cytotoxic chemotherapy, radiation therapy sepsis, chronic illness, or increased red cell destruction such as in hypersplenism. Blood loss may be acute or chronic, due to bleeding from a tumor's raw surface.

The signs and symptoms of anemia include malaise and increased fatigue, tachycardia, dyspnea, or headache. These indications are nonspecific and should not be ascribed to anemia unless other possible causes have been excluded. When deciding whether to transfuse a patient, the total medical picture must be taken into account; in general, the hemoglobin level should be kept at 10g/100c, using packed red cells as necessary in order to maintain adequate oxygenation.

Platelet therapy is used when there is a risk of spontaneous hemorrhage, a risk which is significant when counts drop below 20,000/mm^3. Spontaneous intracranial hemorrhage increases substantially when platelet counts of 10,000/mm^3 or less are present.

NAUSEA AND VOMITING

Nausea and vomiting may be complications of any cancer treatment, whether it is surgery, radiation, or chemotherapy. Prophylactic therapy for vomiting is much more effective than after-the-fact treatment. The physiology of vomiting is now well understood, as is the pharmacology of the numerous drugs which are used for the prevention and treatment of nausea and vomiting. Oral therapy, suppository administration, or intermittent IV therapy can be used in selected patients. The phenothiazines are the most effective of the antiemetic drugs; the dosage must be individualized in each patient, depending on the response. The newest group of antiemetic agents includes metoclopramide (Reglan),

which is used most commonly in chemotherapy treatment protocols.

SUMMARY

There are nearly 1 million new patients with cancer each year in the United States, and there is significant variability in the quality of care they receive. Cancer teams may render good or poor therapy depending on their medical knowledge and experience, whether the therapy is multidisciplinary, and whether cancer therapy is the team's full-time activity.

Excellent cancer care is a team effort that includes not only the scientific application of medical knowledge, but supportive, compassionate care for the individual patient. Patients know that cancer can recur and that it can be fatal; they seek a quality of life comparable to that which existed before their diagnosis. Few can adapt to the stresses of treatment without good communication with a compassionate physician and the cancer team. Too often, cancer care is rendered impersonally, but supportive care that recognizes the patient's fears and dreams, hopes and worries makes for a better-tolerated illness and a more-satisfied patient.

***

REFERENCES

American Cancer Society. 1979. *Report on the social, economic and psychological needs of patients in California, major findings and implications.* San Francisco: American Cancer Society. California Division.

Foley, K.M. 1986. The treatment of pain in the patient with cancer. *CA* 36:194-212.

Hudnut, R. 1971. In *The sleeping giant.* p. 127. New York: Harper & Row.

Jacob, G.A. 1984. Hospice, what it is not. *CA* 34:191-201.

McCorkle, R. 1987. Complications of early discharge from the hospital. In *Proceedings of the Fifth National Conference on Human Values in Cancer.* pp. 67-74. San Francisco: American Cancer Society.

McKenna, R.J., and Toghia, N. 1989. Maximizing the productive activities of the cancer patient: policy issues in work and illness. In Borofsky, I. ed. *The cancer patient.* New York: Praeger.

Ota, D.M.; Kleman, G.; and Diamond, K. 1986. Practical considerations in the nutritional management of the cancer patient. *Curr. Probs. Cancer* 10:347-98.

Peterson, M.B. 1987. The potential of the clergy in cancer rehabilitation programs. In *Proceedings of the Fifth National Conference on Human Values in Cancer.* pp. 122-28. San Francisco: American Cancer Society.

Rainey, L.C.; Crane, L.A.; Breslow, D.M., and Ganz, P.A. 1984. Cancer patients' attitudes toward hospice services. *CA* 34:191-201.

Sutherland, A.S. 1951. In *Archives of the Memorial Sloan Kettering Cancer Center Quadrennial Report 1948-1950.* p. 52. Memorial Hospital, New York City.

Yancik, R., and Yates, J.W. 1986. Quality of life assessment of cancer patients: conceptual and methodological challenges and constraints. *Cancer Bull.* 38:217-22.

Chapter 38

DIAGNOSIS AND TREATMENT OF CANCER PAIN

Kathleen M. Foley, M.D.

Chief, Pain Service
Department of Neurology
Memorial Sloan-Kettering Cancer Center
Professor of Neurology and Neuroscience
Professor of Clinical Pharmacology
Cornell University Medical College
New York, New York

INTRODUCTION

Assessment of public attitudes toward cancer reveal that, for the patient, pain is the most feared consequence (Daut and Cleeland 1982; Levin, Cleeland, and Dar 1985). For the clinician, pain represents one of the most difficult diagnostic and therapeutic medical problems in oncology. Existing studies suggest that moderate-to-severe pain occurs in one-third of cancer patients receiving active therapy and in 60% to 90% of patients with advanced disease (Foley 1985). Management of cancer pain requires an organized approach in a framework of knowledge that encompasses the different types of pain and patients with cancer pain; the common pain syndromes; and the use of available pharmacological, psychological, anesthetic, and neurosurgical approaches.

TYPES OF PAIN

Cancer pain can be defined by its temporal aspects: acute, chronic, or incidental; or on the basis of its physiological mechanisms: somatic, visceral, or neuropathic pain (Payne 1987).

Acute pain is characterized by a well-defined temporal onset, of limited duration, and is usually amenable to a wide variety of analgesic treatments. *Chronic pain* is pain lasting for more than three months and is often further complicated by psychological factors of depression and demoralization. *Incident pain* is pain on movement, usually due to mechanical factors such as an unstable spine secondary to vertebral body collapse or a fracture in a bone metastasis. On a physiologic basis, three categories of cancer pain have been recognized:

1. *Somatic pain,* which occurs as a result of activation of nociceptors in cutaneous and deep tissues, and is characterized as aching, gnawing pain. Bone metastases and postsurgical pains are examples of somatic pain.

2. *Visceral pain* results from infiltration, compression, distension, or stretching of thoracic and abdominal viscera. The pain is poorly localized and often described as deep, or squeezing, and is referred to cutaneous sites that may be remote from the site of the lesion, such as shoulder pain from diaphragmatic irritation.

3. *Neuropathic pain* results from injury to the peripheral and/or central nervous system as a consequence of tumor growth or cancer therapy. The resultant pain is associated with loss of motor and sensory function, and is characterized as burning, or vice-like with paroxysms of pain. Brachial and lumbosacral plexopathy are examples of this type of pain. *Somatic pain* and *visceral pain* are amenable to treatment with analgesic, anesthetic, and neurosurgical approaches; whereas *neuropathic pain* responds to these approaches only in part, making pain management in certain cancer patients very difficult.

TYPES OF PATIENTS WITH PAIN

The types of patients who experience pain have also been identified, and although these categories are artificial, they are useful in discussing specific therapeutic approaches (Foley 1982; Foley 1985).

GROUP I: PATIENTS WITH ACUTE CANCER-RELATED PAIN

This group includes patients with tumor-associated pain, in which pain is the major symptom prompting medical consultation and the diagnosis of cancer. Pain has a special significance as the harbinger of cancer. Recurrent pain during the course of illness or following successful therapy has the immediate implication of recurrent disease. Defining the cause of pain may present a diagnostic problem, but effective treatment of the cause of the pain, e.g., radiation therapy for bone metastases, is usually associated with dramatic pain relief. A second subset in this group are those patients with pain associated with cancer therapy — for example, patients with postoperative pain or patients with pain secondary to oral ulceration from chemotherapy, or myalgias secondary to steroid withdrawal. In this group, the cause of the pain is readily identifiable, and its course is predictable and self-limiting. These patients are not difficult to diagnose, and pain treatment directed at the cause of their pain is used to manage the transient symptoms. These patients endure significant pain for the promise of a successful outcome.

GROUP II: PATIENTS WITH CHRONIC CANCER-RELATED PAIN

In contrast to those patients with acute pain, these patients present as difficult diagnostic and therapeutic clinical problems. They can be subdivided into two groups: patients with chronic pain from tumor progression, and patients with chronic pain related to cancer treatment. Both share a characteristic pain symptom that has persisted for more than three months. In those patients with chronic pain from tumor progression (e.g. patients with carcinoma of the pancreas, metastatic melanoma, or Pancoast syndrome), the pain escalates in intensity secondary to tumor infiltration of adjacent bone, nerve, or soft tissue. Multiple antitumor and analgesic approaches have varying degrees of success. Psychological factors play a significant role for this group of patients, in whom palliative therapy may be of little value and is physically debilitating. The sense of hopelessness and fear of impending death may further add to and exaggerate the complaint. Pain becomes an aspect of global suffering. Identifying both the pain and the suffering component is essential to developing adequate therapy for this group of patients (Foley 1982; Fishmen et al. 1987; Twycross and Lack 1984; Twycross and Fairfield 1982). The chronic nature of the pain is associated with a series of psychological signs, including disturbances in sleep or appetite, impaired concentration, and irritability often mimicking a depressive disorder. Management must be directed at controlling the pain, and analgesic therapy combined with a wide range of alternative approaches is necessary to provide adequate analgesia.

A second group of patients with chronic pain are those with pain associated with cancer therapy. These patients commonly have all of the syndromes described in table 38.1. Treatment of the pain for this group of patients is often limited by the lack of available methods to remove the cause of pain. Again, treatment is directed at the symptoms, not the cause. This group closely parallels those patients in the general population with chronic, intractable pain syndromes. Psychological factors play a significant role in how these patients adapt to, and function with, chronic pain. Although it is consoling to both the patient and the physician to realize that the pain does not represent recurrent or progressive disease, the pain's persistence is a constant reminder of the previous diagnosis of cancer. All approaches must be aimed at maintaining the patient's functional status.

Table 38.1
SPECIFIC PAIN SYNDROMES IN PATIENTS WITH CANCER

A. PAIN SYNDROMES ASSOCIATED WITH DIRECT TUMOR INVOLVEMENT
  1. *Tumor infiltration of bone*
    a. Base of skull syndromes
      1) Jugular foramen metastases
      2) Clivus metastases
      3) Sphenoid sinus metastases
    b. Vertebral body syndromes
      1) C2 metastases
      2) C7-T1 metastases
      3) L1 metastases
    c. Sacral syndrome
  2. *Tumor infiltration of nerve*
    a. Peripheral nerve
      1) Peripheral neuropathy
    b. Plexus
      1) Brachial plexopathy
      2) Lumbar plexopathy
      3) Sacral plexopathy
    c. Root
      1) Leptomeningeal metastases
    d. Spinal cord
      1) Epidural spinal cord compression
B. PAIN SYNDROMES ASSOCIATED WITH CANCER THERAPY
  1. *Postsurgery syndromes*
    a. Post-thoracotomy syndrome
    b. Postmastectomy syndrome
    c. Postradical neck syndrome
    d. Phantom limb syndrome
  2. *Postchemotherapy syndromes*
    a. Peripheral neuropathy
    b. Aseptic necrosis of the femoral head
    c. Steroid pseudorheumatism
    d. Postherpetic neuralgia
  3. *Postradiation syndromes*
    a. Radiation fibrosis of brachial and lumbar plexus
    b. Radiation myelopathy
    c. Radiation-induced second primary tumors
    d. Radiation necrosis of bone
C. PAIN SYNDROMES NOT ASSOCIATED WITH CANCER OR CANCER THERAPY
  1. Cervical and lumbar osteoarthritis
  2. Thoracic and abdominal aneurysms
  3. Diabetic neuropathy

GROUP III: PRE-EXISTING CHRONIC PAIN AND CANCER-RELATED PAIN

This group includes those patients with a history of chronic nonmalignant pain, who develop cancer and pain. For this group, psychological factors are significant. These patients are at high risk for developing further functional incapacity and escalating chronic pain symptoms. Their history should not be used in a punitive way to minimize or deny their complaints. Identifying this group of patients as a high-risk group helps to improve their psychological assessment and intervention.

GROUP IV: PATIENTS WITH A HISTORY OF DRUG ADDICTION AND CANCER-RELATED PAIN

Three subgroups can be identified: patients actively involved in illicit drug use and drug-seeking behavior; patients receiving methadone in a maintenance program; and patients who have not used drugs for several years. Under-treatment with analgesic drugs occurs most commonly in this group of patients. Assessment of reported pain by physicians and nurses is colored by the fact that the pain symptoms are confused with drug-seeking behavior. Attention to the medical and psychological needs of these patients requires individualized assessment and consultation with experts in drug-related problems. The first subgroup represents a major management problem, straining the most tolerant of medical care systems. Pain in the other two subgroups is readily managed with the recognition that the psychological stresses consequent to the pain and cancer may place the patient at a high risk for recidivism.

GROUP V: DYING PATIENTS WITH CANCER-RELATED PAIN

Group V includes dying patients with pain. Maintaining the patient's comfort should be the therapeutic goal. The issues of hopelessness, death, and dying become prominent, and the suffering component of the illness must be addressed. Inadequate pain control exacerbates the patient's suffering and demoralizes both family and medical personnel, who feel that they have failed in treating the patient's pain at a time when adequate treatment may matter most. The risk-benefit ratios associated with analgesic approaches become less of an issue when the goal of pain therapy is comfort.

COMMON PAIN SYNDROMES IN PATIENTS WITH CANCER

Careful analysis of patients with cancer and pain has led to a series of descriptions of common pain syndromes unique to this disease process. These pain syndromes are often misdiagnosed because health care professionals are unfamiliar with their clinical presentation. There are three major categories of pain syndromes (Foley 1979).

The first and most important category is pain associated with direct tumor involvement. This group accounts for 78% of pain problems in an inpatient cancer pain population, and 62% of the pain problems in an outpatient cancer pain population surveyed. Metastatic bone disease, nerve compression or infiltration, or hollow viscus involvement are the most common causes of pain from direct tumor involvement.

The second category includes those pain syndromes associated with cancer therapy. This group accounted for approximately 19% of pain problems in an inpatient cancer pain population, and 25% of pain problems in an outpatient cancer pain clinic. It includes those patients in whom pain occurred during the course of, or as a result of, chemotherapy, surgery, or radiation therapy; each of these primary therapeutic modalities is associated with a series of specific pain syndromes with a characteristic pattern and clinical presentation.

The third major category of pain syndromes consists of pain not related to the cancer or the cancer therapy. Approximately 3% of patients have pain unrelated to their cancer or their cancer therapy. This figure increases to 10% in an outpatient cancer pain population surveyed.

Accurate diagnosis in this group of patients clearly alters both therapy and prognosis.

PAIN SYNDROMES ASSOCIATED WITH DIRECT TUMOR INVOLVEMENT

TUMOR INVASION OF BONE

Pain from invasion of bone, by either primary or metastatic tumors, is the most common cause of pain in both adults and children with cancer. The underlying neurophysiologic and neuropharmacologic mechanisms of bone pain are poorly understood. Anatomic studies reveal that both myelinated and, occasionally, unmyelinated nerve fibers are present in bone, most densely in the region of compact bones. The periosteum and all of the components of joints, except for the articular cartilage, are pain-sensitive structures, whereas the cortex and bone marrow are considered to be pain-insensitive bone structures. Pathologically, metastatic tumor in bone is associated with two processes: active bone destruction and new bone formation. The current hypotheses for the origin of bone pain relate to the role of prostaglandins in the metastatic process. Drugs that inhibit prostaglandin synthesis inhibit pain, and, in some instances, tumor growth in both clinical and experimental studies.

Clinically, metastatic tumor involvement of bone produces pain either by direct involvement of the bone and activation of the nociceptors locally or by compression of adjacent nerves, soft tissues, or vascular structures.

METASTASES TO THE BASE OF SKULL

The syndromes associated with metastases to the base of skull have been previously described (Greenberg et al. 1981). They are common in patients with nasopharyngeal tumors, but can occur with any tumor type that can metastasize to bone. The syndromes in this group all share two common features: pain is the earliest complaint and often precedes neurologic signs and symptoms by several weeks to months; and documentation by plain radiography is often difficult, requiring the use of tomography, CT scanning, and MRI. At the current time, both CT scan and MRI are superior to conventional radiological techniques to evaluate these patients. In patients with predominantly bony disease, the CT scan appears to be more sensitive, whereas in those with soft-tissue extension, MRI seems to be more sensitive in assessing the base of the skull.

JUGULAR FORAMEN SYNDROME

This syndrome is characterized by the onset of occipital pain, referred to the vertex of the head and ipsilateral shoulder and arm. Head movement often exacerbates the pain with associated local tenderness over the occipital condyle. The patient's signs and symptoms vary with cranial nerve involvement, and can include hoarseness, dysarthria, dysphasia, neck and shoulder weakness, and ptosis. Neurologic examination can help localize the lesion by determining the functioning of the ninth, tenth, eleventh, and twelfth cranial nerves. Involvement of all four of these nerves suggests jugular foramen and hypoglossal canal involvement with secondary nerve dysfunction. Horner's syndrome suggests sympathetic involvement extracranially but in close proximity to the jugular foramen.

CLIVUS METASTASES
Pain characterized by vertex headache and exacerbated by neck flexion is a common mode of presentation. Lower cranial nerve dysfunction from sixth to twelfth usually begins unilaterally but often progresses to bilateral lower cranial nerve dysfunction. MRI is particularly helpful in evaluating diseases of the clivus.

SPHENOID SINUS METASTASES
Bifrontal headache, radiating into both temples with intermittent retro-orbital pain, is a common symptom of this syndrome. Patients often complain of nasal stuffiness, a sense of fullness in the head, and associated diplopia. Neurologic sign of unilateral or bilateral sixth nerve palsy further suggest this diagnosis.

METASTASES TO VERTEBRAL BODIES
These syndromes share two common features: pain is an early symptom preceding neurologic signs and symptoms; and if the nature of the pain is not accurately diagnosed, irreversible neurologic deficits, including paraplegia and quadriplegia, may develop. Numerous studies have documented that greater than 85% of patients with epidural spinal cord compression have vertebral body metastases, and in 10% of patients with cord compression, pain was the only complaint in the absence of any neurologic findings.

Odontoid fractures. Pain in this region can result from pathologic fracture and secondary subluxation with resulting spinal cord or brain stem compression. Fractures of the odontoid process are most often secondary to destruction of the atlas. The pain characteristically radiates over the posterior aspect of the skull to the vertex and is exacerbated by neck movement, particularly neck flexion. Neurologic signs include progressive sensory and motor findings, beginning in the upper extremities with associated autonomic dysfunction; but pain is the earliest symptom. Neck manipulation is dangerous. MRI scans are most helpful to confirm the diagnosis. Early diagnosis of tumor in the vertebral body before subluxation or fracture allows therapy to be directed at the control of tumor growth (Sundaresan, Galicich, and Lane 1981).

C7-T1 vertebral metastases. This is a common site for metastatic disease originating from lung, breast, and lymphoma. Pain originating because of metastatic disease in the C7-T1 vertebral bodies is usually localized to the adjacent spinal area and characterized by a constant, dull, aching pain radiating bilaterally to both shoulders. Percussion may elicit tenderness over the spinous process at this level. With nerve-root compression, radicular pain in the C7, C8, T1 distribution is most often unilateral in the posterior arm, elbow, and ulnar aspect of the hand. The neurologic symptoms include paresthesia and numbness in the fourth and fifth fingers, with progressive hand and triceps weakness. Horner's syndrome suggests paravertebral sympathetic involvement. Metastatic bone disease at this level results from either hematogenous spread to bone, or, more commonly, from tumor originating in the brachial plexus or paravertebral space spreading along the nerves to the contiguous vertebral body and epidural space. CT scan is the diagnostic procedure of choice and with MRI can help define the presence of metastatic disease in bone and soft tissue. In patients with bilateral radicular signs and symptoms of spinal cord dysfunction, myelography should be performed to rule out associated epidural spinal cord compression (Kanner, Martini, and Foley 1982).

Lumbar metastases L1. Dull, aching midback pain, exacerbated by lying or sitting, and relieved by standing is the usual presenting complaint. Movement exacerbates the pain, particularly when the patient goes from the recumbent to standing position. The pain is referred to the sacroiliac regions or the superior iliac crest, unilaterally or bilaterally. Lack of knowledge of these referred points for L1 disease often confuses the diagnostic workup.

Sacral metastases. Aching pain beginning insidiously in the back or coccygeal region, exacerbated by lying or sitting and relieved by walking, is the common clinical complaint for tumor infiltration of the sacrum. Increasing pain with neurologic signs and symptoms of perianal sensory loss, bowel and bladder dysfunction, and impotence, can help localize the site of the disease. Some patients may complain of specific tenderness over the sciatic notch and radicular symptoms in the sciatic nerve distribution associated with nerve compression from local bony changes in the sacrum. Plain radiographs are inadequate to assess the region fully, and CT scan is the most useful initial diagnostic procedure, with MRI clearly of further value. In certain instances, barium enema, IVP and/or lymphangiogram may help to define the presence of presacral tumor not visualized on other studies.

TUMOR INFILTRATION OF NERVE, PLEXUS, MENINGES AND SPINAL CORD
Pain syndromes in this group are caused by direct tumor infiltration of nerve, by progressive compression of nerve structures, or by sudden compression by metastatic fractures of bone adjacent to nerves or nerve roots. The neuropathology of these lesions has not been correlated with the nature of pain, but neurophysiologic evidence suggests that persistent mechanical and

noxious stimulation of nociceptors, combined with the partial damage of axons and nerve membranes, may account for the types of pain seen in this group of syndromes. The types of pain are most typically somatic and neuropathic. The high percentage of patients with nerve injury and neuropathic pain may account for some of the difficulties physicians encounter in managing this group of patients.

Tumor infiltration of peripheral nerve. Constant, burning pain with hypesthesia and dysesthesia in an area of sensory loss is the typical clinical presentation. The most common cause of infiltration of the peripheral nerve is from tumors that invade the paravertebral or retroperitoneal space. The pain is commonly radicular and unilateral, and a careful sensory examination can often delineate the site of nerve compression. The most common example of infiltration of the peripheral nerve is metastatic tumor involvement of the rib, producing intercostal nerve entrapment. The use of the CT scan to diagnose these syndromes can help to document the anatomic region of compression and rule out the presence of associated root or epidural compression of nerve.

Tumor infiltration of the brachial plexus. Pain in the shoulder or arm is the earliest presenting symptom with tumor infiltration of the brachial plexus. The lower plexus, C7-T1, is the most common site for tumor infiltration, but the site may vary with the tumor type. For example, in patients with breast cancer and/or lymphoma, infiltration of the upper plexus in the C5-C6 distribution commonly occurs. However, in patients with carcinoma of the lung, infiltration of the lower plexus predominates. The patterns of pain also vary with the site of plexus involvement. Tumor infiltration

of the upper plexus is usually associated with pain in the paraspinal space as far down as lateral to the T4 vertebral body, with radicular pain in the shoulder and anterior aspect of the upper arm. Pain from lower plexus involvement is characterized by referred pain to the infrascapular area and the posterior aspect of the arm and elbow. The neurologic symptoms of pain and paresthesia in the fourth and fifth fingers may precede objective clinical signs for several weeks to months. Typically, pain precedes motor or sensory changes, and objective motor signs occur before distinct sensory signs. The supraclavicular and axillary regions may be normal on exam, particularly in those patients with a lower plexopathy. Horner's syndrome suggests sympathetic involvement in the paravertebral space and is commonly associated with involvement of the lower plexus. Tumor in the brachial plexus commonly spreads along the nerve root into the epidural space, so the incidence of epidural spinal cord compression in this group of patients is as high as 50%.

One problem encountered in evaluating patients with pain in the distribution of the brachial plexus arises in the patient who has previously received radiation therapy. In this case, the differential diagnosis must include radiation fibrosis of the plexus (Foley 1987). Table 38.2 describes the characteristics of the pain symptomatology seen in patients with tumor and radiation therapy. Current data would suggest that careful attention to the pattern of pain and neurologic deficit combined with CT scans of the plexus can provide sufficient information to diagnose tumor infiltration from radiation fibrosis and obviate the need for surgical exploration or a biopsy (Cascino et al. 1983). Other differential diagnoses include brachial neuritis, rotator cuff tear at the shoulder joint, and cervical disc disease. These common pain syndromes are often misdiagnosed.

Table 38.2
CLINICAL FEATURES OF BRACHIAL PLEXUS SYNDROMES IN PATIENTS WITH BREAST CANCER

	Tumor Infiltration	Radiation Fibrosis	Reversible Radiation Injury
Incidence of pain	89%	18%	40%
Location of pain	Shoulder, upper arm, elbow, radiating to 4th and 5th fingers	Shoulder, wrist, hand	Hand, forearm
Nature of pain	Dull aching in shoulder; lancinating pain in elbow and ulnar aspect of hand; occasional dysesthesia, burning, or freezing sensations	Aching pain in shoulder; paresthesia in C5-C6 distribution in hand	Aching pain in shoulder and ulna; paresthesia in hand and forearm
Severity of pain	Moderate to severe (severe in 98% of patients)	Mild to moderate; severe in 35% of patients	Mild
Course	Progressive neurologic dysfunction; atrophy and weakness with C7-T1 distribution; persistent pain; Horner's syndrome	Progressive weakness with C5-C6 distribution; stabilizing pain with appearance of weakness	Transient weakness and atrophy affecting C6-C7, T1; complete resolution of motor findings
CT scan findings	Circumscribed mass with diffuse infiltration of tissue planes	Diffuse infiltration of tissue planes	Normal
EMG findings	Segmental slowing; no myokymia	Myokymia	Segmental slowing; no myokymia

(Reprinted from: Stillman, M., and Foley, K.M. [1987].)

Tumor infiltration of the lumbosacral plexus. This is most common in patients with genitourinary, gynecologic, and colonic cancers but it can occur from any tumor that metastasizes to this anatomic region. Local tumor extension into adjacent lymph nodes and bone produces pain that varies with the site of plexus involvement. In a review of 85 patients with lumbosacral plexopathy, 67% of patients had direct tumor extension, 22% had metastases to the lumbosacral plexus, and in 11% the primary site of tumor was unknown (Jaeckle, Young, and Foley 1985). Pain was the presenting symptom in 91% of patients, with weakness in 60%, and numbness in 42%. The pain is typically of two types: local pain in the sacrum or sacroiliac joint, low back, or groin; and radicular pain in the lateral, posterior, or anterior leg. Table 38.3 describes the typical pain syndromes seen with lumbosacral plexopathy. CT scanning is the most useful diagnostic study to define a soft-tissue mass and/or bony abnormality in the lumbosacral and pelvic regions. At the current time, MRI has not been fully tested to determine if it is more sensitive than CT scans in this region. The differential diagnosis includes lumbar neuritis, postsurgical lumbar plexopathy, radiation fibrosis, and lumbar disc disease. Again, each of these entities has a characteristic presentation that is different from that described for tumor infiltration.

Leptomeningeal metastases. In this clinical entity, tumor infiltrates the cerebrospinal leptomeninges with or without concomitant invasion of the nervous system (Olson, Chirnik, and Posner 1978). Pain occurs in 40% of patients and can be of two types: headache, with or without neck stiffness, characterized by constant pain; and back pain, most commonly localized to the low back and buttock region. Pain results from traction on tumor-infiltrated nerves and meninges. Lumbar puncture is the procedure of choice to detect neoplastic cells in the cerebrospinal fluid (CSF) of such patients. An elevated CSF protein and low glucose concentration are often associated findings. The more recent use of CSF markers including beta-2 microglobulin and LDH can help clarify the diagnosis in those patients with minimal cytological changes. Myelography can be particularly helpful in delineating tumor nodules along nerves and cauda equina. The differential diagnosis varies with the site of neurologic involvement. Signs and symptoms of neurologic dysfunction at several levels of the neural axis in a patient with cancer suggest this diagnosis.

Epidural spinal cord compression. Severe neck and back pain is the hallmark of this entity (Portenoy, Lipton, and Foley 1986). Pain is the initial symptom in over 95% of patients, and in 10% of patients it may be the only neurologic symptom in a patient with a complete block. Pain occurs from local bone or root compression and is generally of two types: local pain over the involved vertebral body; or radicular pain, unilaterally in patients with cervical or lumbosacral compression, and bilaterally in those with thoracic cord compression. The neurologic symptoms vary with the site of epidural disease and commonly include motor weakness progressing to paraplegia, a level of sensory loss, and loss of bowel and bladder function. Eighty-five percent of patients have associated vertebral body tumors. Algorithms have been developed to assess patients with back pain without signs of myelopathy. The presence of a greater than 50% collapse on plain radiographs in a patient with severe back pain and a normal neurologic examination is associated with as much as an 87% chance of epidural spinal cord compression. Therefore, the complaint of pain in this patient population is serious, and should lead the physician to the appropriate diagnosis.

Table 38.3
SYMPTOMS AND SIGNS BY LEVEL OF PLEXUS INVOLVEMENT: PROSPECTIVE PATIENTS (N = 34)

Clinical level	Upper	Lower	Pan
Number of patients	12	16	6
Most common tumor	Colorectal	Sarcoma	Genitourinary
Pain distribution			
Local	Lower abdomen	Buttock, perineum	Lumbosacral
Radicular	Anterolateral thigh	Posterolateral thigh, leg	Variable
Referred	Flank, iliac crest	Hip and ankle	Variable
Numbness/paresthesias	Anterior thigh	Perineum, thigh, sole	Anterior thigh, leg, foot
Motor and reflex changes	L2-L4	L5-S1	L2-S2
Sensory loss	Anterolateral thigh	Posterior thigh, sole	Esp. anterior thigh, leg
Tenderness	Lumbar	Sciatic notch, sacrum	Lumbosacral
Positive SLRT*			
Direct	6/12	8/16	5/6
Reverse	2/12	8/16	5/6
Leg edema	5/12	6/16	5/6
Rectal mass	3/12	7/16	1/6
Sphincter weakness	0/12	8/16	0/6

(Reprinted from: Jaeckle, Young, and Foley [1985].)

PAIN SYNDROMES ASSOCIATED WITH CANCER THERAPY

Two types of clinical pain syndromes occur in the course of, or subsequent to, the treatment of cancer patients with surgery, chemotherapy, or radiation therapy.

The first type occurs acutely, within weeks after the specific therapy, and include the immediate postoperative pain syndromes, the mucositis of chemotherapy, and the radiation-induced esophagitis. These syndromes are readily recognized and the associated pain is self-limited.

The second type of pain occurs several weeks to months later, in certain instances years later, and presents the clinical problem: Is the pain a complication of therapy, or a sign of recurrent disease? The incidence of these late pain syndromes is not known, but they represent an important aspect of the differential diagnosis in this group of patients.

POSTSURGICAL PAIN SYNDROMES

POST MASTECTOMY PAIN SYNDROME

Four percent to 10% of women having any surgical procedure on the breast, from lumpectomy to radical mastectomy, develop this syndrome (Granek, Ashikari, and Foley 1983). Pain can occur immediately or several months following surgery and is characterized as a tight, constricting, burning pain in the posterior arm, axilla, and anterior chest wall. Often a trigger point area in the axilla recreates the pain on palpation. Movement exacerbates the pain and patients often posture their arm in a flexed position, close to the chest wall. This posturing can lead to the development of a frozen shoulder and secondary pain from disuse atrophy of the arm and shoulder muscles. Postmastectomy pain results from interruption of the intercostobrachial nerve, a cutaneous sensory branch of T1-T2, and subsequent formation of a traumatic neuroma at the end of the severed nerve.

POST THORACOTOMY PAIN SYNDROME

The clinical features include pain in the distribution of the intercostal nerve following surgical injury or interruption (Kanner, Martini, and Foley 1982). The pain is of two types: the immediate postoperative pain, which clears in 75% of patients in three months and is associated with sensory loss in the area of scar; and persistent postoperative pain, which persists for longer than three months, or recurs in the surgical area, following resolution of the initial postoperative pain. The persistence of postoperative pain or the recurrence of pain in the surgical area are both statistically associated with recurrent tumor or infiltration in the chest wall, paraspinal, or epidural space. The CT scan, rather than a chest radiograph, is the diagnostic procedure to assess this particular pain problem. In less than 5% to 10% of patients on follow-up the cause of this clinical pain syndrome alone was a development of a traumatic neuroma or nerve injury. Therefore, in patients with recurrent tumor, therapy directed at the tumor is the treatment of choice for the pain. For those patients with nerve injury alone, local rubbing, transcutaneous nerve stimulation, and amitriptyline have been used with varied success.

POST-RADICAL NECK SYNDROMES

Surgical interruption of the cervical nerves following radical neck dissection is characterized by a constant burning sensation in the area of sensory loss. Dysesthesia and intermittent shock-like pain may also be present. Carbamazepine is particularly useful for this group of patients, to manage the pain's dysesthetic component. A second type of pain syndrome in patients with radical neck dissection includes a series of musculoskeletal pain problems resulting from surgical injury to motor nerves innervating the shoulder and upper arm. These syndromes are characterized by aching pain in the shoulder and neck, and are exacerbated by sitting up and walking around, and relieved by lying down. They usually include the suprascapular nerve entrapment syndrome, and pain secondary to thoracic outlet compression. Local nerve blocks and support slings can markedly relieve these muscle-tension complaints and prevent progressive motor and sensory signs and symptoms.

PHANTOM LIMB AND STUMP PAIN

Pain following surgical amputation of a limb is of two types: phantom limb pain and stump pain (Sherman, Sherman, and Parker 1984). These painful clinical entities are distinct from normal phantom limb sensation experienced by all patients following limb amputation.

The phantom limb pain is usually characterized by a burning, cramping pain in the phantom limb, which is often identical in nature and location to the preoperative pain.

Stump pain can be triggered by local pressure on the stump and is associated with the presence of a traumatic neuroma. The stump pain is exacerbated by movement and pressure and relieved by rest, in contrast to phantom limb pain, which is unaffected by mechanical stimuli. Phantom limb pain frequently clears within two months of the surgical procedure. Its recurrence may be the first sign of disease recurrence at a proximal nerve root, mimicking the original phantom limb pain.

POSTCHEMOTHERAPY PAIN SYNDROME

PERIPHERAL NEUROPATHY

The painful dysesthesia following treatment with vinca alkaloids are part of a symmetric polyneuropathy. They are usually localized to the hands and feet and characterized as a burning pain, exacerbated by superficial stimuli. In children, a more diffuse syndrome occurs characterized by generalized myalgia and arthralgia, often beginning with jaw pain and progressing to a symmetric polyneuropathy including cranial nerve dysfunction. This syndrome is self-limited, usually lasting four to six weeks, with resolution of the pain along with partial resolution of nerve function.

STEROID PSEUDORHEUMATISM

This entity occurs after both rapid and slow withdrawal of steroid medication in patients taking these drugs for any length of time. The syndrome is characterized by prominent diffuse myalgia and arthralgia, with muscle and joint tenderness on palpation but without objective inflammatory signs. Generalized malaise and fatigue are common features of this entity. This syndrome is commonly seen in patients who are being pulsed with steroids as part of their chemotherapy regimen. Steroid withdrawal markedly exacerbates pain from bony metastases or epidural spinal cord compression.

ASEPTIC NECROSIS OF BONE

Aseptic necrosis of the humeral and more commonly the femoral head are often known complications of cancer therapy, especially chronic steroid therapy (Ihde and Devita 1975). Pains in the shoulder, knee, and leg are the common presenting complaints with radiographic changes occurring several weeks to months after the onset of pain. Limitation of joint movement with progressive inability to use the arm or hip functionally is the natural history of this illness. It is most common in patients with Hodgkin's disease, but can occur in any patient on chronic steroid therapy. The bone scan and MRI are the most useful diagnostic procedures. The appropriate treatment is the replacement of the diseased joint, with dramatic resolution of the pain.

POSTHERPETIC NEURALGIA

This well-described clinical entity is dramatized by persistent pain after cutaneous eruption from herpes zoster infection has cleared (Portenoy, Duma, and Foley 1987; Watson et al. 1982). In patients with cancer, herpes zoster infection commonly occurs in the area of tumor pathology or in the port of previous radiation therapy. The true incidence of postherpetic neuralgia in patients with cancer is unknown but appears to be more common in patients who develop the infection after the age of 50. The pain is of three types: continuous burning pain in the area of sensory loss; painful dysesthesia; and shock-like pain. Management of patients with postherpetic neuralgia has been recently reviewed. Careful attention to the patient's complaint and to the motor and sensory examination is imperative, because although the site of postherpetic pain does not necessarily correspond to the site of the previous tumor, the presence of pain often obscures underlying pathology. If the sensory loss is more extensive than the scarring, or if the motor findings are out of the distribution of the nerve involved, future workup of the patient may be necessary in order to rule out some other cause, such as metastatic disease in bone, paraspinal space, or epidural space.

POSTRADIATION PAIN SYNDROMES

RADIATION FIBROSIS OF THE BRACHIAL PLEXUS

As previously discussed, pain in the distribution of the brachial plexus following radiation therapy results from fibrosis of surrounding connective tissue and secondary injury to nerve (Foley 1987). It may occur as early as six months or as late as 20 years (table 38.2). The typical clinical symptoms include complaints of numbness or paresthesia in the hand, usually in a C5-C6 distribution. The pain occurs late in the course of the clinical entity and is characterized as diffuse arm pain. Lymphedema in the arm, radiation skin changes, and induration of the supraclavicular and axillary areas are often present. Neurologic signs include sensory changes in the C5-C6 distribution and motor weakness in the deltoid and biceps muscles. These signs progress to the development of a painful, useless, swollen extremity.

RADIATION FIBROSIS OF THE LUMBOSACRAL PLEXUS

Radiation fibrosis of the lumbosacral plexus is much less common than that of the brachial plexus (Thomas, Cascino, and Earle 1985). The lower incidence appears to be related to the tumor type, which does not have the comparable long survival rate of breast cancer. Pain in the leg or perineum from radiation fibrosis of the lumbar plexus presents a diagnostic problem. A history of radiation treatment, local skin changes, lymphedema of the leg, or radiologic changes consistent with radiation necrosis of hip or sacrum can help establish the diagnosis.

RADIATION MYELOPATHY

Pain is an early symptom in 15% of patients with this entity (Jellinger and Sturm 1971; Thomas, Cascino, and Earle 1985). The pain may be localized to the area of spinal cord damage or may be referred with dysesthesia below the level of injury. The neurologic symptoms and signs are those of a Brown-Sequard syndrome characterized by a ipsilateral motor paresis with a contralateral sensory loss at the cervico-thoracic level. Myelography and MRI can be helpful to rule out metastatic disease. No effective therapy has been reported to be useful to reverse the myelopathy of radiation injury.

RADIATION-INDUCED PERIPHERAL NERVE TUMORS

A painful enlarging mass in an area previously irradiated suggests this diagnosis (Foley et al. 1980). These tumors develop four to 20 years following radiation therapy in patients cured of their previous tumors. Both malignant peripheral nerve tumors and second primary tumors in a previously irradiated site have been described.

In summary, table 38.4 outlines the approach to the patient with cancer pain and includes: its temporal aspects (acute, subacute, chronic, and incidental); an understanding of the type of pain (somatic, visceral, and neuropathic); and the types of patients with pain and the specific pain syndromes (see table 38.1). Recognizing the physical and psychological components and assessing these in an orderly fashion can provide the physician with sufficient data to plan a comprehensive approach (table 38.5). Critical to this approach is the development of a trusting relationship between the

Table 38.4
APPROACH TO THE PATIENT WITH PAIN AND CANCER

1. Knowledge of the temporal aspects of pain: acute, chronic, incident
2. Understanding of the physiological mechanisms of cancer pain: somatic, visceral, neuropathic
3. Identification of the types of patients with pain: patients with acute cancer-related pain, patients with chronic cancer-related pain, patients with pre-existing chronic pain and cancer-related pain, patients with a history of drug addiction and cancer-related pain, dying patients with cancer-related pain
4. Diagnosis of the cancer pain syndromes: pain syndromes associated with direct tumor involvement, pain syndromes associated with cancer therapy, pain syndromes not associated with cancer or cancer therapy

patient and family and a physician, who respects the complaint of pain and provides treatment of both pain and suffering. The goal of successful pain therapy is to provide patients with adequate pain relief that allows them to function as they choose and to die relatively free of pain.

The use of pharmacologic therapy should be within the armamentarium of the practicing physician. Drug therapy with opioid, nonopioid, and adjuvant drugs is the mainstay of treatment. Other interventions include the use of anesthetic, surgical, and behavioral approaches, and usually involve referral to appropriate experts.

PHARMACOLOGIC APPROACHES

The fundamental concept that underlies the appropriate and successful management of pain by a pharmacological approach in patients with cancer is individualization of analgesic therapy. Table 38.6 details guidelines for the use of analgesics in the management of cancer pain. These guidelines stress individualization of therapy and provide a systematic approach (Foley 1986; Foley and Inturrisi 1987; Foley 1987).

Analgesic drugs are classified according to their chemical receptor and pharmacologic properties, their sites and mechanisms of analgesia, and the intensity of pain for which they are generally used. Based on this last concept, analgesics can be separated into three broadly defined groups: the mild analgesics, including the nonopioid analgesics and certain weak opioid analgesics, such as codeine, oxycodone, and propoxyphene; the strong opioid analgesics, including morphine and related opioids; and the adjuvant analgesic drugs, which include those that may enhance the analgesic effects of the opioids, and those which have intrinsic analgesic activity in certain situations, e.g., amitriptyline.

MILD ANALGESICS

Mild analgesics include both the nonopioids and the weak opioid analgesics, whose common therapeutic indication is to relieve mild-to-moderate pain. This group represents the first-line approach to the management of cancer pain and includes: acetaminophen, aspirin, and the nonsteroidal anti-inflammatory drugs (NSAIDs) (Kantor 1982). These drugs are most commonly used orally, and tolerance and physical dependence do not occur with repeated administration. However, their analgesic effectiveness is limited by ceiling effects, i.e., escalation of the dose beyond a certain level (for aspirin, 900 mg to 1300 mg per dose) does not produce additive analgesia. Aspirin and the NSAIDs have analgesic, antipyretic, and anti-inflammatory actions. As an analgesic, acetaminophen is as potent as aspirin and is an antipyretic, but it is much less effective than aspirin in inflammatory conditions. Aspirin and acetaminophen are the drugs of first choice because of their proven efficacy for mild-to-moderate pain, and because of their relatively low cost. Acetaminophen has certain advantages over aspirin and the NSAIDs as a mild analgesic. Patients allergic to aspirin do not exhibit cross-sensitivity to acetaminophen. The NSAIDs have an analgesic effectiveness equal to or greater than that of aspirin. They share with aspirin adverse effects on the gastrointestinal, hematopoietic, hepatic, and renal systems.

These drugs differ in their pharmacokinetic profile and duration of analgesic action. Ibuprofen and fenoprofen, the short half-life NSAIDs, have the same duration of action as aspirin. Diflunisal and naproxyn have longer half-lives and are longer acting. Aspirin and the NSAIDs have a specific role to play in the management of metastatic bone pain. Studies have shown that aspirin inhibits tumor growth in an animal model of metastatic bone tumor, and dramatic pain relief has

Table 38.5
ASSESSMENT APPROACH TO THE MANAGEMENT OF THE PATIENT WITH CANCER PAIN

1. Believe the patient's complaint of pain
2. Take a careful history of the pain complaint to place it temporally in the patient's cancer history
3. Assess the characteristics of the pain including its site, its pattern of referral, its aggravating and relieving factors
4. Clarify the temporal aspects of the pain: acute, subacute, chronic, intermittent, or incident
5. Assess the type of patient with pain (table 38.2), evaluating the prior and existing psychological state of the patient, and the degree of suffering
6. Perform a careful medical and neurological examination
7. Order and personally review the appropriate diagnostic procedures
8. Know the limitations of the diagnostic procedures employed
9. Evaluate the patient's extent of disease
10. Define the specific pain syndrome and outline a therapeutic approach (table 38.3)
11. Treat the pain to facilitate the necessary workup
12. Provide continuity of care from evaluation to treatment to ensure patient compliance and to reduce anxiety
13. Individualize the management approach to the needs of the patient

Table 38.6
GUIDELINES FOR THE PRACTICAL USE OF OPIOID ANALGESICS

1. Start with a specific drug for a specific type of pain
2. Know the pharmacology of the drug prescribed
   a. Know the difference between potency and efficacy
   b. Know the duration of the analgesic effect
   c. Know the pharmacokinetics of the drug
   d. Know the equianalgesic doses for the drug and its route of administration
3. Administer analgesic on a regular basis
4. Use a combination of drugs to provide additive analgesia
   a. Opioid plus nonopioid (aspirin, acetaminophen, NSAIDs)
   b. Opioid plus antihistamine (hydroxycine)
   c. Opioid plus amphetamine (dexedrine)
5. Gear the route of administration to the patient's needs
6. Treat the side-effects appropriately
   a. Sedation
   b. Respiratory depression
   c. Nausea and vomiting
   d. Constipation
   e. Multifocal myoclonus and seizures
7. Watch for the development of tolerance
8. Taper drugs slowly
9. Respect individual differences among patients
10. Do not use placebos to assess the nature of the pain
11. Anticipate complications
    a. Overdose
    b. Psychological dependence

been reported anecdotally in several series of patients receiving NSAIDs for management of severe, metastatic bone pain. However, the response of individual cancer patients to a particular NSAID is not easily predictable. It is therefore recommended that each patient be given an adequate trial of one drug on a regular basis before switching to another drug. If analgesia is not adequate, a trial of another NSAID, one at a time, is appropriate. The concurrent use of two different NSAIDs is discouraged because of the available *in vitro* data suggesting that such combinations compete with each other for protein binding and therefore have diminished analgesic effectiveness.

WEAK OPIOID ANALGESICS

When a nonopioid analgesic is ineffective or poorly tolerated, an opioid analgesic is considered as an alternative drug to manage mild-to-moderate pain. Codeine, oxycodone, and propoxyphene are classified as the mild opioid analgesics, and they all share the same spectrum of pharmacologic action as morphine. They are most often used with a nonopioid in a fixed oral dose mixture. Because these drugs possess a higher analgesic potential than the nonopioid drugs, they serve as a second step in the analgesic ladder that has been promoted by the World Health Organization (fig. 38.1) (WHO 1986). The major advantage of using a combination of a weak opioid with a nonopioid is that there is additive analgesia. The opioid mediates analgesia by binding to opiate receptors in the central nervous system, whereas the nonopioid acts to inhibit the biosynthesis of prostaglandins and acts on peripheral receptors.

Currently, many of the fixed-dose combinations of opioids and nonopioids contain less than the full dose of a nonopioid agent. To individualize the dose better, it is recommended that each component be administered separately. This is particularly important in the patient who becomes tolerant to the opioid portion of the

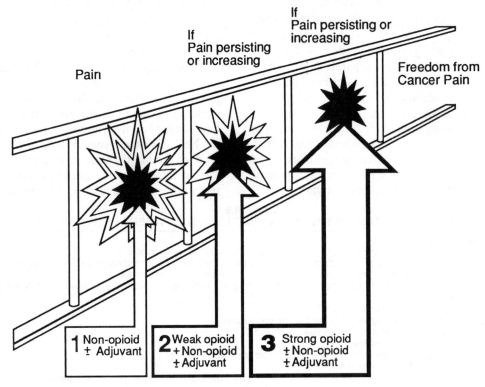

Fig. 38.1. The WHO 3-step ladder for cancer pain relief.

fixed-dose combination, or who has increased pain. When escalation of the fixed-dose combination is required, the additional NSAID may become excessive. If the patient has had a sufficient trial of a nonopioid analgesic with adequate doses on a regular basis, and has obtained minimal pain relief, or experienced excessive side effects, the use of a weak opioid in combination with a nonopioid is the treatment approach of choice.

In those patients with moderate-to-severe pain, it is often more appropriate to start with a weak opioid and to titrate the patient to a strong opioid, particularly if pain relief is inadequate.

STRONG OPIOID ANALGESICS

The opioid analgesics are characterized by important pharmacologic differences derived from their interaction with multiple CNS opioid receptors. The morphine-like agonist drugs present one end of the spectrum. They bind to discrete opiate receptors and produce analgesia. The opioid antagonist drugs represent the other end of the spectrum. These drugs also bind to opioid receptors, but block the effect of morphine-like agonists and do not have analgesic properties of their own. Between these two groups are the mixed-agonist/antagonist drugs that can demonstrate agonist or antagonist properties. Tables 38.7 and 38.8 list the commonly available agonist, mixed-agonist/antagonist, and partial-agonist drugs, as well as their plasma half-life, relative potency, usual starting dose, and current pharmacologic facts.

In choosing an opioid analgesic, it is essential to understand the pharmacology of the specific drug. It is also essential to distinguish between the terms *potency* and *efficacy* when comparing one opioid analgesic to another.

Relative analgesic *potency* is the ratio of the doses of two analgesics required to produce the same analgesic effect. Increased potency alone does not provide any selective advantage, because the more potent drugs also exhibit a parallel increase in their ability to produce undesirable effects. Analgesic *efficacy* refers to the level or degree of analgesia that can be achieved by increasing the dose of the drug to the point of limiting side effects. Relative potency estimates allow calculation of the equianalgesic dose, which provides a rational basis for selecting the appropriate dose when changing the drug or the route of administration of the same drug. The equianalgesic dose is the recommended starting dose. The optimal dose for each patient is determined by the adjustment of that dose. The values in table 38.8 are based upon relative potency studies, in which 10 mg of morphine was the starting dose. When selecting an equianalgesic dose, this table can be quite useful but its limitations need to be understood. Table 38.7 provides relative potency studies for the drugs used for mild-to-moderate pain, and table 38.8 for moderate-to-severe pain. The equianalgesic tables provide a relationship between the various opioid analgesics and a starting point for the physician when recommending analgesic doses. It is strongly recommended that each dose be titrated to the needs of the individual patient because of

the wide variation in a patient's pain, as well as in the pharmacokinetic profile of each of these drugs.

The third group of drugs, referred to as the adjuvant analgesic drugs, are used either as coanalgesics in specific types of pain, or are used to counteract the adverse effects of the opioids. Their specific use is considered within the discussion of the guidelines for the rational use of nonopioid and opioid analgesics. Specific guidelines for the treatment of cancer pain have been developed as part of the World Health Organization's Cancer Pain Relief Program (WHO 1986). These guidelines are based on the use of a three-step analgesic ladder combining the use of nonopioids, opioids, and adjuvant drugs.

GUIDELINES FOR THE USE OF DRUG THERAPY IN CANCER PAIN MANAGEMENT

START WITH A SPECIFIC DRUG FOR A SPECIFIC TYPE OF PAIN

In those patients with mild-to-moderate pain who have not responded or could not tolerate a nonopioid analgesic, an oral opioid analgesic such as codeine or oxycodone is the appropriate first choice. Each drug should be given an adequate trial on a regular basis before it is considered to be ineffective. The next step is to use oral morphine. For acute, severe pain, parenteral morphine is the drug of choice. Oral morphine has been considered the first-line drug of choice for the management of patients with pain and cancer for several reasons: it has a short half-life; its pharmacokinetics remain linear over repeated administration; it is widely available; and there is a large clinical experience in its chronic use in both the English and American hospice movements (Ventafridda, Ripamonti, and Bianchi 1986; Ventafridda, Tamburini, and Caraceni 1987).

Other choices for an opioid analgesic include hydromorphone and levorphanol, both congeners of morphine. Because of its short half-life hydromorphone is a useful alternative to both levorphanol and methadone in elderly patients who do not tolerate morphine. Levorphanol, with its long plasma half-life, is also a useful alternative to morphine, but it must be used cautiously. For patents who are unable to tolerate either morphine or hydromorphone, levorphanol represents a useful medication with a good oral-to-parenteral ratio of 2:1.

In cancer pain management, methadone is a second-line opioid analgesic. The bioavailability of methadone is 85%, and its oral-to-parenteral ratio is 1:2. However, although its plasma half-life averages 24 hours, with a range from 13 to 50 hours, its duration of analgesia is often only four to eight hours. Repetitive analgesic doses of methadone lead to drug accumulation because of this discrepancy. Methadone is a useful alternative to morphine but requires greater sophistication in its clinical use (Ventafridda, Ripamonte, and Bianchi

Table 38.7
ANALGESICS COMMONLY USED ORALLY FOR MILD-TO-MODERATE PAIN

DRUG	DOSE* (MG)	DOSE RANGE (MG)	COMMENTS	PRECAUTIONS
A. Non-Narcotics				
Aspirin	650	650	Often used in combination with opioid-type analgesics	Renal dysfunction; avoid in hematologic disorders and in combination with steroids
Choline magnesium trisalicylate	ND+	1500-3000	Longer duration of action than aspirin	Minimal gastrointestinal side effects; no effect on platelets
Acetaminophen	650	650	No significant anti-inflammatory effects	Minimal gastrointestinal side effects; no effect on platelets
Ibuprofen (Motrin)	ND	200-400	Anti-inflammatory and analgesic effects	
Fenoprofen (Nalfon)	ND	200-400	Like ibuprofen	Like aspirin
Diflunisal (Dolobid)	ND	500-1000	Longer duration of action than ibuprofen; higher analgesic potential than aspirin	Like aspirin
Naproxen (Naproxyn)	550	250-500	Like diflunisal	Like aspirin
B. Morphine-Like Agonists				
Codeine	32-65	32-65	Often used in combination with nonopioid analgesics; biotransformed in part to morphine	Impaired ventilation; bronchial asthma increased intracranial pressure
Oxycodone	5	5-10	Shorter acting; also in combination with nonopioid analgesics (Percodan, Percocet) which limits dose escalation	Like codeine
Meperidine (Demerol)	50	50-100	Shorter acting; biotransformed to normeperidine, a toxic metabolite	Normeperidine accumulates with repetitive dosing causing CNS excitation; not for patients with impaired renal function or receiving monoamine oxidase inhibitors
Propoxyphene HCL (Darvon) Propoxyphene napsylate (Darvon-N)	65-130	65-130	"Weak" narcotic; often used in combination with nonopioid analgesics; long half-life; biotransformed to potentially toxic metabolite (norpropoxyphene)	Propoxyphene and metabolite accumulate with repetitive dosing; overdose complicated by convulsions
C. Mixed Agonist-Antagonists				
Pentazocine (Talwin)	50	50-100	In combination with nonopioids; in combination with naloxone to discourage parenteral abuse	May cause psychotomimetic effects; may precipitate withdrawal in opioid-dependent patients

For these equianalgesic doses (see also comments) the time of peak analgesia ranges from 1.5 to 2 hours and the duration from 4 to 6 hours. Oxycodone and meperidine are shorter-acting (3-5 hours) and diflunisal and naproxen are longer-acting (8 to 12 hours).
* These are the recommended starting doses from which the optimal dose for each patient is determined by titration and the maximal dose limited by adverse effects.
+ ND = not determined.

Table 38.8
ORAL AND PARENTERAL OPIOID ANALGESICS FOR MODERATE-TO-SEVERE PAIN

	Route*	Dose+ (mg)	Duration(hr)	Plasma Half-life(hr)	Comments
A. Narcotic Agonists					
Morphine	IM	1060	4-6	2-3.5	Standard for comparison; also available in slow-release tablets and rectal suppositories
	PO		4-7		
Codeine	IM	130	4-6	3	Biotransformed to morphine; useful as initial opioid analgesic
	PO	200+	4-6		
Oxycodeine	IM	15		—	Short-acting; available as 5 mg dose in combination with aspirin and acetominophen
	PO	30	3-5		
Heroin	IM	5	4-5	0.5	Illegal in United States; high solubility for parenteral administration
	PO	(60)	4-5		
Levorphanol (Levocromoran)	IM	2	4-6	12-16	Good oral potency, requires careful titration in initial dosing because of drug accumulation
	PO	4	4-7		
Hydromorphone (Dilaudid)	IM	1.5	4-5	2-3	Available in high-potency injectable form (10 mg/mL) for cachetic patients and as rectal suppositories; more soluble than morphine
	PO	7.5	4-6		
Oxymorphone (Numorphan)	IM	1	4-6	2-3	Available in parenteral and rectal suppository form only
	PR	10	4-6		
Meperdine (Demerol)	IM	75	4-5	3-4	Contraindicated in patients with renal disease; accumulation of active toxic metabolite normeperidine; produces CNS excitation
	PO	300+	4-6	12-16	
Methodone (Dolophine)	IM	10		15-30	Good oral potency; requires careful titration of the initial dose to avoid drug accumulation
	PO	20			
B. Mixed Agonist-Antagonists					
Pentazocine (Talwin)	IM	60	4-6	2-3	Limited use in cancer pain; psychotomimetic effects with dose escalation; available only in combination with naloxone; aspirin or acetaminophen may precipitate withdrawal in tolerant patients
	PO	180+	4-7		
Malbuphine (Mybalm)	IM	10	4-6	5	Not available orally; less severe psychotomimetic effects than pentazocine; may precipitate withdrawal in physically dependent patients
	PO	—			
Butorphanol (Stadol)	IM	2	4-6	2.5-3.5	Not available orally; produces psychotomimetic effects; may precipitate withdrawal in physically dependent patients
	PO	—			
C. Partial Agonists					
Buprenorphine (Tengesic)	IM	0.4	4-6	7	Not available in United States; no psychotomimetic effects; may precipitate withdrawal in tolerant patients
	SL	0.8	5-6		

*IM denotes intramuscular, PO oral, PR rectal, and SL sublingual.
+Based on single-dose studies in which an intramuscular dose of each drug listed was compared with morphine to establish the relative potency. Oral doses are those recommended when changing from a parenteral to an oral route. For patients without prior narcotic exposure, the recommended oral starting dose is 30 mg for morphine, 5 mg for methadone, 2 mg for levorphanol, and 4 mg for hydromorphone.

1986). It is most useful in the patient who has developed some degree of tolerance to morphine, or who has had a prior opioid experience. In the opioid-naive patient, initial doses should be titrated carefully and not on a fixed regimen.

Opioid mixed agonist/antagonist drugs such as pentazocine, nalbuphine, and butorphanol have a limited role. In therapeutic doses these drugs may produce certain self-limiting psychotomimetic effects. Patients receiving opioid agonist drugs on a long-term basis may experience an opioid withdrawal reaction when given a mixed agonist/antagonist drug. Therefore, these drugs should be tried before prolonged administration of an opioid agonist is initiated. Pentazocine is available only in combination with naloxone, and nalbuphine and butorphanol are only available in parenteral preparations, making long-term use in the cancer patient unfeasible. A newer drug in this class, the partial agonist buprenorphine, may also precipitate narcotic withdrawal in patients receiving narcotic analgesics for prolonged periods. Buprenorphine, however, does not produce psychotomimetic effects. It is currently available in Europe in a sublingual preparation, and has been demonstrated to be effective as a first-line agent in the management of patients with mild-to-moderate cancer pain (Ventafridda, DeConno, and Guarise 1983).

KNOW THE PHARMACOLOGY OF THE DRUG PRESCRIBED

DURATION OF ANALGESIC EFFECT
The duration of analgesic effect is the result of many factors including the dose, the intensity of pain, the criteria for analgesia, the individual pharmacokinetic variation, and the patient's prior opioid experience. Table 38.8 lists the relative duration for each analgesic at the dose which produces the peak equivalent to that of morphine. Drugs which are administered by mouth have a slower onset of action and a longer duration of effect. Drugs given parenterally have a rapid onset of action but a shorter duration of effect. Recognition of these differences allows for appropriate prescribing of each agent.

PHARMACOKINETICS OF THE DRUG
The plasma half-lives of the opioid analgesics vary widely and do not correlate with the analgesic time course (Inturrisi et al. 1984). As has been previously discussed, the drugs methadone and levorphanol produce analgesia for four to six hours but accumulate with repetitive dosing, and such accumulation accounts for the untoward effects of sedation and respiratory depression. Adjustment of dose and dosing interval based on the plasma half-life may be necessary during the introduction of these drugs. More importantly, plasma half-life can be altered by compromised liver and kidney function, and dose adjustments and dosing intervals must be individualized.

EQUIANALGESIC DOSE AND ROUTE OF ADMINISTRATION
Knowledge of the equianalgesic doses ensures more appropriate drug use, particularly when switching from one opioid analgesic to another, and from one route of administration to another. Lack of attention to differences in drug dose is the most common cause of undermedication of pain patients and can lead to overmedication as well.

Patients who have been receiving one opioid analgesic for a long period and who are then switched to another opioid analgesic to provide better analgesia should receive half the equianalgesic dose of the new drug as the initial starting dose. This is based upon the concept that cross-tolerance is not complete, and that the relative potency of some of the opioid analgesics may change with repetitive doses.

ADMINISTER ANALGESICS REGULARLY
Medication should be administered regularly, and the patient should be awakened from sleep if necessary. The purpose of this is to maintain the patient's pain at a tolerable level. The development of steady-state level may allow reduction in the total amount of drug taken in a 24-hour period. Once they reach a steady-state, patients receiving methadone require a smaller amount of the drug than that initially prescribed to control pain. The pharmacologic rationale for this approach is to maintain the plasma level of the drug above the minimal effective concentration for pain relief. Before determining that an opioid analgesic is ineffective in a particular patient, the drug should be given regularly with the interval between the doses based upon the known duration of drug effect. The time to reach a steady-state level depends upon the half-life of the drug, e.g., with morphine, steady-state levels can be reached with five to six doses within a 24-hour period, whereas it may take five to seven days to reach steady-state with methadone. Full assessment of the analgesic efficacy of a drug cannot be completed in a 1- or 2-day period.

USE OF COMBINATIONS OF DRUGS
A combination of drugs can provide additive analgesia, may reduce side effects, and can reduce the rate of dose escalation of the opioid portion of the combination. There are several combinations that produce additive analgesic effects. These include an opioid plus a nonopioid, such as aspirin, acetaminophen, or ibuprofen; an opioid plus an antihistamine, specifically, hydroxyzine 100 mg; or an opioid plus an amphetamine, intramuscular dexedrine. Studies have demonstrated the efficacy of these combinations for single-dose studies, using larger doses than are commonly used. In clinical practice, 25 mg of oral hydroxyzine has been used on a regular basis, with anecdotal observations of its effectiveness. Similarly, dextroamphetamine in 2.5 mg to 5 mg oral doses given twice a day, and methylphenidate in 5 mg to 10 mg doses twice a day, have been reported to reduce the sedative effects of opioids in patients

receiving adequate analgesia but with excessive sedation. Several adjuvant drugs that appear to have analgesic properties on their own include the corticosteroids, the anticonvulsants, the tricyclic antidepressants, the phenothiazines, and the butyrophenones. Controlled studies now demonstrate that both cocaine and the benzodiazepines do not provide additive analgesia to patients receiving opioid analgesics.

CORTICOSTEROIDS

Corticosteroids have been reported to have specific and nonspecific benefits in managing acute and chronic cancer pain. Their ability to provide euphoria, increased appetite, and weight gain greatly contributes to the cancer patient's sense of well-being. Corticosteroids are reported to reduce bone pain of metastatic origin, and are commonly used as oncolytic agents for certain types of tumors. Several studies demonstrate prolonged survival time and reduced opioid dosage requirements in terminal cancer patients with benefits outweighing the potential risks. The recent data suggests that the corticosteroid effect is short-lived and not maintained in controlled studies. In particular instances, the dose of corticosteroids depends upon the clinical situation. For the treatment of patients with severe headache and increased intracranial pressure, doses of dexamethasone of 16 mg/day ameliorate the pain and other neurologic symptoms. For patients with epidural spinal cord compression, the regimen of initial treatment with 100 mg of dexamethasone given intravenously, followed by a tapering schedule and maintenance dose of 16 mg of dexamethasone during radiation therapy, has been associated with significant pain reduction. For patients with tumor infiltration of the peripheral nerve or plexus, 16 mg of dexamethasone as an initial bolus, followed by a tapering schedule during radiation therapy, is associated with significant pain reduction. In patients receiving corticosteroids, nonsteroidal anti-inflammatory drugs should be avoided because these drugs may place the patient at greater risk for gastrointestinal side effects.

ANTICONVULSANTS

This group of adjuvant analgesic drugs have specific analgesic effects in certain pain syndromes. Phenytoin and carbamazepine are most useful in the management of patients with pain of neuropathic origin such as occurs in brachial and lumbosacral plexopathy and postherpetic neuralgia. In patients with phantom limb pain, secondary to traumatic neuromas, and in patients with postsurgical neuropathic pain syndromes, carbamazepine has been anecdotally reported to be useful. The minimal effective dose for analgesia from these drugs has not been determined. The dose of carbamazepine is typically 100 mg/day and slowly increased to 800 mg/day over a 7- to 10-day period. Similarly for phenytoin, the initial starting dose is 100 mg slowly titrated up to 300 mg/day. Side effects for each of these drugs can be significant, and they should be watched carefully. With carbamazepine, blood counts should be taken before drug therapy is started, two weeks after initiation of therapy, and at regular intervals to assess the degree, if any, of neutropenia.

TRICYCLIC ANTIDEPRESSANTS

The tricyclic antidepressants have analgesic properties in specific pain conditions of neuropathic origin. The mechanism of analgesic efficacy is thought to be mediated by increasing levels of serotonin in the CNS. Amitriptyline has been most widely studied and has been demonstrated to be effective in controlling neuropathic pain in both postherpetic neuralgia and diabetic neuropathy. It is commonly used in the management of patients with brachial and lumbosacral plexopathy because of the underlying nature of the neuropathic pain (Walsh 1983). The doses of amitriptyline as an analgesic vary from 10 mg to 75 mg. The starting dose is 25 mg, and 10 mg for the elderly patient. The dose is slowly titrated to 75 mg daily, using a single bedtime dose. There is increasing evidence to suggest that dose escalations may provide the patient with additive analgesia, and increases should be made to 150 mg/day if the patient is able to tolerate the drug. Imipramine has also been reported to enhance morphine analgesia in cancer patients with pain.

PHENOTHIAZINES

Methotrimeprazine (Levoprome) is a phenothiazine drug with significant analgesic efficacy. In single-dose studies in patients with postoperative pain and chronic pain, 15 mg given intramuscularly is equivalent to 10 mg of intramuscular morphine. Methotrimeprazine is useful in managing the patient who is tolerant to opioid analgesics, because its analgesia is not produced through an opiate receptor mechanism. It is also useful in the patient with bowel obstruction and pain because unlike the opioids, it does not produce significant constipation. In the patient with respiratory compromise, methotrimeprazine avoids the selective respiratory depressant effects of the opioids. Because of its antiemetic and antianxiety properties, it can be helpful in managing the patient with hepatic-induced nausea, vomiting, and anxiety. Treatment should begin with the initial test dose of 5 mg given parenterally to assess both its sedative and hypotensive effects. Doses of 10 mg to 20 mg parenterally are most commonly used. The drug is recommended for intermittent, not chronic, administration and for the management of patients with acute abdominal obstruction in whom opioids would only add to the problems of obstruction.

Prochlorperazine and metoclopramide are commonly used to manage the emetic effects of the opioid analgesics. They are used in combination with an opioid and can often be discontinued once a patient is on a stable dose of opioid and has developed tolerance to the drug's emetic properties. Metoclopramide also increases gastric emptying time, which is commonly delayed by opioid drugs.

BUTYROPHENONES

Haloperidol has been anecdotally reported to be useful in cancer patients with pain (Brevik and Rennemo 1982), but its major role is as the first-line drug in the management of acute psychosis and delirium with doses ranging from 1 mg to 3 mg, one to three times a day.

GEAR THE ROUTE OF ADMINISTRATION TO THE PATIENT'S NEEDS

The route of administration should be geared to the patient's needs. The oral route is the most practical, but in patients who require immediate pain relief parenteral administration, either intramuscular or intravenous, is the route of choice (Aker 1979). The rectal route of administration should be considered for patients who cannot take oral drugs or for whom parenteral administration is contraindicated (Beaver and Feise 1977). Several of the more novel routes of drug administration, including sublingual (Weinberg et al. 1988), continuous subcutaneous (Bruera et al. 1987; Coyle et al. 1986), continuous intravenous, and continuous epidural and intrathecal infusions (Coombs, Saunders, and Gaylor 1982; Cousins and Bridenbaugh 1987; Moulin, Inturrisi, and Foley, 1986), provide cancer patients with a variety of alternatives. The use of continuous subcutaneous and continuous intravenous infusions have allowed patients to return home during the terminal phases of their illness, with adequate pain control by the parenteral route of administration that can be easily managed by family and home care agency. Specific guidelines for the use of these techniques have been developed (Bruera et al. 1987; Coyle et al. 1986; Coombs, Saunders and Gaylor 1982; Portenoy et al. 1985).

TREAT THE SIDE EFFECTS APPROPRIATELY

The use of opioid analgesics can have both desirable and undesirable side effects; it is the adverse effects that markedly limit their use. The limiting components of these side effects have been the major impetus for the development of novel routes of administration. The most common side effects are respiratory depression, nausea and vomiting, sedation, constipation, urinary retention, and multifocal myoclonus. A host of other side effects including confusion, hallucinations, nightmares, dizziness, and dysphoria have been reported by patients acutely and chronically receiving these drugs.

RESPIRATORY DEPRESSION

Respiratory depression is potentially the most serious adverse effect. Therapeutic doses of morphine may depress all phases of respiratory activity (rate, minute/volume, tidal exchange). However, as carbon dioxide accumulates it stimulates the respiratory center, resulting in a compensatory increase in respiratory rate that masks the degree of respiratory depression. At equianalgesic doses, the morphine-like drugs produce an equivalent degree of respiratory depression. For obvious reasons, individuals with impaired respiratory function or bronchial asthma are at greater risk of experiencing clinically significant respiratory depression in response to usual doses of these drugs. When respiratory depression occurs, it is usually in opioid-naive patients following acute administration of an opioid, and is associated with signs of CNS depression including sedation and mental clouding. Tolerance to this effect develops rapidly with repeated drug administration, allowing opioid analgesics to be used in the management of chronic cancer pain without significant risk of respiratory depression.

In patients chronically receiving opioids who develop respiratory depression, naloxone diluted 1 part to 10 should be titrated carefully to prevent the precipitation of severe withdrawal symptoms while reversing the respiratory depression. In the comatose patient, an endotracheal tube should be placed before administering naloxone to prevent aspiration-associated respiratory compromise with excessive salivation and bronchial spasm.

In patients receiving meperidine chronically, naloxone may produce seizures by blocking the depressant action of meperidine and allowing the convulsant activity of the metabolite normeperidine to be manifest.

SEDATION

Sedation and drowsiness vary with the drug and dose and may occur after both single and repetitive administration of opioid drugs. Although these effects may be useful in certain clinical situations, they are not desirable components of analgesia, particularly in the ambulatory patient. Management includes reducing the individual drug dose and prescribing the drug more frequently or switching to an analgesic with a shorter plasma half-life. Amphetamines and methylphenyldate in combination with an opioid can be used to counteract the sedative effects, as well as discontinuing all other drug therapy that might exacerbate the sedative effects of the opioid analgesics.

NAUSEA AND VOMITING

The opioid analgesics produce nausea and vomiting by an action limited to the medullary chemoreceptor trigger zone. The incidence of nausea or vomiting is markedly increased in ambulatory patients. Tolerance develops to these side effects with repeated administration of the drugs. Nausea caused by one drug does not mean that all drugs will produce similar symptoms. To obviate this effect, switch the patient to an alternative opioid analgesic or prescribe an antiemetic, e.g., prochlorperazine or metoclopramide, in combination with the opioid.

CONSTIPATION

The opioid analgesics act at multiple sites in the gastrointestinal tract and spinal cord and produce a decrease in intestinal secretions and peristalsis, resulting in a dry stool and constipation. At the time opioid analgesics are started, provisions for regular bowel regimen including cathartics and stool softeners should be instituted. Anecdotal survey data suggests that doses far above those used for routine bowel management are necessary and that careful attention to dietary factors combined with the use of a bowel regimen can reduce patient complaints dramatically. Tolerance to the constipatory effects of these drugs develops very slowly over time.

MULTIFOCAL MYOCLONUS AND SEIZURES

Multifocal myoclonus and seizures have been reported in patients receiving multiple doses of meperidine, although signs and symptoms of CNS hyperirritability may occur with toxic doses of all the opioid analgesics (Kaiko et al. 1983). Management of this CNS hyperirritability includes discontinuing the meperidine, using intravenous Valium if seizures occur, and substituting morphine to control the persistent pain. Because the half-life of normeperidine is 16 hours, it may take two or three days for the signs of CNS hyperirritability to completely clear.

WATCH FOR THE DEVELOPMENT OF TOLERANCE

The earliest sign of the development of tolerance is the patient's complaint that the duration of effective analgesia has decreased. In such instances, increase the frequency of drug administration or increase the amount of drug at each dose. It has been well-demonstrated that tolerance occurs in all patients receiving opioid analgesics on a chronic basis. More importantly, it is recognized that tolerance to each of the desirable and undesirable effects of the opioid drugs occurs at different rates. For example, tolerance to the respiratory depressant effects of the opioid occur quite rapidly. Tolerance to the constipatory effects of the drugs develops very slowly, if at all. There is no limit to tolerance, and escalation of drug dose often requires doubling the dose to produce a better analgesic effect. The dose of the drug should not be the major concern of the prescribing physician. Studies of the patterns of opioid use in patients with cancer pain reveal that the majority of cancer patients increased their opioid requirements from their initial dose to the time of death. However, one-third of patients maintain a stable dose of drug throughout the entire course of their pain therapy and a small percentage of patients, approximately 20%, reduce their opioid requirements (Foley 1986; Kanner and Foley 1981). It is particularly important to recognize that the development of tolerance is multifactorial. It is not only related to the drug itself, but to a series of other factors including progression of disease, psychological state of the patient, prior opioid exposure, and route of administration.

Because cross-tolerance among the opioid analgesics is incomplete, switching from one opioid drug to another is best done by using half the equianalgesic dose and then titrating the patient up to effective pain control. Escalation or reduction of the dose then follows according to the patient's response. An alternative way to manage tolerance is the use of adjuvant analgesic drugs. Similarly, in tolerant patients with pain localized to the buttocks or lower extremities, continuous epidural infusions of a local anesthetic may provide significant temporary analgesia, thereby allowing the reduction of the opioid analgesic. Tolerance develops to this anesthetic approach as well.

TAPER DRUGS SLOWLY

The long-term administration of opioid analgesics is associated with the development of physical dependence, a state in which the sudden cessation of the opioid analgesic produces signs and symptoms of withdrawal. Abrupt withdrawal is characterized by agitation, tremors, insomnia, fear, marked autonomic nervous system hyperexcitability, and exacerbation of pain. A slow tapering of the dose of the opioid prevents such symptoms. The appearance of abstinence symptoms from the time of drug withdrawal is related to the elimination half-life curve for the particular drug. The type of abstinence symptoms similarly varies with the individual drug. For example, with morphine, withdrawal symptoms occur within six to 12 hours after cessation of the drug. Reinstituting the drug in doses of approximately 25% of the previous daily dose suppresses these symptoms.

DO NOT USE PLACEBOS TO ASSESS THE NATURE OF PAIN

The placebo response is a potent phenomenon in clinical medicine and has been well-described in patients with cancer pain. A positive analgesic response from intramuscular saline suggests that the patient is a placebo responder. It does not suggest that the pain is unreal or less severe than reported by the patient. Such misuse of placebos encourages the development of distrust between the patient and physician and interferes with adequate pain control.

ANTICIPATE COMPLICATIONS

Overdose occurs either intentionally, when a patient takes an excessive amount of opioid drug in a suicide attempt, or unintentionally, when the recommended dosage accidentally produces excessive sedation or respiratory depression. In both instances, the complication can be treated effectively with naloxone. Intentional overdose in cancer patients occurs rarely, and concern for this is overemphasized. Overdose in patients previously stabilized on an opioid regimen rarely is caused by drug intake alone. More commonly, it is the medical deterioration of the patient with a superimposed metabolic encephalopathy. Patients who develop unintentional drug overdose should be scrutinized carefully to rule out other causes of excessive sedation, confusion, or respiratory depression. In such cases, a reversal of these effects with naloxone is not necessarily diagnostic.

PHYSICAL AND PSYCHOLOGICAL DEPENDENCE

Physical dependence has been previously described. This is in contrast to psychological dependence or addiction, which is characterized as a concomitant behavioral pattern of drug abuse characterized by craving a drug for more than pain relief and by overwhelming involvement in procurement of the drug. This is a state distinct from tolerance and from physical dependence, which are responses to the pharmacologic effect of long-term opioid administration. The profound fear of causing psychological dependence plays a major role in the physician's reluctance to prescribe opioid analgesics, particularly in cancer patients in the early phase of their disease (Marks and Sachar 1973). This same fear is shared by patients who consistently take less analgesic drug than is effective to control their pain. There is increasing evidence to suggest that cancer patients with pain can take opioid analgesics for prolonged periods and can discontinue such drugs when adequate pain relief is achieved by other approaches. In almost all instances, dramatic escalation of drug intake is associated with progression of disease and subsequent death. A very small percentage of patients with cancer and pain may become psychologically dependent upon drugs and may participate in drug-seeking behavior and illicit drug use. However, clinical experience demonstrates that this group has had a prior experience with drug abuse behavior before the diagnosis of their cancer. Careful evaluation of patients who might be at risk for the development of this complication is necessary, but such concern should not be punitive to the patient with severe cancer pain.

Effective use of pharmacologic approaches can manage pain in 85% to 95% of patients with pain and cancer. However, it is important to recognize that multiple approaches can be combined with pharmacologic approaches to help improve symptoms in patients with pain and cancer. These approaches include psychological, anesthetic, and neurosurgical approaches.

PSYCHOLOGICAL APPROACHES

Psychological approaches should be an integral part of the care of the cancer patient with pain (Massie and Holland 1987). The major goal of these interventions is to promote an increased sense of control, by reducing the sense of hopelessness and helplessness that many cancer patients with pain experience. Comparative effectiveness of any one of these techniques to medical or surgical therapy is impossible. These varied techniques are especially useful in three clinical situations: in the management of patients with intermittent predictable pain, such as pain associated with procedures; in the management of incidental pain of patients with metastatic bone disease, controlled at rest but markedly exacerbated by movement; and in the management of chronic cancer pain by providing patients with specific coping and behavioral techniques to help them live with their chronic pain. These techniques include hypnosis, relaxation training, biofeedback, psychotherapy, and cognitive and behavioral training (Fishman and Loscalzo 1987).

ANESTHETIC APPROACHES

Anesthetic approaches consist of five major types: myofascial trigger point injections, peripheral nerve blocks, autonomic nerve blocks, intrathecal nerve blocks, and the use of nitrous oxide. The techniques for each of these procedures are described in detail in standard textbooks (Cousins and Bridenbaugh 1987). Short-acting and long-acting anesthetics are used for temporary and diagnostic nerve blocks, e.g., trigger point injections, whereas phenol, alcohol, and freezing of the nerves are the common agents used for permanent blocks. The principle pathologic effect produced by these chemical agents is demyelination and secondary nerve degeneration. The block produced by phenol tends to be less profound and of shorter duration than that of alcohol, and phenol is more commonly used to its advantage when the risk of motor paresis or loss of bowel or bladder control is high. Local freezing of the nerve produces a functional loss in the nerve that only lasts for several weeks. In most instances a permanent nerve block is performed only when a temporary nerve block has demonstrated some efficacy. The available anesthetic and neurosurgical approaches are listed in tables 38.9 and 38.10.

NEUROSURGICAL APPROACHES

Neurosurgical approaches can be divided into two major categories: neurodestructive procedures in which surgical or radiofrequency lesions are made along pain pathways; and neurostimulatory procedures, in which electrodes are stereotactically placed to activate pain-inhibitory pathways. These procedures have been used in the management of cancer pain with varying success (Nathan 1963; Rosomoff, Carroll, and Brown 1975; Sundaresan and DiGiacinto 1987; Ventafridda and Bonica 1979). The available data suggests that these procedures are more effective for cancer pain than for chronic nonmalignant pain. In part this reflects the fact that most of the procedures are useful for somatic pain and not for neuropathic pain. Again, reviews of the neurosurgical management of pain contain details of the types of procedures and technical approaches. Certain guidelines apply to the use of these procedures for the cancer patient. The selection of the appropriate procedure should be individualized for the patient and the specific pain problem. An adequate trial of analgesics and antitumor therapy should be initiated, and both the referring physician and the patient should be aware of the potential risks and benefits of the planned procedure.

Of all of the neurosurgical procedures for pain relief, cordotomy remains the most useful and durable. The major goal is to interrupt the anterolateral spinothalamic tract in the cervical or thoracic region. This procedure may be performed as a percutaneous, stereotactic procedure, or by an open surgical approach. It is most useful in managing unilateral pain below the level of the mandible, and is most enduring in unilateral pain below the waist. This procedure is most commonly used

Table 38.9
TYPES OF ANESTHETIC PROCEDURES COMMONLY USED IN CANCER PAIN

TYPE	MOST COMMON INDICATIONS
I. NERVE BLOCKS	
Peripheral	Pain in discrete dermatomes in chest and abdomen
Epidural	Unilateral lumbar or sacral pain Midline perineal pain Bilateral lumbosacral pain
Intrathecal	Midline perineal pain Bilateral lumbosacral pain
Autonomic: Stellate ganglion	Reflex sympathetic dystrophy, e.g., frozen shoulder Arm pain
Lumbar sympathetic	Reflex sympathic dystrophy Lumbosacral plexopathy Vascular insufficiency of the lower extremity
Coeliac plexus	Midabdominal pain
II. CONTINUOUS EPIDURAL INFUSION WITH LOCAL ANESTHETICS	Unilateral and bilateral lumbosacral pain Midline perineal pain
III. CHEMICAL HYPOPHYSECTOMY	Diffuse bone pain
IV. INHALATION THERAPY	Generalized pain Incident pain
V. TRIGGER POINT INJECTION	Focal muscle pain

in cancer patients with pain, providing patients with adequate analgesia for several months prior to death.

All of the neurosurgical approaches are most effective in treating patients with well-defined localized pain. However, diffuse rather than focal pain problems are more common in cancer patients, so the role of neurosurgery is limited. These clinical limitations are magnified further by the fact that patients, as they become more aware of their disease and treatment options, are hesitant to undergo neurodestructive procedures. They consider the pain an important marker for their disease and are concerned about the potential complications of these procedures. As a result, the procedures are performed late, rather than early, during a patient's illness, and full evaluation of their effectiveness and duration of action is limited by the patient's overriding medical problems.

In summary, a multidisciplinary approach to managing pain in cancer patients is currently feasible, and effective use of a wide range of modalities is the rule rather than the exception.

Table 38.10
NEUROABLATIVE, NEUROSTIMULATORY, NEUROPHARMACOLOGIC PROCEDURES
FOR CANCER PAIN MANAGEMENT

SITE	NEUROABLATIVE	NEUROSTIMULATORY	PHARMACOLOGIC
Peripheral nerve	Neurectomy	Transcutaneous and percutaneous electrical nerve stimulation	Local anesthetics
Nerve Root	Rhizotomy		Local anesthetics Neurolytic agents
Spinal Cord	Dorsal root entry zone lesions Cordotomy Myelotomy	Dorsal column stimulation	Epidural and intrathecal local anesthetics and opiates
Brainstem	Mesencephalic tractotomy	Periaqueductal stimulation	Intraventricular opiates
Thalamus	Thalamotomy	Thalamic stimulation	
Cortex	Cingulumotomy Frontal lobotomy		
Pituitary	Transphenoidal hypophysectomy	Chemical hypophysectomy	

REFERENCES

Aker, S.N. 1979. Oral findings in the cancer patient. *Cancer* 43:2103-107.

Beaver, W.T., and Feise, G.A. 1977. A comparison of the analgesic effects of oxymorphone by rectal suppository and intramuscular injection in patients with postoperative pain. *J. Clin. Pharmacol.* 17:276-91.

Brevik, H., and Rennemo, F. 1982. Clinical evaluation of combined treatment with methadone and psychotropic drugs in cancer patients. *Acta Anesthesiol. Scand.* 74(Suppl):135-40.

Bruera, E.; Chadwick, S.; and Brenneis, C. et al. 1987. Subcutaneous infusion of narcotics using a disposable portable device. *Ca. Treat. Rep.* 71:635-37.

Cascino, T.L.; Kori, S.; and Krol, G. et al. 1983. CT scanning of the brachial plexus in patients with cancer. *Neurology* 33:1553-57.

Coombs, D.W.; Saunders, R.L.; and Gaylor, M.S. 1982. Epidural narcotic infusion reservoir: implantation technique and efficacy. *Anesthesiology* 56:469-73.

Cousins, M.J., and Bridenbaugh, P.O. eds. 1987. *Neural blockade in clinical anesthesia and management of pain.* 2nd ed. Philadelphia: J. B. Lippincott.

Coyle, N.; Mauskop, A.; and Maggard, J. et al. 1986. Continuous subcutaneous infusions of opiates in cancer patients with pain. *Oncol. Nurs. Forum* 13:53-57.

Daut, R.L., and Cleeland, C.S. 1982. The prevalence and severity of pain in cancer. *Cancer* 50:1913-18.

Fishman, B.; Pasternak, S.; and Wallenstein, S.L. et al. 1987. The Memorial pain assessment card: a valid instrument for the evaluation of cancer pain. *Cancer* 60:1151-58.

Fishman, B., and Loscalzo, M. 1987. Cognitive-behavioral interventions in management of cancer pain: principles and applications. In Payne, R., and Foley, K.M. eds. *Medical Clinics of North America: cancer pain.* 71(2):271-88. Philadelphia: W.B. Saunders.

Foley, K.M. 1982. Clinical assessment of pain. *Acta Anesth. Scand.* 74(Suppl):91-96.

Foley, K.M. 1986. Current controversies in opioid therapy. In Foley, K.M., and Inturrisi, C.E. eds. *Advances in pain research and therapy: opioid analgesics in the management of clinical pain.* pp. 3-11. New York: Raven Press.

Foley, K.M. 1987. Brachial plexopathy in patients with breast cancer. In Harris, J.R.; Hellman, S.; and Henderson, I.C. et al. eds. *Breast diseases.* pp. 532-37. Philadelphia: J. B. Lippincott.

Foley, K.M.; Woodruff, J.M.; and Ellis, F. et al. 1980. Radiation-induced malignant and atypical peripheral nerve sheath tumors. *Ann. Neurol.* 7:311-18.

Foley, K.M., and Inturrisi, C.E. 1987. Analgesic drug therapy in cancer pain: principles and practice. In Payne, R., and Foley, K.M. eds. *Medical Clinics of North America: cancer pain.* 71(2): 207-32. Philadelphia: W.B. Saunders.

Foley, K.M. 1985. The treatment of cancer pain. *N. Engl. J. Med.* 313:84-95.

Foley, K.M. 1979. Pain syndromes in patients with cancer. In Bonica, J.J., and Ventafridda, V. eds. *Advances in pain research and therapy.* vol. 2. pp. 59-75. New York: Raven Press.

Granek, I.; Ashikari, R.; and Foley, K.M. 1983. Postmastectomy pain syndrome: clinical and anatomical correlates. *Proc. ASCO* 3:122.

Greenberg, H.S.; Deck, M.D.; and Vikram, B. et al. 1981. Metastasis to the base of the skull: clinical findings in 43 patients. *Neurology* 31:530-37.

Ihde, D.C., and Devita, V.T. 1975. Osteonecrosis of the femoral head in patients with lymphoma treated with intermittent combination chemotherapy (including corticosteroids). *Cancer* 36:1585-88.

Inturrisi, C.E.; Max, M.; and Foley, K.M. et al. 1984. The pharmacokinetics of heroin in patients with chronic pain. *N. Engl. J. Med.* 310:1213-17.

Jaeckle, K.A.; Young, D.F.; and Foley, K.M. 1985. The natural history of lumbosacral plexopathy in cancer. *Neurology* 35:8-15.

Jellinger, K., and Sturm, K.W. 1971. Delayed radiation myelopathy in man. *J. Neurol. Sci.* 14:389-408.

Kaiko, R.F.; Foley, K.M.; and Grabinski, P.Y., et al. 1983. Central nervous system excitatory effects of meperidine in cancer patients. *Ann. Neurol.* 13:180-85.

Kaiko, R.F.; Wallenstein, S.L.; and Rogers, A.G. et al. 1981. Analgesic and mood effects of heroin and morphine in cancer patients with postoperative pain. *N. Engl. J. Med.* 304:1501-05.

Kanner, R.M., and Foley, K.M. 1981. Patterns of narcotic drug use in a cancer pain clinic. *In research developments in drug and alcohol use.* Ann. N.Y. Acad. Sci. 362:161-72.

Kanner, R.M.; Martini, N.; and Foley, K.M. 1982. Incidence of pain and other clinical manifestations of superior pulmonary sulcus tumor (Pancoast's tumors). In Bonica, J.J.; Ventafridda, V.; and Pagni, C.A. eds. *Advances in pain research and therapy.* vol. 4. pp.27-38. New York: Raven Press.

Kanner, R.M.; Martini, N.; and Foley, K.M. 1982. Nature and incidence of post-thoracotomy pain. *Proc. ASCO* 1:152.

Kantor, T.G. 1982. Control of pain by nonsteroidal anti-inflammatory drugs. *Med. Clin. North Am.* 66:1053-59.

Levin, D.; Cleeland, C.S.; and Dar, R. 1985. Public attitudes toward cancer pain. *Cancer* 56:2337-39.

Marks, R.M., and Sachar, E.J. 1973. Undertreatment of medical inpatients with narcotic analgesics. *Ann. Intern. Med.* 78:173-81.

Massie, M.J., and Holland, J.C. 1987. The cancer patient with pain: psychiatric complications and their management. In Payne, R., and Foley, K.M. eds. *Medical Clinics of North America: cancer pain.* 71(2):243-58. Philadelphia: W.B. Saunders.

Moulin, D.E.; Inturrisi, C.E.; and Foley, K.M. 1986. Epidural and intrathecal opioids: cerebrospinal fluid and plasma pharmacokinetics in cancer pain patients. In Foley, K.M., and Inturrisi, C.E. eds. *Advances in pain research and therapy: opioid analgesics in the management of clinical pain.* vol. 8. pp. 369-84. New York: Raven Press.

Nathan, P.W. 1963. Results of anterolateral cordotomy for pain in cancer. *J. Neurol. Neurosurg. Psychiatry* 26:353-62.

Olson, M.E.; Chirnik, N.L.; and Posner, J.B. 1978. Infiltration of the leptomeninges by systemic cancer: a clinical and pathological study. *Arch. Neurol.* 30:122-37.

Pasternak, G.W. 1988. Multiple morphine and enkephalin receptors and the relief of pain. *JAMA.* 259:1362-67.

Payne, R. 1987. Anatomy, physiology, and neuropharmacology of cancer pain. In Payne, R., and Foley, K.M. eds. *Medical Clinics of North America: cancer pain.* 71(2):153-68. Philadelphia: W.B. Saunders.

Payne, R.; and Foley, K.M. 1984. Advances in the management of cancer pain. *Ca. Treat. Rep.* 68:173-83.

Portenoy, R.K.; Duma, C.; and Foley, K.M. 1987. Acute herpetic and postherpetic neuralgia: review of clinical features and current therapy. *Ann. Neurol.* 20:651-64.

Portenoy, R.K.; Lipton, R.B.; and Foley, K.M. 1986. Back pain in the cancer patient: an algorithm for evaluation and management. *Neurology* 37:134-38.

Portenoy, R.K.; Moulin, D.E.; and Rogers, A. et al. 1985. Intravenous infusion of opioids in cancer pain: clinical review and guidelines for use. *Ca. Treat. Rep.* 70:575-81.

Posner, J.B. 1987. Back pain and epidural spinal cord compression. In Payne, R., and Foley K.M. eds. *Medical Clinics of North America: cancer pain.* 71:185-205. Philadelphia: W.B. Saunders.

Rosomoff, H.L.; Carroll, F.; and Brown, J. 1975. Percutaneous radiofrequency cervical cordotomy: technique. *J. Neurosurg.* 23:639-44.

Rotstein, J., and Good, R.A. 1957. Steroid pseudo-rheumatism. *Arch. Intern. Med.* 99:545-55.

Schell, H.W. 1966. The risk of adrenal corticosteroid therapy with far-advanced cancer. *Am. J. Med. Sci.* 252:641-49.

Sherman, R.A.; Sherman, C.J.; and Parker, L. 1984. Chronic phantom and stump pain among American veterans: results of a survey. *Pain* 18:83-95.

Sundaresan, N., and DiGiacinto, G.V. 1987. Antitumor and antinociceptive approaches to control cancer pain. In Payne, R., and Foley, K.M. eds. *Medical Clinics of North America.* 71:329-48. Philadelphia: W.B. Saunders.

Sundaresan, N.; Galicich, J.H.; and Lane, J. 1981. Treatment of odontoid fractures in cancer patients. *J. Neurosurg.* 54:468-72.

Thomas, J.E.; Cascino, T.E.; and Earle, J.D. 1985. Differential diagnosis between radiation and tumor plexopathy of the pelvis. *Neurology* 35:1-7.

Twycross, R.G., and Lack, S.A. 1984. Symptom control in far-advanced cancer. In *Pain relief.* London: Pittman Books, Ltd.

Twycross, R.G., and Fairfield, S. 1982. Pain in far-advanced cancer. *Pain* 14:303-10.

Ventafridda, V.; DeConno, F.; and Guarise, G. et al. 1983. Chronic analgesic study on buprenorphine action in cancer pain: comparison with pentazocine. *Drug Res.* 33:587-90.

Ventafridda, V.; Ripamonti, C.; and Bianchi, M. et al. 1986. A randomized study on oral administration of morphine and methadone in the treatment of cancer pain. *J. Pain Symp. Mgt.* 1:203-207.

Ventafridda, V.; Tamburini, M.; and Caraceni, A. et al. 1987. A validation study of the WHO method for cancer pain relief. *Cancer* 59:850-56.

Ventafridda, V., and Bonica, J.J. eds. 1979. *Advances in pain research and therapy.* vol.2. New York: Raven Press.

Walsh, T.D. 1983. Antidepressants and chronic pain. *Clin. Neuropharmacol.* 6:271-95.

Watson, C.P.; Evan, R.J.; and Reed, K. et al. 1982. Amitriptyline vs. placebo in postherpetic neuralgia. *Neurology* 32:671-73.

Weinberg, D.S.; Inturrisi, C.E.; and Reidenberg, B. et al. 1988. Sublingual absorption of selected opioid analgesics. *Clin. Pharm. Therap.* 44:335-42.

World Health Organization. 1986. *Cancer pain relief.* Geneva: World Health Organization.

Chapter 39

PSYCHIATRIC COMPLICATIONS IN CANCER PATIENTS

Mary Jane Massie, M.D.
Eric Heiligenstein, M.D.
Marguerite S. Lederberg, M.D.
Jimmie C. Holland, M.D.

Mary Jane Massie, M.D.
Associate Attending Psychiatrist
Memorial Sloan-Kettering Cancer Center
New York, New York

Eric Heiligenstein, M.D.
Pediatric Psychiatry Service
Dean Medical Clinic
Madison, Wisconsin

Marguerite S. Lederberg, M.D.
Associate Attending Psychiatrist
Memorial Sloan-Kettering Cancer Center
New York, New York

Jimmie C. Holland, M.D.
Chief, Psychiatry Service
Memorial Sloan-Kettering Cancer Center
New York, New York

INTRODUCTION

HISTORICAL BACKGROUND

Cancer is a group of diseases that for centuries has struck fear in the hearts of people. Its previously certain fatal outcome, absence of known cause or cure, and association with pain and disfiguring lesions made it particularly frightening and loathsome. Physicians long avoided telling patients they had cancer, believing the diagnosis would be too painful to hear. The press avoided printing the word and the family colluded with the physician to keep the diagnosis a secret from the patient.

Several factors have contributed to attitude changes in the United States. The American Cancer Society, founded in 1913, began to educate the public about early diagnosis and treatment. In the 1950s and 1960s, physicians and patients became less pessimistic about cancer as radiation therapy and chemotherapy altered the pattern of outcome for several neoplasms in children and young adults. Clinicians began discussing more openly all aspects of the illness with patients and families.

The hospice movement in Europe and the pioneering work of Dr. Elisabeth Kübler-Ross in the United States led to a re-examination of and improvement in care for dying patients. Far more attention was given to symptom control, particularly pain. Patients who wished to discuss their fears of advanced cancer and death could do so because the situation's reality could be acknowledged.

Cancer's transition from a group of neglected and hopeless diseases to one of potential cures, increased treatment efforts, and extensive research generated more interest in the disease's psychosocial aspects. The field of psycho-oncology was developed to deal with the human dimensions of cancer and its impact on the psychological and social functioning of patients, their families, and treating staff.

PSYCHOLOGICAL IMPACT OF CANCER

Persons who receive diagnoses of cancer exhibit characteristic normal responses (table 39.1). A period of initial disbelief, denial, or despair is common and generally lasts two to five days. Patients may state "this must be the wrong diagnosis," "pathology must have mixed up my slides," "I knew it all along," or "there is no reason to take treatment, it won't work." The second phase, dysphoric mood, lasts one to two weeks. Patients report anxiety, depressed mood, anorexia, insomnia, and irritability. The ability to concentrate and carry out

Table 39.1
NORMAL RESPONSES TO CRISES ENCOUNTERED
WITH CANCER

Symptoms	Duration
PHASE 1: INITIAL RESPONSE	
Disbelief or denial	2-5 days
("wrong diagnosis";	
"mixed up slides")	
Despair	
("I knew it all along";	
"no reason to take treatment")	
PHASE 2: DYSPHORIA	
Anxiety	7-14 days
Depressed mood	
Anorexia	
Insomnia	
Irritability	
Poor concentration	
Disruption of daily activities	
PHASE 3: ADAPTATION	
Adjusts to new information	>14 days,
Confronts the issues presented	but can
Finds reasons for optimism	extend for
"Gets on" with activities	months
(e.g., new or revised treatment plan,	
other goals)	

usual daily activities is impaired and intrusive thoughts of the illness and uncertainty about the future are present. Adaptation usually begins after several weeks as patients integrate new information, confront reality issues, find reasons for optimism, and resume activities (Massie and Holland 1987a).

The patient's perceptions of the disease, its manifestations, and the stigma commonly attached to cancer contribute to these responses. For adults, fear of a painful death is a primary concern. Most children fear serious illness because of separation from and loss of loved ones. All patients fear the potential for disability, dependence, altered appearance, and changed body function. The new role of being sick or different involves a change in nearly every aspect of the adult's or child's life. The fear of being abandoned by family and friends is common.

Although such concerns are pervasive, the initial level of psychologic distress is highly variable and accounted for by three factors (table 39.2): *medical factors* (tumor site, stage at diagnosis, associated pain, treatment(s) required, rehabilitation, clinical course of illness, associated medical conditions); *patient-related factors* (level of cognitive development, ability to cope with stressful events, emotional maturity, ability to accept altered or unachieved life goals, concurrent life stresses, support of family and others); and *societal factors* (attitudes toward cancer and treatment, stigma associated with diagnosis, health care policies) (Holland 1982). Consideration of these factors enables the physician to better evaluate the patient.

Although most patients adjust well to the stress of cancer, a persistent, severe, or intolerable level of distress that prohibits the patient's usual functioning is not normal and requires evaluation by a mental health professional.

Cancer treatment, often lengthy and arduous, necessitates flexibility in patterns of emotional adaptation. Beyond the initial adjustment, the possibility of cure changes the threat of death to a focus on uncertainty and management of treatment side effects. Simultaneously, the patient must also meet normal work and family obligations, maintain confidence in the outcome and a sense of control, and manage financial burdens. Critical events such as relapse or treatment failure are more traumatic than the initial diagnosis because the outcome is known to be more guarded. Anxiety and depression may recur with greater severity.

The effects of childhood cancer on the family include reactions of anger, grief, hostility, guilt, mourning for possible loss, and disbelief (Lascari and Stehberns 1973; Chodoff, Friedman, and Hamburg 1964; Powazek et al. 1980). For most parents, the diagnosis of cancer in their child means "death" despite recent changes in prognosis of many neoplasms. The intellectual understanding that many medical advances have occurred does little to decrease parents' distress and fears; they must accept the rigors of treatment without any guarantee of success.

The illness alters all aspects of family life. The parents' goals, wishes, and expectations for the ill child are forever changed. The diagnosis of cancer in a child will most likely aggravate existing family problems. However, contrary to popular belief, the likelihood of divorce is not increased, nor are couples usually brought closer together (Lansky et al. 1978).

Childhood cancer has a significant impact on siblings. Numerous behavioral and school problems have been documented (Kagen-Goodheart 1977). Many concerns of siblings are strikingly similar to those of the sick child: symptoms of anxiety, social isolation, decreased self-esteem, and a sense of vulnerability to illness and injury are prominent. Because parents must devote time to the ill child's clinic visits and hospitalizations, there may be inadvertent parental neglect of the siblings.

Table 39.2
FACTORS THAT INFLUENCE PATIENTS'
PSYCHOLOGICAL ADAPTATION TO CANCER

MEDICAL
  Tumor site, stage at diagnosis
  Predicted outcome
  Symptoms, functional loss(es)
  Treatment(s) required
  Rehabilitation available
  Clinical course of illness
  Associated medical conditions
PATIENT-RELATED
  Level of cognitive and psychological development
  Ability to cope with life crises
  Emotional maturity and ability to accept altered or unachieved life goals
  Prior experiences with cancer (family member's death from cancer)
  Concurrent life crises (divorce, grief, other illness)
  Support of family and others
SOCIETAL
  Attitudes towards cancer and treatment
  Stigma associated with diagnosis
  Health care policy (insurance for care, disability, protection from job discrimination)

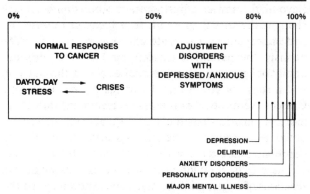

SPECTRUM OF PSYCHIATRIC DISORDERS IN CANCER
(Derived from PSYCOG Prevalence Data)

Fig. 39.1. Prevalence of psychiatric disorders in 215 adult cancer patients indicated that slightly more than half were adjusting normally to the crisis of illness. Adjustment disorder with depressed and/or anxious mood was the most common psychiatric disorder diagnosed (Derogatis et al. [1983]).

PREVALENCE OF PSYCHIATRIC DISORDERS IN CANCER PATIENTS

The many myths about psychologic problems in cancer patients vary from "all patients are distressed and need psychiatric help" to "none are upset and no one needs help." One of the first efforts in psycho-oncology was to obtain objective data on the type and frequency of emotional problems in cancer patients. Using criteria from the *Diagnostic and Statistical Manual of Mental Disorders (DSM-III)* classification of psychiatric disorders, the Psychosocial Collaborative Oncology Group at three cancer centers determined the prevalence of psychiatric disorders in 215 randomly assessed hospitalized and ambulatory adult patients with cancer (fig. 39.1) (Derogatis et al. 1983). Slightly more than half (53%) were adjusting normally to the crisis of illness. The remainder (47%) had sufficient distress to receive a diagnosis of a psychiatric disorder. Adjustment disorder with depressed and/or anxious mood was by far the most common (68%). Major depressive disorder was next (13%), followed by organic mental disorder (8%), personality disorder (7%), and pre-existing anxiety disorder (4%). Nearly 90% of the psychiatric disorders (adjustment disorders, organic mental disorders, and major depression) were related to responses to disease or treatment. Only 11% represented prior psychiatric problems, primarily personality and anxiety disorders. The physician who treats cancer patients can expect to find a group of psychologically healthy individuals who are responding to the stresses posed by cancer and its treatment. Comparable research in children is lacking, but clinical data appear to reflect a similar spectrum of problems.

SPECIFIC PSYCHOLOGICAL PROBLEMS AND THEIR MANAGEMENT

There are six psychiatric conditions that frequently occur in cancer patients and require specific interventions. Three are direct responses to illness: adjustment disorders with anxiety and/or depression, major depressive disorder, and organic mental disorders. The remaining three—primary anxiety disorders, personality disorders, and major mental illness—are pre-existing conditions often exacerbated by illness (table 39.3).

ADJUSTMENT DISORDERS

The most common psychiatric disorder diagnosed in adults and children with cancer is an adjustment disorder in reaction to the stress of illness. The characteristic symptoms are anxiety and depression. The key features of adjustment disorders are the persistence of symptoms and interference with occupational or school functioning. When symptoms are severe, adjustment disorders are difficult to differentiate from major depression and generalized anxiety disorders. Regular follow-up of these patients can often clarify these diagnostic questions.

TREATMENT OF ADJUSTMENT DISORDERS

Interventions are directed at helping the patient adapt to the stresses of cancer and resume successful coping. Individual psychotherapy focuses on clarifying the medical situation, the meaning of illness, and on reinforcing positive defense mechanisms. It is often desirable to include a spouse, partner, or family member to enhance support at home. Group therapy is often helpful, as are behavioral methods such as relaxation and hypnosis. The decision to prescribe psychotropic medication is based on a high level of distress, an inability to carry out daily activities, or poor response to psychotherapeutic support. A therapeutic trial of benzodiazepines may effectively control symptoms and facilitate other therapeutic interventions. Although the common fear of causing addiction to psychotropic drugs in both adult and pediatric cancer patients is unfounded, these drugs are underprescribed and patients experience distress that could be controlled by judicious use of medication.

Table 39.3
COMMON PSYCHIATRIC DISORDERS IN CANCER PATIENTS

DISORDERS DIRECTLY RELATED TO ILLNESS
  Adjustment disorders
    Anxiety
    Depression
    Mixed features
  Major depression
  Organic mental disorder (delirium)
  Post-traumatic stress disorder (PTSD)
PRE-EXISTING DISORDERS EXACERBATED BY ILLNESS
  Anxiety disorders
    Phobias of needles, hospitals, enclosed spaces
    Panic disorder
    Agoraphobia
    Generalized anxiety
  Personality disorders
    Paranoid, obsessive, dependent
    Borderline, histrionic
    Schizophrenia
    Bipolar disorder

DEPRESSIVE DISORDERS

The overlap of physical illness and symptoms of depression is widely recognized. Diagnosis of depression in physically healthy adults and children requires the presence of somatic complaints, insomnia, anorexia, fatigue, and weight loss. These symptoms, however, are common to both cancer and depression. In cancer patients, the diagnosis of depression must depend on dysphoric mood or appearance, crying, anhedonia, feelings of helplessness, decreased self-esteem, guilt, social withdrawal, and thoughts of "wishing for death" or suicide.

Several studies utilizing patient self-report and observer ratings found major depression in approximately one-fourth of hospitalized adult cancer patients (Bukberg, Penman, and Holland 1984; Evans et al. 1986; Plumb and Holland 1977). This prevalence is similar to equally ill patients with other medical diagnoses, suggesting that the level of illness, not the specific diagnosis, is the primary determinant (Moffic and Paykel 1975; Schwab et al. 1967). Factors associated with higher prevalence of depression in cancer patients are: greater level of physical impairment, more advanced stages of illness, pancreatic cancer, pain, and prior history of depression (Holland et al. 1986).

The clinical evaluation includes a careful assessment of symptoms and history of emotional problems, particularly depressive episodes; family history of depression; concurrent life stresses; and level of social support. Exploring the patient's understanding of the medical situation and meaning of illness is essential. The contribution of pain to depressive symptoms needs to be clarified because a depressive disorder cannot be diagnosed with certainty until pain is controlled.

Symptoms of depression can be produced by numerous commonly prescribed medications, including methyldopa, reserpine, barbiturates, diazepam, and propranolol. Of the many cancer chemotherapeutic agents, depressive symptoms are produced by relatively few: prednisone, dexamethasone, vincristine, vinblastine, procarbazine, asparaginase, amphotericin-B, and interferon (Young 1982; Weddington 1982; Holland, Fasanello, and Ohnuma 1974). Many metabolic, nutritional, endocrine, and neurologic disorders produce depressive symptoms (Hall et al. 1978). Cancer patients with abnormal levels of potassium, sodium, or calcium may become depressed, as can patients with a variety of nutritional deficiencies (folate, B_{12}). Hypo- or hyperthyroidism and adrenal insufficiency can also be responsible for depressive symptoms.

Suicidal ideation always requires careful assessment. Cancer patients who are at higher risk are those with poor prognosis or advanced stages of illness, a prior psychiatric history, substance abuse, previous suicide attempts, or a family history of suicide. A recent death of friends or spouse, few social supports, extreme hopelessness, major depression, poorly controlled pain, delirium, and recent information of a grave prognosis are significant risk factors (Breitbart 1989).

TREATMENT OF DEPRESSIVE DISORDERS

Prolonged and severe depression usually requires treatment that combines psychotherapy with somatic treatment, either medication or electroconvulsive therapy. In depressed children and adolescents, individual psychotherapy is the primary treatment modality. Antidepressants should only be prescribed for children and adolescents if other types of treatment have failed, as evidence is lacking for definite therapeutic effect in these age groups (Campbell and Spencer 1988).

Pharmacologic treatments appropriate for use in adult cancer patients (table 39.4) are: the tricyclics; second-generation and heterocyclic antidepressants; monoamine oxidase inhibitors; psychostimulants; lithium carbonate; and benzodiazepines (Massie and Lesko 1989).

Tricyclic antidepressants (TCAs). The tricyclic compounds are used as the first-line antidepressants because of their established effectiveness, relative safety, and ease of administration. There are several reports of the efficacy of antidepressants in depressed adults with serious physical illness including cancer (Lipsey et al. 1984; Rifkin et al. 1985). The precise mechanism by which the TCAs work is unknown, although there is pharmacologic evidence that they affect the monoamine neurotransmitter systems in the brain.

Tricyclic compounds are largely similar in efficacy and side-effect profiles. The choice of an antidepressant depends on the patient's specific medical problems and the TCA's side-effect profile. The agitated depressed patient with insomnia may benefit from a TCA that has anticholinergic-mediated sedative effects, such as amitriptyline or doxepin. The patient with stomatitis secondary to chemotherapy or radiation therapy, slowed intestinal motility, or urinary hesitancy should receive a TCA with the least anticholinergic effects, such as desipramine or nortriptyline.

In debilitated patients, TCAs are started at low doses. Ten mg to 25 mg can be given at bedtime and increased by 25 mg every one to two days. Depressed cancer patients often show a therapeutic response to TCA at lower total dose (25-125 mg/d) than physically healthy, depressed patients (150-300 mg/d). The precise mechanism(s) for this effect is unclear but may represent increased end-organ sensitivity to these compounds. Patients are usually maintained on a TCA for four to six months after symptoms improve.

Imipramine, doxepin, nortriptyline, and amitriptyline are used in the management of cancer pain. These compounds have been shown to be effective often at lower doses (10-25 mg/d) than those used for depression. Although initially it was felt that analgesic effects resulted from treatment of depression, it now appears that there is a direct effect, independent of effect on mood, on specific analgesic systems in the brain and spinal cord.

Table 39.4
ANTIDEPRESSANT MEDICATIONS USED IN CANCER PATIENTS*

Drug	Starting Daily Dosage (mg) (PO)	Therapeutic Daily Dosage (mg) (PO)
Tricyclic antidepressants		
Amitriptyline	25	75-100
Doxepin	25	75-100
Imipramine	25	75-100
Desipramine	25	75-100
Nortriptyline	25	100-150
Second-generation antidepressants		
Bupropion	15	200-450
Fluoxetine	20	20-60
Trazodone	50	150-200
Heterocyclic antidepressants		
Maprotiline	25	50-75
Amoxapine	25	100-150
Monoamine oxidase inhibitors		
Isocarboxazid	10	20-40
Phenelzine	15	30-60
Tranylcypromine	10	20-40
Lithium carbonate	300	600-1200
Psychostimulants		
Dextroamphetamine	2.5 at 8 AM and Noon	5-30
Methylphenidate	2.5 at 8 AM and Noon	5-30
Pemoline	18.75 at 8 AM and Noon	37.5-150
Benzodiazepine		
Alprazolam	0.25-1.00	0.75-6.00

*(Adapted from Massie and Holland [1987].)

Second-generation and heterocyclic antidepressants. If a patient does not respond to a trial of TCAs, or cannot tolerate side effects, a second-generation (trazodone, fluoxetine, or bupropion) or a heterocyclic (amoxapine or maprotiline) antidepressant should be considered. The starting dose and therapeutic range of these agents are shown in table 39.4. The side effect profile of the heterocyclic compounds is similar to the TCAs. The second-generation agents appear to be less cardiotoxic. Early clinical experience with bupropion suggests it may have an activating effect in withdrawn medically ill patients.

Monoamine oxidase inhibitors (MAOIs). If a patient has responded well to a monoamine oxidase inhibitor for depression prior to treatment for cancer, its continued use is warranted. Most psychiatrists are reluctant to initiate treatment with MAOIs in cancer patients because further dietary restriction is often poorly received. MAOIs are usually reserved for patients in whom a TCA has failed or has not been well tolerated.

Psychostimulants. The psychostimulants, dextroamphetamine, methylphenidate, and pemoline, are increasingly being used in depressed patients with advanced cancer in whom low energy, withdrawal, or narcotic-associated lethargy is present. Psychostimulants in low dose stimulate appetite, potentiate the analgesic effect of narcotics and promote a sense of well-being. A common starting dose is 2.5 mg of dextroamphetamine or methylphenidate given at 8:00 AM and noon; a starting dose of pemoline is 18.75 mg at 8:00 AM and noon. Most adults can be treated for one to two months, followed by discontinuation of the medication without a recurrence of depressive symptoms. Due to less prom-

ising results in the treatment of depression in children with TCAs, the psychostimulants may be an alternative.

Lithium carbonate. Patients who were receiving lithium carbonate prior to beginning cancer treatment should be maintained on their therapeutic dose. Maintenance doses of lithium may need adjustment in seriously ill patients in whom dehydration is a risk, and serum levels should be followed. Lithium should be prescribed with caution in patients receiving cisplatin because of both drugs' potential nephrotoxicity.

Several authors have reported a granulocyte-stimulating property of lithium in neutropenic cancer patients (Cantane et al. 1977; Lyman, Williams, and Preston 1980). However, the functional capabilities of these leukocytes have not been determined and the stimulation effect appears to be transient.

Benzodiazepines. The triazalobenzodiazepine alprazolam has both anxiolytic and antidepressant effects. Alprazolam is particularly useful in cancer patients who have mixed symptoms of anxiety and depression (Feighner et al. 1983; Rickels, Feighner, and Smith 1985).

ELECTROCONVULSIVE THERAPY (ECT)

Occasionally, ECT must be considered for adult cancer patients whose depression is resistant to other interventions and in whom it represents a life-threatening complication of treatable cancer. When prominent psychotic features are present or treatment with antidepressants poses unacceptable side effects, ECT should be considered.

ANXIETY DISORDERS

Many types of anxiety are experienced by cancer patients. Situational anxiety is common and most patients are anxious while waiting to hear their diagnosis; before stressful or painful procedures (bone-marrow aspiration, chemotherapy, radiation therapy, wound debridement); prior to surgery; and while awaiting test results. Anxiety is expected at these times and most patients manage with the reassurance and support from their physicians. At times further treatment is necessary. Extreme fearfulness, inability to cooperate or understand procedures, a prior history of panic attacks, or needle phobia or claustrophobia may require an anxiolytic medication to reduce symptoms to a manageable level. These are particularly useful on the night before surgery or prior to a painful procedure.

The differential diagnosis of anxiety in the cancer patient can be complex. Patients in severe pain are anxious and agitated and respond to adequate pain control with analgesics. The anxiety that accompanies respiratory distress, while eventually relieved by medical intervention, often requires an anxiolytic. Many patients on corticosteroids experience insomnia and anxiety, which should be treated with benzodiazepines. Patients developing metabolic encephalopathy (delirium) can appear restless or anxious and treatment with neuroleptics is often required as determination and correction (if possible) of the cause(s) is begun. Anxiety symptoms are also features of withdrawal from narcotics, benzodiazepines, and barbiturates. Patients who abuse alcohol commonly underreport alcohol intake prior to admission. The physician needs to consider alcohol withdrawal in all patients who develop otherwise unexplained anxiety symptoms during the first week of hospitalization. Other medical conditions that may have anxiety as a prominent feature or presenting symptom are hyperthyroidism, pheochromocytoma, carcinoid, and mitral valve prolapse.

Anxiety disorders that antedate the onset of cancer can compromise medical treatment. Phobias and panic disorders are the most common types. Occasionally patients have their first episode of panic while being treated in a medical setting. Psychiatric evaluation prior to undertaking cancer treatment is essential in patients with a history of panic disorder or phobia. Patients with claustrophobia may have extreme anxiety in the confined spaces of diagnostic scanning devices or radiation therapy treatment rooms. Patients with needle phobias report having avoided medical evaluations for years because of their fears. Patients with agoraphobia often are unable to tolerate hospital admission unaccompanied by a family member.

Post-traumatic stress disorder (PTSD) is a specific type of anxiety disorder due to the effects of traumatic experiences, including military combat, natural catastrophes, assault, rape, accidents, and life-threatening illness. Recall of prior painful or frightening treatment are common causes of PTSD in cancer patients, especially children. Illness can also exacerbate feelings about earlier traumas. This has been noted in cancer patients who are Holocaust survivors. In the adult and pediatric cancer patient, symptoms can develop at various stages of illness but are frequent at the time of diagnosis.

Important variables in the disorder's development are the patient's personality traits, the biological vulnerability to stressful events, and the severity of the stressor. In general, pediatric and geriatric populations have more difficulty coping with stressful events and are at risk for PTSD. The underdeveloped emotional state of children prevents them from using various adaptive strategies, and the elderly are likely to have fixed coping mechanisms that minimize their flexibility in dealing with trauma.

The typical presenting symptoms include periods of intrusive repetition of the stressful event (nightmares, flashbacks, and intrusive thoughts) along with denial, emotional numbness, and depression. Children rarely experience a numbing response to the environment and often respond to trauma with anxiety, restlessness, hyperalertness, and difficulty concentrating. In both adults and children, use of denial is prominent and minimizes the painful event. The nonspecific emotional symptoms can make the diagnosis difficult to distinguish from a generalized anxiety disorder, depression, or panic disorder. Questions about intrusive phenomena help to determine the specific diagnosis. Many patients are relieved to understand their symptoms are an expected response to severe stress.

TREATMENT OF ANXIETY DISORDERS

Many patients with intermittent anxiety, simple phobias, or PTSD find relaxation therapy and distraction techniques helpful. When the need for a diagnostic procedure or treatment is urgent, benzodiazepines should be used (e.g., prior to venipuncture, intravenous chemotherapy administration, a scanning procedure, or radiation therapy treatment).

Benzodiazepines with rapid onset of action (diazepam, clorazepate) and long half-life have been used for patients with acute anxiety. In recent years, short-acting benzodiazepines (alprazolam, lorazepam, oxazepam) are preferentially used in medically ill patients. These medications are rapidly metabolized and are better tolerated by patients with impaired hepatic function and by those taking other medications with sedative effects.

The starting dose of an anxiolytic is determined by the severity of the anxiety, the patient's physical status (respiratory and hepatic impairment), and the concurrent use of other medications (antidepressants, analgesics, antiemetics). Table 39.5 lists the usual initial dose of benzodiazepines, elimination half-life, and presence or absence of active metabolites.

Dose schedule depends on the patient's tolerance and the anxiolytic's duration of action. When a long-acting benzodiazepine is used in patients with chronic anxiety, the dose should not exceed twice a day. The shorter-acting benzodiazepines are given three to four times a day. It is best to increase the dose before switching to another agent in patients with persistent symptoms.

Patients who experience severe anticipatory anxiety (i.e., anxiety before chemotherapy administration) are

Table 39.5
COMMONLY PRESCRIBED BENZODIAZEPINES IN CANCER PATIENTS

Drug	Approximate Dose Equivalent	Initial Dosage PO (mg)	Elimination Half-Life Drug Metabolites (hr)	Active Metabolite
SHORT ACTING				
Alprazolam	0.5	0.25-0.5 mg TID	10-15	Yes
Oxazepam	10.0	10-15 mg TID	5-15	No
Lorazepam	1.0	0.5-2.0 mg TID	10-20	No
INTERMEDIATE ACTING				
Chlordiazepoxide	10.0	10-25 mg TID	10-40	Yes
LONG ACTING				
Diazepam	5.0	5-10 mg BID	20-100	Yes
Clorazepate	7.5	7.5-15 mg BID	30-200	Yes

given an anxiolytic the night before and immediately prior to the treatment. Patients with chronic anxiety states require anxiolytics daily or intermittently for months or years. Cancer patients, even those with chronic anxiety, usually do not take more medication than they absolutely require and eagerly discontinue medications as soon as their symptoms remit.

The most common side effects of the benzodiazepines are dose-dependent and include drowsiness, confusion, and motor incoordination. When the dose is lowered, uncomfortable sedation often disappears while the antianxiety effects continue. Sedation is most common and most severe in patients with impaired liver function. Physicians should be aware of the synergistic effects of the benzodiazepines with other medications with central nervous system depressant properties, such as narcotics.

Low-dose neuroleptics are effective in patients with severe anxiety that is not controlled with maximal therapeutic doses of benzodiazepines. The low efficacy of the antihistamines for anxiety limits their general usefulness, although they are prescribed for control of anxiety in patients with respiratory impairment or other conditions where benzodiazepines are contraindicated.

PTSD is most often treated with tricyclic antidepressants, which appear to be effective in reducing the panic and depressive symptoms in most adult patients. In children, benzodiazepines are useful because of their effect on the often-noted anxiety and restlessness.

ORGANIC MENTAL DISORDERS (DELIRIUM)

Delirium related to disease or treatment was the third most common psychiatric diagnosis among cancer patients in one series. Posner (1978) has reported that 15% to 20% of hospitalized cancer patients have cognitive function abnormalities unrelated to structural disease. Approximately one-fifth of psycho-oncology consultations are for assistance in the diagnosis and management of delirium (Massie and Holland 1987a). Delirium is usually due to one or more causes: medications, electrolyte imbalance, failure of a vital organ or system, nutritional deficiencies, infections, vascular diseases, or hormone-producing tumors (Lipowski 1980).

Early symptoms of delirium are often unrecognized. Any patient who shows acute onset of agitation, behavioral changes, impaired cognitive function, altered

attention span, or a fluctuating level of consciousness should be evaluated for presence of delirium. In children, mood changes, irritability, social withdrawal, and apathy are noted. Medical staff concerns are consequently focused on depression or behavior problems, but formal mental status examination reveals changes in attention, memory, and concentration characteristic of delirium.

Corticosteriods are a frequent cause of delirium. Psychiatric disturbances range from common minor mood disturbance to infrequent psychosis (Hall et al. 1979). Characteristic symptoms include affective changes (emotional lability, euphoria, depressed mood), anxiety, fears, paranoid interpretation of events, suspiciousness, delusions, and hallucinations. More severe symptoms develop within four to five days of high-dose steroid treatment (60 mg/day in adults or 60 mg/m^2 in children) or with rapidly tapered doses. Psychiatric symptoms can also develop while patients are on maintenance dose. No relationship has been shown between the development of steroid-induced mental status changes and premorbid personality or psychiatric history.

Many analgesics cause acute confusional states. Levorphanol, morphine sulfate, and meperidine, commonly used in the treatment of cancer pain, often cause delirium. Among the more than 285 chemotherapeutic agents now available for cancer, CNS symptoms are not generally a prominent feature. Those most apt to cause delirium are methotrexate, fluorouracil, vincristine, vinblastine, bleomycin, carmustine (BCNU), cisplatin, asparaginase, and procarbazine.

TREATMENT OF ORGANIC MENTAL DISORDERS (DELIRIUM)

Organic mental disorders require corrective medical interventions but interim symptomatic treatment may be necessary. Patients with quiet delirium do not require psychopharmacologic management. General care should include sensory stimulation to avoid deprivation effects, provision of familiar stimuli such as family, use of companions to ensure safety, and adequate nursing care.

Delirious adult and pediatric patients with psychotic symptoms or agitation respond to neuroleptic medication. Haloperidol is the most commonly prescribed agent. It has an excellent safety record with little effect on heart rate, blood pressure, respiration, or cardiac output. Haloperidol can be given orally in tablet or concentrate, or parenterally (IM or IV). Peak plasma concentrations are achieved in two to four hours after an oral dose, and measurable plasma concentrations occur in 15 to 30 minutes after parenteral administration.

The initial dose of haloperidol for both adult and child cancer patients is low, starting with 0.5 mg to 1.0 mg administered by mouth or 0.25 mg to 0.5 mg parenterally. The dose can be repeated at 30-minute intervals until symptoms are controlled. If psychotic symptoms are reduced but agitation remains, low-dose benzodiazepines can be added. Dystonic reactions, though uncommon, are treated with anticholinergic agents such as diphenylhydrazine or benzitropine.

PERSONALITY DISORDERS

Patients with difficult personalities often are worse under the stress of cancer. These patients usually have personality disorders that cause their maladaptive and frustrating behavior. The disorders are characterized by the exaggeration of normal personality styles to a pathological point: the paranoid who is suspicious and constantly threatens litigation; the obsessive whose excessive attention to details is accompanied by repeated criticism; the dependent personality who demands care far beyond objective needs; the patient with borderline personality disorder who is unable to conform to rules and who manipulates, divides, and disturbs other patients and staff; and the histrionic personality who overdramatizes symptoms and distress and demands attention. These patients have coping strategies and defenses that are fixed in a single, rigid pattern that denies them flexibility in adapting to illness. The disorders are rarely modified by psychotherapy in the medical setting and are best treated as outlined below.

TREATMENT OF PERSONALITY DISORDERS
The following principles apply to most patients with personality disorders who require cancer treatment.

1. Psychiatric evaluation should be requested to determine the patient's own complaints and the specific problems that are causing management difficulties. The interview should identity prior adjustment and previous ways of coping with stress. It should be followed by a multidisciplinary staff meeting in which the problems are described from a psychodynamic perspective in order to form a rational basis for management.

2. All information about diagnosis, studies, test results, and treatments should be given to the patient by one person, preferably the patient's physician.

3. Bedside rounds should include the primary nurse and house officer to assure communication and diminish misunderstanding. Clinic visits should include family and nurse to ensure plans are clear when instructions are given.

4. Certain hospital rules may need to be modified to allow these patients a sense of control. Relenting on minor restrictions (e.g., extending visiting hours 30 minutes more) may permit the patient to accept other requirements necessary for treatment.

5. Patients with poor impulse control are often less anxious when a companion is present during difficult treatments. Close patient observation decreases staff's concern about self-destructive behavior. Psychotropic medication may be indicated and should be prescribed with close psychiatric supervision.

SCHIZOPHRENIA

Schizophrenia is the most feared mental illness and bears the greatest social stigma. When schizophrenia and cancer occur together, the burden is particularly great for the person, his or her family, and those who must manage the medical and psychiatric care.

There are several problem areas. First, patients with schizophrenia may respond inappropriately to cancer's warning symptoms and appear initially with a more advanced stage of disease. Second, because delusional beliefs may compromise understanding of illness and proposed treatment, physicians must give special attention to issues of informed consent and competence. Third, paranoid distrust may interfere with expression of appropriate complaints of pain or discomfort. Fourth, they may have limited ability to participate in their care, especially at home where compliance is difficult to manage.

Rarely, a first episode of schizophrenia appears in a young adult during treatment for cancer. Central nervous system complications of the disease or its treatment are by far the most common causes of psychotic symptoms in a cancer patient. Other disorders with psychotic features must be considered in the differential diagnosis: drug intoxication (cocaine, hallucinogens, amphetamines, phencyclidine); temporal lobe epilepsy; bipolar disorder; major depression; and schizoaffective disorder.

TREATMENT OF SCHIZOPHRENIA
Patients with schizophrenia are best managed by one doctor and one nurse. A social worker is a useful liaison between hospital staff, family, and patient. Psychiatric evaluation should be obtained prior to or early in treatment to assess potential problems, provide the treating staff with an understanding of the illness, and to monitor antipsychotic medication.

Work with the family is critical because they may need to assume responsibility for care at home, administer medication, schedule clinic visits, and monitor medical symptoms. Home visits from a psychiatric nurse can provide support.

Pharmacologic treatment for schizophrenia depends on the nature and severity of the psychiatric symptoms, which may be influenced by a variety of medical variables. Frequent psychiatric assessment is required throughout the course of treatment. Appropriate medications include perphenazine, trifluoperazine, or thioridazine.

BIPOLAR DISORDER

Patients who have pre-existing bipolar disorder are at risk for relapse of their psychiatric symptoms under the stress of physical illness. Continuation of prophylactic lithium treatment is necessary during cancer treatment. Episodes of acute mania often require the addition of an antipsychotic agent. Regular psychiatric care with appropriate psychopharmacological intervention can effectively reduce the morbidity and disruption caused by manic episodes.

THERAPEUTIC INTERVENTIONS IN CANCER

The cornerstone of psychological interventions in cancer is emotional support. Psychoeducational counseling focusing on advice and information about illness can be helpful to both patient and family and can be carried out by different members of the treatment team. Religious counseling is meaningful for many patients during the existential crisis created by cancer. A one-to-one visit by a "veteran" patient who has successfully negotiated the same cancer treatment often helps. Psychotherapy provided by a mental health professional usually consists of short-term, crisis-oriented therapy to assist the patient to strengthen adaptive defenses and better cope with the problems of illness.

Group therapy for cancer patients is useful in several ways. First, groups have an educational function in orienting and teaching patients. Second, groups encourage emotional learning and can relieve anxiety by allowing individuals to share similar problems and solutions. Third, the support they provide often becomes a voice for social awareness and change, giving participants a valuable sense of strength. Behavioral therapies emphasize self-regulatory interventions and are well-received by patients. Many learn relaxation exercises, visual imagery for distraction, and self-hypnotic suggestions. Although these techniques do not have antitumor effect, such techniques are particularly effective in reducing anticipatory nausea and vomiting in patients receiving chemotherapy.

LONG SURVIVORS AND CURED PATIENTS

Cured cancer patients have special medical and psychiatric concerns. Preoccupation with disease recurrence, a sense of greater vulnerability to illness (the Damocles syndrome), pervasive awareness of mortality, and a permanent sense of physical inferiority can diminish self-esteem and confidence. Concern about infertility, often submerged at the time of diagnosis and treatment, can reappear when patients marry.

The survivor's intellectual functioning is a major concern. Children and adults with brain tumors are at risk from both their disease and treatment. Most have residual deficits, with mild to marked decline in IQ scores and a dementia-like syndrome. Children with acute lymphoblastic leukemia (ALL) who received more than 25 Gy of cranial irradiation scored lower on a range of cognitive tests in several long-term follow-up studies (Copeland et al. 1985; Tamaroff et al. 1982). As a consequence, CNS prophylaxis for ALL currently uses 18 Gy and/or intrathecal methotrexate. This regimen produces less cognitive impairment and protocols are structured so that only children with high-risk leukemia receive this treatment (Anderson and Stehbens 1985).

As the number of cancer survivors grows, more attention is being given to societal attitudes. The newly formed National Coalition of Cancer Survivorship is an outgrowth of the need for and value of support. The issues surrounding health and life insurance policies are a prime example of an area where research is needed to delineate problems and develop solutions. Many centers around the country are developing survivor clinics that incorporate a multidisciplinary approach to the cured child, adolescent, or adult.

MANAGEMENT OF GRIEF

Grief is frequently encountered in the oncology setting and staff management can affect the nature of bereavement and influence the family's long-term adjustment. Once death has occurred, grieving has acute and chronic components (Osterweis, Solomon, and Green 1984). Reminders of the deceased precipitate waves of an overwhelming sense of loss, crying, and agitation. The intense distress of the first few months are characterized by social withdrawal, preoccupation with the deceased, diminished concentration, restlessness, depressed mood, anxiety, insomnia, and anorexia. The bereaved spouse or parent repeatedly recalls how the final days were handled, how the painful news of grave prognosis and death were conveyed, and how sensitively the final moments were managed. The surviving relatives or parents usually search for fault and will tend to blame both themselves and staff. The physician must recognize his or her special meaning to survivors and understand their reactions in this context. A meeting held one to two months after the death is a valuable setting where autopsy findings and any troubling questions can be discussed.

Over several months, grief usually diminishes in intensity. The duration of normal grieving is much more variable than originally assumed and often extends well beyond a year. Parents, for example, often report that they are "never the same again"; some never really recover. Older spouses from a long union often grieve acutely for two to four years or longer (Parkes and Weiss 1983).

STRESSES ON
HEALTH-CARE PROVIDERS

Recent studies have helped clarify the picture of emotional reaction of patients and their relatives to cancer, but few studies have addressed the stresses on the oncologist and its effect on personal and professional life (Mount 1986; Kash and Holland 1988; Lederberg 1989). Studies show that, despite recent criticism of medicine as uncaring, patients still accept treatment largely because they trust their doctors and his or her recommendations (Penman et al. 1984). The harried, stressed oncologist is compromised in his or her ability to give attention to the art of medicine, yet seldom is this human aspect of care more important than in oncology.

Most physicians generally tolerate work stresses well and have characteristics of the hardy personality that are known to buffer stress: strong commitment to work, a sense of control of their work without letting the magnitude of the problems become overwhelming, and a view of daily problems as a challenge (Kobasa and Puccetti 1983). Physicians also have the characteristics that predispose them to chronic stress. Many work long hours and seek little recreation; many have trouble saying no to requests for additional work. Beeper and telephone intrusions into private moments strain friendships, marital relationships, and upset children. The need to care for patients while pursuing research and scholarly activities adds special strains to the academic setting. Frequent sleep loss is an additional stressor; chronic fatigue is more insidious.

The practice of oncology carries specific additional strains. There is the uncertainty inherent in most treatment decisions and the repeated impact of patients' deaths. Some personal stress inevitably accompanies decisions about withholding or stopping life-sustaining treatment amid all the medical, social, and ethical ambiguities that abound in the current climate. Discussing these issues with patient and family is difficult and painful.

The incidence of serious psychiatric problems in physicians is probably underreported. Alcohol and drug abuse are the most common psychiatric problems seen in physicians, followed by depression and suicide.

The physician with symptoms of emotional fatigue or burnout notices he or she has less zest and enthusiasm for work; may feel chronically tense, easily angered, and easily frustrated; and depressed moods may frequently ensue. The need for a few drinks after work or experimenting with drugs to relax are ominous signs. On the physical side, insomnia is common. Appetite change may lead to weight gain or weight loss. The stressed physician reports feeling exhausted and tired all the time. Headaches or somatic pains are indicators of distress. At this point, the physician may tune out and feel detached from his or her patients. This is an early sign of stress in house staff who say they feel less able to care and are cynical and pessimistic about the meaning of their work. They may begin to work longer hours and have a sense that "nobody can do it right but me" and "nobody works around here but me," when in fact they are less efficient and less effective.

Monitoring symptoms of emotional fatigue and acknowledging stress are important for anyone working in oncology. Survival tactics must be instituted that include recognizing limitations, developing a comfortable perspective on self and work, accepting personal and medical inadequacies, using gallows humor to lighten the meaning of painful events, working a normal workday for a few weeks, stopping when others do, taking a long weekend, and regular exercise. When symptoms do not remit, psychiatric consultation should be sought.

REFERENCES

Anderson, B.L., and Stehbens, J.A. 1985. Intellectual functioning of children with leukemia by age at diagnosis. Presented at the American Psychological Association Convention.

Breitbart, W. 1989. Suicide in cancer patients. In Holland, J.C., and Rowland, J.H. eds. *Handbook of psycho-oncology: psychological care of the patient with cancer.* New York: Oxford University Press.

Bukberg, J.; Penman, D.; and Holland, J.C. 1984. Depression in hospitalized cancer patients. *Psychosom. Med.* 46:199-212.

Campbell, M., and Spencer, E.K. 1988. Psychopharmacology in child and adolescent psychiatry: review of the past five years. *J. Am. Acad. Child Adolesc. Psychiatry* 27:269-79.

Cantane, R.L.; Kaufman, J.; and Mittelman, A. et al. 1977. Attenuation of myelosuppression with lithium. *N. Engl. J. Med.* 297:452-53.

Chodoff, P.; Friedman, S.B.; and Hamburg, D.A. 1964. Stress defenses and coping behavior: observations in parents of children with malignant diseases. *Am. J. Psychiatry* 120: 743-49.

Copeland, D.R.; Fletcher, J.M.; and Pfefferbaum-Levine, B. et al. 1985. Neuropsychological sequelae of childhood cancer in long-term survivors. *Pediatrics* 75:745-53.

Derogatis, L.R.; Morrow, G.R.; and Fetting, J. et al. 1983. Prevalence of psychiatric disorders among cancer patients. *JAMA* 249:751-57.

Evans, D.L.; McCartney, C.F.; and Nemeroff, C.B. et al. 1986. Depression in women treated for gynecological cancer: clinical and neuroendocrine assessment. *Am. J. Psychiatry* 143:447-52.

Feighner, J.P.; Aden, G.C.; and Fabre, L.F. et al. 1983. Comparison of alprazolam, imipramine, and placebo in the treatment of depression. *JAMA* 249:3057-64.

Hall, R.C.W.; Popkin, M.K.; and Devaul, R.A. et al. 1978. Physical illness presenting as psychiatric disease. *Arch. Gen. Psychiatry* 35:1315-20.

Hall, R.C.W.; Popkin, M.K.; and Stickney, S.K. et al. 1979. Presentation of the steroid psychosis. *J. Nerv. Ment. Dis.* 167:229-36.

Holland, J.C. 1982. Psychological aspects of cancer. In Holland, J.F., and Frei, E. eds. *Cancer medicine.* 2nd ed. pp. 1175-1203, 2325-31. Philadelphia: Lee & Febiger.

Holland, J.C.; Fasanello, S.; and Ohnuma, T. 1974. Psychiatric symptoms associated with L-asparaginase administration. *J. Psychiatric Res.* 10:165.

Holland, J.C.; Hughes-Korzun, A.; and Tross, S. et al. 1986. Comparative psychological disturbance in pancreatic and gastric cancer. *Am. J. Psychiatry* 143:982-86.

Kagen-Goodheart, L. 1977. Reentry: living with childhood cancer. *Am. J. Orthopsychiatry* 47:651-58.

Kash, K., and Holland, J.C. 1989. Special problems of physicians and house staff. In Holland, J.C., and Rowland, J.H. eds. *Handbook of psycho-oncology: psychological care of the patient with cancer.* New York: Oxford University Press.

Kobasa, S.C., and Puccetti, M.D. 1983. Personality and social resources in stress-resistance. *J. Person. Soc. Psycho.* 45: 839-50.

Lansky, S.B.; Cairns, N.U.; and Hassannein, R. et al. 1978. Childhood cancer: parent discord and divorce. *Pediatrics* 62:184-88.

Lascari, A.D., and Stehberns, J.A. 1973. Reactions of families to childhood leukemia. *Clin. Pediatr.* 12:210-14.

Lederberg, M.S. 1989. Psychological problems of staff and their management. In Holland, J.C., and Rowland, J.H. eds. *Handbook of psycho-oncology: psychological care of the patient with cancer.* New York: Oxford University Press.

Lipowski, Z.J. 1980. *Delirium: acute brain failure in man.* Springfield, Ill.: Charles C. Thomas.

Lipsey, J.R.; Robinson, R.G.; and Pearlson, G.D. et al. 1984. Nortriptyline treatment of poststroke depression: double-blind study. *Lancet* I:297-300.

Lyman, G.H.; Williams, C.C.; and Preston, D. 1980. Use of lithium carbonate to reduce infection and leukopenia during systemic chemotherapy. *N. Engl. J. Med.* 302:257-60.

Massie, M.J., and Holland, J.C. 1987a. Consultation and liaison issues in cancer care. *Psychiatric Med.* 5:343-59.

Massie, M.J., and Holland, J.C. 1987b. The cancer patient with pain: psychiatric complications and their management. *Med. Clin. North Am.* 71:243-58.

Massie, M.J., and Lesko, L.M. 1989. Psychopharmacological management. In Holland, J.C., and Rowland, J.H. eds. *Handbook of psycho-oncology: psychological care of the patient with cancer.* New York: Oxford University Press.

Moffic, H., and Paykel, E.S. 1975. Depression in medical inpatients. *Br. J. Psychiatry* 126:346-53.

Mount, B.M. 1986. Dealing with our losses. *J. Clin. Oncol.* 4:1127-34.

Osterweis, M.; Solomon, F.; and Green, M. eds. 1984. *Bereavement reactions, consequences, and care.* Washington, D.C.: National Academy Press.

Parkes, C.M., and Weiss, R. 1983. *Recovery from bereavement.* New York: Basic Books.

Penman, D.; Holland, J.C.; and Bahna, G. et al. 1984. Informed consent for investigational chemotherapy: patients' and physicians' perceptions. *J. Clin. Oncol.* 2: 849-55.

Plumb, M., and Holland, J.C. 1977. Comparative studies of psychological function in patients with advanced cancer 1.: self-reported depressive symptoms. *Psychosom. Med.* 39: 264-76.

Posner, J.B. 1978. Neurologic complications in systemic cancer. *Disease a Month* 2:7-60.

Powazek, M.; Schijving, J.; and Goff, J.R. et al. 1980. Psychosocial ramifications of childhood leukemia: one year postdiagnosis. In Schulman, J.L., and Kupat, M.J. eds. *The child with cancer.* pp. 143-55. Springfield, Ill: Charles C. Thomas.

Rickels, K.; Feighner, J.P.; and Smith, W.T. 1985. Alprazolam, amitriptyline, doxepine, and placebo in the treatment of depression. *Arch. Gen. Psychiatry* 42:134-41.

Rifkin, A.; Reardon, G.; and Siris, S. et al. 1985. Trimipramine in physical illness with depression. *J. Clin. Psychiatry* 46[2, Sec 2]:4-8.

Schwab, J.J.; Bialow, M.; and Brown, J.M. et al. 1967. Diagnosing depression in medical inpatients. *Ann. Intern. Med.* 67:695-707.

Tamaroff, M.; Miller, D.R.; and Murphy, M.L. et al. 1982. Immediate and long-term post-therapy neuropsychologic performance in children with acute lymphoblastic leukemia treated without central nervous system radiation. *J. Pediatr.* 101:524-29.

Weddington, W.W. 1982. Delirium and depression associated with amphotericin-B. *Psychosomatics* 23:1076-78.

Young, D.F. 1982. Neurological complications of cancer chemotherapy. In Silverstein, A. ed. *Neurological complications of therapy: selected topics.* pp. 57-113. New York: Futura Publishing.

Chapter 40

PRINCIPLES OF ONCOLOGY NURSING

Teresa Ades, R.N., B.S.N.
Patricia Greene, R.N., M.S.N.

Teresa Ades, R.N., B.S.N.
Coordinator of Nursing Programs
American Cancer Society
Atlanta, Georgia

Patricia Greene, R.N., M.S.N.
Vice President for Nursing
American Cancer Society
Atlanta, Georgia

"The unique function of the nurse is to assist the individual, sick or well, in the performance of those activities contributing to health or its recovery (or peaceful death) that he/she would perform unaided if he/she had the necessary strength, will or knowledge. And to do this in such way as to help him/her gain independence as rapidly as possible."

INTRODUCTION

This frequently cited definition of nursing, quoted above, offered by Virginia Henderson in 1966 still aptly describes the functional role of nursing. Another interpretation, by Madeline Leininger, defines the caring nature of professional nursing as "those cognitively learned humanistic and scientific modes of helping or enabling an individual, family, or community to receive personalized services through specific culturally defined or ascribed modes of caring processes, techniques, and patterns to improve or maintain a favorable healthy condition for life or death" (Leininger 1981). This definition of nursing care sets the stage for nursing intervention across the health-illness continuum. It speaks of helping behaviors that are both scientific and humanistic.

In her book, *From Novice to Expert*, Patricia Benner describes professional nursing practice domains and competencies identified through a series of interviews and observations of beginning and experienced nurses. The nurses were asked to describe patient-care episodes, which were analyzed; the nurses' interventions and outcomes led to the identification of 31 competencies in seven categories, or domains (Benner 1984). These domains (table 40.1) identify the caring component for all nursing specialties.

In oncology nursing, caring interventions are provided at all stages of the health-illness continuum. A description of the nurses' role in each stage follows.

THE NURSE'S ROLE IN PRIMARY PREVENTION

Nurses today are viewed by the public as authorities on cancer and are becoming leaders in primary cancer prevention by providing information and education, serving as role models, assessing individuals for risk factors, and suggesting interventions to change behavior. Nurses who are well-versed in the subject of cancer are both educators and role models for patients and their families, peers, and friends, as well as for the general public. These roles enable nurses to influence individuals to change behavior (Nevidjon 1986).

Increasing public awareness about cancer challenges all nurses today, not just oncology nurses. The Oncology Nursing Society, a specialty organization of more than 15,000 professional nurses, has long recognized the importance of cancer prevention in nursing practice. The society's original *Outcome Standards for Public Education* published in 1982 reflects the expectation that nurses will be involved in educating the public about health practices and behavior to prevent cancer or to detect it early (Frank-Stromborg 1986).

As role models and educators, nurses are finding opportunities to provide cancer education in the community as hospitals and volunteer organizations increasingly call on them for input in planning programs on such subjects as breast cancer awareness. Teachers may utilize nurses as educational resources to supplement their teaching (McIntire and Cioppa 1984). The American Cancer Society and other groups seek nurse volunteers to present their educational programs to the public. For example, a popular American Cancer Society program with nurse participation is the yearly Great American Smokeout.

Emphasis on cancer prevention has increased dramatically with the realization that many forms of cancer are the direct result of lifestyle practices and/or exposure to certain occupational or environmental agents. If the National Cancer Institute's goal of a 50% reduction in mortality by the year 2000 is to be accomplished, primary cancer prevention may be the best and most challenging means for reducing cancer mortality.

Nurses are assuming more responsibility in cancer risk assessment. Since "knowing what causes cancer is not enough to reduce the risk of cancer" (White 1986), nurses are educating and counseling individuals about risk factors and ways to reduce their risk.

A cancer risk assessment enables nurses to counsel individuals about the relationship between risk factors and cancer development. Risk assessment is particularly significant when it stimulates an individual to take actions aimed at changing his or her behavior.

Changing health behaviors and sustaining those changes is an important key to effective cancer prevention. Once it is determined that a person is at risk for the development of a particular cancer, the nurse works with other health-care providers to minimize anxiety and maximize sound decision making regarding behavior change (McIntire and Cioppa 1984).

To accomplish behavior changes, the nurse must make repeated efforts using a combination of interventions: teaching individuals and families about risk factors and what they can do to minimize them; utilizing both group and individual efforts; involving mass media to reach large groups; and supporting legislative regulation to facilitate health promotion.

Table 40.1
DOMAINS OF NURSING PRACTICE

DOMAIN: THE HELPING ROLE

The healing relationship: creating a climate for and establishing a commitment to healing
Providing comfort measures and preserving personhood in the face of pain and extreme breakdown
Presencing: being with a patient
Maximizing the patient's participation and control in his or her own recovery
Interpreting kinds of pain and selecting appropriate strategies for pain management and control
Providing comfort and communication through touch
Providing emotional and informational support to patients' families
Guiding a patient through emotional and developmental change; providing new options, closing off old ones; channeling, teaching, mediating
Acting as a psychological and cultural mediator
Using goals therapeutically
Working to build and maintain a therapeutic community

DOMAIN: THE DIAGNOSTIC AND MONITORING FUNCTION

Detecting and documenting significant changes in a patient's condition
Providing an early warning signal; anticipating breakdown and deterioration prior to explicit confirming diagnostic signs
Anticipating problems: future think
Understanding the particular demands and experiences of an illness; anticipating patient care needs
Assessing the patient's potential for wellness and for responding to various treatment strategies

DOMAIN: EFFECTIVE MANAGEMENT OF
RAPIDLY CHANGING SITUATIONS

Skilled performance in extreme, life-threatening emergencies: rapid grasp of a problem; contingency management; rapid matching of demands and resources in emergency situations
Identifying and managing a patient crisis until physician assistance is available

DOMAIN: THE TEACHING-COACHING FUNCTION

Timing: capturing a patient's readiness to learn
Assisting patients to integrate the implications of illness and recovery into their lifestyles
Eliciting and understanding the patient's interpretation of his or her illness
Providing an interpretation of the patient's condition and giving a rationale for procedures
The coaching function: making culturally avoided aspects of an illness approachable and understandable

DOMAIN: ADMINISTERING AND MONITORING THERAPEUTIC
INTERVENTIONS AND REGIMENS

Starting and maintaining intravenous therapy with minimal risks and complications
Administering medications accurately and safely: monitoring untoward effects, reactions, therapeutic responses, toxicity, and incompatibilities
Combating the hazards of immobility: preventing and intervening with skin breakdown, ambulating and exercising patients to maximize mobility and rehabilitation, preventing respiratory complications, creating a wound management strategy that fosters healing, comfort, and appropriate drainage

DOMAIN: MONITORING AND ENSURING THE QUALITY OF
HEALTH CARE PRACTICES

Providing a backup system to ensure safe medical and nursing care
Assessing what can be safely omitted from or added to medical orders
Getting appropriate and timely responses from physicians

DOMAIN: ORGANIZATIONAL AND WORK-ROLE COMPETENCIES

Coordinating, ordering, and meeting multiple patient needs and requests: setting priorities
Building and maintaining a therapeutic team to provide optimum therapy
Coping with staff shortages and high turnover: contingency planning
Anticipating and preventing periods of extreme work overload within a shift
Using and maintaining team spirit; gaining social support from other nurses
Maintaining a caring attitude toward patients even in absence of close and frequent contact
Maintaining a flexible stance toward patients, technology, and bureaucracy

(Source: Benner [1984]. Used with permission.)

THE NURSE'S ROLE
IN SECONDARY PREVENTION

Secondary prevention refers to the steps taken to diagnose a cancer as early as possible after the cancer has developed. According to the American Cancer Society, a significant number of lives can be saved each year if cancer is detected early. Oncology nurses knowledgeable about cancer risk factors and screening principles play an important role in early detection. Through the Oncology Nursing Society's *Standards of Oncology Nursing Practice,* the nurse is challenged to ensure that the patient and family have adequate information about cancer prevention and detection.

Screening and early detection are important aspects of cancer prevention and cancer control. Early detection, or the diagnosis of cancer when it is localized and curable, contributes to increased survival in many common cancers (Frank-Stromborg 1986). Cancers particularly amenable to early detection and hence increased survival include colorectal, breast, uterine, prostate, skin, oral, and testicular cancers.

According to the U.S. Commission on Chronic Illness, screening refers to the presumptive identification of unrecognized disease or defect by the application of tests, examinations, or other procedures that can be applied rapidly. Screening tests sort out persons who, though apparently well, probably have a disease from those who probably do not (Commission on Chronic Illness 1957). Obviously, all individuals cannot be screened for all cancers, but it is reasonable to focus screening efforts on those individuals at high risk and on those cancers best suited for early detection and screening.

Traditionally, the physician's office has been the site of early detection. As nurses have expanded their roles, they are now providing services for which the physicians find less time. Gradually, the medical and nursing communities have become partners in cancer screening and early detection; now nurses receive specialized training in early detection techniques, such as oral, breast, pelvic, and skin examinations.

Stromborg and Nord in 1979 showed that 91% of patients who received a cancer-detection physical examination at a cancer detection clinic conducted by a nurse were satisfied, highly satisfied, or very highly satisfied with the examination. When nurses were compared with physicians, a significantly higher percentage of people perceived the nurse examiner as a caring person who took time to explain procedures.

Nurses can provide cancer screening in any clinical setting, not only in cancer-screening clinics or comprehensive cancer centers (Frank-Stromborg 1986). Neither should cancer screening be limited to oncology nurses. Today nurses in outpatient, acute-care and long-term-care settings, schools, and community environments use their skills to assist with the early detection of all types of cancer for a variety of populations.

Nevidjon summarized cancer prevention and early detection activities as reported by oncology nurses. Many screening programs were described, such as:

1. Comprehensive screening clinics for people at high risk. A questionnaire, stool blood test, and physical were accompanied by comprehensive teaching with use of models to learn breast self-examination and testicular self-examination techniques.
2. Breast cancer screening programs.
3. A pigmented lesion clinic where moles or lesions were assessed and sunscreen samples and education were provided.

These screening programs were integrated with patient and public education programs, risk assessments to identify high-risk groups, and recommendations for behavior change (Nevidjon 1986).

The nurse also plays a critical role in providing support during the diagnostic process and assisting the patient and his or her family with obtaining information once the diagnosis is made.

The cancer diagnosis may be established quickly or it may involve a lengthy process. During this time patients and family members experience much apprehension over "not knowing." By explaining all diagnostic procedures and assuring the maintenance of open communication, the nurse helps to minimize fear and apprehension.

Once a cancer diagnosis is made, varied emotional responses occur: anger, denial, depression, fear. The nurse is aware of these responses and is able to encourage effective coping by the patient and can initiate appropriate intervention.

As the physician discloses information to the patient, the nurse is in an ideal position to reinforce, clarify, and assess the patient's understanding and response. Key questions asked by the nurse are:

1. What do the patient and family know?
2. What does the cancer diagnosis mean to the patient and family?
3. What is the patient's and family's response?
4. What is the social impact of cancer on the patient and family?

Once this information is collected, the nurse can begin to educate the patient and family about the disease and treatment, potential risks and benefits, and long-term effects.

THE NURSE'S ROLE
IN CANCER TREATMENT

As treatments rapidly change, become increasingly complex, and offer new forms of cancer management, nurses are faced with one of the most challenging and potentially rewarding dimensions of cancer nursing practice. Among the new areas are educating the patient and family about the disease, treatment, and care; providing emotional support to the patient and family; minimizing treatment-related morbidity to improve the quality of life; coordinating care throughout the course of treatment; and assisting with the administration of treatment regimens.

Educating patients and their families is an integral part of cancer treatment and a recognizable component of cancer nursing practice. *Standards of Oncology Nursing Practice,* coauthored by the Oncology Nursing Society and the American Nurses Association, describes the work of the oncology nurse as being responsible for assuring that the patient and family understand enough about the disease process and treatment to attain self-management and to participate in treatment (Oncology Nursing Society and American Nurses Association 1987). To achieve this outcome, the nurse collects data regarding what the patient knows and understands about the disease and treatment, assesses the data, then formulates a nursing diagnosis; develops a plan of care based on that diagnosis, implements the nursing care plan, then regularly evaluates achievement of the outcome; and revises the care plan when necessary.

The nurse's initial contact with the patient and family establishes the basis for education, counseling, and supportive intervention. In addition to a physical assessment, the nurse identifies the information needs of the patient and family. The homecare-provider—the person responsible for the patient's care after returning home—is identified and involved any time the patient is given instructions.

Regardless of the treatment selected, the nurse frequently repeats information given to patients and families in order to assure that the patients understand and retain the information. Throughout the treatment phase, the nurse constantly assesses patient and family needs. Interventions are revised or new ones planned involving teaching and emotional support. A teaching plan is developed based on assessment data and addresses the disease process, treatment options, and potential toxicities and benefits. Once decisions regarding treatment have been made, the nurse provides specific information about the treatment, side effects, and measures to minimize or prevent toxicity. Individualized teaching strategies, based on specific patient needs, include verbal instructions by the nurse; use of audiovisual and written materials to reinforce verbal information for ongoing education at home; use of both individual and group format; and use of a patient network allowing patients to talk to other patients and thereby promote emotional as well as educational support. In this way the nurse increases the patient's comfort and competence in the ability to manage symptoms. To facilitate symptom management, the nurse provides written information for easy referral while at home.

Minimizing treatment-related morbidity to improve the patient's quality of life offers the nurse new challenges and rewards. Today, patients are living longer while receiving multiple, complicated treatment modalities with numerous potential side effects and toxicities. Research in the areas of treatment-related morbidity

and methods to decrease untoward effects has provided the nurse with a better understanding of treatment side effects and effective nursing intervention and observation to minimize negative aspects.

Effective nursing care of the patient receiving cancer treatment involves four components: providing emotional support to facilitate coping with the cancer diagnosis and treatment; managing toxicities; teaching the patient and family to identify and manage the expected side effects of therapy; and assisting with the administration of the therapy.

The focus of care is the same for surgery, chemotherapy, radiation therapy, or any combination. The teaching component requires the nurse to understand the prescribed treatment. The ability to identify and anticipate patients' needs and problems during therapy is contingent upon the nurse's knowledge of the principles, actions, and potential effects of the various treatment modalities (Walter 1982). Most side effects of therapy occur after the patient leaves the treatment facility and their management is likely to take place at home. Teaching patients what side effects to watch for and how to manage them allows patients to participate actively in their care and provides them with a sense of control.

Common side effects of chemotherapy such as bone marrow suppression, nausea and vomiting, stomatitis, and alopecia can often be managed in the home. The patient and family are taught how to recognize signs and symptoms of infection, measures to minimize risk of infection, and when to notify the physician or nurse. Bleeding precautions for thrombocytopenia are taught, with instructions to notify the physician or nurse immediately should any evidence of bleeding occur. The nurse can anticipate and control nausea and vomiting with effective antiemetic regimens as well as diversional or relaxation techniques. Early education with appropriate emotional support by the nurse can minimize the profound effects that alopecia often has on patients' perceptions of themselves. Stomatitis is best managed by including measures to minimize infections, relieve oral pain, and maintain adequate nutrition and hydration.

The common side effects of surgery relate to the loss of an organ or body part and the development of postoperative complications such as infection and bleeding. Teaching is initiated preoperatively by the nurse to prepare the patient and family for the procedure to be performed, any functional limitations, and potential postoperative complications. In addition to patient teaching, the nurse addresses the emotional needs of both patient and family.

All patients undergoing radiation therapy are likely to experience to some degree side effects that include fatigue and a skin reaction within the treatment area. The nurse discusses general skin care guidelines with the patient and family before treatment is begun. The treatment area is assessed regularly for early identification of potential problems. Fatigue is best managed by instructing patients to pace their activities throughout the day depending on their energy level. Frequent rest periods, going to bed early, and getting up late are suggested to help minimize the treatment-related fatigue.

Numerous other side effects can occur with both treatment modalities and are determined by either the specific area being irradiated, as with radiation therapy, or the specific drug being administered, as with chemotherapy. Effective management is facilitated by patient education and identification of appropriate interventions. In all cases it is extremely important that patients know when to notify the physician or nurse.

Nurses are assuming increasing responsibility in the administration of chemotherapeutic agents. Oncology clinical nurse specialists, nurse clinicians, and staff nurses in oncology units who have received specialized education and training in caring for patients undergoing chemotherapy are providing the necessary expertise and skills for the safe administration of all chemotherapeutic regimens. Regardless of how or by whom the agents are administered, nurses caring for cancer patients are aware of drug reactions and potential effects. This familiarity permits nurses to assess and monitor patients, plan appropriate nursing interventions, and educate patients and families for self-care.

Finally, the nurse is identified today as a coordinator of patient care throughout the treatment phase. As treatments extend over a lengthy period, in both hospital and outpatient settings, the nurse maintains communication with all members of the health-care team to assure continuity of care.

THE NURSE'S ROLE IN REHABILITATION

Today, the future for people diagnosed with cancer is vastly different from that of 15 years ago when a cancer diagnosis for many meant certain, and often imminent, death. Until recently little thought was given to the cancer patient's rehabilitative needs, with the exception of certain physical disabilities. Advances in earlier diagnosis and treatment have resulted in individuals living longer with a chronic illness, requiring care that will assure the development of each individual to the fullest physical, psychological, social, vocational, and educational potential.

The goal of rehabilitation is the readaptation of the individual to his or her environment. This goal parallels the goal of cancer nursing which, as stated by Marino, seeks to promote adaptation and maximal rehabilitation of the person with cancer (Marino 1981). Though the patient cannot be restored to the pre-illness state, he or she may be able to live a full or nearly normal life. The oncology nurse is an ideal person to assist with rehabilitative needs.

Rehabilitation is complex and requires the combined efforts of a multidisciplinary health-care team consisting of physician, nurse, physical therapist, occupational therapist, social worker, psychiatrist, dietitian, prosthetic services, and homecare team. Often the nurse coordinates care for the patient in the hospital and in the home, helping to identify needs and assuring that all rehabilitative needs are met.

Rehabilitation begins at the time of diagnosis when the patient's potential needs are assessed; the team then includes the patient and family in the process of setting realistic goals. This participation assures patients of a sense of control in their lives. Rehabilitative goals are both short- and long-term. An example of a short-term goal is regaining arm and shoulder mobility after a mastectomy. Long-term goals may include returning to work or mastering a limb prosthesis. Other goals are established for both the physical and psychosocial needs of the patient and family.

Preoperative teaching includes discussions about changes to expect. The nurse focusing on rehabilitation can help with such specific issues as stoma placement for the patient about to undergo a colostomy, or communication alternatives for the patient with a head and neck cancer. The nurse also focuses on general care issues such as postoperative complications caused by prolonged bedrest and immobility.

When some definite physical change has resulted from the cancer and its treatment, the nurse is available to assure early intervention by the rehabilitation team to promote maximal adjustment. Many physical changes may result from the cancer itself or from its treatment: amputation of a body part, such as a breast or limb; alteration in communication, such as that occurring with a laryngectomy or glossectomy; loss of muscle strength or coordination resulting from surgery or radiation; loss of joint mobility due to radiation fibrosis or muscle contracture; lymphedema; and removal of part or all of an organ, such as bladder or colon. Early assessment and appropriate intervention enables the rehabilitation team to assure maximal adaptation for the patient and family.

The nurse's assessment of a patient's coping skills, use of defense mechanisms, and communication patterns with family and significant others is ongoing throughout all phases of the cancer illness (Groenwald 1987). While the diagnosis of cancer requires that decisions be made regarding treatment, decisions must also be made regarding work, finances, child care, maintaining the home, and care at home. Each decision and its potential to change lifestyle creates additional stress for the patient and family. Early assessment of the impact of lifestyle changes and the patient's ability to cope with them will permit the nurse and patient to set realistic goals for maximizing readaptation.

Nurses and other health professionals are increasingly participating in group efforts to improve the quality of the cancer patient's life. Cancer support groups such as self-help, counseling/therapy, or education/discussion groups assist patients and families in reducing feelings of anxiety and depression, increase their sense of control, and help them learn more about themselves. Support groups can help to break down barriers and solve mutual problems. The nurse's role in these groups varies tremendously, depending on the group's specific function and structure. The nurse usually acts as resource person, speaker, or referral source in a self-help group. In educational groups, the nurse is often teacher, organizer, and evaluator. Newly established groups frequently seek direction from a nurse who is perceived as a knowledgeable group leader. Experience in group dynamics with careful attention to the group process, assessment of learner needs, and careful evaluation after each session are helpful tools for the nurse initiating a group.

Identification and coordination of services available in the community is often the responsibility of the nurse, who is likely to have the most patient contact. Initiating services prior to discharge from the acute-care setting will maximize continuity of care and minimize patient and family apprehension and anxiety over returning home. The American Cancer Society offers several popular rehabilitation programs that include Reach to Recovery, International Association for Laryngectomies, United Ostomy Association, CanSurmount, I Can Cope, and Road to Recovery. Nurses interested in cancer care may serve as volunteers for some of these rehabilitation programs, which are available to cancer patients and their families.

THE NURSE'S ROLE IN ADVANCED DISEASE

Patients with advanced disease have disseminated or widespread disease, occurring at the time of diagnosis, or, more likely, recurring after being treated with some type of cancer therapy. Improved cancer treatment and the availability of more treatment options mean that cancer patients are living longer and experiencing frequent remissions or exacerbations. This large group of patients presents numerous opportunities for nurses as cancer care focuses on continued rehabilitation or assisting patients to achieve the maximum potential.

Once cancer recurs the likelihood for a cure is lessened, but there is still a hope for the cancer patient as treatment is reinitiated. As it becomes apparent to the patient that anticipation of a cure is no longer realistic, hope must be refocused and maintained, because hopefulness remains an essential component of this advanced disease process. As efforts shift from cure to palliation, the nurse helps maintain hope by focusing on the patient's needs, especially the need to be made comfortable and assured of continued comfort.

Comfort involves providing care for both the physical and psychoemotional needs of the patient and family. The nurse's approach addresses four areas of care: maintaining whatever function the patient already has; preventing or minimizing complications of the disease; recovering lost functions; and improving the patient's health status through counseling and support. By setting realistic goals, the nurse encompasses aspects of each area (Baird 1980).

To promote emotional comfort, the nurse assesses the individual's coping behavior, available support networks for both patient and family, perceptions of the illness and outcome, and expectations of care. The nurse remains alert for signs of ineffective coping behavior, including marked anxiety, denial, depression, or withdrawal.

The physical dimensions of comfort for the patient with advanced disease include pain, nutrition, safety, oxygenation, activity and rest, hygiene, and elimination. Nursing actions promote the prevention or control of physical symptoms, especially pain control. Because nurses are the health professionals most frequently and consistently in contact with the cancer patient, they have become significantly more involved in the pain assessment and management.

Grief and a sense of loss become more intense when a patient is dying. The five major losses experienced by the dying patient are loss of control, loss of identity, loss of achievement, loss of social worth, and loss of relationships. With loss of control, patients often fear becoming a burden to others. The nurse minimizes these fears by maintaining contact, keeping communication open, and discussing these fears. Loss of social worth, which leads to isolation, is best handled by the nurse who sets an example of continued open and honest interaction with the patient and who promotes continued communication between the patient and others.

Today, many cancer patients receive care at home during the terminal phase. In this situation, the family becomes the primary caregiver. The homecare nurse assumes an increasingly essential role, that of assessing the patient and family, planning appropriate interventions, and communicating to other health team members.

Care of the patient with advanced disease means care of the family. Assessment of coping includes family members' ability to cope with the crisis of dying. Such care measures include identifying physical signs of exhaustion, supplying information about what to expect, encouraging family members to eat and sleep, encouraging the family's interaction with the patient, and encouraging their expression of feelings.

The nurse, as patient advocate, has a responsibility to make the patient and family aware of alternatives available for terminal care. Hospice programs are available in many communities today. The goal of hospice care is to help a person continue life in a way significant to that individual (Baird 1980). This goal is achieved by relieving distressing symptoms, providing a caring and loving environment, assuring the patient and family that they will not be abandoned, and delivering expert care.

Nurses have a variety of roles in hospice programs; providing direct bedside care is the most obvious. Others include functioning as team member, program coordinator, or role model for volunteers and other care providers.

Throughout the terminal phase, the nurse attempts to preserve the dignity and identity of the patient and family. Trust is encouraged through open communication, and support is provided to the family as they anticipate the consequences of the impending death.

Bereavement coincides with the patient's imminent death and continues through the actual death event and the period of time immediately thereafter. Bereavement is the objective state of deprivation secondary to a loss (Snyder 1986). Separation and mourning are aspects of the bereavement process. The focus of nursing during this phase is twofold and involves providing meticulous, quality nursing care to the dying patient and simply listening to the mourning family member who must repeatedly verbalize feelings to make sense of the loss (Snyder 1986).

CONCLUSIONS

The role of the oncology nurse has evolved over the last two decades. Prior to the 1970s there was not a nursing specialty devoted to cancer. A number of developments in both nursing practice and cancer treatment and care led to the development of the specialty as it is known today. Nurses with specialized education and experience care for cancer patients at all points along the health-illness continuum from prevention and detection through rehabilitation or death from advanced disease.

The development of specialized knowledge and skills has become necessary as new diagnostic techniques and treatments are introduced. The intensive multimodal therapy used today requires a coordination of care often provided by nurses, with patients and their families taking an active role in treatment. Nurses must assess their ability to assume this responsibility and provide them with the knowledge and support they need to carry it out.

For economic reasons, and also because many patients prefer it, much care is now delivered in the home. Though oncology nurses formerly practiced primarily in hospitals, they are now needed in many settings including ambulatory care centers, private medical practice groups, home health agencies, and hospices.

Primary care nurses are assuming a key role in cancer prevention, screening, and early detection, but oncology nurses need professional support and specialized educational opportunities.

Cancer is a complex disease. Its management demands a comprehensive team of health care professionals performing a variety of functions. The practice of nursing has evolved to assist patients and their families in many ways: through education, by providing psychosocial support, by skillfully delivering therapy, by selecting and administering interventions to minimize the adverse effects of therapy, by assisting with rehabilitation, and by providing comfort and care.

REFERENCES

Baird, S.B. 1980. Nursing roles in continuing care: home care and hospice. *Semin. Oncol. Nurs.* 7(1):28-38.

Benner, P. 1984. *From novice to expert.* pp. 47-161. Menlo Park, Calif.: Addison-Wesley.

Commission on Chronic Illness. 1957. *Chronic illness in the United States: prevention of chronic illness.* vol 1. Cambridge, Mass: Harvard University Press.

Frank-Stromborg, M. 1986. Promotion of cancer prevention/early detection activities by the ONS Board of Directors. *Oncol. Nurs. Forum* 13(4):12.

Frank-Stromborg, M. 1986. The role of the nurse in cancer detection and screening. *Semin. Oncol. Nurs.* 2(3):191-99.

Groenwald, S. 1987. *Cancer nursing: principles and practice.* Boston: Jones and Bartlett.

Henderson, V. 1966. *The nature of nursing: a definition and its implications, practice, research, and education.* p. 15. New York: MacMillan.

Leininger, M. 1981. *Caring: an essential human need.* p. 9. New Jersey: CB Slack.

Marino, L.B. 1981. *Cancer nursing.* St. Louis: C.V. Mosby.

McIntire, S.N., and Cioppa, A.L. eds. 1984. *Cancer nursing.* New York: Wiley Medical.

Nevidjon, B. 1986. Cancer prevention and early detection: reported activities of nurses. *Oncol. Nurs. Forum* 13(4): 76-80.

Oncology Nursing Society and American Nurses Association. 1987. *Standards of oncology nursing practice.* Kansas City, MO: American Nurses Association.

Snyder, C.C. 1986. *Oncology nursing.* Boston: Little, Brown.

Stromborg, M., and Nord, S. 1979. Nurse practitioner acceptance in a cancer detection clinic. *The Nurse Practitioner: Am. J. Primary Health Care* 4:110-12.

Walter, J. 1982. Care of the patient receiving antineoplastic drugs. *Nurs. Clin. North Am.* 17:4.

White, L.N. 1986. Cancer risk assessment. *Semin. Oncol. Nurs.* 2(3):184-90.

Chapter 41

PRINCIPLES OF ONCOLOGY SOCIAL WORK

Grace Christ, C.S.W., A.C.S.W.

Grace Christ, C.S.W., A.C.S.W.
Director of Social Work
Memorial Sloan-Kettering Cancer Center
New York, New York

INTRODUCTION

The functions of oncology social workers fall into three broad categories: clinical practice, education, and research. The first two functions are already well-developed within the field of oncology social work, whereas psychosocial research is still evolving. The focus of this chapter is on the clinical practice functions, since they occupy the majority of the social worker's time and are most frequently used by the health-care staff. Professional education in oncology social work and new directions in social work research will also be addressed.

Oncology social workers traditionally have assisted patients in coping with the stresses of cancer diagnosis, treatment, rehabilitation, and terminal illness (Abrams 1976). However, in recent years, the oncology social-work role has become more complex due to changes that have occurred in the disease, in the treatment process, and in the delivery of health-care services. In addition, increasing numbers of patients need social-work services. These changes have dramatically altered the patient's experience of illness, and consequently their need for support services. The following examples illustrate the changes that have affected the oncology social-work role and increased the need for these services.

Large numbers of patients are now living with cancer as a chronic illness, or they are cured. However, they most cope with lasting effects of the disease and treatment and an increased chance of recurrence or development of a second cancer. Therefore, psychosocial interventions are aimed at supporting patients not only at times of acute crisis but during long periods of chronic illness as well. These changes in the disease process have led to a greater concern with the patients' quality of life over this longer time span and a need for services that specifically address quality-of-life issues.

The advances of high technology cancer treatments have also increased the complexity of patients' needs. Bone marrow transplantations, limb sparing procedures, and infusion pumps challenge health professionals to find new ways to bridge the gap between high technology and the human experience of it. Patients require help in understanding the technology, in making informed decisions about undergoing these treatments, and in living with treatment effects. While such treatments may offer advantages over traditional approaches in some areas of functioning, they may result in more compromised functioning in others. For example, limb-sparing procedures for patients with osteosarcoma preserve an intact body and body image, but may result in problems of mobility and require additional surgery. The oncology social-work role has become more complex as it encompasses these new challenges of high technology.

Massive changes in the health-care delivery system and the introduction of the prospective payment system have shortened inpatient stays and dramatically increased the number of individuals treated as outpatients. Unfortunately, community support services such as physical therapy, home care, equipment, transportation, and counseling are often inadequate to meet the needs of cancer patients. Community services are also expensive and many are not covered by insurance. Social workers devote increasing amounts of time helping patients plan for their care at home, coordinating individualized services from numerous agencies, developing new resources in the community, and advocating with insurance companies to cover additional outpatient treatment and care.

Because of the chronic nature of the disease process and the new trend toward outpatient treatment, the patient's family members or friends now have more responsibility for the patient's treatment and care at home. Supporting the caregiver has become a major focus of supportive intervention, in addition to providing services for the patient.

SOCIAL-WORK CLINICAL FUNCTIONS

In their clinical role, oncology social workers provide a broad range of practical and financial assistance services, counsel patients and families, and help them with the complex plans and decisions that often must be made during times of extraordinary stress.

COORDINATION OF CARE AND THE PROVISION OF COMMUNITY RESOURCES

Oncology social workers often coordinate the multidisciplinary discharge planning process to ensure an uninterrupted flow of health services that will maximize the patient's chance of recovering functional status and minimize health expenditures (New York Times 1988). The growing emphasis on discharge planning has heightened the awareness of oncology health professionals to the importance of careful coordination of posthospital care for cancer patients.

Practical services and community resources have never been more essential to the adequate treatment and care of cancer patients. Unfortunately, the medical insurance system has not responded to the shift from hospital-based care to community-based care by providing greater coverage for outpatient treatment or home care. Thus, most of the outpatient costs either are not covered or are inadequately reimbursed. In addition, home-care services that traditionally have been covered by Medicare, Medicaid, and Blue Cross have been severely curtailed; in some cases, nursing care is reimbursed for only two hours a day. Moreover, health insurance policies rarely cover the custodial care often required by cancer patients and focus instead on skilled nursing care.

In some communities, the few resources that exist are often overwhelmed by the demand from many medical institutions. The community resources that cancer patients need may be divided into the following five categories: (1) financial assistance for treatment and income maintenance; (2) home care, including personal care and household assistance (*personal care* includes injections, catheter care, stoma management, nasogastric tube feeding, pain management, medical monitoring, grooming, bathing, dressing, and physical or occupational therapy [Parsons 1977; Googe and Varricchio 1981]; *household assistance* includes housecleaning, meal preparation, laundering, and shopping [Grobe, Bhmann, and Alstrup 1982]; (3) equipment, such as wheelchairs, walkers, bath benches, bed pans, urinals, commodes, hospital beds, alternating pressure mattresses, intravenous poles and pumps, and stoma bags (Grobe, Bhmann, and Alstrup 1982; Googe and Varricchio 1981); (4) transportation, including ambulances, ambulettes, taxis, car services, and volunteer drivers (Putnam et al. 1980); and (5) emotional support and planning, including psychological counseling, financial counseling, recreation, companionship, legal advice, and nutritional counseling (Grobe, Bhmann, and Alstrup 1982).

OBTAINING COMMUNITY RESOURCES
Patients who are receiving inpatient or outpatient care from a hospital may receive information and referral for practical services from a member of the hospital's social work department. The particular expertise of hospital-based social workers is to assess and enhance the problem-solving abilities of patients and families in relation to the medical plan as well as to link them with the appropriate health resources in the community that will provide the services. Patients who are not being treated by the hospital system can be helped with home care and other practical services by social workers in community agencies or in private practice or by a local unit of the American Cancer Society.

To help patients gain access to these services, the oncology social worker develops a large network of agencies and community services. This enables the social worker to match individual patients quickly with the appropriate resources in the patient's locale (Polinsky et al. 1987). Unique services are also part of the social workers' resource network. For example, the Make-a-Wish Foundation grants special wishes of a seriously or terminally ill child; the Corporate Angel Network provides free transportation on a corporate jet to and from treatment centers.

Because patients tend to focus on their immediate needs rather than on those still to come, it is necessary to enhance the awareness of services that will meet future needs in a timely way. Unfortunately, it is becoming increasingly difficult to obtain services in the community because of bureaucratic complications. Thus, even the most sophisticated patients and families often need professional help in gaining access to services.

PROBLEMS RELATED TO THE CHRONIC NATURE OF CANCER
Most practical services for cancer patients are provided by the oncology social worker at the time of the patients' discharge from the hospital after an acute episode of illness (Hunter and Johnson 1980; Sharagen et al. 1978; Wellisch et al. 1983), or at home or in a hospice during the terminal phase of the illness (Amado, Cronk, and Mileo 1979; Cassileth and Donovank 1983; Market and Simon; Putnam et al. 1980; Rosenbaum and Rosenbaum 1980). Increasingly, however, these services are needed by patients during the chronic phase of cancer, that is, when the progression of the disease and the intensified treatment make the patient increasingly debilitated, but not yet in need of acute hospitalization or hospice care (Dwyer and Held 1982; Edstrom and Miller 1981; Parsons 1977).

In this chronic phase, patients may not only suffer from the symptoms of the disease, but also from the sequelae of chemotherapy and radiation therapy, such as nausea and vomiting, anorexia, weight loss, pancytopenia, and weakness (Edstrom and Miller 1981). Because of variations in the course of the disease and the unpredictability of the side effects of chemotherapy and radiation, medical crises may arise suddenly and create concomitant changes in the types of home care the patients need (Dwyer and Held 1982). Discharge plans made by the oncology social worker immediately after hospitalization cannot always anticipate the patient's future needs as the disease progresses. Thus, when further deterioration occurs months later, the patient is an outpatient and is not as easily identified as in need of services (Lindenberg and Coulton 1980). Fewer screening mechanisms are in place for determining the needs of this outpatient population.

A range of new interventions are being developed to deal with the problems of obtaining practical resources for cancer patients and in monitoring their care. For example, the Social Work Department at the Memorial Sloan-Kettering Cancer Center tested the feasibility and acceptability of using a computer-automated telephone outreach system to assess the needs of chemotherapy outpatients for a range of practical services (Siegel et al. 1989). The fully automated system was programmed to place telephone calls to 79 patients; to conduct a question survey in a high-quality, digitally stored voice; to interpret, confirm, and record the patients' answers; and to flag patients who identified one or more unmet needs so that they could receive prompt, direct professional attention.

The results of the pilot study indicated that computer-automated surveys are likely to have broad-based acceptance among cancer outpatients, and that the outpatients are able to comply with instructions for completing the interview. Research efforts should continue to focus on developing those methods that have the potential of providing a cost-effective, universal, and ongoing assessment of patients' needs that would facilitate timely intervention and the efficient use of professional staff.

DEVELOPING NEW RESOURCES

Because of recent shortages in community resources for cancer patients, there has been an increased emphasis on developing new resources and on using existing agencies and foundations more creatively. One important new resource involves advocacy on behalf of patients who have survived cancer and need help in finding employment and insurance. The increasing numbers of cured and chronically ill patients highlight the need to remove the social barriers that hinder patients from leading productive lives.

THE ONCOLOGY SOCIAL WORKER AS COUNSELOR AND THERAPIST

As a counselor, the social worker's primary goal is to help patients and family members adapt to the stresses of diagnosis and treatment within today's complex health-care system. These individuals may be psychologically healthy or disturbed, or have a different cultural background. Social workers can and do treat psychopathology, but their major focus is to support the optimal adaptation of all patients to their cancers. To achieve this goal, they rely on a broad range of counseling modalities and therapeutic techniques: individual, group, and family therapy; education; behavior modification; crisis intervention; supportive techniques; and insight-oriented

interventions. Clearly, the counseling role includes the role of therapist, but social workers also often have to assume the more active roles of broker and patient advocate. In recent years, special emphasis has been placed on counseling strategies that focus on stress management and decision-making.

STRESS MANAGEMENT

Stress management involves helping patients develop ways of handling specific stresses related to diagnosis, treatment, the side effects of treatment, and the impact of treatment on body image, emotional state, and personal and social relationships. As more and more patients have been effectively treated, health professionals — especially mental health professionals — have had to shift from focusing exclusively on survival to improving quality of life by identifying and minimizing the effect of impairments, enhancing the ability to function independently, and mitigating the impact of social barriers (Dobkin and Morrow 1985; 1986). This shift has led to new stress management interventions such as sex therapy, social skills training, hypnosis, relaxation, behavior modification, and social and political advocacy.

PLANNING AND DECISION-MAKING

Helping patients with the complex planning and decision-making that confront them during periods of extreme stress (for example, at diagnosis, when the disease recurs locally, or metastasizes, or becomes chronic or terminal) is a relatively new clinical function in oncology social work. For example, there are several treatments for breast cancer that can produce excellent results. Although each treatment may have an equal effect on the patient's chances for survival, each can affect the quality of life differently; it may lead to better functioning in some areas, and to compromised functioning in other areas. The patient must make the complex treatment decisions often at diagnosis, a time when her ability to make decisions is severely compromised.

Strategies have also been developed for helping patients make decisions throughout the course of the illness. For example, after a mastectomy, the woman must decide whether she wants breast reconstruction, which necessitates weighing the value of an improved appearance against the cost and risks of additional surgery. Another difficult decision is whether to participate in an experimental treatment program. As the disease progresses, patients must weigh the impact of the effects and side effects of research treatment against the possibility of longer survival. Given such options, patients and families are frequently left wondering whether they fought hard enough to extend life or compromised too much of the patient's quality of life for an increase in survival time. Patients also can choose where they will be treated and by whom, and often must decide what kind of care they need at home, and whether they can afford it. Finally, if their treatment is unsuccessful, they must choose how they wish to die and where — in a hospital, in a hospice, or at home.

The social worker helps patients make these decisions by informing them about options, clarifying their misconceptions and misunderstandings, encouraging them to evaluate the outcomes of different choices, identifying and mitigating the barriers to decision-making, facilitating family communication about the patient's decisions, and helping patients understand, accept, and adapt to the outcomes of their choices.

INTEGRATING THE DISCHARGE PLANNING AND COUNSELING FUNCTIONS OF THE SOCIAL WORK ROLE

Other health professionals often tend to differentiate medical social work from psychiatric social work, viewing medical social workers as discharge planning technicians and psychiatric social workers as nondisease-related therapists. For example, medical social workers are not expected to understand psychiatric issues, while psychiatric social workers are not expected to appreciate medical issues or the need for discharge planning (Goldberg et al. 1984). This dichotomy tends to reinforce the notion that the two social-work specialties require different skills rather than represent different emphases within the general framework of social-work practice. In fact, misperceptions about the social-work role occur, in part, because of the enormous diversity and multiple dimensions of the role, which is required by the diverse and complicated needs of the patients.

In actual practice, the oncology social worker must assess both the psychosocial and medical situations in order to plan adequately for a patient's care after discharge. Similarly, the social worker often must deal with the patient's emotional state so that he or she will be able to follow through on treatment and participate actively in recovery or rehabilitation. In other words, patients' thoughts and plans regarding the practical aspects of their care and their emotional reactions constantly interact. Many patients are unable to separate the facts from their need for help in planning for their posthospital care, their need for an accurate understanding of the stage of their disease, and their emotional reactions.

Social workers cannot provide effective psychological treatment unless they are knowledgeable about the disease process and have a clear idea of how to help the patients adapt to the disease and how it is treated. Knowledge of the disease process includes in-depth understanding of the biological aspects of cancer, the continuum of the disease experience, and the differences in how patients and family members react to each stage of the disease and to each aspect of treatment.

Oncology social work reflects an ecological systems perspective — the social worker's focus is to change the environment and the context in which patients experience stress and to help them cope with that stress more effectively (Germain 1977). This perspective requires the social worker to be involved in all aspects of a patient's treatment and care and perform a broad range of functions.

STAGES OF THE DISEASE: THE ONCOLOGY SOCIAL-WORK PRACTICE MODEL

The oncology social-work clinical-practice model includes the organization of the disease process into a series of stages or crisis points, a multimodality approach to treatment, and the identification of individuals at high risk for social breakdown.

ILLNESS STAGES

An essential function of the oncology social worker is to help patients cope effectively with the social and psychological tasks confronting them at each stage of the illness. With improved technology and medical treatment, more and more cancer patients are either cured or living with cancer as a chronic disease. The fact that the preterminal and terminal phases of cancer have been prolonged places new demands on both caregivers and patients.

In this effort, the oncology social worker must be truly "Janus-faced"; that is, he or she must help patients solve problems related to disease progression, terminal illness, and death, and at the same time prepare other patients to live with long-term chronic illness and cure. The social worker monitors the adaptive challenges facing patients and families at each stage of illness and attempts to develop educational and supportive interventions that will help them master those challenges.

While the whole course of the disease is stressful, there are certain times when all patients have more difficulty coping and around which interventions can be organized. Each stage has specific adaptive tasks that challenge either the patient or the family. Some of these stages are very familiar, such as diagnosis and terminal illness. Others are less well-known, such as the stresses of treatment termination that have been identified more recently. This stage has been reported by many recovered patients as a time of significant anxiety because they are unable to continue something active to control the disease and must live with less medical surveillance (Christ 1984). These include, but are not limited to the following: diagnosis, treatment induction, treatment side effects, treatment termination, normalization, survivorship, recurrence/metastases, research treatment, and terminal illness.

The adaptive tasks of each stage are listed below, followed by a description of some of the interventions used by oncology social workers to help patients fulfill these important adaptive challenges.

DIAGNOSIS: ADAPTIVE TASKS
   1. Coping with the confrontation of one's own mortality.
   2. Coping with overwhelming emotional reactions.
   3. Moving from denial of the reality of the disease to constructive processing of disease and treatment information.
   4. Making decisions about the appropriate treatment.

All patients report that the diagnostic process involves a confrontation with the reality of one's mortality, even if the biopsy is negative for cancer. Patients are emotionally overwhelmed and often say that for them life will never be the same again; that is, they will always have a heightened sense of their own personal vulnerability. Interventions need to be aimed at ways of quickly reducing anxiety in order to enable cancer patients to integrate the information they need to make vital treatment decisions.

One such intervention at diagnosis is the Sunday admissions program at the Memorial Sloan-Kettering Cancer Center (MSKCC). Social workers conduct group sessions to orient family members to the hospital system and medical procedures by informing them about where to wait for the results of surgery, how to obtain information about visiting hours, housing, parking, the availability of support services, and other details. This begins to restore a sense of control over their environment and helps to contain anxiety.

Patient-to-patient volunteers also attend these group sessions. These are recovered patients who have regained a good deal of their former level of functioning and who are trained to share their experiences effectively with other patients. Their very presence reduces family member's anxiety because they demonstrate the potential to survive and continue life much the same as before. They provide information about the illness and treatment experience, what a patient thinks and feels, and make suggestions about useful ways of communicating. Both the information and the experience of talking with a recovered patient are reassuring to families and lead to a better understanding of the issues.

In addition to supportive and educational techniques, the oncology social worker often uses crisis intervention techniques to assist patients and/or family members who are in acute emotional crisis during the diagnostic process. The first 100 days following diagnosis have been identified as a time of intense emotional turmoil for most patients (Weisman and Worden 1976-1977), some of whom require brief therapeutic interventions to regain a sense of control.

INITIATION OF TREATMENT: ADAPTIVE TASKS
   1. Understanding the treatment plan.
   2. Moderating the patient's distressed mood.
   3. Reorganizing the family to incorporate the demands of treatment and offer support to the patient.

As treatment begins, patients require much more specific information—for example, does the treatment involve radiation, surgery, chemotherapy, or a combination of these? If this information is provided before treatment begins, the patient feels less anxious and is better able to participate with the staff in meeting the treatment goals. The medical staff also demonstrate their competence through providing reassuring information to the patient that enables him or her to become an active participant in treatment.

Patients also often want information about usual and unusual emotional reactions to assess their own ways of coping. With the beginning of treatment, many patients experience a greater ability to control their emotions because they feel they are doing something active to treat the disease. They are able to feel good when they are physically well and emotionally upset only when physically distressed. This general lifting of mood is less likely with treatments such as chemotherapy, which may cause side effects that are difficult to control.

Family members also want guidance about how to help the patient deal with the stress of treatment. At the same time, they are concerned about how they will be able to fulfill their own ongoing responsibilities while the patient is being treated. If the patient is the family's major wage earner or emotional supporter, the shifting of these functions to other family members can be quite disruptive and stressful. Often family members can be reassured that the disruption is temporary and the patient will recover and be able to assume usual family functions. They may also need help in continuing to involve the patient in vital family roles and decision-making.

SIDE EFFECTS: PSYCHOSOCIAL TASKS
   1. Rebuilding self-esteem when there is loss of a body part, hair loss, weight loss, and fatigue.
   2. Coping with the ambivalence about treatment caused by disturbing side effects of treatment.
   3. Developing ways to have some control over side effects.
   4. Incorporating the physical demands of treatment into ongoing personal and family life.

Oncology social workers have found that patients often need to learn specific strategies for coping with the impact of disturbing treatment side effects on their physical and psychological functioning. These side effects may cause the patient to become ambivalent about continuing treatment, and hence the patient may fail to comply with treatment requirements or terminate treatment altogether. Interventions used at this stage include group and individual emotional support of the patient and the use of relaxation and other behavioral techniques.

The Breast Surgery Rehabilitation Group developed by social workers at Memorial Sloan-Kettering Cancer Center is an example of a group intervention program designed to help patients cope with the side effects of treatment. Ninety-five percent of all patients undergoing breast surgery attend this group. It meets three times a week and its leaders are a nurse, a physical therapist, and a Reach to Recovery volunteer (Christ, Bowles, and Bownam 1987). The group's goal is to inform patients of the physical and psychological tasks of recovery from their surgery and to assure them that many of their reactions and concerns are normal. In addition to information about physical recovery, patients learn about common reactions, such as fears of recurrence, changes in body image, reluctance to communicate with others about the surgery, and problems with depression and emotional control. In this way patients are encouraged to become active participants in their physical and psychological rehabilitation.

Groups have also been developed for patients undergoing adjuvant therapy, radiation, and chemotherapy to help in coping with the specific side effects of these treatments. When social workers cannot use groups because of small numbers of patients with a given diagnosis or because of their geographic distance from the institution, the same content can be provided in individual counseling sessions and with the use of printed materials and audio- and videotapes.

Oncology social workers also help patients adjust to treatment effects by obtaining practical assistance, such as prostheses, wigs, home care, child care, transportation, and financial support. These services often ease discomfort and stress.

Relaxation and other behavioral techniques recently have been found to be effective in controlling the nausea and vomiting caused by chemotherapy (Redd 1985-1986), reducing anxiety associated with a range of treatment effects, and controlling pain (Loscalzo 1985). Oncology social workers increasingly use these techniques to help patients cope.

TERMINATION OF TREATMENT: PSYCHOSOCIAL TASKS

1. Recognizing the fear of having less medical surveillance.

2. Recognizing the continuation of some problems that predated the diagnosis.

3. Adapting to remaining physical impairments and psychological stress.

4. Changing expectations of support from family and friends.

The patient's reaction to the end of treatment varies, depending on the reason for ending treatment. For example, it may have been a successful course of treatment, or the patient may have had toxic reactions and been unable to continue, or the patient may have completed the treatment, but the treatment does not appear to have affected the disease. Even when treatment has clearly been successful, patients may report feeling apprehensive about the decreased contact with medical staff and returning to normal living. Because they expect to feel more positive emotions, patients often think this anxiety is abnormal.

Family members and friends often expect the patient to return to normal life quickly following treatment, not realizing that psychosocial recovery often takes much longer than physical recovery. The patient must now return to work and to the personal and social challenges

he or she had prior to the diagnosis, but with a changed body and new psychological concerns. Patients worry about physical symptoms and yet struggle to keep up with colleagues to prove they have recovered.

The oncology social worker can help patients cope with the stresses of treatment termination by informing other staff, patients, and families about these specific challenges and by creating opportunities for patients to maintain communication with the treatment team.

For example, a patient-to-patient program is one way for recovered patients to maintain contact with the institution while off treatment (Mastrouito 1989). In these programs, patients volunteer to meet with other patients who have similar diagnoses or treatment courses. They may also offer educational programs around topics related to post-treatment adaptation, such as employment and insurance problems, ways of maintaining health, and opportunities for socializing. Newsletters for recovered patients are another way of maintaining reassuring contact. Such patient-oriented programs are often supervised and managed by social workers. For those patients who have a high likelihood of recurrence following treatment, such as in leukemia, monthly group sessions are another way for these individuals to have communication with health-care staff while off treatment. Some patients attend such groups regularly, but most attend only when they feel the need for reassuring contact or when they have an adjustment problem they wish to discuss. Individual patient communication with the social worker around psychosocial counseling issues is often used by patients to help contain their anxiety about distance from the treatment team.

SURVIVORSHIP: PSYCHOSOCIAL TASKS

1. Resuming normal activities and relationships with a changed body and a changed sense of lifetime.

2. Coping with a sense of emptiness — "the crisis is over."

3. Coping with the fear of recurrence.

4. Confronting stigma and social barriers to normalization.

One of the most difficult issues for cancer survivors is their social and psychological rehabilitation (Siegel and Christ 1986; Gotay 1987; Tebbi and Mallon 1987; Mellentte and Franco 1987; Teeter et al. 1987; Christ 1987). The powerful, life-threatening impact of a diagnosis of cancer and its treatment makes the return to preexisting roles and responsibilities with new personal and social expectations enormously difficult. Survivors often have remaining physical effects of the disease or treatment, such as hair loss; loss of a breast, limb, or other body part; loss of energy; and limitations in sexual or cognitive functioning (Fobair et al. 1986). These effects may be temporary, or the patient may confront permanent body changes. The idea that cancer survivors can resume where they left off following successful treatment, is simply inconsistent with the experience of the majority of survivors. Instead, the illness often creates a major discontinuity in their lives that brings about lasting changes in the way they perceive themselves and their future (Fobair et al. 1986; Cella et al. 1987). Many people develop extraordinary expectations of their performance, feeling they need to pay back for surviving, or they need to make up for lost "life time" and keep up with their healthy peers. They may become intensely focused on bringing their lives back to normal, believing they must function even better than before to prove they have indeed recovered. Yet they fear the body changes they have experienced might lessen their ability to feel equal to others or to feel normal.

Anna, age 55, recovered well from surgical removal of her shoulder for osteosarcoma with resulting loss of independent motion of her arm. She made extraordinary efforts to keep a beautiful appearance, be overly responsible for her two adult daughters, return to work with her husband, and find ways to compensate for painful, less gratifying sexual intercourse due to vaginal dryness caused by her treatment. Exhausted and depressed, she finally asked the social worker for help when her parents both died and she felt she could not take the time to mourn.

Survivors often describe conflicting feelings of joy of having survived and the mourning of lost potential.

The 42-year-old wife of a 10-year lymphoma survivor spoke of her constant, acute awareness that her husband's disease could recur. They made plans for no more than four months ahead for fear of having to face recurrent cancer. Most difficult for them was their inability to have children because of his earlier chemotherapy. Children would have enabled them to invest their energies in life and would have given them a promise of a future even if he did become ill again.

Fears of recurrence are heightened by the ambiguity that surrounds cancer in a society that demands the appearance of strength and certainty. Cancer survivors, especially those engaged in highly competitive jobs, often fear that disclosure of their diagnosis and treatment will be a barrier to full social acceptance and participation. The very perception of physical vulnerability can preclude employment in certain professions.

Steve, a 27-year-old man treated successfully for Hodgkin's disease, had planned to be a New York City police detective. Two years after completing treatment, he applied to the police academy. Despite receiving a high test score, he was told that he did not qualify due to his history of cancer. He was told he could be a transit patrolman, a much lesser assignment with little possibility of advancement. With the support of the oncology social worker he took his case to court. The police department decided to settle the case out of court and to allow him to join the department. However, the out-of-court settlement meant that this situation could not be used as a test case that would have provided more long-term security and perhaps have led to greater acceptance for other cancer survivors.

Cancer survivors often have difficulty obtaining employment or commercial insurance coverage due to real or imagined physical vulnerabilities. At times, survivors are passed over for promotions. Although their company may value them for their competence, they may be thought of as a risk in a management position. As a result, the survivor may wish to withhold information about his or her disease from a new employer, but then may have to confront the possibility of being fired if it is later disclosed.

Patients in this stage of recovery often require less medical information and more guidance and support in the areas of social, psychological, and sexual adaptation; genetic counseling; and in confronting barriers such as societal stigma and difficulty in obtaining insurance.

The oncology social worker serves as an advocate for the rights of cancer survivors and works with the American Cancer Society and with self-help groups such as the Coalition of Cancer Survivors and other recovered patient groups to press for legislation that will protect them from discrimination and increase their ability to live full and meaningful lives.

These recovered-patient groups also provide useful social contacts and are valuable sources of updated information. However, coordinating self-help groups, advocating for an individual patient, and assisting with problems in returning to a normal way of life following treatment often require professional skill. Because these are new services, additional staff are needed in order to effectively implement them.

RECURRENCE/METASTASIS: PSYCHOSOCIAL TASKS

1. Understanding information about the new situation.

2. Regaining a life focus and time perspective appropriate to the changed prognosis.

3. Alleviation of guilt or self-blame.

4. Decision-making about the new treatment course and resolution of practical problems related to initiation of treatment again.

The specific meaning of recurrence to the patient depends on the availability of effective treatments and the expected life span of the patient with recurrence or metastasis. This can vary considerably—from months, as in the case of some melanoma recurrences, to years, as is true for many patients with breast cancer. If the patient's expected life span has been drastically shortened by the recurrence of metastasis then the emotional reactions can be as strong as those experienced during terminal illness (Weisman and Worden 1985-1986). The multidisciplinary team must now work closely with each other and the patient to provide the necessary information with which he or she will decide on the next treatment steps.

Most patients experience significant disappointment, anger, and especially guilt; for example, could they have taken better care of themselves in a way that would have prevented the progression of the disease? The oncology social worker often uses crisis intervention techniques with those patients and families who become immobilized by feelings of helplessness, hopelessness, and grief. He or she identifies the next steps in the process of planning for the patient's care and the family's well-being. Patients and families are reassured by reminding them of how they coped effectively with previous illness and by encouraging them to actively engage in the tasks of planning and decision-making. In this way, they again experience their personal strengths and abilities. At Memorial Sloan-Kettering Cancer Center, families at this stage often benefit from the inpatient groups, led by a floor nurse and social worker, where they hear from other patients and families about various options for coping when recurrence appears, and later as the disease progresses. Such groups are available in most oncology units or community hospitals.

RESEARCH TREATMENT: PSYCHOSOCIAL TASKS

1. Processing information about treatment options.

2. Coping with ambivalence about continuing treatment.

3. Resolving differences between patient, family, and staff about treatment decisions.

4. Maintaining hope while making realistic decisions.

5. Solving practical problems involved in managing treatment.

6. Managing anxiety about unpredictable side effects of treatment and symptoms of disease progression.

To help the patient accomplish these difficult tasks, the social worker develops a process of continuing clarification of the information the patient needs about treatment options, treatment goals, possible side effects, financial costs of different options, and available support services. Many patients fear that research means they will be treated without regard for quality of life, and they are unclear about how much control they have once they have made the decision to have research treatment. Importantly, the social worker facilitates the patient's communication about treatment reactions to the research staff; increases the patient's comprehension of the research; enables the patient to make informed decisions about continuing treatment; advocates with patients for protocol modifications that might enhance the quality of life; and obtains ongoing information from the patient about how the treatment is affecting him or her, and how to proceed. Treatment reactions are often very individual, so a well-coordinated approach among members of the research team and the patient is required to enhance patient compliance and assure effective patient communication about treatment side effects.

TERMINAL ILLNESS: PSYCHOSOCIAL TASKS

1. Maintaining a meaningful quality of life.

2. Coping with a deteriorating physical condition.

3. Confronting relevant existential and spiritual issues.

4. Planning for surviving family members.

The social worker provides intensive interventions with increasing numbers of patients as their illness progresses and the patients need more help to manage a loss of function (Moynihan, Christ, and Gallo-Silver 1988). Terminal illness now often extends over a period of months rather than weeks, challenging both patient and family with the task of maintaining a meaningful quality of life during the often long and arduous process of dying. While the patient is engaged in such life-focused tasks, he or she rarely wishes to confront death directly. In fact, fears of talking about death and the difficulty of maintaining open communication with loved ones in the midst of such emotional intensity are the kind of psychosocial problems addressed by the social worker during this terminal stage.

As during earlier stages, the patient must make decisions about treatment and care, but during terminal illness he or she also faces deteriorating physical functioning. The patient must decide how and where treatment will take place and with what modality, weighing the benefits of prolonged survival against the possibility of unpleasant side effects.

The patient must also cope with symptoms like severe weight loss, energy loss, and pain, often in the home with limited home-support services. Insurance companies tend to view prolonged terminal illness as a chronic stage of treatment, and may refuse to reimburse needed home care. This forces the patient to be hospitalized when he or she would prefer to die at home.

The oncology social worker helps the patient clarify information, arranges for home care and financial support, interprets emotional reactions in the context of progressive disease, facilitates communication between the patient and caregivers, and helps with pain and other symptom control with the use of hypnosis and other behavioral interventions.

Patients also need to clarify the meaning and significance of their lives during this time. They ask what they have contributed to family, friends, society, and how their efforts will continue after their death. They may also confront negative feelings, such as guilt about smoking or other lifestyle behaviors that may have contributed to the disease, and anger and sadness about lost opportunities and potential. The social worker helps the patient and family cope with the impending separation and loss, using clergy and others who can also help bring comfort and a sense of completion.

Whether young or old, patients have responsibilities to children, partners, other family members, friends, and colleagues. Helping the patient, family, and significant others plan for the future of the survivors can be very supportive to all concerned. Completing tasks helps the patient to confront the reality of separation, provides a sense of control over a devastating experience, and creates a sense of resolution and completion.

The social worker may help with specific tasks like making out a will, contacting other members of the family, assisting with formal job termination to secure health and financial benefits, or prearranging a funeral. The social worker may also help with interpersonal tasks, such as repairing ruptured family relationships, working on lifestyle and value differences, arranging foster care or adoption of children, and appointing a family member to carry on the patient's responsibilities after death. Patients often are relieved by the completion of such tasks and show an increased ability to share feelings and thoughts about their condition.

Oncology social workers have developed special programs for dependent children of dying cancer patients. These programs provide help during the parent's terminal illness as well as during the bereavement period (Christ et al. 1988). The aim of the programs is to prevent or reduce the development of pathological symptoms in these psychologically high-risk children.

BEREAVEMENT: PSYCHOSOCIAL TASKS

1. To accept the reality of the loss.

2. To experience the pain of grief.

3. To adjust to an environment in which the deceased is missing.

4. To withdraw emotional energy and reinvest in another relationship.

The tasks of bereavement, identified by Worden (1982), focus strongly on the psychological needs of the individual who has lost a close friend or family member. Currently, bereavement counseling is being developed in some acute-care centers to provide more comprehensive and continuous services to patients and families. This trend also reflects greater recognition of the need to assist widows, widowers, and children in order to prevent their social and psychological breakdown. If such services do not exist in acute-care institutions, social workers can refer the individual to bereavement counseling through the American Cancer Society, local family service agencies, or specific bereavement counseling centers.

THE MULTIMODALITY APPROACH

Oncology social workers have responded to the increasing complexity of patients' needs by developing new modalities of treatment that enable them to meet the needs over the long course of the illness. These methods of intervention include, but are not limited to, the following: individual therapy, group therapy, resource provision or case management, patient education, crisis intervention, behavioral interventions such as hypnosis and relaxation methods, supportive counseling, insight-oriented therapy, play therapy, and patient advocacy.

Fig. 41.1 indicates which interventions are used most frequently at various stages.

IDENTIFYING HIGH-RISK PATIENTS

Although patients often experience social and emotional disturbances in response to a diagnosis of cancer, few request counseling, supportive interventions, psychiatric consultation, or even self-help. Most patients are unable to request psychological support for a variety of reasons. Some are psychologically immobilized and cannot exert the emotional energy needed to get help. Others think a request for support indicates an inability to cope, a loss of independence, or mental illness. Furthermore, most patients are unaware that counseling may help assuage the existential terror that is evoked by a diagnosis of cancer or alleviate grief over the loss of body function or appearance. Unfortunately, these same patients often later resent not receiving emotional support from the health-care team. Because patients have difficulty requesting and using these services, it is useful to have them prescribed by physicians and to make sure they are available and readily accessible.

Patients are at different points along a continuum of need for social work counseling services, from those who are seriously mentally ill, to those who are psychologically vulnerable, to those who are resilient and well-supported. Although most cancer patients can benefit from some counseling, others must receive it to maintain their functioning and to prevent a social and emotional breakdown.

Cancer patients with a history of mental illness or psychiatric treatment generally have an ongoing relationship with a number of supportive services in the community that may need information about their medical condition. Such patients should be urged to communicate with their therapists or other mental health counselors about their medical condition, or a social worker can transmit this information and arrange for continuing psychological treatment. The diagnosis of cancer may exacerbate a pre-existing mental illness or seriously affect day-to-day functioning. Early social work intervention may prevent a functional breakdown that can have lasting adverse consequences like the loss of a job, the severance of important social relationships, and the alienation of friends and relatives.

A much larger group of patients has a variety of social and psychological characteristics that place them at risk for having adaptational problems when confronting a diagnosis of cancer, but they are not mentally ill. However, these patients' difficulties in coping may interfere with daily functioning and treatment compliance. Such vulnerable patients include, for example, those who are:

- living alone or who have few friends or relatives available to help them;
- over age 75;
- children or young adults;
- financially stressed, e.g., having very limited or no insurance coverage;
- parents of dependent children;
- multiple stressed—who have experienced a great deal of life stress or who are in the midst of other life crises, such as the recent loss of a job or a divorce;
- members of family situations characterized by high levels of conflict, like a previous history of violence or abuse; or

INTERVENTIONS

	Resource Provision		Education		Cognitive Skills		Crisis Intervention		Supportive Intervention		Insight Oriented	
	C	A	C	A	C	A	C	A	C	A	C	A
Stage I Diagnosis	IF †		IFG †††				IF †††		IF	IFG ††		
Stage II Treatment Induction	IF ††		IFG †††	IG			IF †		IFG ††	IG		
Stage III Treatment Side Effects	IF †		IF ††	I	IF †††	IG	IF †		IF ††	I		
Stage IV Treatment Termination	IF †		IF †				IF †		IF †††	I	IF ††	
Stage V Survivorship							IF †		IFG †††		IF ††	
Stage VI Recurrence/Metastasis	IF ††		IF ††				IF †††		IF ††			
Stage VII Research Treatments	IF ††		IF †††				IF ††		IF †††		IF †	
Stage VIII Terminal Illness	IF †††		IF ††		IF †††		IF †††		IF	IFG †††	IF ††	IFG
Stage IX Bereavement			IFG †						IFG †††		IFG †††	

††† - Most frequently used intervention
†† - Frequently used intervention
† - Sometimes used intervention
C = Child; A = Adult; I = Individual; F = Family; G = Group

Fig. 41.1 Interventions used most frequently at various stages.

● ill with other disease or whose family members are ill, especially with cancer, and therefore they may have difficulty being realistic about their own diagnosis and prognosis.

Often a higher-risk patient is more difficult to identify than one with a previously diagnosed mental illness. The oncology social worker develops a method for early identification of such higher-risk patients when they are admitted to the hospital. All patients with these characteristics will benefit when the physician recommends that they obtain social work services.

At the other end of the continuum from patients with diagnosed mental illness are those individuals who appear to be resilient and psychologically strong and have numerous personal, social, practical, and financial resources. They may be considered lower risk on the psychological continuum. Unfortunately, their psychological and support needs are often overlooked by professionals. Such individuals must be informed of available support services so that they can make rapid and highly effective use of them. Patients often resent not having access to these services. As one patient stated, "I knew I could cope well with a cancer diagnosis and I did, but I might have coped better with some help and would have liked to have known about counseling that could have been available to me."

SOCIAL-WORK PROFESSIONAL EDUCATION

Oncology social workers have developed innovative programs for educating social workers to the specialty of oncology, and provided training to other mental health professionals in oncology. In 1973, the Social Work Department of Memorial Sloan-Kettering Cancer Center in New York, assisted by a grant from the American Cancer Society, developed a postgraduate training program for social workers that has provided a week-long course 10 times a year for over 15 years. More than 100 social workers and other mental health professionals from cancer centers and other health-care institutions throughout the country participate in this training each year. In 1975 the Social Work Oncology Group (SWOG) was developed out of the Sidney Farber Cancer Institute in response to the expressed needs and interests of social workers in Boston. This program expanded, with support from the National Cancer Institute in 1978, to provide continuing education programs, peer support, and communication networks to social workers throughout New England.

Similar programs have been developed in other geographic areas. A mid-Atlantic SWOG functions out of the Fox Chase Cancer Center in Philadelphia. The California division of the American Cancer Society conducts ongoing professional education programs for social workers and other mental-health professionals. In addition, many social-work oncology support groups have been developed in rural and urban areas throughout the United States.

In 1985, oncology social workers from postgraduate training programs, social-work organizations, cancer centers, and treatment institutions and agencies throughout the country joined together to form the National Association of Oncology Social Workers (NAOSW).* This organization is now well-established with over 700 members. The stated purpose of the NAOSW is to: (1) promote the members' clinical, educational, and research development; (2) devise and maintain professional standards for oncology social workers; and (3) serve as an advocate for the rights of patients and their families to obtain necessary services. These purposes are carried out through an annual conference, quarterly newsletter, and established network communication.

RESEARCH IN ONCOLOGY SOCIAL WORK

Social work research in oncology is a new but growing area of expertise. Its goal is to enhance the ability of social workers to provide the most efficient and timely service to cancer patients, family members, and caregivers. The problems investigated usually emerge from social workers' daily contact with patients and family.

A unique feature of social work research is a strong collaboration between the research and clinical staff. Social workers and the research staff formulate problems into empirically researchable questions, and when the answers are available, they can be quickly integrated into clinical services.

Oncology social workers have traditionally supported medical research and have participated in multidisciplinary mental-health research. More recently, social-work initiated research has developed in the following areas: (1) the identification of patients in need of various kinds of material and emotional assistance; (2) facilitating patient of family-member adaptation, survival, or loss; (3) promoting preventive-health behavior; and (4) understanding more about the informal (i.e., nonprofessional) sources of support that patients may

receive, and the burden that primary caregivers may experience in promoting such support and assistance.

Because service delivery has changed dramatically in recent years, research in this area focuses increasingly on the practical and administrative needs of patients and families and identifying patients who are most likely to have difficulty having their needs met. For example, Berkman et al. (1983) investigated the characteristics of elderly cancer patients who require institutional care. Siegel et al. (1989) identified the prevalence of unmet needs of ambulatory patients undergoing chemotherapy. The goal of this research is to develop interventions for ongoing monitoring of patients' needs that will improve the quality of service.

Oncology social workers are especially concerned about the impact of diagnosis and treatment on quality of life at all stages of illness. Examples of such research include the studies of Fobair et al. (1986), which examined the consequences of long-term treatment on survivors of cancer. In recent years, social workers have also undertaken research on the psychosocial impact of AIDS (Siegel 1988). The AIDS epidemic has provided a unique opportunity for interdisciplinary studies on a major public health problem as it develops, with a special focus on prevention.

It is well-documented in the psychosocial oncology and gerontological literature that family members and friends provide most of the practical and emotional assistance needed by individuals being treated as outpatients. While a considerable body of research conducted over the past two decades documents the benefits for patients who are the recipients of social support, only more recently has there been a growing awareness of the costs (emotional, social, physical, and financial) that may be associated with being a provider of care. Therefore, the burden experienced by family members and friends who provide care to cancer patients at home are another principal focus for social-work research.

REFERENCES

Abrams, R. 1976. *Not alone with cancer: a guide for those who care: what to expect, what to do.* Springfield, Ill.: Charles C. Thomas.

Adams-Greenly, M.; Moynihan, R.; and Christ, G. 1986. Helping children when a parent is dying. In Billings, J.A. ed. *Advanced cancer: symptom control, support, and hospice in the home.* chap. 10. Chelsea, Mass.: J.B. Lippincott.

Amado, A.; Cronk, B.A.; and Mileo, R. 1979. Cost of terminal care: home hospice vs. hospital. *Nursing Outlook* 27:522-26.

Berhoman, B.; Stalberg, C.; and Parker, E. et al. 1983. Elderly cancer patients: factors predictive of risk for institutionalization. *J. Psychosoc. Oncol.* 1(1):85-100.

Cassileth, B.R., and Donovank, J.A. 1983. History and implications of the new legislation. *J. Psychosoc. Oncol.* 1:59-69.

Cella, D.F.; Tan, C.; and Sullivan, M. et al. 1987. Identifying survivors of pediatric Hodgkin's disease who need psychological interventions. *J. Psychosoc. Oncol.* 5:1-3.

---

*Contact the national office by writing: Linda Sibila, Administrative Secretary, 1233 York Ave., Apt. 12N, New York, N.Y. 10021.

Christ, A.E. 1984. Psychosocial challenges in childhood cancer. In *Childhood cancer impact on the family.* vol. 5. New York: Plenum Press.

Christ, G.H.; Bowles, M.E.; and Bowman, L.J. 1987. Educational and support groups for breast cancer patients and their families. In Harris, J. et al. eds. *Breast diseases.* pp. 648-55. Boston: J.B. Lippincott.

Christ, G.; Loscalzo, M.; and Weinstein, L. et al. 1988. Community resources for cancer patients. In DeVita, V.T. Jr.; Hellman, S.; and Rosenberg, S.A. eds. *AIDS: etiology, diagnosis, treatment, and prevention.* 2nd ed. Philadelphia: J.B. Lippincott.

Christ, G.H. 1987. Social consequences of the cancer experience. *Am. J. Pediatr. Hematol. Oncol.* 9(1):84-88.

Dobkin, P.L., and Morrow, G.R. 1985/86. Long-term side effects in patients who have been treated successfully for cancer. *J. Psychosoc. Oncol.* 23-51.

Dwyer, J.E., and Held, D.M. 1982. Home management of the adult patient with leukemia. *Nurs. Clin. North Am.* 17: 665-75.

Edstrom, S., and Miller, M.W. 1981. Preparing the family to care for the cancer patient at home: a home care course. *Cancer Nursing* 4:49-53.

Fobair, P.; Hoppe, R.T.; and Bloom, J. et al. 1986. Psychosocial problems among survivors of Hodgkin's disease. *J. Clin. Oncol.* 4:805-14.

Germain, C.B. 1977. An ecological perspective on social work practice in health care. *Social work in health care* 3:67-76.

Goldberg, R.J.; Tull, R.; and Sullivan, N. et al. 1984. Defining discipline role in consultation psychiatry: the multidisciplinary team approach to psychosocial oncology. *Gen. Hosp. Psychiatry* 6:17-23.

Googe, M.D., and Varricchio, C.G. 1981. A pilot investigation of home health care needs of cancer patients and their families. *Oncol. Nurs. Forum* 8:24-28.

Gotay, C.C. 1987. Quality of life among survivors of childhood cancer: a critical review and implications for intervention.

Grobe, M.E.; Bhmann, D.L.; and Alstrup, D.M. 1982. Needs assessment for cancer patients and their families. *Oncol. Nurs. Forum* 9:26-30.

Hunter, G., and Johnson, S.H. 1980. Physical support systems for the homebound oncology patient. *Oncol. Nurs. Forum* 7:21-23.

Lindenberg, R.E., and Coulton, C. 1980. Planning for posthospital care: a follow-up study. *Health and Social Work* 5:45-50.

Loscalzo, M. 1985. Management of cancer pain: behavioral and cognitive approaches to pain control. *Syll. Postgrad. Course Pain Serv.* New York: Department of Neurology, Memorial Sloan-Kettering Cancer Center.

Market, W.M., and Simon, V.B. The hospice concept. *Cancer* 28:225-37.

Mastrouito, R.; Moynihan, R.T.; and Parsonnet, L. 1989. Self-help and mutual support programs in *Handbook of Psycho-oncology,* Holland, J., and Rowland, G, eds. New York: Oxford University Press.

Mellenette, S.J., and Franco, P.C. 1987. Psychosocial barriers to employment of the cancer survivor. *J. Psychosoc. Oncol.* 5.

Moynihan, R.; Christ, G.; and Gallo-Silver, L. 1988. Psychosocial, spiritual and bereavement issues in the treatment of terminally ill people with AIDS. *Social Casework* 68(6): 360-87.

Parsons, J. 1977. A descriptive study of intermediate stage terminally ill cancer patients at home. *Nurs. Dig.* 5:1-26.

Polinsky, M.L.; Ganz, P.A.; Randofessart-O'Berry, J. et al. 1987. Developing a comprehensive network of rehabilitation resources for referral of cancer patients. *J. Psychosoc. Oncol.* 5:1-10.

Putnam, S.T.; McDonald, M.M.; and Miller, M.M. et al. 1980. Home as a place to die. *Am. J. Nurs.* 80:1451-53.

Redd, W.H. 1985/86. Use of behavioral methods to control the aversive effects of chemotherapy. *J. Psychosoc. Oncol.* No. 4, 1985/86, pp. 17-22.

Rosenbaum, E.H., and Rosenbaum, D.R. 1980. Principles of home care for the patient with advanced cancer. *JAMA* 244:1484-89.

Sharagen, J.; Halman, M.; and Myers, D. et al. 1978. Impediments to the cause and effectiveness of discharge planning. *Social Work in Health Care* 4:65-80.

Siegel, K., and Christ, G. 1986. Psychosocial consequences of long-term survival of Hodgkin's disease. In Redman, J., and Lacker, M. eds. *Hodgkin's disease: the consequences of survival.* Philadelphia: Lea and Feiberger.

Siegel, K.; Bauman, L.G.; and Christ, G. 1988. Patterns of change in sexual behavior among gay men in New York City. *Arch. Sex. Behav.* 17(6):481-97.

Siegel, K.; Mesagno, F.P; and Chen, J.Y. et al. 1989. Computerized telephone assessment of the needs of chemotherapy outpatients: a feasibility study. *Am. J. Clin. Oncol.* 28(6): 561-69.

Tebbi, C.K., and Mallon, J.C. 1987. Long-term psychosocial outcome among cancer amputees in adolescence and early adulthood. *J. Psychosoc. Oncol.* 5.

Teeter, M.A.; Holmes, G.E.; and Holmes, F.F. et al. 1987. Decisions about marriage and family among survivors of childhood cancer. *J. Psychosoc. Oncol.* 5.

The New York Times. 1988. Hospital expanding procedures to assist patients for discharge. Feb. 11, 1988.

Weisman, A.D., and Worden, J.W. 1976/77. The existential plight in cancer: significance of the first 100 days. *Psychiatry Med.* 1:1-15.

Weisman, A.D., and Worden, J.W. 1985/86. The emotional impact of recurrent cancer. *J. Psychosoc. Oncol.* 3(4):5-16.

Wellisch, D.K.; Fawzy, F.I.; and Landsverk, J. et al. 1983. Evaluation of psychosocial problems of the homebound cancer patient: the relationship of disease and the sociodemographic variables of patients to family problems. *J. Psychosoc. Oncol.* 1:1-15.

Worden, J.W. 1982. *Grief counseling and grief therapy: a handbook for the mental health practitioner.* New York: Springer.

Chapter 42

SEXUALITY AND CANCER

Barbara L. Andersen, Ph.D
Gretchen Schmuch, M.S.W.

Barbara L. Andersen, Ph.D.
Associate Professor
Department of Psychology and Department of Obstetrics and Gynecology
The Ohio State University
Columbus, Ohio

Gretchen Schmuch, M.S.W.
Research Associate
Department of Psychology
University of Iowa
Iowa City, Iowa

Research for this chapter was supported by Grant PRB-27 from the American Cancer Society.

INTRODUCTION

Cancer and cancer treatments produce significant sexual disruption. Sexual morbidity has been documented across all disease sites and following all therapies (Andersen 1985). Although the effects of the disruption are influenced by the extent of the disease and treatment, even patients with *in situ* disease receiving comparatively lesser therapies are not immune. National conferences have addressed this issue by describing the problems and highlighting the future directions for research (American Cancer Society 1987; National Institutes of Health 1987).

OVERVIEW OF SEXUAL FUNCTION AND DYSFUNCTION

Appreciation of cancer patients' sexual difficulties begins with an understanding of sexual functioning in normal, healthy women and men. The health care provider needs to be comfortable with and confident in his or her ability to assess at least three important areas with the cancer patient. First, it is important to understand and quantify sexual behavior. Kinsey and colleagues included the following types of sexual activity in their research: preadolescent heterosexual and homosexual play, masturbation, nocturnal sex dreams, premarital petting, marital and extramarital coitus, homosexual contacts, and, finally, the "total sexual outlet," defined as the sum of the various types of sexual activity culminating in orgasm (Kinsey, Pomroy, and Martin 1948). For heterosexual individuals, the frequency of intercourse is perhaps the most important, as this behavior is significantly correlated with other important activities (Andersen and Broffitt 1988), and is significantly related to sexual satisfaction and adjustment. It is also necessary to include a range of sexual activities, as intercourse and its frequency become vulnerable following cancer treatment. Many individuals will find it necessary to engage in other sexual activities (e.g., body caressing) if they wish to maintain sexual activity with their partner.

The second and third important areas are the phases of the sexual response cycle (including desire, excitement, orgasm, and resolution) and the corresponding sexual dysfunctions. Masters and Johnson and others have described the physiologic aspects of sexual responding (Masters and Johnson 1966; Kaplan 1979). This work provided a useful framework for other investigators to integrate psychological and behavioral responses during sexual activity.

Of all the phases of sexual responding, sexual desire is the least understood. It is most often thought of as a biologic drive or urge for sexual activity. In individuals with a life-long lack of sexual interest, sexual drive or urges are not blocked but seem not to occur (Leiblum and Rosen 1988). Some hypothesize that for male sexual desire, adequate amounts of testosterone are needed, with androgen providing the hormonal basis for female sexual desire. Others view sexual desire as a subjective feeling that may be triggered by internal cues (e.g., fantasy, erection, or vaginal lubrication) or external ones (e.g., pornography, or the presence of an interested partner). The diagnosis (Madorsky, Ashamalla, and Schussler et al. 1976) of inhibited sexual desire or hypoactive sexual desire characterizes individuals who are generally uninterested in sexual activity (American Psychiatric Association 1980). Such an attitude can be manifest behaviorally by avoidance of sexual contexts or refusal of sexual activity. These behaviors, however, are not presumed to be due to highly negative responses (aversions) to interpersonal or genital contact. Instead, individuals with a desire disorder are believed to be indifferent or neutral towards sexual activity. They report no sexual fantasies or other pleasant, arousing sexual cognitions. Emotionally, they describe themselves as not feeling sexy or sexual and they report no interest in initiating or responding to a partner's initiations for sexual activity. Individuals with sexual desire dysfunction can presumably experience normal sexual excitement and/or orgasm when engaging in sexual activity; however, disruption in the focus, intensity, or duration of sexual activity is probable, and thus secondary disruption of excitement or orgasm is common.

The phase of sexual excitement begins with sexual stimulation, either physiologic or psychologic. The physiologic responses are widespread vasocongestion, either superficial or deep, and myotonia, as evidenced by either voluntary or involuntary muscle contractions. Other changes include increased heart rate and blood pressure and deeper, more rapid respiration. For men, the most obvious sign of sexual excitement is penile erection. The scrotum changes with vasocongestion, producing a smoothing out of the skin ridges of the scrotal sac. The testes are partially elevated toward the perineum by shortening of the spermatic cords. For women, sexual excitement is characterized by the appearance of vaginal lubrication, produced by vasocongestion in the vaginal walls leading to transudation of fluid. Other changes include a slight enlargement of the clitoris and uterus, caused by engorgement. The uterus also rises in position and the vagina expands and balloons out. Maximal vasocongestion of the vagina produces a congested orgasmic platform in the lower one-third of the vaginal barrel. These physiologic changes are generally accompanied by heightened interest in sexual activity and, when possible, lead to initiating or responding to another's initiations of sexual activity.

Sexual dysfunction during the excitement phase inhibits or disrupts the predominant physiologic responses and leads to subjective distress. For men, erectile dysfunction, an inability to achieve or maintain an erection of sufficient strength or duration to allow for satisfactory intercourse, may occur. For women, insufficient vaginal engorgement or lubrication may make penetration difficult or impossible. As with desire-phase difficulties, subsequent orgasmic disruption can easily occur due to dysfunctional arousal.

The specific neurophysiologic mechanisms of orgasm are not presently known, although Masters and Johnson (1966) proposed that orgasm is triggered by a neural reflex arc once a plateau of excitement has been reached or exceeded. Orgasm has been described as a total body response, including facial grimacing, generalized myotonia, carpopedal spasms, and contractions of the gluteal and abdominal muscles. The subjective experience of orgasm includes feelings of intense pleasure with a peaking and rapid, exhilarating release. Awareness of the physical experience of orgasm typically focuses on pelvic sensations, concentrated in the clitoral body, vagina, and uterus for women; and in the penis, prostate, and seminal vesicles for men. In the first state of the ejaculatory process, seminal emission, men experience a sensation of inevitability and a perception of a change in pressure. During this period there is a smooth-muscle contraction of the prostate, seminal vesicle, and vas deferens, and partial closure of the bladder neck resulting in seminal emission into the posterior urethra. Further neural control is needed for the second stage, ejaculation, during which there is striated muscle contraction of the perineum, complete bladder closure, and projectile ejaculation through the urethra. If the internal sphincter at the neck of the urinary bladder is open the ejaculate spills into the bladder (retrograde ejaculation), which can be documented with post-masturbation urine and semen studies. The sensations of orgasm can be present without the second stage of projectile ejaculate, and the ejaculation is considered "dry." Some men are psychologically distressed by the absence of this semen, while others are not.

Orgasm in the female is marked by rhythmic contractions of the uterus, the orgasmic platform, and the rectal sphincter, beginning at 0.8-second intervals and then diminishing in intensity, duration, and regularity. Women are unique in their capacity to be multiorgasmic; that is, capable of a series of distinguishable orgasmic responses without a lowering of excitement between them. Men instead enter a refractory period (from several hours to days, depending on the man's age), during which another ejaculation is not possible, although partial erections can be maintained.

In either sex, if effective stimulation ends (with or without orgasm), the anatomic and physiologic changes reverse. In women, the orgasmic platform disappears as the orgasmic response pumps blood away from the tissues. The uterus moves back into the true pelvis and the vagina shortens and narrows. In men, erection diminishes markedly following orgasm, although further detumescence occurs more slowly with normal vascular outflow. The testes decrease in size and descend into the scrotum.

Two forms of male orgasmic dysfunction are currently recognized. One is rapid or premature ejaculation, which occurs too quickly or with minimal stimulation. Such a rapid response is accompanied by the man's subjective sense that he has no control over the timing of ejaculation, and behavioral efforts (e.g., stopping stimulation before it becomes too intense, cognitive distraction) are of little or no use in postponing ejaculation. The other form of ejaculatory difficulty is delayed or retarded ejaculation. Here ejaculation fails to occur, or is very difficult to achieve despite prolonged stimulation and effort. Subtypes of orgasmic dysfunction among women have also been noted. Primary orgasmic dysfunction includes women who have never experienced orgasm under any circumstances except sleep or fantasy. If the woman has experienced orgasm but expresses concern with its frequency or circumstances of occurrence, then the difficulty is described as secondary. A common complaint is orgasm occurring randomly or not with coitus.

The final phase of the sexual response cycle refers to the immediate postorgasm period, which is marked by sensations of bodily relaxation and feelings of sexual contentment and satisfaction. A filmy sheet of perspiration covers the body, and the elevated heart rate and respiration gradually return to normal. Sexual distress during the resolution period usually occurs following excitement and orgasm-phase problems; individuals report symptoms of continued pelvic vasocongestion and residual sexual tension. Complaints with resolution following unimpaired excitement and orgasm are infrequent; when they occur, they are typically prompted by such inhibitory, emotional factors as guilt, marital discord, and fear of pregnancy.

SEXUAL MORBIDITY FOR CANCER PATIENTS

Tables 42.1 and 42.2 provide summaries of the specific behavioral and sexual response cycle disruptions that have been studied. While many difficulties are pathognomonic for certain diseases or treatments, there are some generalities; for the most part, these characteristics differ from those of sexual dysfunction among healthy individuals.

First, the sexual problems of cancer patients typically have an acute onset, appearing immediately after treatment and recovery. Prior to their diagnosis, most cancer patients have had reasonably satisfactory sexual adjustment, and thus the suddenness and unexpectedness of the difficulties are distressing, particularly if the patients have not been forewarned about the likelihood or nature of the problems. Some people, for example

prostate or gynecologic cancer patients, may experience sexual difficulties as an early sign of their disease prior to diagnosis (Andersen et al. 1986). However, even these men and women may have had satisfactory sexual functioning prior to the appearance of the disease. In contrast, healthy individuals often come to sexual therapy bringing long-standing sexual complaints that may have worsened or become more distressing over time. They may also have a history of satisfactory sexual functioning that is only recently problematic in particular contexts (e.g., coital inorgasmia, or premature ejaculation after a lengthy period of sexual inactivity).

Second, the sexual difficulties are usually pervasive, with major alterations in the frequency or range of sexual behavior with or without the disruption of more than one phase of the sexual response cycle. The sexual difficulties are severe and, in combination with their pervasiveness, patients are often concerned about their ability to maintain any form of sexual activity. The sexual difficulties of healthy individuals are usually most severe for a particular phase of the sexual response cycle (for example, orgasmic disruption) with little or no impairment of the other phases (such as unimpaired arousal with orgasmic dysfunction).

Third, the sexual difficulties are often worsened by disease or treatment side effects that are, in themselves, difficult to treat. Fatigue or low energy, and pain are particularly troublesome. After the acute effects of treatment have subsided, many cancer patients report residual and activity-disrupting fatigue (Devlen et al. 1987), which may be a factor in much of the disrupted sexual desire. Pain, either coital (dyspareunia) or otherwise, is an obvious deterrent to desire for and arousal during sexual activity.

General characteristics of the response-cycle disruptions that occur in cancer patients differ from those of healthy individuals. Disruption of sexual desire may be the primary problem, but more typically the loss is

Table 42.1
SEXUAL MORBIDITY ESTIMATES FOR MEN

Site Subgroup	Method Rating[a]	General Disruption (%)	No Sexual Activity (%)	Desire (%)	Excitement (%)	Orgasm (%)
				Area of Sexual Functioning Difficulty		
Colon-Rectum	3			30-60	30-75	65-85
Bladder	4		30-50	30-70	90	
Prostate						
(A) Retropubic	3				83	78
(B) Perineal	3				88	100
A or B with hormonal						
therapy	3				100	100
Radiotherapy	3				37	
Interstitial therapy with						
lymphadenectomy	4				15-25	30
Testicular						
Seminoma:						
Orch + RT	4			12	15	10
Nonseminoma:						
Orch + RL +/− chemo	4			15-20	5-15	20-40
Orch + RL + RT						
+/− chemo	4			50	24	55
Hodgkin's disease	4	20-30				

[a] Methodology rating scale for prior emperical literature: 1 = Longitudinal trials; 2 = Longitudinal investigations +/− control(s); 3 = More than 3 retrospective studies; 4 = Only 1-2 retrospective studies.

Table 42.2
SEXUAL MORBIDITY ESTIMATES FOR WOMEN

Site Subgroup	Method Rating[a]	Area of Sexual Functioning Difficulty					
		General Disruption (%)	No Sexual Activity (%)	Desire (%)	Excitement (%)	Orgasm (%)	Dysparunia (%)
Breast							
Radical and modified radical	2	30-40					
Modified radical	1	15-25					
Lumpectomy + RT	1	5					
Colon-Rectum	4			28			21
Cervix	2	30-40	12	29	29	29	29
Pelvic exenteration	3		90	50	100	100	
Vulvar disease							
In situ	4		15	15	36	28	
Invasive	4		70-80		90-100	90-100	
Hodgkin's disease	4	20	32				

[a] Methodology rating scale for prior empirical literature: 1 = Longitudinal trials; 2 = Longitudinal investigations +/− control(s); 3 = More than 3 retrospective studies; 4 = Only 1-2 retrospective studies.

concomitant with other sexual problems (e.g., erectile failure, orgasmic dysfunction). However, many cancer patients maintain sexual desire despite significant disruption in their ability to perform, or they continue sexual relations even when there are significant deterrents (e.g., dyspareunia). This fact underscores the importance accorded to the maintenance of a sexual life by many individuals successfully treated for cancer.

For cancer patients, difficulty with sexual excitement, both in terms of bodily responses (erection, or lubrication) and subjective feelings of arousal, is a common problem. In turn, orgasmic dysfunctions are also frequent, either because of lowered excitement or specific impairment.

Orgasmic dysfunction is usually complete rather than situational, as is often the case for healthy individuals. For example, a woman who was regularly orgasmic during intercourse prior to treatment for cervical cancer discovers that she is nonorgasmic following treatment. Also, she reports not feeling sufficiently aroused to even get close to experiencing orgasm.

Problematic resolution among cancer patients is varied. Those who experience pain during intercourse often have residual discomfort during resolution. Those without pain *per se,* but who lack desire or have lowered excitement and/or orgasmic disruption, may feel residual sexual tension, disappointment, or the concern that sexual responsiveness is permanently changed. These feelings are all disruptive to the resolution phase.

Finally, unlike sexual dysfunctions for healthy individuals that may be readily and effectively treated, the sexual problems of cancer patients will be difficult to treat, and perhaps refractory. Prevention through provision of the least disruptive but comparably curative treatment is the single most important strategy in addressing cancer patients' sexual difficulties. Research has demonstrated that breast-saving treatments, as opposed to radical surgeries, result in significantly better psychological and sexual adjustment. Similar findings are emerging for treatment of *in situ* vulvar disease, prostate cancer, and disease at other sites. Interventions to reduce the incidence and severity of problems would

be most effective if delivered during the diagnostic, treatment, and early post-treatment periods. This would enable patients to anticipate possible sexual difficulties, and to be provided with specific suggestions to facilitate the resumption of sexual activity. Interventions would need to be tailored to disease and treatment effects. However, an accurate and detailed explanation of the anticipated sexual disruptions is necessary for all patients. The latter important step can be taken by the health care professional during treatment planning.

BREAST CANCER

Women with breast cancer have been the most well-studied cancer patient group. Small-sample retrospective studies to randomized clinical trials have provided sufficient data to clarify the sexual adjustment outcomes that might be expected for the woman awaiting treatment.

Most of the early retrospective and prospective investigations were conducted with women who received modified radical mastectomy or, in some cases, radical mastectomy. The strongest data comes from controlled longitudinal studies indicating that 30% to 40% of these women would report significant sexual problems (e.g., loss of desire, reduced frequency of intercourse, or reduction in excitement) from one to two years post-treatment, in comparison to 10% of women with benign disease receiving diagnostic biopsy (Maguire et al. 1978; Morris, Greer, and White 1977). Body image, while it is a difficult concept to measure, was also significantly disrupted.

The most recent studies have come from clinical trials in which psychological or behavioral endpoints have been examined along with disease endpoints in the comparison of modified radical mastectomy vs. lumpectomy and radiotherapy. With few exceptions (Fallowfield, Baum, and Maguire, 1986) studies have reported a clear benefit to the less disfiguring treatment (Beckmann et al. 1983; Dettaes and Welvaart 1985; Sarger and Reznikoff 1981; Steinberg, Juliano, and Wise, 1985) for women studied in the United States, England, the

Netherlands, and Denmark. For the lumpectomy patients, such differences include less alteration in body image and greater comfort with nudity and in discussing sexuality with one's partner; no or few changes in the frequency of intercourse; and a lower incidence of sexual dysfunction. Thus, there is apt to be less sexual disruption with lumpectomy and radiotherapy than with modified radical mastectomy.

COLON AND RECTAL CANCER

Several retrospective studies have been conducted on the effects of colon and rectal cancer on sexual function. For men, estimates of sexual dysfunction range from 30% to 60% for sexual desire, 30% to 75% for erectile difficulties, and from 65% to 85% for ejaculation disruption (Aso and Yasutami 1974; Bernstein and Bernstein 1966; Druss et al. 1969; Goligher 1951; Sutherland et al. 1952; Weinstein and Roberts 1977). Estimates for women come from a single investigation, which reported that 28% of the women had reduced desire and 21% had dyspareunia (Druss et al. 1969). These rates are approximately twice that found for individuals receiving related surgical treatments for benign conditions such as ulcerative colitis treated with ileostomy (Kuchenoff et al. 1981). When the tumor is low, patients are treated with resection and colostomy rather than anastomosis. Sexual functioning is significantly more impaired, particularly for males, who report less frequent intercourse, erectile difficulties, and dry ejaculation more readily than their nonstoma counterparts (Wirsching, Druner, and Herrmann 1975). Thus, predictors for postoperative sexual functioning are the patient's age, tumor site, and gender.

BLADDER CANCER

Superficial bladder tumors are treated by transurethral resection and fulguration and may result in minimal sexual disruption; however, documenting data are not available. Men and women undergoing repeated cystoscopies have been noted to report reduced sexual desire and may have pain with intercourse due to urethral irritation (Schover et al. 1984).

Treatment for invasive bladder cancer results in substantial sexual difficulties. As the average bladder cancer patient is in his or her late 60s, lower frequencies of sexual activity and frequent lapses in functioning (e.g., erectile failure) would be expected. Not surprisingly treatment for men, which includes cystectomy and concomitant prostatectomy, vesiculectomy, and urethrectomy, produces further decreases in desire, erectile failure, and orgasmic difficulty (e.g., retrograde ejaculation). Twenty-nine percent of the men studied by Bergman, Nilsson, and Peterson (1979) and 50% of the men studied by Schover, Evans, and von Echenbach (1986) reported stopping all sexual activity postoperatively. Of those attempting to remain sexually active, desire decreased for 30% to 70% of patients. Inadequately rigid, or only brief, erections occurred for the majority, with less than 10% having erections of sufficient rigidity or duration to permit intercourse. Orgasm, if experienced, is reported by approximately one-half of the patients as less intense and without ejaculate. Substantial changes occur for men following bladder cancer, and even the men most motivated to maintain sexual activity other than intercourse may have only limited success. The sexual outcomes for women with bladder cancer have not been studied; however, it would be expected that they would be similar to those of women receiving an anterior pelvic exenteration where the vagina is narrowed instead of removed. The few women who might remain sexually active would be expected to have impaired sexual excitement and orgasm during intercourse due to difficult penetration.

Finally, in an effort to prevent outcomes such as these, several steps have been taken, including nerve sparing cystoprostatectomy with urethrectomy, continent diversions, and penile prosthesis surgery. Schlegel and Walsh (1987) reported that 40% of men capable of erections prior to surgery retained their functioning with continent diversions to reduce urinary incontinence and obtain satisfactory voiding. Steven et al. (1986) modified the surgical procedure by leaving the apical prostatic capsule. This procedure facilitated the anastomosis of a segment of intestine to the urethra, making it possible to create an internal urinary diversion. Of the eight sexually active patients studied, erectile capacity was preserved in four with three of these able to continue intercourse. Other authors have described related surgical procedures with intra-abdominal reservoirs for urinary diversions which patients are able to empty with self-catheterization. Mansson et al. (1988) compared two patient groups, one receiving the standard conduit diversion and the other with reservoir. Both groups had substantial sexual difficulties; however, the reservoir group had better overall adjustment. The latter finding was attributed to the absence of odor, leakage, and embarrassment, common problems for patients with urinary conduits. Boyd and Schiff (1989) have reported 19 patients with diffuse transitional cell carcinoma who had undergone cystoprostatectomy with urethrectomy and been implanted with inflatable penile prostheses. Sexual functioning was satisfactory with acceptable function and appearance for those for whom the glandular urethra could remain intact. When total urethrectomy was necessary, the glans penis would collapse, with attendant difficulties with orgasm and appearance.

MALE GENITAL CANCER

Men with prostate cancer have been the most widely studied. Cancer treatment produces substantial sexual change, but even the diagnostic biopsy may result in sexual difficulties. For example, approximately 24% of open perineal biopsy (Dahlen and Goodwin 1957; Finkle and Moyers 1960) and 32% of transurethral resection (Finkle and Prian 1966; Gold and Hotchkiss 1969;

Holtgrewer and Volk 1964; Madorsky et al. 1976) patients report erectile failure. In addition, approximately 57% of the patients report a complete loss, or at least a reduced amount, of seminal fluid ejaculated.

Radical surgical prostatectomy for cancer is performed by the perineal, retropubic, or transpubic routes. Surveys of patients with Dukes' stages A, B, or C disease undergoing these approaches have reported diminished or complete erectile failure for 90% of those surveyed (Andersen 1985). The estimated incidence of ejaculation difficulties is 78% of the retropubic prostatectomy patients (Kopecky, Laskowski, and Scott, 1970), and 100% of the perineal prostatectomy patients (Ormond 1947). (These rates are three to four times higher than those for patients treated with less extensive surgery for benign prostate disease.) If hormone therapy and/or orchiectomy is also included, virtually all of the patients experience both erectile failure and ejaculation difficulty (Scott and Boyd 1969; Veenema, Gursel, and Lattimer 1981).

It is thus not surprising that some patients with local disease opt for supervoltage irradiation, which is also used for patients with regional disease. When patients with either limited or extracapsular extension have been treated with definitive courses, approximately 37% experience significant erectile difficulties (Loh, Brown, and Beiler 1971; Mollenkamp, Cooper, and Kagen 1975; Ray, Cassady, and Bagshaw 1973; Rhamy, Wilson, and Caldwell 1972). Again the incidence of sexual difficulties is high, but it is less than one-half the estimates reported for radical surgery.

Another treatment considered for localized prostatic cancer has been interstitial implantation (usually with a retropubic approach) of the prostate with iodine 125 (^{125}I) or gold (^{198}Au) combined with pelvic lymphadenectomy. The lowest estimates of sexual difficulties have been found with these treatments, with erectile difficulties in the range of 15% to 25% and retrograde ejaculation in the range of 30% (Carlton et al. 1976; Fowler et al. 1979; Herr 1979).

Patients with metastatic disease or extensive regional spread are treated with regimens such as bilateral orchiectomy, estrogen administration, or both. The majority of patients who receive estrogen develop gynecomastia (the excessive development of male mammary glands), a troubling side effect for many men. Ellis and Greyheck (1963) estimated that erectile difficulties occur for 47% of the patients who receive orchiectomy alone, 22% for estrogen alone, and 73% for malaise, weight loss, anemia, and pain that patients with metastatic cancer experience.

Testicular cancer accounts for only 1% of cancer in males, but it is the most common site for disease among those aged 15 to 35 years. The surge of studies of the sexual and fertility outcomes for these men is perhaps due to two reasons. First, dramatic improvements in cure rates, particularly for disseminated tumors, have recently been achieved with chemotherapy. Second, the disease strikes men in the prime of their fatherhood and sexual-functioning years, and as men survive, fertility and sexuality will be increasingly important concerns.

Testicular cancer is either classified as pure seminoma (accounting for roughly 40% of the cases) or nonseminoma. Treatment for the two differs markedly and results in differential sexual outcomes. Pure seminoma is radiosensitive, with the usual treatment consisting of radical orchiectomy of the testicle (occurrence of disease in both testicles is rare), followed by retroperitoneal and homolateral iliac node irradiation to the level of the diaphragm. Chemotherapy is used for cases that fail to respond. Nonseminomas are treated with radical orchiectomy followed by a difficult chemotherapy regimen, usually consisting of cisplatin, vinblastine, bleomycin, and actinomycin D. Whether a retroperitoneal lymphadenectomy (RL) is done between orchiectomy and chemotherapy is a point of some controversy. As the data indicate that RL has a significant negative impact on sexual functioning and fertility (due to permanent difficulty with ejaculation), clarification of the medical indications for RL would be important. Men who are refractory to either course, or who relapse, can be treated with salvage chemotherapy. Because of their importance in predicting outcome, only studies providing histopathology and treatment information will be reviewed.

Schover, Gonzales, and von Eschenbach (1986) provided a retrospective report on the sexual outcomes for 84 men who received orchiectomy and radiotherapy for seminoma. In terms of sexual behavior, 19% of the sample reported none or only low rates of sexual activity (i.e., one episode of sexual activity less than once per month). In terms of disruption of the sexual response cycle, 12% of the sample reported low desire, 15% reported erectile dysfunction, and 10% reported difficulty with orgasm (particularly lowered intensity). As the mean age of this sample was 45 years, such estimates would not be unexpected. However, 49% of the sample also reported reduced semen volume, which has been hypothesized to occur from radiation scatter to the prostate and seminal vesicles. Correlational analyses suggested that higher radiation dosages to the para-aortic field was predictive of greater erectile and orgasmic difficulties.

Three retrospective studies have provided data for nonseminoma patients (Bracken and Johnson 1976; Nijman et al. 1987; Schover and von Eschenbach 1985). In these studies, all patients received orchiectomy and RL, with or without other therapies. Reduced ejaculate volume (none in most cases) occurred for 90% to 100% of the men across studies and therapies. These data in combination with those for seminoma patients point to the instrumental role of RL in reducing or eliminating semen outflow. Sexual outcomes for patients receiving orchiectomy and RL, with or without chemotherapy, appear similar. An estimated 15% to 20% of such patients report lowered desire, 5% to 15% report erectile difficulties, and 20% to 40% report orgasmic disruption. In contrast, if orchiectomy, RL, and radiotherapy are given, with or without chemotherapy, sexual outcomes are worsened. More than 50% of the patients report lowered desire, 24% report erectile difficulties, and 55% report difficulties with orgasm. In summary, the addition of RL adds a significant decrement to the sexual and fertility outcomes for nonseminoma patients, though its effect on semen outflow and radiotherapy appears to significantly worsen sexual-response-cycle functioning as well.

Cancer of the penis usually results in extreme sexual difficulties. When the disease is confined to the organ, total penectomy obviously leaves patients significantly impaired; however, stimulation of the remaining genital tissue, including the mons pubis, the perineum, and the scrotum, can produce orgasm for some (Witkin and Kaplan 1989). Ejaculation can occur through the perineal urethrostomy, with the accompanying sensations of the bulbocavernosus and ischiocavernosus musculature. Patients with partial excisions can remain capable of erection, orgasm, and ejaculation (Bracken and Johnson 1976).

FEMALE GENITAL CANCER

The primary sites for disease are the cervix, endometrium, ovary, vulva, and vagina. Most of the data comes from studies of cervical-cancer patients, with a major focus on treatment alternatives of radical hysterectomy, radiotherapy, or combination therapy for those with early stage disease. The widespread belief that radiotherapy is the most sexually disruptive comes from findings of poorly controlled retrospective studies. In fact, Vincent (1975) randomized women with cervical cancer to receive either radiotherapy or radical hysterectomy, and found comparable rates of sexual difficulties (approximately 30%) for each group. Andersen, Anderson, and deProsse (1989a) confirmed these data and also documented the patterns of sexual functioning for each group. Women treated surgically experience diminished excitement and, possibly, orgasmic disruption; women treated with radiotherapy experience diminished excitement and significant dyspareunia, a further deterrent to arousal. Women treated with combination therapy resemble radiotherapy patients in their pattern of difficulty. The significant change in sexual behavior that occurs for all women is a reduction in the frequency of intercourse; however, this change is likely due to disease and treatment to the pelvis, rather than to cancer *per se*. All groups experience transitory loss of sexual desire in the immediate (i.e., 0 to 6 months) post-treatment period, although later during the post-treatment year desire returns to pretreatment levels. Despite these changes, significant marital distress does not occur and relationships remain intact.

Pelvic exenteration for recurrent or extensive cervical disease is a radical surgery that produces permanent and pervasive sexual changes. The surgery involves the removal of the uterus, tubes, and ovaries; the urinary bladder and/or the rectum, depending on tumor location and pattern of spread; and the vagina. Clinical reports are uniform in their report of the end of all sexual activity for 80% to 90% of women surveyed (Andersen and Hacker 1983b; Brown et al. 1972; Dempsey, Buchsbaum, and Morrison 1975; Knorr 1967; Vera 1981). Various surgical procedures have been used for vaginal reconstruction. Women without such surgery obviously cannot resume intercourse due to vaginal closure, and when intercourse becomes difficult or impossible for couples, all sexual activity (the one exception being kissing) ceases. Vaginal reconstruction is not a panacea and should never be portrayed as such to the woman considering the surgery. Surgical technique and adequate healing are important; for some women the cavity may be too large, too small, or may result in a constant, annoying discharge. Still other women might not resume intercourse following reconstruction because of realistic fears of pain or bleeding. Pelvic exenteration, regardless of whether vaginal reconstruction is included, is the most sexually disfiguring, dysfunction-producing, and debilitating cancer surgery a woman can undergo.

Treatments for *in situ* vulvar disease include wide local excision of the lesion, skinning procedures, CO_2 laser, combination therapy, and, in rare cases, total (simple) vulvectomy. A large-sample retrospective study of over 100 women treated for *in situ* disease revealed few sexual differences between these treatment groups (Andersen et al. 1988). Sexual outcome was directly correlated with the magnitude of sexual disruption, such that women with greater genital change experienced the greatest sexual disruption.

Treatment for invasive vulvar disease produces even greater genital disfigurement, including surgical removal of all labial tissue and usually the clitoris (radical vulvectomy). While the capacity for intercourse remains, substantial bodily disfigurement and reductions in pelvic and genital sensitivity are incurred. Like pelvic exenteration patients, it is not surprising that 70% to 80% of women report the end of all sexual activity (Andersen and Hacker 1983a; Moth et al. 1983; Tamburini et al. 1986).

The remaining sites for gynecologic disease — the endometrium, ovary, and vagina — have not been studied, but there are some generalities regarding sexual outcomes that can be stated. For women with localized endometrial or ovarian disease, sexual responses would be similar to women receiving comparable treatments for cervical cancer. Chemotherapy is often included for women with regional or disseminated disease, and with it the interests in and ability to engage in sexual activity decline. Although sexuality probably remains important to individuals and couples, little is known about their sexual circumstances. Primary therapy for vaginal cancer is usually pelvic and vaginal radiotherapy. Sexual outcomes would be similar to those for the cervical-cancer patient treated with radiotherapy, and arousal difficulties and severe dyspareunia would be anticipated. For women with a central vaginal recurrence, pelvic exenteration and its resultant outcomes might be anticipated.

HODGKIN'S DISEASE

In the past 35 years, the survival rate of patients with this disease has increased dramatically. Five-year average survival rates have risen from approximately 13% to 19%, to 80% to 90%. The typical patient is a young adult male; 50% of the cases occur in people between the ages of 20 and 40 years. Survival rates are the highest in this age range and younger (69% to 76%, for men) and significantly poorer for those over 45 years (10% to 41%, for men) at diagnosis (Axtell, Asire, and Myers 1976). The significant improvements in outcome have resulted from the use of complex chemotherapeutic modalities and extended field radiation.

Irradiation is the primary modality for treating the majority of localized stages. Chemotherapy with or without consolidation irradiation for disseminated disease can take many forms, but the MOPP regimen (nitrogen mustard, vincristine [Oncovin], procarbazine, and prednisone) has been an important standard. Fertility and sexual morbidity with the therapy is high, as is the risk of second tumors. As long-term follow-up data on the new survivors accumulate, other therapies with lesser morbidity may possibly be chosen.

General survey (Fobair et al. 1986) and interview and questionnaire assessments (Cella and Tross 1986) indicate that decreased energy for and interest in sexual activity, with resultant lowered activity levels, may be problems for at least 20% of men and women. Similar rates (32%) for loss of desire have also been reported for combined samples of Hodgkin's disease and non-Hodgkin's lymphoma patients (Devlen et al. 1987). Specific sexual dysfunctions (e.g., erectile failure) have not been reported, but with treatment-induced ovarian failure, reports of dyspareunia would not be unexpected. Correlates of sexual disruption include continued low energy and depression. There is also data to suggest that Hodgkin's disease patients may be at greater risk for marital disruption, possibly due to the extended strain on families during the lengthy treatment period and the difficulties with impaired fertility (Fobair et al. 1986).

Data suggest that the current treatment regimens result in permanent infertility for most patients. For men, the effects of combination chemotherapy with MOPP or MVPP for patients completing hormonal studies from 12 months to 12 years after the completion of therapy have found azoospermia and testicular biopsies indicating complete loss of the germinal epithelium, and less than 10% of such patients achieve sperm densities above minimal range (Waxman et al. 1987; Whitehead et al. 1982). However, approximately one-third of patients with advanced Hodgkin's disease have been found to manifest gonadal dysfunction prior to therapy (Chapman, Sutcliffe, and Malpas 1981). For women, parallel decrements have been reported. With radiation only, a dose-response relationship appears to interact with age, such that younger women generally require a higher dose to produce permanent amenorrhea. In a study of 41 women with advanced Hodgkin's disease receiving MVPP (21 of whom also received MVPP as a maintenance therapy or had other agents because of relapse), Chapman et al. (Chapman, Sutcliffe, and Malpas 1979; Chapman, Sutcliffe, and Malpas 1981) reported that only 17% of the women had functioning ovaries at a mean of three years after therapy. Also, ovarian failure (as reflected by amenorrhea) occurred after fewer cycles of therapy in older women. Hodgkin's disease *per se* does not appear to impair ovarian functioning, as 27% of the women in the latter study conceived in the presence of active disease. In contrast to these data, a report on a trial of radiation therapy and TVVPP therapy (thiotepa, vinblastine, vincristine, procarbazine, and prednisone) for 34 women that followed the woman for a mean of seven years has reported that 100% of the women less than 35 years at treatment and 50% of the women over 35 years continued to menstruate, with a third of the sample subsequently becoming pregnant (Lacker and Toner 1986). It does not appear that efforts to "down regulate" the gonads are effective at preventing impaired fertility in both men and women (Waxman et al. 1987).

BRIEF ASSESSMENT OF SEXUAL FUNCTIONING

For cancer patients, the diagnostic period is a crisis and is the most stressful period they will endure (Andersen, Anderson, and deProsse, 1989b). Despite this, patients must process complex information and instructions as they undergo diagnostic studies and learn of treatment possibilities. Survival is a central concern. As this issue is clarified, concerns regarding impending treatments and their short- and long-term effects become paramount. This is the context in which assessment of the patient's previous sexual functioning and explanation of the sexual morbidity from the disease and treatment(s) becomes important. Assessment of a patient's predisease sexual functioning will: (1) enable the health care provider to individualize the explanation of the anticipated sexual difficulties for each patient (e.g., disruption in fertility may be important to a heterosexual male but not to a homosexual male); (2) provide important baseline information for understanding any post-treatment sexual problems; and (3) establish a context and precedent for patients to voice their sexual concerns. Table 42.3 provides a brief assessment model designed to assess both important sexual behaviors (e.g., intercourse) and the sexual response cycle. The acronym ALARM used in this table refers to the assessment of the following: sexual activities, libido/desire, arousal and orgasm, resolution, and any medical history relevant to sexual functioning. Although many important areas such as marital adjustment are omitted, the model covers the central areas. Sample questions are provided for illustration. The examples used are for heterosexual individuals; some modification would be necessary for homosexual individuals.

Table 42.3
ALARM MODEL FOR THE ASSESSMENT OF SEXUAL FUNCTIONING AREA AND SAMPLE QUESTIONS

(A)	Activity: Frequency of current sexual activities (e.g., intercourse, kissing, masturbation).

Example:
1. Prior to the appearance of any signs/symptoms of your illness, how frequently were you engaging in intercourse (specific weekly or monthly estimate)?
2. On occasions other than when having intercourse (or an equivalent intimate activity), do you share other forms of physical affection with your partner, such as kissing and/or hugging on a daily basis?
3. In the recent past (e.g., last 6 months) have you masturbated? If so, estimate how often this has occurred (specific weekly or monthly estimate).

(L)	Libido/Desire: Desire for sexual activity and interest in initiating or responding to partner's initiations for sexual activity.

Example:
1. Prior to the appearance of your illness, would you have described yourself as generally interested in having sex?
2. Considering your current regular sexual relationship, who usually initiates sexual activity?
3. You indicated that your current frequency for intercourse is x times per week/month. Would you personally prefer to have intercourse more often, less often, or at the current frequency?

(A)	Arousal and Orgasm: Occurrence of erection/lubrication and ejaculation/vaginal contractions, accompanied by feelings of sexual excitement.

Example (for men):
1. When you are interested in having sexual activity, with your partner or alone, do you have any difficulty in achieving an erection? Do you feel emotionally aroused?
2. If there is erectile difficulty: When did this problem start, how often does it occur, are there particular circumstances for its occurrence (e.g., with partner only), and what do you understand to be the cause for the difficulty?
3. During sexual activity, either alone or with a partner, do you have any difficulty with ejaculation, such as coming "too soon" or only after an extended period of time?
4. If premature/delayed ejaculation is suggested: While it is difficult to estimate precisely, how long would you estimate that it takes on the average to ejaculate after intensive stimulation begins?

Example (for women):
1. When you are interested in engaging in sexual activity do you notice that your genitals become moist?
2. If postmenopausal: Has there been any change in vaginal lubrication during sexual activity since the menopause? Are you currently taking hormonal replacement therapy?
3. If there is arousal deficit: Do you experience any pain with intercourse? How long have you had problems with becoming aroused during sexual activity, and are there particular circumstances during which you have felt more arousal than others?
4. During sexual activity, either alone or with a partner, can you experience a climax or orgasm?
5. If orgasm does not occur: Are you bothered at all by the absence of orgasm?

(R)	Resolution: Feelings of release of tension following sexual activity and satisfaction with current sexual life.

Example:
1. Following intercourse or masturbation do you feel that there has been a release of sexual tension?
2. On a scale from 1 (indicating that it could not be worse) to 10 (indicating that it could not be better) how would you rate your current sexual life?
3. Do you have any feelings of discomfort or pain immediately after sexual activity?
4. If there is resolution difficulty: Describe the problems you are having after sexual activity, how long they have occurred, and your understanding of their cause(s).

(M)	Medical history relevant to sexuality: Current age and medical history (e.g., have you had diabetes, hypertension?), psychiatric history (e.g., have you had emotional difficulties in the past for which you have sought treatment?), and substance use history (e.g., how much alcohol [or drugs] do you consume on weekly basis?), what do you drink (e.g., beer, wine, alcohol?) which may have caused acute or chronic disruption of sexual activity or responses.

Two important aspects of conducting a brief assessment like the one suggested here are to understand sexual behavior and sexual functioning in healthy individuals and to have the ability to discuss sexual functioning in a frank, open, and nonevaluative manner. To the extent that the health care provider is informed, comfortable, and interested in addressing these patient concerns, cancer patients will begin to feel more hopeful and confident in coping with the sexual difficulties they may face.

REFERENCES

American Cancer Society. 1987. Workshop on psychosexual and reproductive issues of cancer patients, January 1967. San Antonio, Texas.

American Psychiatric Association. 1980. *DSM-III: Diagnostic and statistical manual of mental disorders.* 3rd ed. Washington, D.C.

Andersen, B.L. 1985. Sexual functioning morbidity among cancer survivors: present status and future research directions. *Cancer* 55:1835-42.

Andersen, B.L.; Anderson, B.; and deProsse, C. 1989a. Controlled prospective longitudinal study of women with cancer. I: Sexual functioning outcomes. *J. Consult. Clin. Psychol.* 57:683-91.

Andersen, B.L.; Anderson, B.; and deProsse, C. 1989b. Controlled prospective longitudinal study of women with cancer. II: psychological outcomes. *J. Consult. Clin. Psychology* 57:692-97.

Andersen, B.L., and Broffitt, B. 1988. Is there a reliable and valid self report measure of sexual behavior? *Arch. Sex. Behav.* 17:509-25.

Andersen, B.L., and Hacker, N.F. 1983a. Psychosexual adjustment after vulvar surgery. *Obstet. Gynecol.* 62:457-62.

Andersen, B.L., and Hacker, N.F. 1983b. Psychosexual adjustment following pelvic exenteration. *Obstet. Gynecol.* 61:331-38.

Andersen, B.L.; Lachenbruch, P.A.; and Anderson, B. et al. 1986. Sexual dysfunction and signs of gynecologic cancer. *Cancer.* 57:1880-86.

Andersen, B.L.; Turnquist, D.; and LaPolla, J.P. et al. 1988. Sexual functioning after treatment of *in situ* vulvar cancer: preliminary report. *Obstet. Gynecol.* 71:15-19.

Aso, R., and Yasutami, M. 1974. Urinary and sexual disturbances following radical surgery for rectal cancer, and pudendal nerve block as a countermeasure for urinary disturbance. *Am. J. Proctol.* 6:60-70.

Axtell, L.M.; Asire, A.J.; and Myers, M. H. eds. 1976. *Cancer patient survival, Rep. No. 5.* Bethesda, Md: National Cancer Institute.

Beckmann, J.; Johansen, L; and Richardt, C. et al. 1983. Psychological reactions in younger women operated on for breast cancer. *Danish Med. Bull.* 30:10-13.

Bergman, B; Nilsson, S; and Petersen, I. 1979. The effect on erection and orgasm of cystectomy, prostatectomy and vesiculectomy for cancer of the bladder: a clinical and electromyographic study. *Br. J. Urol.* 51:114-20.

Bernstein, W.C., and Bernstein, E.F. 1966. Sexual dysfunction following radical surgery for cancer of the rectum. *Dis. Colon Rectum* 9:328-32.

Boyd, S.D., and Schiff, W.M. 1989. Inflatable penile prostheses in patients undergoing cystoprostatectomy with urethrectomy. *J. Urol.* 141:60-62.

Bracken, R.B., and Johnson, D.E. 1976. Sexual function and fecundity after treatment for testicular tumors. *Urology* 7:35-38.

Brown, R.S.; Haddox, V.; and Posada, A. et al. 1972. Social and psychological adjustment following pelvic exenteration. *Am. J. Obstet. Gynecol.* 114:162-71.

Carlton, C.E.; Hudgins, P.T.; and Guerriero, W.G. et al. 1976. Radiotherapy in the management of stage C carcinoma of the prostate. *J. Urol.* 116:206-10.

Cella, D.F., and Tross, S. 1986. Psychological adjustment to survival from Hodgkin's disease. *J. Consult. Clin. Psychol.* 54:616-22.

Chapman, R.M.; Sutcliffe, S.B.; and Malpas, J.S. 1979a. Cytotoxic-induced ovarian failure in women with Hodgkin's disease. I: hormone function. *JAMA* 242:1877-81.

Chapman, R.M.; Sutcliffe, S.B.; and Malpas, J.S. 1979b. Cytotoxic-induced ovarian failure in Hodgkin's disease. II: effects on sexual function. *JAMA* 242:1882-99.

Chapman, R.M.; Sutcliffe, S.B.; and Malpas, J.S. 1981. Male gonadal dysfunction in Hodgkin's disease: a prospective study. *JAMA* 245:1323-28.

Dahlen, C.P., and Goodwin, W.E. 1957. Sexual potency after perineal biopsy. *J. Urol.* 77:660-69.

deHaes, J.C.J.M., and Welvaart, K. 1985. Quality of life and breast cancer surgery. *J. Surg. Oncol.* 18:123-25.

Dempsey, G.M.; Buchsbaum, H.J.; and Morrison, J. 1975. Psychosocial adjustment to pelvic exenteration. *Gynecol. Oncol.* 3:325-34.

Devlen, J.; Maguire, P.; and Phillips, P. et al. 1987. Psychological problems associated with diagnosis and treatment of lymphomas. II: prospective study. *Br. Med. J.* 295:955-57.

Druss, R.G.; O'Connor, J.F.; and Prudden, J.F. et al. 1969. Psychologic response to edectomy II. *Arch. Gen. Psychiatry* 20:419-27.

Ellis, W.J., and Grayheck, J.T. 1963. Sexual function in aging males after orchiectomy and estrogen therapy. *J. Urol.* 89:895-99.

Fallowfield, L.J.; Baum, M.; and Maguire, P. 1986. Effects of breast conservation on psychological morbidity associated with diagnosis and treatment of early breast cancer. *Br. Med. J.* 293:1331-34.

Finkle, A.L., and Moyers, T.G. 1960. Sexual potency in aging males. V: coital ability following open perineal prostatic biopsy. *J. Urol.* 84:649-53.

Finkle, A.L., and Prian, D. 1966. Sexual potency in elderly men before and after prostatectomy. *JAMA* 196:394.

Fobair, P.; Hoppe, R.T.; and Bloom, J. et al. 1986. Psychosocial problems among survivors of Hodgkin's disease. *J. Clin. Oncol.* 4:805-14.

Fowler, J.E.; Barzell, W.; and Hilaris, B.S. et al. 1979. Complications of 125 iodine implantation and pelvic lymphadenectomy in the treatment of prostatic cancer. *J. Urol.* 121:447-51.

Gold, F.M., and Hotchkiss, R.S. 1969. Sexual potency following simple prostatectomy. *N.Y. State J. Med.* 1:2987-89.

Goligher, J.C. 1951. Sexual function after excision of the rectum. *Proc. Royal Soc. Med.* 44:824-27.

Herr, H.W. 1979. Preservation of sexual potency in prostatic cancer patients after pelvic lymphadenectomy and retropubic ^{125}I implantation. *J. Urol.* 121:621-23.

Holtgrewer, H.L., and Volk, W.L. 1964. Late results of transurethral prostatectomy. *J. Urol.* 91:51-55.

Kaplan, H.S. 1979. *Disorders of sexual desire.* New York: Brunner/Mazel.

Kinsey, A.C.; Pomroy, W.C.; and Martin, C.E. 1948. *Sexual behavior in the human male.* Philadelphia: W. B. Saunders Co.

Knorr, N.J. 1967. A depressive syndrome following pelvic exenteration and ileostomy. *Arch. Surg.* 94:258-60.

Kopecky, A.A.; Laskowski, T.Z.; and Scott, R. 1970. Radical retropubic prostatectomy in the treatment of prostatic carcinoma. *J. Urol.* 103:641-44.

Kuchenhoff, J.; Wirsching, M.; and Druner H.V. et al. 1981. Coping with a stoma: a comparative study of patients with rectal carcinoma or inflammatory bowel diseases. *Psychother. Psychosom.* 36:98-104.

Lacher, M.J., and Toner, K. 1986. Pregnancies and menstrual function before and after combined radiation (RT) and chemotherapy (TVPP) for Hodgkin's disease. *Cancer Investig.* 4:93-100.

Leiblum, S.R., and Rosen, R.C. eds. 1988. *Sexual desire disorders.* New York: Guilford Press.

Loh, E.S.; Brown, H.E.; and Beiler, D.D. 1971. Radiotherapy of carcinoma of the prostate: preliminary report. *J. Urol.* 106:906-909.

Madorsky, M.L.; Ashamalla, M.G.; and Schussler, I. et al. 1976. Post-prostatectomy impotence. *J. Urol.* 1154:401-403.

Maguire, G.P.; Lee, E.G.; and Bevington, D.J. et al. 1978. Psychiatric problems in the first year after mastectomy. *Br. Med. J.* 1:963-65.

Mansson, A.; Johnson, G.; and Mansson, W. 1988. Quality of life after cystectomy: comparison between patients with conduit and those with caeca reservoir diversion. *Br. J. Urol.* 62:240-45.

Masters, W.H., and Johnson, V.E. 1966. *Human sexual response.* Boston: Little, Brown.

Mollenkamp, J.S.; Cooper, J.F.; and Kagen, A.R. 1975. Clinical experience with supervoltage radiotherapy in carcinoma of the prostate: a preliminary report. *J. Urol.* 113:374-77.

Morris, T.; Greer, H.S.; and White P. 1977. Psychological and social adjustment to mastectomy: a two-year follow-up study. *Cancer* 40:2381-87.

Moth, I.; Andreason, B.; and Jensen, S.B. et al. 1983. Sexual function and somatopsychic reactions after vulvectomy. *Danish Med. Bull.* 30:27-30.

National Institutes of Health. 1987. International Conference on Reproduction and Human Cancer. Bethesda, Md.

Nijman, J.M.; Koops, H.S.; and Oldhoff, J. et al. 1987. Sexual function after bilateral retroperitoneal lymph node dissection for nonseminomatous testicular cancer. *Arch. Androl.* 18:255-67.

Ormond, J.K. 1947. Radical perineal prostatectomy for carcinoma. *J. Urol.* 58:61-67.

Ray, G.R.; Cassady, J.R.; and Bagshaw, M.A. 1973. Definitive radiation therapy of carcinoma of the prostate. *Radiology* 106:407-18.

Rhamy, R.K.; Wilson, S.K.; and Caldwell, W.L. 1972. Biopsy-proved tumor following definitive irradiation for resectable carcinoma of the prostate. *J. Urol.* 107:627-30.

Sanger, C.K., and Reznikoff, M. 1981. A comparison of the psychological effects of breast-saving procedures with the modified radical mastectomy. *Cancer* 48:2341-46.

Schover, L.R.; Gonzales, M.; and von Eschenbach, A.C. 1986. Sexual and marital relationships. *Urology* 17:117-23.

Schover, L.R.; Evans, R.; and von Eschenbach, A.C. 1986. Sexual rehabilitation and male radical cystectomy. *J. Urol.* 136:1015-17.

Schover, L.R., and von Eschenbach, A.C. 1985. Sexual and marital relationships after treatment for nonseminomatous testicular cancer. *Urology* 25:251-55.

Schover, L.R.; von Eschenbach, A.C.; and Smith, D.B. et al. 1984. Sexual rehabilitation of urologic cancer patients: a practical approach. *CA* 34:3-11.

Scott, W.W., and Boyd, H.L. 1969. Combined hormonal control therapy and radical prostatectomy in the treatment of selected cases of advanced carcinoma of the prostate: a retrospective study based upon 25 years of experience. *J. Urol.* 101:86-92.

Steinberg, M.D.; Juliano, M.A.; and Wise, L. 1985. Psychological outcome of lumpectomy versus mastectomy in the treatment of breast cancer. *Am. J. Psychiatry* 142:34-39.

Steven, K.; Klarskov, P.; and Jakobsen, H. et al. 1986. Transpubic cystectomy and ileocecal bladder replacement after preoperative radiotherapy for bladder cancer. *J. Urol.* 135:470-75.

Sutherland, A.M.; Orbach, C.F.; and Dyk, R.B. et al. 1952. The psychological impact of cancer and cancer surgery. I: adaptation to the dry colostomy. *Cancer* 5:857-72.

Tamburini, M.; Filiberti, A.; and Ventafridda, V. et al. 1986. Quality of life and psychological state after radical vulvectomy. *J. Psychosom. Obstet. Gynecol.* 5:263-69.

Veenema, R.J.; Gursel, E.O.; and Lattimer, J.K. 1977. Radical retropubic prostatectomy for cancer: a 20-year experience. *J. Urol.* 117:330-31.

Vera, M.I. 1981. Quality of life following pelvic exenteration. *Gynecol. Oncol.* 12:355-66.

Vincent, C.E.; Vincent, B.; and Greiss, F.C. et al. 1975. Some marital-sexual concomitants of carcinoma of the cervix. *South. Med. J.* 68:551-58.

Waxman, J.H.; Ahmen, R.; and Smith, D. et al. 1987. Failure to preserve fertility in patients with Hodgkin's disease. *Cancer Chemother. Pharmacol.* 19:159-62.

Weinstein, M., and Roberts, M. 1977. Sexual potency following surgery for rectal carcinoma. *Ann. Surg.* 185:195-300.

Whitehead, E.; Shaiet, S.M.; and Blackledge, G. et al. 1982. The effects of Hodgkin's disease and combination chemotherapy on gonadal function in the adult male. *Cancer* 49:418-22.

Witkin, M.H., and Kaplan, H.S. 1982. Sex therapy and penectomy. *J. Sex. Marital Ther.* 8:209-21.

Wirsching, M.; Druner, H.U.; and Herrmann, G. 1975. Results of psychosocial adjustment to long-term colostectomy. *Psychother. Psychosom.* 26:245-57.

Chapter 43

DENTAL ONCOLOGY

Norman G. Schaaf, D.D.S.
William Carl, D.D.S.

Norman G. Schaaf, D.D.S.
Chief of Dentistry and Maxillofacial Prosthetics
Department of Dentistry and Maxillofacial Prosthetics
Roswell Park Memorial Institute
Buffalo, New York

William Carl, D.D.S.
Senior Cancer Dental Surgeon
Department of Dentistry and Maxillofacial Prosthetics
Roswell Park Memorial Institute
Buffalo, New York

INTRODUCTION

The role of dentistry in the care of the cancer patient falls into two areas: (1) oral care of patients as it relates to secondary effects of cancer treatment, such as radiation therapy for head and neck lesions and/or chemotherapy for cancers distant from the oral cavity such as leukemias, lymphomas, or sarcomas; and (2) prosthetic reconstruction of the head and neck surgical patient.

PART I: ORAL MANIFESTATIONS AND MANAGEMENT OF LOCAL RADIATION THERAPY AND SYSTEMIC CHEMOTHERAPY

The treatment of head and neck cancers by radiation therapy and the treatment of cancer in sites distant from the oral cavity by systemic chemotherapy precipitate oral side effects; if uncontrolled, they may lead to serious local and systemic consequences.

This section covers the oral complications of cancer therapy and the appropriate oral control measures.

ORAL MANIFESTATIONS AND MANAGEMENT OF RADIATION THERAPY FOR CANCER IN THE HEAD AND NECK AREA

Of the approximately 30,500 new patients with oral cancer each year in the United States, more than 9,000 receive head and neck irradiation either as primary treatment or as an adjunct to surgery (American Cancer Society 1990; Engelmeier and King 1983). Because of the success achieved by combined therapy, more head and neck cancer patients survive for longer periods of time, and the number of irradiated patients who need specific oral care constantly increases. The primary goal of oral care of the irradiated head and neck cancer patient is modification of the oral environmental changes that therapy precipitated.

LOCAL SIDE EFFECTS OF RADIATION THERAPY

The therapeutic dose of radiation therapy for most intraoral and other head and neck tumors is 50 Gy to 70 Gy to the lesion and surrounding area. The lymph nodes of the neck may receive an additional 40 Gy to 50 Gy. The therapy is usually administered in increments of 2 Gy per day until the designated accumulative dose has been attained (Chen 1986).

MUCOSITIS

Mucositis, a troublesome soft-tissue reaction, sometimes develops during radiation therapy. Its severity is related to the quality of radiation, the total dosage, and the length of treatment. After approximately 20 Gy have been administered, the mucosa in the field of radiation takes on a whitish appearance. Continuing treatment renders the mucosa thin and friable, and it also appears reddish in color. Eventually a pseudomembrane forms; when the membrane peels off, a bleeding, ulcerated surface appears. Mucositis may be focal at first, but as treatment reaches the 30 Gy to 40 Gy level, the condition may involve the entire mucosa (Carl 1986; Sapp 1972; Beumer, Curtis, and Harrison 1979).

The soft palate, the floor of the mouth, and the lateral borders and the ventral surface of the tongue are particularly sensitive to irradiation (fig. 43.1). Sometimes the mucositis is so severe that treatment must be interrupted. The patient may be unable to take food or even liquids by mouth, and may require the insertion of a nasogastric feeding tube until the acute reactions

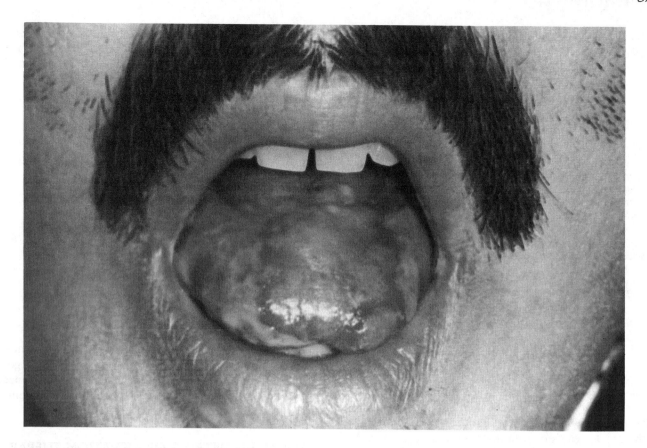

Fig. 43.1. Severe generalized muscositis in a patient who has received 50 Gy for squamous cell carcinoma of the floor of the mouth. Note the desquamation of the lateral borders of the tongue.

subside. Mucositis usually persists for two to three weeks after treatment.

SALIVARY CHANGES

Within the first two weeks of radiation therapy, patients begin to notice changes in the quantity and the quality of saliva. The saliva becomes ropy, and patients encounter difficulties in managing it (Carl 1986). The sensitivity of the various salivary glands located in different areas of the mouth is related to this initial shift in saliva quality. For example, the change initially affects the parotid glands more than the mucous glands (Awward and Habib 1962; Ben-Aryeh et al. 1975). The net result is an abundance of undiluted mucus.

The severity of xerostomia (dry mouth) is related to the dosage of radiation and the area in the radiation field. If the portals are located over the parotid and submandibular glands, xerostomia eventually becomes severe. Patients often lose all desire for food, which initiates a vicious cycle of nutritional deficiency at a time when the body can least afford it. Xerostomia seldom reverses in adult patients if the dosage has been above 40 Gy. Young patients may experience some improvement in saliva flow and quality (Carl 1986).

The decreased saliva flow is readily visible during clinical examination. The negative changes in the quality of saliva that is still being generated are more subtle. The pH of saliva usually ranges from 6.5 to 7, but the saliva of irradiated patients frequently has a pH range of

5 to 5.5. Saliva normally buffers and lubricates, but it loses those protective qualities after radiation therapy (Frank, Herdly, and Phillipe 1965).

CHANGES IN THE ORAL MICROFLORA

Radiation-induced environmental changes lead to a shift in the microbial balance of the mouth. There is often an increase in the relative number of *Candida albicans* organisms. The signs and symptoms of this increase are a burning sensation and the accumulation of grayish-white plaques with peripheral zones of erythema. Other microbial changes include increases of the relative numbers of cariogenic aerobic organisms such as *Streptococcus mutans* and *Lactobacillus*. In the anaerobic bacterial population, there is an increase in *Actinomyces sp.* (Brown et al. 1975). Generalized dryness, the absence of buffering and lubricating saliva, the presence of oral fluids with low pH, and an abundance of cariogenic organisms in accumulated plaque probably contribute the most to radiation-induced caries (Beumer, Curtis, and Harrison 1979).

RADIATION-INDUCED CARIES

Doctors initially attributed radiation-induced caries to the direct effect of radiation on the teeth. However, observers later noted that teeth decayed more readily after radiation whether they were in the field of treatment or not (Del Regato 1939). Radiation-induced caries begin as spotty white demineralizations on the buccal and lingual surfaces (Carl, Schaaf, and Chen 1972). If the teeth are left untreated, caries will even- tually circle the cervical area and the crown may break off at the gingival margin (figs. 43.2 and 43.3). Exposed

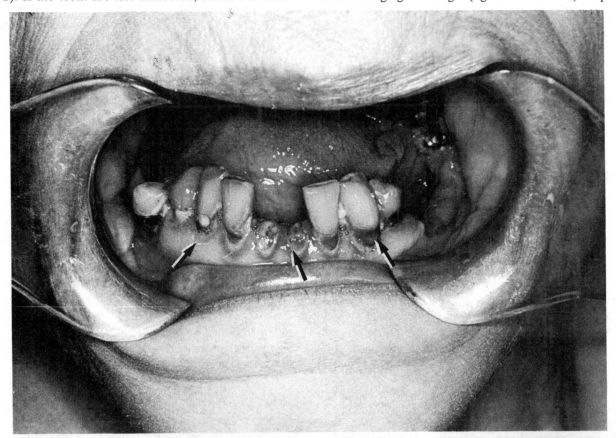

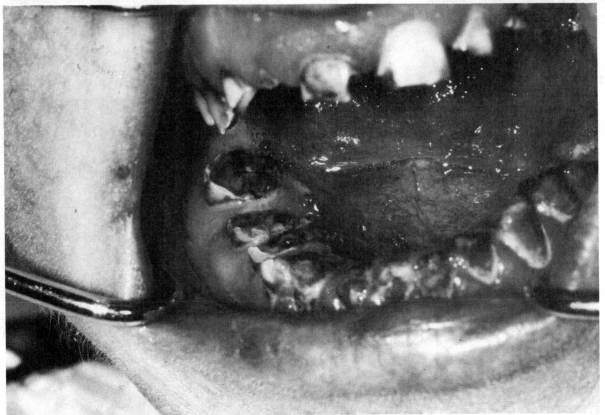

Fig. 43.2 and 43.3. Radiation caries in patients who received more than 60 Gy of radiation for intraoral tumors. The patients did not have the benefit of specific instructions in oral care.

dentin on the incisal and occlusal surfaces softens, and the enamel is gradually undermined.

EFFECTS OF RADIATION THERAPY ON THE PERIODONTIUM

When teeth are in the direct line of the primary radiation beam, the periodontium is often affected. The radiation leads to the disorientation in direction and attachment of the ligament fibers. The membrane widens and results in a loss of vascularity (Silverman and Chierici 1965). These changes reduce the capacity of periodontium repair and regeneration, which dictates caution in periodontal treatment of irradiated patients. As the periodontal ligament fibers lose their vascularity and cellularity, they may not reattach after scaling, curettage, and mucogingival surgery.

BONE CHANGES AND OSTEORADIONECROSIS

Bone absorbs more radiation than does an equal volume of soft tissue. The mandible, because it has higher bone density and lower vascularity, is more vulnerable to osteoradionecrosis than is the maxilla (Beumer, Curtis, and Harrison 1979; Mainous and Boyne 1974).

Radiation reduces the number of bone cells, and causes progressive fibrosis and an imbalance in the osteoclastic-osteoblastic relationship. The vascularity gradually decreases through edema, endarteritis, and hyalinization of small vessels (Ewing 1926; Bedwinek et al. 1926). Bone, like other tissues with reduced blood supply and cellularity, heals slowly after trauma and infection. This must be considered when dental extractions are done after radiation therapy.

The development of osteoradionecrosis is related to the dosage of radiation, the condition of the bone and the mucosa before radiation, and the changes that take place during and after therapy. Osteoradionecrosis occurs more frequently in patients who have natural teeth, probably because the periodontium structure provides more opportunities for initial infections (Carl 1986).

The first signs of osteoradionecrosis include pain, exfoliation of bone segments, and continued suppuration. Radiographically, osteoradionecrosis shows as diffuse osteolysis with irregular borders and/or scattered islands of radiolucency (fig. 43.4). The incidence of osteoradionecrosis has decreased since the advent of megavoltage radiation.

DENTAL AND ORAL CARE OF THE IRRADIATED PATIENT

The secondary reactions of radiation are unavoidable, but with proper care and patience, many treatment effects can be modified and reduced to a tolerable level. The patient must be aware of the implications of treatment and the penalties of neglect. The dentist who treats irradiated patients must also realize that they have a chronic situation that requires attention at relatively short intervals (Carl 1986).

INFORMATION AND INSTRUCTION

The treatment's oral side effects must be explained to the patient in simple terms. Patients must understand that they have to keep the oral tissues lubricated, and that good oral hygiene is the cornerstone of oral health (Carl 1986). This clarification applies to those who have natural teeth as well as those who are edentulous. All dentulous patients about to undergo radiation therapy in the head and neck area should be instructed in the Bass method of brushing and flossing (Bass 1948) and irrigation with 5% solutions of sodium bicarbonate. If flossing is a problem, the use of Stim-U-Dents® (Johnson & Johnson Dental Products Co., East Windsor, N.J.

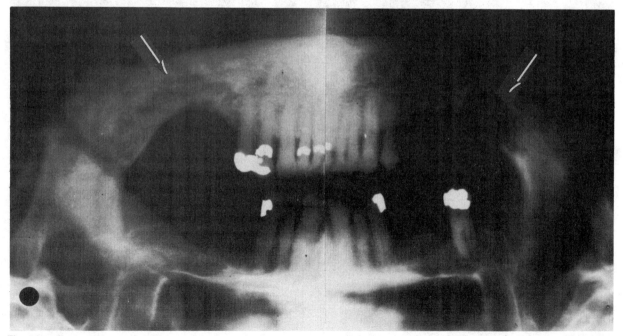

Fig. 43.4. Osteoradionecrosis in a patient who received 70 Gy of radiation for carcinoma of the tonsils. Osteoradionecrosis developed several years after therapy.

08250) or proxabrushes (John O. Butler Co., Chicago, Ill. 60630) is recommended; most patients find it easier to use Stimu-U-Dents® or proxabrushes because they require only one hand. In addition to an oral hygiene demonstration, patients should receive written instructions that explain the side effects of radiation and illustrate the proper method of oral hygiene. Soft brushes such as Right Kind® (John O. Butler Co., Chicago, Ill. 60630) or Oral B Sulcus Brush® (Oral B Company, Wayne, N.J. 07470) are recommended.

The Bass method of brushing emphasizes cleaning the cervical areas of teeth and the gingival crevices, where radiation caries and periodontal disease begins.

The edentulous patient, whether or not a denture wearer, also needs to exhibit correct oral hygiene. Daily irrigation and debridement are essential because dehydration and retention of mucous stimulate *Candida albicans* and other, bacterial infections.

Changing the patients' habits is difficult. Many soon forget the implications of their cancer treatment and continue their original oral hygiene patterns. On the other hand, preventive measures, if carried out conscientiously, considerably modify the unfavorable side effects of radiation therapy. Good care of the mouth during and after therapy contributes significantly to the success of cancer treatment.

PREIRRADIATION DENTAL EXTRACTIONS

Historically, the main reasons for full-mouth dental extractions before radiation therapy were the assumptions that the teeth would decay after radiation therapy and that later dental extractions would cause osteoradionecrosis. Fortunately, this approach has been replaced with a more conservative one. However, there are indications for preirradiation extractions. The most important of these include advanced periodontal disease, high caries index, and poor oral hygiene (fig. 43.5).

Advanced periodontal disease and a large number of caries usually indicate poor oral hygiene. When radiation in and around the oral cavity enters the picture, the stakes are high. The primary concern is to create a clean field and an environment that can be more easily maintained.

Preirradiation dental extractions differ from extractions under normal conditions in that the dentist must consider the potential bone changes associated with radiation therapy. These changes disturb the balance between bone resorption and bone deposition, reduce the capacity of bone to remodel, and necessitate contouring the alveolar bone at the time of extraction to remove spicules, sharp edges, and other unattached segments. The extraction sites should be sutured without tension of the tissue to expedite healing. Studies have shown that the time interval between dental extractions and the start of radiation is not as critical as doctors once believed (Starcki and Shannon 1977).

POSTIRRADIATION EXTRACTIONS

Dental extractions after radiation therapy have long been regarded as a cause of osteoradionecrosis, yet

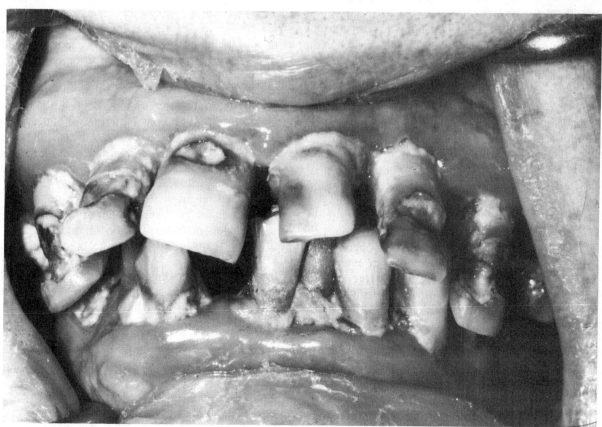

Fig. 43.5. Poor oral hygiene, advanced caries, and periodontal disease, as in this patient, are indications for preirradiation dental extractions.

evidence exists that the procedure involves minimal risks (Carl, Schaaf, and Sako 1973; Carl 1975). However, this does not mean that extractions can be done without regard for tissue and without certain precautions. The following factors should be considered: the amount of radiation received; the location of the tumor; the number of extractions at any given time; premedication; suturing; previous major surgery; and the possible time span between radiation and extractions (Carl 1986).

When dental extractions are necessary after irradiation, the patient should be premedicated with antibiotics. Penicillin is the antibiotic of choice (500 mg every 6 hours for four to five days) unless there is sensitivity, in which case erythromycin is an alternative. The alveolar process must be contoured, and the soft tissue over the extraction sites should be sutured.

The time span between therapy and dental extractions can be regarded in two ways: (1) radiation-induced bone and vascular changes are irreversible and progressive, therefore the length of time will hardly provide a margin of safety; and (2) during a short period between radiation and extractions, the tissue changes are in their early phases and the healing capacity is still relatively high.

ORAL MAINTENANCE AND FOLLOW-UP CARE

Maintaining the teeth and other oral cavity tissues in a relatively healthy condition after radiation therapy requires the patient's continuous attention and frequent follow-ups by the dentist. When the patient neglects oral hygiene and other care instructions, the development of dental caries and periodontal disease is inevitable. A 6-month recall visit is not appropriate for the irradiated patient; three months is a more proper period of time because the oral condition can deteriorate rapidly. Rarely does a patient's oral hygiene remain high all the time.

TOPICAL FLUORIDE

Daily application of topical fluoride on clean tooth surfaces reduces the incidence of radiation caries considerably (Dreizen at al. 1977). Patients can apply fluoride gel in flexible custom-made applicators once a day for five to six minutes. The experience with this method has been disappointing, however, because patients fail to comply consistently. Also, if teeth drift, the applicators no longer fit intimately to the tooth surfaces. Topical fluoride uptake is a surface phenomenon confined to the outer 30 to 50 microns of enamel (Knutson, Armstrong, and Feldman 1947). More success has been achieved with a 0.4% stannous fluoride gel applied once a day with a toothbrush. If the gel application is coupled with the Bass method of brushing, an appreciable level of periodontal protection is achieved at the same time. Above all, patients must understand that fluoride is no substitute for regular plaque removal with a toothbrush, floss and/or Stim-U-Dents® and proxabrushes. Teeth must be clean for fluoride to have an effect. Indefinite daily application is necessary because most of the fluoride is lost from the surface within 24 hours (Gron 1977).

RESTORATIVE DENTISTRY

The success of restorative dentistry for all patients depends on good oral hygiene. Although the same is true, in part, for irradiated patients, the clinician has to deal with the additional hostile factors of dryness, reduced pH of oral fluids, and microbial changes. These factors, as well as the patient's ability to tolerate lengthy and involved procedures, dictate the choice of restorative materials and methods (Carl, Schaaf, and Chen 1972).

DENTURES FOR IRRADIATED PATIENTS

For irradiated patients, the fabrication and wearing of dentures is still controversial. Some clinicians believe that patients should not wear dentures during radiation therapy; others feel that it takes at least one year before the mucosa has recovered sufficiently to tolerate dentures with impunity (Rahn, Matalon, and Drake 1968; Daley and Drake 1972).

Considering the fact that radiation-induced tissue changes are progressive and irreversible, a safety-time factor to the fabrication of dentures cannot be assigned. We do not hesitate to fabricate dentures once the acute soft-tissue reactions to the radiation have resolved. Approximately four to six weeks after radiation therapy, patients enter a phase where the oral conditions appear relatively normal. Later, fibrosis and submental edema frequently develop.

When fabricating dentures for irradiated patients, the principles of good prosthodontics with additional considerations must be followed. Impressions must be made with particular care and with materials that do not stress or displace soft tissue. Overextended flanges may perforate the mucosa and ultimately expose bone. Custom trays must be border-molded to register the functional periphery without pressure. The clinician must consider the sensitivity of the irradiated tissue in selecting wash materials. Zinc oxide and eugenol (ZOE) may cause a burning sensation. Patients can better tolerate light-body rubber base or reversible hydrocolloid (alginate) diluted to 1.5 times its normal impression consistency. The objective is to obtain an impression with minimal tissue displacement.

The occlusion must be distributed equally and balanced without lateral displacement of the bases. Edema of the tongue and buccal mucosa often dictate the position and overlap of the buccal and lingual cusps (Carl 1986).

Postinsertion adjustments and continued care of dentures and tissues are as important in the edentulous patient as is oral care for the dentulous patient.

ORAL MANIFESTATIONS OF CANCER CHEMOTHERAPY AND THEIR MANAGEMENT

Many current anticancer drugs can damage cancer cells and normal cells alike, especially normal cells that have high replacement rates. Cells that are vulnerable to the toxic side effects of chemotherapy compose the oral mucosa, salivary glands, and bone marrow. Damaged mucosa and salivary glands directly affect the oral cavity; compromised bone marrow indirectly makes the oral cavity an easy target for infections.

The chemotherapeutic agents that may cause stomatitis and bone marrow depression include methotrexate, cyclophosphamide, daunorubicin, doxorubicin hydrochloride, 5-fluorouracil, bleomycin, nitrogen mustard, cytarabine hydrochloride, 6-mercaptopurine, busulfan, and L-phenylalanine mustard.

STOMATITIS

Stomatitis may develop when the chemotherapeutic agents interfere with the maturation cycle of the cells that compose the oral epithelium. The epithelium becomes thin and friable; sometimes desquamation occurs. The condition may be focal or generalized and involve the buccal mucosa, palate, tongue, floor of the mouth, and the gingiva (fig. 43.6). Jagged teeth, the accumulation of calculus and plaque, defective dental restorations, and dental prostheses may all aggravate stomatitis (Hickey, Toth, and Lindquist 1982; Carl 1986; Carl 1983).

Stomatitis is painful and may require systemic analgesics; patients often neglect oral hygiene, because of the pain involved. In a short time, plaque accumulation, dehydrated mucus, and other debris precipitate a chain reaction of secondary infections and dental pathoses.

Patients under active treatment for acute leukemia and those with bone marrow transplants (BMT) may develop particularly severe stomatitis (fig. 43.7). The combination of total body irradiation and intensive chemotherapy reduces the granulocyte and platelet counts to very low levels that may persist for weeks (Carl and Higby 1985). The compromised epithelial barrier facilitates invasion of potentially lethal bacteria and fungi that may lead to local infections and, possibly, septicemia (Dreizen 1978; McElroy 1984).

MYELOSUPPRESSION AND IMMUNOSUPPRESSION

Drug-related destruction of stem cells that normally mature into granulocytes and lymphocytes deprives patients of the normal protection of the immune system. Chemotherapy greatly compromises phagocytic activity, reduces production of B lymphocytes, delays hypersensitivity by T lymphocytes, and blocks the mononuclear phase of the inflammatory reaction. The patient may develop bacterial, fungal, viral, and mixed infections. The risk of infection increases proportionally to the degree and duration of drug-induced leukopenia (Dreizen, Bodey, and Brown 1978; Dreizen, Bodey, and Rodriguez 1975). When the granulocyte or lymphocyte counts fall below 1,000/mm^3, patients have a greater than 50% chance of developing an infection. Seventy percent

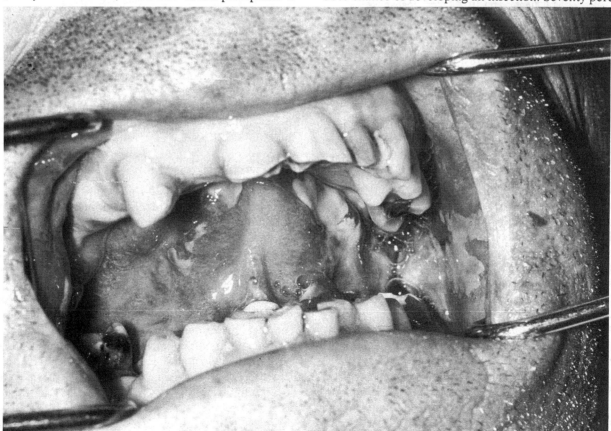

Fig. 43.6. Generalized stomatitis in a patient who received chemotherapy for acute leukemia. The tongue and the buccal mucosa are severely involved.

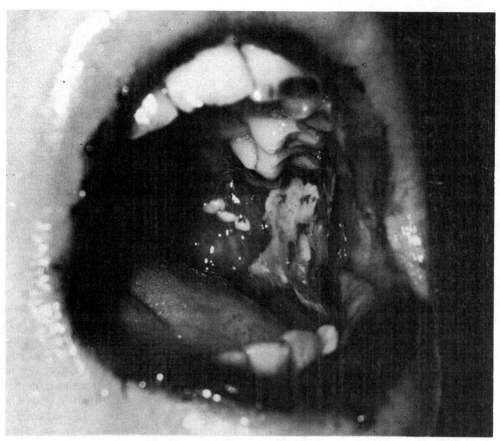

Fig. 43.7. Generalized stomatitis in a patient who received a bone marrow transplant for treatment of leukemia. At this time, the patient's white blood cell count (WBC) and platelet count are below 1,000/mm³ and 10,000/mm³, respectively.

of patients with acute leukemia and 50% of patients with solid tumors and lymphomas die of infections (Bodey 1977; Rodriguez 1978).

The chemotherapeutic agents that depress the bone marrow at therapeutic doses cause thrombocytopenia and leukopenia and disturb the patient's hemostatic and immune mechanisms. Chronic periodontal disease and chronic pulpitis may become acute (Carl 1986; Peterson and Sonis 1983). Severe myelosuppression may also precipitate spontaneous bleeding from the periodontium, especially in patients with existing periodontal disease (fig. 43.8). The normal platelet count in adults ranges from 150,000/mm³ to 300,000/mm³; the severely myelosuppressed patient may have a platelet count below 5,000/mm³ (Carl 1986).

Periodontal disease is, in most cases, an inflammatory response to the metabolites of microorganisms in plaque and calculus adhering to subgingival tooth structures; thus, the deposits that collect subgingivally must be removed. Periodontal pockets deeper than 4 mm or 5 mm are difficult to keep free of plaque and often become the foci of acute infection and septicemia in patients with compromised immune mechanisms. The simple act of chewing can introduce thousands of potentially pathogenic organisms into the bloodstream when periodontal disease is present.

Several factors influence the susceptibility of patients. Among them are: (1) malignancy- and chemotherapy-induced hematopoietic and immune deficiencies; (2) tumor necrosis and nidus for pathogen growth; (3) obstruction of the lymphatic and venous system because of tumor involvement; (4) medications that promote development of resistant pathogen growth; (5) physical debility; (6) nosocomial acquisition of pathogens; (7) nutritional deficiencies; and (8) neglected hygiene (Dreizen 1978; Aubertin et al. 1978; Bodey et al. 1975).

INFECTIOUS AGENTS

Bacteria are responsible for most infections in patients receiving antineoplastic drugs. Antibiotics usually control staphylococci and other gram-positive organisms; however, gram-negative organisms such as *Pseudomonas, Klebsiella,* and *Escherichia* cause approximately 20% of severe bacterial infections in compromised patients. Although *Candida albicans* is responsible for a smaller number of infections, if the organism persists for a long time it may become invasive and cause death. The incidence of fungal infections may be as high as 40% in patients with hematologic malignancies (Dreizen 1978). In a study of adult patients with leukemia, approximately 30% had severe oral infections, 25% of which were due to gram-negative organisms. Viruses and gram-positive bacteria accounted for the rest (Dreizen et al. 1982).

The potential of the normal oral flora to cause disease is apparently related to the quantity of the organisms present. When periodontal disease sets in the

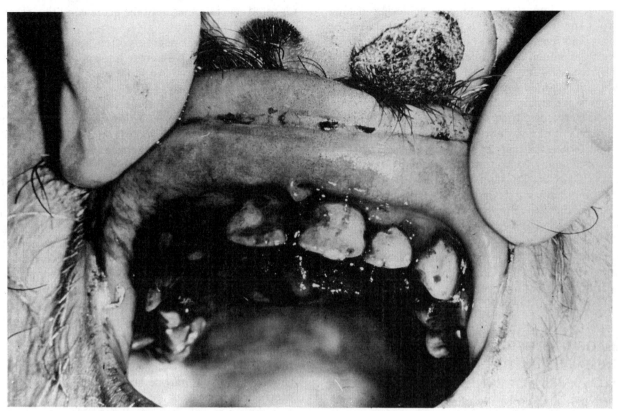

Fig. 43.8. Gingival bleeding in a patient with acute leukemia. This patient had advanced periodontal disease before he became myelosuppressed through chemotherapy.

oral cavity harbors anaerobes, enteric gram-negative bacteria, spirochetes, *Actinomyces*, and fungi (Dreizen 1978). Enteric gram-negative bacteria predominate in the oral cavity of patients with acute leukemia (Brown, Dreizen, and Bodey 1973). Supragingival plaque in immunodeficient patients has higher levels of catalase-negative diphtheroids and *Candida sp.* than plaque in healthy individuals (Brown et al. 1979).

OTHER ORAL CHANGES
ASSOCIATED WITH CHEMOTHERAPY

The quantity and quality of saliva often decrease during and after cancer chemotherapy. Doctors have identified salivary gland lesions comparable to those seen in patients with Sjoegren's syndrome (Rodu and Gockerman 1983). Patients have reported reduction in the saliva flow as early as two days after administration of chemotherapy. As is the case with radiation therapy, the existing saliva no longer flows freely, but has a ropy, adhesive quality. Prolonged xerostomia and reduced salivary pH promote imbalance in the oral flora, accelerate periodontal deterioration, and precipitate dental caries.

PREVENTIVE AND MAINTENANCE
ORAL AND DENTAL CARE FOR
PATIENTS RECEIVING CHEMOTHERAPY

Oncologists, dentists working with cancer patients, and other health-care professionals should be aware of the importance of oral care, especially under compromised conditions. Yet, in light of the urgency of a patient's cancer treatment, practitioners often overlook oral care (Lindquist, Hickey, and Drane 1978). Many authors have described the potential dangers of infections and have emphasized the need for plaque control and reduction of bacterial populations. It is important to give a patient instructions on how to achieve good oral hygiene under conditions that apply to his or her case. For example, a patient with a platelet count below 20,000/mm^3 and a lymphocyte count of less than 1,000/mm^3 cannot tolerate the same oral-hygiene procedures with a brush and floss as a patient with normal hematologic functions.

The patient's preparatory workup for treatment should include prechemotherapy dental evaluation, preventive care and oral-care instructions, in the same way as oral-care procedures are now applied to patients who undergo radiation therapy in the head and neck area.

Teeth with carious lesions should have immediate treatment, at least to the point of arresting the carious process. Periodontitis remains a local problem in a patient with an intact immune mechanism, but a myelosuppressed patient is at greater risk for developing more extensive local disease and septicemia through the persisting inflammatory process.

Only effective oral hygiene methods that concentrate on the areas most vulnerable, namely the cervical areas of the teeth and the gingival crevices, can control plaque

(Carl 1986). The type of toothbrush and the method of brushing are important factors in achieving plaque control. The Bass method is also recommended for patients who receive chemotherapy (Bass 1948).

Once the patient has adopted an effective method of oral hygiene and has achieved a reasonable degree of oral health, maintenance is easier even in periods when conditions are unfavorable. As the patient's myelosuppression increases during the course of chemotherapy, conventional oral and dental hygiene methods must be adjusted. When the platelet count decreases to 20,000/mm^3, disposable Toothettes® (Halbrand, Inc., Willoughby, Ohio 44094) should replace the toothbrush. Toothettes® have soft foam-rubber tips at the end of a handle, and they can remove most of the plaque that accumulates on teeth and soft-tissue surfaces.

Constant modification of the oral environment is absolutely necessary, especially during active cancer treatment, to reduce the population of the oral microflora and to reduce the severity and duration of stomatitis (Carl 1986; Dreizen 1978).

MANAGEMENT OF ACUTE DENTAL EMERGENCIES IN THE MYELOSUPPRESSED PATIENT

Cancer patients, especially those with hematologic malignancies, are often in an already compromised condition when admitted to the hospital. To complicate matters, many have poor oral hygiene and advanced dental disease. Their malignancy demands immediate treatment, and dental care under those conditions seems a luxury.

The most common dental complications include bleeding from the gingival tissues; acute periapical infections; pericoronitis involving partially erupted teeth, especially third molars; periodontal infections with marginal gingival necrosis; and aggravation of stomatitis by dental restorations and/or prostheses.

Acute periapical infections usually result from pulp necrosis. In a patient with a platelet count above 50,000/mm^3, uncomplicated extractions usually incur minimal risk. The risks of bleeding make dental extractions inadvisable in severely myelosuppressed patients. Removal of infected pulp and drainage of the periapical abscess can, however, aid in managing pulp pathosis and acute periapical infections. This procedure will take care of the immediate problem, but more definitive treatment, either root canal therapy or extraction, is necessary for follow-up care.

Pericoronitis usually occurs around mandibular third molars. The soft-tissue remnant overlying the tooth's occlusal surface is traumatized by the cusps of the opposing tooth and/or by plaque collected in the deep gingival crevice that surrounds the tooth. To control the infection, the soft-tissue pocket must be cleaned to reduce bacterial activity. The pocket should be irrigated with warm saline and 3% hydrogen peroxide, and then carefully packed for five to ten minutes with cotton saturated with Betadine. The procedure may have to be repeated several times until the acute condition resolves (Carl 1986).

Marginal gingival necrosis often appears in myelosuppressed patients with acute leukemia. The degree of gingival pathology in these situations is inversely related to the white blood cell (WBC) count (fig. 43.9). The condition is painful and progressive, and limits almost any personal oral hygiene. Daily careful irrigation of the gingival areas with 5% sodium bicarbonate, coupled with careful suction, will reduce and neutralize the organisms responsible for the condition.

Conservative treatment at times fails and a dentist may have to extract teeth in leukemic patients. Potential complications include bleeding, further infections, osteomyelitis, and septicemia. Preoperative planning in such circumstances should be done with the cooperation of the oncologist. The surgery must be performed in a hospital. Arrangements for possible blood transfusions are necessary, and the patient must take antibiotics until the danger of an open-wound infection has passed. Penicillin G is the preferred antibiotic, unless the patient is allergic in which case erythromycin may be used. The platelet count usually accurately indicates the patient's homeostatic capacity, but it is not always reliable. The count may be near normal, but qualitative defects in the platelets and abnormal adhesiveness and fibrinolysis may still cause prolonged bleeding. A coagulation profile of prothrombin time, partial thromboplastin time, thrombin time, fibrinogen levels, and template bleeding time should be obtained (Segelman and Doku 1977; Carl 1978).

The extraction site itself should be closed with sutures. Sometimes the socket requires packing with resorbable hemostatic material, but this may at times become a nidus for infection. In most cases healing time is prolonged and the tissue over the extraction site remains thin and friable for several weeks. No platelet-suppressing pain medication should be prescribed.

PART II: MAXILLOFACIAL PROSTHETICS AND THE HEAD AND NECK CANCER PATIENT

With significant numbers of patients surviving cancer, rehabilitation and a return to an appropriate lifestyle have increased in importance in recent decades. Non-living substitutes or prosthetics frequently correct aesthetic and functional disabilities resulting from surgical defects in the head and neck area. The surgeon and/or radiation therapist and others providing head and neck cancer treatment should have the services of a maxillofacial prosthodontist available to enable a complete and well-rounded reconstruction.

By definition, "Maxillofacial Prosthetics is the branch of prosthodontics concerned with the restoration and/or replacement of the stomatognathic and associated facial structures with prostheses that may be removed on a

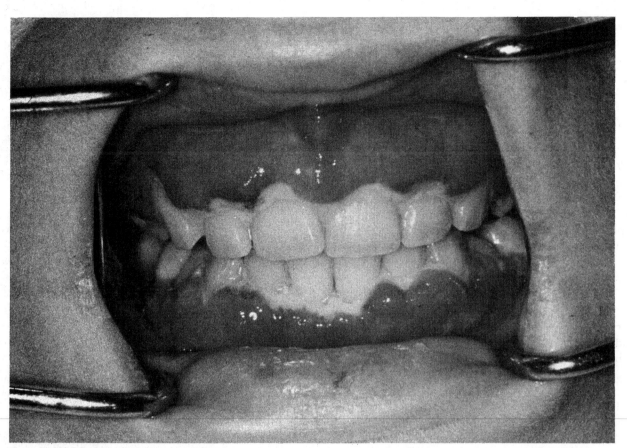

Fig. 43.9. Gingivitis in a patient with acute leukemia. At this time, the patient's WBC count was below 500/mm³. Note the necrotic gingival margin.

regular or elective basis" (*J. Pros. Dent: Glossary of Prosthodontic Terms* 1987). The maxillofacial prosthodontist is usually a dentist with two years of postgraduate training in prosthodontics (the study of prostheses for the oral cavity) plus one additional hospital-oriented year of experience in the use of prostheses for the head and neck area in general (maxillofacial prosthetics). Accelerated training of these specialists and of laboratory technicians in recent years has made them available in most metropolitan areas. They are increasingly being integrated into head and neck cancer treatment and rehabilitation teams.

CLASSIFICATION

One method of classifying prostheses for the patient with head and neck cancer is presented in table 43.1. To clarify this classification, a discussion of each type of prosthesis follows.

FACIAL PROSTHESES

These extraoral restorations help return the patient's appearance to an acceptable state and negate dressings or patches. The most commonly used materials for facial prostheses include silicone rubber (MDX4-4210, Dow Corning, Midland, Mich.), ethyl or methyl methacrylate (acrylic), or polyurethane. In practice, all of the materials have certain shortcomings, but can be used successfully. The prostheses

are usually attached by the use of skin adhesives, but occasionally they can be retained by undercuts in the facial defect or by mechanical means, such as elastics or attachment with eyeglasses.

NASAL

The loss of external nasal tissue is common because of the frequent occurrence and necessary treatment of basal cell carcinoma in this exposed area. Although

Table 43.1
CLASSIFICATION OF PROSTHESES FOR PATIENTS WITH HEAD AND NECK CANCER

Facial Prostheses
    Nasal
    Orbital and ocular
    Auricular
    Composite
Intraoral Prostheses
    Obturators (postoperative)
    Speech aids
    Complete and partial dentures (modified)
    Feeding prostheses
Treatment Prostheses
    Obturators (surgical)
    Stents
    Splints
    Flange prostheses
    Prosthetic dressings
    Mandibular exercisers
Implants
    Mandibular (metal)
    Facial (silicone rubber)

surgical reconstruction is usually possible, the surgeon frequently delays reconstruction for a time because of possible recurrence of disease. A prosthesis is generally acceptable because the nose is a rather discrete portion of the face (figs. 43.10 and 43.11) (Schaaf 1970). Eyeglasses help hide the prosthesis-skin margins and generally detract from the prosthetic nature of the nose.

ORBITAL AND OCULAR

The orbital prosthesis restores the appearance when all of the orbital contents have been removed, including the eyelids. As yet, no surgical reconstructive procedure can replace the total eye with its attachments and further restore sight. The patient with an orbital exenteration is suited for a prosthesis because of the definitely outlined margins. These prostheses are frequently successful; however, the patient must accept certain limitations. The globe will not move in harmony with the other eye, nor will the eyelids blink. Eyeglasses with heavy rims, and, possibly, tinted lenses help to enhance the overall appearance (figs. 43.12 and 43.13). The ocular prosthesis is used when an enucleation of the globe is necessary. Because an implant and sufficient tissues are available, including the eyelids, this facial prosthesis is the most successful. The residual tissue often affords some movement, further enhancing the overall effect. Color matching of the iris and sclera to the remaining eye can provide a restoration that is often undetectable.

AURICULAR

When cancer surgery has necessitated the removal of the entire external ear, the area is not easily reconstructed surgically. On the other hand, the prosthetic ear is probably the most readily accepted facial prosthesis. Adjacent hair partially masks prosthesis margins and increases patient acceptance. This facial prosthesis is also the one which skin adhesives retain most often. When feasible, surgically prepared skin loops are also possible (figs. 43.14 and 43.15)

COMPOSITE

More extensive surgery engenders larger facial defects. Although larger prostheses are not as aesthetically acceptable, they are necessary in situations where surgical reconstruction is not possible. The larger facial defects also frequently compromise vital functions such as speech and mastication, so patients usually accept the prosthesis as an integral part of their rehabilitation (figs. 43.16 and 43.17).

INTRAORAL PROSTHESES

This class of prosthesis complements or restores resected portions of the oral cavity or nearby anatomic sites, such as the nasopharyngeal area or nasal fossa. Most prostheses in the oral cavity depend upon the teeth or a stable denture for overall stability. For this reason, it is important that every tooth possible is saved for retaining the prosthesis. Consultation with the

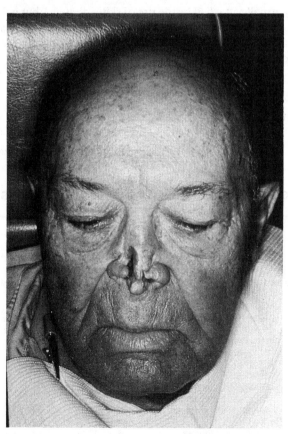

Fig. 43.10. Nasal defect after resection for basal cell carcinoma.

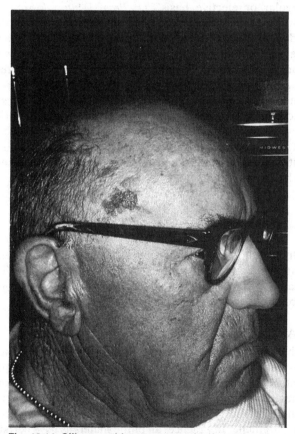

Fig. 43.11. Silicone-rubber nose prosthesis retained by a skin adhesive.

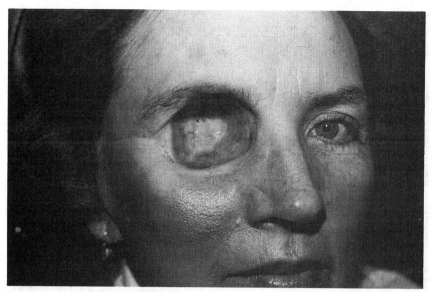

Fig. 43.12. Orbital exenteration and skin graft to treat melanoma of the eyelid.

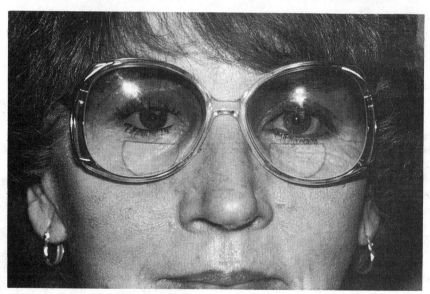

Fig. 43.13. Appearance of the orbital prosthesis is enhanced by the use of eyeglasses.

prosthodontist prior to cancer surgery can be helpful in getting the patient in the best possible dental and oral condition to receive a prosthesis after surgery.

OBTURATORS (POSTOPERATIVE)

A surgical defect that is an extension of the oral cavity disturbs numerous oral functions. The uncontrolled air flow into other cavities impairs speech; food travelling into the surgical defect renders mastication difficult; difficulty in managing the defect disturbs deglutition. An obturator is a prosthesis that closes an opening. Palatal obturators are most commonly prepared for patients who have had a maxillectomy. The restoration of appropriate speech frequently gives the patient a significant psychological boost. The return of oral function with the removal of the nasogastric tube places the patient in a more socially acceptable situation for returning home from the hospital (figs. 43.18, 43.19, and 43.20).

SPEECH AIDS

With the loss of proper function of the palatopharyngeal opening due to a pharyngectomy or soft palate surgery, the patient exhibits nasal emission of air and nasality of speech. The speech aid is an extension of an oral prosthesis (complete denture or partial denture) and functionally reacts with residual pharyngeal musculature to return speech to normal. This prosthesis also aids swallowing by preventing the regurgitation of food into the nasopharynx during the deglutition process.

COMPLETE AND PARTIAL DENTURES (MODIFIED)

The varied surgical procedures carried out in the oral cavity necessitate construction of unusual modifications of oral prostheses. Dentists commonly prepare dentures that plump the lips after surgery and supply missing portions of the alveolar process and teeth. A maxillary prosthesis that lowers the hard palate to facilitate function of the restricted tongue can aid patients who

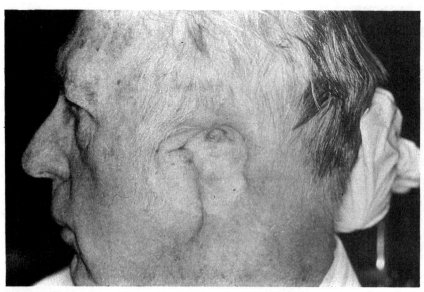

Fig. 43.14. Resection of the ear to treat basal cell carcinoma.

have had a partial glossectomy, and, as a result, improve speech and deglutition (figs. 43.21 and 43.22).

FOOD GUIDES

Difficulties in deglutition result from surgical procedures that involve the floor of the mouth, base of the tongue, and the epiglottis. Surgical or prosthetic reconstructions of the tongue have not been very successful, but it is possible to construct protheses that will guide liquids and semiliquids into the esophagus. In these instances, the patient cannot chew because the tongue is not available to continually replace the food onto the chewing surfaces of the teeth. However, in patients in whom food guides are possible, this method of taking food is preferable over tube feedings (figs. 43.23, 43.24, and 43.25).

TREATMENT PROSTHESES

Although the definition of maxillofacial prosthetics states that the prosthetic reconstruction replaces portions of the head and neck that are missing or defective, many prostheses are actually necessary in the active treatment of the patient. Most often, these prostheses fill out tissue spaces or hold two tissue fragments in relation to each other. In this way, the prosthesis promotes healing, prevents dysfunction, and generally offers patients the benefit of rehabilitation procedures before debilitation.

OBTURATORS (SURGICAL)

Like the postoperative obturator, the surgical obturator most commonly closes an opening in the palate. However, it is put in place while the patient is in the operating room. Thus, it also serves to hold packs in place and support the face on the side being operated on. With such a prosthesis the defect does not immediately confront the patient upon awakening from anesthesia or removal of the surgical pack, and the patient frequently does not require a nasogastric tube for feeding (figs. 43.26 and 43.27).

STENTS

Acting as a tissue positioner (figs. 43.28 and 43.29) or guide, as in radiation therapy (figs. 43.30, 43.31, and 43.32), a stent may be an extension of another oral prosthesis that serves to carry a split-thickness skin graft to place, such as into the floor of the mouth after hemiglossectomy or into the maxillary area after a partial maxillectomy.

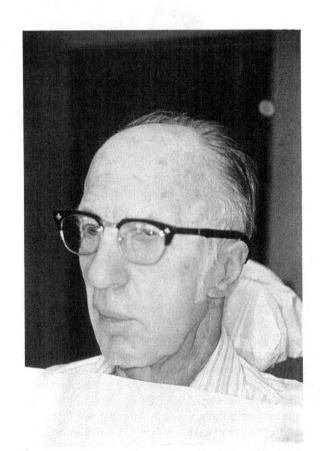

Fig. 43.15. Silicone-rubber ear prosthesis is retained by silicone rubber.

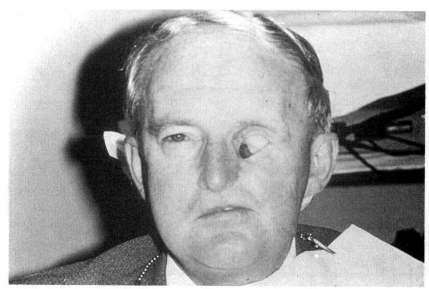

Fig. 43.16. Maxillectomy and orbital exenteration result in a larger area to be restored.

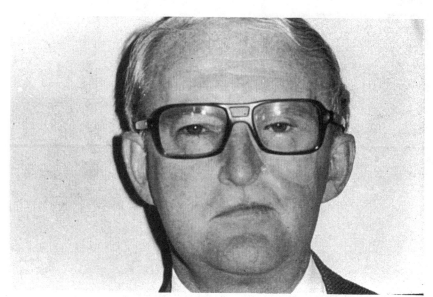

Fig. 43.17. Composite prosthesis restores the orbital and adjacent facial area.

SPLINTS

When it has been necessary to split the mandible during cancer surgery, a dental splint is useful to maintain contact between the mandibular segments until their union is completed. The splint can be accurately attached to the teeth or screwed or wired to the bony segments for rigid stability.

FLANGE PROSTHESES

Frequently, when one side of the mandible has been resected, the remaining segment deviates toward the affected side because of the muscle pull. The patient then has difficulty in chewing and speech. When the patient has a sufficient number of stable teeth, it is possible to construct a prosthesis that will return the mandibular segment to a proper relationship with the maxilla and maintain it there while the patient functions in a nearly normal fashion (figs. 43.33, 43.34, and 43.35).

PROSTHETIC DRESSINGS

Immediately after surgery, when it is impractical to construct a definitive facial prosthetic because of rapid tissue change, a simulated dressing is a useful adjunct to the patient's treatment. It does not require complicated adhesive and gauze dressings, but allows the dressing to be removed in one piece. This treatment prosthesis is also useful for patients who work in dusty environments where a delicate facial prosthesis would be impractical.

MANDIBULAR EXERCISERS

For those patients who have sufficient stable natural teeth, a simple prosthesis that employs the principle of the screw and inclined plane can combat the trismus that frequently occurs after radiation and surgery. With this prosthesis, patients can increasingly put the mandibular musculature under stress to improve their ability to depress the mandible.

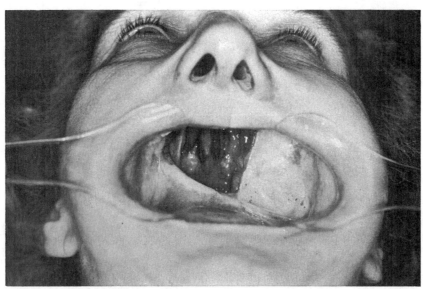

Fig. 43.18. Maxillary defect after surgical treatment for squamous cell carcinoma of the palate.

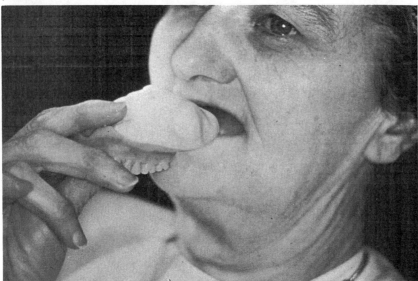

Fig. 43.19. The obturator will restore midface support and supply superior midface structures.

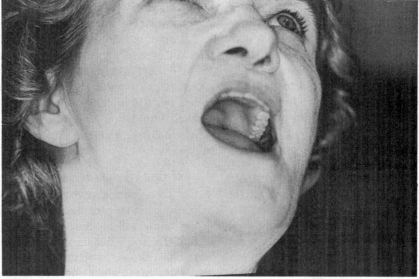

Fig. 43.20. Prosthetic restoration of the maxilla allows the patient to speak, masticate, and swallow normally.

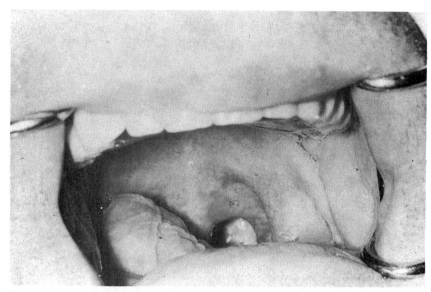

Fig. 43.21. Partial glossectomy leaves little tongue for speaking and swallowing.

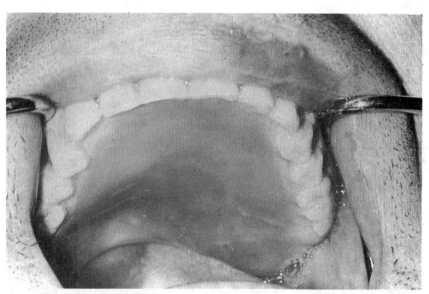

Fig. 43.22. The prosthetic palate is shaped to a lower level to improve tongue function.

IMPLANTS

The use of prostheses or nonliving substitutes to supplement tissues of the head has been well established. The availability of inert metals that the body tolerates (vitallium, ticonium, titanium, and tantalum) and other materials that do not cause a foreign body reaction (medical-grade silicone and rubber) has allowed plastic surgeons and maxillofacial prosthodontists to enhance the rehabilitation of the patient who has undergone head and neck cancer surgery.

MANDIBULAR IMPLANTS (METAL)

Metal implants, prepared in a tray form, can be custom-cast to fit a particular patient or prepared from available preformed sections. Because loss of continuity of the mandible is debilitating, these implants offer a definite opportunity for reconstructing the mandible and recontouring the patient's face (figs. 43.36, 43.37, and 43.38).

FACIAL IMPLANTS (SILICONE RUBBER)

The placement of custom-prepared medical-grade silicone rubber implants can recontour the facial defects resulting from loss of bony support of the face. The body readily accepts this material, and it does not resorb with time (Bessette et al. 1981).

INDICATIONS FOR THE USE OF A PROSTHESIS

The patient who has a large surgical defect, has undergone heavy irradiation, and is a poor risk for additional surgery because of advanced age or poor health has all the contraindications for plastic and reconstructive surgery.

An interim prosthesis is advisable in cases where a disease recurrence is possible, where radiation or chemotherapy is under consideration, or where surgical reconstruction of the anatomic part is simply not possible.

The prosthesis does not place physical stress on the patient, takes less time than reconstructive surgery, and can achieve more aesthetically pleasing results depending upon

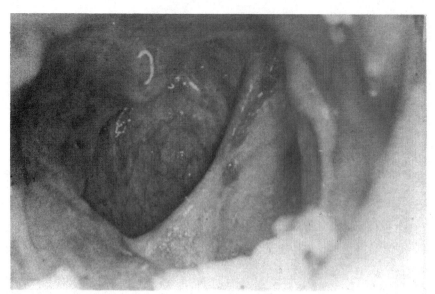

Fig. 43.23. Complete glossectomy with airway and hypopharynx in the floor of the mouth.

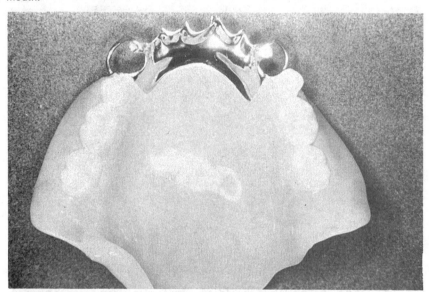

Fig. 43.24. Mandibular oral prosthesis guides for the hypopharyngeal area.

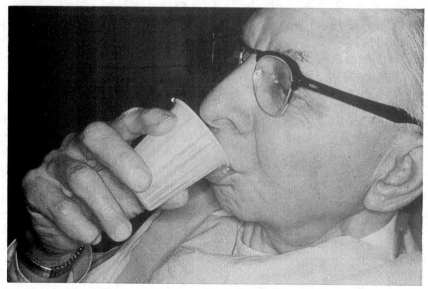

Fig. 43.25. This patient is able to take a liquid diet orally.

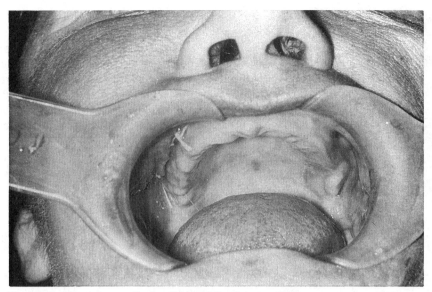

Fig. 43.26. Edentulous patient scheduled for right maxillectomy.

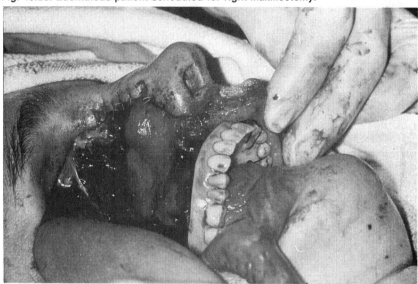

Fig. 43.27. Surgical obturator is wired to the opposite maxilla and immediately restores the palate.

the anatomic site. No prosthesis, however, is permanent; gradual changes in the patient or deterioration of the prosthetic material require replacement or adjustment every two to three years. The patient must contend with its daily removal and cleansing.

THE FUTURE

As long as surgery and radiation therapy remain the primary treatments for cancer of the head and neck, maxillofacial prostheses will be necessary. The techniques and materials for preparing these prostheses continue to improve and exciting and innovative ideas have surfaced recently. Udagama and King (1983) have developed methods for making the edges of facial prostheses difficult to detect. A Swedish method (Branemarket al. 1969) of using osseointegrated titanium fixtures to

retain extraoral and intraoral prostheses has proven highly successful. Presently, more and more North American centers are replacing less desirable adhesives with these fixtures. Albrektsson and associates (1981) have further perfected osseointegrated metal implants that can support and retain both intraoral or facial prostheses. Our own experience in this area has resulted in an excellent success rate using ultraviolet light-treated titanium implants (BUD Implant System). These innovations will enhance the appearance and functional usefulness of maxillofacial prostheses (figs. 43.39, 43.40, and 43.41.) Parel and colleagues (1983) suggested that donor parts can be remade into prostheses by using plastinated facial structures. These ideas and techniques on the horizon give insight into the exciting future of maxillofacial prostheses for head and neck cancer patients.

CONCLUSION

At times, the head and neck surgeon is not fully aware of the many primary and supportive services that the maxillofacial prosthodontist can perform with the aid of prostheses. Such a specialist should be on the surgical team or should be available for consultation with the surgeon before any head and neck cancer surgery takes place. Not only can these measures smooth the course of the cancer patient's treatment, they can also simplify the surgeon's treatment plan and facilitate nursing care.

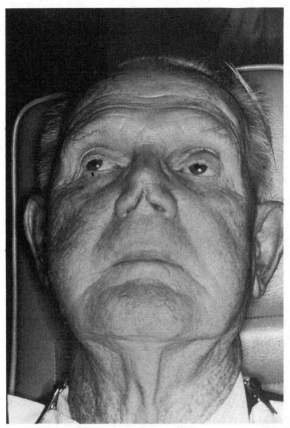

Fig. 43.28. Effects of nose tip surgery.

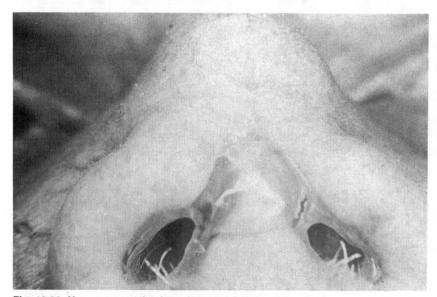

Fig. 43.29. Nares stent maintains adequate airway.

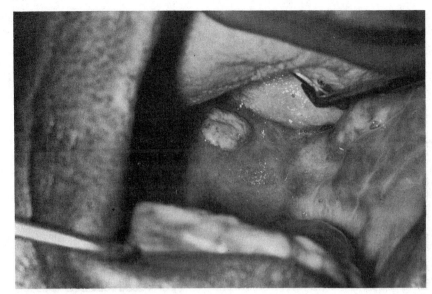

Fig. 43.30. Lesion on soft palate.

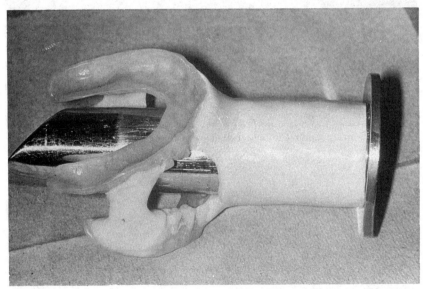

Fig. 43.31. Stent acts as a guide for radiation therapy.

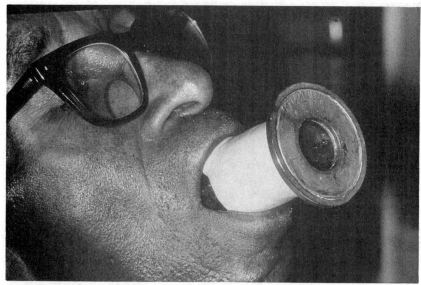

Fig. 43.32. Daily therapy is easily reduplicated using radiation stent.

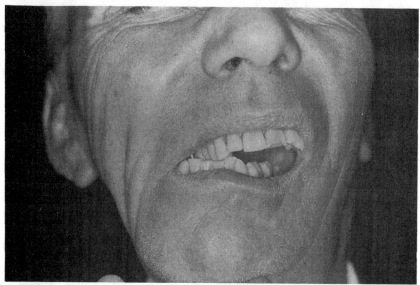

Fig. 43.33. Partial mandibulectomy results in deviation toward the surgical side.

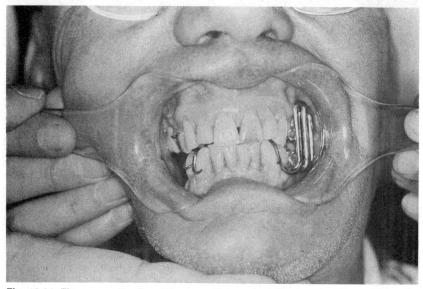

Fig. 43.34. Flange prosthesis returns mandible and maxilla to a proper relationship.

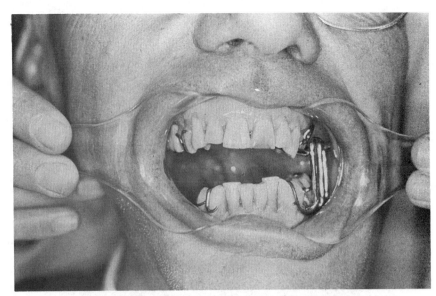

Fig. 43.35. Vertical movement of the mandible is possible.

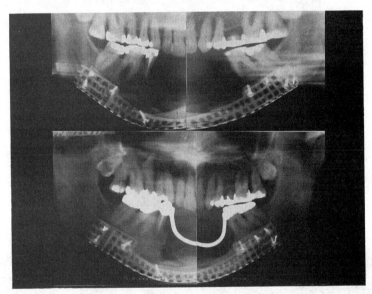

Fig. 43.36. A titanium implant restores the continuity of the mandible.

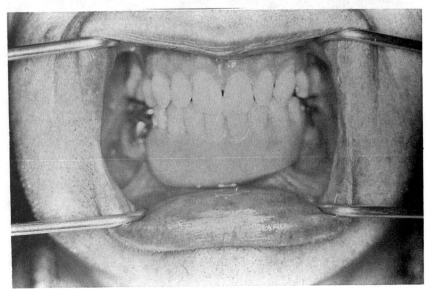

Fig. 43.37. An oral prosthesis restores the continuity of the mandible.

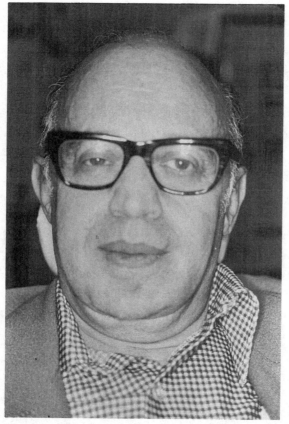

Fig. 43.38. Chin and mandibular contours are restored.

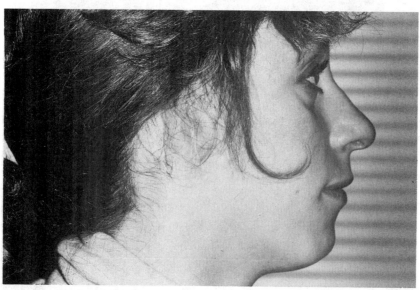

Fig. 43.39. Totally missing external ear.

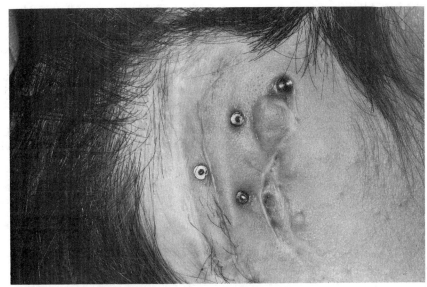

Fig. 43.40. Percutaneous osseointegrated titanium implants.

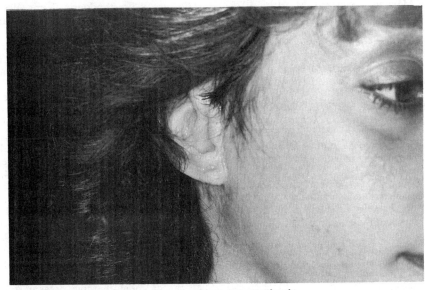

Fig. 43.41. Magnet-retained silicone rubber ear prosthesis.

REFERENCES

American Cancer Society. 1990. *Cancer facts and figures.* Atlanta: American Cancer Society.

Albrektsson, T.; Branemark, P.I.; and Hansson, H.A. et al. 1981. Osseointegrated titanium implants. *Acta Orthop. Scand.* 52:155-70.

Aubertin, J.; Lacut, J.Y.; and Hoerni, B. et al. 1978. *Opportunistic infections in cancer patients.* pp. 29-41. New York: Masson.

Awward, H.K., and Habib, Y.A. 1962. Effect of x-irradiation on NA and K secretion by human parotid gland. *J. Appl. Physiol.* 17:677.

Bass, C.C. 1948. The optimum characteristics of toothbrushes for personal oral hygiene. *Dent. Items Interest* 70:696-718.

Bedwinek, J.M. et al. 1926. Osteoradionecrosis in patients treated with definitive radiotherapy for squamous cell carcinoma of the oral cavity and naso- and oropharynx. *Radiology* 119:665-67.

Ben-Aryeh, H. et al. 1975. Effects of irradiation on saliva in cancer patients. *Int. J. Oral Surg.* 4:205-10.

Bessette, R.W.; Casey, D.M.; and Shatkin, S.S. et al. 1981. Customized silicone rubber maxillofacial implants. *Ann. Plastic Surg.* 7:453.

Beumer, J. III; Curtis, T.; and Harrison, R.E. 1979. Radiation therapy of the oral cavity: sequelae and management. *Head Neck Surg.* 1:301-12.

Bodey, G.P.; Hersh, E.M.; and Valdivieso, M. et al. 1975. Immunosuppressive agents on the immune system. *Postgrad. Med.* 58:67-74.

Bodey, G.P. 1977. Infectious complications in the cancer patient. *Curr. Prob. Cancer* 1(12):3-63.

Branemark, P.I. et al. 1969. Intraosseous anchorage of dental prostheses I: experimental studies. *Scand. J. Plast. Reconstr. Surg.* 3:81-100.

Brown, L.R.; Dreizen, S.; and Bodey, G.P. 1973. Effect of immunosuppression on the human oral flora. In Mergenhagen, S.E., et al. eds. *Comparative immunology of the oral cavity.* pp. 204-20. Washington, D.C.: U.S. Government Printing Office.

Brown, L.R. et al. 1975. The effect of radiation induced xerostomia on human oral microflora. *J. Dent. Res.* 54:740-50.

Brown, L.R.; Macklev, B.F.; and Levy, B.M. et al. 1979. Comparison of the plaque microflora in immunodeficient and immunocompetent dental patients. *J. Dent. Res.* 58:2344-352.

Carl, W. 1975. Oral surgery and radiation therapy. *Quint. Int.* 6:9-14.

Carl, W. 1978. Dental treatment for patients with leukemia. *Quint. Int.* 11:9-14.

Carl, W. 1983. Oral complications in cancer patients. *Am. Fam. Physician* 27:61-170.

Carl, W. 1986. Oral and dental care of patients receiving radiation therapy for tumors in and around the oral cavity. In Carl, W., and Sako, K. eds. *Cancer and the oral cavity.* pp. 167-83. Chicago: Quintessence Publishing Co.

Carl, W. 1986. Role of oral hygiene practices in oral health and general health. In Loe and Kleinman eds. *Dental plaque control measures and oral hygiene practices.* pp.23-38. Oxford, Washington: IRL Press.

Carl, W. 1986. Oral and dental care of patients receiving chemotherapy. In Carl, W., and Sako, K. eds. *Cancer and the oral cavity.* pp. 151-65. Chicago: Quintessence Publishing Co.

Carl, W., and Higby, D.J. 1985. Oral manifestations of bone marrow transplantation. *Am. J. Clin. Oncol.* 8:31-87.

Carl, W.; Schaaf, N.G.; and Chen, T.Y. 1972. Oral care of patients irradiated for cancer of the head and neck. *Cancer* 30:448-53.

Carl, W.; Schaaf, N.G.; and Sako, K. 1973. Oral surgery and the patient who has had radiation therapy for head and neck cancer. *Oral Surg.* 36:651-57.

Chalian, U.A.; Drane, J.B.; and Standish, S.M. 1972. *Maxillofacial prosthetics.* 1st ed. Baltimore: Williams & Wilkins.

Chen, T.Y. 1986. Radiation. In Carl, W., and Sako, K. eds. *Cancer and the oral cavity.* pp. 109-17. Chicago: Quintessence Publishing Co.

Daley, T.E., and Drake. J.B. 1972. *Management of dental problems in irradiated patients.* Houston: University of Texas Press.

Del Regato, J.A. 1939. Dental lesions observed after roentgen therapy in cancer of the buccal cavity, pharynx, or larynx. *Am. J. Roentgenol.* 42:404-10.

Dreizen, S. 1978. Stomatoxic manifestations of cancer chemotherapy. *J. Prosthet. Dent.* 40:650-55.

Dreizen, S.J. et al. 1977. Prevention of xerostomia-related dental caries in irradiated cancer patients. *J. Dent. Res.* 56:99-104.

Dreizen, S.; Bodey, G.P.; and Brown, L.R. 1978. Opportunistic gram-negative bacillary infections in leukemia: oral manifestations during myelosuppression. *Postgrad. Med.* 55:133-39.

Dreizen, S.; Bodey, G.P.; and Rodriguez, V. 1975. Oral complications of cancer chemotherapy. *Postgrad. Med.* 58:75-82.

Dreizen, S.; McCredie, W.B.; and Keatins, M.J. et al. 1982. Oral infections associated with chemotherapy in adults with acute leukemia. *Postgrad. Med.* 71(6):133-46.

Engelmeier, R.L., and King, G.E. 1983. Complications of head and neck radiation therapy and their management. *J. Prosthet. Dent.* 49:514-22.

Ewing, J. 1926. Radiation osteitis. *ACTA Radiol.* 6:339-412.

Frank, R.M.; Herdly, J.; and Phillipe, E. 1965. Acquired dental defects and salivary gland lesions after irradiation for carcinoma. *J. Am. Dent. Assoc.* 70:868-83.

Glossary of Prosthodontic Terms. 1987. *J. Pros. Dent.* 58:6.

Gron, P. 1977. Chemistry of topical fluoride caries. *Res.* (Suppl. 1):172-204.

Hickey, A.J.; Toth, B.B.; and Lindquist, J.B. 1982. Effect of intravenous hyperalimentation and oral care on the development of oral stomatitis during cancer chemotherapy. *J. Prosthet. Dent.* 47:188-93.

Knutson, J.W.; Armstrong, W.; and Feldman, F.M. 1947. The effect of topically applied sodium fluoride and dental caries experience IV: report findings with two, four, and six applications. *Public Health Rep.* 62:425-30.

Lindquist, J.; Hickey, A.J.; and Drane, J.B. 1978. Effect of oral hygiene on stomatitis in patients receiving cancer chemotherapy. *J. Prosthet. Dent.* 40:312-14.

Mainous, G.E., and Boyne, P.J. 1974. Hyperbaric oxygen in total rehabilitation of patients with mandibular osteoradionecrosis. *Int. J. Oral Surg.* 3:297-301.

McElroy, T.H. 1984. Infection in the patient receiving chemotherapy for cancer: oral considerations. *JADA* 109:454-56.

Parel, S.M.; Bickely, H.; and Holt, G.R. et al. 1983. Prosthetic use of plastinated facial structures. *J. Prosthet. Dent.* 49:529-31.

Peterson, D.E., and Sonis, J.T. 1983. Oral complications of cancer chemotherapy: present status and future studies. *Cancer Treat. Rep.* 66:1251-56.

Rahn, A.O.; Matalon, V.; and Drake. J.B. 1968. Prosthetic evaluation of patients who have received irradiation to the head and neck region. *J. Prosthet. Dent.* 19:174-79.

Rodriguez, V. 1978. Acute infections in cancer patients. *Univ. Texas System Cancer Center News* 23:4.

Rodu, B., and Gockerman, J.P. 1983. Oral manifestations of the chronic graft-vs.-host reaction. *JAMA* 249:504-07.

Sapp, J.P. 1972. The role of the dentist in the management of patients irradiated for oral cancer. *J. Can. Dent. Assoc.* 38:104-10.

Schaaf, N.G. 1970. Color characterizing silicone rubber facial prostheses. *J. Prosthet. Dent.* 24:198-202.

Segelman, A.E., and Doku, H.C. 1978. Treatment of the oral complications of leukemia. *J. Oral Surg.* 35:469-77.

Silverman, S., and Chierici, G. 1965. Radiation therapy of oral carcinoma I: effects on oral tissues and management of the periodontium. *J. Periodontol.* 36:478-84.

Starcki, E.N., and Shannon, I.L. 1977. How critical is the interval between extraction and irradiation in patients with head and neck malignancy? *Oral Surg.* 43:333-37.

Udagama, A., and King, G.E. 1983. Mechanically retained facial prostheses: helpful or harmful? *J. Pros. Dent.* 49:85-86.

Chapter 44

ONCOLOGIC IMAGING

William R. Hendee, Ph.D.
B.J. Manaster, M.D., Ph.D.
H. Ric Harnsberger, M.D.
David G. Bragg, M.D.
William M. Thompson, M.D.
Bruce L. McClennan, M.D.

William R. Hendee, Ph.D.
Vice President for Science and Technology
American Medical Association
Chicago, Illinois

B.J. Manaster, M.D., Ph.D.
Associate Professor of Radiology
Director of Musculoskeletal Radiology
Department of Radiology
University of Utah
School of Medicine
Salt Lake City, Utah

H. Ric Harnsberger, M.D.
Associate Professor of Radiology
Department of Radiology
University of Utah
School of Medicine
Salt Lake City, Utah

David G. Bragg, M.D.
Professor and Chairman
Department of Radiology
University of Utah
School of Medicine
Salt Lake City, Utah

William M. Thompson, M.D.
Professor and Chairman
Department of Radiology
University of Minnesota Medical School
Minneapolis, Minnesota

Bruce L. McClennan, M.D.
Professor of Radiology
Director, Abdominal Imaging Section
Mallinckroist Institute of Radiology
St. Louis, Missouri

PART I: STATE OF THE ART

INTRODUCTION

The clinical imaging of cancer has progressed dramatically over the past two decades. Before then, oncologic imaging depended principally on traditional x-ray techniques. In several regions of the body, tumors were difficult to visualize in early stages of development. For some cancers, ultrasound (US) occasionally was helpful, as was nuclear medicine; but nuclear medicine was generally more useful as a tool for detection of liver, lung, and bone metastases once cancer had been diagnosed by other means.

In the early 1970s, computed tomography (CT) was introduced into clinical medicine and revolutionized the field of diagnostic imaging, including that applicable to oncology. The technology offered several clinical advantages that complemented traditional imaging methods. For the first time, x-ray images of the cross-sectional anatomy of patients were available. These images revealed subtle differences in tissue densities that had been undetectable by traditional imaging methods, especially in the brain, where conventional x-ray techniques were not very helpful. Computed tomography greatly enhanced the physician's ability to visualize tumors in a variety of organs and tissues. Frequently, with CT the physician could detect and verify the presence of cancer to a greater degree of certainty than had been possible before.

Computed tomography offered other advances beyond its ability to reveal subtle differences in tissue densities. It employed the principle of reconstruction mathematics in computing images from thousands of measurements of x-ray transmission through the body. These computations required the use of a digital computer to convert the transmission measurements into computed attenuation coefficients that could be displayed as gray-scale cross-sectional images of the body. Computed tomography was the first general application of computers to diagnostic imaging, and it opened the way for application of this technology to other imaging methods.

Following the lead of computed tomography in the use of computers as an integral part of the imaging process, nuclear medicine quickly moved into the arena of physiological imaging. Through the use of computers, real-time and gray-scale ultrasound imaging quickly followed, as did digital subtraction angiography and, more recently, digital radiography. In the early 1980s, magnetic resonance imaging (MRI) was developed by applying the techniques of reconstruction mathematics to produce images from radiofrequency signals elicited from the body. Similar applications in nuclear medicine led to the techniques of single photon emission computed tomography (SPECT) and positron emission tomography (PET). Potential imaging techniques utilizing measurements of the electrical waves (electroencephalographic imaging) and magnetic waves (magnetoencephalographic imaging) of the brain, are being explored. Diagnostic imaging, including its use in oncology, has been forever changed by these technologies, all pioneered by the introduction of computed tomography.

Possibilities for improved cancer detection and diagnosis are no longer limited exclusively by imaging technology. They also now challenge our fundamental understanding of how cancers arise and evolve, and how this understanding can be exploited to produce images at an earlier stage in a cancer's development. In addition, they challenge our understanding of how physicians detect subtle abnormalities in images, and how physicians interpret those findings to arrive at diagnoses. Finally, they force the issue of how accurately diagnoses can be made, and how the accuracy can be verified efficiently for new technologies and procedures.

These are among the frontiers of research for the next decade of diagnostic imaging—including its applications to the detection of cancer.

DETECTION OF CANCER

A promising area of basic research in oncologic imaging is that of tagged antibodies. During the course of a cancer's development, distinctive tumor antigens are produced by the cancer cells. Frequently, these antigens are present on the surfaces of the cancer cells and are accessible to agents that bind to the antigens (Woo et al. 1988). Receptor antigens of cancer cells include carcinoembryonic antigens (CEAs) characteristic of colon, lung, breast, and pancreatic tumors (AMA 1988); interleukin-2 receptors of malignant T-cells (Uchiyama, Brodor, and Waldmann 1981); transferrin receptors found in a variety of tumor cells (Goding and Burns 1981); and epidermal growth factor (EGF) receptors found in several others (Masui, Moroyama, and Mendelsohn 1981). The latter receptors attract growth factors secreted by tumors to stimulate the growth of cancer cells.

Antibodies are substances produced by the body to react with antigens in an effort to neutralize them. Each antibody is designed to react with one or more of the seemingly endless variety of antigens present in nature; millions of different antibodies are possible (Hendee 1985). The research challenge is the identification and production of a single antibody that targets a single antigen in a predictable and reproducible manner. If this challenge could be met, then the antibody could be tagged with radioactivity and administered to the patient. After enough time had elapsed to permit the antibody to react with the antigen, a nuclear medicine study could be performed to determine the location of the radioactive antibody. Dense concentrations of radioactivity would reflect the presence of antigens, and therefore cancer cells.

The specificity of antibodies for antigens was improved greatly by Kohler's and Milstein's development of the technique for producing monoclonal antibodies (Kohler and Milstein 1975). This technique involves the fusion (hybridization) of a mouse lymphocyte with a mouse myeloma cell to yield a hybrid cell line (hybridoma) with several desirable properties, including the reproductive characteristics and indefinite life span of a cancer cell (contributed by the myeloma cell), and the production of a specific antibody (contributed by the lymphocyte). Once a hybridoma is identified that produces a desired monoclonal antibody, it can be isolated and grown indefinitely and continuously in culture, or be injected into the peritoneal cavity of a mouse to produce ascitic fluid containing large amounts of the antibody (Alazraki and Taylor 1988). Hence, an ongoing supply of antibody can be produced once it is isolated and identified as specific for a particular tumor antigen.

A single cancer cell may have up to one million antigen sites on its surface, and a cubic millimeter of tumor may contain a million or more cancer cells. Consequently, the potential exists theoretically for tagging a microscopic cancer with up to a trillion radioactive antibodies. If each antibody contains a single radioactive atom of technetium 99m (^{99m}Tc), this potential translates to almost a millicurie (37 million becquerels) of radioactivity per cubic millimeter of cancer. For several reasons, this theoretical potential cannot be realized in practice. If only 1/1000 of the potential is realized, however, the possible advantages for cancer detection with monoclonal antibodies are exciting.

Targeting a cancer with an antibody is not easy. The shedding of antigens from cancer cells into the general circulation traps the antibodies and prevents them from reaching the tumor. Also, antibodies may cross-react with antigens in other tissues, creating high background activities and confusing images. Tumors tend to be heterogeneous, with some cancer cells containing high concentrations of antigens and others having significantly lower concentrations. In some situations, labeling antibodies with radioactivity may diminish their reactivity with tumor antigens.

Monoclonal antibodies have been produced for several types of cancer; however, their use for cancer detection so far has focused principally on malignant melanoma (Brown et al. 1981; Larson et al. 1985; Halpern, Dillman, and Hagen 1983; Murray et al. 1987). In these studies, antibody fragments rather than whole antibodies usually are used to reduce the body's tendency to produce its own antibodies in response to administered antibodies. Both iodine 131 and indium 111 have been used as the radioactive tag for the antibody fragments, with indium 111 offering favorable gamma rays (174 keV and 247 keV) compared to iodine 131 for imaging nuclear medicine. Antibodies for a variety of other tumor antigens are being studied as possible imaging agents.

More knowledge is needed about cancer cells' expression of antigens and affinity for antibody accumulation. Furthermore, additional insight is needed into the production of antibodies with greater sensitivity and specificity for tumor antigens. These needs will be satisfied through basic research into the characteristics of tumor cells and their immunologic properties. This level of research offers a frontier of great promise for future developments in oncologic imaging.

UNDERSTANDING THE DIAGNOSTIC PROCESS

Radiology involves the detection and diagnosis of disease and injury from images of anatomic structures and physiologic and metabolic processes in the body. These images are visual patterns that reveal information about the underlying conditions of health, disease, and injury to the patient. For optimal conversion of patterns into information, images should be presented in a manner closely matched to the sensitivity characteristics of the human visual system. These characteristics are poorly understood at present.

Although conventional film radiography continues to be an important imaging technology in medicine, every current method of imaging can provide digital information, and digital expression of radiologic data is sure to expand in the future. Digital information can be smoothed, sharpened, inverted, reversed, contrast-enhanced, and "windowed" to yield images with almost any desired set of visual characteristics. Because so little is known about the human visual process, however, it is difficult to say what images are of greatest use to the radiologist.

Various models have been proposed to describe the human visual system. These models can be generalized into three categories: the signal-to-noise model, the computational model, and the signal channel model (Hendee 1988). Each of these models fits certain visual tasks. The signal channel model is the most general and is favored today by most researchers studying the psychophysics of vision.

The *signal-to-noise model* describes the ability of an observer to extract simple signals from a uniform visual background. The model proposes an "ideal observer" who can detect signals that differ from background by some amount (e.g., a factor of 4 in amplitude). Under these simplistic conditions, the performance of an actual observer can be compared to the ideal in an effort to understand how the human functions as an observer of visual patterns. Using this approach, several investigators have shown that human performance often differs substantially from the ideal, especially when the patterns to be interpreted are complex. These results suggest that the processes of detecting and interpreting visual signals are substantially more complex than those incorporated into the signal-to-noise model.

The *computational model* proposes that the first stage in "seeing" an image is the rapid assembly of visual stimuli into a "primal sketch" of the visual scene. This sketch is then refined into a complete image by comparison to *a priori* knowledge about the scene and identification of further information in the image. The computational model is an interesting theoretical concept, but has been of limited practical significance to date. Current understanding of psychophysical processes of human vision are simply too rudimentary to permit the evolution of this approach into a satisfactory working model.

In the *signal channel model*, the visual system is presumed to consist of different parallel channels for receiving visual information, with each channel "tuned" to a specific frequency range of information. In this manner, information about the visual scene (e.g., shape, color, size, contrast, and orientation) is acquired simultaneously through a network of parallel receptivity channels. This model has been reasonably successful in predicting the response of observers to visual scenes containing relatively complex information. It also has contributed to an increased appreciation of the importance of contrast sensitivity of the eye to detection of subtle details in images.

These models do not completely describe the process of detection, the simplest of the stages of evaluating visual information. The procedures for recognizing and then interpreting detected information are far more complex and poorly understood. All of these processes are used in arriving at a medical diagnosis from review of diagnostic images. That is to say, these processes are pivotal to the interpretive procedure in radiology, and further understanding of them is essential to improving this procedure.

Radiology is a difficult discipline to learn, in part because the range of information is so great, and in part because it requires intimate knowledge of the technology of radiology matched with detailed knowledge of anatomy, physiology, metabolism, and, increasingly, biochemistry. Superimposed on these requirements is the need to understand how radiologic diagnoses are arrived at, especially in circumstances where various imaging techniques are combined with other information about the patient. Currently, the student is taught radiology through an apprentice relationship with experienced radiologists; the student learns by "doing radiology" under the guidance of those experienced in the discipline. This approach is an inefficient way to teach and learn. However, improved understanding of the cognitive aspects of radiology is required before the apprentice method can be replaced by more efficient approaches. To satisfy this requirement, an enhanced research effort is being applied to studies of the psychophysics of vision and the interpretation of visual patterns.

VERIFICATION OF EFFECTIVENESS

The evolution of diagnostic imaging methods that depict subtle tissue abnormalities enhances the likelihood that these abnormalities can be detected and intercepted early enough to reduce the mortality and morbidity associated with a variety of diseases. These methods also increase the possibilities for using imaging methods and related techniques for screening asymptomatic individuals for cancer and other diseases. For example, several professional organizations have recommended x-ray mammography as a routine screening technique for early detection of breast cancer. As another example, measurements of x-ray absorption in selected skeletal areas have been proposed as an effective screening method for early detection of osteoporosis. The use of chest x-ray examinations for detecting lung cancer in asymptomatic males with a history of cigarette smoking has also been investigated. Ultrasonic searches for prostatic cancer are being explored as potential screening methods. Further improvements in imaging techniques will lead to new techniques for cancer screening. The use of imaging methods to detect and verify the presence of suspected cancers in symptomatic patients also is likely to expand in the future (Seidman et al. 1987; Tabar and Dean 1987). This enthusiasm for these techniques should be accompanied by thorough analysis of their clinical- and cost-effectiveness, and of their ultimate contribution to reduced mortality and morbidity from cancer.

Evaluation of the clinical impact and cost-effectiveness of imaging technologies is not an easy task. Five criteria have been proposed for the evaluation of any new medical technology. All five criteria must be satisfied by a technology before its ultimate value can be determined. These criteria are described below in terms of an imaging technology (Russell 1983):

1. *Information.* A new technology might be judged useful if it contributes information that is not obtainable by existing imaging methods. This information might consist of images that yield new ways of looking at tissue properties, or improved images of tissue properties that are accessible by more traditional methods. "Prettier" pictures available with a new technology satisfy this criterion only if they convey new information or present the same information with a greater degree of certainty. The criterion is not satisfied by a technology that presents "nicer" images but no new information or no improvement in confidence in the information.

2. *Diagnosis.* A new technology must not only present new or improved information; it must also lead to an improvement in diagnostic accuracy. This criterion can be evaluated only by comparison of the new technology to a standard of diagnosis. In oncologic imaging, this standard should be a surgical biopsy or some other well-accepted method of diagnosis. The standard could be another imaging technique only if the accuracy of that technique has been well established by comparison to a standard.

3. *Therapeutic impact.* A new technology that improves diagnostic accuracy is helpful only if it influences the patient's treatment following diagnosis. It is of little value if it improves the differential diagnosis for a condition that is approached with a universal treatment protocol regardless of the differential diagnosis. It should be recognized that an improved diagnosis may lead ultimately to improvements in therapy, even if no changes in the therapeutic approach are available immediately.

4. *Patient improvement.* A diagnostic technology may be of little value even if it affects patient treatment, if the treatment has little impact on the patient's overall well-being. Impact on morbidity and mortality are the ultimate goals of therapy, and they should also be the ultimate goals of any new diagnostic technology proposed for adoption. A diagnostic technology could satisfy this criterion if it yields the same therapeutic outcome, but produces less morbidity than alternate diagnostic strategies. For example, computed tomography is preferred over pneumoencephalography, in part because it produces less patient morbidity during the diagnostic process.

5. *Cost-effectiveness.* If the other four criteria are satisfied, then an imaging technology should be evaluated in terms of cost-effectiveness before it is implemented clinically (Eddy et al. 1988). Resources for health care are not unlimited, and wise decisions are required to utilize these resources to provide optimum health benefits for the greatest number of people. For example, widespread adoption of a screening technique that detects cancer early and reduces morbidity and

mortality in a small number of patients may not be economically justifiable if it replaces another public health measure that would provide a similar health benefit to a larger number of people.

Evaluation of an oncologic imaging procedure by these criteria is a considerable challenge to researchers in radiology that has not always been addressed satisfactorily. With increasing cost constraints facing health care, the presence of this challenge will become increasingly apparent. Evaluation of new technologies in radiology according to these criteria represents a fruitful area of investigation for radiology researchers.

CONCLUSIONS

Oncologic imaging has experienced spectacular successes in research breakthroughs and clinical improvements over the past two decades. This evolution in the technology of imaging applied to cancer detection and diagnosis promises to continue beyond this decade, provided that attention is devoted to an improved understanding of the science of oncology, the diagnostic process, and the evaluation of imaging technologies. Each of these areas presents challenges to the radiologist that can be met only if the dedication to research in radiology continues.

PART II: MUSCULOSKELETAL TUMOR IMAGING

INTRODUCTION

Most tertiary centers prefer to do their own radiographic workups and biopsies for three reasons. First, the radiographic workup should be tailored to the individual patient and be designed to answer specific questions; all available imaging modalities need not be used in each case. Second, computed tomography (CT) or magnetic resonance (MR) after biopsy can be at best confusing, and at worst drastically misleading, due to bleeding or edema. Finally, an incorrectly planned biopsy on either a bony- or soft-tissue lesion may convert a case calling for limb salvage to one requiring amputation.

MUSCULOSKELETAL TUMOR IMAGING

A properly tailored radiographic workup is essential to adequate treatment of musculoskeletal lesions. Before operation, musculoskeletal tumors cannot always be correctly labeled histologically; but they should be identified as belonging to one of the following categories:

1. A benign "leave me alone" lesion that it is best to ignore;
2. A lesion that is almost certainly benign and can safely be "watched" for confirmation of the diagnosis;
3. A benign symptomatic lesion to be treated with elective surgery and no further workup;

4. A lesion with uncertain diagnosis regarding its benign or malignant nature; and
5. A clearly malignant lesion that requires a preoperative radiologic workup followed by surgery for confirmation of histology and definitive treatment.

If the lesion belongs to either category 4 or 5, the next step is to stage the tumor; Enneking (1985) developed a staging methodology that is accepted in the orthopaedic community. This system uses both histologic and radiographic information and serves as a guideline for both prognosis and treatment. The radiographic features of the staging system include site; encapsulated or not encapsulated; intra- or extracompartmental, with compartments defined as subcutaneous, parosseous, bone, and muscle; involvement of major neurovascular structures; and metastatic disease (usually by hematogenous spread to lung or, occasionally, to bone). The information used in this system is similar to that used for the American Joint Committee on Cancer's clinical staging recommendations (1983).

The biopsy site should also be guided by the radiographic workup. The biopsy must include the most aggressive, viable portion of the lesion; this region is typically somewhat peripheral, since the center of an aggressive lesion may be necrotic. The biopsy, whether percutaneous or open, should be planned so that the site can be included during the definitive surgical procedure. Vital tissue planes must not be compromised by possible tumor spill during biopsy, and skin needed to close over the resected area must also not be violated. The biopsy should be within a single compartment and should not approach neurovascular structures.

Once surgical staging is accomplished, surgical treatment options must be considered. Communication between the surgeon and radiologist is essential so that the correct questions are addressed and answered by the diagnostic procedures. For example, if amputation is the only surgical option, the workup need only be directed toward defining the proximal extent of the lesion. If, on the other hand, limb salvage is considered, both proximal and distal extent of bone and muscle involvement must be determined, as well as involvement of the vital neurovascular structures.

Bearing in mind the need to arrive at a logical differential diagnosis, and the need to assist in biopsy and treatment planning, the radiographic workup should begin with plain film (see fig. 44.1). This is the best method for assessing bone detail and aggressiveness of the lesion. Several determinants are assessed in order to arrive at the correct diagnosis, or at least to properly categorize the lesion. These determinants include the age of the patient, soft-tissue involvement, pattern of bone destruction (geographic vs. permeative), location of the lesion (which particular bone is involved, as well as the site of involvement along the long and axial axes of that bone), zone of transition from abnormal to normal bone, and size of lesion. The nature of the lesion is often diagnosed on the plain film using

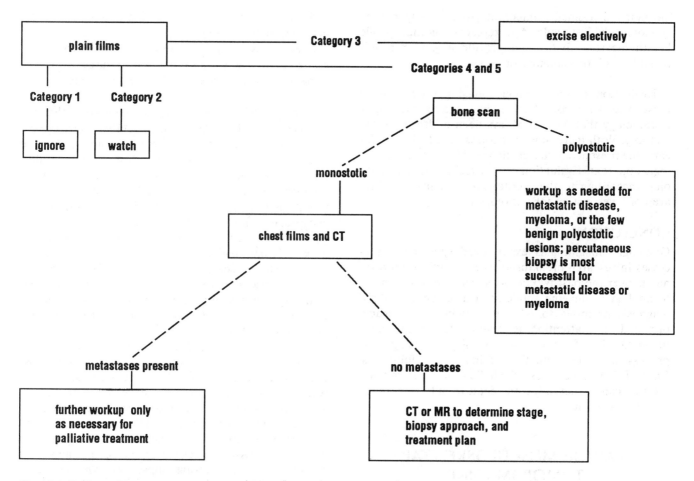

Fig. 44.1. Radiographic workup for musculoskeletal lesions begins with plain films.

these parameters. For example, in a child, a destructive lesion in the metaphysis of a long bone that produces bone matrix is an osteosarcoma, while a similarly destructive lesion in the diaphysis of a long bone that produces only reactive sclerosis has a high probability of being Ewing's sarcoma. Location of the lesion is extremely important in other diagnoses. For example, giant-cell tumor is often subarticular and chondroblastoma is virtually always epiphyseal in location. If definite histologic diagnosis is not achieved, the determinants are extremely helpful in assessing whether further workup is required.

If the lesion on plain film corresponds to category 4 or 5, the next study should be a bone scan: ^{99m}Tc MDP scans are used primarily to determine whether a lesion is monostotic or polyostotic. A polyostotic lesion is more likely to represent metastatic disease or myeloma, though a few benign bone lesions may be polyostotic, and occasionally a malignant primary bone lesion will metastasize to bone. The degree of abnormal uptake does not correlate with histologic grade of the lesion; the extent of the bone lesion may also not be accurately reflected by the bone scan.

If the lesion is monostotic by bone scan and thought to represent a primary bone tumor, posteroanterior (PA) and lateral chest films and a chest CT should be obtained to assess metastatic disease. If there are no

lung metastases, CT or MR of the lesion is obtained to determine stage, biopsy approach, and treatment plan. Both studies should not be obtained because of the high cost relative to benefit. An entirely intraosseous lesion may be examined by CT because it clearly defines both extent of lesion and matrix, whereas an entirely extraosseous lesion is far more clearly delineated by MR because of its superb soft-tissue contrast. An intraosseous lesion extending into the soft tissues may be examined by either modality, but many researchers believe that MR more easily answers the pertinent staging and surgical treatment queries (Pettersson et al. 1987). Both CT and MR are nonspecific for histology. Moreover, it is very difficult in either method to differentiate tumor from peritumoral edema; soft-tissue involvement may be overestimated.

After definitive therapy, imaging follow-up is required to monitor for tumor recurrence or complications of therapy. Radiation therapy may be complicated by tumor recurrence, infection, radiation osteonecrosis, and radiation-induced sarcomas (4 to 20 years post-therapy). Each of these complications may show destructive changes on plain film and have abnormal uptake on bone scan, and may be very difficult to differentiate from one another. Chemotherapy may be complicated by tumor recurrence and increased incidence of infection. Limb salvage with allograft may be complicated by tumor recurrence, infections, hardware or graft failure, and delayed union. It often takes up to two years for union with the graft to be demonstrated; union with vascularized fibular grafts may progress considerably faster. In general, follow-up of limb salvage cases with hardware is accomplished by plain film; exceptional circumstances should be tailored to the individual patient's problem and may require other imaging modalities. Soft tissue sarcomas are best followed by MRI.

PART III: IMAGING OF CENTRAL NERVOUS SYSTEM (CNS) NEOPLASIA

INTRODUCTION

Although central nervous system (CNS) tumors constitute only 2% of all reported cases of cancer in the United States, poor long-term survival rates accompanied by devastating clinical manifestations combine to amplify the societal impact of this relatively rare tumor group. Presenting symptoms vary from headache and nausea to more ominous ones such as seizures and hemiparesis. A diagnostic examination is needed to screen these patients into structural and non-structural groups.

Until recently, computed tomography (CT) has functioned as the primary radiologic examination used to detect the presence of intracranial neoplasm. Early CNS neoplasia that did not cause mass effect or blood-brain barrier leak were not detected by CT. Larger tumors in the posterior fossa and lower temporal lobes of the brain occasionally remained hidden from CT's view.

Magnetic resonance imaging (MRI) has now become the imaging modality of choice for detection of CNS neoplasia. As a tool exquisitely sensitive to abnormal foci of brain water, MR is able to detect tumors in the early, subcentimeter size range. The goals of diagnostic imaging with MR in patients with intracranial tumor are early detection, stereotactic biopsy guidance, precise tumor delineation for assessment of resectability, and multiplanar images for radiation therapy port planning.

COMMON PATHOLOGY

Benign and malignant intracranial tumors are commonly divided into two broad anatomic categories, intra-axial and extra-axial; most intra-axial tumors are gliomas. Primary glial neoplasms may arise from astrocytes (astrocytoma, anaplastic astrocytoma, glioblastoma multiform); oligodendrocytes (oligodendroglioma); and ependocytes (ependymoma). Unfortunately, over one-half of glial tumors are of the more malignant glioblastoma variety. Common extra-axial tumors include meningiomas, Schwannomas, and neurofibromas. This report will focus on the imaging issues of the intra-axial glioma group only.

DETECTION AND PATHOLOGICAL DIAGNOSIS

Magnetic resonance imaging has replaced CT as the principal imaging modality for the detection of CNS tumor. Its inherent sensitivity to abnormal collections of water in the brain has allowed the identification of CNS neoplasia in the subcentimeter size range. However, this sensitivity to the presence of an abnormal area of brain is not matched by an equivalent level of specificity as to the lesion's histologic nature. The poor specificity of MR has produced an increased need for a safe means of obtaining a pathologic diagnosis from the smaller, deep lesions seen on MR. Consequently, stereotactic biopsy has become the primary technique employed to obtain tissue from these lesions. This technique has become extremely accurate, permitting the routine biopsy of 5-mm lesions.

Because MR identifies both the tumor and tumor-related edema as an abnormal signal, stereotactic biopsy for histologic diagnosis has been done with CT guidance. Gadolinium, a paramagnetic intravenous contrast agent, now permits MR to localize a biopsy site by identifying the tumor nidus as an area where the contrast leaks across an injured blood-brain barrier. A nonferromagnetic MR-compatible stereotactic biopsy frame used in conjunction with gadolinium permits both detection and pathologic diagnosis to be completed in the MR suite.

TREATMENT AND FOLLOW-UP

Multiplanar images of near-precise tumor margins seen on MR help the neurosurgeon decide if the tumor can be resected for cure. Fewer attempts are now made at curative surgery as a result of MR's ability to predict tumor involvement of brain, which, if resected, would result in severe impairment or death of the patient.

Stereotactic biopsy is now usually followed by external beam or implant radiation therapy. The graphic delineation of tumor margins depicted on the sagittal and coronal MR scan planes allows the MR information to be precisely translated onto external beam radiation therapy simulation films. Both the stereotactic technology and the three-dimensional anatomic information available from MR multiplanar images have greatly improved radiation therapy implant techniques.

Once detection and treatment of the CNS neoplasm is completed, follow-up imaging becomes important, given the propensity of this tumor to recur. A follow-up, post-treatment, baseline gadolinium-enhanced MR scan or enhanced CT scan at three to six months is recommended. This baseline MR or CT study allows differentiation of radiation change from recurrent tumor by providing a comparison image to decide if the lesion has grown. Any increase in size of the lesion or extent of gadolinium (MR) or iodinated contrast (CT) enhancement of the nidus can then be construed to represent tumor recurrence. Even with the use of baseline MR or CT scans, it may at times be impossible to differentiate recurrent tumor from treatment-related changes.

SUMMARY

Gadolinium-enhanced MR serves as the pivotal diagnostic imaging examination in the detection and follow-up of primary brain tumor (fig. 44.2). Information derived from multiplanar MR images directs stereotactic biopsy, surgery, and radiation treatment of CNS neoplasia.

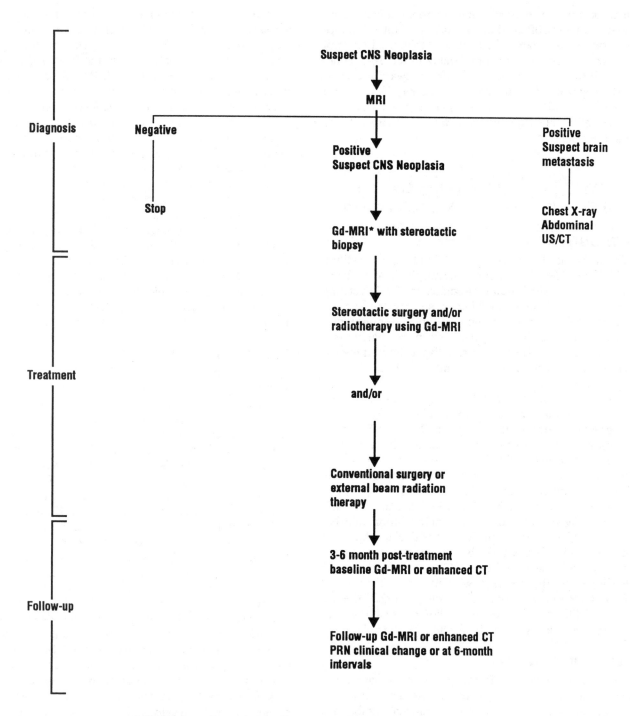

* Gadolinium-enhanced magnetic resonance imaging

Fig. 44.2. Decision tree in central nervous system neoplasia. (Adapted with permission from: Bragg and Harnsberger [1985].)

PART IV: IMAGING IN EXTRACRANIAL HEAD AND NECK MALIGNANCY

INTRODUCTION

The principal tumor type found in the extracranial head and neck is squamous cell carcinoma (SCC). Originating on the mucosal surfaces of the upper aerodigestive tract, SCC spreads along both mucosal and deep-tissue planes. Often the surgeon's mucosal appraisal of primary tumor stage will not objectively represent tumor extent because the deep-tissue aspects of the tumor may not be visible or palpable. However, combining the surgeon's endoscopic assessment of the mucosal extent of primary SCC with the deep-tissue extent as defined by CT or MRI renders an accurate pre-treatment tumor stage.

Both CT and MRI are effective in addressing the clinical problem of primary and nodal SCC staging.

Each modality graphically delineates the precise deep-tissue anatomy of the extracranial head and neck. The choice of examination for staging of SCC in this region of the body should be based on the radiologist's expertise, modality availability, and relative cost. In addition to SCC primary and nodal tumor staging, CT or MR can help to solve the clinical-radiologic problems of recurrent tumor evaluation, "unknown primary" search, and treatment assessment.

STAGING OF PRIMARY SCC WITH CT OR MRI

Primary tumor classification (T) for SCC used by the American Joint Committee on Cancer is based on the size and anatomic extent of the tumor mass. The clinician bases this T-stage estimation on his or her impression of the tumor from inspection and palpation. Treatment decisions are based entirely on this clinical impression unless CT or MR is done to examine more thoroughly the tumor's deep-tissue extent.

Tumor below the mucous membrane and tumor in areas difficult to palpate, such as the high oropharynx and nasopharynx, often will have more extensive deep-tissue components than suspected from clinical examination. Computed tomography findings in patients with T2 or greater SCC have been shown to alter treatment planning up to 25% of the time as a result of identifying unsuspected deep-tissue tumor. The objective information on deep-tissue extent of tumor obtained from CT or MR, in combination with the objective mucosal extent derived from endoscopic examination, provides the most accurate pretreatment staging assessment (fig. 44.3). Armed with a clear understanding of tumor stage, the clinician can make educated treatment decisions.

The application of CT or MR to each primary site in the head and neck is beyond the scope of this section. However, in each of the common primary sites of the extracranial head and neck, radiologic examination poses specific questions that can help provide the clearest picture of the primary tumor. The answers to these site-specific questions direct the patient's treatment-decision algorithm.

STAGING OF NODAL SCC WITH CT OR MRI

The detection of nodal metastases at the time of presentation of primary SCC in the head and neck will affect both the mode of treatment and the patient's general prognosis. The overall 5-year survival for patients with malignant adenopathy at tumor presentation is less than 30%, regardless of primary tumor location. Obviously, it is important that an objective nodal stage (N) exist prior to initial treatment.

Simultaneous primary tumor (T) and nodal (N) staging can be done with either CT or MRI. Radiologic criteria for the diagnosis of malignant adenopathy include a lymph node greater than or equal to 1.5 cm in size and/or any lymph node with central inhomogeneity (mixed density on CT and mixed intensity on MR) regardless of size. Extranodal tumor can be diagnosed when the soft-tissue planes around the abnormal lymph node are obscured. When imaging is done methodically, radiologic evaluation will change clinical nodal stage in 15% to 20% of cases.

Radiologic and clinical nodal staging are limited by their lack of tissue specificity and reliance on size criteria for the diagnosis of malignant adenopathy. Reactive hyperplasia enlarges lymph nodes as well, although only rarely greater than 1.5 cm. Fine-needle aspiration biopsy can be used in selected cases to minimize false-positive results. Small tumor deposits in normal-size nodes will not be appreciated by clinical or radiologic examination.

RECURRENT TUMOR EVALUATION

The treated patient with new symptoms is clinically difficult to evaluate because dermal fibrosis and underlying treatment-related soft-tissue plane disturbance prevent adequate physical examination. CT or MR "sees through" these barriers, often diagnosing recurrent tumor when it cannot be seen or felt. In about 25% of cases of clinically suspected tumor recurrence, radiologic examination will be the only method of diagnosing recurrence. In one-third of patients in whom the recurrent tumor is clinically apparent, radiologic evaluation will show the recurrence to be more extensive than appreciated by clinical examination alone.

Radiologic examination in the setting of suspected or apparent recurrent SCC of the head and neck has both a diagnostic role and a part in planning salvage surgery and radiation therapy. The best results with follow-up scanning are found when a post-treatment baseline scan is available for comparison purposes. In patients with an initial tumor with known high recurrence rates or poor surgical results, this baseline scan is best obtained at three to six months after treatment. With this scan in hand, a clinician can separate any development of a mass from treatment changes and identify the growth as recurrent tumor.

THE SEARCH FOR THE UNKNOWN (OCCULT) PRIMARY TUMOR

A patient with an unknown primary tumor is not defined as a patient with malignant adenopathy by needle-aspiration biopsy, but as one with a clinically occult primary tumor. These patients represent a small but problematic group, and radiologic evaluation with CT or MR can be of great assistance. Three possible situations exist in a patient with an occult SCC in the head and neck: the primary tumor site is very small, it has regressed after metastasizing to the cervical lymph nodes, or it is primarily submucosal and hidden from view. Radiologic evaluation will be helpful in the latter situation.

The goals of scanning a patient with an occult primary tumor are to identify the occult tumor, to suggest suspicious areas for deep-tissue biopsy at the time of endoscopy, and to stage (N) the nodal disease in the neck. Special attention must be given to the nasopharynx, faucial and lingual tonsils, and the pyriform sinus areas, as these are the common sites in which occult SCC is found.

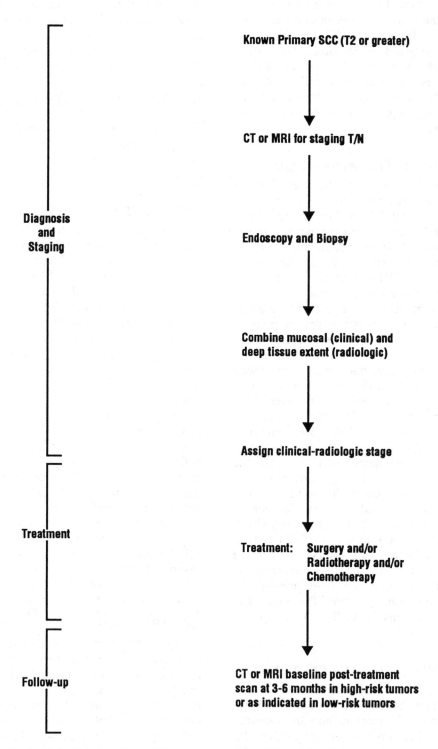

Diagnosis and Staging

Known Primary SCC (T2 or greater)

↓

CT or MRI for staging T/N

↓

Endoscopy and Biopsy

↓

Combine mucosal (clinical) and deep tissue extent (radiologic)

↓

Assign clinical-radiologic stage

Treatment

Treatment: Surgery and/or Radiotherapy and/or Chemotherapy

↓

Follow-up

CT or MRI baseline post-treatment scan at 3-6 months in high-risk tumors or as indicated in low-risk tumors

Fig. 44.3. Imaging decision algorithm in patients with head and neck squamous cell carcinoma. (Adapted with permission from: Bragg and Harnsberger [1985].)

PART V: IMAGING IN LUNG CANCER

INTRODUCTION

With more than 150,000 new cases of lung cancer estimated in the United States for 1990, this disease represents the most common cause of cancer mortality in both males and females. No screening technique can as yet satisfactorily detect lung cancer at an early enough stage to effect improved survivals. Chest radiography represents the mainstay in diagnosis, even though physicians are unable to consistently and accurately identify the lung cancer until its size approaches 1 cubic centimeter, by which time it is already late in its natural history. The National Lung Cancer Trial Programs determined that the majority of both peripheral and central lung cancers could be recognized in retrospect on earlier 4-month screening radiographs, in some instances for as long as two years (Fontana et al. 1984). The present goals for diagnostic imaging in the patient with lung cancer should address the issue of recognizing the primary tumor site, accurately defining mediastinal node involvement, and defining symptomatic extrathoracic metastatic sites of disease.

PRIMARY LUNG CANCER

At present, chest radiographic screening of patients at high risk for the development of primary lung cancer is not recommended. Nonetheless, the chest radiograph is the most effective technique currently available for the detection process and is complemented by sputum cytology in the patient with central lung cancer. The World Health Organization (WHO) recognizes four basic histologic types of primary lung cancers: squamous cell carcinoma, adenocarcinoma (including bronchioloaveolar cell carcinoma), and large-cell and small-cell anaplastic cancers. Squamous cell and small-cell anaplastic tumors (including oat cell cancers) usually present initially as central lung cancers (occurring in the inner third of the lung, adjacent to the hilum). Adenocarcinomas and large-cell anaplastic carcinomas (some researchers believe these tumors are alike) share the same tendency for a peripheral location (developing in the outer third of the lung). Small-cell anaplastic carcinomas are usually disseminated at the time of presentation, so staging discussions should separate primary lung cancers into nonsmall-cell and small-cell carcinomas.

There are no pathognomonic plain film characteristics of primary lung cancers. The most common presenting features are those of a noncalcified, solitary nodular lesion in the lung with an ill-defined outer margin. Squamous cell cancers have a greater tendency to cavitate, a feature rarely found with adenocarcinomas and small-cell anaplastic tumors.

Technical factors necessary for adequate chest x-ray screening should include high kilovoltage chest x-rays that allow better penetration, shorter radiographic exposure times, and improved nodule detection. Previous chest radiographs are essential in recognizing significant change. They are often the only means by which the subtle, slow growth characteristic of non-oat cell primary lung cancers can be identified. Any solitary nodular lesion in a person at risk for lung cancer should be presumed to represent a primary lung cancer until proven otherwise. Initial confirmation should include fluoroscopy or a shallow, oblique, repeat chest x-ray to confirm intrathoracic location of the nodule and absence of any intrinsic calcifications—a radiographic hallmark of benign disease. If a nodular lesion has not changed in size over a period of more than two years, it can be safely assumed to be benign (Bragg, Rubin, and Youker 1985).

The use of CT in verification and characterization of the solitary pulmonary nodule has been the subject of considerable debate. In some opinions, CT seldom helps to further characterize the solitary pulmonary nodule; however,

recent articles can be reviewed to further explore this technique (Siegelman et al. 1986; Zerhouni et al. 1986).

IMAGING FOR PRETREATMENT STAGING

The primary goal of imaging in staging the lung cancer patient prior to definitive treatment should be the avoidance of unnecessary surgical morbidity, mortality, and expense. Another goal should be the definition of radiation-therapy treatment ports, if that therapeutic modality is indicated.

Physicians dealing with the patient at risk for primary lung cancer should be familiar with the new International Staging System for Lung Cancer, modified in 1986 (Mountain 1986). This system is based on the T, N, and M system and subsequent stage groupings based on these categories. In most instances, the plain chest x-ray can adequately define the T-compartment, and a physician can make an assessment based on the size of the tumor, or its proximity to a lobar bronchus, the carina, the chest wall, and the mediastinum. Computed tomography (CT) is the best means of assessing the nodal or N-compartment. The plain chest x-ray can only recognize grossly enlarged nodes; the x-ray will only have a sensitivity of approximately 50%, yet will be quite specific when the findings are abnormal. Computed tomography (CT) and magnetic resonance imaging (MRI) both utilize the enlarged node (>1 cm) as the nonspecific criterion for abnormality. Lymph nodes detected as abnormal by CT or MRI must be histologically verified prior to assuming they are involved by the lung cancer (Baron et al. 1988; Staples et al. 1988). The recent MRI consensus conference reported that MRI had no imaging advantage over CT in staging lung cancer, with the possible exception of definition of chest wall and mediastinal invasion (Marx 1987).

The primary goals of imaging techniques in the staging of the nodal compartment are to identify abnormally enlarged lymph nodes, which need further verification through biopsy; to find no enlarged lymph nodes and allow the patient to proceed directly to thoracotomy, avoiding mediastinal exploration prior to anticipated surgical resection; to plan treatment; to recognize additional, unsuspected lung nodules suggesting the lesion may be metastatic rather than primary; and to define invasion of the chest wall or mediastinum (both of these tasks are difficult challenges with both CT and MRI). Evaluation of the hilum is relatively unimportant, as the presence or absence of hilar nodal disease does not preclude surgery, but merely modifies the surgical approach. Metastatic involvement of lymph nodes in the mediastinum that are less than 10 mm in size by CT or MR is reported to occur in approximately 7% to 10% of cases (Baron et al. 1982), even though normal lymph-node size varies inversely with the distance of the lymph node from the pulmonary hilum. The positive predictive value of the enlarged lymph node containing cancer therefore increases in size.

In the patient with non-oat cell cancer, random extrathoracic imaging in search of metastatic involvement in the asymptomatic patient with normal laboratory findings is not justified. In the patient with small-cell anaplastic cancer, however, imaging of the brain, liver, and skeleton usually is indicated.

Imaging techniques as applied to the treated patient with primary lung cancer must be tailored to the tumor histology and the mode of treatment. Specific recommendations are beyond the scope of this section.

IMAGING REQUIREMENTS IN METASTATIC LUNG CANCER

The two most common radiologic-pathologic patterns of metastatic pulmonary parenchymal disease are hematogenous or nodular metastases and lymphangitic spread of tumor. It is believed that, in both instances, the blood-borne route is the pathway of spread to the lung, regardless of the pattern of tumor expression.

Hematogenous lesions are usually represented by a nodular pattern; the nodules are more numerous and sizable in the dependent portion of the lung, corresponding to the zone of greatest perfusion. Metastatic lesions from sarcomas are generally sharply outlined, as the host lung parenchyma does not react to their presence. These deposits are usually found in a subpleural location upon CT evaluation and pathologic examination. Metastatic adenocarcinomas are more often poorly defined and outlined on both radiologic and pathologic examination.

Lymphangitic metastatic lesions are difficult to identify specifically on plain chest x-rays. The manifestations of lymphangitic spread are secondary to an increase in the linear pattern in the lung as a reflection of distention of the parenchymal lymphatics; occasionally there is an ill-defined nodular pattern, pleural effusions, and enlargement of the central, hilar lymph nodes.

Computed tomography is useful in the identification and characterization of metastatic pulmonary disease. This technique will allow far more nodular metastatic lesions to be detected, and it is able to more accurately access the character of the often nonspecific plain-film findings in lymphangitic tumor spread. The CT criteria of lymphangitic tumor spread typically involves the bronchovascular bundles and the peripheral portion of the lung (Munk et al. 1988).

Rarely, a patient will initially present with radiographic evidence of pulmonary metastases and an unknown or unidentified primary tumor site; such cases call for abbreviated clinical and radiographic workups. Biopsy confirmation of the presumed pulmonary metastases can be performed with fluoroscopic or CT guidance. In asymptomatic patients, lymphangitic metastases in women more commonly result from breast cancers. The metastases in men are almost always from primary cancers in the upper gastrointestinal tract or pancreas. Unilateral lymphangitic metastases are virtually always associated with a primary lung cancer.

In the patient with a primary tumor that is known to metastasize to the lung prior to definitive treatment, the radiologist should direct a coordinated imaging approach for the assessment of the thorax. In instances where the identification of the occult pulmonary tumor would lead to a modification of the anticipated treatment of the primary tumor, CT should be utilized in screening the lungs to detect unsuspected metastatic lesions, as well as to serve as a baseline for follow-up.

PART VI: IMAGING GASTROINTESTINAL CANCER

INTRODUCTION

The advantages and limitations of the various imaging procedures, as well as their appropriate application to detecting and staging gastrointestinal malignancies, have not been well defined. The new imaging modalities developed over the past 15 years have gone through many evolutions. The changing technology and significant differences in experience and expertise have not allowed sufficient time to evaluate these imaging modalities in the field of cancer.

This section discusses some of these problems and explains tumor detection, tumor staging, and general imaging decision trees.

GASTROINTESTINAL TRACT NEOPLASIA

Most malignant neoplasms of the gastrointestinal (GI) tract originate from the mucosa, so barium studies are sensitive in detecting these tumors (Rosenberg et al. 1985; Thompson 1983; Suzuki et al. 1972; Zornoza and Lindell 1980; Huang 1981; Wong and Goldberg 1985; Montagne, Moss, and Margulis 1978; Freeny and Marks 1982; Shirakabe and Maruyama 1983; Sindelar 1985; Sellink 1983; Herlinger 1983; Sugarbaker, Gunderson, and Wittes 1985; Otto et al. 1980; Laufer, Smith, and Mullens 1976; Laufer 1979; Evers et al. 1981; Johnson and Carlson 1983; Kelvin et al. 1981; Robbins 1979). Because of its ability to directly visualize the mucosa and to permit biopsy of suspicious lesions, some clinicians advocate fiberoptic endoscopy as the study of choice to screen the patient population at risk of developing malignancies of the esophagus, stomach, and colon (Showstack, Schroeder, and Steinberg 1981). Due to the problems of performing fiberoptic endoscopy— including patient sedation, cost, a limited number of endoscopists, and a large number of patients—single- and double-contrast barium examinations remain the most widely accepted screening procedures for GI malignancies. The overall accuracy rate for tumor detection using these barium techniques ranges from 70% to over 90% (Thompson 1983; Wong and Goldberg 1985; Montagne, Moss, and Margulis 1978; Freeny and Marks 1982; Otto et al. 1980; Laufer, Smith, and Mullens 1976; Laufer 1979; Evers et al. 1981; Johnson and Carlson 1983; Kelvin et al. 1981). A negative aspect of these statistics is that many GI tumors are detected late, when they have already metastasized. Also, the barium techniques are not efficacious in the staging of

GI tract malignancies because they rarely provide information concerning depth of tumor penetration and metastatic disease. While the cross-sectional imaging modalities (ultrasound [US], and especially computed tomography [CT]) have a relatively minor role in the detection of GI cancers, they can be important in preoperative staging and/or follow-up. The role of magnetic resonance (MR) in staging GI malignancies is still evolving.

STAGING OF GI MALIGNANCIES

The American Joint Committee Task Force has developed classification and staging systems for squamous cell and adenocarcinomas of the esophagus, adenocarcinoma of the stomach, and adenocarcinoma of the colon (American Joint Committee 1978). These tumors make up over 90% of GI cancers (Robbins 1979). No TNM staging system has been devised for tumors of the small bowel.

The current imaging modalities cannot stage tumors using the TNM system because they have a limited ability to determine the depth of bowel wall penetration, which is one of the criteria for the primary tumor, T. Also, they cannot accurately determine metastatic disease in lymph nodes, the N criterion of the TNM system. Because of these limitations a CT classification has been devised for the esophagus, stomach, and colon (tables 44.1, 44.2, and 44.3) (Moss et al. 1981a; Moss et al. 1981b; Theoni et al. 1981).

Computed tomography has been shown to be accurate in staging esophageal cancer (Moss et al. 1981a; Daffner et al. 1979; Thompson et al. 1983; Picus et al. 1983; Heiken, Balfe, and Roper 1984; Becker et al. 1987). One group reported poor results, but there were some differences in their study compared to other reports (Quint et al. 1985; Quint, Glazer, and Orringer 1985; Halvorsen and Thompson 1986). Computed tomography is the best imaging technique for following the results of therapy (Heiken, Balfe, and Roper 1984; Becker et al. 1987).

Only a limited number of clinicians have reported using CT to stage gastric cancer (Moss et al. 1981b; Moss et al. 1980; Balfe, Koehler, and Karstaedt 1981). The most recent report indicated that CT is not an accurate staging technique and, therefore, it is not needed for preoperative staging of gastric cancer (Sussman et al. 1988).

Table 44.1
CT STAGING OF ESOPHAGEAL CARCINOMA

Stage I	Intraluminal mass without wall thickening or metastases
Stage II	Thickened esophageal wall (>5 mm) without invasion of adjacent structures or distant metastases
Stage III	Thickened esophageal wall with direct extension to adjacent structures; no distant metastases but local or regional mediastinal adenopathy may or may not be present
Stage IV	Any tumor with distant metastases

(Source: Moss, Theoni, and Schnyder et al. [1981].)

Table 44.2
CT STAGING OF GASTRIC ADENOCARCINOMA

Stage I	Intraluminal gastric mass without gastric wall thickening; no evidence of local or distant metastases
Stage II	Thickened gastric wall (>1 cm) without invasion of adjacent structures or distant metastases
Stage III	Thickened gastric wall with direct extension to adjacent structures, without distant metastases
Stage IV	Any tumor with distant metastases

(Source: Moss, Schnyder, and Marks et al. [1981].)

The initial reports indicated that CT was accurate in staging colorectal cancers (Theoni et al. 1981; Ellert and Kreel 1980; Husband, Hodson, and Parsons 1980; Mayes and Zornoza 1980; Dixon et al. 1981; Zaunbauer, Haertel, and Fuchs 1981; Van Wees, Koehler, and Feldberg 1983). More recently, a number of authors (Grabbe, Lierse, and Winkler 1983; Adalsteinsson et al. 1985; Freeny et al. 1986; Thompson et al 1986) found that CT cannot accurately stage colorectal cancer preoperatively because it lacks the ability to determine the depth of bowel wall extension or to accurately detect metastases to lymph nodes. These are two major criteria of the Dukes staging system (Dukes 1938). Thus, except in special circumstances, preoperative CT is not recommended in patients with colorectal cancer. However, CT can accurately evaluate the liver, and can determine the amount of extracolonic involvement in large tumors and perforated tumors. Computed tomography is recommended as a routine follow-up procedure in rectosigmoid cancer patients (Zelas et al. 1980; Adalsteinsson et al. 1981; Moss et al. 1981; Clark et al. 1984; Butch et al. 1985; McCarthy et al 1985; Grabbe and Winkler 1985; Butch et al. 1986).

ROLE OF IMAGING PROCEDURES IN DETECTING, STAGING, AND FOLLOW-UP

A decision imaging tree for patients with suspected or known gastrointestinal malignancies is shown in fig. 44.4. This refers primarily to patients with squamous cell carcinomas of the esophagus and adenocarcinomas of the stomach, small bowel, colon, and rectum. Other GI malignancies are not included because they are rare.

The role and impact of magnetic resonance imaging in the detection and staging of GI malignancies is unknown. Initial reports have not been favorable for using MRI to examine patients with carcinoma of the

Table 44.3
CT STAGING OF PRIMARY AND RECURRENT COLON TUMORS

Stage I	Intraluminal mass without thickening of colon wall
Stage II	Thickened colon wall (>0.5 cm) or pelvic mass without invasion of adjacent structures or extension to pelvic sidewalls
Stage IIIA	Thickened colon wall or pelvic mass with invasion of adjacent structures but not to pelvic sidewalls or abdominal wall
Stage IIIB	Thickened colon wall or pelvic mass extending to pelvic sidewalls and/or abdominal wall without distant metastases
Stage IV	Metastatic disease with or without local abnormality

(Source: Theoni, Moss, and Schnyder et al. [1981].)

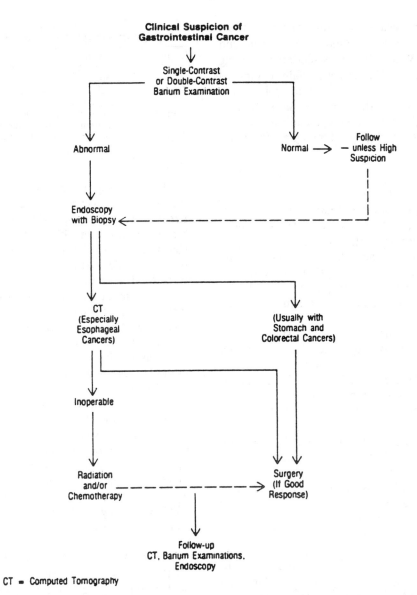

Fig. 44.4. Imaging decision tree for patients with suspected gastrointestinal malignancy: squamous cell and adenocarcinoma of the esophagus and adenocarcinoma of the stomach, small bowel, colon, and rectum. Most patients with stomach and colorectal tumors require surgery, so routine preoperative staging with CT is not recommended. CT may help define extent of small bowel tumors prior to surgery and is best for follow-up of GI tumors. (Reproduced with permission from: Thompson [1987].)

esophagus and upper gastrointestinal tract (Quint, Glazer, and Orringer 1985b). However, its inherent ability to examine the abdomen, in particular the pelvis in sagittal, coronal, and axial projections, may provide a better degree of tumor evaluation, particularly in terms of extension, than CT can determine (Butch et al. 1986).

PANCREATIC CARCINOMA

Ductal adenocarcinoma accounts for over 75% of all pancreatic malignancies (Cubilla and Fitzgerald 1979). The results of surgical treatment of this tumor are poor, and pancreatic carcinoma does not respond well to other forms of therapy (Hermann and Cooperman 1979; Sindelar, Kinsolla, and Mayer 1985). The operative mortality for both partial and total pancreatectomy has averaged 20%, with a 5-year survival rate of only 4% (Sindelar, Kinsolla, and

Mayer 1985). Despite advances in pancreatic imaging and early diagnosis, overall survival of patients with pancreatic carcinoma has not increased (Sindelar, Kinsolla, and Mayer 1985). However, the combination of the new imaging modalities coupled with percutaneous fine-needle aspiration biopsy (FNAB) has dramatically diminished the time required to establish the diagnosis (Lawson, Berland, and Foley 1985; Clark et al. 1985; Freeny and Ball 1978; Freeny and Lawson 1982). This is important because patients with pancreatic cancer have a mean survival time after diagnosis of 4.3 months (Statistical Research Service 1970).

STAGING OF PANCREATIC CARCINOMA

Accurate tumor staging is more important now than in the past because of improved combined diagnostic modalities leading to an earlier diagnosis. The current staging is based on the TNM classification as defined by the American Joint Committee on Cancer (1978). In this system, T1 and T2 tumors are arbitrarily designated as surgically resectable; T1 tumors are confined to the pancreas, while T2 tumors may extend to local structures but resection is still possible. Lesions classified as T3 and T4 are extensive and incompatible with surgical resection. Current diagnostic imaging modalities can detect ductal pancreatic carcinoma with an 85% to 95% accuracy, and they can differentiate resectable from unresectable tumors in 75% to 80% of patients (Sindelar, Kinsolla, and Mayer 1985; Lawson, Berland, and Foley 1985; Clark et al. 1985; Freeny and Ball 1978; Freeny and Lawson 1982).

ROLE OF IMAGING PROCEDURES IN DETECTION, STAGING, AND FOLLOW-UP

Conventional radiographs are rarely of any help. However, they are useful under the following conditions: the pancreatic tumor is quite large; there is diffuse metastatic disease throughout the chest, abdomen, and skeleton; or there is calcification in the primary tumor, which occurs rarely (Freeny and Lawson 1982; Eaton and Ferrucci 1973).

The increasing utilization of the new cross-sectional imaging modalities has decreased the use of barium studies for evaluation of patients with suspected pancreatic tumors. Prospective detection of pancreatic cancer by routine upper GI series is possible in only 25% of cases. The development of hypotonic duodenography resulted in a three-fold increase in diagnostic accuracy for tumors in the head of the pancreas (Eaton and Ferrucci 1973; Op den Orth 1973). However, most of these tumors were large and metastatic disease was already present.

Ultrasound is a low-cost, noninvasive screening procedure (fig. 44.5) that should be the initial evaluation technique for patients with jaundice (Lawson, Berland, and Foley 1985; Freeny and Lawson 1982; Lee et al. 1979; Cotton et al. 1980; Marks, Filly, and Callen 1980; Simeone, Wittenberg, and Ferrucci 1980; Lawson et al. 1982; Hessel et al. 1982; Ferrucci et al. 1983). An ultrasound demonstration of intrahepatic ducts of any size and/or a common hepatic duct greater than 6 mm to 7 mm is highly suggestive of biliary obstruction (Eaton and Ferrucci 1973; Op den Orth 1973). The accuracy of US for differentiating obstructive from nonobstructive jaundice is over 95% (Lawson, Berland, and Foley 1985; Clark et al. 1985; Cotton et al. 1980; Simeone, Wittenberg, and Ferrucci 1980) In many patients, overlying bowel gas obscures the extrahepatic ducts and head of the pancreas, so demonstration of the exact level and cause of the patient's obstructive jaundice by US is only 60% to 80% accurate (Lawson, Berland, and Foley 1985;Freeny and Lawson 1982; Hessel et al. 1982). In approximately 50% to 75% of patients, US can detect enlargement of the pancreatic head, a change in parenchymal textural pattern, and/or pancreatic ductal dilation (Lawson, Berland, and Foley 1985). Ultrasound can also help evaluate the liver for metastatic lesions.

Many radiologists rely on CT for more accurate detection of the level and cause of biliary obstruction as well as evaluation of local and distant metastases (Lawson, Berland, and Foley 1985; Clark et al. 1985; Freeny and Ball 1978; Freeny and Lawson 1982; Ferrucci et al. 1983; Stanley, Sagel, and Levitt 1977; Hauser, Battikha, and Wettstein 1980; Megibow et al. 1981 Shimizu et al. 1981). When pancreatic carcinoma is highly suspected, CT is the procedure of choice; however, because of CT's limited accessibility and higher cost, ultrasound, particularly in jaundiced patients, is used as the initial screening procedure (Ferrucci et al. 1983). In 85% to 95% of cases, computed tomography can make an accurate diagnosis of carcinoma of the pancreas without any additional imaging procedures. It can reliably assess resectability and precisely guide FNAB (Lawson, Berland, and Foley 1985; Clark et al. 1985; Freeny and Ball 1978; Freeny and Lawson 1982). For both US and CT, pancreatic masses usually must be at least 2 cm in diameter to produce a recognizable contour abnormality and, hence, a detectable tumor. Smaller tumors may distort the contour of the pancreas and, therefore, be detectable by CT, particularly if high-resolution contrast-enhanced CT is performed (Wittenberg et al. 1982).

The surgeon's most important problem is to determine the exact level of bile-duct obstruction (Pedrosa, Casanova, and Rodriguez 1981; Baron et al. 1982; Baron et al. 1983). As fig. 44.5 shows, some patients can go straight to surgery from US and/or CT after precise identification of the level and cause of the obstructive jaundice. The surgeon decides whether or not to perform FNAB and/or pancreatic angiography (Eisenberg 1973). If CT defines metastases, and these can be confirmed by FNAB, the patient can undergo palliation with percutaneous, peroral, or surgical decompression of the biliary tree (Hoevels, Lunderquist, and Ihse 1978; Gobien et al. 1984; Bonnel et al. 1984). Some patients will require operative treatment of gastric outlet obstruction from metastases.

If CT cannot determine the exact level of biliary obstruction, then percutaneous cholangiogram (PTC) or endoscopic retrograde cholangiopancreatography (ERCP) should be performed, usually with biliary drainage and occasionally with FNAB. Patients can then be treated either with surgery or palliative procedures depending upon tumor stage (Hoevels, Lunderquist, and Ihse 1978; Gobien et al. 1984; Bonnel et al. 1984).

Jaundiced patients with nondilated ducts detected by US will usually undergo a liver biopsy to confirm diffuse liver disease (see fig. 44.5).

Nonjaundiced patients with ductal adenocarcinomas of the body and tail will usually be first evaluated using CT (fig. 44.6). If a pancreatic mass is detected and found to be operable, the patient normally will go straight to surgery. Some surgeons may request preoperative angiography and FNAB (Eisenberg 1973). Inoperable patients can have their diagnosis confirmed by FNAB and undergo palliation. If CT fails to identify a mass in the pancreas and there is still a high suspicion of a tumor, a situation which might occur in a patient with a suspected functioning endocrine

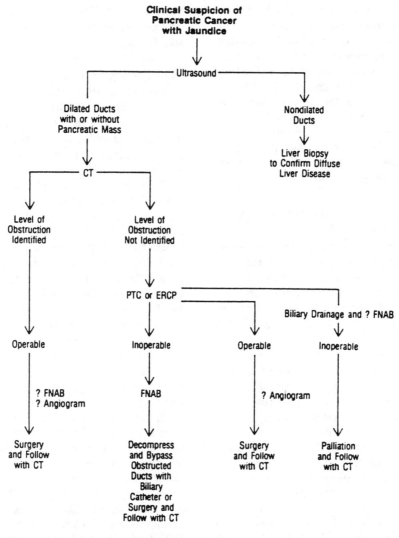

ERCP = Endoscopic Retrograde Cholangiopancreatography
FNAB = Fine-Needle Aspiration Biopsy
PTC = Percutaneous Transhepatic Cholangiography
CT   = Computed Tomography

Fig. 44.5. Imaging decision tree for jaundiced patients suspected of having pancreatic cancer. If CT confirms obstructive jaundice and shows level of obstruction and pancreatic head mass, many patients can go to surgery from CT. Some surgeons may request FNAB (fine-needle aspiration biopsy) to confirm the diagnosis and an arteriogram to define the peripancreatic blood vessels. Follow-up of pancreatic tumors is best performed by CT. US = ultrasound; PTC = percutaneous cholangiogram; ERCP = endoscopic retrograde cholangiopancreatography. (Reproduced with permission from: Thompson [1987].)

tumor, angiography coupled with portal vein sampling may localize a functioning tumor (Krudy et al. 1984). The overall results of angiographic localization of gastrinomas in patients with Zollinger-Ellison syndrome has been disappointing, as these tumors are usually small and hypovascular (Lawson, Berland, and Foley 1985; Marks, Filly, and Callen 1980) and are best localized using venous sampling (Krudy 1984). Insulinomas, however, are frequently hypervascular and, while small (1 cm in diameter), they may be diagnosed with a 75% to 80% accuracy, particularly if subselective arterial injections and magnification techniques are used (Lawson, Berland, and Foley 1985; Freeny and Lawson 1982).

The cross-sectional imaging modalities are useful in following patients with pancreatic tumors once they have been treated (Heiken et al. 1984). Unfortunately, most patients have such a short life expectancy that follow-up is of little practical value.

Preliminary evaluation of the pancreas with MRI has been promising (Stark et al. 1984b; Haaga 1984; Simeone et al. 1985) because the imaging modality can easily identify the pancreas and retroperitoneal structures and detect pathological changes. However, whether MRI has any potential for improving the overall survival of patients with pancreatic carcinoma is unknown.

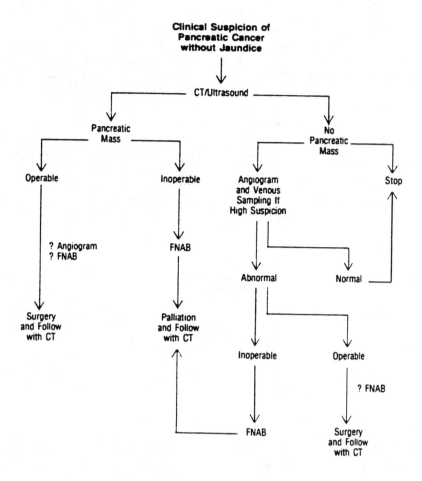

CT   = Computed Tomography
FNAB = Fine-Needle Aspiration Biopsy

Fig. 44.6. Imaging decision tree for nonjaundiced patients with suspected pancreatic cancer. Most prefer CT as the initial examination procedure. Some surgeons will request FNAB and arteriogram prior to surgery. FNAB can confirm that the tumor is inoperable for cure. (Reproduced with permission from: Thompson [1987].)

PRIMARY AND METASTATIC CARCINOMA OF THE LIVER

The goal of hepatic imaging is threefold: to detect tumors, to discriminate malignancy from benign disease, and to find early lesions amenable to resectability (Lawson, Berland, and Foley 1985). Imaging techniques are also valuable in assessing the response of various therapeutic regimens. The techniques for detecting primary and metastatic liver tumors have undergone tremendous changes during the past 15 years (Berk et al. 1978; Zeman et al. 1985; Cady, McDonald, and Gunderson 1985; Bernardino and Green 1979) and further significant advances in diagnosis are on the horizon. To date, however, the improved ability to detect malignant liver tumors with the new imaging techniques has had little effect on survival statistics.

STAGING OF HEPATIC MALIGNANCIES

No staging system has been developed for hepatocellular carcinoma, undoubtedly due to the extensive nature of the tumor when it is first detected and to the poor survival statistics. Metastatic disease to the liver for primary tumors are indicated as M1 lesions, which automatically increase the tumor stage of any primary neoplasm.

ROLE OF IMAGING PROCEDURES IN DETECTION, STAGING, AND FOLLOW-UP

Several biochemical tests have been used to screen for liver dysfunction; however, liver function tests may not be sufficiently sensitive to detect hepatic involvement by tumor and are often not specific enough to distinguish between hepatic tumor, biliary obstruction, or diffuse hepatic parenchymal disease. Several imaging studies are available to evaluate the liver (fig. 44.7). These include radionuclide liver/spleen scan (Snow, Goldstein, and Wallace 1979; McCarty et al. 1979; Knopf et al. 1982; Alderson, Adams, and McNeil 1983; McClees and Gedgaudas-McClees 1984), ultrasonography (Green et al. 1977; Scheible, Gosnik, and Leopold 1977; Yeh and Rabinowitz 1980; Bernardino, Thomas, and Maklad 1982; Lewis 1984; LaBerge et al. 984), and computed tomography (LaBerge et al. 1984; Moss et al. 1979; Prando et al. 1979; Young, Turner, and Castellino 1980; Marchal, Baert, and Wilms 1980; Zornoza and Ginaldi 1981; Burgener and Hamlin 1981). In the past the significantly more invasive procedure of angiography was also used (Chuang 1984). Radionuclide imaging has

been a standard screening test for patients suspected of having metastatic disease to the liver. However, the procedure has low spatial resolution and is unable to detect lesions under 2 cm in diameter. Technetium Tc 99m sulfur colloid scintigraphy (RN) has a sensitivity of 67% to 86% for detecting focal liver lesions (Snow, Goldstein, and Wallace 1979; McCarty et al. 1979; Knopf et al. 1982; Alderson, Adams, and McNeil 1983; McClees and Gedgaudas-McClees 1984). These figures are lower than those reported for CT and similar to those reported for US. McClees reported that scintigraphy was as good as CT and better than US (McClees and Gedgaudas-McClees 1984). Scintigraphy does not provide any specific information about the space-occupying lesion

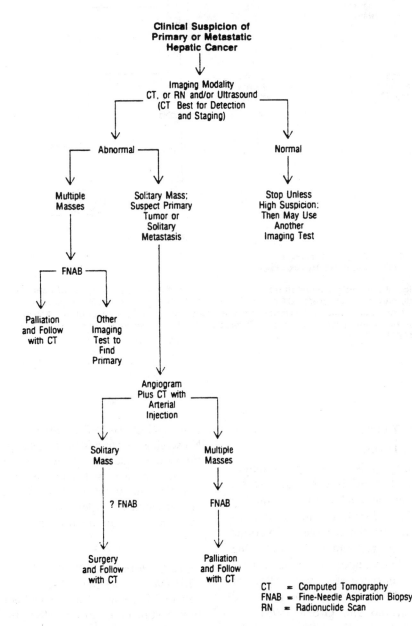

Fig. 44.7. Imaging decision tree for patients with suspected primary or metastatic hepatic tumor. CT is the best examination for detection, but cost and limited availability in some cases will dictate the use of radionuclide scan (RN) and/or ultrasound (US). Fine-needle aspiration biopsy is helpful in confirming metastases. (Reproduced with permission from: Thompson [1987].)

in the liver, thus the false-positive rate for scintigraphy is higher than for CT or US. Despite these problems, scintigraphy's lower cost and easier accessibility keep it an important screening test for patients with suspected hepatic malignancy. Currently, CT is considered the best modality for tumors with a high predilection for hepatic involvement (Zeman et al. 1985).

Ultrasound is the preferred screening test for differentiating biliary obstruction from hepatic parenchymal disease in the jaundiced patient (Lawson, Berland, and Foley 1985; Ferrucci et al. 1983; Pedrosa, Casanova, and Rodriguez 1981; Pedrosa et al. 1981; Baron et al. 1982; Baron et al. 1983), but is less accurate than CT for detecting hepatic tumors (Lawson, Berland, and Foley 1985; Alderson, Adams, and McNeil 1983). The sensitivity for detecting space-occupying lesions of the liver reportedly ranges from 70% to 80% (Lawson, Berland, and Foley 1985; Alderson, Adams, and McNeil 1983). Nevertheless, some advocate US for screening because of its lower expense and wider availability compared to high-resolution CT. Ultrasound is a very useful complementary technique, particularly when coupled with FNAB (Grant et al. 1983). The accuracy of ultrasound depends significantly more than scintigraphy or CT upon the technical expertise of the operator and radiologist interpreting the scans.

Computed tomography is the preferred technique for evaluating the liver (see fig. 44.7). Of the current imaging modalities, CT has the highest degree of accuracy, sensitivity, and specificity, and it can also provide important additional information about other organ systems (Berk et al. 1978; Zeman et al. 1985; Snow, Goldstein, and Wallace 1979; McCarty et al. 1979; Knopf et al. 1982; Alderson, Adams, and McNeil 1983; LaBerge et al. 1984; Moss et al. 1979; Prando et al. 1979; Young, Turner, and Castellino 1980; Marchal, Baert, and Wilms 1980). Intravenous contrast enhancement must be utilized to evaluate the liver in most patients. This is a disadvantage compared to the other imaging techniques, as the patients are at risk for allergic reactions from the contrast material. Computed tomography also does not accurately detect diffuse diseases of the liver such as cirrhosis, hepatitis, and some diffuse primary and metastatic tumors (Harbin et al. 1983). Scintigraphy may better identify these entities and their severity (McClees and Gedgaudas-McClees 1984). Computed tomography may not be able to differentiate benign vs. neoplastic space-occupying lesions in all patients, but it can identify cysts and cavernous hemangiomas with a high degree of accuracy (Lawson, Berland, and Foley; Zeman et al. 1985; Glazer et al. 1985). Some patients may require fine-needle aspiration biopsy, hepatic arteriography, or a red-blood-cell radionuclide scan to establish the diagnosis.

Accurate identification of hepatic segmental and subsegmental anatomy is extremely important when contemplating extensive hepatic resection for either primary or metastatic disease. Computed tomography and ultrasonography can localize the tumor to a specific

segment or lobe; most surgeons, however, also request arteriography prior to surgical intervention (Lawson, Berland, and Foley 1985; Zeman et al. 1985).

Computed tomography is the most frequently used modality for following patients with malignant hepatic masses because it accurately and specifically demonstrates the lesions, provides easier comparison between examinations, and demonstrates subtle changes. Scintigraphy and US can also be used, particularly if the patient has numerous surgical clips in place following surgery and/or cannot cooperate well enough to obtain an adequate CT scan.

Due to fundamentally differing properties from radionuclides, roentgenography, and ultrasound, MRI is likely to define and characterize lesions not seen by other imaging modalities (Glazer et al. 1985; Moss et al. 1984; Heiken et al. 1985; Ohtomo et al. 1985; Edelman et al. 1986; Stark et al. 1986; Ferrucci 1988; Bronskill et al. 1988). Recent advances in pulse sequences are now providing high-quality scans that are detecting hepatic lesions not shown by even the most advanced CT scanning techniques (Edelman et al. 1986; Stark et al. 1986). The use of specific tissue variables and higher resolution may mean that a definitive diagnosis can be made (Glazer et al. 1985; Ohtomo et al. 1985).

GALLBLADDER AND BILE DUCT MALIGNANCY

Carcinoma of the gallbladder spreads locally to invade the liver bed and metastasizes to regional lymph nodes (Fahim et al. 1962; Edmonson 1958; Gupta, Udupa, and Gupta 1980). Despite recent advances in cancer detection and management, no improvement in survival has resulted for patients with gallbladder carcinoma, and 5-year survival is rare. The poor prognosis associated with this tumor results from advanced patient age, lack of early specific symptoms and inability to establish an early diagnosis, and the propensity for early invasion.

Cholangiocarcinomas are usually slow-growing, with death secondary to liver failure and cholangitis secondary to the biliary obstruction (Takasan et al. 1980; Lees et al. 1980). Because of the slow growth rate and the difficulties posed by resection of these tumors, surgical treatment usually consists of exploration for palliative decompression. No improvement in survival has been noted in these patients despite the improved method of diagnosis.

STAGING OF GALLBLADDER AND BILE DUCT MALIGNANCY

To date, no tumor staging pattern has been developed for carcinoma of the gallbladder or cholangiocarcinoma. This undoubtedly is due to the very poor prognosis of these tumors at the time of initial detection.

ROLE OF IMAGING IN DETECTING, STAGING, AND FOLLOW-UP

Gallbladder cancer is usually not detected until late in the course of the patient's disease, so routine radiographs are of little help unless the tumor has eroded into the gastrointestinal tract and produces air in the biliary system (Berk, Ferrucci, and Leopold 1983).

Patients with bile duct or gallbladder cancer frequently are jaundiced, and US is an excellent modality for detecting the presence of biliary obstruction (Berk et al. 1982; Lee, Henderson, and Ehrlich 1977; Neiman and Mintzer 1977; Conrad, Landay, and Jones 1978; Weill, Eisencher, and Zelther 1978; Sample et al. 1978; Taylor and Rosenfeld 1977) (see fig. 44.5). With gallbladder carcinoma, ultrasound may show a large mass in the gallbladder fossa or a thickening of the focal gallbladder wall (Crade et al. 1979; Allibone, Fagan, and Porter 1981; Ruiz et al. 1980; Yum and Fink 1980; Weiner et al. 1984; Yeh 1979). Gallstones are invariably present. The site of the obstruction is at the level of the cystic duct. Unfortunately, the findings may mimic chronic and/or acute cholecystitis. Ultrasound evaluation of cholangiocarcinoma is not specific, and usually demonstrates dilation of the biliary system proximal to the obstructing tumor (Levine et al. 1979). Because of a lack of associated soft-tissue mass, a physician can only infer the correct diagnosis.

Computed tomographic evaluation of patients with gallbladder cancer will usually demonstrate widespread disease, with a bulky mass in the gallbladder bed and evidence of extension into the liver or along the hepatoduodenal ligament into the head of the pancreas and retroperitoneum (Itai et al. 1980; Thorsen et al. 1984; Mathers, Lee, and Heiken 1984). The findings are not specific, but the diagnosis usually can be suggested in the presence of obstructive jaundice and a mass in the gallbladder bed (Smathers, Lee, and Heiken 1984). In patients with cholangiocarcinoma, CT will demonstrate the biliary obstruction proximal to the tumor. However, in most patients, a focal mass will not be identified (Ruiz et al. 1980; Itai et al. 1983). Occasionally, using intravenous contrast administration and fine, detailed thin-section CT, a small primary tumor may be identified. Metastases to the liver and regional lymph nodes may be identified in advanced disease (Thorsen et al. 1984). Percutaneous fine-needle aspiration biopsy directed by CT frequently provides a correct diagnosis. Percutaneous cholangiography or ERCP will usually be needed for definition of the bile ducts and complete delineation of the tumor involvement and the exact point of obstruction (Lawson, Berland, and Foley 1985; Berk, Ferrucci, and Leopold 1983; Berk et al. 1982). This provides the surgeon with the necessary information, as many of these tumors are at the junction of the right and left hepatic ducts and are not amenable to surgical resection. The surgeon may call on the interventional radiologist to place biliary catheters for palliation and possible internal radiation.

The majority of gallbladder cancer patients do not survive long enough for follow-up imaging studies to assume major importance. Computed tomography is the preferred technique for following the results of treatment.

Patients with cholangiocarcinomas are best followed with a combination of modalities. Computed tomography may be helpful in evaluating metastatic disease to the liver and upper abdominal structures. Cholangiography via biliary catheters is used to evaluate the bile ducts.

To date, experience with MRI as a diagnostic modality in patients with carcinoma of the gallbladder and bile ducts has been limited. Whether MRI will prove useful in these patients is unknown. Magnetic resonance imaging is not likely to have a significant impact in patients with gallbladder cancer because the tumor is detected so late. It may not prove helpful in patients with cholangiocarcinoma, since these tumors are quite small and the resolution of MRI is not as good as that of CT.

PART VII: IMAGING TUMORS OF THE KIDNEY

INTRODUCTION

Malignant tumors of the kidney make up only 2% to 3% of all human neoplasms; of these, renal cell carcinoma accounts for over 85% of all kidney cancers (McClennan and Balfe 1985). The American Cancer Society statistics for 1990 estimated 24,000 new cases of renal or ureteral cancer and 9,600 cancer-related deaths (Silverberg, Boring, and Squires 1990). At initial diagnosis, about one-third of all patients have metastases, often involving only a single organ site. Renal cell carcinoma and transitional cell carcinoma of the kidney are relatively radioinsensitive tumors whose treatment is largely surgical, with or without adjuvant medical therapy. The stage and grade are the most significant prognostic factors. Survival is related to the extent of tumor and the presence or absence of metastatic disease.

The imaging strategy for real or suspected renal neoplasms should follow a logical (oncologic) progression from detection to definition (staging) to evaluation for metastases. This imaging progression should also consider accepted criteria for treatment. Computed tomography has become the major cross-sectional imaging study for the evaluation of renal neoplasms (McClennan and Rabin 1988). While intravenous urography (IVU) remains the primary test for detection of renal cancers, CT has commanded the preeminent role for further definition and staging. The accuracy of CT scanning with intravenous contrast enhancement is extremely high, between 90% and 96% (McClennan and Rabin 1988; Johnson et al. 1987). Excellent discrimination can be achieved with CT in distinguishing low-stage (stage I or II—PT1-PT3a) from higher-stage disease. Computed tomographic scanning is best for imaging local extrarenal spread as well as other abdominal organ involvement and distant disease. The technique has replaced diagnostic angiography for staging renal cell carcinoma and performs much better than ultrasound alone for detecting and staging disease (Mauro et al. 1982). Angiography is now reserved for so-called road mapping, prior to renal sparing surgery (i.e., cancer in solitary kidneys) or therapeutic embolization with alcohol or particulate embolic materials such as balloons or coils. Doppler US with color flow techniques can be useful for evaluation of the major renal veins or inferior vena cava for presence and extent of tumor thrombosis (Dubbins and Wells 1986). The predictive value of CT scanning for malignant neoplasia when typical features are present (e.g., calcification, solid mass, contrast enhancement) can be as high as 96% (Curry et al. 1984). Because not all solid renal parenchymal masses are malignant tumors, careful image analysis and contrast enhancement are necessary to avoid equivocal or indeterminate diagnosis.

Increasingly, reports confirm the utility of magnetic resonance imaging for the evaluation of renal neoplasms (Fein et al. 1987; Hricak et al. 1988). Currently, the role of MRI for screening for renal neoplasia is limited because small cancers (<3 cm) may remain undetected. The use of gd-DTPA significantly improves the ability of MRI to detect and characterize small tumors. Overall accuracy for MRI reportedly ranges from 74% to 87%. MRI is an effective adjunctive imaging test for evaluating large bulky neoplasms, lymph node metastases, and major vascular involvement. A negative predictive value of 98% for tumor vascular extension and 99% for adjacent organ involvement have been reported using MRI in patients with renal cancers (Hricak et al. 1988).

PRETREATMENT STAGING

The indications for CT scanning in renal cancer patients are listed in table 44.4. Contrast-enhanced renal CT is the best imaging test for pretreatment staging and determination of resectability. CT is more accurate and sensitive than angiography for detection of perinephric tumor extent and regional lymph-node involvement. It detects main renal venous invasion and inferior vena cava involvement as accurately as angiography and venography. MRI may further obviate angiography or venography because multiplanar MRI images allow for accuracy in the range of 95% to 100%. The advent of better T1-T2 tumor tissue discrimination, MRI contrast media, and MRI bowel contrast agents will make MRI a more clinically efficacious imaging modality for evaluation of renal cancers.

Consideration of tumor stage is critical to the decision regarding surgical resection and curability. A thorough knowledge of Robson's classification system and

Table 44.4
INDICATIONS FOR CT SCANNING IN RENAL CANCER PATIENTS

1. Patients with urographic evidence of renal neoplasia
2. Patients with normal IVU but suspicious signs (i.e., hematuria) or symptoms
3. Patients with paraneoplastic syndromes
4. Patients with unknown primary and metastatic disease (e.g., lytic bone destruction)
5. Patients with syndromes associated with renal cancers (e.g., von Hippel Lindau disease and acquired cystic disease of dialysis)
6. Patients with previous renal cancer therapy (rule out recurrence)

Table 44.5
RELATIONSHIP BETWEEN ROBSON SYSTEM AND TNM SYSTEM

Robson	Disease Extent	TNM
I	Tumor confined to kidney (small, intrarenal)	T1
	Tumor confined to kidney (large)	T2
II	Tumor spread to perinephric fat but within Gerota's fascia	T3a
IIIA	Tumor spread to renal vein or cava	T3ab
IIIB	Tumor spread to local lymph nodes (LN)	N1-N3
IIIC	Tumor spread to local vessels and LN	T3b, N1-N3
IVA	Tumor spread to adjacent organs (excluding ipsilateral adrenal)	T4
IVB	Distant metastasis	M1a-d; N4

its relationship to the TNM system is essential (see table 44.5). Approximately 33% of all patients with renal cell carcinoma present with stage I disease, while 12% present with stage II, 24% with stage III, and 31% with stage IV disease (McClennan and Balfe 1985). Five-year and 10-year survival rates are much higher for stage I (PT1) and stage II (PT2) disease compared with stage III (PT3a,b,c) and stage IV (PT4) disease (Bassill, Dosouretz, and Prout 1985). The clinician should weigh evaluation of any imaging test against both clinical and pathologic staging criteria while also considering patient age and other comorbid conditions. Evaluation of CT or MRI scans should include evaluation of tumor size, shape, renal capsular extension, perinephric extension, tumor vascularity (contrast enhancement features), local and distant lymph node metastases (N stage), and major vascular involvement (table 44.6). Contiguous organ involvement and metastatic disease (M stage) also must be evaluated. In addition, individual tumoral characteristics—particularly size and degree of necrosis and hemorrhage, vascularity, and calcification (McClennan and Rabin 1988)—can be important to the prognosis or to the disease-free interval after therapy. For patient follow-up or evaluation for recurrent tumor, CT scanning and/or MRI are the best imaging procedures. Patients with positive lymph nodes or adrenal metastases at the time of surgery have the highest incidence of postnephrectomy local recurrence.

CURRENT IMAGING RECOMMENDATIONS

Modern generation high-resolution fast (sub-5 second) CT scanning is the best means for pretreatment evaluation

Table 44.6
CT FEATURES OF RENAL CELL CARCINOMA

1. Mass with attenuation similar to or less than renal parenchyma
2. Poor definition from parenchyma
   a. "Pseudocapsule"
3. Contrast enhancement—marked or transient
4. Calcification
   a. Central
   b. Peripheral
5. Secondary signs
   a. Lymph nodes
   b. Venous invasion
   c. Metastases

Table 44.7
IMAGING METHODS FOR EVALUATION OF RENAL CANCER

METHOD	CAPABILITY	COST/BENEFIT	ROUTINE RECOMMENDATION
NONINVASIVE			
1. Chest radiography	Limited usefulness; tomography required for detection of metastases	High	Yes
2. Skeletal radiography	Limited usefulness except to confirm positive bone scan for metastases	Low	No
3. Ultrasound (Doppler and color flow)	Useful to exclude simple cysts; limited staging information available; less sensitive and less specific than CT for tumor extent; Doppler may be of use for vascular invasion	Fair	Not usually
4. MRI	Promising role for tumor staging; comparable utility fair for tumor detection with contrast enhancement	Fair	Not usually
NEARLY NONINVASIVE			
1. Urography	Best screening test available; limited ability for precise staging	High	Yes
2. Radionuclide studies			
a. Bone scans	Best screening test for skeletal mass	High	Yes
b. Liver-spleen scan	Limited use if liver chemistries normal	Low	No
3. CT	Most useful test for T, N, M staging information; requires IV contrast media	High	Always
INVASIVE			
1. Angiography (digital)			
a. Arteriography	Limited diagnostic and staging information compared with CT; arteriography is required for embolization	Low	No
b. Venography	Useful if CT indeterminate for renal vein/cava involvement (many arteriographic and most venographic studies can be done digitally)	Low	No
2. Lymphography	Limited or no utility	None	No
3. Biopsy (CT, US, fluoroscopy)	Percutaneous biopsy requires US, CT, or fluoroscopy; open biopsy rarely needed; not necessary for T-stage confirmation; may be useful to confirm metastases and determine operability	Low	No

of real or suspected renal cancers. It has effectively replaced angiography as a preoperative staging technique, and only MRI provides comparable anatomic information regarding tumor characteristics and stage. Table 44.7 outlines currently available imaging techniques and their real or potential benefits.

PART VIII: IMAGING CARCINOMA OF THE BLADDER

INTRODUCTION

Malignant tumors of the bladder are the most common urinary tract neoplasms. The American Cancer Society statistics estimated 49,000 new cases (mostly in males) in 1990 (Silverberg, Boring, and Squires 1990). Curiously, male age-adjusted death rates (approximately 7 out of 100,000) have remained relatively stable for more than 50 years (Silverberg, Boring, and Squires 1990; Whitmore 1988). Concluding his editorial on bladder cancer, George Prout, M.D., commented, "It seems there is more to learn about bladder carcinoma now than there was 25 years ago" (Prout 1982).

This statement is still clinically applicable today, as significant dilemmas in the management of patients with bladder cancer remain largely unresolved. One major problem is a lack of sufficient diagnostic techniques to

help predict which patients are at risk for the development of invasive carcinoma from pre-existing superficial bladder tumors. About two-thirds of all patients will develop recurrent tumors after treatment for superficial carcinoma of the bladder (Catalona 1980). These new neoplasms can be more anaplastic or invasive in up to 25% of cases. The clinical staging process for invasive carcinoma of the bladder can be in error in up to 66% of patients, and clinical stage directly relates to therapeutic choice and prognosis (Whitmore 1988; Catalona 1980; Balfe, Heiken, and McClennan 1985). The most important prognostic factor for patients with invasive bladder cancer is the degree of bladder wall invasion (Balfe, Heiken, and McClennan 1985). With current therapies, treatment failures generally stem from distant metastases, not pelvic (local) recurrences. Therefore, the major goals of an appropriate imaging strategy are to refine pretreatment staging by optimally defining local tumor extent, e.g., bladder wall invasion; to assess adequately the lymph node drainage areas and common sites for metastases; and to maintain follow-up with patients after treatment in order to detect recurrence (Balfe, Heiken, and McClennan 1985).

Radiologic imaging techniques do not contribute significantly to the detection of bladder cancer, so their primary impact is to provide more precise pretreatment staging information and methods for serial post-treatment surveillance. Urography, ultrasound (US), computed tomography (CT), magnetic resonance imaging (MRI), angiography, and lymphangiography have all been used for these purposes (Balfe, Heiken, and McClennan 1985; Hatch and Barry 1986; Amendola et al. 1986; Bryan et al. 1987; Dershaw and Scher 1988; Heiken and Lee 1988; Lee and Rholl 1986; Consensus Conference 1988). To date, no single imaging technique successfully meets all the goals. However, noninvasive cross-sectional imaging techniques, such as US and MRI, hold great promise and are the current leaders in the growing field of available imaging modalities (Dershaw and Scher 1988; Consensus Conference 1988).

PRETREATMENT STAGING

Accurate staging is critical to selection of optimal treatment, and is an important prognostic indicator of patient survival. With increasing bladder wall invasion, the incidence of lymph node metastases increases and overall patient survival diminishes, no matter what form of therapy is chosen (Balfe, Heiken, and McClennan 1985). From the therapeutic point of view, it is clear that the basic imaging strategy for staging is to find those patients who may benefit from curative therapy, be that radical cystectomy or radiation therapy. This strategy would require identification of patients with tumors still confined to the bladder, with only microscopic metastases to a small number of lymph nodes. Those patients not selected for radical surgery do not require as extensive an imaging evaluation of pelvic or retroperitoneal lymph nodes.

The imaging approach to bladder cancer should also consider the typical presentations and the common patterns of spread: local extension (T-stage); lymphatic involvement (N-stage); and metastases (M-stage). Approximately 70% of bladder cancers present as superficial tumors (Tis, Ta, and T1) (Whitmore 1988; Balfe, Heiken, and McClennan 1985). For such tumors, urography is performed routinely to screen the upper urinary tracts after cystoscopic evaluation of the bladder has provided a diagnosis. Infiltrating tumors (T2-4) account for about 25% of carcinomas of the bladder at presentation (Whitmore 1988). Urography, CT, MRI, or US can be utilized to refine T-stage information and detect occult metastases. Only about 5% of bladder cancers have overt metastases at the time of presentation (Whitmore 1988; Balfe, Heiken, and McClennan 1985). Therefore, urography and radionuclide skeletal imaging are usually all that are indicated. However, 10% to 40% of all invasive cancers will have positive lymph nodes, and as many as 55% will develop distant metastases (Whitmore 1988). The utility of radiologic imaging studies for the detection and staging of bladder cancer follows.

DETECTION

Signs and symptoms of bladder carcinoma are often vague or absent. Cystoscopic biopsy is the method of choice for confirmation. Urography detects most large bladder tumors (i.e., >1.5-2 cm in size); the post-void film is the most sensitive portion of the urogram (Balfe, Heiken, and McClennan 1985; Hatch and Barry 1986). Urography fulfills largely a screening role for the rest of the urothelium and aids in overall patient assessment regarding findings that may alter the treatment plan, such as hydronephrosis or congenital anomalies. Computed tomographic scanning does not detect bladder cancer. Retrospective reviews have shown that both MRI and US are able to detect neoplasms larger than 1.5 cm in size (Heiken and Lee 1988; Consensus Conference 1988). Detection rates for transabdominal ultrasound (TAUS) range from 58% to 94% for larger tumors (Dershaw and Scher 1988). Screening for metastases at the time of diagnosis is usually not performed for superficial carcinomas of the bladder; it is usually reserved for infiltrating tumors or high-grade lesions (Balfe, Heiken, and McClennan 1985).

LOCAL TUMOR EXTENT (T-STAGE)

Imaging modalities for evaluation of local tumor extent include CT, MRI, and US (transrectal ultrasound [TRUS], transurethral ultrasound [TUUS], and transabdominal ultrasound [TAUS]). Angiography rarely, if ever, is useful today. CT scanning and MRI are nearly equal on overall accuracy for tumor staging, although no large prospective comparative series yet exists (Heiken and Lee 1988; Consensus Conference 1988). The ability of CT to accurately assess depth of muscle invasion and extent of perivesical involvement remains limited. Overall, accuracy for CT has been variable, with reports ranging from 40% to 83% for distinguishing extravesical tumor stages from other stages (Amendola et al. 1986; Bryan et al 1987). Furthermore, CT cannot reliably differentiate superficial (stage A; Tis-T1) lesions from B1-B2 (T2-T3) disease (Balfe, Heiken, and McClennan 1985). A critical impact point for radiologic imaging appears to be between stages T2 (B1) and T3a (B2). Magnetic resonance imaging and US reportedly perform more accurately than CT for the evaluation of bladder wall invasion; accuracies of MRI and US range from 64% to 85%. A greater sensitivity for wall invasion exists for MRI compared with CT (Heiken and Lee 1988; Consensus Conference 1988). Still, CT, MRI, or US cannot reliable distinguish edema, inflammation, and fibrosis. Ultrasound is a useful adjunct to cystoscopy for surveillance; transrectal ultrasound is good for evaluation of the bladder trigone and immediate environs, but poor for other parts of the bladder such as the dome. The accuracy of the staging information of transabdominal ultrasound and transurethral ultrasound continues to increase, and this improvement coincides with that in technology, transducer design, and operator experience.

NODAL STATUS (N-STAGE)

Accurate evaluation of lymph node status is crucial to optimal therapeutic selection in patients with invasive bladder cancer (Balfe, Heiken, and McClennan 1985).

For surgical candidates this evaluation is largely performed by surgical (staging) lymph node dissection. Lymphangiography successfully has detected lymph node metastases; however, reported inconsistent opacification of major lymph node drainage routes, and inconsistent accuracies (range 48% to 92%) have limited the widespread use of lymphangiography today (Balfe, Heiken, and McClennan 1985). Accuracy may improve with percutaneous fine-needle aspiration biopsy (PFNAB) in combination with lymphangiography for preoperative staging. The major advantage of both CT and MRI over lymphangiography is that they are noninvasive and may demonstrate enlarged lymph nodes in nodal areas not adequately opacified by bipedal lymphangiography (Amendola et al. 1986; Bryan et al 1987; Heiken and Lee 1988; Lee and Rholl 1986; Consensus Conference 1988). A unique ability of MRI is that it can identify large lymph nodes and separate them from blood vessels without the need for intravenous contrast material, which CT does require. However, neither cross-sectional imaging technique can identify metastases in normal-sized lymph nodes, but CT can be used for percutaneous fine-needle aspiration biopsy if required. Neither US nor angiography adequately images the lymph node drainage areas of the bladder.

METASTATIC DISEASE (M-STAGE)

Screening techniques by their nature have a high sensitivity, but low specificity. Therefore, positive findings usually need histologic confirmation. The sites with the highest risk for metastases include the bones, lungs, and liver (Balfe, Heiken, and McClennan 1985). Patients considered candidates for radical curative therapy benefit from screening imaging studies such as radionuclide bone scanning, chest CT, and occasionally CT or MRI of the liver, when liver involvement is highly suspected.

CURRENT IMAGING RECOMMENDATIONS

In the detection phase, intravenous urography plays a major role for screening of the urothelium, but not in identifying carcinoma of the bladder. Screening for metastases is best performed on those patients considered to be curable, but whose subsequent workup depends on initial T-stage information. Deeply invasive (T3) lesions may be locally uresectable; therefore, further delineation of their T-stage is required. At this point, CT, MRI, or TUUS may be considered, if appropriate imaging studies have been performed and correctly interpreted. The impact of the newer imaging methods — CT and MRI — is most marked when they

Table 44.8
IMAGING METHODS FOR CARCINOMA OF THE BLADDER

METHOD	STAGING CAPABILITY	COST/BENEFIT RATIO	RECOMMENDED/ROUTINE STAGING PROCEDURE
Noninvasive			
1. Chest imaging			
a. Plain films	Capable of detecting large lesions; screen technique	High	Yes
b. Tomography	Capable of detecting smaller lesions (metastases)	Medium	No
c. CT	High sensitivity; moderate specificity for pulmonary lesions	Medium	No; only selected operative candidates
2. Radionuclide studies			
a. Bone scan	Sensitive to skeletal metastases	Medium	No; only in patients clinically at risk for widespread metastases
b. Liver-spleen scan	Sensitivity for large intrahepatic metastases	Low	No
3. Bone films	May document skeletal metastases (complements bone scan)	Medium	Only to document lesions detected by RN scanning
4. Magnetic resonance imaging (MRI)	Equal to or greater than that of CT	Medium	May replace CT
MINIMALLY INVASIVE			
1. Urography	Urothelial screening examination	High	Yes
2. Cystography	May demonstrate fixation of bladder wall, but insensitive to minimal invasion	Low	No
3. CT	Sensitive to local invasion if macroscopic	Medium	No; only in operative candidates
4. Sonography (Transurethral)	Capable of imaging local invasion	Medium	As alternative to CT
5. Retrograde ureteropyelography	Screens urothelium, evaluates suspicious urographic lesions	High	Yes
6. MRI	Equal to that of CT; may become preferred method	Moderate	Unknown
INVASIVE			
1. Lymphangiography	Identifies lymph node metastases in external iliac, common iliac, and para-aortic areas	Low	No; selected operative candidates only
2. Angiography	May identify gross extravesical extent by abnormal vascularity	Low	No
3. Percutaneous needle aspiration	Documents presence and character of tumor detected by other methods	Medium	Selected patients

demonstrate regional extension or lymph node metastases not clinically evident. However, there are still significant problems in the oncologic imaging evaluation of patients with carcinoma of the bladder: detection of cancer below the spatial resolution of current technology (CT, MRI, and US); and an inability to consistently differentiate edema, inflammation, and fibrosis from tumor, whether primary or recurrent. Table 44.8 summarizes the currently available oncologic imaging procedures and displays recommendations for their use.

PART IX: BREAST CANCER SCREENING AND DIAGNOSIS

INTRODUCTION

The therapeutic options available to patients with breast cancer have changed dramatically during the past two decades. Prior to this time, radical surgery was the only acceptable treatment approach, and patients' fear of this procedure was almost as great as their concern about the disease. In conjunction with an evolving debate about the appropriate treatment for breast cancer, the role of screening and diagnosis has commanded equal attention.

BACKGROUND INFORMATION AND SCREENING CONTROVERSIES

Mass screening is currently the only way to reduce breast cancer mortality rates in those with cancer in an early stage and in those with more favorable prognoses. The application of imaging to breast examination significantly reduces the size of threshold for detection. Theoretically, the smaller the lesion size, the lower the likelihood of axillary metastases and disseminated disease at the time of initial presentation.

The initial application of x-ray mammography occurred over 70 years ago, but practical mammographic techniques did not become available until the 1950s. Gros, in France, developed the first dedicated mammographic system (Bassett and Gold 1988). Wolfe and others popularized xerography as an alternative x-ray imaging technique for breast cancer diagnosis in the late 1960s (Wolfe 1968). During the 1970s, mammographic systems became more sophisticated and film-intensifying screen mammography improved considerably, with lowered radiation doses and improved resolution.

The Health Insurance Plan (HIP) study began in 1962 as a controlled study of 62,000 women divided equally into a study group and a control group. This randomized trial offered four annual mammographic screening and physical examinations, and has at this point followed many of these patients for 18 years. Approximately nine years after the beginning of this study, a 40% reduction in breast cancer mortality was shown to be present in the study group evaluated by mammography; however, this improvement was confined to women age 50 and older. Subsequent follow-up has shown a gradual reduction in that mortality advantage, but also a mortality advantage in the 40- to 49-year age group which now appears similar to the 50- to 59-year-old patients (Feig 1988).

In 1973, the Breast Cancer Detection Demonstration Project (BCDDP) screened 280,000 volunteer women in 28 centers across the United States. The BCDDP uncontrolled trial documented the role of screening mammography in detecting a clinically occult yield of breast cancers (nearly 50% of cancers were detected only by mammography) in all age groups studied, from age 35 to age 74. Other trials in Europe and Canada have validated the role of screening mammography, while fueling the debate as to the benefit of screening in the patient under age 50.

During the 1970s, a concern developed over the

Table 44.9
BREAST IMAGING TECHNIQUES

TECHNIQUE	ADVANTAGES/DISADVANTAGES	COMMENT
Film screen mammography	Most commonly used breast imaging technique Requires technical training and experience More time-consuming to interpret than xeromammogram Does not visualize chest wall	Should be the standard for the field Radiation dose should be less than 0.001 Gy
Xeromammography	Allows a greater technical latitude Visualizes chest wall Easier to interpret (does not require magnification/bright light examination) Greater radiation exposure dose	Similar diagnostic accuracy as film/screen mammography New systems may reduce exposure dose
Ultrasound	Useful for young, premenopausal, dense breast May be helpful in differentiating a cystic from a solid *palpable* mass Not useful in fatty or postmenopausal breast	Dedicated ultrasound units not acceptable for screening
Diaphanography (light scanning)		Not acceptable for screening
Thermography		Not acceptable for screening
Computed tomography		Not acceptable for screening
Magnetic resonance imaging		Not acceptable for screening

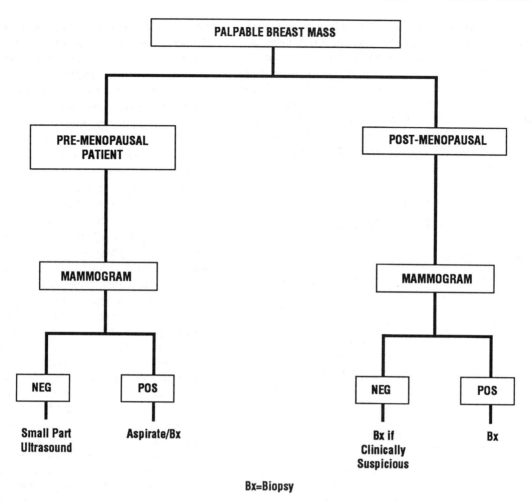

Bx=Biopsy

Fig. 44.8. Diagnostic study of patient with a palpable breast mass.

potential risk of the low doses of radiation associated with mammography in increasing the natural rate of breast cancer development. This hypothesis resulted from a linear extrapolation of higher-dose studies. A conservative, cautious analysis of these data would suggest the risk, if any, is small, and is focused on the patient who is under age 30 when exposed to the radiation. In appreciation of this potential hazard, and in light of the fact that the denser, more glandular breast of the young patient requires a higher radiation dose to penetrate, x-ray mammography should be limited to women over age 35 unless unusual indications justify the presumed risk of radiation at a younger age.

EXAMINATION TECHNIQUES
Mammographic screening should be reserved for the patient without symptoms or palpable signs of breast abnormalities. A diagnostic study (fig. 44.8) is a problem-solving technique tailored to the symptomatic patient or to the individual with a specific complaint that needs clarification (Sickels 1988)

Table 44.9 summarizes the various imaging techniques applied to breast cancer screening and diagnosis. The only proven, acceptable breast screening techniques at present are film-screen mammography and xeromammography. The choice between the two techniques is dependent on the radiology operator; there is

no significant difference in accuracy between the two procedures. Ultrasound should be reserved for the dense breast or for the younger individual with a palpable lesion that needs further clarification by imaging. The US beam does not readily pass through the fatty, postmenopausal breast tissue. Transmission of the US beam more readily occurs through the glandular, dense breast of the younger patient. There is no role for the use of ultrasound, transmission light scanning, or thermography as a free-standing, screening-diagnostic technique for the detection of breast cancer.

MAMMOGRAPHIC ABNORMALITIES: LOCALIZATION TECHNIQUES

The primary mammographic signs of breast cancer are nonspecific, and relate to the presence of a poorly marginated, dominant (visible on the 2-view mammographic study) mass with or without associated clustered microcalcifications. These tiny calcifications appear in approximately 40% of breast cancers. Their minute size, variability in shape, and number characterize them. Ancillary or secondary signs of malignancy include asymmetrical breast density, distortion of normal breast architecture, duct or vessel enlargement, and skin thickening or retraction (Lanyi 1986).

Nearly 50% of breast cancers are not palpable and will

be detected only by mammography; therefore, the radiologist must identify the lesion for the surgeon. This requires radiographic localization to guide surgical biopsy. Many of these procedures involve the placement of a needle-wire, under x-ray guidance. These needles, or wires, are left in place to direct the surgeon to the mammographic site of abnormality. If microcalcifications are present, specimen x-rays must confirm their presence in the biopsy material. A follow-up mammogram is necessary approximately four to six months following the biopsy, to make certain that the mammographic abnormality has been sampled and appropriately removed. More recent stereoscopic aspiration biopsy procedures have been introduced and appear to show comparable accuracy to open biopsy. However, these procedures require special equipment and trained cytologists.

PART X: ONCOLOGIC IMAGING OF THE PROSTATE

INTRODUCTION

Prostate cancer is the most common malignant tumor in older men, increasing sharply in incidence after the age of 50 (Koss 1988). For 1990, the American Cancer Society estimated 106,000 new cases and 30,000 cancer-related deaths in adult males (Silverberg, Boring, and Squires 1990). Carcinoma of the prostate is the leading cause of death in males over the age of 75; nearly 34% of men in the eighth decade of life harbor the disease. Clinically obvious disease presents only a fraction of the cases of prostate carcinoma, so early detection and optimal staging are the current challenges for the new imaging technologies. Mindful of the fact that disease prevalence (latent cancer) is in excess of that which is clinically significant (overt cancer), the problem revolves around the detection of prostate cancers that have the biologic potential to produce disease and harm the patient (Balfe, Heiken, and McClennan 1985). With up to 35% of men having locally advanced carcinoma of the prostate at the time of diagnosis and up to 45% having metastases, there is a critical need for more adequate clinical and imaging techniques directed at detection and initial staging. The digital rectal exam, carefully performed, can detect palpable prostate cancer in the peripheral zone of the gland with a high degree of sensitivity (69%) and specificity (89%) (Chodak et al. 1986). Technological advances in serum analyses, such as prostate specific antigen (PSA) and prostatic acid phosphatase (PAP) have been useful adjuncts in the patient with clinically overt disease (Ercole et al. 1987). However, radiologic imaging tests designed either to detect or refine staging criteria for prostate cancer have not had a major impact on its diagnosis and treatment, but this is changing. As the mean age of our male population increases, attention will continue to focus on early detection and treatment for cure as well as on long-term surveillance (McClennan 1988).

In the past, radiologic imaging modalities played little, if any, role in the early detection of prostate cancer. Intravenous urography evaluates the upper tracts—occasionally detecting incidental disease—but only reveals the imprint of the prostate on the base of the contrast-filled bladder. Intravenous urography is a poor indicator of overall gland size and is insensitive to all but the most aggressive cancers. Ultrasound (US), specifically transrectal ultrasound (TRUS), offers an encouraging future as a noninvasive technique capable of providing excellent anatomic detail, imaging early cancers in the peripheral zone of the prostate and providing valuable staging information in conjunction with TRUS-guided needle biopsy (McClennan 1988; Lee et al. 1988) Transabdominal ultrasound (TAUS) and transurethral ultrasound (TUUS), like urography, provide little useful staging information. Computed tomography (CT) has been an extensive part of the pretreatment evaluation process in patients with prostate cancer (Platt, Bree, and Schwab 1987; Salo et al. 1987; Friedman et al. 1988). Published series have been small, however, and clouded by the fact that calculated accuracy figures (47% to 75% accurate) were based on clinical rather than pathologic staging. Magnetic resonance imaging (MRI) has no useful role as a screening test at this juncture, nor is it reliable for the diagnosis of prostate cancer because it is difficult to separate prostate cancer from benign prostatic hypertrophy (BPH) (Lee and Rholl 1986; Phillips et al. 1987; Heiken and Lee 1988; Biondetti et al. 1987; Consensus Conference 1988). However, with the exquisite contrast resolution and multiplanar imaging capability, MR can provide valuable information regarding local tumor extent (seminal vesicle, bladder, rectum, and levator ani muscle invasion). For this process, MRI holds a distinct advantage CT scanning; volume averaging and limitations of transaxial imaging plane diminish the usefulness of CT for local staging (Lee and Rholl 1986; Heiken and Lee 1988). For lymph node assessment, both MR and CT perform competitively because neither can as yet detect microscopic metastases in normal-sized lymph nodes; MR has the advantage of being able to distinguish between blood vessels and lymph nodes without the need for intravenous contrast material. However, CT can better survey the rest of the pelvis and abdomen and is more widely available with fewer environmental constraints on patient access (Lee and Rholl 1986; Phillips et al. 1987; Heiken and Lee 1988).

PRETREATMENT STAGING

The challenge of pretherapy staging is to select those men with disease confined to the prostate gland because they benefit the most from radical surgery or radiation therapy performed for cure. Extracapsular extension and metastases are associated with poor survival and shorter disease-free intervals, but excellent results are possible still in some patients with stage C or D1 disease, particularly when no metastases are present at the time of diagnosis. Unfortunately, clinical staging that relies on a digital rectal examination, physical examination, and prostate biopsy is not sufficiently accurate for an adequate therapeutic management decision. Clinical understaging occurs, and even determining tumor grade from biopsy specimens can lead to underestimation of the aggressiveness of prostate cancer when compared to the whole prostatectomy specimen. In view of these clinical difficulties, a variety of imaging modalities have been brought to bear on the early detection, local extent at the time of diagnosis, and lymph node status in patients with carcinoma of the prostate.

DETECTION

Transrectal ultrasound is gaining in stature as a useful tool in the early detection of prostate cancer (Lee et al. 1988; Platt, Bree, and Schwab 1987). Questions remain as to the efficacy of TRUS as a screening tool or as an improvement over the time-honored digital rectal exam (McClennan 1988; Platt, Bree, and Schwab 1987). Furthermore, there is controversy over whether the early detection of asymptomatic prostate (latent) cancer will have a significant effect on morbidity and mortality from this common disease. It is not yet universally accepted that small foci of prostate cancers are really early, large cancers, or that all small cancers progress to lethal cancers (Platt, Bree, and Schwab 1987). A conjoint approach which includes digital rectal exam, TRUS, biopsy, and even PSA seems to offer the best combination of clinical-pathological and imaging tools for optimal detection efficacy. Still, the positive predictive value for biopsy of suspicious areas in the prostate gland detected by TRUS and/or rectal examination ranges from 23% to 41% (Chodak et al. 1986; McClennan 1988). The process of detecting prostate cancer will continue to combine the well-performed digital rectal examination, advances in US equipment design and operator expertise, and improvements in biopsy techniques. Patient and clinician awareness of the biological vicissitudes of the disease and the need for periodic examinations in men over age 50 years will improve the overall patient survival statistics.

LOCAL EXTENSION (T-STAGE)

Accurate assessment of local tumor stage is essential to the proper therapeutic choice. The choice of radical surgery, implantation, or external beam radiation therapy depends on the total volume of disease and local intraglandular as well as extraglandular extension. One goal of noninvasive imaging is to separate stage B (T2) from more extensive C and D (T3-4) disease. Computed tomography, MRI, and US have been extensively studied, and are all accurate methods for determining prostate size as a rough index of total tumor volume. However, CT has been limited by volume averaging and transaxial imaging plane for the accurate depiction of seminal vesicle invasion and subtle extracapsular extension (Platt, Bree, and Schwab 1987; Salo et al. 1987). Detection of seminal vesicle invasion is key, because it represents stage C (T3) disease and usually carries a high incidence of lymph node metastases. Significant false-positive and false-negative readings do occur

even with good-quality CT scans. Imaging of local periprostatic fat or venous plexus involvement with CT is also fraught with the same difficulties encountered in imaging the seminal vesicles. Overall accuracy of only 67% for CT staging for carcinoma of the prostate was recently reported (Platt, Bree, and Schwab 1987). More useful than CT for local extension is TRUS, with sensitivities in the range of 86%, specificity of 94%, and overall accuracy of 90% for local extracapsular extension (Salo et al. 1987). However, the same study reported poor sensitivity of 29% and accuracy of only 77% for seminal vesicle invasion. MRI staging accuracies range from 83% to 89% with multiplanar images (Lee and Rholl 1986; Heiken and Lee 1988). Microscopic capsular or early extracapsular invasion results in understaging with all techniques. Periprostatic tumor extension into periprostatic fat carries an overall accuracy of 85% (Biondetti et al. 1987), and is best depicted on T1-weighted images, while invasion of periprostatic venous plexus with an accuracy of 80% is better appreciated on T2-weighted images (Lee and Rholl 1986; Heiken and Lee 1988; Biondetti et al. 1987). Magnetic resonance imaging is superior to CT or TRUS for seminal vesicle invasion, and overall it performs at 90% accuracy rates for differentiating stage B (T2) from stages C-D (T3-4) disease. Improvements in TRUS accuracy will result from refinement in diagnostic criteria, selective biopsy of suspicious areas of extraprostatic involvement, and improvements in equipment (transducer) design. TRUS and MRI are competitive imaging techniques for accurate T-stage evaluation of patients with prostate cancer.

LYMPH NODE STATUS (N-STAGE)

The gold standard for evaluation of lymph node status is surgical lymph node dissection. The widespread utilization of radical prostatectomy with staging lymph node dissection or radiation therapy by implantation has obviated the need for elaborate attempts at imaging. Lymphangiography (LAG) does opacify the major nodal groups at risk for metastases from prostate cancer. A low false-positive rate exists for LAG, but a prohibitively high false-negative (sensitivity 33% to 75%) has precluded LAG as part of the standard imaging evaluation (Balfe, Heiken, and McClennan 1985). Three major reasons for the poor predictive performance of lymphangiography are: microscopic intranodal metastases are missed; nonfilling of lymph nodes occurs with complete lymph node replacement; and lymph node metastases occur in lymph nodes not routinely opacified by the bipedal route. The first of these three deficiencies currently plagues all imaging modalities. However, CT and MRI may perform better in the other two categories. CT and MRI offer comparable information when evaluating lymph node status in patients with real or suspected prostate cancer. CT scanning has high specificity (96%) for enlarged lymph node metastases (Balfe, Heiken, and McClennan 1985; Platt, Bree, and Schwab 1987; Salo et al. 1987). MRI, while studied less extensively than CT for the evaluation of lymph node metastases, can perform at a similar level of accuracy, with an improved ability to distinguish enlarged nodes from blood vessels or contiguous

Table 44.10
IMAGING METHODS FOR CARCINOMA OF THE PROSTATE

MODALITY	STAGING CAPABILITY	COST/BENEFIT RATIO	RECOMMENDED ROUTINE STAGING PROCEDURE
A. NONINVASIVE			
1. Chest films	Detects hematogenous of lymphatic spread	High	Yes
2. Bone films	Detects lytic, blastic, or mixed metastases in advanced disease	Medium	No; confirms and follows bone scan findings
3. Radionuclide studies			
a. Bone scan	a. Detects early skeletal metastases	High	Yes
b. Liver-spleen scan	b. Detects liver metastases	Low	No; low-yield study
4. Magnetic resonance	Capable of imaging extracapsular spread; intraglandular anatomy reasonably well displayed; cannot tell BPH from cancer; as good or better than CT, especially for lymph node assessment	High	Yes; may replace CT
B. MINIMALLY INVASIVE			
1. Computed tomography			
a. Chest	Capable of assessing lesions seen on chest film; may detect deposits not seen on chest film	Medium	No; selected patients at high risk for widespread metastases
2. CT or MRI			
a. Pelvis	Capable of imaging local tumor volume and extension; capable of imaging pelvic lymph node metastases	High	No; selected patients at risk for extracapsular and/or lymph node metastases
3. Urography	Screens urinary tract for obstruction or coexistent abnormalities	Medium	Yes
4. Transrectal sonography	Capable of assessing T-stage; excellent for detection	High	Maybe
5. Lymphoscintigraphy	Capable of assessing gross lymphatic involvement	Low	No
C. INVASIVE			
1. Lymphangiography	Capable of assessing nodes in external iliac, common iliac, and para-aortic groups	Low	No; selected patients at risk for nodal metastases may benefit
2. Prostatography	Theoretically capable of showing direct lymphatic drainage of diseased lobe	Low	No
3. Transrectal or transperineal aspiration biopsy	Documents presence and character of tumors seen by other methods	High	May become routine

(From: Balfe, Heiken, and McClennan [1985].)

muscle. Both CT and MR are most useful when they demonstrate clinically unsuspected lymph node disease, which fine-needle aspiration biopsy can confirm if necessary, and thus spare patients needless attempts at radical therapy. Ultrasound, even endorectal ultrasound, has little or no utility for the evaluation of pelvic lymph nodes. Like LAG, CT or MRI do not provide sufficiently accurate information on which to base all therapeutic decisions (Balfe, Heiken, and McClennan 1985).

METASTATIC DISEASE (M-STAGE)
The skeletal system is the most common site for metastatic disease in men with carcinoma of the prostate. Common target areas include lumbar spine, pelvis, femur, and ribs. Radionuclide bone imaging is the most sensitive test for detection of skeletal metastases. False-negative bone scans are uncommon. Careful correlation with conventional radiographs is required, however, because healing and tumor progression may appear

similar. Homogenous spread often involves the lungs, but radiographic evidence is often lacking, even when autopsy studies have revealed that 25% of patients with prostate cancer have pulmonary metastases (Balfe, Heiken, and McClennan 1985). Surveillance of the skeletal system after estrogen therapy or radiation therapy may require serial radionuclide imaging. Positive laboratory tests, like PAP or PSA, may also require radionuclide skeletal imaging.

CURRENT IMAGING RECOMMENDATIONS

The focus of optimal imaging strategies should be to select patients with the best chance for survival and then enter them into radical treatment protocols. Table 44.10 summarizes the various imaging techniques applied to prostate cancer screening and diagnosis. Patients with low-stage disease should undergo aggressive imaging evaluation, as survival is highest when tumor volume is low and confined to the prostate gland. Some high-grade tumors have a higher incidence of lymph node metastases; therefore, tumor grade, in addition to stage, may prompt oncologic imaging studies. Accurate follow-up information from MRI or transrectal ultrasound can be valuable to the therapist regarding tumor volume and the therapeutic response. Further improvements in imaging equipment, particularly transrectal ultrasound and MRI, will enable more optimal clinical pretreatment staging with a positive outcome on patient survival.

REFERENCES

Adalsteinsson, B.; Glimelius, B.; and Graffman, S. et al. 1985. Computed tomography in staging rectal carcinoma. *Acta Radiol. Diagn.* (Stockholm) 26:45-50.

Adalsteinsson, B.; Glimelius, B.; and Graffman, S. et al. 1981. Computed tomography of recurrent rectal carcinoma. *Acta Radiol. Diagn.* (Stockholm) 22:669-72.

Alazraki, N.P., and Taylor, A.T. 1988. Radioimmunodiagnosis through imaging: prospects for tumor imaging using labeled monoclonal antibodies. *Invest. Radiol.* 23:414-20.

Alderson, P.O.; Adams, D.F.; and McNeil, B.J. 1983. Computed tomography, ultrasound, and scintigraphy of the liver in patients with colon or breast carcinoma: a prospective comparison. *Radiology* 149:225-30.

Allibone, G.W.; Fagan, C.J.; and Porter, S.C. 1981. Sonographic features of carcinoma of the gallbladder. *Gastrointest. Radiol.* 6:169-73.

Amendola, M.A.; Glazer, G.M.; and Grossman, H.B. et al. 1986. Staging of bladder carcinoma: MRI-CT-surgical correlation. *AJR* 146:1179-83.

American Joint Committee for Cancer Staging and End Result Reporting. 1978. *Manual for staging of cancer.* Chicago: National Cancer Institute.

American Joint Committee on Cancer. 1983. *Manual for staging of cancer.* 2nd ed. New York: J. B. Lippincott.

Baker, H.L.; Houser, O.W.; and Cambell, J.K. 1980. National Cancer Institute study: evaluation of CT in the diagnosis of intracranial neoplasms I: overall results. *Radiology* 136:91-96.

Balfe, D.M.; Koehler, R.E.; and Karstaedt, N. 1981. Computed tomography of gastric neoplasms. *Radiology* 140:431-36.

Balfe, D.M.; Heiken, J.D.; and McClennan, B.L. 1985. Bladder cancer. In Bragg, D.; Rubin, P.; and Youker, J. eds. *Oncologic imaging.* chap. 17. pp. 389-404. New York: Pergamon Press.

Balfe, D.M.; Heiken, J.D.; and McClennan, B.L. 1985. Prostatic cancer. In Bragg, D.; Rubin, P.; and Youker, J. eds. *Oncologic imaging.* pp. 405-24. New York: Pergamon Press.

Barnett, P.H.; Zehouni, E.A.; and White, R.I. 1980. Computed tomography in the diagnosis of cavernous hemangioma. *AJR* 134:439-47.

Baron, R.L.; Leavitt, R.G.; and Sagel, S.S. et al. 1982. Computed tomography in the preoperative evaluation of bronchogenic carcinoma. *Radiology* 145:727-32.

Baron, R.L.; Stanley, R.J.; and Lee, J.K.T. et al. 1983. Computed tomographic features of biliary obstruction. *AJR* 140:1173-78.

Baron, R.L.; Stanley, R.J.; and Lee, J.K.T. et al. 1982. A prospective comparison of the evaluation of biliary obstruction using computed tomography and ultrasonography. *Radiology* 145:91-98.

Bassill, B.; Dosouretz, D.E.; and Prout, G.R. 1985. Validation of the tumor, nodes, and metastases classification of renal cell carcinoma. *J. Urol.* 134:450-54.

Becker, C.D.; Barbier, P.A.; and Terrier, F. et al. 1987. Patterns of recurrence of esophageal carcinoma after transhiatal esophagectomy and gastric interposition. *AJR* 148:273-77.

Berk, R.N.; Ferrucci, J.T. Jr.; and Leopold, G.R. 1983. *Radiology of the gallbladder and bile ducts: diagnosis and intervention.* Philadelphia: W.B. Saunders.

Berk, R.N.; Ferrucci, J.T. Jr.; and Goldstein, H.M. et al. 1978. Progress in clinical radiology: diagnostic imaging of the liver and bile ducts. *Invest. Radiol.* 13:265-78.

Berk, R.N.; Cooperberg, P.L.; and Gold, R.P. et al. 1982. Radiology of the bile ducts. *Radiology* 145:1-9.

Berland, L.L.; Lawson, T.L.; and Foley, W.D. et al. 1982. Comparison of pre- and post-contrast CT in hepatic masses. *AJR* 238:853-58.

Bernardino, M.E., and Green, B. 1979. Ultrasonographic evaluation of chemotherapeutic response in hepatic metastases. *Radiology* 133:437-41.

Bernardino, M.E.; Thomas, J.L.; and Maklad, N. 1982. Hepatic sonography: technical considerations, present applications, and possible future. *Radiology* 142:249-51.

Biondetti, P.R.; Lee, J.K.T.; and Ling, D. et al. 1987. Clinical stage B prostate carcinoma: staging with MR imaging. *Radiology* 162:325-29.

Bonnel, D.; Ferrucci, J.T. Jr.; and Muller, P.R. et al. 1984. Surgical and radiological decompression in malignant biliary obstruction: a retrospective study using multivariate risk factor analysis. *Radiology* 152:347-51.

Bragg, D.G.; Rubin, P.; and Youker, J. 1985. Thoracic neoplasms: imaging requirements for diagnosis and staging. In *Oncologic imaging.* chap. 10. New York: Pergamon Press.

Bragg, D.G., and Harnsberger, H.R. 1985. Newer radiologic techniques. In DeVita, V.T.; Hellman, S.; and Rosenberg, S.A. eds. *Cancer: principles and practice of oncology.* Philadelphia: J.B. Lippincott.

Brant-Zawadski, M.; Badami, J.P.; and Mills, C.M. et al. 1984. Primary intracranial tumor imaging: a comparison of magnetic resonance and CT. *Radiology* 150:435-40.

Brant-Zawadski, M.; Norman, D.; and Newton, T.H. et al. 1984. Magnetic resonance of the brain: the optimal screening technique. *Radiology* 152:71-77.

Bronskill, M.J.; Henkelman, R.M.; and Poon, P.Y. et al. 1988. Magnetic resonance imaging, computed tomography, and radionuclide scintigraphy in detection of liver metastases. *J. Can. Assoc. Radiol.* 39:3-9.

Brown, J.P.; Nishiyama, K.; and Hellstrom, I. et al. 1981. Structural characterization of human melanoma-associated antigen p97 using monoclonal antibodies. *J. Immunol.* 127:539-46.

Bryan, P.J.; Butler, H.E.; and LiPuma, J.P. et al. 1987. CT and MR imaging in staging bladder neoplasms. *J. Comput. Assist. Tomogr.* 11(1):96-101.

Burgener, F.A., and Hamlin, D.J. 1981. Contrast enhancement in abdominal CT: bolus vs. infusion. *AJR* 137:351-58.

Butch, R.J.; Stark, D.D.; and Wittenberg, J. et al. 1986. Staging rectal cancer by MR and CT. *AJR* 146:1155-60.

Butch, R.J.; Wittenberg, J.; and Mueller, P.R. et al. 1985. Presacral masses after abdominoperineal resection for colorectal carcinoma: the need for needle biopsy. *AJR* 144:309-12.

Cady, B.; McDonald, J.S.; and Gunderson, L.L. 1985. Cancer of the hepatobiliary system. In DeVita, V.; Hellman, S.; and Rosenberg, S. eds. *Cancer: principles and practice of oncology.* 2nd ed. pp. 741-70. Philadelphia: J. B. Lippincott.

Catalona, W.J. 1980. Bladder carcinoma (editorial). *J. Urol.* 123:35.

Chodak, G.W.; Wald, V.; and Parmer, E. et al. 1986. Comparison of digital examination and transrectal ultrasonography for diagnosis of prostatic cancer. *J. Urol.* 135:951-54.

Chuang, V.P. 1984. Hepatic tumor angiography: a subject review. *Radiology* 148:633-39.

Clark, J.; Bankoff, M.; and Carter, B. et al. 1984. The use of computerized tomography scan in the staging and follow-up study of carcinoma of the rectum. *Surg. Gynecol. Obstet.* 159:335-42.

Clark, L.R.; Jaffe, M.H.; and Choyke, P.L. et al. 1985. Pancreatic imaging. *Radiol. Clin. North Am.* 23:489-501.

Clausen, C.; Laniado, and Schorner, W. et al. 1985. Gadolinium-DPTA in MR imaging of glioblastomas and intracranial metastases. *AJNR* 6:669-74.

Conrad, M.R.; Landay, M.J.; and Jones, J.O. 1978. Sonographic "parallel channel" sign of biliary tree enlargement in mild to moderate obstructive jaundice. *AJR* 130:279-86.

Consensus Conference. 1988. Magnetic resonance imaging. *JAMA* 259:2132-38.

Cotton, P.B.; Lees, W.R.; and Wallon, A.G. et al. 1980. Gray-scale ultrasonography in pancreatic diagnosis. *Radiology* 134:453-59.

Council on Scientific Affairs, American Medical Association. 1988. Positron emission tomography in oncology. *JAMA* 259:2126-31.

Crade, M.; Taylor, K.J.W.; and Rosenfeld, A.T. et al. 1979. The varied ultrasonic character of gallbladder tumor. *JAMA* 241:2195-96.

Cubilla, A.L., and Fitzgerald, P.J. 1979. Classification of pancreatic cancer (nonendocrine). *Mayo Clinic Proc.* 54:449-58.

Curry, N.S.; Reinig, J.; and Schabel, S.I. et al. 1984. An evaluation of the effectiveness of CT vs. other imaging modalities in the diagnosis of atypical renal masses. *Invest. Radiol.* 19:447-52.

Daffner, R.H.; Halber, M.D.; and Postlethwait, R.W. et al. 1979. CT of the esophagus II: carcinoma. *AJR* 133:1051-55.

Dershaw, D.D., and Scher, H.I. 1988. Serial transabdominal sonography of bladder cancer. *AJR* 150:1055-59.

Dillon, W.P.; Mills, K.M.; and Kjos, B. et al. 1984. Magnetic resonance imaging of the nasopharynx. *Radiology* 152:731-38.

Dixon, A.K.; Fry, I.K.; and Morson, B.C. et al. 1981. Preoperative computed tomography of carcinoma of the rectum. *Br. J. Radiol.* 54:655-59.

Drayer, B.P.; Johnson, P.C.; and Bird, C.R. et al. 1988. Magnetic resonance imaging and glioma. *BNI Quarterly* 3:44-55.

Dubbins, P.A., and Wells, I. 1986. Renal carcinoma: duplex Doppler evaluation. *Br. J. Radiol.* 59:231-36.

Dukes, C.E. 1938. The classification of cancer of the rectum. *J. Pathol.* 35:323-32.

Earnest, F.; Kelly, P.J.; and Scheiterhauer, B.W. et al. 1988. Cerebral astrocytomas: histopathologic correlation of MR and CT contrast enhancement with stereotactic biopsy. *Radiology* 166:823-27.

Eaton, S.B. Jr., and Ferrucci, J.T. Jr. 1973. *Radiology of the pancreas and duodenum.* Philadelphia: W.B. Saunders.

Eddy, D.M.; Hasselbad, V.; and McGivney, W. et al. 1988. The value of mammography screening in women under age 50 years. *JAMA* 259:1512-19.

Edelman, R.R.; Hahn, P.F.; and Buxton, R. et al. 1986. Rapid MR imaging with suspended respiration: clinical application in the liver. *Radiology* 161:125-31.

Edmonson, H.A. 1958. *Tumors of the liver and intrahepatic bile ducts.* sect. VII, fasc. 25. Washington, D.C.: Armed Forces Institute of Pathology.

Eisenberg, H. 1973. Pancreatic angiography. In Hilal, S.K. ed. *Small vessel angiograph: imaging, morphology, physiology, and clinical application.* pp. 405-33. St. Louis: C.V. Mosby.

Ellert, J., and Kreel, L. 1980. The value of CT in malignant colonic tumors. *J. Comput. Tomogr.* 4:225-40.

Enneking, W.F. 1985. Staging of musculoskeletal neoplasm. *Skeletal Radiol.* 13:183-94.

Ercole, C.J.; Lange, P.H.; and Mathisen, M. et al. 1987. Prostatic specific antigen and prostatic acid phosphatase in the monitoring and staging of patients with prostatic cancer. *J. Urol.* 1181-84.

Friedman, A.C.; Seidmon, E.J.; and Radecki, P.D. et al. 1988. Relative merits of MRI, transrectal endosonography and CT in diagnosis and staging of carcinoma of the prostate. *Urology* 31:530-37.

Evers, K.; Laufer, I.; and Gordon, R.L. et al. 1981. Double-contrast enema examination for detection of rectal carcinoma. *Radiology* 140:635-39.

Fahim, R.B.; McDonald, J.R.; and Richards, J.C. et al. 1962. Carcinoma of the gallbladder: a study of its modes of spread. *Ann. Surg.* 156:114-24.

Feig, S.A. 1988. Decreased breast cancer mortality through mammographic screening: results of clinical trials. *Radiology* 167:659-65.

Fein, A.B.; Lee, J.K.T.; and Balfe, D.M. et al. 1987. Diagnosis and staging of renal cell carcinoma: a comparison of MR and CT. *AJR* 148:749-53.

Ferrucci, J.T. Jr. 1988. MR imaging of the liver. *AJR* 147:1103-16.

Ferrucci; J.T. Jr.; Adson, M.A.; and Mueller, P.R. et al. 1983. Advances in the radiology of jaundice: a symposium and review. *AJR* 141:1-20.

Foley, W.D.; Berland, L.L.; and Lawson, T.L. et al. 1983. Contrast enhancement technique for dynamic hepatic computed tomographic scanning. *Radiology* 147:797-803.

Fontana, R.S.; Sanderson, D.R.; and Taylor, W.F. et al. 1984. Early lung cancer detection: results of the initial (prevalence) radiology and cytologic screening at the Mayo Clinic. *Am. Rev. Resp. Dis.* 130:549-61.

Freeny, P.C.; Marks, W.M.; and Ryan, J.A. et al. 1986. Colorectal carcinoma evaluation with CT: preoperative staging and detection of postoperative recurrence. *Radiology* 158:347-53.

Freeny, P.C.; Marks, W.M.; and Ball, T.J. 1982. Impact of high-resolution computed tomography of the pancreas on utilization of endoscopic retrograde cholangiopancreatography and angiography. *Radiology* 142:35-40.

Freeny, P.C., and Marks, W.M. 1982. Adenocarcinoma of the gastroesophageal junction: barium and CT examination. *AJR* 138:1077-84.

Freeny, P.C., and Lawson, T.L. 1982. Adenocarcinoma of the pancreas. In Freeny, P.C., and Lawson, T.L. eds. *Radiology of the pancreas.* pp. 397-496. New York: Springer-Verlag.

Freeny, P.C., and Ball, T.J. 1978. Rapid diagnosis of pancreatic carcinoma: an algorithmic approach. *Radiology* 130:683-91.

Freeny, P.C., and Marks, W.M. 1983. Computed arteriography of the liver. *Radiology* 148:193-97.

Gatenby, R.A.; Mulhern, C.B.; and Strawitz, J. et al. 1985. Comparison of clinical and CT staging of head and neck tumors. *AJNR* 6:399-401.

Glazer, H.S.; Niemeyer, J.H.; and Balfe, D.M. et al. 1986. Neck neoplasms: MR imaging I: initial evaluation. *Radiology* 160:343-48.

Glazer, G.M.; Aisen, A.M.; and Francis, I.R. et al. 1985. Hepatic cavernous hemangioma: magnetic resonance imaging. *Radiology* 155:417-20.

Gobien, R.P.; Stanley, J.H.; and Soucek, C.K. et al. 1984. Routine preoperative biliary drainage: effect on management of obstructive jaundice. *Radiology* 152:353-56.

Goding, J.W., and Burns, G.F. 1981. Monoclonal antibody OKT9 recognizes the receptor for transferrin on human acute lymphocytic leukemia cells. *J. Immunol.* 127:1256-58.

Grabbe, E.; Lierse, W.; and Winkler, R. 1983. The perirectal fascia: morphology and use in staging of rectal carcinoma. *Radiology* 149:241-46.

Grabbe, E., and Winkler, R. 1985. Local recurrence after sphincter-saving resection for rectal and rectosigmoid carcinoma. *Radiology* 155:305-10.

Grant, E.G.; Richardson, J.D.; and Smirniotopoulos, J.G. et al. 1983. Fine-needle biopsy directed by real-time sonography: technique and accuracy. *AJR* 141:29-32.

Green, B.; Bree, R.L.; and Goldstein, H.M. et al. 1977. Gray-scale ultrasound evaluation of hepatic neoplasms: patterns and correlations. *Radiology* 124:203-208.

Gupta, S.; Udupa, K.N.; and Gupta, S. 1980. Primary carcinoma of the gallbladder: a review of 328 cases. *J. Surg. Oncol.* 14:35-44.

Haaga, J.R. 1984. Magnetic resonance imaging of the pancreas. *Radiol. Clin. North Am.* 22:869-77.

Halpern, S.E.; Dillman, R.O.; and Hagen, P.L. 1983. The problem and promise of monoclonal antitumor antibodies in diagnostic imaging. *Diagn. Imag.* 5:40-47.

Halvorsen, R.A., and Thompson, W.M. 1986. Critical review of esophageal carcinoma by Quint, L.E.; Glazer, G.M.; and Orringer, M.B. et al. (1985) in *Radiology* 155:171-75. *Invest. Radiol.* 20.

Halvorsen, R.A. Jr. and Thompson, W.M. 1987. CT for staging gastrointestinal cancer I: esophagus and stomach. *Invest. Radiol.* 22:2-16.

Harbin, W.P.; Robert, N.J.; and Ferrucci, J.T. Jr. 1983. Diagnosis of cirrhosis based on regional changes in hepatic morphology. *Radiology* 135:273-83.

Harnsberger, H.R.; Mancuso, A.A.; and Muraki, A.S. 1983. The upper aerodigestive tract and neck: CT evaluation of recurrent tumors. *Radiology* 149:503-509.

Hatch, T.R., and Barry, J.M. 1986. The value of excretory urography in staging bladder cancer. *J. Urol.* 136:49.

Hauser, H.; Battikha, J.G.; and Wettstein, P. 1980. Computed tomography of the dilated main pancreatic duct. *J. Comput. Assist. Tomogr.* 4:53-58.

Heiken, J.P.; Balfe, D.M.; and Roper, C.L. 1984. CT evaluation after esophagogastrectomy. *AJR* 143:550-60.

Heiken, J.P., and Lee, J.K.T. 1988. MR imaging of the pelvis. *Radiology* 166:11-16.

Heiken, J.P.; Lee, J.R.T.; and Glazer, H.S. et al. 1985. Hepatic metastases studied with MR and CT. *Radiology* 156:423-27.

Heiken, J.P., and Lee, J.K.T. 1988. MR imaging of the pelvis. *Radiology* 166:11-16.

Heiken, J.P.; Balfe, D.M.; and Picus, D. et al. 1984. Radical pancreatectomy: postoperative evaluation by CT. *Radiology* 153:211-15.

Hendee, W.R. 1988. (The human visual system and its application to perception of radiologic images *Invest. Radiol.* 24:25.

Hendee, W.R. 1985. The impact of future technology on oncologic diagnosis. In Bragg, D.G.; Rubin, P.; and Youker, J.E. eds. *Oncologic imaging.* pp. 629-44. New York: Pergamon Press.

Herlinger, H. 1983. Double-contrast enterolysis. In Margulis, A.R., and Burhenne, H.J. eds. *Alimentary tract radiology.* 3rd ed. pp. 890-902. St. Louis: C.V. Mosby.

Hermann, R.E., and Cooperman, A.M. 1979. Current concepts in cancer: cancer of the pancreas. *N. Engl. J. Med.* 301:482-85.

Hessel, S.J.; Siegelman, S.S.; and McNeil, B.J. et al. 1982. Prospective evaluation of computed tomography and ultrasound of the pancreas. *Radiology* 143:129-33.

Hoevels, J.; Lunderquist, A.; and Ihse, I. 1978. Percutaneous transhepatic intubation of bile ducts for combined internal-external drainage in preoperative and palliative treatment of obstructive jaundice. *Gastrointest. Radiol.* 3:23-31.

Hricak, H.; Thoeni, R.F.; and Carroll, P.R. et al. 1988. Detection and staging of renal neoplasms: a reassessment of MR imaging. *Radiology* 166:643-49.

Huang, G.J. 1981. Early detection and surgical treatment of esophageal carcinoma. *Jap. J. Surg.* 11:399-405.

Husband, J.E.; Hodson, N.J.; and Parsons, C.A. 1980. The use of computed tomography in recurrent rectal tumors. *Radiology* 134:677-82.

Institute of Medicine. 1977. *A policy statement: computed tomographic scanning.* Washington, D.C.: National Academy of Sciences.

Itai, Y.; Araki, T.; and Tasaka, A. et al. 1982. Computed tomographic appearance of resectable pancreatic carcinoma. *Radiology* 143:719-26.

Itai, Y.; Araki, T.; and Yoshikawa, K. et al. 1980. Computed tomography of the gallbladder carcinoma. *Radiology* 137:713-18.

Itai, Y.; Araki, T.; and Furui, S. 1983. Computed tomography of primary intrahepatic biliary malignancy. *Radiology* 147:485-90.

Johnson, C.D.; Dunnick, N.R.; and Cohan, R.M. et al. 1987. Renal adenocarcinoma: CT staging of 100 tumors. *AJR* 148:59-63.

Mauro, M.A.; Wadsworth, D.E.; and Stanley, R.J. et al. 1982. Renal cell carcinoma: the utility of angiography in the CT era. *AJR* 139:1135-38.

Johnson, C.D., and Carlson, H.C. 1983. Barium enemas of carcinoma of the colon: sensitivity of double- and single-contrast studies. *AJR* 140:1143-49.

Kelvin, F.M.; Gardiner, R.; and Vas, W. et al. 1981. Colorectal carcinoma missed on double-contrast barium enema study: a problem in perception. *AJR* 137:307-13.

Knopf, D.R.; Torres, W.E.; and Fajman, W.J. et al. 1982. Liver lesions: comparative accuracy of scintigraphy and computed tomography. *AJR* 138:623-27.

Kohler, G., and Milstein, C. 1975. Continuous culture of fused cells secreting antibody of predefined specificity. *Nature* 256:495-97.

Koss, L.G. 1988. The puzzle of prostatic carcinoma. *Mayo Clinic Proc.* 63:193-97.

Krudy, A.G.; Doppman, J.L.; and Jensen, R.T. et al. 1984. Localization of islet cell tumors by dynamic CT: comparison with plain CT, arteriography, sonography, and venous sampling. *AJR* 143:585-89.

LaBerge, J.M.; Laing, F.C.; and Federle, M.P. et al. 1984. Hepatocellular carcinoma: assessment of resectability by computed tomography and ultrasound. *Radiology* 152:485-90.

Lanyi, M. 1986. *Diagnosis and differential diagnosis of breast calcifications.* Berlin: Springer-Verlag.

Larson, S.M.; Carrasquillo, J.A.; and McGuffin, R.W. et al. 1985. Use of ^{131}I-labeled murine Fab against a high molecular weight antigen of human melanoma: primary experience. *Radiology* 155:487-92.

Laufer, I. 1979. Tumors of the colon. In Laufer, I. ed. *Double-contrast gastrointestinal radiology with endoscopic correlation.* pp. 517-560. Philadelphia: W.B. Saunders.

Laufer, I.; Smith, N.C.W.; and Mullens, J.E. 1976. The radiological demonstration of colorectal polyps undetected by endoscopy. *Gastroenterology* 70:167-70.

Lawson, T.L.; Berland, L.L.; and Foley, W.D. 1985. Malignant neoplasms of the pancreas, liver, and biliary tract. In Bragg, D.G.; Rubin, P.; and Youker, J. eds. *Oncologic imaging.* pp. 287-342. New York: Pergamon Press.

Lawson, T.L.; Berland, L.L.; and Foley, W.D. et al. 1982. Ultrasonic visualization of the pancreatic duct. *Radiology* 144:865-71.

Lee, J.K.T.; Stanley, R.J.; and Melson, G.L. et al. 1979. Pancreatic imaging by ultrasound and computed tomography: a general review. *Radiol. Clin. North Am.* 16:105-17.

Lee, J.K.T., and Rholl, K.S. 1986. MRI of the bladder and prostate. *AJR* 147:732-36.

Lee, J.K.T., and Rholl, K.S. 1986. MRI of the bladder and prostate. *AJR* 147:732-36.

Lee, F.; Littrup, P.J.; and Torp-Pedersen, S.T. et al. 1988. Prostate cancer: comparison of transrectal US and digital rectal examination for screening. *Radiology* 168:389-94.

Lee, T.G.; Henderson, S.C.; and Ehrlich, R. 1977. Ultrasound diagnosis of common bile duct dilation. *Radiology* 124:792-97.

Lees, C.D.; Zapolanski, A.; and Cooperman. A.M. et al. 1980. Carcinoma of the bile ducts. *Surg. Gynecol. Obstet.* 151:193-98.

Levine, E.; Maklad, N.F.; and Wright, C.H. et al. 1979. Computed tomographic and ultrasonic appearances of primary carcinoma of the common bile duct. *Gastrointest. Radiol.* 4:147-51.

Lewis, E. 1984. Screening for diffuse and focal liver disease: the case for hepatic sonography. *J. Clin. Ultrasound* 12:67-73.

MacCarthy, R.L.; Stephens, D.A.; and Hattery, R.R. et al. 1979. Hepatic imaging by computed tomography: a comparison with ^{99m}Tc-sulfur colloid, ultrasonography, and angiography. *Radiol. Clin. North Am.* 17:137-55.

Mancuso, A.A.; Harnsberger, H.R.; and Muraki, A.S. et al.

1983. CT of cervical and retropharyngeal lymph nodes I: normal anatomy; II: pathology. *Radiology* 148:709-23.

Marchal, G.J.; Baert, A.L.; and Wilms, G.E. 1980. CT of noncystic liver lesions: bolus enhancement. *AJR* 135:57-65.

Marks, J.E., and Gado, M. 1977. Serial CT of primary brain tumors following surgery, irradiation, and chemotherapy. *Radiology* 125:119-25.

Marks, W.M.; Filly, R.A.; and Callen, P.W. 1980. Ultrasonic evaluation of normal pancreatic echogenicity and its relationship to fat deposition. *Radiology* 137:475-79.

Marx, J. Imaging technique passes muster. *Science* 238:888-89.

Masui, H.; Moroyama, T.; and Mendelsohn, J. 1986. Mechanism of antitumor activity in mice for antiepidermal growth factor receptor monoclonal antibodies with different isotopes. *Cancer Res.* 46:5592-98.

Mayes, G.B., and Zornoza, J. 1980. Computed tomography of colon carcinoma. *AJR* 135:43-46.

McCarthy, S.M.; Barnes, D.; and Deveney, K. et al. 1985. Detection of recurrent rectosigmoid carcinoma: prospective evaluation of CT and clinical factors. *AJR* 144:577-79.

McClees, E.C., and Gedgaudas-McClees, R.K. 1984. Screening for diffuse and focal liver disease: the case for hepatic scintigraphy. *J. Clin. Ultrasound* 12:75-81.

McClennan, B.L. 1988. Transrectal US of the prostate: is the technology leading the science? *Radiology* 168:571-75.

McClennan, B.L., and Rabin, D.N. 1988. In Lee, J.K.T.; Sagel, S.S.; and Stanley, R.J. eds. *Computed body tomography with MRI correlation.* New York: Raven Press.

McClennan, B.L., and Balfe, D.M. 1985. Kidney and ureter. In Bragg, D.; Rubin, P.; and Youker, J. eds. *Oncologic imaging.* chap. 16. pp. 363-87. New York: Pergamon Press.

Megibow, A.J.; Bosniak, M.A.; and Ambos, M.A. et al. 1981. Thickening of the celiac axis and/or superior mesenteric artery: a sign of pancreatic carcinoma on computed tomography. *Radiology* 141:449-53.

Montagne, J.P.; Moss, A.A.; and Margulis, A.R. 1978. Double-blind study of single and double-contrast upper gastrointestinal examinations using endoscopy as a control. *AJR* 130:1041-45.

Moss, A.A.; Schnyder, P.; and Thoeni, R.F. et al. 1981a. Esophageal carcinoma: pretherapy staging by computed tomography. *AJR* 136:1051-56.

Moss, A.A.; Schnyder, P.; and Marks, W. et al. 1981b. Gastric adenocarcinoma: a comparison of the accuracy and economics of staging by computed tomography and surgery. *Gastroenterology* 80:45-50.

Moss, A.A.; Schnyder, P.; and Grandardjis, G. et al. 1980. Computed tomography of benign and malignant gastric abnormalities. *J. Clin. Gastroenterol.* 44:401-409.

Moss, A.A.; Thoeni, R.F.; and Schnyder, P. et al. 1981. Value of computed tomography in the detection and staging of recurrent rectal carcinomas. *J. Comput. Assist. Tomogr.* 5:870-74.

Moss, A.A.; Schrumpf, J.; and Schnyder, P. et al. 1979. Computed tomography of focal hepatic lesions: a blind clinical evaluation of the effect of contrast enhancement. *Radiology* 131:427-30.

Moss, A.A. 1982. Computed tomography in the staging of gastrointestinal carcinoma. *Radiol. Clin. North Am.* 20:761-80.

Moss, A.A.; Dean, P.B.; and Axel, L. et al. 1982. Dynamic CT of hepatic masses with intravenous and intra-arterial contrast material. *AJR* 238:847-52.

Moss, A.A.; Goldberg, H.I.; and Stark, D.B. et al. 1984. Hepatic tumors: magnetic resonance and CT appearance. *Radiology* 150:141-47.

Mountain, C.F. 1986. A new international staging for lung cancer. *Chest* 89S:225-33.

Munk, E.L.; Muller, N.L.; and Miller, R.R. et al. 1988. Pulmonary lymphangitic carcinomatosis: CT and pathologic findings. *Radiology* 166:705-709.

Murray, J.L.; Rosenblum, M.G.; and Lamki, L. et al. 1987. Clinical parameters related to optimal tumor localization of indium 111-labeled mouse antimelanoma monoclonal antibody ZME-018. *J. Nucl. Med.* 28:25-33.

Neiman, H.L., and Mintzer, R.A. 1977. Accuracy of biliary duct ultrasound comparison with cholangiography. *AJR* 129:979-82.

Norman, D.; Enzmann, D.R.; and Levin, V.A. et al. 1976. CT in the evaluation of malignant glioma before and after therapy. *Radiology* 121:85-88.

Ohtomo, K.; Itai, Y.; and Furui, S. et al. 1985. Hepatic tumors: differentiation by transverse relaxation time (T2) of magnetic resonance imaging. *Radiology* 155:421-23.

Op den Orth, J.O. 1973. Hypotonic duodenography without the use of a stomach tube. *Radiol. Clin. Biol.* 42:173-74.

Otto, D.J.; Gelfand, D.W.; and Wu, W.C. et al. 1980. Sensitivity of double-contrast barium enema: emphasis on polyp detection. *AJR* 135:327-30.

Pedrosa, C.S.; Casanova, R.; and Lezana et al. 1981. Computed tomography in obstructive jaundice II: the cause of obstruction. *Radiology* 139:635-45.

Pedrosa, C.S.; Casanova, R.; and Rodriguez, R. 1981. Computed tomography in obstructive jaundice I: the level of obstruction. *Radiology* 139:627-34.

Perkerson, R.B. Jr.; Erwin, B.C.; and Baumgartner, B.R. et al. 1985. CT densities in delayed iodine hepatic scanning. *Radiology* 155:445-56.

Pettersson, H.; Gillespy, T.; and Hamlin, D. et al. 1987. Primary musculoskeletal tumors: examination with the MR imaging compared with conventional modality. *Radiology* 164:237.

Phillips, M.E.; Kressel, H.Y.; and Spritzer, C.E. et al. 1987. Prostatic disorders: MR imaging at 1.5 T. *Radiology* 164:386-92.

Platt, J.F.; Bree, R.L; and Schwab, R.E. 1987. The accuracy of CT in the staging of carcinoma of the prostate. *AJR* 149:315-18.

Picus, D.; Balfe, D.M.; and Koehler, R.E. et al. 1983. Computed tomography in the staging of esophageal carcinoma. *Radiology* 146:433-38.

Prando, A.; Wallace, S.; and Bernardino, M.E. et al. 1979. Computed tomographic arteriography of the liver. *Radiology* 130:697-701.

Prout, G.R. 1982. Bladder cancer. *J. Urol.* 128:284.

Quint, L.E.; Glazer, G.M.; and Orringer, M.B. et al. 1985a. Esophageal carcinoma: CT findings. *Radiology* 155:171-75.

Quint, L.E.; Glazer, G.M.; and Orringer, M.B. 1985b. Esophageal imaging by MR and CT: study of normal anatomy and neoplasm. *Radiology* 156:727-31.

Robbins, S.L. 1979. The gastrointestinal tract. In Robbins, S.L., and Contran, R.S. eds. *Pathologic basis of disease.* 2nd ed. pp. 946-52. Philadelphia: W.B. Saunders.

Rosenberg, J.C. et al. 1985. Cancer of the esophagus. In DeVita, V.T.; Hellman, S.; and Rosenberg, S.A. eds. *Cancer: principles and practice of oncology.* 2nd ed. pp. 621-57. Philadelphia: J.B. Lippincott.

Ruiz, R.; Teyssou, H.; and Fernandez, N. et al. 1980. Ultrasonic diagnosis of primary carcinoma of the gallbladder: a review of 16 cases. *J. Clin. Ultrasound* 8:489-95.

Russell, I. 1983. The evaluation of computerized tomography: a review of research methods. In Culyer, A.J., and Horisberger, B. eds. *Economic and medical evaluation of health care technologies.* New York: Springer-Verlag.

Salo, J.O.; Kivisaari, L.; and Rannikko, S. et al. 1987. Computerized tomography and transrectal ultrasound in the assessment of local extension of prostatic cancer before radical retropubic prostatectomy. *J. Urol.* 137:435-38.

Sample, W.F.; Sarti, D.A.; and Goldstein, L.I. et al. 1978. Gray-scale ultrasonography of the jaundiced patient. *Radiology* 128:719-25.

Scheible, W.; Gosink, B.B.; and Leopold, G.R. 1977. Gray-scale echographic patterns of hepatic metastatic disease. *AJR* 129:983-87.

Seidman, H.; Gelb, S.K.; and Silverberg, E. et al. 1987. Survival experience in the Breast Cancer Detection Demonstration Project. *CA* 37:258-90.

Sellink, J.L. 1983. Single-contrast enterolysis. In Margulis,

A.R., and Burhenne, H.J. eds. *Alimentary tract radiology*. 3rd ed. pp. 871-89. St. Louis: C.V. Mosby.

Shimuzi, H.; Ida, M.; and Takayama, S. et al. 1981. Diagnostic accuracy of computed tomography in obstructive biliary disease: a comparative evaluation with direct cholangiography. *Radiology* 138:411-16.

Shirakabe, J., and Maruyama, M. 1983. Neoplastic disease of the stomach. In Margulis, A.R., and Burhenne, H.J. eds. *Alimentary tract radiology*. 3rd ed. pp. 721-65. St. Louis: C.V. Mosby.

Showstack, J.A.; Schroeder, S.A.; and Steinberg, H. 1981. Evaluating the costs and benefits of a diagnostic technology: the case of upper gastrointestinal endoscopy. *Med. Care* 19:498.

Sickels, E.A. 1988 Detection and diagnosis of breast cancer with mammography. *Persp. Radiol.* 1(2).

Siegelman, S.S.; Khouri, N.F.; and Leo, F.P. et al. 1986. Solitary pulmonary nodules: CT assessment. *Radiology* 160:307-12.

Staples, C.A.; Muller, N.L.; and Miller, R.R. et al. 1988. Mediastinal nodes in bronchogenic carcinoma: comparison between CT and mediastinoscopy. *Radiology* 167:367-72.

Silverberg, E.; Boring, C.C.; and Squires, T.S. 1990. Cancer statistics 1990. *CA* 40:9-26.

Simeone, J.F.; Wittenberg, J.; and Ferrucci, J.T. Jr. 1980. Modern concepts of imaging of the pancreas. *Invest. Radiol.* 15:6-18.

Simeone, J.F.; Edelman, R.R.; and Stark, D.D. et al. 1985. Surface coil MR imaging of abdominal viscera III: the pancreas. *Radiology* 157:437-41.

Sindelar, W.F. 1985. Cancer of the small intestine. In DeVita, V.; Hellman, S.; and Rosenberg, S.A. eds. *Cancer: principles and practice of oncology*. 2nd ed. pp. 771-94. Philadelphia: J. B. Lippincott.

Sindelar, W.F.; Kinsolla, T.J.; and Mayer, R.J. 1985. Cancer of the pancreas. In DeVita, V.T.; Hellman, S.; and Rosenberg, S.A. eds. *Cancer: principles and practice of oncology*. 2nd ed. pp. 691-740. Philadelphia: J. B. Lippincott.

Smathers, R.L.; Lee, J.K.T.; and Heiken, J.P. 1984. Differentiation of complicated cholecystitis from gallbladder carcinoma by computed tomography. *AJR* 143:225-59.

Snow, J.H.; Goldstein, H.M.; and Wallace, S. 1979. Comparison of scintigraphy, sonography, and computed tomography in the evaluation of hepatic neoplasms. *AJR* 132:915-18.

Som, P.M. 1987. Lymph nodes of the neck. *Radiology* 165:593-600.

Stanley, R.J.; Sagel, S.S.; and Levitt, R.G. 1977. Computed tomography of the pancreas. *Radiology* 124:705-12.

Stark, D.D.; Wittenberg, J.; and Middleton, M.S. et al. 1986. Liver metastases: detection by phase contrast MR imaging. *Radiology* 158:327-32.

Stark, D.P.; Moss, A.A.; and Goldberg, H.I. et al. 1984a. CT of pancreatic islet cell tumors. *Radiology* 150:491-94.

Stark, D.P.; Moss, A.A.; and Goldberg, H.I. et al. 1984b. Magnetic resonance and CT of the normal and diseased pancreas: a comparative study. *Radiology* 150:153-62.

Statistical Research Service. 1970. *Cancer mortality statistics*. New York: American Cancer Society.

Stevens, M.H.; Harnsberger, H.R.; and Mancuso, A.A. 1985. CT of cervical lymph nodes: staging and management of head and neck cancer. *Arch. Otolaryngol.* 11:735-73.

Sugarbaker, P.H.; Gunderson, L.L; and Wittes, R.E. 1985. Colorectal cancer. In DeVita, V.; Hellman, S.; and Rosenberg, S.A. eds. *Cancer: principles and practice of oncology*. 2nd ed. pp. 795-84. Philadelphia: J. B. Lippincott.

Sussman, S.K.; Halvorsen, R.A. Jr.; and Illescas, F.F. et al. 1988. Gastric adenocarcinoma: CT vs. surgical staging. *Radiology* 167:335-49.

Suzuki, H.; Kobayashi, S.; and Endo, M. et al. 1972. Diagnosis of early esophageal cancer. *Surgery* 71:99-103.

Tabar, L., and Dean, P.B. 1987. The control of breast cancer through mammography screening: what is the evidence? *Radiol. Clin. North Am.* 25:993-1005.

Takasan, H.; Kim, C.I.; and Arii, S. et al. 1980. Clinicopatho-logic study of 70 patients with carcinoma of the biliary tract. *Surg. Gynecol. Obstet.* 150:721-26.

Taylor, K.J.W., and Rosenfeld, A.T. 1977. Gray-scale ultrasonography in the differential diagnosis of jaundice. *Arch. Surg.* 112:820-25.

Thoeni, R.F.; Moss, A.A.; and Schnyder, P. et al. 1981. Detection and staging of primary rectal and rectosigmoid cancer by computed tomography. *Radiology* 141:135-38.

Thompson, W.M. 1983. Esophageal cancer. *Int. J. Radiat. Oncol. Biol. Phys.* 9:1533-65.

Thompson, W.M.; Halvorsen, R.A.; and Foster, W.L. Jr. et al. 1986. Preoperative and postoperative CT staging of rectosigmoid carcinoma. *AJR* 146:703-10.

Thompson, W.M., and Halvorsen, R.A. Jr. 1987. CT for staging gastrointestinal cancer II: small bowel and colon. *Invest. Radiol.* 22:96-105.

Thompson, W.M.; Halvorsen, R.A.; and Foster, W.L. Jr. et al. 1983. Computed tomography for staging esophageal and gastroesophageal cancer: a re-evaluation. *AJR* 141:951-58.

Thorsen, M.K.; Quiroz, F.; and Lawson, T.L. et al. 1984. Primary biliary carcinoma: CT evaluation. *Radiology* 152:479-83.

Uchiyama, T.; Broder, S.; and Waldmann, T.A. 1981. A monoclonal antibody (anti-TAC) reactive with activated and functionally mature human T-cells I: production of anti-TAC monoclonal antibody and distribution of TAC-positive cells. *J. Immunol.* 126:1393-97.

Van Waes, P.F.G.M.; Koehler, P.R.; and Feldberg, M.A.M. 1983. Management of rectal carcinoma: impact of computed tomography. *AJR* 140:1137-42.

Ward, E.M.; Stephens, D.H.; and Sheedy, P.F. II. 1983. Computed tomographic characteristics of pancreatic carcinoma: an analysis of 100 cases. *RadioGraphics* 3:547-65.

Weill, F.; Eisencher, A.; and Zelther, F. 1978. Ultrasonic study of the normal and dilated biliary tree: the "shotgun" sign. *Radiology* 127:221-24.

Weiner, S.N.; Koenigsberg, M.; and Morehouse, H. et al. 1984. Sonography and computed tomography in the diagnosis of carcinoma of the gallbladder. *AJR* 142:735-39.

Weinstein, M.A.; Modic, M.T.; and Pavlicek, W. et al. 1984. Nuclear magnetic resonance for the examination of brain tumors. *Semin. Roentgenol.* 19:139-47.

Whitmore, W.F. Jr. 1988. Bladder cancer: an overview. *CA* 38:213-23.

Wittenberg, J.; Simeone, J.F.; and Ferrucci, J.T. Jr. et al. 1982. Nonfocal enlargement in pancreatic carcinoma. *Radiology* 144:131-35.

Wolfe, J. 1968. Xerography of the breast. *Radiology* 91:231-40.

Wong, W.S., and Goldberg, H.I. 1985. Gastric, small bowel, and colorectal cancer. In Bragg, D.G.; Youker, J.; and Rubin, P. eds. *Oncologic imaging*. pp. 243-85. New York: Pergamon Press.

Woo, D.V.; Markoe, A.M.; and Brady, L.W. et al. 1988. Monoclonal antibodies for use in radiotherapy and diagnosis. *Am. J. Clin. Oncol.* 11:355-61.

Yeh, H.C. 1979. Ultrasonography and computed tomography of carcinoma of the gallbladder. *Radiology* 133:167-73.

Yeh, H., and Rabinowitz, J.G. 1980. Ultrasonography and computed tomography of the liver. *Radiol. Clin. North Am.* 18:321-38.

Young, S.W.; Turner, R.J.; and Castellino, R.A. 1980. A strategy for contrast enhancement of malignant tumors using dynamic computed tomography and intravascular pharmacokinetics. *Radiology* 137:137-47.

Yum, H.Y., and Fink, A.H. 1980. Sonographic findings in primary carcinoma of the gallbladder. *Radiology* 134:693-96.

Zaunbauer, W.; Haertel, M.; and Fuchs, W.A. 1981. Computed tomography in carcinoma of the rectum. *Gastrointest. Radiol.* 6:79-84.

Zelas, P.; Haaga, J.R.; and Lavery, I.C. et al. 1980. The diagnosis by percutaneous biopsy with computed tomography of a recurrence of carcinoma of the rectum in the pelvis. *Surg. Gynecol. Obstet.* 151:525-27.

Zeman, R.K.; Paushter, D.M.; and Schiebler, M.L. et al. 1985. Hepatic imaging: current status. *Radiol. Clin. North Am.* 23: 473-87.

Zerhouni, E.A.; Stitik, F.P.; and Siegelman, S.S. et al. 1986. CT of the pulmonary nodule: a cooperative study. *Radiology* 160:319-27.

Zornoza, J., and Ginaldi, S. 1981. Computed tomography in hepatic lymphoma. *Radiology* 138:405-10.

Zornoza, J., and Lindell, M.M. Jr. 1980. Radiologic evaluation of small esophageal carcinoma. *Gastrointest. Radiol.* 5:107-11.

Chapter 45

PRINCIPLES OF CANCER BIOLOGY

Dennis J. Templeton, M.D., Ph.D.
Robert A. Weinberg, Ph.D.

Dennis J. Templeton, M.D., Ph.D.
Department of Pathology
Case Western Reserve University School of Medicine
Cleveland, Ohio

Robert A. Weinberg, Ph.D.
Professor of Biology
Massachusetts Institute of Technology
Cambridge, Massachusetts
Member, Whitehead Institute for Biomedical Research
Cambridge, Massachusetts

INTRODUCTION: STUDY OF TUMOR CELLS GROWN IN CULTURE

The biological traits of cancer cells are known largely from experiments in which these cells are grown *in vitro* under a variety of culture conditions. This permits the study of a number of cancer cell traits that are not readily observed when cells are growing in the midst of a tumor mass *in vivo*. Since the 1950s, when routine *in vitro* culturing of mammalian cells was first achieved, a large number of tumor cells have been adapted to grow in culture as permanent cell lines.

Although culturing techniques have created a number of distinct tumor-cell lines, cells derived from recent biopsies do not always grow well upon initial introduction into cultures. Instead, the explanted tumor-cell population must undergo extensive adaptation during which variant tumor-cell clones grow out and show traits beyond those exhibited by their recently explanted progenitors. Accordingly, the knowledge of the biology of human tumor cells is often distorted by studying the traits of variants that may deviate substantially from tumor cells growing *in vivo*.

An alternative to studying cultured cells deriving from spontaneous human tumors arises from experiments designed to transform normal cultured cells into tumor cells during their growth *in vitro*. Such experiments utilize several types of oncogenic agents, notably carcinogenic chemicals and oncogenes. By inducing malignant conversion with precisely defined reagents, researchers have hoped to clearly delineate the changes that accompany the conversion of a normal cell into a tumor cell.

With rare exceptions, attempts at transforming normal human cells *in vitro* have been notably unsuccessful. For reasons that remain unclear, human cells are refractory to agents that are able to induce readily the neoplastic conversion of rodent cells; thus, the great bulk of what is understood about the mechanisms of neoplastic transformation derives from rodent models. Implicit in the following discussions of rodent cells is the notion that they represent very good models of the processes that intervene to create human cancer.

Rodent models of cancer offer additional advantages, perhaps most importantly the ability to grow rodent tumor cells in culture and introduce these into fully syngeneic, immunocompetent hosts at will. The ensuing tumor-host interactions presumably mirror many of the interactions that occur in a human bearing a tumor of endogenous origin. Most studies of *in vitro* transformation have utilized fibroblasts or closely related mesenchymal cells, which can be readily grown *in vitro*. Mesenchymal cells have some, but hardly all, of the attributes of the epithelial cells that are the precursors to the common human tumors, the carcinomas.

THE PLEIOTROPIC NATURE OF MALIGNANT CONVERSION

A comparison of normal cells and their transformed, tumorigenic derivatives reveals a large number of distinct shifts in cell phenotype. These encompass traits as diverse as morphology, energy metabolism, and response to growth-stimulatory factors; a thorough cataloguing of these differences might include changes in hundreds of cell parameters. A central problem in tumor biology over the past century has been to explain how cancer cells can acquire so many different, novel phenotypes.

A partial answer to this quandary is provided by the notion of the multistep progression of tumor cells (Foulds 1969). A favored model states that cells pass through a number of distinct intermediate stages during their evolution from normalcy to full malignancy. The notion of ongoing evolution is central to this model, which depicts tumors as large, heterogeneous populations of cells from which rare variants emerge that have selective growth advantage; clones of these favored cells then expand and ultimately dominate the tumor-cell population. This process is repeated in successive cycles to yield the endstage—highly evolved tumor cells that differ substantially from their normal ancestors.

The kinetics of tumor formation in experimental animals and in humans suggest a rather small number of distinct stages occurring during tumor progression. The estimates range between three and six, but the small number of stages is dwarfed by the large number of cellular changes associated with malignant transformation. This gives rise to the concept of *pleiotropy*, in which changes in a small number of central regulators are able to elicit a large number of distinct changes in cell phenotype.

TUMOR CELLS HAVE AN ALTERED CELL STRUCTURE

Tumor cells usually can be distinguished from their normal counterparts by an examination of their morphology in microscopic sections. In many cases, the diagnosis of malignant cells can be made by examining the appearance of isolated tumor cells; diagnostic cytologists use the features of increased nuclear size, increased nuclear-cytoplasmic ratio, irregular chromatin distribution, and prominent nucleoli to formulate a diagnosis. When isolated tumor cells are examined on cytologic smears, they retain most of the features of tumor cells growing within a tumor mass.

When studied in culture, normal untransformed cells growing in monolayers make many contacts with the substratum, often displaying a flattened "fried egg" appearance. Tumor cells make fewer contacts, and frequently these are in the form of long processes that extend from the cell body and cross over the extended processes of adjacent cells.

Cells in culture are usually observed using phase-contrast microscopy through which the tumor-cell body is often seen to be rounded, having either a spheroid or a spindle shape. The rounded shape causes tumor cell bodies to refract light, producing a bright highlight at the rounded edge. In contrast, the edges of the flattened, normal cells refract little light.

The cell's overall shape is dictated by its internal architecture in the form of its cytoskeleton. A major component of the cytoskeleton is the protein actin, which is present in normal fibroblasts as linear polymers called actin cables or microfilaments. Actin cables can be visualized in intact cells by using fluorescent antibodies directed against the protein. In normal cells this process demonstrates actin cables spanning nearly the entire length of the cell. The actin cables are believed to be anchored to the inner surface of the cell membrane, where the cell makes contact with the culture dish.

Transformed cells also contain actin, but immunofluorescence staining does not demonstrate the organized cables found in normal cells (Verderame et al. 1980). Disruption of this cytoskeletal component can produce significant changes in the cell's external morphology. It is not clear whether the ultrastructural changes represented by actin cable disruption are a result of overall metabolic alterations in the tumor cell, or whether the architectural changes effect the metabolic changes found in tumor cells. The cytoskeletal alterations may be a very early event in the sequence of changes that lead to a transformed cell. The cytoskeletal protein vinculin, which serves to anchor the termini of actin cables to the cell surface, has been shown to be modified directly by the transforming protein encoded by the *src* oncogene (Sefton et al. 1981).

TUMOR CELLS DISPLAY ALTERED INTERACTIONS WITH NEIGHBORING CELLS

Cells growing in normal tissues have an ordered growth pattern, characterized by regular and predictable relationships with their neighbors. The structural order characteristic of each tissue is dependent upon each component cell conforming to a precise growth pattern. The predominant growth pattern in body tissues is that of a two-dimensional sheet of cells (albeit often rolled or convoluted), which is one or several cell layers thick. This is true at both the macroscopic and microscopic levels, as evidenced by the orderly sheets of cells that make up the skin or intestinal mucosa and the single layer of cells that encircle the tiny follicles that make up the thyroid gland. Even a bulky organ like the liver is organized at the microscopic level as cells adjoined to their neighbors at their sides, forming a single-layer sheet; in the liver, it is rolled into a convoluted tube called an *acinus*.

Cells explanted from the body and grown in culture mimic the tendency of their progenitors to form a single layer (monolayer) of cells. Cells taken from mouse embryos (largely fibroblasts and other mesenchymal cells) will adhere to glass or some plastic surfaces and will divide until each cell is touching neighbors on all sides. These cells then will stop dividing (Abercrombie and Heaysman 1954). Within such a confluent cell monolayer, each cell maintains contact to the substratum (the culture dish) and will not grow over adjacent cells. Further cell division is inhibited by contacts made with other cells; this is the phenomenon of *contact inhibition*.

Tumor cells have escaped the controls that normally regulate orderly tissue growth. In the organism, this is evidenced by the formation of tumor masses that displace adjacent normal tissue. When grown in culture, tumor cells also display a disordered growth pattern. They grow until contact is made with their neighbors and then they continue to divide, forming jumbled piles of cells upon cells. Unless they are divided into subcultures and placed in fresh medium, the tumor cells will continue to divide until they have exhausted the culture medium and die. This loss of contact inhibition can help to identify agents that induce cell transformation in culture. Thus, normal cells can be grown in culture dishes and treated with chemical carcinogens or cancer-causing viruses. When a cell becomes transformed, it will acquire the altered growth behavior that allows it to continue to divide long after the cell monolayer has grown to confluence; its progeny will pile up upon their neighbors and siblings to form a thick clump of cells that can be distinguished from the normal monolayer by staining (Temin and Rubin 1958). These piles of trans-formed cells are termed *foci*. This change of behavior *in vitro* usually serves as a good predictor of *in vivo* behavior. Thus, cells purified from foci obtained in culture usually exhibit attributes of naturally arising tumor cells, such as the ability to form tumors and metastases in appropriate host animals. This suggests that the attributes of transformed cells seen *in vitro* and *in vivo* are mechanistically linked to one another.

The mechanism that maintains contact inhibition is uncertain, but it clearly involves the passage of signals induced upon cell-to-cell contact. At least two kinds of contacts are made between normal cells in culture: (1) tight junctions, also called *desmosomes* by the electron microscopist; and (2) gap junctions, which allow passage of small molecules between the cytoplasm of two adjoining cells. Passage of small molecules between cells may explain how a cell is able to announce its presence to its neighbors, thus preventing growth once the confluent monolayer is formed. Tumor cells grown in culture (and tumors observed microscopically) usually retain the tight junctions found in nontransformed cells. Gap junctions, however, are frequently reduced or absent, suggesting again that intercellular communication may be important for maintenance of normal growth patterns (Weinstein et al. 1976; Lowenstein 1979).

With the exception of cells from hematopoietic lineages, normal cells grown in culture must have a solid substrate upon which to grow. The presence of a basement membrane, which underlays epithelial cell layers, may represent an analogous phenomenon in the intact tissue. If normal cells are prevented from adhering to a substrate by being suspended in a viscous medium or a semisolid medium containing agar, they stop dividing and are said to exhibit *anchorage-dependent* growth. The reason for this dependence on substrate is unclear, but it is possible that cells require contact with extracellular proteins or glycoproteins (often mimicked by serum proteins coating the tissue-culture plate surface) to organize their growth pattern and to continue dividing. Transformed cells grown in culture frequently grow even when they are deprived of association with substrate, by being suspended in a semisolid medium (Macpherson and Montagnier 1964). This *anchorage independence* displayed by many tumor cells leads to the conclusion that transformed cells do not require the same level of external stimulation as normal cells in order to maintain a state of active growth.

In addition to growth in a semisolid medium, many tumor cells can grow in a fluid medium without attach-ment to a substrate. These cells grow singly or in small clumps; in the laboratory they are usually agitated gently to keep them from settling to the bottom of the culture vessel. This phenomenon has a counterpart to the behavior of tumor cells in the cancer patient; many types of tumors tend to grow along the pleural surfaces of the thorax or abdomen, producing a suspension of tumor cells in a protein-rich fluid that may seriously compromise the patient's respiratory or circulatory function.

Normal cells produce proteins that are exported to the outer cell surface and are used to coat the cells and their immediate surroundings. The best studied of these proteins is *fibronectin*, which, by itself, is sufficient to promote the adhesion of cells to the surface of a culture dish. Signals from extracellular proteins are not required for the growth of many types of tumor cells in culture, so it may not be surprising that tumor cells usually make significantly less fibronectin and other extracellular matrix proteins than do normal cells (Vaheri and Mosher 1978).

TUMOR CELLS HAVE REDUCED REQUIREMENTS FOR GROWTH

Growing body tissues are bathed in a complex mixture of nutrients including amino acids, minerals, and vita-mins, and uncounted types of growth-stimulatory and growth-inhibitory substances. When *in vitro* culture methods were being formulated, nutrient mixtures (cell culture media) of defined chemical composition were devised that provided many of the compounds necessary for cell growth. Nevertheless, it was always necessary to supplement the mixtures with blood serum (usually from calves or fetal calves) in order to optimize growth rate and cell survival. These sera contain a complex, and still poorly defined, mixture of growth-stimulatory factors. Recently, rodent cells have been found to grow in a chemically defined medium supplemented at its simplest with three peptide growth factors: insulin, transferrin, and epidermal growth factor.

Normal human cells typically require fetal calf serum for growth, presumably because some essential factor is present in fetal calf serum and absent or reduced in calf serum. The growth of human cancer cells is usually much less dependent upon serum factors; tumor cells frequently can be grown in reduced concentrations of fetal calf or calf serum. When normal cells are placed in medium containing reduced levels (<1%) of serum, they become arrested in the G_0 phase of the cell growth cycle and stop dividing. Tumor cells often will continue to grow even under conditions of reduced serum levels.

The reduced dependence of tumor cells on serum growth factors may be explained, in part, by the discovery that some genetic alterations that occur in human and animal tumors are changes in the production of, or response to, polypeptide growth factors.

CANCER CELLS ARE "IMMORTAL"

When normal rodent cells are explanted from an animal and grown in culture, they will divide for a finite number of generations and then experience a so-called crisis of senescence, in which most cells stop dividing and die. In such rodent cell cultures, a few of the cultured cells may undergo a poorly defined change that enables them to continue to divide. The descendants of these cells can then be cultured through an unlimited number of passages. Such cultures, established to grow indefinitely in culture, are termed *cell lines* (Todaro and Green 1963).

Normal human cells undergo a crisis similar to rodent cells, but for unknown reasons no cells survive to establish permanent cell lines. Explanted human tumor cells (though they are frequently difficult to adapt to tissue culture in the first place) do not exhibit this phenomenon; they usually have an unlimited potential for growth and are said to be immortalized. Similarly, human tumors transplanted experimentally into immunodeficient mice exhibit an apparently unlimited potential to regenerate tumors after repeated transplantation.

Although established rodent cell lines share the phenotype of immortality with tumor cells, they exhibit few other characteristics of malignant cells. Established cell lines retain contact inhibition and are anchorage dependent. Most will not form tumors when injected into appropriate host animals. Thus, the phenotype of immortality in culture is only one of several phenotypes of tumorigenic cells. Immortalization may be necessary for tumorigenesis, but it is hardly sufficient. This conclusion is corroborated by studies of transformation genetics. Thus, specific genes carried by some oncogenic viruses are known to promote the establishment of immortal cell lines at high frequency. In nearly all cases, these immortalizing genes are not capable of converting a cell to the fully tumorigenic state; yet other changes are required to achieve this ability.

TUMOR CELLS MUST ESCAPE IMMUNE SURVEILLANCE

Experimental tumors arising from treatment of animals or cultured cells with carcinogenic chemicals or oncogenic viruses frequently express on their surfaces novel antigens that are not present on the surfaces of their untransformed progenitors. One type of novel antigen may be common to many kinds of tumor cells and may be recognized by a class of lymphocytes called natural killer (NK) cells (Herberman and Ortaldo 1981). NK cells can recognize some tumor cell antigens even without a specific prior immunization, and may be able to destroy tumor cells bearing this type of antigen.

In other instances, novel antigens specific to a particular type of tumor may be displayed. When animals are immunized with killed tumor cells bearing such an antigen, they subsequently may be protected from the growth of injected viable cells bearing the same antigen. These antigens are referred to as tumor-specific transplantation antigens (TSTAs). The molecules constituting TSTAs are usually not involved causally in cell transformation, but are best regarded as markers or sequelae to the central transforming event or events (Old 1981). Tumors arising in humans rarely express this type of antigen, although developmental antigens are common.

One model for the development of tumors in humans states that all individuals develop, over the course of their lives, numerous transformed cells, but that most of these are recognized as foreign and are killed by one or another component of the host's immune system. Proponents of this model of immune surveillance point to the fact that some tumors evoke a lymphocytic response (as evidenced by the lymphocytic infiltrates seen in microscopic sections of some testicular seminomas and medullary carcinomas of the breast), and that the clinical severity of these tumors is inversely correlated with the degree of lymphocytic involvement. The increased frequency of B-cell neoplasms and the otherwise rare Kaposi's sarcoma in AIDS patients frequently is explained by a lowered efficiency of immune surveillance in these immunocompromised hosts (Ziegler 1982). Immunocompromised individuals experience almost 200-fold more malignancies than that of the population as a whole (Vaheri and Mosher 1978).

One mechanism by which the tumor cell may escape the host immune response is to down-regulate the expression of HLA antigens, which normally serve to assist lymphocyte recognition of the target cell. Among the many effects produced by oncogenic adenoviruses, one is a reduction in the expression of HLA antigens in the transformed cell. In certain types of naturally occurring human tumors, such as neuroblastomas, cells from advanced tumor stages often have reduced levels of HLA antigens.

TUMOR CELLS EXHIBIT SOME FEATURES OF CELL DIFFERENTIATION

Many tumor cells display some characteristic features of the normal cells found in their tissue of origin. Thus, cells from breast tumors may make duct-like tubules; those from thyroid tumors, tiny colloid-filled follicles; and cells of rhabdomyosarcomas, cross-striations similar to those found in skeletal muscle. The distinction between the common adenocarcinoma and squamous or epidermoid carcinoma is dependent upon the features of glandular mucosa (mucus secretion and tubule formation) in the former, and squamous mucosa (keratin production) in the latter. In general, the tumors that express more of the features of the mature tissue (so called well-differentiated tumors) have a less malignant clinical course than do their poorly differentiated counterparts. Some tumors, notably the neuroblastomas of infancy, spontaneously differentiate into a more benign tumor type and may actually regress without treatment.

Although most tumors have some attributes of differentiation, the initial transforming event probably takes place in a dividing and still-undifferentiated stem cell, the precursor of the differentiated cells within a tissue. Part of the process that creates a transformed cell may involve a partial or complete block in the normal developmental pathways leading to full differentiation. A well-differentiated tumor retains most of the program for cell development, and a poorly differentiated tumor retains only some.

These concepts offer some explanations for the origin of tumors. Growth of tissues is normally limited by the fact that as cells differentiate, they lose the proliferative ability of their stem-cell precursors. Tumor cells become blocked in this differentiation pathway and retain the potential for unlimited growth. As an example, cells of the epidermal layer of the skin originate from stem cells in the basal layer and begin to express keratin. These cells are displaced outwardly by the newer cells which follow them, and as their cytoplasm fills with keratin, the cells elongate and become metabolically inactive until they are eventually sloughed from the surface. Tumor cells arising from the epidermis do not exhibit the features of mature skin cells (they may make little keratin) and retain the proliferative activity which, in the normal skin, is restricted to the stem cells in the basal layer. With this model in mind, recent attempts have been made to induce tumor-cell differentiation by treating patients with chemicals (e.g., retinoic acid, a relative of vitamin A) known to induce differentiation in culture (Gouvera 1982). To date, however, no conclusive evidence of their therapeutic value has been shown.

In addition, many tumor cells express proteins that are not found in the mature tissue, but which are a part of the normal pattern of protein expression from the corresponding embryonic tissue. For example, the embryonic liver produces and secretes alpha-feto-protein (AFP), which is analogous to serum albumin produced by the adult liver. Alpha-fetoprotein is not found in mature liver tissue, except under conditions in which the organ is injured and is actively regenerating. Hepatocellular carcinoma, the common cancer of liver-cell origin, frequently expresses large quantities of AFP, which is found both in the tumor cells and in the circulation of patients bearing hepatocellular tumors (Abelev 1971). Similarly, an embryonic protein aptly termed carcinoembryonic antigen (CEA) is secreted by many tumors of lung and gastrointestinal tract origin; the circulating level of CEA is a rough indicator of the tumor burden carried by the patient (Concannon et al. 1974).

Tumor cells frequently express proteins or metabolic products that might or might not be expected from the tissue in which the tumor arose. Frequently, this is a hormonally active product that may announce the tumor's presence long before it becomes evident on the basis of its size. One example is the insulinoma, an insulin-secreting pancreatic islet-cell tumor. Patients with these tumors will usually present with symptoms of hypoglycemia resulting from insulin excess. Another tumor that produces an active hormone is choriocarcinoma, which arises from the placenta and is retained by the uterus after delivery. This tumor expresses into the circulation a large quantity of the hormone HCG (human chorionic gonadotropin), which is a normal product of the placenta. Fortunately, choriocarcinoma is quite sensitive to the chemotherapeutic agent methotrexate. Patients who have undergone chemotherapy for this tumor are regularly monitored for the appearance of HCG in their serum, as an early indicator of recurrence. Tumors may also express products that are not typical of their tissue of origin. Such inappropriate or "ectopic" hormone production is exemplified by certain lung carcinomas that produce parathyroid hormone and renal cell carcinomas that elaborate erythropoietin.

TUMOR CELLS HAVE AN ALTERED METABOLISM

Tumor cells exhibit a vast array of metabolic differences that distinguish them from their untransformed counterparts. The overall trend is toward simplified metabolic activities and an increased synthesis of material necessary for cell division. This generalization is understandable in light of the process of selection that has taken place over the tumor's lifetime. Tumor cells have no need to express proteins relevant to the specialized functions of the original tissue, and their growth is favored when they divert much of their resources to the purposes of cell division.

One very apparent metabolic change in culture-grown tumor cells is their production of large amounts of acid, which results at least in part because tumor cells tend to utilize anaerobic pathways of glycolysis even in the presence of oxygen. This was observed decades ago by Warburg (1930), but has since been shown to occur as well in rapidly growing untransformed cells. An increased rate of glucose transport is another striking feature of tumor cells.

The increased metabolic rate and the rapid rate of cell growth cause an increased demand for blood-borne nutrients in the expanding tumor. Since the diffusion of solutes and oxygen is limited to a few millimeters, many rapidly growing, poorly vascularized neoplasms suffer necrosis of their central portions. This is seen in tissue sections as poorly defined cell bodies with degenerated nuclear material and with infiltrating granulocytes, surrounded by a ring of viable tumor tissue. Some tumors manage to stimulate the growth of non-neoplastic blood vessels that grow from the surrounding normal tissue into the expanding tumor, a result of the action of polypeptide angiogenic growth factors released by the tumor cells.

Recently, much attention has been given to investigation of the metabolic pathways of phosphatidylinositol (PI) in normal and transformed cells. PI is a phospholipid present as a minor component of the membranes of normal and transformed cells. In normal cells, the intracellular concentrations of the phosphorylated forms of PI and its metabolite inositol are known to be raised in response to several polypeptide growth factors. Cells transformed by certain oncogenes (particularly *ras* genes) contain elevated levels of these compounds. This raises the interesting possibility that growth factors and at least some oncogenes may promote cell division by stimulation of the same pathway. To date there has been no proof that the protein products of any oncogenes directly catalyze the phosphorylation of inositol, but a phosphatidylinositol kinase has been reported to be bound to at least one kind of oncogene-encoded protein (Kaplan et al. 1987).

TUMOR CELLS ARE CAPABLE OF INVASION AND METASTASIS

Invasion of adjacent tissue and metastasis to distant organs are the most ominous features of a malignant tumor. Without these features, surgical resection could control most cancers. A tumor's ability to metastasize is a complex phenomenon, which requires at the minimum the following features: (1) invasion of tumor cells through adjacent tissues and through blood or lymphatic vessel walls, with release of tumor cells into the circulation (intravasation); (2) survival of tumor cells within the circulation and escape of immune surveillance; and (3) escape from the circulation (extravasation) and implantation in a tissue with establishment of a new tumor locus.

Invasion is a feature common to nearly all types of malignant tumors. Microscopically, this is apparent when tumor cells are seen to be admixed with nonmalignant cells in the adjacent tissue. In some tumors, malignant cells mingle with or replace adjacent normal cells, but remain confined to the original plane of cells from which the tumor cells originated. For example, tumor cells arising in breast ducts may fill the lumen of the duct and replace the normal duct cells for several millimeters without penetrating through the basement membrane into the adjacent tissue. These tumors are referred to as *in situ* ductal carcinomas, and they metastasize infrequently. Invasive breast carcinomas include those that have penetrated the wall of the duct and are found growing in the adjacent stromal tissue. These tumors are thought to arise from earlier *in situ* carcinomas, although their pattern of invasiveness may have developed very early in the course of tumor progression.

Another example concerns the highly malignant skin cancer, melanoma. The superficially spreading form of melanoma initially grows in a radial pattern, i.e., it spreads laterally through the skin but remains confined to the epidermal cell layer. The vertical growth phase is a later stage in which the tumor invades the dermis and develops a propensity to metastasize.

Most carcinomas arise in epithelial cells that are underlaid by a basement membrane composed of dense proteoglycans; the basement membrane may represent a barrier to early tumor-cell invasion. Tumor cells frequently secrete enzymes, including several types of collagenase, heparanase, and stromolysin, that are capable of degrading this type of physical barrier (Recklies et al. 1980). Expression of these enzymes may be a critical step in the invasion of tumor cells into adjacent tissues and into the circulation.

Once a tumor has eroded through the wall of the blood or lymphatic vessel, individual tumor cells or a small clump may detach and circulate through the body as an embolus. These cells can become encased in fibrin or aggregates of platelets, which may protect them from destruction by the cell's immune system. The presence of tumor cells in the circulation does not guarantee the establishment of metastatic tumor loci, since the survival of tumor cells in the circulation appears to be quite low. Only about 0.1% of tumor cells injected intravenously into mice survive for over 24 hours (Fisher and Fisher 1959).

Cells of many tumor types demonstrate the ability to "home" to a specific target organ. Clinically, this is demonstrated by the tendency of certain tumors to preferentially metastasize to specific organs. Sometimes the pattern of metastasis may reflect the pattern of the blood circulation; thus, the major site of blood-borne metastasis from the colon is the liver, which is the recipient of blood flow from the colon through the portal vein. However, most patterns of metastasis are not readily explainable on the basis of blood flow patterns; examples of this are the frequent metastasis of gastric carcinoma to the ovary and of lung carcinomas to the adrenal gland. These target organs receive less than 1% of the total blood circulation but the frequency of metastasis to them is much higher than to the kidneys, which receive about 10% of the circulation.

The ability of some tumors to develop a mechanism for homing to target organs has been demonstrated experimentally with B16 murine melanoma cells. Mice injected with these tumor cells develop tumor metastases in several organs. For example, when tumor cells are recovered from metastases to the lung and then regrown in culture, these cells have a much higher tendency subsequently to form metastases in the lungs of newly injected mice (Brunson et al. 1979). Thus, the tumor cells are capable of expressing a certain pattern of metastasis which, at least in these cases, is genetically determined. It is not clear how these patterns of metastasis arise, but some evidence suggests that tumor cells can respond to specific chemotactic signals released by certain organs. A tumor cell may therefore pass through the circulation until it receives an appropriate signal, and then be stimulated to attach to the vessel wall and extravasate into the tissue bed.

GENETIC MUTATION AS A BASIS OF NEOPLASTIC TRANSFORMATION

A variety of experimental data accumulated over more than one-half of a century have suggested that the many neoplastic changes in cell phenotype occur as a direct consequence of alterations to the cell genome. The derived genetic theories of cancer contrast with an alternative theory: that cancer results because of changes in nongenetic (epigenetic) regulatory circuits that occur without alteration of the cellular genome.

The strongest support for the genetic origins of cancer derives from observations that agents known to damage DNA (mutagens) have often been found to act as carcinogens. An awareness of this association first came from work with x-rays. Early experimenters succumbed to cancer at high rates. Several decades later it was realized that x-rays could act as potent agents for inducing genetic damage. In the 1970s, the work of Bruce Ames focused attention on a wide variety of chemicals that exhibit both mutagenic and carcinogenic properties. The correlation between their relative mutagenic and carcinogenic potencies suggested that these agents induce cancer through their ability to damage DNA (McCann and Ames 1976).

A corollary to these findings was the notion that the progenitors of tumor cells sustain a number of genetic alterations that create mutant genes, the expression of which then dictates the cell's malignant phenotype. These genetic changes occur in cells of the target organs in which tumors eventually appear and are called *somatic mutations* to distinguish them from the mutations that occur in germ cells and are transmitted from one generation to the next.

The search for the hypothesized mutant cancer-causing genes proceeded slowly. Their number and mode of action were initially totally obscure. The first progress in understanding such cancer genes came from work with several small DNA viruses, SV40 and the mouse polyoma virus. In the early 1960s, these viruses were found to be able to infect and transform cultured rodent cells into a tumorigenic state. This showed that the process of neoplastic conversion of a cell, hitherto thought to occur only in the tissues of an animal, could be induced *in vitro*. Moreover, such transformation was achieved by small, relatively simple biological agents (Dulbecco 1969). The resulting transformed cells were found to retain several viral genes in their DNA, and their presence was found to be essential for the cells' continued display of cancer traits. It was clear that the viral oncogenes were orchestrating the malignant properties of these cells: they initiated the process of transformation and their continued presence was required for maintenance of the transformed state.

The viral oncogenes retained in these cells were relatively simple and small in size. This led to the realization that a small number of genes, in this case viral oncogenes, can induce a large number of concordant shifts in cell phenotype. Thus, oncogenes could act pleiotropically to elicit multiple changes, apparently through an ability to trip central regulatory controls within the cell. Some speculated that this logic could be transferred to human tumor cells in which no viral oncogenes were apparent; perhaps a small number of mutant cell genes could also act as oncogenes to induce the many behavioral aberrancies associated with malignant cells.

THE SEARCH FOR CELLULAR ONCOGENES

Substantial progress was made in the late 1970s in the search for oncogenes within cancer cells prepared from human tumors or from chemically induced rodent tumors. The cancerous state of these particular cells did not appear to derive from infection by oncogene-bearing tumor viruses.

One strategy to detect oncogenes within the nonviral tumors was to extract DNA from cancer cells and introduce it into normal nontransformed recipient cells via the procedure known variously as gene transfer or transfection. The transfected recipient cells were then studied to detect any changes in their phenotype. In a number of cases, the recipients took on some of the neoplastic traits that had been exhibited by the donor cells from which DNA had been prepared (Shih et al. 1979). This yielded a simple yet important conclusion: that the information encoding cancerous behavior could be passed from cell to cell via DNA molecules. This meant that among the transfected DNA molecules, there must be several carrying cancer-inducing genes: oncogenes. As oncogenes were not detectable in the DNA of normal cells, it was clear that they appeared in cancer cells as part of the processes that led to the malignant state.

With the advent of gene cloning technologies, it was possible to isolate these cellular oncogenes in the early 1980s. One well-studied example stemmed from a human bladder carcinoma cell line termed EJ/T24 (Krontiris and Cooper 1981). This oncogene was relatively small, encompassing only 6,000 base pairs of DNA; the cell nucleus by contrast contains about 6 billion base pairs of human DNA. Nonetheless, this small oncogene could exert profound effects on a cell by inducing concomitant changes in cell shape, secretion of growth factors, loss of contact inhibition, anchorage independence, increased glucose transport, and a host of other changes—including in many cell types, tumorigenicity and metastasis.

This bladder carcinoma oncogene was found to arise from a normal cellular gene of very similar structure. Such a normal antecedent is often termed a *proto-oncogene*, which implies the ability of a normal gene to exhibit oncogenic powers following appropriate mutations in its DNA sequence. This and other proto-oncogenes are present in a wide variety of organisms (Shilo and Weinberg 1981). Their ubiquitous presence in many distantly related life forms is a testimonial to the essential role they play in normal cellular and organismic physiology. Such an essential role has ensured that they have been conserved over vast evolutionary distances in relatively unchanged form. The involvement of proto-oncogenes in cancer occurs only as a consequence of rare genetic accidents that cause a deregulation of their function and with this, a resulting deregulation in the complex apparatus responsible for governing cell growth.

Many of the oncogenes detected in human tumors were known from earlier work on RNA tumor viruses (retroviruses), many of which carry oncogenes in their genomes. Like SV40 and polyoma, retroviruses use their oncogenes to transform cells that they infect. The retroviral oncogenes were found to derive ultimately from normal cellular genes, proto-oncogenes. It is now realized that during their infectious passage through cells, retroviruses are capable of picking up and mobilizing proto-oncogenes residing in the genomes of infected host cells. These acquired genes, carried now in the viral genome, assume the role of oncogenes and are responsible for the tumorigenic properties of these hybrid viruses.

Many of the oncogenes originally detected by virtue of their association with various retroviruses were then found to be activated through nonviral mutational mechanisms in human tumors (table 45.1). The Ha-*ras* oncogene, associated initially with a rat sarcoma retrovirus, was seen to be closely related to the EJ/T24 bladder carcinoma oncogene (Der, Krontiris, and Cooper 1982; Parada et al. 1982). The *myc* oncogene, discovered in the context of the avian myelocytomatosis virus genome, was seen as activated in many Burkitt's lymphomas (Taub et al. 1982). The *abl* oncogene of mouse Abelson leukemia virus was discovered as an activated oncogene in many, if not all, chronic myelogenous leukemias (de Klein et al. 1982).

MECHANISM OF ONCOGENE ACTIVATION

A variety of somatic mutational mechanisms are responsible for creating activated cellular oncogenes. The mutation responsible for the bladder carcinoma oncogene was surprisingly subtle, a single base change out of the 6,000 bases constituting the original proto-oncogene. This *point mutation* affected, in turn, the amino acid sequence of the protein that the gene specified (Tabin et al. 1982). The structurally altered protein is the molecule that ultimately affects cell metabolism, thereby inducing malignancy.

Other oncogenes arise through mutations that affect the structure of their encoded proteins. In chronic myelogenous leukemia, the oncogenicity of the *abl* gene derives from the fact that this gene has fused with a fully unrelated gene, *bcr* (Groffen et al. 1984). The *bcr-abl* hybrid protein encoded by these fused genes differs substantially in structure and function from the normal *abl* proto-oncogene protein.

Oncogenes like *myc* or the related N-*myc* acquire their malignant properties through mechanisms that affect the level of expression of their encoded proteins but leave their protein structures intact. These deregulations of protein quantity are achieved through several distinct mechanisms. In childhood neuroblastomas, the copy number of the N-*myc* gene frequently is amplified from its usual diploid number to many dozens per cell (Seeger et al. 1985). Because this amplified state is often correlated with poor prognosis, it is thought that N-*myc* amplification is an important cause of the aggressiveness of such tumors. In mammary carcinomas, the HER-2/*neu* oncogene is amplified in tumors having a high metastatic potency (Slamon et al. 1987). This amplification provides a useful diagnostic index and a possible explanation of the tumor cells' metastatic aggressiveness.

In Burkitt's lymphomas, the deregulation of *myc* gene expression is due to chromosomal translocations that fuse the *myc* proto-oncogene with immunoglobulin genes. This unusual juxtaposition places the *myc* gene under the control of the immunoglobulin gene regulatory elements. Expression of the *myc* gene is normally modulated by a complex array of physiological stimuli; its control by elements of the immunoglobulin gene leads to a steady expression that is uncoupled from normal regulatory circuits.

ONCOGENES AND TUMOR PROGRESSION

As oncogene action was explored in detail, it became clear that single oncogenes were unable to induce the

Table 45.1
CELL ONCOGENES INVOLVED IN HUMAN TUMORS

Oncogene	Retrovirus Association	Example of Human Tumor Involvement	Subcellular Localization of Protein	Nature of Protein
abl	Abelson murine leukemia virus	Myelogenous leukemia	Myelogenous plasma membrane	Tyrosine kinase
erb-B	Avian erythroblastosis virus	Mammary carcinoma, glioblastoma	Plasma membrane	Tyrosine kinase
erb B-2/ HER-2/*neu*		Mammary and ovarian carcinoma	Plasma membrane	Tyrosine kinase
Ha-*ras*	Harvey murine sarcoma virus	Wide variety	Cytoplasmic membranes	GDP/GTP binding
Ki-*ras*	Kirsten murine sarcoma virus	Wide variety	Cytoplasmic membranes	GDP/GTP binding
N-*ras*		Wide variety	Cytoplasmic membranes	GDP/GTP binding
myc	MC-29 avian myelocytomatosis virus	Lymphoma	Nucleus	Possible transcription factor
N-*myc*		Neuroblastoma	Nucleus	Possible transcription factor
L-*myc*		Small cell lung carcinoma	Nucleus	Possible transcription factor
hst		Stomach carcinoma	Secreted	Related to fibroblast growth factor
bcl-2		Follicular lymphoma	Not known	Not known
dbl		B-cell nodular lymphomas	Not known	Not known

transformation of fully normal cells into fully malignant cells. Instead, the actions of a single oncogene usually induce only partial conversion to malignancy. This point is made most graphically by introducing single oncogenes into normal cells recently explanted from a normal tissue or embryo. For example, when a *ras* oncogene, originating from a human tumor, is introduced into rat embryo fibroblasts growing in monolayer culture, the recipient cells may show anchorage independence but are unable to form tumors when inoculated in host animals. Moreover, these cells soon die after several passages in culture, unlike well-established tumor cells. A *myc* oncogene has distinct, but incomplete, effects on the cellular phenotype. *Myc*-bearing cells may be able to grow indefinitely in culture, but they too are nontumorigenic. However, full tumorigenicity ensues when both the *myc* and *ras* oncogenes are introduced concomitantly into these embryo cells (Land, Parada, and Weinberg 1983). Analogous results have been reported with other oncogene pairs acting in other cell types.

While human tumors bearing both a *myc* and a *ras* oncogene have been observed only rarely, this experimental model teaches a number of lessons that appear to be widely applicable to cancer cell biology. Growth regulation of the mammalian cell appears to be organized in such a way that single oncogenes are unable to induce full conversion to malignancy. This serves as a protective mechanism operating in normal cells by acting to prevent the outgrowth of tumors whenever single oncogenes arise through isolated genetic accidents.

The observed oncogene cooperation also shows that different oncogenes act in distinct ways on cell metabolism. Each oncogene may induce only a subset of the changes associated with full malignancy; several acting in concert can achieve the end result of creating a highly malignant cell. In the case of the *ras-myc* pair, the *ras* oncogene can induce anchorage independence and growth factor secretion while the *myc* oncogene can immortalize cells. The sum of these traits reflects many of the important aspects of a fully tumorigenic cell.

Yet a third point derives from attempts to reconcile the phenomenon of multistep carcinogenesis with the observed complementary effects of various oncogenes. It would appear that each of the steps through which cells pass during the progression from normalcy to malignancy is demarcated by a distinct genetic change, often one that creates an oncogene like *myc* or *ras*. The precise number of distinct steps is poorly documented in human tumorigenesis, and in most cases the precise nature of the gene mutations involved in delineating these steps is also unknown. Nevertheless, it is already clear that a very small number of genes, often oncogenes, can orchestrate the large number of changes that are associated with neoplastic transformation.

ANTI-ONCOGENES AND TUMOR PROGRESSION

Oncogenes represent only one of several classes of genetic elements that play critical roles in tumorigenesis. Another group of genes, known variously as tumor-

suppressors or anti-oncogenes, may be equally important. Unlike oncogenes and antecedent proto-oncogenes, all of which function as growth-promoting elements in the cell, anti-oncogenes appear to function in the normal cell to restrict or repress cellular proliferation (Klein 1987).

Proto-oncogenes participate in cancer through their hyperactive or deregulated alleles. In contrast, growth-suppressing genes are involved in tumorigenesis when they suffer genetic inactivation. Loss-of-function mutations affecting both copies of an anti-oncogene serve to remove a normally existing barrier to cell growth, unleashing the clonal proliferation that leads to a tumor mass. Inactivating mutations occur much more readily than the precisely targeted mutations that activate proto-oncongenes, so it is likely that anti-oncogenes are as frequently involved in cancer as the much-studied oncogenes.

Inactive alleles of tumor-suppressor genes can be acquired in two ways: they may be created through somatic mutation occurring in a target organ, or they may be passed through the germline, being present in the conceptus and all body tissues. The latter situation may create a congenital predisposition to cancer because one of the two required mutational events needed to knock out both homologous copies of the gene has already occurred in all cells of the target organ (Knudson 1971). This well describes the origins of retinoblastoma. When a defective allele of the Rb gene is acquired congenitally, then a familial retinoblastoma ensues involving multiple, independent tumor foci in both eyes of the afflicted child. In the sporadic form of the disease, both alleles are inactivated somatically in a single cell—a rare constellation of events that leads to only a single tumor-cell focus.

The easiest mechanism for inactivation of both copies of an anti-oncogene involves an initial inactivation of one allele and the subsequent replacement of the surviving wild-type allele with a duplicated copy of the mutant allele. The processes creating homozygosity of this allele may also lead to homozygosity of other closely linked genes on the chromosome. Accordingly, workers have searched the genomes of tumor cells for regions that were initially heterozygous for different genetic markers prior to tumorigenesis and have been reduced to a homozygous condition during the course of tumor progression (Cavenee et al. 1985). Homozygous regions indeed have been found in a number of distinct tumor types, and in each case changes in a specific chromosomal region are associated with a specific form of cancer (table 45.2). Although largely unproven, it is assumed that these reductions to homozygosity reflect loss of function of specific anti-oncogenes whose absence triggers cancer.

Oncogenes and tumor-suppressor genes together may represent the two most important genetic elements in cancer formation. Their study may make it possible to correlate distinct pathological stages of tumor formation with identifiable changes in the cell genome. Attempts at making such a correlation have been most successful

Table 45.2
IDENTIFIED OR SUSPECTED
TUMOR-SUPPRESSOR GENES

Name	Tumor Involvement	Chromosomal Site
	Neuroblastoma	1p
	Small cell lung carcinoma	3p
	Colon carcinoma	5q
	Wilms' tumor	11p
	Bladder carcinoma	11p
	Retinoblastoma, osteosarcoma	13q
	Ductal breast carcinoma	13q
p53	Astrocytoma, colon carcinoma	17p
DCC	Colon carcinoma	18q
	Meningioma, acoustic neuroma	22q

when studying human colon carcinogenesis. Most early premalignant lesions, known as adenomatous polyps, carry activated *ras* oncogenes. The carcinomatous derivatives of these often carry homozygosities in chromosome 5 or 17 (Bos et al. 1987). This suggests that the inactivation of an anti-oncogene accompanies, and indeed may cause, the progression of the premalignant adenoma to a frank carcinoma. Such descriptions represent only the beginning of understanding human tumor progression in terms of discrete, well-defined lesions occurring in the genome of the evolving tumor cell clone.

TUMOR CELLS AND GROWTH FACTORS

A hallmark of tumor cells is their reduced dependence on mitogenic growth factors. For example, as mentioned earlier while normal cells will often require the addition of 10% serum to their culture medium, tumor cells will often grow well in only 1% serum. The serum functions essentially as a source of factors, so these observations indicate that tumor cells have acquired a measure of growth factor autonomy.

This has important implications for understanding the essential nature of cancer. The disease is best characterized as a breakdown of communication and interdependence between cells. Since much of the cell-to-cell communication is mediated by transmission of growth factors, a loss of growth-factor dependence represents an important breakdown in the regulatory network that maintains normal tissue architecture.

Oncogenes represent important means through which tumor cells acquire growth-factor independence. They possibly mediate such independence in at least four distinct ways. The first mechanism depends upon the observation that tumor cells often secrete mitogenic growth factors. Sporn and Todaro (1980) postulated that these secreted growth factors may feed back on and stimulate the growth of the same cell that has just released them, which results in an autostimulatory or *autocrine* positive feedback loop. Equally significant, the endogenous production of growth factor renders their importation from elsewhere in the tissue unnecessary. Oncogenes participate in autocrine stimulation in two ways. Some oncogenes, like *ras* and *src*, may turn on the expression of normally tightly regulated growth-factor

genes. Alternatively, growth-factor genes may themselves suffer alterations that cause their uncontrolled expression (Doolittle et al. 1983). A growth-factor gene so altered takes on the role of an oncogene.

Tumor cells have been found to secrete a great variety of growth factors. Among these are TGF-α, which acts like the related epidermal growth factor (EGF), platelet-derived growth factor (PDGF), and TGF-β. As long as the secreting cell also displays cell-surface receptors that bind the secreted product, then these released factors can drive autocrine growth.

A second mechanism of growth-factor autonomy stems from the growth-factor receptors that are displayed on the surface of normal cells. These receptors release growth-stimulatory signals into the cell when they bind their cognate ligands. Recent work suggests that alterations in receptor number or structure can result in the release of gratuitous mitogenic signals into the cell, even in the absence of any encountered growth factor ligands (Downward et al. 1984). These aberrantly expressed or structured receptors then function as oncogene proteins. Aggressively growing mammary carcinomas often display enormous numbers of a receptor-like protein encoded by the HER-2/*neu* proto-oncogene (Slamon et al. 1987). Cells of the human epidermoid carcinoma-cell line A431 display versions of the EGF receptor that are both truncated and present in several-hundred-fold increased amounts (Ulrich 1984).

A third mechanism of growth factor autonomy derives from components of the cytoplasmic signalling pathway responsible for picking up signals from surface receptors and transducing them to central growth-regulatory switches within the cell. Although the details of these pathways are still poorly understood, it appears that proteins of genes like *ras* and *src* participate in signal-transducing events in these pathways. When these proteins undergo certain structural alterations, they may operate constitutively, even in the absence of prior prompting by upstream components in their signalling pathway. Growth factors are rendered unnecessary because mitogenic signals are generated through an alternative mechanism—in this case through the misfiring of cytoplasmic signal transducers.

A final route to growth factor autonomy stems from the behavior of nuclear proto-oncogenes that are regulated through wide ranges of expression. For example, genes like *fos* and *myc* may be virtually silent in nongrowing cells and increase their expression 20-fold to 50-fold when the cell encounters appropriate growth factors such as PDGF. The mutations that convert these genes into active oncogenes often allow their constitutive expression in a way that is no longer dependent upon growth factor stimulation. One striking example of this is the translocation seen in Burkitt's lymphomas that removes the *myc* gene from its normal regulatory sequences and places it under control of immunoglobulin gene regulatory elements. Similar end results may be obtained in childhood neuroblastomas, in which amplification of the N-*myc* proto-oncogene results in its vast overexpression.

THE METABOLIC BASIS OF ONCOGENE ACTION

While oncogenes have been found to induce many of the distinctive traits of neoplastic cells, a fundamental puzzle remains: How do the oncogene proteins succeed in altering the cell in such profound ways? This question must ultimately be reduced to these proteins' biochemical mechanisms of action. The progress in understanding this has been slow, but it is now clear that a number of oncogene proteins, exemplified by the pp60 protein of the *src* oncogene, act as tyrosine kinases and, as such, serve to phosphorylate tyrosine residues on target proteins (Collett, Purchio, and Erikson 1980). Other oncogene proteins, such as those of the *fos* and *jun* oncogenes, act as transcription regulators (Franza et al. 1988; Vogt, Bos, and Doolittle 1987).

Even these insights leave the major questions unanswered. In the case of the tyrosine kinases, a decade of work has provided little insight into how protein phosphorylation can induce cancer-specific phenotypes. The nuclear oncogene proteins acting as transcriptional regulators may well modulate the expression of banks of important genes, but the identities of these genes are elusive.

A further aspect of cancer biochemistry addresses the small molecules, known as second messengers, that function as intracellular hormones by conveying mitogenic signals from one part of the cell to another. A number of second messengers have been found within cells that include elements as diverse as calcium ions and cyclic AMP. Perhaps the most critical of these are the breakdown products of the phosphatidylinositol phosphates, compounds that act as pharmacologically potent intracellular growth agonists. It is widely suspected that many oncogene proteins act through their ability to deregulate the PI pathway.

The understanding of the biochemical basis of oncogene action remains incomplete and, in many respects, highly speculative. This will change rapidly; within a decade, many of these puzzles will be worked out in great detail. With this progress will come insight into how oncogenes act pleiotropically to induce a multitude of cancer cell phenotypes. Such insights may be applicable to the causal mechanisms of many types of cancer. In addition, the understanding of the biochemistry of the cancer cell may lead to the first perception of molecular targets within the cancer cell that can be attacked by totally new types of therapeutics. In the end, this faith drives much of contemporary cancer research: By understanding the cause, we can create the cure.

REFERENCES

Abelev, G.I. 1971. Alpha-fetoprotein in oncogenesis and its association with malignant tumors. *Adv. Cancer Res.* 14:295.

Abercrombie, M., and Heaysman, J.E.M. 1954. Observations on the social behavior of cells in tissue culture II: "monolayering" of fibroblasts. *Exp. Cell Res.* 6:293-306.

Bos, J.L.; Fearon, E.R.; and Hamilton, S.R. et al. 1987. Prevalence of *ras* gene mutations in human colorectal cancers. *Nature* 327:293-97.

Brunson, K.W. et al. 1979. Selection and altered tumor cell properties of brain-colonizing metastatic melanoma cells selected from B16 melanoma. *Int. J. Cancer* 23:854.

Cavenee, W.K.; Hansen, M.F.; and Nordenskjold, M. et al. 1985. Genetic origin of mutations predisposing to retinoblastoma. *Science* 228:501-503.

Collett, M.S.; Purchio, A.F.; and Erikson, R.L. 1980. Avian sarcoma virus transforming protein, pp60 *src*, shows protein kinase activity specific for tyrosine. *Nature* (London) 285:167-69.

Concannon, J.P.; Dalbow, M.H.; and Liebler, G.A. et al. 1974. The carcinoembryonic antigen assay in bronchogenic carcinoma. *Cancer* 34:184-92.

de Klein, A.; Geurts van Kessel, A.; and Grosveld, G. et al. 1982. A cellular oncogene is translocated to the Philadelphia chromosome in chronic myelocytic leukaemia. *Nature* 300:765-67.

Der, C.J.; Krontiris, T.G.; and Cooper, G.M. 1982. Transforming genes of human bladder and lung carcinoma cell lines are homologous to the *ras* genes of Harvey and Kirsten sarcoma virus. *Proc. Natl. Acad. Sci.* 79:3637-40.

Doolittle, R.F.; Hunkapillar, M.W.; and Hood, L.E. et al. 1983. Simian sarcoma virus oncogene, v-*sis*, is derived from the gene (or genes) encoding a platelet-derived growth factor. *Science* 221:275-77.

Downward, J.; Yarden, Y.; and Mayer, E. et al. 1984. Close similarity of epidermal growth factor receptor and v-*erb* B oncogene protein sequences. *Nature* 307:521-27.

Dulbecco, R. 1969. Cell transformation by viruses. *Science* 166:962-68.

Fisher, B., and Fisher, E.R. 1959. Experimental studies of factors influencing hepatic metastases I: the effect of number of tumor cells injected and time of growth. *Cancer* 12:926-41.

Foulds, L. 1969. *Neoplastic development.* vol. 1. New York: Academic Press.

Franza, B.R. Jr.; Rauscher, F.J. III; and Josephs, S.F. et al. 1988. The *fos* complex and *fos*-related antigens recognize sequence elements that contain AP-1 binding sites (con't). *Science* 239:1150-53.

Gouvera, J. 1982. Degree of bronchial metaplasia in heavy smokers and its regression after treatment with a retinoid. *Lancet* I:710.

Groffen, J.; Stephenson, J.R.; and Heisterkamp, N. et al. 1984. Philadelphia chromosomal breakpoints are clustered within a limited region, *bcr*, on chromosome 22. *Cell* 36:93-99.

Herberman, R.B., and Ortaldo, J.R. 1981. Natural killer cells: their role in defenses against disease. *Science* 214:24.

Kaplan, D.R.; Whitman, M.; and Schaffhausen, B. et al. 1987. Common elements in growth factor stimulation and oncogenic transformation: 85 kd phosphoprotein and phosphatidylinositol kinase activity. *Cell* 50:1021-29.

Klein, G. 1987. The approaching era of the tumor suppressor genes. *Science* 238:1539-45.

Knudson, A.G. 1971. Mutation and cancer: statistical study of retinoblastoma. *Proc. Natl. Acad. Sci.* 68:820-23.

Krontiris, T.G., and Cooper, G.M. 1981. Transforming activities of human tumor DNAs. *Proc. Natl. Acad. Sci.* 78:1181-84.

Land, H.; Parada, L.F.; and Weinberg, R.A. 1983. Cellular oncogenes and multistep carcinogenesis. *Science* 222:771-78.

Lowenstein, W.R. 1979. Junctional intercellular communication and the control of growth. *Biochem. Biophys. Acta* 560:1.

Macpherson, I., and Montagnier, L. 1964. Agar suspension culture for the selective assay of cells transformed by polyoma virus. *Virology* 23:291-94.

McCann, J., and Ames, B.N. 1976. Detection of carcinogens as mutagens in the salmonella/microsome test—assay of 300 chemicals: discussion. *Proc. Natl. Acad. Sci.* 73:950-55.

Old, L.J. 1981. Cancer immunology: the search for specificity. (GHA Clowes Memorial Lecture.) *Cancer Res.* 41:361.

Parada, L.F.; Tabin, C.J.; and Shih, C. et al. 1982. Human EJ bladder carcinoma oncogene is homologue of Harvey sarcoma virus *ras* gene. *Nature* 297:474-78.

Recklies, A.D.; Tiltman, K.J.; and Stoker, T.A.M. et al. 1980. Secretion of proteinases from malignant and nonmalignant human breast tissue. *Cancer Res.* 40:550-55.

Seeger, R.C.; Brodeur, G.M.; and Sather, H. et al. 1985. Association of multiple copies of the N-*myc* oncogene with rapid progression of neuroblastomas. *N. Engl. J. Med.* 313:1111-16.

Sefton, B.M.; Hunter, T.; and Ball, E.H. et al. 1981. Vinculin: a cytoskeletal target of the transforming protein of Rous sarcoma virus. *Cell* 24:165-74.

Shih, C.; Shilo, B.Z.; and Goldfarb, M.P. et al. 1979. Passage of phenotypes of chemically transformed cells via transfection of DNA and chromatin. *Proc. Natl. Acad. Sci.* 76:5714-18.

Shilo, B.Z., and Weinberg, R.A. 1981. DNA sequences homologous to vertebrate oncogenes are conserved in *Drosophila melanogaster. Proc. Natl. Acad. Sci.* 78:6789-92.

Slamon, D.J.; Clark, G.M.; and Wong, S.G. et al. 1987. Human breast cancer: correlation of relapse and survival with amplification of the HER-2/*neu* oncogene. *Science* 235:177-82.

Sporn, M.B., and Todaro, G.J. 1980. Autocrine secretion and malignant transformation of cells. *N. Engl. J. Med.* 303:878-80.

Tabin, C.J.; Bradley, S.M.; and Bargmann, C.I. et al. 1982. Mechanism of activation of a human oncogene. *Nature* 300:143-49.

Taub, R.; Kirsch, I.; and Morton, C. et al. 1982. Translocation of the c-*myc* gene into the immunoglobulin heavy chain locus in human Burkitt's lymphoma and murine plasmacytoma cells. *Proc. Natl. Acad. Sci.* 79:7837-41.

Temin, H.M., and Rubin, H. 1958. Characteristics of an assay for Rous sarcoma virus and Rous sarcoma cells in tissue culture. *Virology* 6:669-88.

Todaro, G.U., and Green, H. 1963. Quantitative studies of the growth of mouse embryo cells in culture and their development into established lines. *J. Cell Biol.* 17:299-13.

Ullrich, A.; Coussens, L.; and Hayflick, J.S. et al. 1984. Human epidermal growth factor receptor cDNA sequence and aberrant expression of the amplified gene in A431 epidermoid carcinoma cells. *Nature* 309:418-25.

Vaheri, A., and Mosher, D.F. 1978. High molecular weight, cell surface-associated glycoprotein (fibronectin) lost in malignant transformation. *Biochem. Biophys. Acta* 516:1.

Verderame, M.; Alcorta, D.; and Egnor, M. et al. 1980. Cytoskeletal F-actin patterns quantitated with fluorescein isothiocyanate-phalloidin in normal and transformed cells. *Proc. Natl. Acad. Sci.* 77:6624-28.

Vogt, P.K.; Bos, T.J.; and Doolittle, R.F. 1987. Homology between the DNA-binding domain of the GCN4 regulatory protein of yeast and the carboxy terminal region of a protein coded for the oncogene *jun. Proc. Natl. Acad. Sci.* 84:3316-19.

Warburg, O.H. 1930. *The metabolism of tumors: investigations from the Kaiser Wilhelm Institute for Biology.* London: Constable.

Weinstein, R.S. et al. 1976. The structure and function of intercellular junctions in cancer. *Adv. Cancer Res.* 23:23.

Ziegler, J.L. et al. 1982. Outbreak of Burkitt's-like lymphoma in homosexual men. *Lancet* II:631.

ACKNOWLEDGEMENTS

The editors wish to extend their appreciation to the following individuals who played key roles in the development and production of this text:

New York: Genell Subak-Sharpe (editorial director), Ann Forer Stockton, Peter Gannon, Everton Lopez, Hope Subak-Sharpe, and Sarah Subak-Sharpe.

Atlanta: Rosemarie Perrin (Director of Professional Education, Audiovisuals, and Materials), Marella Synovec, Mary Jo Bumpers, Jane Zanca, and Marisa Rothman.

Boston: Diane Forti.

INDEX

CHARTERED DIVISIONS OF THE AMERICAN CANCER SOCIETY, INC.

Alabama Division, Inc.
504 Brookwood Boulevard
Homewood, Alabama 35209
(205) 879-2242

Alaska Division, Inc.
406 West Fireweed Lane
Suite 204
Anchorage, Alaska 99503
(907) 277-8696

Arizona Division, Inc.
2929 East Thomas Road
Phoenix, Arizona 85016
(602) 224-0524

Arkansas Division, Inc.
901 North University
Little Rock, Arkansas 72207
(501) 664-3480

California Division, Inc.
1710 Webster Street
P.O. Box 2061
Oakland, California 94612
(415) 893-7900

Colorado Division, Inc.
2255 South Oneida
P.O. Box 24669
Denver, Colorado 80224
(303) 758-2030

Connecticut Division, Inc.
Barnes Park South
14 Village Lane
Wallingford, Connecticut 06492
(203) 265-7161

Delaware Division, Inc.
92 Read's Way
New Castle, Delaware 19720
(302) 324-4227

District of Columbia Division, Inc.
1825 Connecticut Avenue, N.W.
Suite 315
Washington, D.C. 20009
(202) 483-2600

Florida Division, Inc.
1001 South MacDill Avenue
Tampa, Florida 33629
(813) 253-0541

Georgia Division, Inc.
46 Fifth Street, NE
Atlanta, Georgia 30308
(404) 892-0026

Hawaii/Pacific Division, Inc.
Community Services Center Bldg.
200 North Vineyard Boulevard
Honolulu, Hawaii 96817
(808) 531-1662

Idaho Division, Inc.
2676 Vista Avenue
P.O. Box 5386
Boise, Idaho 83705
(208) 343-4609

Illinois Division, Inc.
77 East Monroe
Chicago, Illinois 60603
(312) 641-6150

Indiana Division, Inc.
8730 Commerce Park Place
Indianapolis, Indiana 46268
(317) 872-4432

Iowa Division, Inc.
8364 Hickman Road, Suite D
Des Moines, Iowa 50325
(515) 253-0147

Kansas Division, Inc.
1315 SW Arrowhead Road
Topeka, Kansas 66604
(913) 273-4114

Kentucky Division, Inc.
701 West Muhammad Ali Blvd.
P.O. Box 1807
Louisville, Kentucky 40201-1807
(502) 584-6782

Louisiana Division, Inc.
Fidelity Homestead Bldg.
837 Gravier Street
Suite 700
New Orleans, Louisiana 70112-1509
(504) 523-4188

Maine Division, Inc.
52 Federal Street
Brunswick, Maine 04011
(207) 729-3339

Maryland Division, Inc.
8219 Town Center Drive
White Marsh, Maryland 21162-0082
(301) 931-6868

Massachusetts Division, Inc.
247 Commonwealth Avenue
Boston, Massachusetts 02116
(617) 267-2650

Michigan Division, Inc.
1205 East Saginaw Street
Lansing, Michigan 48906
(517) 371-2920

Minnesota Division, Inc.
3316 West 66th Street
Minneapolis, Minnesota 55435
(612) 925-2772

Mississippi Division, Inc.
1380 Livingston Lane
Lakeover Office Park
Jackson, Mississippi 39213
(601) 362-8874

Missouri Division, Inc.
3322 American Avenue
Jefferson City, Missouri 65102
(314) 893-4800

Montana Division, Inc.
313 N. 32nd Street
Suite #1
Billings, Montana 59101
(406) 252-7111

Nebraska Division, Inc.
8502 West Center Road
Omaha, Nebraska 68124-5255
(402) 393-5800

Nevada Division, Inc.
1325 East Harmon
Las Vegas, Nevada 89119
(702) 798-6857

New Hampshire Division, Inc.
360 Route 101, Unit 501
Bedford, New Hampshire 03102-6800
(603) 472-8899

New Jersey Division, Inc.
2600 Route 1, CN 2201
North Brunswick, New Jersey 08902
(201) 297-8000

New Mexico Division, Inc.
5800 Lomas Blvd., NE
Albuquerque, New Mexico 87110
(505) 260-2105

New York State Division, Inc.
6725 Lyons Street
P.O. Box 7
East Syracuse, New York 13057
(315) 437-7025

☐ **Long Island Division, Inc.**
145 Pidgeon Hill Road
Huntington Station, New York 11746
(516) 385-9100

☐ **New York City Division, Inc.**
19 West 56th Street
New York, New York 10019
(212) 586-8700

☐ **Queens Division, Inc.**
112-25 Queens Boulevard
Forest Hills, New York 11375
(718) 263-2224

☐ **Westchester Division, Inc.**
30 Glenn St.
White Plains, New York 10603
(914) 949-4800

North Carolina Division, Inc.
11 South Boylan Avenue
Suite 221
Raleigh, North Carolina 27603
(919) 834-8463

North Dakota Division, Inc.
123 Roberts Street
P.O. Box 426
Fargo, North Dakota 58107
(701) 232-1385

Ohio Division, Inc.
5555 Frantz Road
Dublin, Ohio 43017
(614) 889-9565

Oklahoma Division, Inc.
3000 United Founders Blvd.
Suite 136
Oklahoma City, Oklahoma 73112
(405) 843-9888

Oregon Division, Inc.
0330 SW Curry
Portland, Oregon 97201
(503) 295-6422

Pennsylvania Division, Inc.
P.O. Box 897
Route 422 & Sipe Avenue
Hershey, Pennsylvania 17033-0897
(717) 533-6144

☐ **Philadelphia Division, Inc.**
1422 Chestnut Street
Philadelphia, Pennsylvania 19102
(215) 665-2900

Puerto Rico Division, Inc.
Calle Alverio #577,
Esquina Sargento Medina,
Hato Rey, Puerto Rico 00918
(809) 764-2295

Rhode Island Division, Inc.
400 Main Street
Pawtucket, Rhode Island 02860
(401) 722-8480

South Carolina Division, Inc.
128 Stonemark Lane
Columbia, South Carolina 29210
(803) 750-1693

South Dakota Division, Inc.
4101 Carnegie Place
Sioux Falls, South Dakota 57106-2322
(605) 361-8277

Tennessee Division, Inc.
1315 Eighth Avenue, South
Nashville, Tennessee 37203
(615) 255-1227

Texas Division, Inc.
2433 Ridgepoint Drive
Austin, Texas 78754
(512) 928-2262

Utah Division, Inc.
610 East South Temple
Salt Lake City, Utah 84102
(801) 322-0431

Vermont Division, Inc.
13 Loomis Street, Drawer C
P.O. Box 1452
Montpelier, Vermont 05601-1452
(802) 223-2348

Virginia Division, Inc.
4240 Park Place Court
Glen Allen, Virginia 23060
(804) 270-0142/(800) ACS-2345

Washington Division, Inc.
2120 First Avenue North
Seattle, Washington 98109-1140
(206) 283-1152

West Virginia Division, Inc.
2428 Kanawha Boulevard East
Charleston, West Virginia 25311
(304) 344-3611

Wisconsin Division, Inc.
615 North Sherman Avenue
Madison, Wisconsin 53704
(608) 249-0487

Wyoming Division, Inc.
2222 House Avenue
Cheyenne, Wyoming 82001
(307) 638-3331

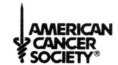

AMERICAN CANCER SOCIETY TOLL FREE: 1-800-ACS-2345